Meyler's Side Effects of Endocrine and Metabolic Drugs

Meyler's Side Effects of Endocrine and Metabolic Drugs

Editor

J K Aronson, MA, DPhil, MBChB, FRCP, FBPharmacolS, FFPM (Hon)
Oxford, United Kingdom

ELSEVIER

AMSTERDAM • BOSTON • HEIDELBERG • LONDON • NEW YORK • OXFORD
PARIS • SAN DIEGO • SAN FRANCISCO • SINGAPORE • SYDNEY • TOKYO

Elsevier
Radarweg 29, PO Box 211, 1000 AE Amsterdam, The Netherlands
The Boulevard, Langford Lane, Kidlington, Oxford OX5 1GB, UK
525 B Street, Suite 1900, San Diego, CA 92101-4495, USA

Notice
No responsibility is assumed by the publisher for any injury and/or damage to persons
or property as a matter of products liability, negligence or otherwise, or from any use or operation
of any methods, products, instructions or ideas contained in the material herein. Because of rapid
advances in the medical sciences, in particular, independent verification of diagnoses and drug
dosages should be made

Medicine is an ever-changing field. Standard safety precautions must be followed, but as new
research and clinical experience broaden our knowledge, changes in treatment and drug therapy
may become necessary or appropriate. Readers are advised to check the most current product
information provided by the manufacturer of each drug to be administered to verify the
recommended dose, the method and duration of administrations, and contraindications. It is the
responsibility of the treating physician, relying on experience and knowledge of the patient, to
determine dosages and the best treatment for each individual patient. Neither the publisher nor the
authors assume any liability for any injury and/or damage to persons or property arising from this
publication.

British Library Cataloguing in Publication Data
A catalogue record for this book is available from the British Library

Library of Congress Catalog Number: 2008933972

ISBN: 978-044-453271-8

For information on all Elsevier publications
visit our web site at http://www.elsevierdirect.com

Typeset by Integra Software Services Pvt. Ltd, Pondicherry, India www.integra-india.com
Printed and bound in the USA

08 09 10   10 9 8 7 6 5 4 3 2 1

Contents

Preface

This volume covers the adverse effects of drugs with endocrine or metabolic effects. The material has been collected from *Meyler's Side Effects of Drugs: The International Encyclopedia of Adverse Drug Reactions and Interactions* (15th edition, 2006, in six volumes), which was itself based on previous editions of *Meyler's Side Effects of Drugs* and *Side Effects of Drugs Annuals*, and from later *Side Effects of Drugs Annuals* (SEDA) 28, 29, and 30. The main contributors of this material were JK Aronson, I Aursnes, A Buitenhuis, LG Cleland, P Coates, J Costa, MNG Dukes, M Farré, JA Franklyn, HMJ Krans, RCL Page, BS True, CJ van Boxtel, and J Weeke. For contributors to earlier editions of *Meyler's Side Effects of Drugs* and the *Side Effects of Drugs Annuals*, see http://www.elsevier.com/wps/find/bookseriesdescription.cws_home/BS_SED/description.

A brief history of the Meyler series

Leopold Meyler was a physician who was treated for tuberculosis after the end of the Nazi occupation of The Netherlands. According to Professor Wim Lammers, writing a tribute in Volume VIII (1975), Meyler got a fever from para-aminosalicylic acid, but elsewhere Graham Dukes has written, based on information from Meyler's widow, that it was deafness from dihydrostreptomycin; perhaps it was both. Meyler discovered that there was no single text to which medical practitioners could look for information about unwanted effects of drug therapy; Louis Lewin's text "Die Nebenwirkungen der Arzneimittel" ("The Untoward Effects of Drugs") of 1881 had long been out of print (SEDA-27, xxv-xxix). Meyler therefore determined to make such information available and persuaded the Netherlands publishing firm of Van Gorcum to publish a book, in Dutch, entirely devoted to descriptions of the adverse effects that drugs could cause. He went on to agree with the Elsevier Publishing Company, as it was then called, to prepare and issue an English translation. The first edition of 192 pages (*Schadelijke Nevenwerkingen van Geneesmiddelen*) appeared in 1951 and the English version (*Side Effects of Drugs*) a year later.

The book was a great success, and a few years later Meyler started to publish what he called surveys of unwanted effects of drugs. Each survey covered a period of two to four years. They were labelled as volumes rather than editions, and after Volume IV had been published Meyler could no longer handle the task alone. For subsequent volumes he recruited collaborators, such as Andrew Herxheimer. In September 1973 Meyler died unexpectedly, and Elsevier invited Graham Dukes to take over the editing of Volume VIII.

Dukes persuaded Elsevier that the published literature was too large to be comfortably encompassed in a four-yearly cycle, and he suggested that the volumes should be produced annually instead. The four-yearly volume could then concentrate on providing a complementary critical encyclopaedic survey of the entire field. The first *Side Effects of Drugs Annual* was published in 1977. The first encyclopaedic edition of *Meyler's Side Effects of Drugs*, which appeared in 1980, was labelled the ninth edition, and since then a new encyclopaedic edition has appeared every four years. The 15th edition was published in 2006, in both hard and electronic versions.

Monograph structure

The monographs in this volume are arranged in eight sections:

- corticosteroids and related drugs;
- prostaglandins;
- sex hormones and related drugs;
- iodine and drugs that affect thyroid function;
- insulin and other hypoglycemic drugs;
- other hormones and related drugs;
- lipid-regulating drugs
- endocrine and metabolic adverse effects of non-hormonal and non-metabolic drugs.

In each monograph in the Meyler series the information is organized into sections as shown below (although not all the sections are covered in each monograph).

DoTS classification of adverse drug reactions

A few adverse effects have been classified using the system known as DoTS. In this system adverse reactions are classified according to the **Dose** at which they usually occur, the **Time-course** over which they occur, and the **Susceptibility factors** that make them more likely, as follows:

- **Relation to Dose**
  - Toxic reactions—reactions that occur at supratherapeutic doses
  - Collateral reactions—reactions that occur at standard therapeutic doses
  - Hypersusceptibility reactions—reactions that occur at subtherapeutic doses in susceptible individuals

- **Time course**
  - Time-independent reactions—reactions that occur at any time during a course of therapy
  - Time-dependent reactions
    - Immediate or rapid reactions—reactions that occur only when a drug is administered too rapidly
    - First-dose reactions—reactions that occur after the first dose of a course of treatment and not necessarily thereafter
    - Early reactions—reactions that occur early in treatment then either abate with continuing treatment (owing to tolerance) or persist
    - Intermediate reactions—reactions that occur after some delay but with less risk during longer term therapy, owing to the "healthy survivor" effect
    - Late reactions—reactions the risk of which increases with continued or repeated exposure
    - Withdrawal reactions—reactions that occur when, after prolonged treatment, a drug is withdrawn or its effective dose is reduced

- Delayed reactions—reactions that occur some time after exposure, even if the drug is withdrawn before the reaction appears

- *Susceptibility factors*
  - Genetic
  - Age
  - Sex
  - Physiological variation
  - Exogenous factors (for example drug–drug or drug–food interactions, smoking)
  - Diseases

Drug names

Drugs have usually been designated by their recommended or proposed International Non-proprietary Names (rINN or pINN); when these are not available, chemical names have been used. In some cases brand names have been used.

Spelling

For indexing purposes, American spelling has been used, e.g. anemia, estrogen, rather than anaemia, oestrogen.

Cross-references

The various editions of *Meyler's Side Effects of Drugs* are cited in the text as SED-l3, SED-14, etc; the *Side Effects of Drugs Annuals* are cited as SEDA-1, SEDA-2, etc.

J K Aronson
Oxford, November 2008

Organization of material in monographs in the Meyler series (not all sections are included in each monograph)

General information
Drug studies
  Observational studies
  Comparative studies
  Drug-combination studies
  Placebo-controlled studies
  Systematic reviews
Organs and systems
  Cardiovascular
  Respiratory
  Ear, nose, throat
  Nervous system
  Neuromuscular function
  Sensory systems
  Psychological
  Psychiatric
  Endocrine
  Metabolism
  Nutrition
  Electrolyte balance
  Mineral balance
  Metal metabolism
  Acid-base balance
  Fluid balance
  Hematologic
  Mouth
  Teeth
  Salivary glands
  Gastrointestinal
  Liver
  Biliary tract
  Pancreas
  Urinary tract
  Skin
  Hair
  Nails
  Sweat glands
  Serosae
  Musculoskeletal
  Sexual function
  Reproductive system
  Breasts
  Immunologic
  Autacoids
  Infection risk

Body temperature
Multiorgan failure
Trauma
Death
Long-term effects
  Drug abuse
  Drug misuse
  Drug tolerance
  Drug resistance
  Drug dependence
  Drug withdrawal
  Genotoxicity
  Cytotoxicity
  Mutagenicity
  Tumorigenicity
Second-generation effects
  Fertility
  Pregnancy
  Teratogenicity
  Fetotoxicity
  Lactation
  Breast feeding
Susceptibility factors
  Genetic factors
  Age
  Sex
  Physiological factors
  Disease
  Other features of the patient
Drug administration
  Drug formulations
  Drug additives
  Drug contamination and adulteration
  Drug dosage regimens
  Drug administration route
  Drug overdose
Interactions
  Drug-drug interactions
  Food-drug interactions
  Drug-device interactions
  Smoking
  Other environmental interactions
Interference with diagnostic tests
Diagnosis of adverse drug reactions
Management of adverse drug reactions
Monitoring therapy
References

CORTICOSTEROIDS AND RELATED DRUGS

Corticorelin (corticotropin-releasing hormone (CRH))

General Information

For complete functional evaluation of the hypothalamic–hypophyseal–adrenal axis one can use synthetic corticorelin (corticotropin-releasing hormone), which is available in both human (hCRH) and ovine (oCRH) forms (1).

Single bolus injections in standard doses (for example 200 µg of hCRH or oCRH), whether given on a single occasion or at fixed intervals, have a very low rate of complications. At higher doses adverse effects occur in almost 40% of patients (2). At a dose of 1 mg/kg they mainly comprise flushing or a feeling of warmth (30%), a sensation of discomfort (5%), palpitation (3%), and dyspnea (1%). Higher doses (more than 200 mg) can cause hypotension or coronary ischemia. Patients with brain injury are more susceptible to adverse reactions (2). No serious allergic reactions have been reported. Continuous infusions of hCRH or oCRH for several hours have also been well tolerated, but adverse effects occurred with cumulative doses of 200–300 µg/hour.

High doses can provoke marked adverse effects in patients with neurological disorders, coronary heart disease, or disorders of the pituitary–adrenal axis, especially if the blood–brain barrier has been damaged (for example by a head injury or during intracranial surgery). Nonstandard doses should only be used in experimental work with well-designed safety precautions.

References

1. Anonymous. Corticorelin: ACTH RF, corticoliberin, corticotrophin-releasing hormone, corticotropin-releasing factor, human corticotropin-releasing hormone, ovine corticotrophin-releasing factor, Xerecept. Drugs R D 2004;5(4):218–9.
2. Nink M, Krause U, Lehnert H, Beyer J. Safety and side effects of human and ovine corticotropin-releasing hormone administration in man. Klin Wochenschr 1991;69(5):185–95.

Corticosteroids—glucocorticoids

General Information

Nomenclature

The two main classes of adrenal corticosteroids are properly known as glucocorticoids and mineralocorticosteroids. The former are often known by shorter names and are commonly referred to as "glucocorticoids", "corticosteroids", "corticoids", or even simply "steroids"; the latter are often referred to as "mineralocorticoids". Here we shall use the terms "glucocorticoids" and "mineralocorticoids". When referring to both we shall use the term "corticosteroids".

Relative potencies

The main human anti-inflammatory corticosteroid, the glucocorticoid cortisol (hydrocortisone), as secreted by the adrenal gland, has generally been replaced by related glucocorticoids of synthetic origin for therapeutic purposes. These Δ^1-dehydrated glucocorticoids are designed to imitate the physiological hormone. They have marked glucocorticoid potency but only minor effects on sodium retention and potassium excretion; the relative glucocorticoid and mineralocorticoid potencies of the best-known compounds, insofar as these potencies are agreed, are compared in Table 1.

Over many years, a great deal of research has been devoted to producing better glucocorticoids for therapeutic use. Those endeavors have succeeded only in part; from the start the mineralocorticoid effects were sufficiently minor to be nonproblematic; the fact that successive synthetic glucocorticoids had an increasing potency in terms of weight was not of direct therapeutic significance; and the most hoped-for aim, that of dissociating wanted from unwanted glucocorticoid effects has not been achieved (1). Most untoward effects, such as those due to the catabolic and gluconeogenic activities of the glucocorticoid family, probably cannot be dissociated entirely from the anti-inflammatory activity (2) it is possible that myopathy and muscle wasting are actually more common when triamcinolone or dexamethasone are used,

Table 1 Relative potencies of glucocorticoids

Compound	Glucocorticoid potency relative to hydrocortisone	Mineralocorticoid potency	Equivalent doses (mg)
Cortisone	0.8	++	25
Hydrocortisone	1.0	++	20
Prednisone	4	+	5
Prednisolone	4	+	5
Methylprednisolone	5	0	4
Triamcinolone	5	0	4
Paramethasone	10	0	2
Fluprednisolone	10	0	1.5
Dexamethasone	30	0	0.75
Betamethasone	30	0	0.6

but this may merely reflect overdosage of these potent drugs. However, some progress in achieving a dissociation of effects has been made. Beclomethasone does have a relatively greater local than systemic effect. Deflazacort, one of the few new glucocorticoids to have been developed in recent years, originally promised reduced intensity of adverse effects, for example on bone mineral density, but the early promise has not held up (SEDA-18, 389). Cloprednol seems to affect the hypothalamic–pituitary–adrenal axis much less than other glucocorticoids, and to cause less excretion of nitrogen and calcium (3).

Uses

Most patients who are treated therapeutically with glucocorticoids do not have glucocorticoid deficiency. Adverse reactions to glucocorticoids depend very largely on the ways in which, and the purposes for which, they are used. There are four groups of uses.

(1) Substitution therapy is used in cases of primary and secondary adrenocortical insufficiency; the aim is to provide glucocorticoids and mineralocorticoids in physiological amounts, and the better the dosage regimen is adapted to the individual's needs, the less the chance of adverse effects (1).

(2) Anti-inflammatory and immunosuppressive therapy exploits the immunosuppressive, anti-allergic, anti-inflammatory, anti-exudative, and anti-proliferative effects of the glucocorticoids (2). The desired pharmacodynamic effects reflect a general influence of these substances on the mesenchyme, where they suppress reactions that result in the symptoms of inflammation, exudation, and proliferation; the non-specific effects of glucocorticoids on the mesenchyme are part of their physiological actions, but they can only be obtained to a clinically useful extent by using dosages at which the more specific (and unwanted) physiological effects also occur. High doses sufficient to suppress immune reactions are used in patients who have undergone organ transplantation.

(3) Hormone suppression therapy can be used, for example, to inhibit the adrenogenital syndrome (3). Higher doses are used. The treatment of the adrenogenital syndrome is only partly substitutive and has to be adapted to the individual case, but doses are needed at which various hormonal effects of the glucocorticoids and mineralocorticoids are likely to become troublesome.

(4) Massive doses of glucocorticoids, far exceeding physiological amounts, are given in the immediate management of anaphylaxis, although their beneficial effects are delayed for several hours. This is because, in severely ill patients, early administration of hydrocortisone 100–300 mg as the sodium succinate salt can gradually enhance the actions of adrenaline (4). Glucocorticoids have been used as an adjunct to the use of inotropic and vasopressor drugs for septic shock. Their efficacy, as well as their proposed mechanisms of action, is controversial; inhibition of complement-mediated aggregation and resultant endothelial injury, and inhibition of the release of beta-endorphin are current theories of their mechanism of action. However, controlled studies have not indicated a beneficial effect of high-dose glucocorticoid therapy in treating septic shock (5,6). Hence, there is no established role for glucocorticoids in the treatment of shock, except shock caused by adrenal insufficiency.

Routes of administration

Glucocorticoids can be given by the following routes:

- oral
- rectal
- intravenous
- intramuscular
- inhalation
- nasal
- topical (skin, eyes, ears)
- intradermal
- intra-articular and periarticular
- intraspinal (epidural, intrathecal)
- intracapsular (breast)

All of these routes are covered in this monograph, except the inhalation route, which is the subject of a separate monograph.

Observational studies

A study has been undertaken to clarify whether glucocorticoid excess affects endothelium-dependent vascular relaxation in glucocorticoid treated patients and whether dexamethasone alters the production of hydrogen peroxide and the formation of peroxynitrite, a reactive molecule between nitric oxide and superoxide, in cultured human umbilical endothelial cells (7). Glucocorticoid excess impaired endothelium-dependent vascular relaxation in vivo and enhanced the production of reactive oxygen species to cause increased production of peroxynitrite in vitro. Glucocorticoid-induced reduction in nitric oxide availability may cause vascular endothelial dysfunction, leading to hypertension and atherosclerosis.

Comparative studies

In another randomized trial, the effects and adverse effects of early dexamethasone on the incidence of chronic lung disease have been evaluated in 50 high-risk preterm infants (8). The treated infants received dexamethasone intravenously from the fourth day of life for 7 days (0.5 mg/kg/day for the first 3 days, 0.25 mg/kg/day for the next 3 days, and 0.125 mg/kg/day on the seventh day). The incidence of chronic lung disease at 28 days of life and at 36 weeks of postconceptional age was significantly lower in the infants who were given dexamethasone, who also remained intubated and required oxygen therapy for a shorter period. Hyperglycemia, hypertension, growth failure, and left ventricular hypertrophy were the transient adverse effects associated with early glucocorticoid administration. Early dexamethasone administration may be useful in preventing chronic lung disease, but its use should be restricted to preterm high-risk infants.

Placebo-controlled studies

Patients taking glucocorticoids have an increased risk of infections, including those produced by opportunistic and rare pathogens. However, it has been suggested that glucocorticoid administration in severe community-acquired pneumonia could attenuate systemic inflammation and lead to earlier resolution of pneumonia and a reduction in sepsis-related complications. In a placebo-controlled study in 46 patients with severe community-acquired pneumonia who received protocol-guided antibiotic treatment hydrocortisone (intravenous 200 mg bolus followed by infusion at a rate of 10 mg/hour) for 7 days produced significant clinical improvement (9). Adverse effects were not described.

Although there have been several trials of early dexamethasone to determine whether it would reduce mortality and chronic lung disease in infants with respiratory distress, the optimal duration and adverse effects of such therapy are unknown. The purpose of one study was: (a) to determine if a 3-day course of early dexamethasone therapy would reduce chronic lung disease and increase survival without chronic lung disease in neonates who received surfactant therapy for respiratory distress syndrome and (b) to determine the associated adverse effects (10). This was a prospective, placebo-controlled, multicenter, randomized study of a 3-day course of early dexamethasone therapy, beginning at 24–48 hours of life in 241 neonates, who weighed 500–1500 g, had received surfactant therapy, and were at significant risk of chronic lung disease or death. Infants randomized to dexamethasone received a 3-day tapering course (total dose 1.35 mg/kg) given in six doses at 12-hour intervals. Chronic lung disease was defined by the need for supplementary oxygen at a gestational age of 36 weeks. Neonates randomized to early dexamethasone were more likely to survive without chronic lung disease (RR = 1.3; CI = 1.0, 1.7) and were less likely to develop chronic lung disease (RR = 0.6; CI = 0.3, 0.98). Mortality rates were not significantly different. Subsequent dexamethasone therapy was less in early dexamethasone-treated neonates (RR = 0.8; CI = 0.70, 0.96). Very early (before 7 days of life) intestinal perforations were more common among dexamethasone-treated neonates (8 versus 1%). The authors concluded that an early 3-day course of dexamethasone increases survival without chronic lung disease, reduces chronic lung disease, and reduces late dexamethasone therapy in high-risk, low birthweight infants who receive surfactant therapy for respiratory distress syndrome. The potential benefits of early dexamethasone therapy in the regimen used in this trial need to be weighed against the risk of early intestinal perforation.

Although dexamethasone is commonly associated with transient adverse effects, several randomized trials have shown that it rapidly reduces oxygen requirements and shortens the duration of ventilation. A randomized study was designed to evaluate the effects of two different dexamethasone courses on growth in preterm infants (11). The first phase included 30 preterm infants at high risk of chronic lung disease, of whom 15 (8 boys) were given dexamethasone for 14 days, from the tenth day of life; they received a total dose of 4.75 mg/kg; 15 babies were assigned to the control group (8 boys). The second phase included 30 preterm infants at high risk of chronic lung disease, of whom 15 babies (7 boys) were treated with dexamethasone for 7 days, from the fourth day of life; they received a total dose of 2.38 mg/kg; 15 babies were assigned to the control group (9 boys). Infants given dexamethasone had significantly less weight gain than controls, but they caught up soon after the end of treatment. At 30 days of life, the gains in weight and length in each group were similar to those in control infants, but those given dexamethasone had significantly less head growth. There were no differences between the groups at discharge. The longer-term impact of postnatal dexamethasone on mortality and morbidity is less clear. Better data, from larger clinical trials with longer follow-up, will determine whether this kind of treatment enhances lives, makes little difference, causes significant harm, or does several of these things (12).

Systematic reviews

A systematic review of glucocorticoid adjunctive therapy in adults with acute bacterial meningitis has been published (13). Five trials involving 623 patients were included (pneumococcal meningitis = 234, meningococcal meningitis = 232, others = 127, unknown = 30). Treatment with glucocorticoids was associated with a significant reduction in mortality (RR = 0.6; 95% CI = 0.4, 0.8) and in neurological sequelae (RR = 0.6; 95% CI = 0.4, 1), and with a reduction in case-fatality in pneumococcal meningitis of 21% (RR = 0.5; 95% CI = 0.3, 0.8). In meningococcal meningitis, mortality (RR = 0.9; 95% CI = 0.3, 2.1) and neurological sequelae (RR = 0.5; 95% CI = 0.1, 1.7) were both reduced, but not significantly. Adverse events were similar in the treatment and placebo groups (RR = 1; CI = 0.5, 2), with gastrointestinal bleeding in 1% of glucocorticoid-treated patients and 4% of the rest. The authors recommended the early use of glucocorticoid therapy in adults in whom acute community-acquired bacterial meningitis is suspected.

A systematic review of randomized controlled trials has been performed to determine whether dexamethasone therapy in the first 15 days of life prevents chronic lung disease in premature infants (14). Studies were identified by a literature search using Medline (1970–97) supplemented by a search of the Cochrane Library (1998, Issue 4). Inclusion criteria were: (a) prospective randomized design with initiation of dexamethasone therapy within the first 15 days of life; (b) report of the outcome of interest; and (c) less than 20% crossover between the treatment and control groups during the study period. The primary outcomes were mortality at hospital discharge and the development of chronic lung disease at 28 days of life and 36 weeks postconceptional age. The secondary outcomes were the presence of a patent ductus arteriosus and treatment adverse effects. Dexamethasone reduced the incidence of chronic lung disease by 26% at 28 days (RR = 0.74; CI = 0.57, 0.96) and 48% at 36 weeks postconceptional age (RR = 0.52; CI = 0.33, 0.81). These reductions were more significant when dexamethasone was started in the first 72 hours of life. The 24% relative risk reduction of deaths was marginally significant (RR = 0.76; CI = 0.56, 1.04). The 27% reduction in patent ductus arteriosus and the 11% increase in infections were not statistically significant, nor were any other changes. The conclusion from this meta-analysis was that systemic dexamethasone given to at-risk infants soon after birth may reduce the incidence of chronic lung disease. There was no evidence of significant short-term adverse effects.

General adverse effects

The incidence and severity of adverse reactions to glucocorticoids depend on the dose and duration of treatment. Even the very high single doses of glucocorticoids, such as methylprednisolone, which are sometimes used, do not cause serious adverse effects, whereas an equivalent dose given over a long period of time can cause many long-term effects.

The two major risks of long-term glucocorticoid therapy are adrenal suppression and Cushingoid changes. During prolonged treatment with anti-inflammatory doses, glucose intolerance, osteoporosis, acne vulgaris, and a greater or lesser degree of mineralocorticoid-induced changes can occur. In children, growth can be retarded, and adults who take high doses can have mental changes. There may be a risk of gastroduodenal ulceration, although this is much less certain than was once thought. Infections and abdominal crises can be masked. Some of these effects reflect the catabolic properties of the glucocorticoids, that is their ability to accelerate tissue breakdown and impair healing. Allergic reactions can occur.

Anyone who prescribes long-term glucocorticoids should have a checklist in mind of the undesired effects that they can exert, both during treatment and on withdrawal, so that any harm that occurs can be promptly detected and countered. The main groups of risks arising from long-term treatment with glucocorticoids are summarized in Table 2.

The adverse reactions that were reported in a study of 213 children are listed in Table 3 (15).

Drug interactions that affect the efficacy of glucocorticoids have been reviewed (16).

Organs and Systems

Cardiovascular

The considerable body of evidence that glucocorticoids can cause increased rates of vascular mortality and the underlying mechanisms (increased blood pressure, impaired glucose tolerance, dyslipidemia, hypercoagulability, and increased fibrinogen production) have been

Table 2   Risks of long-term glucocorticoid therapy

1. Exogenous hypercorticalism with Cushing's syndrome
Moon face (facial rounding)
Central obesity
Striae
Hirsutism
Acne vulgaris
Ecchymoses
Hypertension
Osteoporosis
Proximal myopathy
Disorders of sexual function
Diabetes mellitus
Hyperlipidemia
Disorders of mineral and fluid balance (depending on the type of glucocorticoid)
2. Adrenal insufficiency
Insufficient or absent stress reaction
Withdrawal effects
3. Unwanted results accompanying desired effects
Increased risk of infection
Impaired wound healing
Peptic ulceration, bleeding, and perforation
Growth retardation
4. Other adverse effects
Mental disturbances
Encephalopathy
Increased risk of thrombosis
Posterior cataract
Increased intraocular pressure and glaucoma
Aseptic necrosis of bone

Table 3 Adverse reactions in 213 children given intravenous methylprednisolone

Adverse effect	Number
Behavioral changes	21
Abdominal disorders	11
Pruritus	9
Urticaria	5
Hypertension	5
Bone pain	3
Dizziness	3
Fatigue	2
Fractures	2
Hypotension	2
Lethargy	2
Tachycardia	2
Anaphylactoid reaction	1
"Grey appearance"	1

reviewed (17). In view of their adverse cardiovascular effects, the therapeutic options should be carefully considered before long-term glucocorticoids are begun; although they can be life-saving, dosages should be regularly reviewed during long-term therapy, in order to minimize complications.

The benefit of glucocorticoid therapy is often limited by several adverse reactions, including cardiovascular disorders such as hypertension and atherosclerosis. Plasma volume expansion due to sodium retention plays a minor role, but increased peripheral vascular resistance, due in part to an increased pressor response to catecholamines and angiotensin II, plays a major role in the pathogenesis of hypertension induced by glucocorticoid excess. However, the molecular mechanism remains unclear.

Long-term systemic administration of glucocorticoids might be expected, because of their effects on vascular fragility and wound healing, to increase the risk of vascular complications during percutaneous coronary intervention. To assess the potential risk of long-term glucocorticoid use in the setting of coronary angioplasty, 114 of 12 883 consecutively treated patients who were taking long-term glucocorticoids were compared with those who were not. Glucocorticoid use was not associated with an increased risk of composite events of major ischemia but was associated with a threefold risk of major vascular complications and a three- to fourfold risk of coronary perforation (18).

Hypertension

The secondary mineralocorticoid activity of glucocorticoids can lead to salt and water retention, which can cause hypertension. Although the detailed mechanisms are as yet uncertain, glucocorticoid-induced hypertension often occurs in elderly patients and is more common in patients with total serum calcium concentrations below the reference range and/or in those with a family history of essential hypertension (SEDA-20, 368; 19).

Hemangioma is the most common tumor of infancy, with a natural history of spontaneous involution. Some hemangiomas, however, as a result of their proximity to vital structures, destruction of facial anatomy, or excessive bleeding, can be successfully treated with systemic glucocorticoids between other therapies. The risk of hypertension is poorly documented in this setting. In one prospective study of 37 infants (7 boys, 17 girls; mean age 3.5 months, range 1.5–10) with rapidly growing complicated hemangiomas treated with oral prednisone 1–5 mg/kg/day, blood pressure increased in seven cases (20). Cardiac ultrasound examination in five showed two cases of myocardial hypertrophy, which was unrelated to the hypertension and which regressed after withdrawal of the prednisone.

Myocardial ischemia

Cortisone-induced cardiac lesions are sometimes reported and electrocardiographic changes have been seen in patients taking glucocorticoids (21). Whereas abnormal myocardial hypertrophy in children has perhaps been associated more readily with corticotropin, it has been seen on occasion during treatment with high dosages of glucocorticoids, with normalization after dosage reduction and withdrawal.

Fatal myocardial infarction occurred after intravenous methylprednisolone for an episode of ulcerative colitis (22).

- A day after a dose of intravenous methylprednisolone 60 mg a 79-year-old woman developed acute thoracic pain and collapsed. An electrocardiogram showed signs of a myocardial infarction and her cardiac enzyme activities were raised. She died within several hours. Autopsy showed an anterior transmural myocardial infarction and mild atheromatous lesions in the coronary arteries.

This report highlights the risk of cardiovascular adverse effects with short courses of glucocorticoid therapy in elderly patients with inflammatory bowel disease, even with rather low-dosage regimens. Acute myocardial infarction occurred in an old man with coronary insufficiency and giant cell arteritis after treatment with prednisolone (SEDA-10, 343) but could well have been coincidental.

Myocardial ischemia has been reportedly precipitated by intramuscular administration of betamethasone (SEDA-21, 413; 23). It has been suggested that long-term glucocorticoid therapy accelerates atherosclerosis and the formation of aortic aneurysms, with a high risk of rupture (SEDA-20, 369; 24).

Patients with seropositive rheumatoid arthritis taking long-term systemic glucocorticoids are at risk of accelerated cardiac rupture in the setting of transmural acute myocardial infarction treated with thrombolytic drugs (25).

- Two women and one man, aged 53–74 years, died after they received thrombolytic therapy for acute myocardial infarction. All three had a long history of seropositive rheumatoid arthritis treated with prednisone 5–20 mg/day for many years.

Cardiomyopathy

Postnatal exposure to glucocorticoids has been associated with hypertrophic cardiomyopathy in neonates. Such an effect has not previously been described in infants born to mothers who received antenatal glucocorticoids. Three neonates (gestational ages 36, 29, and 34 weeks), whose mothers had been treated with betamethasone prenatally in doses of 12 mg twice weekly for 16 doses, 8 doses, and 5 doses respectively, developed various degrees of hypertrophic cardiomyopathy diagnosed by echocardiography (26). There was no maternal evidence of diabetes, except for one infant whose mother had a normal fasting and postprandial blood glucose before glucocorticoid therapy, but an abnormal 1-hour postprandial glucose after 8 weeks of betamethasone therapy, with a normal HbA$_{1C}$ concentration. There was no family history of hypertrophic cardiomyopathy, no history of maternal intake of other relevant medications, no hypertension, and none of the infants received glucocorticoids postnatally. Follow-up echocardiography showed complete resolution in all infants. The authors suggested that repeated antenatal maternal glucocorticoids might cause hypertrophic cardiomyopathy in neonates. These changes appear to be dose- and duration-related and are mostly reversible.

Transient hypertrophic cardiomyopathy is a rare sequel of the concurrent administration of glucocorticoid and insulin excess (SEDA-21, 412; 27). The heart is also almost certainly a site for myopathic changes analogous to those that affect other muscles.

Transient hypertrophic cardiomyopathy has been attributed to systemic glucocorticoid administration for a craniofacial hemangioma (28).

- A 69-day-old white child presented with a rapidly growing 2.5 × 1.5 cm hemangioma of the external left nasal side wall. He was normotensive and there was no family history of cardiomyopathy or maternal gestational diabetes. Because of nasal obstruction and possible visual obstruction, he was given prednisolone 3 mg/kg/day. After 10 weeks his weight had fallen from 7.6 to 7.1 kg and 2 weeks later he became tachypneic with a respiratory rate of 40/minutes. A chest X-ray showed cardiomegaly and pulmonary venous congestion. An echocardiogram showed hypertrophic cardiomyopathy. The left ventricular posterior wall thickness was 10 mm (normal under 4 mm), and the peak left ventricular outflow gradient was 64 mmHg. He was given a beta-blocker and a diuretic and the glucocorticoid dose was tapered. The cardiomyopathy eventually resolved.

Dilated cardiomyopathy caused by occult pheochromocytoma has been described infrequently.

- A 34-year-old woman had acute congestive heart failure 12 hours after administration of dexamethasone 16 mg for an atypical migraine (29). The authors postulated that the acute episode had been induced by the dexamethasone, which increased the production of adrenaline, causing beta$_2$-adrenoceptor stimulation, peripheral vasodilatation, and congestive heart failure.

In an addendum the authors reported another similar case.

Obstructive cardiomyopathy has been attributed to a glucocorticoid in a child with subglottal stenosis (30).

- A 4-month-old boy (weight 4 kg) developed fever, nasal secretions, and stridor due to a subglottal granuloma. Dexamethasone 1 mg/kg/day was started and

tapered over 1 week. The mass shrank to 25% of its original size but the symptoms recurred 2 weeks later. The granuloma was excised and dexamethasone 1 mg/kg/day was restarted. After 5 days he developed a tachycardia (140/minute) and a new systolic murmur. Echocardiography showed severe ventricular hypertrophy with dynamic left ventricular outflow tract obstruction. The dexamethasone was weaned over several days. Over the next 3 weeks several echocardiograms showed rapid resolution of the outflow tract obstruction and gradual improvement of the cardiac hypertrophy. After 8 months there was no further problem.

Cardiac dysrhythmias

Serious cardiac dysrhythmias and sudden death have been reported with pulsed methylprednisolone. Oral methylprednisolone has been implicated in a case of sinus bradycardia (31).

- A 14-year-old boy received an intravenous dose of methylprednisolone 30 mg/kg for progressive glomerulonephritis. After 5 hours, his heart rate had fallen to 50/minute and an electrocardiogram showed sinus bradycardia. His heart rate then fell to 40/minutes and a temporary transvenous pacemaker was inserted and methylprednisolone was withdrawn. His heart rate increased to 80/minutes over 3 days. After a further 3 days, he was treated with oral methylprednisolone 60 mg/m^2/day and his heart rate fell to 40/minutes in 5 days. Oral methylprednisolone was stopped on day 8 of treatment and his heart rate normalized.

Hypokalemia, secondary to mineralocorticoid effects, can cause cardiac dysrhythmias and cardiac arrest.

Recurrent cardiocirculatory arrest has been reported (32).

- A 60-year-old white man was admitted for kidney transplantation. Immediately after reperfusion and intravenous methylprednisolone 500 mg, he developed severe bradycardia with hypotension and then cardiac arrest. After resuscitation, his clinical state improved quickly, but on the morning of the first postoperative day directly after the intravenous administration of methylprednisolone 250 mg, he had another episode of severe bradycardia, hypotension, and successful cardiopulmonary resuscitation. A third episode occurred 24 hours later after intravenous methylprednisolone 100 mg, again followed by rapid recovery after resuscitation. Two weeks later, during a bout of acute rejection, he was given intravenous methylprednisolone 500 mg, after which he collapsed and no heartbeat or breathing was detectable; after cardiopulmonary resuscitation he was transferred to the intensive care unit, where he died a few hours later.

If patients at risk are identified, glucocorticoid bolus therapy should be avoided or, if that is not possible, should only be done under close monitoring.

Pericarditis

- Disseminated *Varicella* and staphylococcal pericarditis developed in a previously healthy girl after a single application of triamcinolone cream 0.1% to relieve pruritus associated with *Varicella* skin lesions (SEDA-22, 443; 33).

Vasculitis

Long-term treatment with glucocorticoids can cause arteritis, but patients with rheumatoid arthritis have a special susceptibility to vascular reactions, and cases of periarteritis nodosa after withdrawal of long-term glucocorticoids have been reported (34).

Respiratory

Local adverse effects are common in patients with asthma who use inhaled glucocorticoids, as suggested by a survey of the prevalence of throat and voice symptoms in patients with asthma using glucocorticoids by metered-dose pressurized aerosol (SEDA-20, 369; 35).

There have been no reports of an increased frequency of lower respiratory tract infections. However, patients with aspiration of gastric material who were treated with glucocorticoids did not have improved survival but had a higher incidence of pneumonia (SED-12, 982).

In cases of pneumothorax with closed thoracotomy tube drainage, chronic glucocorticoid treatment has been reported to delay and impede re-expansion of the lung (SED-8, 820).

Hiccup is a rare complication of glucocorticoid therapy; five cases have been published at various times (36).

- A 59-year-old man had intractable hiccups during treatment with dexamethasone for multiple myeloma (37).
- Persistent hiccupping has been described in a 30-year-old man after the administration of a single intravenous dose of dexamethasone (16 mg) (38). The symptom was resistant to metoclopramide and resolved spontaneously after 4 days. On rechallenge, the hiccups recurred within 2 hours and disappeared after 36 hours.

Low-dose metoclopramide can be effective and may allow a patient to continue beneficial therapy without the discomfort and exhaustion that can accompany intractable hiccups.

Ear, nose, throat

Atrophic changes and fungal and other infections can alter the nasal mucosa after aerosol treatment (39), and since most systematic published documentation on these intranasal products is limited to 1–2 years of experience (although they have been in use for a far longer period), some reserve is warranted with respect to their long-term safety and the wisdom of continual use.

Nervous system

Cerebral venous thrombosis associated with glucocorticoid treatment has rarely been reported. A relation between glucocorticoids and venous thrombosis has already been suggested but has never been clearly understood. Three young patients, two women (aged 28 and 45)

and one man (aged 38 years), developed cerebral venous thrombosis after intravenous high-dose glucocorticoids (40). All presented with probable multiple sclerosis according to clinical, CSF, and MRI criteria. All had a lumbar puncture and were then treated with methylprednisolone 1 g/day for 5 days. All the usual causes of cerebral venous thrombosis were systematically excluded. The authors proposed that glucocorticoids interfere with blood coagulation and suggested that the administration of glucocorticoids after a lumbar puncture carries a particular risk of complications.

Dexamethasone is widely used for the prevention and treatment of chronic lung disease in premature infants, in whom follow-up studies have raised the possibility of an association with alterations in neuromotor function and somatic growth. In 159 survivors (mean age 53 months) of a previous placebo-controlled study, the children who had received dexamethasone had a significantly higher incidence of cerebral palsy (39/80 versus 12/79; OR = 4.62; 95% CI = 2.38, 8.98) (41). The most common form of cerebral palsy was spastic diplegia. Developmental delay was more frequent in the dexamethasone group (44/80 versus 23/79; OR = 2.9; CI = 1.5, 5.4). In a systematic review the authors concluded that postnatal dexamethasone at currently recommended doses should be avoided because of long-term neurological adverse effects (42). Lower doses of dexamethasone or inhaled glucocorticoids might be indicated for ill ventilator-dependent infants with chronic lung disease after the age of 2 weeks.

In 146 children who participated in a placebo-controlled trial of early postnatal dexamethasone therapy for the prevention of the chronic lung disease of prematurity, follow-up at school age (mean age 8 years old) showed that the children who had received dexamethasone were significantly shorter than the controls (mean height 122.8 cm versus 126.4 cm for boys and 121.3 cm versus 124.7 cm for girls) and had a significantly smaller head circumference (49.8 cm versus 50.6 cm) (43). They also had significantly poorer motor skills, motor coordination, and visuomotor integration. Compared with the controls, the children who had received dexamethasone had significantly lower IQ scores, including full scores (mean 78.2 versus 84.4), verbal scores (84.1 versus 88.4), and performance scores (76.5 versus 84.5). The frequency of clinically significant disabilities was higher among the children who had received dexamethasone than among the controls (39% versus 22%). The authors did not recommend the routine use of dexamethasone therapy for the prevention or treatment of chronic lung disease.

Long-term treatment with glucocorticoids can cause cerebral atrophy (44).

Severe organic brain syndrome has been seen in six patients taking long-term glucocorticoids (SEDA-3, 304). The manifestations included confusion, disorientation, apathy, confabulation, irrelevant speech, and slow thinking; the symptoms occurred abruptly.

Latent epilepsy can be made manifest by glucocorticoid treatment. Seizures in patients with lung transplants were related to glucocorticoids, which had been used in high dosages to prevent organ rejection. There was an increased risk of seizures in younger patients (under 25 years) and with intravenous methylprednisolone (SEDA-21, 413) (45).

Long-term glucocorticoid treatment can result in papilledema and increased intracranial pressure (the syndrome of pseudotumor cerebri or so-called "benign intracranial hypertension"), particularly in children.

- Benign intracranial hypertension occurred in a 7-month-old child after withdrawal of topical betamethasone ointment and in a 7-year-old boy treated with a 1% cortisol ointment in large amounts.
- A 6-year-old girl, who had taken prednisone for 2.5 years for nephrotic syndrome with seven relapses in 3 years, developed symptoms of benign intracranial hypertension after oral glucocorticoid dosage reduction over 10 months from 30 mg/day to 2.5 mg/every other day (46). Laboratory studies and head CT scan were normal, but there was bilateral papilledema and the cerebrospinal fluid pressure was increased. She was given prednisone 1 mg/kg/day initially, with acetazolamide, and 25 ml of cerebrospinal fluid was removed. All her symptoms resolved and treatment was gradually withdrawn. She developed no further visual failure.

The symptoms can simulate those of an intracranial tumor. All patients taking large doses of glucocorticoids who complain of headache or blurred vision, particularly after a reduction in dosage, should have an ophthalmoscopic examination to exclude this complication. Paradoxically, cerebral edema occurring during a surgical procedure can be partly prevented by glucocorticoids (47).

An encephalopathy can occur at any age (SEDA-18, 387), not necessarily in association with intracranial hypertension.

There have been repeated reports of epidural lipomatosis, which can lead to spinal cord compression (48,49) or spinal fracture (50); in one instance, the excised lipomata contained brown fat, a phenomenon that may prove to be not unusual in glucocorticoid-induced lipomata (SEDA-16, 451).

- A 40-year-old woman with ulcerative colitis took cortisone 20 mg/day and developed progressive paraplegia (50). There was kyphosis of the thoracic spine from T7 to T9, with pathological fractures. An MRI scan showed massive epidural fat extending from T1 to T9. She recovered 3 months after surgical removal of the epidural fat.
- A 78-year-old man was given methylprednisolone (60 mg/day reducing to 8 mg/day) for temporal arteritis (51). After 4 months, he developed numbness and paresis of the legs and hyperalgesia at dermatomes T3 and T4. After 10 months he had marked disturbance of proprioception combined with spinal ataxia and an increasing loss of motor bladder control. There was an intraspinal epidural lipoma in the dorsal part of the spine from T1-10. The fat was removed surgically and within 4 weeks his gait disturbance and proprioception improved, the sensory deficit abated, and the bladder disorder disappeared completely.
- A 57-year-old man took prednisone 20–30 mg/day for 13 years for rheumatoid arthritis (52). He had been

treated unsuccessfully with gold, azathioprine, hydroxychloroquine, and sulfasalazine; tapering his glucocorticoid dosage had been unsuccessful. He developed worsening back pain in his thoracic spine and lateral leg weakness. He was unable to walk. He was Cushingoid and had marked thoracic kyphosis associated with multiple vertebral body fractures in T5-8. An MRI scan at T5-6 showed displacement and compression of the spinal cord by high-signal epidural fat, which had caused anterior thecal displacement and total effacement of cerebrospinal fluid.

The authors of the last report commented on the high dose of prednisone used.

Glucocorticoid-induced spinal epidural lipomatosis is not very common in children. Spinal magnetic resonance imaging was performed in 125 children with renal diseases (68 boys); they either had back pain or numbness, were obese, or had taken a cumulative dose of prednisone of more than 500 mg/kg; there was lipomatosis in five patients (53).

In the past there was reason to think that glucocorticoids might precipitate multiple sclerosis. However, this has not been confirmed, and there is evidence that a special glucocorticoid regimen can actually be capable of retarding deterioration in multiple sclerosis (SEDA-18, 387).

A Guillain–Barré-like syndrome occurred in a patient receiving high-dose intravenous glucocorticoid therapy (SEDA-16, 449). Although glucocorticoids have been used successfully to treat weakness due to chronic inflammatory demyelinating sensorimotor neuropathy, other types of acquired chronic demyelinating neuropathies can be impaired by these drugs.

- In four patients with a pure motor demyelinating neuropathy treated with oral prednisolone (60 mg/day) motor function rapidly deteriorated within 4 weeks of starting prednisolone (SEDA-19, 375; 54). Intravenous immunoglobulin some months later in two of them produced clear improvement in strength and motor nerve conduction.

Sensory systems

The eye can be involved in generalized adverse reactions to systemically administered glucocorticoids. For example, conjunctivitis can occur as part of an allergic reaction and infections of the eye can be masked as a result of anti-inflammatory and analgesic effects. Ophthalmoplegia can occur as one of the consequences of glucocorticoid myopathy (SEDA-16, 450). Two complications that require special discussion are cataract and glaucoma.

Cataract

Oral glucocorticoid treatment is a risk factor for the development of posterior subcapsular cataract. A review of nine studies including 343 asthmatics treated with oral glucocorticoids showed a prevalence of posterior subcapsular cataracts of 0–54% with a mean value of 9% (55). In a 1993 study in children taking low-dose prednisone there were cataracts in seven of 23 cases (56). Some studies have shown a clear correlation with the duration of treatment and total dosage, others have not (SEDA-17, 449). The use of inhaled glucocorticoids was associated with a dose-dependent increased risk of posterior subcapsular and nuclear cataracts in 3654 patients aged 49–97 years (SEDA-22, 446; 57). Data on glucocorticoid use were available for 3313 of these patients; glucocorticoid use was classified as none in 2784 patients, inhaled only in 241, systemic only in 177, and both inhaled and systemic in 111. Compared with nonuse, current or prior use of inhaled glucocorticoids was associated with a significant increase in the prevalence of nuclear cataracts (adjusted relative prevalence = 1.5; 95% CI = 1.2, 1.9) and posterior subcapsular cataracts (1.9; 1.3, 2.8), but not cortical cataracts. The increased prevalence of posterior subcapsular cataracts was significantly associated with current use of inhaled glucocorticoids (2.6; 1.7, 4.0); there was no association with past use. Current use of inhaled glucocorticoids was also associated with an increased prevalence of cortical cataracts (1.4; 1.1, 1.7). The highest prevalences of posterior subcapsular and grade 4 or 5 nuclear cataracts were found in patients who had taken a cumulative dose of beclomethasone over 2000 mg.

It has been suggested that the risk of cataract is higher in patients with rheumatoid arthritis than in patients with bronchial asthma, and it is also higher in children. The reversibility of the lenticular changes has often been discussed (58,59), but even without glucocorticoid withdrawal regression has been found in children taking long-term treatment (60). Nevertheless, some 7% of the patients who develop cataract caused by glucocorticoid treatment have to be operated on. A change in permeability of the lens capsule, followed by altered electrolyte concentrations in the lens and a change in the mucopolysaccharides in the lens have been advanced as reasons for the development of cataract.

Increased intraocular pressure and glaucoma
Ocular hypertension and open-angle glaucoma are well-known adverse effects of ophthalmic administration of glucocorticoids (SEDA-17, 449).

Frequency
A total of 113 patients with angiographically proven subretinal neovascularization were enrolled into a prospective study of the effects of intravitreal triamcinolone (61). About 30% developed a significant rise in intraocular pressure (at least 5 mmHg) above baseline during the first 3 months.

A large case-control study, in which 9793 elderly patients with ocular hypertension or open-angle glaucoma were compared with 38 325 controls, has shown an increased risk of these complications with oral glucocorticoids (SEDA-22, 446; 62). The risk of ocular hypertension or open-angle glaucoma increased with increasing dose and duration of use of the oral glucocorticoid. There was no significant increase in the risk of ocular hypertension or open-angle glaucoma in patients who had stopped taking oral glucocorticoids 15–45 days before. The authors estimated that the excess risk of

ocular hypertension or open-angle glaucoma with current oral glucocorticoid use is 43 additional cases per 10 000 patients per year. However, in patients taking over 80 mg/day of hydrocortisone equivalents, the excess risk is 93 additional cases per 10 000 patients per year. Monitoring of intraocular pressure may be justified in long-term users of oral glucocorticoids, as it is in long-term users of topical glucocorticoids.

Prolonged use of high doses of inhaled glucocorticoids also increases the risk of ocular hypertension and open-angle glaucoma (SEDA-22, 446; 63). In a case-control study of the records of 9793 elderly patients with ocular hypertension or open-angle glaucoma over a 6-year period, there was a significantly increased risk of ocular hypertension and open-angle glaucoma in patients who had taken high doses of inhaled glucocorticoids (1500–1600 micrograms) for 3 months or longer (OR = 1.44; 95% CI = 1.01, 2.06). Both a high dosage of inhaled glucocorticoid and prolonged continuous duration of therapy had to be present to increase the risk.

Glaucoma and ocular hypertension have been reported after dermal application of glucocorticoids for facial atopic eczema (SEDA-19, 376) (64), and after treatment with beclomethasone by nasal spray and inhalation (SEDA-20, 373; 65).

The effects of topical dexamethasone on intraocular pressure have been compared with those of fluorometholone (SEDA-22, 446; 66). The ocular hypertensive response to topical dexamethasone in children occurs more often, more severely, and more rapidly than that reported in adults. It should be avoided in children if possible and it is desirable to monitor the intraocular pressure when it is being used. Fluorometholone may be more acceptable.

Pathogenesis
The pathogenesis of glucocorticoid-induced glaucoma is still unknown, but there is reduced outflow, and excessive accumulation of mucopolysaccharides may be a major factor. An association with cataract and papilledema has often been observed. The rise in intraocular pressure is variable: in the pediatric study of low dose cited above there was a reversible effect in only two of 23 subjects compared with controls, but in other studies serious increases in pressure have occurred, with a risk of blindness.

There is almost certainly a genetic predisposition to glucocorticoid-induced glaucoma, as there is to glaucoma in general.

Susceptibility factors
Children have more frequent, more severe, and more rapid ocular hypertensive responses to topical dexamethasone than adults. In one case a systemic glucocorticoid caused significant but asymptomatic ocular hypertension in a child (67).

- A 9-year-old girl with acute lymphoblastic leukemia received a 5-week course of oral prednisolone 60 mg/day (2.3 mg/kg/day). She did not receive any other systemic medications that have a known effect on intraocular pressure. Her baseline pressures in the right and left eyes were 16 and 17 mmHg with visual acuities of 20/20 and 20/15 respectively. The cup-to-disk ratio was 0.5 in both eyes, with normal visual fields. She was not myopic and had no family history of glaucoma or glucocorticoid responsiveness. After 8 days of systemic glucocorticoid therapy, her intraocular pressures increased to 39 mmHg and 38 mmHg in the right and left eyes respectively. Gonioscopy confirmed an open drainage angle in both eyes. She was given topical betaxolol 0.25% and dorzolamide 2% bd. However, her intraocular pressure continued to increase to 52 mmHg in the right eye and 47 mm Hg in the left eye on day 10. Topical latanoprost 0.001% od and brimonidine 0.2% bd were added, and the intraocular pressures fell to 38 mmHg and 36 mmHg. Two days after withdrawal of the prednisolone, the intraocular pressure returned rapidly to 17 mm Hg in both eyes. Over the next 6 weeks, this was maintained despite stepwise withdrawal of all glaucoma medications. Four months later, she was given a 4-week course of oral dexamethasone 10 mg/day and had similar patterns of changes in intraocular pressure. Oral acetazolamide was prescribed. She remained largely asymptomatic throughout, except for one episode of reduced visual acuity from 20/20 to 20/40 in the right eye when the intraocular pressure reached 52 mmHg.

Chorioretinopathy

Systemic glucocorticoid treatment can cause severe exacerbation of bullous exudative retinal detachment and lasting visual loss in some patients with idiopathic central serous chorioretinopathy (SEDA-20, 374; 68). The atypical presentation of this condition can include peripheral retinal capillary nonperfusion and retinal neovascularization. The treatment of choice in patients with idiopathic central serous chorioretinopathy is laser photocoagulation.

In a prospective, case-control study 38 consecutive patients (28 men and 10 women), aged 28–63 years with central serous chorioretinopathy, were compared with 38 age- and sex-matched controls (28 men and 10 women) aged 27–65 years (69). Eleven patients (29%; eight men and three women) with central serous chorioretinopathy were taking glucocorticoids, compared with two patients (5.2%; one man and one woman) in the control group (OR = 7.33, 95% CI = 1.49, 36).

Subtenon local injection of a glucocorticoid is effective in the treatment of certain forms of uveitis. Central serous chorioretinopathy, confirmed by optical coherence tomography, developed after a single local subtenon glucocorticoid injection to treat HLA-B27-associated iritis (70).

- A healthy 37-year-old man developed progressive blurred vision, photophobia, and floaters in the left eye. Best-corrected visual acuity was 20/20 in the right eye and 20/50 in the left eye. The intraocular pressures were 21 mmHg in the right eye and 16 mmHg in the left eye. The anterior and posterior segments of the right eye were normal, but the anterior segment of the left eye showed 2+ conjunctival injection and mild keratitic

precipitates. There was a 2+ anterior chamber cellular reaction with a 1 mm hypopyon, engorged iris vessels, and fibrinous iris posterior synechiae that were released after pupillary dilatation. Binocular and indirect ophthalmoscopy of the left eye showed a normal optic nerve, macula, retinal vasculature, and periphery. There was no evidence of retinal or vitreous inflammation, vasculitis, or cystoid macular edema. The fovea was well visualized after pupillary dilatation, with a normal and distinct foveal reflex. HLA-B27 iritis was suspected and subsequently confirmed with positive serotyping. He was given prednisolone acetate 1% every hour, cycloplegic eye drops, and a 1.0 ml periocular injection of triamcinolone acetonide (40 mg/ml) into the subtenon space of the left eye. Within 1 week, there was a marked therapeutic response, with complete resolution of the hypopyon and fibrin deposition and partial improvement in acuity to 20/40 in the left eye. There were only occasional residual anterior chamber inflammatory cells. Macular biomicroscopy showed the new development of subretinal fluid and serous pigment epithelial detachment at the fovea. Fluorescein angiography confirmed an enlarging pinpoint spot of hyperfluorescence. Optical coherence tomography confirmed the subretinal location of this fluid collection, consistent with a diagnosis of central serous chorioretinopathy. The topical glucocorticoid drops were rapidly tapered and withdrawn over 5 days. There was progressive reduction in subretinal fluid and gradual improvement in visual acuity. By 12 weeks the fluid had resolved and visual acuity recovered to 20/20 in the left eye.

Endophthalmitis

Intravitreal triamcinolone injection is safe and effective for cystoid macular edema caused by uveitis, diabetic maculopathy, and central retinal vein occlusion, and for pseudophakic cystoid macular edema. Potential risks include glaucoma, cataract, retinal detachment, and endophthalmitis. Infectious endophthalmitis is extremely rare when appropriate sterile technique is practised. Seven patients developed a clinical picture simulating endophthalmitis after intravitreal injection of triamcinolone (71). The authors believed that this effect was a toxic reaction to the injected material and explained that the differential diagnosis of infectious endophthalmitis in eyes that have been injected with triamcinolone under sterile conditions includes a sterile toxic endophthalmitis that requires careful monitoring, perhaps every 8-12 hours, in order to determine whether the inflammation is worsening or improving. Resolution occurs spontaneously, and in the absence of eye pain unnecessary intervention can be avoided.

Hypopyon associated with non-infectious endophthalmitis after intravitreal injection of triamcinolone has been described previously (72). Pseudohypopyon and sterile endophthalmitis after intravitreal injection of triamcinolone for pseudophakic cystoid macular edema has been reported (73).

- An 88-year-old woman underwent phacoemulsification surgery, which was complicated by posterior capsule rupture. Anterior vitrectomy was performed, with implantation of a silicone intraocular lens into the sulcus. Postoperatively, she developed cystoid macular edema, which failed to respond to topical dexamethasone, topical ketorolac, and posterior subtenon injection of triamcinolone, limiting visual acuity to 6/24 at 7 months after the surgery. An intravitreal injection of triamcinolone acetonide (4 mg in 0.1 ml) (Kenalog®, Bristol-Myers Squibb, Middlesex, UK) was administered through the pars plana with a 30-gauge needle using a sterile technique. Three days later she reported painless loss of vision, which had developed immediately after the injection. Visual acuity was reduced to perception of hand movements. There was minimal conjunctival injection and the cornea was clear. A 3 mm pseudohypopyon, consisting of refractile crystalline particles, was visible in the anterior chamber, associated with 3+ anterior chamber cells (or particles). Severe vitreous haze prevented visualization of the retina. Because infectious endophthalmitis could not be excluded, she was treated with intravitreal injections of ceftazidime and vancomycin. Vitreous and aqueous taps were performed and the pseudohypopyon was completely aspirated from the anterior chamber. The next day a 2 mm pseudohypopyon had reformed. The position of the pseudohypopyon depended on gravity and shifted with changes in head position. Aqueous and vitreous cultures were negative. Microscopy of the aspirated pseudohypopyon showed triamcinolone particles with no cells. The pseudohypopyon, vitreous haze, and cystoid macular edema (as demonstrated on optical coherence tomography) resolved spontaneously over 6 weeks and visual acuity recovered to 6/12.

The pseudohypopyon was a unique feature of this case and was due to the presence of a posterior capsule defect enabling the passage of triamcinolone from the vitreous cavity into the anterior chamber. The authors commented that presumably the triamcinolone crystals had been carried into the anterior chamber by currents generated by saccadic eye movements in the partially vitrectomized vitreous cavity. In this case the pseudohypopyon was distinguishable from an infective or inflammatory hypopyon by its ground glass appearance, the presence of refractile particles, and its shifting position, which depended on the patient's head position. The absence of ocular pain, photophobia, ciliary injection, or iris vessel dilatation suggested a non-inflammatory response and perhaps it would be appropriate to monitor such patients closely rather than administering intravitreal antibiotics.

Keratopathy and keratitis
Band-shaped keratopathy is caused by the deposition of calcium salts in the basement membrane of the corneal epithelium and superficial stroma. It is typically a chronic process that develops over a period of months and years, and is associated with chronic corneal or intraocular inflammation.

- Infectious crystalline keratopathy developed in a 73-year-old woman with noninsulin-dependent diabetes mellitus after the use of topical prednisolone 1% eye-drops, for conjunctival injection over 12 months (SEDA-20, 372; 74).
- Acute-onset calcific band keratopathy has been reported in a woman using topical prednisolone (SEDA-20, 372; 75).

Patients with severe keratoconjunctivitis sicca are at definite risk of this complication, and the addition of phosphate-containing eye-drops tilted the precariously balanced situation toward precipitation of calcium in the cornea and bandage contact lens. Acetate-containing rather than phosphate-containing glucocorticoid eye drops may be a safer alternative in patients with such predisposing factors.

Bacterial keratitis is one of the most frequent ophthalmic infections. In a meta-analysis of publications from 1950 to 2000, the use of a topical glucocorticoid before the diagnosis of bacterial keratitis significantly predisposed to ulcerative keratitis in eyes with pre-existing corneal disease (OR = 2.63; 95% CI = 1.41, 4.91). Previous glucocorticoid use significantly increased the risk of antibiotic failure or other infectious complications (OR = 3.75; 95% CI = 2.52, 5.58). The use of glucocorticoids with an antibiotic for the treatment of bacterial keratitis did not increase the risk of complications, but neither did it improve the outcome of treatment.

Retinal damage
An apparent association between severe retinopathy of prematurity and dexamethasone therapy has been shown in a retrospective study (SEDA-20, 372; 76). Infants treated with dexamethasone required longer periods of mechanical ventilation (44 versus 26 days), had a longer duration of supplemental oxygen (57 versus 29 days), had a higher incidence of patent ductus arteriosus (28/38 versus 18/52), and required surfactant therapy more often for respiratory distress syndrome (17/38 versus 11/52). Prospective, randomized, controlled studies are needed to correct for differences in severity of cardiorespiratory disease. Until such studies are available, careful consideration must be given to indications, dosage, time of initiation, and duration of treatment with dexamethasone in infants of extremely low birthweight.

Retinal hemorrhage occurred in four women after they had received epidural methylprednisolone for chronic back and hip pain (SEDA-20, 373; 77). Retinal and choroidal vascular occlusions are a serious and sometimes lasting complication of periocular and facial injections of glucocorticoids (SEDA-21, 416).

Toxic optic neuropathy
Toxic optic neuropathy can occur and may underlie various reports of sudden blindness in patients taking glucocorticoids. In one case, transient visual loss occurred on several occasions, each time after administration of a glucocorticoid (SEDA-17, 447). In another case, blindness occurred suddenly and paradoxically after glucocorticoid injections into the nasal turbinates (78). Although glucocorticoids are sometimes used successfully to relieve

pre-existing optic neuritis, a number of such patients react adversely with increased episodes of visual loss.

Exophthalmos

Exophthalmos has been described incidentally as a complication of long-term glucocorticoid therapy and there has been a series of 21 cases (79).

Psychological

The psychostimulant effects of the glucocorticoids are well known (80), and their dose dependency is recognized (SED-11, 817); they may amount to little more than euphoria or comprise severe mental derangement, for example mania in an adult with no previous psychiatric history (SEDA-17, 446) or catatonic stupor demanding electroconvulsive therapy (81). In their mildest form, and especially in children, the mental changes may be detectable only by specific tests of mental function (82). Mental effects can occur in patients treated with fairly low doses; they can also occur after withdrawal or omission of treatment, apparently because of adrenal suppression (83,84).

- A 32-year-old woman developed irritability, anger, and insomnia after taking oral prednisone (60 mg/day) for a relapse of ileal Crohn's disease (85). The prednisone was withdrawn and replaced by budesonide (9 mg/day), and the psychiatric adverse effects were relieved after 3 days. A good clinical response was maintained, with no relapse after 2 months of budesonide therapy.

Seventeen patients taking long-term glucocorticoid therapy (16 women, mean age 47 years, mean prednisone dose 16 mg, mean length of current treatment 92 months) and 15 matched controls were assessed with magnetic resonance imaging and proton magnetic resonance spectroscopy, neurocognitive tests (including the Rey Auditory Verbal Learning Test, Stroop Colour Word Test, Trail Making Test, and estimated overall intelligent quotient), and psychiatric scales (including the Hamilton Rating Scale for Depression, Young Mania Rating Scale, and Brief Psychiatric Rating Scale) (86). Glucocorticoid-treated patients had smaller hippocampal volumes and lower N-acetylaspartate ratios than controls. They had lower scores on the Rey Auditory Verbal Learning Test and Stroop Colour Word Test (declarative memory deficit) and higher scores on the Hamilton Rating Scale for Depression and the Brief Psychiatric Rating Scale (depression). These findings support the idea that chronic glucocorticoid exposure is associated with changes in hippocampal structure and function.

Development

Dexamethasone has been used in ventilator-dependent preterm infants to reduce the risk and severity of chronic lung disease. Usually it is given in a tapering course over a long period (42 days). The effects of dexamethasone on developmental outcome at 1 year of age has been evaluated in 118 infants of very low birthweights (47 boys and 71 girls, aged 15–25 days), who were not weaning from assisted ventilation (87). They were randomly assigned double-blind to receive placebo or dexamethasone (initial

dose 0.25 mg/kg) tapered over 42 days. A neurological examination, including ultrasonography, was done at 1 year of age. Survival was 88% with dexamethasone and 74% with placebo. Both groups obtained similar scores in mental and psychomotor developmental indexes. More dexamethasone-treated infants had major intracranial abnormalities (21 versus 11%), cerebral palsy (25 versus 7%; OR = 5.3; CI = 1.3, 21), and unspecified neurological abnormalities (45 versus 16%; OR = 3.6; CI = 1.2, 11). Although the authors suggested an adverse effect, they added other possible explanations for these increased risks (improved survival in those with neurological injuries or at increased risk of such injuries).

Behavioral disorders

Children have marked increases in behavioral problems during treatment with high-dose prednisone for relapse of nephrotic syndrome, according to the results of a study conducted in the USA (88). Ten children aged 2.9–15 years (mean 8.2 years) received prednisone 2 mg/kg/day, tapering at the time of remission, which was at week 2 in seven patients. At baseline, eight children had normal behavioral patterns and two had anxious/depressed and aggressive behavior using the Child Behaviour Checklist (CBCL). During high-dose prednisone therapy, five of the eight children with normal baseline scores had CBCL scores for anxiety, depression, and aggressive behavior above the 95th percentile for age. The two children with high baseline CBCL scores had worsening behavioral problems during high-dose prednisone. Behavioral problems occurred almost exclusively in the children who received over 1 mg/kg every 48 hours. Regression analysis showed that prednisone dosage was a strong predictor of increased aggressive behaviour.

Intravenous methylprednisolone was associated with a spectrum of adverse reactions, most frequently behavioral disorders, in 213 children with rheumatic disease, according to the results of a US study (12). However, intravenous methylprednisolone was generally well tolerated. The children received their first dose of intravenous methylprednisolone 30 mg/kg over at least 60 minutes, and if the first dose was well tolerated they were given further infusions at home under the supervision of a nurse. There was at least one adverse reaction in 46 children (22%) of whom 18 had an adverse reaction within the first three doses. The most commonly reported adverse reactions were behavioral disorders (21 children), including mood changes, hyperactivity, hallucinations, disorientation, and sleep disorders. Several children had serious acute reactions, which were readily controlled. Most of them were able to continue methylprednisolone therapy with premedication or were given an alternative glucocorticoid. The researchers emphasized the need to monitor treatment closely and to have appropriate drugs readily available to treat adverse reactions.

Large doses are most likely to cause the more serious behavioral and personality changes, ranging from extreme nervousness, severe insomnia, or mood swings to psychotic episodes, which can include both manic and depressive states, paranoid states, and acute toxic psychoses. A history of emotional disorders does not necessarily preclude glucocorticoid treatment, but existing emotional instability or psychotic tendencies can be aggravated by glucocorticoids. Such patients as these should be carefully and continuously observed for signs of mental changes, including alterations in the sleep pattern. Aggravation of psychiatric symptoms can occur not only during high-dose oral treatment, but also after any increase in dosage during long-term maintenance therapy; it can also occur with inhalation therapy (89). The psychomotor stimulant effect is said to be most pronounced with dexamethasone and to be much less with methylprednisolone, but this concept of a differential psychotropic effect still has to be confirmed.

Memory

The effects of prednisone on memory have been assessed (SEDA-21, 413; 90). Glucocorticoid-treated patients performed worse than controls in tests of explicit memory. Pulsed intravenous methylprednisolone (2.5 g over 5 days, 5 g over 7 days, or 10 g over 5 days) caused impaired memory in patients with relapsing-remitting multiple sclerosis, but this effect is reversible, according to the results of an Italian study (91). Compared with ten control patients, there was marked selective impairment of explicit memory in 14 patients with relapsing-remitting multiple sclerosis treated with pulsed intravenous methylprednisolone. However, this memory impairment completely resolved 60 days after methylprednisolone treatment.

Glucocorticoids can regulate hippocampal metabolism, physiological functions, and memory. Despite evidence of memory loss during glucocorticoid treatment (SEDA-23, 428), and correlations between memory and cortisol concentrations in certain diseases, it is unclear whether exposure to the endogenous glucocorticoid cortisol in amounts seen during physical and psychological stress in humans can inhibit memory performance in otherwise healthy individuals. In an elegant experiment on the effect of cortisol on memory, 51 young healthy volunteers (24 men and 27 women) participated in a double-blind, randomized, crossover, placebo-controlled trial of cortisol 40 mg/day or 160 mg/day for 4 days (92). The lower dose of cortisol was equivalent to the cortisol delivered during a mild stress and the higher dose to major stress. Cognitive performance and plasma cortisol were evaluated before and until 10 days after drug administration. Cortisol produced a dose-related reversible reduction in verbal declarative memory without effects on nonverbal memory, sustained or selective attention, or executive function. Exposure to cortisol at doses and plasma concentrations associated with physical and psychological stress in humans can reversibly reduce some elements of memory performance.

Prednisone, 10 mg/day for 1 year, has been evaluated in 136 patients with probable Alzheimer's disease in a double-blind, randomized, placebo-controlled trial (93). There were no differences in the primary measures of efficacy (cognitive subscale of the Alzheimer Disease Assessment Scale), but those treated with prednisone had significantly greater memory impairment (Clinical Dementia sum of boxes), and agitation and hostility/suspicion (Brief Psychiatric Rating Scale). Other adverse effects in those who took prednisone were reduced bone density and a small rise in intraocular pressure.

In healthy individuals undergoing acute stress, there was specifically impaired retrieval of declarative long-term memory for a word list, suggesting that cortisol-induced impairment of retrieval may add significantly to the memory deficits caused by prolonged treatment (94).

In 52 renal transplant recipients (mean age 45 years, 34 men and 18 women) taking prednisone (100 mg/day for 3 days followed by 10 mg/day for as long as needed; mean dose 11 mg/day) there was a major reduction in immediate recall but not delayed recall (95). However, there was a significant correlation between mean prednisone dose and delayed recall. In animals, phenytoin pretreatment blocks the effects of stress on memory and hippocampal histology.

In a double blind, randomized, placebo-controlled trial 39 patients (mean age 44 years, 8 men) with allergies or pulmonary or rheumatological illnesses who were taking prednisone (mean dose 40 mg/day) were randomized to either phenytoin (300 mg/day) or placebo for 7 days (96). Those who took phenytoin had significantly smaller increases in a mania self-report scale. There was no effect on memory. Thus, phenytoin blocked the hypomanic effects of prednisone, but not the effects on declarative memory.

Sleep

The effects of acute systemic dexamethasone administration on sleep structure have been investigated. Dexamethasone caused significant increases in REM latency, the percentage time spent awake, and the percentage time spent in slow-wave sleep. There were also significant reductions in the percentage time spent in REM sleep and the number of REM periods (SEDA-21, 413; 97).

Psychiatric

Use of glucocorticoids is associated with adverse psychiatric effects, including mild euphoria, emotional lability, panic attacks, psychosis, and delirium. Although high doses increase the risks, psychiatric effects can occur after low doses and different routes of administration. Of 92 patients with systemic lupus erythematosus (78 women, mean age 34 years) followed between 1999 and 2000, psychiatric events occurred in six of those who were treated with glucocorticoids for the first time or who received an augmented dose, an overall 4.8% incidence (98). The psychiatric events were mood disorders with manic features (delusions of grandiosity) (n = 3) and psychosis (auditory hallucinations, paranoid delusions, and persecutory ideas) (n = 3). Three patients were first time users (daily prednisone dose 30–45 mg/day) and three had mean increases in daily prednisone dose from baseline of 26 (range 15–33) mg. All were hypoalbuminemic and none had neuropsychiatric symptoms before glucocorticoid treatment. All the events occurred within 3 weeks of glucocorticoid administration. In five of the six episodes, the symptoms resolved completely after dosage reduction (from 40 mg to 18 mg) but in one patient an additional 8-week course of a phenothiazine was given. In a multivariate regression analysis, only hypoalbuminemia was an independent predictor of psychiatric events (HR = 0.8, 95% CI = 0.60, 0.97).

Although mood changes are common during short-term, high-dose, glucocorticoid therapy, there are virtually no data on the mood effects of long-term glucocorticoid therapy. Mood has been evaluated in 20 outpatients (2 men, 18 women), aged 18–65 years taking at least 7.5 mg/day of prednisone for 6 months (mean current dose 19 mg/day; mean duration of current prednisone treatment 129 months) and 14 age-matched controls (1 man, 13 women), using standard clinician-rated measures of mania (Young Mania Rating Scale, YMRS), depression (Hamilton Rating Scale for Depression, HRSD), and global psychiatric symptoms (Brief Psychiatric Rating Scale, BPRS, and the patient-rated Internal State Scale, ISS) (99). Syndromal diagnoses were evaluated using a structured clinical interview. The results showed that symptoms and disorders are common in glucocorticoid-dependent patients. Unlike short-term prednisone therapy, long-term therapy is more associated with depressive than manic symptoms, based on the clinician-rated assessments. The Internal State Scale may be more sensitive to mood symptoms than clinician-rated scales.

Psychoses

Mania has been attributed to glucocorticoids (100).

- A 46-year-old man, with an 8-year history of cluster headaches and some episodes of endogenous depression, took glucocorticoids 120 mg/day for a week and then a tapering dosage at the start of his latest cluster episode. His headaches stopped but then recurred after 10 days. He was treated prophylactically with verapamil, but a few days later, while the dose of glucocorticoid was being tapered, he developed symptoms of mania. The glucocorticoids were withdrawn, he was given valproic acid, and his mania resolved after 10 days. Verapamil prophylaxis was restarted and he had no more cluster headaches.

The authors commented that the manic symptoms had probably been caused by glucocorticoids or glucocorticoid withdrawal. They concluded that patients with cluster headache and a history of affective disorder should not be treated with glucocorticoids, but with valproate or lithium, which are effective in both conditions. Lamotrigine, an anticonvulsive drug with mood-stabilizing effects, may prevent glucocorticoid-induced mania in patients for whom valproate or lithium are not possible (101).

Glucocorticoids can cause neuropsychiatric adverse effects that dictate a reduction in dose and sometimes withdrawal of treatment. Of 32 patients with asthma (mean age 47 years) who took prednisone in a mean dosage of 42 mg/day for a mean duration of 5 days, those with past or current symptoms of depression had a significant reduction in depressive symptoms during prednisone therapy compared with those without depression (102). After 3–7 days of therapy there was a significant increase in the risk of mania, with return to baseline after withdrawal.

The management of a psychotic reaction in an Addisonian patient taking a glucocorticoid needs special care (SED-8, 820). Psychotic reactions that do not abate promptly when the glucocorticoid dosage is reduced to the lowest effective value (or withdrawn) may need to be treated with neuroleptic drugs; occasionally these fail and antidepressants are needed (SEDA-18, 387). However, in other cases, antidepressants appear to aggravate the symptoms.

- Two patients with prednisolone-induced psychosis improved on giving the drug in three divided daily doses. Recurrence was avoided by switching to enteric-coated tablets.

This suggests that in susceptible patients the margin of safety may be quite narrow (SED-12, 982). It is possible that reduced absorption accounted for the improvement in this case, but attention should perhaps be focused on peak plasma concentrations rather than average steady-state concentrations.

Two women developed secondary bipolar disorder associated with glucocorticoid treatment and deteriorated to depressive–catatonic states without overt hallucinations and delusions (103).

- A 21-year-old woman, who had taken prednisolone 60 mg/day for dermatomyositis for 1 year developed a depressed mood, pessimistic thought, irritability, poor concentration, diminished interest, and insomnia. Although the dose of prednisolone was tapered and she was treated with sulpiride, a benzamide with mild antidepressant action, she never completely recovered. After 5 months she had an exacerbation of her dermatomyositis and received two courses of methylprednisolone pulse therapy. Two weeks after the second course, while taking prednisolone 50 mg/day, she became hypomanic and euphoric. She improved substantially with neuroleptic medication and continued to take prednisolone 5 mg/day. About 9 months later she developed depressive stupor without any significant psychological stressor or changes in prednisolone dosage. She had mutism, reduction in contact and reactivity, immobility, and depressed mood. Manic or mixed state and psychotic symptoms were not observed. She was initially treated with intravenous clomipramine 25 mg/day followed by oral clomipramine and lithium carbonate. She improved markedly within 2 weeks with a combination of clomipramine 100 mg/day and lithium carbonate 300 mg/day. Prednisolone was maintained at 5 mg/day.
- A 23-year-old woman with ulcerative colitis and no previous psychiatric disorders developed emotional lability, euphoria, persecutory delusions, irritability, and increased motor and verbal activity 3 weeks after starting to take betamethasone 4 mg/day. She improved within a few weeks with bromperidol 3 mg/day. After 10 months she became unable to speak and eat, was mute, depressive, and sorrowful, and

responded poorly to questions. There were no neurological signs and betamethasone had been withdrawn 10 months before. She was treated with intravenous clomipramine 25 mg/day and became able to speak. Intravenous clomipramine caused dizziness due to hypotension, and amoxapine 150 mg/day was substituted after 6 days. All of her symptoms improved within 10 days. Risperidone was added for mood lability and mild persecutory ideation.

In one case, glucocorticoid-induced catatonic psychosis unexpectedly responded to etomidate (104).

- A 27-year-old woman with myasthenia gravis taking prednisolone 100 mg/day became unresponsive and had respiratory difficulties. She was given etomidate 20 mg intravenously to facilitate endotracheal intubation. One minute later she became alert and oriented, with normal muscle strength, and became very emotional. Eight hours later she again became catatonic and had a similar response to etomidate 10 mg. Glucocorticoid-induced catatonia was diagnosed, her glucocorticoid dosage was reduced, and she left hospital uneventfully 4 days later.

The effect of etomidate on catatonia, similar to that of amobarbital, was thought to be due to enhanced GABA receptor function in patients with an overactive reticular system.

A case report has suggested that risperidone, an atypical neuroleptic drug, can be useful in treating adolescents with glucocorticoid-induced psychosis and may hasten its resolution (105).

- A 14-year-old African-American girl with acute lymphocytic leukemia was treated with dexamethasone 24 mg/day for 25 days. Four days after starting to taper the dose she had a psychotic reaction with visual hallucinations, disorientation, agitation, and attempts to leave the floor. Her mother refused treatment with haloperidol. Steroids were withdrawn and lorazepam was given as needed. Nine days later the symptoms had not improved. She was given risperidone 1 mg/day; within 3 days the psychotic reaction began to improve and by 3 weeks the symptoms had completely resolved.

Obsessive-compulsive disorder

Obsessive-compulsive behavior after oral cortisone has been described (106).

- A 75-year-old white man, without a history of psychiatric disorders, took cortisone 50 mg/day for 6 weeks for pulmonary fibrosis and developed severe obsessive-compulsive behavior without affective or psychotic symptoms. He was given risperidone without any beneficial effect. The dose of cortisone was tapered over 18 days. An MRI scan showed no signs of organic brain disease and an electroencephalogram was normal. His symptoms improved 16 days after withdrawal and resolved completely after 24 days. Risperidone was withdrawn without recurrence.

Endocrine

The endocrine effects of the glucocorticoids variously involve the pituitary–adrenal axis, the ovaries and testes, the parathyroid glands, and the thyroid gland.

Pituitary gland

Empty sella syndrome occurred in a boy who developed hypopituitarism after long-term pulse therapy with prednisone for nephrotic syndrome (107).

- A 16-year-old Japanese boy's growth and development was normal until the age of 2 years. He then developed nephrotic syndrome and was treated with pulsed glucocorticoid therapy nine times over the next 14 years. After the age of 3 years, his rate of growth had fallen. At 16 years, when he was taking prednisone 60 mg/m^2/day he was given prednisone on alternate days and the dose was gradually tapered. The secretion of pituitary hormones, except antidiuretic hormone, was impaired and an MRI scan of his brain showed an empty sella and atrophy of the pituitary gland.

When markedly impaired growth is noted in patients treated with glucocorticoids long-term or in pulses, it is necessary to assess pituitary function and the anatomy of the pituitary gland. Children who receive glucocorticoid pulse therapy may develop an empty sella more frequently than is usually recognized.

Pituitary–adrenal axis

Raised glucocorticoid plasma concentrations usually result, after 2 weeks, in the first signs of iatrogenic Cushing's syndrome. The characteristic symptoms can occur individually or in combination. Whereas in Cushing's disease or corticotropin–induced Cushing's syndrome, the predominant symptoms are in part determined by hyperandrogenicity and tend to comprise hypertension, acne, impaired sight, disorders of sexual function, hirsutism or virilism, striae of the skin, and plethora, Cushing's syndrome due to glucocorticoid therapy is likely to cause benign intracranial hypertension, glaucoma, subcapsular cataract, pancreatitis, aseptic necrosis of the bones, and panniculitis. Obesity, facial rounding, psychiatric symptoms, edema, and delayed wound healing are common to these different forms of Cushing's syndrome.

It has been said that Cushing-like effects are to be expected if the function of the adrenal cortex is suppressed by daily doses of more than 50 mg hydrocortisone or its equivalent. However, pituitary–adrenal suppression has been described at lower dosage equivalents, for example during prolonged intermittent therapy with dexamethasone (108). The secondary adrenal insufficiency caused by therapeutically effective doses can be observed even after giving prednisone 5 mg tds for only 1 week; after withdrawal, adrenal suppression lasts for some days. If one continues this treatment for about 20 weeks, maximal atrophy of the adrenal cortex results, and lasts for some months. This effect begins with inhibition of the hypothalamus, and culminates in true atrophy of the adrenal cortex. It can occur even with glucocorticoids given by inhalation (109). Inhaled fluticasone is associated with at least a twofold greater suppression of adrenal function than inhaled budesonide microgram for microgram, according to the results of a crossover study (SEDA-21, 415; 110). Patients with liver disease may experience adrenal suppression with lower doses of glucocorticoids (111). It is advisable to use alternate-day therapy to avoid suppression of corticotropin secretion in patients who will need long-term therapy; it will produce the same therapeutic effect as daily dosage. It can be helpful to measure the degree of suppression of corticotropin secretion during long-term glucocorticoid treatment of asthmatic children, as a means of optimizing therapy and avoiding excessive dosage (112). The period of time during which the patient should be considered at risk of adrenal insufficiency after withdrawal of oral prednisolone treatment in childhood nephrotic syndrome is still controversial. A study in such patients has suggested that adrenal insufficiency may occur up to 9 months after treatment has ended (SEDA-19, 376; 113).

Many protocols for treating children with early B cell acute lymphoblastic leukemia involve 28 consecutive days of high-dose glucocorticoids during induction. The effect of this therapy on adrenal function has been prospectively evaluated (114) in 10 children by tetracosactide stimulation before the start of dexamethasone therapy and every 4 weeks thereafter until adrenal function returned to normal. All had normal adrenal function before dexamethasone treatment and impaired adrenal responses 24 hours after completing therapy. Each child felt ill for 2–4 weeks after completing therapy. Seven patients recovered normal adrenal function after 4 weeks, but three did not have normal adrenal function until 8 weeks after withdrawal. Thus, high-dose dexamethasone therapy can cause adrenal insufficiency lasting more than 4 weeks after the end of treatment. This problem might be avoided by tapering doses of glucocorticoids and providing supplementary glucocorticoids during periods of increased stress.

Tolerance to glucocorticoids in this, as in some other respects, varies from individual to individual; some patients tolerate 30 mg of prednisone for a long time without developing Cushing's syndrome, while others develop symptoms at 7.5 mg; the doses recommended today to avoid Cushing's syndrome in most patients are usually equivalent to hydrocortisone 20 mg. Cushing's syndrome and other systemic adverse effects can occur not only from oral and injected glucocorticoids, but also from topical and intranasal treatment (115) and intrapulmonary or epidural administration (SEDA-19, 376; SEDA-20, 370; 116,117).

- Two patients developed hypopituitarism and empty sella syndrome during glucocorticoid pulse therapy for nephrotic syndrome (SEDA-22, 444; 118).

Glucocorticoid-treated patients with inadequate adrenal function who have an intercurrent illness or are due to undergo surgery will have an inadequate reaction to the resulting stress and need to be temporarily protected by additional glucocorticoid (119).

Iatrogenic Cushing's syndrome after a single low dose is exceptional (120).

- A 45-year-old woman was given a single-dose of intramuscular triamcinolone acetonide 40 mg for acute laryngitis and 1 month later was noted to have a cushingoid appearance. Endocrinological tests confirmed hypothalamic–pituitary–adrenal (HPA) axis suppression. Eight months later, the cushingoid appearance had completely disappeared and HPA function had spontaneously recovered.

Pseudohyperaldosteronism has been reported even after intranasal application of 9-alpha-fluoroprednisolone (SEDA-11, 340).

Parathyroid function

There is antagonism between the parathyroid hormone and glucocorticoids (121). Latent hyperparathyroidism can be unmasked by glucocorticoids (122).

Thyroid function

Even a single dose of corticotropin briefly inhibits the secretion of thyrotrophic hormone. The uptake of radioactive iodine is also suppressed by corticotropin and by glucocorticoids, but this has no clinical relevance. Pathological changes in thyroid function induced by glucocorticoid treatment are reportedly rare.

Metabolism

Glucose metabolism

All glucocorticoids increase gluconeogenesis. The turnover of glucose is increased, more being metabolized to fat, and blood glucose concentration is increased by 10–20%. Glucose tolerance and sensitivity to insulin are reduced, but provided pancreatic islet function is normal, carbohydrate metabolism will not be noticeably altered. So-called "steroid diabetes," a benign diabetes without a tendency to ketosis, but with a low sensitivity to insulin and a low renal threshold to glucose, only develops in one-fifth of patients treated with high glucocorticoid dosages. Even in patients with diabetes, ketosis is not to be expected, since glucocorticoids have antiketotic activity, presumably through suppression of growth hormone secretion.

Glucocorticoid treatment of known diabetics normally leads to deregulation, but this can be compensated for by adjusting the dose of insulin. The increased gluconeogenesis induced by glucocorticoids mainly takes place in the liver, but glucocorticoid treatment is especially likely to disturb carbohydrate metabolism in liver disease.

When hyperglycemic coma occurs it is almost always of the hyperosmolar nonketotic type. After termination of glucocorticoid treatment, steroid diabetes normally disappears. An apparent exception to these findings is provided by the case of a patient in whom glucocorticoid treatment was followed by severe diabetes with diabetic nephropathy, but this was a seriously ill individual who had already undergone renal transplantation (SEDA-17, 449). Gestational diabetes mellitus was more common in women who had received glucocorticoids with or without beta-adrenoceptor agonists for threatened preterm delivery compared with controls (SEDA-22, 445; 123).

Glucocorticoids probably have more than one effect on carbohydrate metabolism. An increase in fasting glucagon concentration has been observed in volunteers given prednisolone 40 mg/day for 4 days, and this effect may be involved, alongside gluconeogenesis, in glucocorticoid-induced hyperglycemia. Some newer glucocorticoids have been claimed to have smaller effects on blood glucose (as well as less salt and water retention), but further studies are needed to confirm whether this interesting therapeutic approach has been successful (SEDA-13, 353).

Deflazacort, an oxazoline derivative of prednisolone, was introduced as a potential substitute for conventional glucocorticoids in order to ameliorate glucose intolerance. In a randomized study in kidney transplant recipients with pre- or post-transplantation diabetes mellitus, 42 patients who switched from prednisone to deflazacort (in the ratio 5:6 mg) were prospectively compared with 40 patients who continued to take prednisone (SEDA-22, 445; 124). During the mean follow-up period of 13 months, neither graft dysfunction nor acute rejection developed in the conversion group, and there was improvement in blood glucose control. When the conversion group was stratified into those with pre- or post-transplantation diabetes, there were promising effects in the patients with post-transplantation diabetes. More than a 50% dosage reduction of hypoglycemic drugs was possible in 42% of those with post-transplantation diabetes.

The risk of hyperglycemia requiring treatment in patients receiving oral glucocorticoids has been quantified in a case-control study of 11 855 patients, 35 years of age or older, with newly initiated treatment with a hypoglycemic drug (SEDA-19, 375; 125). The risk for initiating hypoglycemic therapy increased with the recent use of a glucocorticoid. The risk grew with increasing average daily glucocorticoid dosage (in mg of hydrocortisone equivalents): 1.77 for 1–39 mg/day, 3.02 for 40–79 mg/day, 5.82 for 80–119 mg/day, and 10.34 for 120 mg/day or more.

Lipid metabolism

High-dose glucocorticoid therapy can cause marked hypertriglyceridemia, with milky plasma (SEDA-15, 421; SEDA-16, 450). It has been suggested that this is caused by abnormal accumulation of dietary fat, reduced post-heparin lipolytic activity, and glucose intolerance (126). An association between glucocorticoid exposure and hypercholesterolemia has been found in several studies (127) and can contribute to an increased risk of atherosclerotic vascular disease.

Most premature neonates need intravenous lipids during the first few weeks of life to acquire adequate energy intake and prevent essential fatty acid deficiency before they can tolerate all nutrition via enteral feeds. Dexamethasone is associated with multiple adverse effects in neonates, including poor weight gain and impairment of glucose and protein metabolism. In ten neonates (four boys, mean age 17.3 days) taking dexamethasone for bronchopulmonary dysplasia, intravenous lipids (3 g/kg/day) caused hypertriglyceridemia in the presence of hyperinsulinemia and increased free fatty acid

concentrations (128). Because of concomitant hyperinsulinemia, the authors speculated that dexamethasone reduced fatty acid oxidation, explaining poor weight gain.

Altered fat deposition has been repeatedly reported. Fat can be deposited epidurally and at other sites. Adiposis dolora, which involves the symmetrical appearance of multiple painful fat deposits in the subcutaneous tissues, has on one occasion been attributed to glucocorticoids (SEDA-16, 451).

Tumor lysis syndrome

Acute tumor lysis syndrome is a life-threatening metabolic emergency that results from rapid massive necrosis of tumor cells. There have been repeated reports of an acute tumor lysis syndrome when glucocorticoids are administered in patients with pre-existing lymphoid tumors (129).

- A 60-year-old woman took dexamethasone 4 mg 8-hourly for dyspnea due to a precursor T lymphoblastic lymphoma-leukemia with bilateral pleural effusions and a large mass in the anterior mediastinum (130). She developed acute renal insufficiency and laboratory evidence of the metabolic effects of massive cytolysis. She received vigorous hydration, a diuretic, allopurinol, and hemodialysis. She recovered within 2 weeks and then underwent six courses of CHOP chemotherapy. The mediastinal mass regressed completely. She remained asymptomatic until she developed full-blown acute lymphoblastic leukemia, which was resistant to treatment.

Electrolyte balance

The severity of potassium loss due to glucocorticoids depends partly on the amount of sodium in the diet; the most widely used synthetic glucocorticoids cause less potassium excretion than natural hydrocortisone does. Prednisone and prednisolone have a glucocorticoid activity 4–5 times that of hydrocortisone, but their mineralocorticoid activity is less (see Table 1); even at high dosages they do not cause noteworthy sodium and water retention. Of the major synthetic glucocorticoids, dexamethasone has the strongest anti-inflammatory, hyperglycemic, and corticotropin-inhibitory activity; sodium retention is completely absent; the degree of glucocorticoid-induced metabolic alkalosis may also be less with dexamethasone than with hydrocortisone or methylprednisolone (SEDA-10, 343).

Mineral balance

There can be increases in calcium and phosphorus loss because of effects on both the kidney and the bowel, with increased excretion and reduced resorption (131). Tetany, which has been seen in patients receiving high-dose long-term intravenous glucocorticoids, has been explained as being due to hypocalcemia, and there are also effects on bone. Tetany has also been reported in a patient with latent hyperparathyroidism after the administration of a glucocorticoid (122).

Hypocalcemic encephalopathy occurred in a 35-year-old woman with hypoparathyroidism. It was believed that the administration of methylprednisolone intramuscularly had precipitated severe hypocalcemia, which had led to a metabolic encephalopathy (SEDA-20, 371; 132).

The administration of large doses of glucocorticoids to patients with major burns presenting with low cardiac output has been reported to produce a reversible drop in serum zinc, which might lead to impaired tissue repair (SED-8, 824), but it is not clear whether this has clinical effects.

Metal metabolism

Glucocorticoids increase chromium losses and glucocorticoid-induced diabetes can be reversed by chromium supplementation (133). Doses of hypoglycemic drugs were also reduced by 50% in all patients when they were given supplementary chromium.

Hematologic

Erythrocytes

Polycythemia is a symptom of Cushing's syndrome, and conversely anemia correlates with Addison's disease, but polycythemia is not generally encountered as a consequence of treatment with glucocorticoids, perhaps because there is no increased secretion of androgens; an increase in hemoglobin was nevertheless the most frequent adverse effect observed in a study over 8 years of 77 patients treated for hyperergic-allergic reactions. At the beginning of treatment more than 40% (and during continuous therapy more than 70%) of patients showed this change in erythrocytes (134). There was leukocytosis in more than 60% in the early phases and in more than 40% later (134). Thrombocytosis occurred in 5–10% during continuous treatment. This report agrees fairly well with some older publications, but it has been noted in the past that in the long run very high-dose glucocorticoid treatment can result in suppression of the activity of the bone marrow with fatty infiltration replacing hemopoietic tissue.

Leukocytes

Not all classes of leukocytes are affected by glucocorticoids in the same way. The total leukocyte count is increased, but the number of eosinophilic leukocytes falls, as does the lymphocyte count. The number of monocytes is reduced, as is their capacity to perform phagocytosis.

In children, a leukemoid reaction has been induced by betamethasone treatment (135); this possibility must always be borne in mind, since glucocorticoids can actually be used to treat leukemia or its complications. A case of very high white blood cell count with neutrophilia in a preterm infant whose mother had received two doses of betamethasone prenatally to enhance fetal lung maturation is one of a short list of leukemoid reactions possibly attributable to antenatal glucocorticoid treatment (136).

It is possible that in children with acute lymphoblastic leukemia, glucocorticoid therapy adversely affects the duration of remissions, and it has therefore been suggested that leukemia should be ruled out in children

before starting long-term therapy with glucocorticoids (SEDA-11, 340). Depression of the lymphocyte count seems to be a general and direct action of the glucocorticoids (137), but the mechanism is still incompletely understood; certainly, lymphocytolysis seems to be increased by glucocorticoids. Studies of lymphocyte subpopulations show a preferential reduction in T cells, while B cells are constant or slightly reduced. B lymphocyte function (measured as immunoglobulin synthesis) falls, suppressor T lymphocyte activity is suppressed, and helper T lymphocyte function is unaffected by glucocorticoids (SEDA-3, 308) (138).

- Fever and leukopenia with methylprednisolone and prednisolone has been reported in a 29-year-old woman with systemic lupus erythematosus (139).

The authors commented that fever associated with glucocorticoids occurs frequently, whereas leukopenia is rare. Fever and leukopenia are important signs of an exacerbation of systemic lupus erythematosus, and it would be difficult to distinguish between an exacerbation of the disease and an adverse effect of glucocorticoids.

Platelets and coagulation

In heart transplant recipients, intramuscular glucocorticoids can impair fibrinolysis, producing susceptibility to thrombotic disease (SEDA-22, 443; 140). They can also increase the platelet count. In one patient the blue toe syndrome occurred repeatedly when glucocorticoids were used to increase the platelet count (SEDA-16, 451).

Mouth

Oral candidiasis is seen in some 5–10% of patients who use inhaled glucocorticoids, particularly when oral hygiene is poor, but is rarely symptomatic. The risk can be reduced by the use of a large-volume spacer (141,142).

Hypertrophy of the tongue has been attributed to inhaled beclomethasone and may have been related to edema of the buccal mucosa and tongue from direct contact with the glucocorticoid, infection, glossitis caused by glucocorticoid therapy, a direct effect of glucocorticoids on the tongue muscle, or excess localized deposition of fat, as is seen in patients given systemic glucocorticoids (SEDA-20, 371; 143).

Gastrointestinal

Peptic ulceration

It is no longer seriously believed that glucocorticoid treatment in adults markedly increases the risk of peptic ulceration (144,145). However, the symptoms of an existing peptic ulcer can certainly be masked. There may also be a genuine risk of ulcerative disorders in premature children. The issue has often been complicated by the simultaneous (sometimes unrecorded) use of ulcerogenic non-steroidal anti-inflammatory agents. A meta-analysis of whether glucocorticoid therapy caused peptic ulcer and other putative complications of glucocorticoid therapy was negative: peptic ulcers occurred in nine of 3267 patients in the placebo group (0.03%) and 13 of 3335 patients in the glucocorticoid group (0.04%).

Peptic ulcer should not be considered a contraindication when glucocorticoid therapy is indicated (SEDA-19, 376) (146). However, the risk of a fatal outcome due to ulcer complications was increased about fourfold in a previous case-control study. Gastrointestinal hemorrhage occurred more often in glucocorticoid-treated patients (2.25%) than in controls (1.6%) (147). The frequency of gastrointestinal bleeding in these studies compares well with earlier observations in the Boston Collaborative Surveillance Program's 1978 report, according to which 0.5% of a large series of medical inpatients taking glucocorticoids had gastrointestinal bleeding sufficiently severe to require transfusions and 28% had minor bleeding (SED-12, 986).

- A 47-year-old woman developed a gastrocolic fistula during treatment with aspirin (dosage and duration of therapy not stated) and prednisone for chronic rheumatoid arthritis (148).

The author commented that 50–75% of gastrocolic fistulas are related to benign gastric ulcers secondary to the use of NSAIDs. The use of aspirin plus prednisone, as in this patient, increases the risk of complication of peptic ulcer disease two- to fourfold.

The mechanism of whatever harm glucocorticoids may do to the stomach is not clear; cortisol neither consistently increases acid or pepsinogen secretion, nor reduces the protective production of mucin by the gastric mucosa. Serum gastrin concentrations are raised in Cushing's syndrome and in patients taking prolonged glucocorticoid treatment. On the other hand, the secretion of prostaglandin E_2 in gastric juice in response to pentagastrin was impaired during glucocorticoid therapy in children. Since PGE_2 has a cytoprotective effect on the gastric mucosa, impaired secretion in response to increased acid secretion during glucocorticoid therapy may be related to the development of peptic ulcer (SEDA-19, 376; 149).

Some reports suggest that people with hepatic cirrhosis or nephrotic syndrome are particularly at risk. Whatever the degree of risk, patients taking long-term glucocorticoids should be regularly checked to detect peptic ulcers, which can bleed and even perforate without producing pain. There do not seem to be differences in gastric tolerance between the various synthetic glucocorticoids.

Regional ileitis

While glucocorticoids may have a beneficial effect on regional ileitis, perforation of the ileum, lymphatic dilatation, and microscopic fistulae have been observed after treatment.

Ischemic colitis

Glucocorticoids should be used with caution in progressive systemic sclerosis, and concomitant administration of anticoagulants to prevent ischemic colitis is recommended when administering glucocorticoids in high doses, especially by pulse therapy (SEDA-21, 415; 150).

Ulcerative colitis

A possible risk of glucocorticoid treatment of ulcerative colitis is the development of toxic megacolon or colonic

perforation. A change from ulcerative colitis to Crohn's disease may have been induced by prolonged treatment with glucocorticoids (SEDA-19, 376; 151). This case provides further evidence for the view that ulcerative colitis and Crohn's disease may represent a continuous spectrum of inflammatory bowel disease and raises the possibility that reduced polymorphonuclear leukocyte function caused by glucocorticoids may have provoked the development of granulomata.

Diverticular disease

Existing diverticula can perforate during glucocorticoid therapy (SEDA-18, 387). Abdominal tenderness is the most common and often the only early sign of perforated diverticula in patients taking glucocorticoids. However, in some cases, even abdominal tenderness is absent (SEDA-22, 445; 152).

- Perforation of the sigmoid colon occurred in a 61-year-old Caucasian man with colonic diverticular disease and rheumatoid arthritis treated with pulses of methylprednisolone 1 g (153).

The authors suggested that methylprednisolone pulses should be used carefully in patients over 50 years of age and/or people with demonstrated or suspected diverticular disease.

The importance of treatment with glucocorticoids and NSAIDs in the development of sigmoid diverticular abscess perforation has been the subject of a case-control study in 64 patients (38 women), median age 70 years (range 39–91) and 320 age- and sex-matched controls (154). Independently of rheumatic diagnosis glucocorticoid treatment was strongly associated with sigmoid diverticular abscess perforation (OR = 32; 95% CI = 6.4, 159).

Liver

The process of gluconeogenesis, which is promoted by glucocorticoids, takes place mainly in the liver. The glycolytic enzymes of the liver are also activated by these glucocorticoids. The synthesis of ribonucleic acid and of enzymes involved in protein catabolism is increased, but the process of protein catabolism takes place outside the liver as well, for example in the muscles. There is experimental evidence for glucocorticoid-induced enhancement of hepatic lipid synthesis (SEDA-3, 308), but the main effect of glucocorticoids in this connection is lipid mobilization from adipose tissue. The influence of long-term glucocorticoid treatment on liver function is still unknown. If pathological changes are diagnosed, the possible influence of the disease which is being treated has to be borne in mind.

Liver damage from glucocorticoids is rarely severe, but fatal liver failure has been reported.

- A 71-year-old white woman with a compressive optic neuropathy was given five cycles of intravenous methylprednisolone 1 g/day for 3 days followed by tapering oral cortisone for 10–14 days (155). The intervals between cycles were 14 days to 6 weeks. She was otherwise healthy and had no history of liver disease. Her liver function tests were normal or only slightly raised during the first five cycles. She then developed raised liver enzymes, a prolonged prothrombin time, and fatal liver failure. Postmortem examination showed necrosis of the liver parenchyma. Hepatitis serology (A, B, and C) was negative as was in situ hybridization for immunohistochemical proof of hepatitis Bs and Bc or delta virus antibodies in the liver.

- A 53-year-old woman who took prednisolone 20 mg/day for systemic lupus erythematosus for 38 days developed increased aspartate transaminase and alanine transaminase activities (175 and 144 IU/l respectively on day 38 and 871 and 658 IU/l on day 69) (156). She denied taking hepatotoxic drugs. Serological tests for hepatitis viruses were all negative. Autoantibodies against mitochondria and smooth muscle were not detected. Ultrasound and CT scan were consistent with fatty infiltration. Histology showed macrovesicular fat infiltration, periportal cell infiltration with fibrosis, and a few Mallory bodies. The glucocorticoid was gradually tapered and the transaminases gradually fell.
- A 67-year-old teetotaler was given intravenous prednisolone 25 mg tds for primary dermatomyositis and 8 days later developed painless icteric hepatitis, with daily progressive marked deterioration of liver biochemistry (157). She had not taken any other hepatotoxic drugs, and serological tests for hepatitis and hepatotropic viruses were all negative. Antinuclear, antimitochondrial, and smooth muscle autoantibodies were negative. Ultrasound and CT scan of the upper abdomen showed liver fatty infiltration. Prednisolone was tapered gradually, and she gradually improved. However, on day 26 she developed pneumonia and died 6 days later.

Glucocorticoid treatment in the early phase of acute viral hepatitis carries the risk of transition to chronic active hepatitis (SEDA-3, 308).

Three children developed hepatomegaly and raised liver enzymes after receiving high-dose dexamethasone therapy (0.66–1.09 mg/kg/day) (158).

There has been a report of seven cases of acute severe liver damage associated with intravenous glucocorticoid pulse therapy in patients with Grave's ophthalmopathy (159).

Pancreas

Pancreatitis and altered pancreatic secretion can occur at any time during long-term glucocorticoid treatment (SED-12, 986; SEDA-14, 339; 160). Necrosis of the pancreas during glucocorticoid treatment has been described and can be lethal. Impairment of pancreatic function can predispose to glucocorticoid-induced pancreatitis. Two other cases of glucocorticoid-induced pancreatitis have been reported (161).

- A 74-year-old woman with seronegative rheumatoid arthritis was given sulfasalazine followed by methotrexate, both of which were withdrawn because of adverse effects. She also took prednisone 10 mg/day. She developed acute abdominal pain and fever (38.7°C) with no chills. Her serum amylase was 269 IU/l, serum lipase

300 IU/l, and urinary amylase 2895 IU/l. There was no evidence of tumor, hypertriglyceridemia, or lithiasis. In addition to prednisone, she was taking amlodipine, bromazepam, and omeprazole, none of which have been reported to cause pancreatitis. A marked improvement was noted after prednisone withdrawal.
- A 68-year-old woman who had taken prednisone 30 mg/day for polymyalgia rheumatica for 6 months developed sharp stabbing abdominal pain, fever (39°C), and vomiting. Her serum amylase was 310 IU/l, serum lipase 340 IU/l, and urinary amylase 1560 IU/l. Other causes of pancreatitis were ruled out. She had been taking a thiazide diuretic therapy for the past 10 years. Her symptoms improved noticeably after prednisone withdrawal.

Although the literature suggests a causal relation between glucocorticoid therapy and these various pancreatic complications there is still no certainty; glucocorticoid treatment is, after all, often given simultaneously with other forms of therapy which can cause pancreatitis (SED-11, 82). The strongest evidence that there is a causal relation is provided by a Japanese report on 52 autopsies, which showed marked changes in pancreatic histology in glucocorticoid-treated patients compared with controls (SEDA-17, 449).

Acute pancreatitis after rechallenge provides direct evidence that hydrocortisone can cause acute pancreatitis in a patient with ulcerative colitis (162).

- An 18-year old youth was admitted with a history of large bowel diarrhea off and on for 6 months before admission. There was a history of passage of blood mixed with stools for the same duration. There was no history of fever, arthralgias, jaundice, or red eyes. At the time of admission he was passing 10-12 stools in 24 hours, and 6-7 of them contained blood. His pulse rate was 100/minute and there was pallor and minimal pedal edema. He was tender in the flanks with exaggerated bowel sounds. Sigmoidoscopy showed ulceration, erythema, friability, and loss of vascular pattern in the rectum and sigmoid colon, suggestive of ulcerative colitis. A rectal biopsy showed crypt atrophy, crypt abscesses, a mixed cellular infiltrate, goblet cell depletion, and submucosal edema. He was given intravenous fluids and injectable hydrocortisone 100 mg six times an hour. Injections of ofloxacin and metronidazole were added later, because his leukocyte count was 15.6 x 10⁹/l. On the second day of treatment he developed epigastric pain radiating to the back. The pain was continuous, associated with vomiting, and relieved by sitting in the knee-chest position. Acute pancreatitis was corroborated by a serum lipase activity of 650 units/l and high serum amylase activity (550 units/l). Ultrasonography showed a bulky, heterogeneous pancreas with ill defined margins, suggestive of pancreatitis. There were no gallstones. Hydrocortisone was withdrawn and the rest of the treatment continued. Mesalazine was added after 1 day. The pancreatitis resolved in 48 hours, as did the diarrhea. After 1 month the patient was readmitted with a relapse of ulcerative colitis. This time his stool frequency was

4–5 stools in 24 hours, and most contained some blood. There was no fever and his total leukocyte count was normal. He was given mesalazine enemas and injectable hydrocortisone. On the second day after admission, he had a similar bout of acute pancreatitis. Hydrocortisone was withdrawn and he recovered.

Urinary tract

Urinary calculi are more likely during glucocorticoid treatment because of increased excretion of calcium and phosphate (131).

Prednisolone can cause an abrupt rise in proteinuria in patients with nephrotic syndrome. A placebo-controlled study in 26 patients aged 18–68 years with nephrotic syndrome has clarified the mechanisms responsible for this (163). Systemic and renal hemodynamics and urinary protein excretion were measured after prednisolone (125 mg or 150 mg when body weight exceeded 75 kg) and after placebo. Prednisolone increased proteinuria by changing the size–selective barrier of the glomerular capillaries. Neither the renin–angiotensin axis nor prostaglandins were involved in these effects of prednisolone on proteinuria.

Changes resembling diabetic nodular glomerular sclerosis have been seen in glucocorticoid-treated nephrosis.

Treatment with glucocorticoids can result in minor increases in the urinary content of leukocytes and erythrocytes without clear renal injury (164).

The use of high doses of glucocorticoids to counter rejection of renal transplants is still a matter of intensive study; the optimal dose to ensure an effect without undue risk of complications has yet to be agreed on (165).

Vasopressin-resistant polyuria induced by intravenous administration of a therapeutic dose of dexamethasone has been reported (SEDA-20, 370; 166) and nocturia is fairly common during glucocorticoid treatment (167).

The administration of glucocorticoids should be undertaken with caution in progressive systemic sclerosis and the concomitant administration of anticoagulants to prevent scleroderma renal crisis is recommended when administering glucocorticoids in high doses, especially by pulse therapy (SEDA-21, 415; 150).

Skin

Acne is common during treatment, particularly after topical application, and is said to be correlated with the use of compounds that have a particularly strong local effect (168), although this is not proven.

Leukoderma can occur, accompanied by normal melanocyte function but reduced phagocytic activity of the keratinocytes to eliminate the melanosomes (169). Depigmentation can occur at the site of injection of glucocorticoids.

Three cases of severe lipoatrophy, one also with leukoderma, occurring within the same family after intramuscular injection of triamcinolone, suggested genetic susceptibility to this adverse effect (SEDA-3, 303).

Inhibition of the function of the sebaceous glands in the skin is caused by glucocorticoids whilst androgens stimulate their function (170).

A delayed hypersensitivity reaction, characterized by a skin rash, due to dexamethasone has been reported (171). These kinds of reactions to systemic glucocorticoids are rarely reported.

- A 59-year-old woman, who had not used glucocorticoids before, developed an exfoliative rash on her face, upper chest, and skin folds after 3 days treatment with oral dexamethasone (dosage not stated) for an acute episode of encephalomyelitis disseminata. Dexamethasone was immediately withdrawn and her skin lesions resolved over several days. Patch tests were positive to dexamethasone, betamethasone, and clobetasol, but negative to other glucocorticoids, including prednisolone, hydrocortisone butyrate, methylprednisolone, and triamcinolone. Prick tests with all of these glucocorticoids were negative. She tolerated oral methylprednisolone without adverse effects.

Reduced skin thickness and bruising

The glucocorticoids reduce subcutaneous collagen and cause atrophic changes in the skin (172). Subcutaneous atrophy after intramuscular and intra-articular injection has often been reported. Ecchymosis and paper-thin skin folds recall those seen in old people. An increased incidence of subcutaneous ecchymosis in older women has been observed during treatment with triamcinolone acetate (173). Purpura has been observed during glucocorticoid treatment and an increased fragility of the capillaries is thought to occur in about 60% of these patients. There have been reports of cutaneous bruising after the use of high doses of inhaled glucocorticoids (budesonide and beclomethasone), suggesting systemic absorption (SEDA-21, 416; 174).

Prednicarbate is a topical glucocorticoid that seems to have an improved benefit–harm balance, as has been shown in 24 healthy volunteers (7 men, 17 women, aged 25–49 years) in a double-blind, randomized, placebo-controlled study of the effects of prednicarbate, mometasone furoate, and betamethasone 17-valerate on total skin thickness over 6 weeks (175). On day 36, total skin thickness was reduced by a mean of 1% in test fields treated with vehicle; the relative reductions were 13, 17, and 24% for prednicarbate, mometasone furoate, and betamethasone 17-valerate respectively. There were visible signs of atrophy or telangiectasia in two subjects each with betamethasone 17-valerate and mometasone furoate, but not with prednicarbate or its vehicle.

Contact allergy

Topical glucocorticoids are well-known contact sensitizers. Immediate allergic or allergic-like reactions to systemic glucocorticoids also occur, but less often. Two atopic patients developed urticaria, possibly IgE-mediated, from a hydrocortisone injection or infusion (176) and other reactions have been reported.

- A 50-year-old woman developed contact dermatitis on her legs after she applied hydrocortisone aceponate cream (Efficort) to psoriatic lesions on her lower back (177). Similar lesions also occurred on her legs after she used topical betamethasone cream (Diprosone). However, no eczema developed on or around the site of application. Patch tests were negative to a range of glucocorticoids, including Efficort and Diprosone creams. However, a repeated open application test was positive with Efficort cream, hydrocortisone aceponate 0.127% in petroleum, and tixocortol pivalate 1% in petroleum.

- A 42-year-old woman developed a nonpigmented fixed drug eruption after skin testing and an intra-articular injection of triamcinolone acetonide, which has not been previously reported (178).

Contact allergy to glucocorticoids was evaluated in 7238 patients in a multicenter multinational study of five drugs: budesonide, betamethasone-17-valerate, clobetasol-17-propionate, hydrocortisone-17-butyrate, and tixocortol-21-pivalate. There was a positive patch-test reaction to at least one of the glucocorticoids in 189 patients (2.6%). The incidence ranged from 0.4% in Spain to 6.4% in Belgium. Positive reactions were more frequent with budesonide (100 results) and tixocortol (98 reactions) (SEDA-21, 415; 179). Contact allergic reactions to intranasal budesonide and fluticasone propionate have been described. Many of these cases were characterized by perinasal eczema, often with vesicles, and edema as the initial symptoms. Lesions sometimes spread to the upper lip, cheeks, and eyelids. For fluticasone propionate, analysis of data on adverse events from the Spontaneous Reporting System of the US FDA Division of Epidemiology and Surveillance showed that, in the first 5 months after its introduction into the USA in 1995, 46 patients reported 89 adverse events suspected to be caused by fluticasone propionate intranasal spray. Central nervous system symptoms occurred in 46%, cardiac symptoms in 28%, dermatological symptoms in 39%, and epistaxis in 6.5%. These numbers may underestimate the problem, since no cases reported by the drug manufacturer were included. These results suggest that safety issues may differentiate budesonide and fluticasone propionate from other intranasal glucocorticoids, such as beclomethasone dipropionate (SEDA-21, 415; 180).

Budesonide is advocated as a marker molecule for glucocorticoid contact allergy. When patch testing glucocorticoids, one must consider both their sensitizing potential and their anti-inflammatory properties, as well as the possibility of different time courses of such properties. The dose–response relation for budesonide has therefore been investigated with regard to dose, occlusion time, and reading time in 10 patients (ages not stated) who were patch tested with budesonide in ethanol in serial dilutions from 2.0% down to 0.0002%, with occlusion times of 48, 24, and 5 hours (181). Readings were on days 2, 4, and 7. The 48-hour occlusion detected most positive reactors (8/10) at a reading time of 4 days and 0.002% detected most contact allergies. The "edge effect" (reactions with a peripheral ring due to suppression of the allergic reaction under the patch because of the intrinsic anti-inflammatory effect of the glucocorticoid itself) was noted with several concentrations at early readings. That lower concentrations can detect budesonide allergy better at early

readings and that patients with an "edge reaction" can have positive reactions to lower concentrations can be explained by individual glucocorticoid reactivity, the dose–response relation, and the time-courses of the elicitation and the anti-inflammatory capacity.

- A 36-year-old man, who had a long history of atopic dermatitis of the neck, chest, and arms, developed allergic contact dermatitis after topical administration of clobetasone ointment 0.05% (Kindavate) and prednisolone ointment 0.3% (Lidomex) (182). Patch tests with both ointments showed a positive reaction only to Kindavate. Further testing with the separate ingredients of Kindavate showed positive reactions to 0.05, 0.01, and 0.005% clobetasone on day 7.
- A 40-year-old woman had a flare-up of her eczema (183). She had had previous negative patch tests 10 years before. She had taken topical glucocorticoids and emollients for a few months, but had not used budesonide. Patch testing with the European standard series showed a positive reaction to budesonide 0.1% at 3 days. All other allergens were negative. The only antecedent exposure was that she had three children with asthma, all of whom regularly used inhaled budesonide and occasionally nebulizers. She had not used the inhaler but had helped her children to manage the devices. A subsequent patch test with powdered budesonide from the inhaler was positive.
- A 14-year-old girl with newly diagnosed systemic lupus erythematosus developed a pruritic bullous eruption while taking prednisone 20 mg/day (184). She was given a single daily dose of intravenous methylprednisolone 60 mg with rapid improvement. In preparation for discharge, the glucocorticoid was changed to oral prednisone 60 mg/day, to which she developed a pruritic bullous eruption consistent with erythema multiforme. She underwent immediate and delayed hypersensitivity tests. Intradermal and patch tests to liquid prednisone were positive. She was given oral methylprednisolone 48 mg/day and has not had recurrence of the skin lesions.
- A 27-year-old woman, a pharmacist, had dermatitis on three separate occasions a few hours after she started to take oral deflazacort 6 mg for vesicular hand eczema (185). On each occasion, her symptoms included a widespread macular rash mainly on the inner aspects of her arms and legs and buttocks. She also had severe scaling, fever, nausea, vomiting, malaise, and hypotension. A skin biopsy was consistent with erythema multiforme, and direct immunofluorescence showed granular deposits at the dermoepidermal junction. Patch tests to the commercial formulation of deflazacort 6 mg (1% aqueous solution) and to pure deflazacort (1% aqueous solution) were positive, but there were no cross-reactions to other glucocorticoids.

The author of the last report commented that the patient probably developed hypersensitivity to deflazacort as a result of occupational exposure.

Other cases of erythema multiforme-like contact dermatitis after topical budesonide have been reported (SEDA-21, 415; 186). In a large case-control study, potential cases of severe forms of erythema multiforme, toxic epidermal necrolysis and Stevens–Johnson syndrome, were collected in four European countries (France, Portugal, Italy, and Germany) (SEDA-20, 371; 187). There was a significant relation with glucocorticoid use in the preceding week (multivariate analysis relative risk = 4.4; 95% CI = 1.9, 10), or when prescribed for long-term therapy (crude relative risk for use less than 2 months = 54; 95% CI = 23, 124). The estimates of excess risks associated with glucocorticoids or sulfonamides (which are well-known to cause these syndromes), expressed as the number of cases attributable to the drug per million users in 1 week, were 1.5 and 4.5 respectively.

Cross-reactivity between glucocorticoids and progestogens has been described (188).

- A 68-year-old woman, with a prolonged history of pityriasis lichenoides chronica treated with topical glucocorticoids, including hydrocortisone, took a formulation containing conjugated estrogens 0.625 mg and hydroxyprogesterone acetate 5 mg (frequency of administration not stated) for late menopausal syndrome. Years later she started to have pruritus, a maculopapular rash, and flu-like symptoms for several days before menstruation. On this occasion, she presented with a severe, pruritic, papulovesicular eruption on her chest, back, abdomen, and legs. The eruption had developed after treatment for 7 days with the estrogen–progestogen formulation; she had developed similar symptoms on several previous occasions after taking the same medication. She was treated with antihistamines and her skin eruption resolved within a few days. Patch tests were positive to 17-OH-progesterone, tixocortol pivalate, and budesonide.

The authors hypothesized that this patient, who had taken topical glucocorticoids for several years, had become sensitive and that the recurrent episodes of autoimmune progestogen dermatitis were related to endogenous progestogen sensitivity following cross-sensitivity to glucocorticoids. This hypothesis was supported by the development of recurrent eczema several times after she took an estrogen–progestogen preparation.

Musculoskeletal

Osteoporosis

The use of glucocorticoids is associated with reduced bone mineral density, bone loss, osteoporosis, and fractures. This has been described during the long-term use of glucocorticoid by any route of administration (SEDA-19, 377; SEDA-20, 374). The effects of glucocorticoids on bone have been reviewed (SEDA-21, 417; 189). Biochemical markers of bone mineral density are listed in Table 4. In patients with secondary hypoadrenalism, hydrocortisone 30 mg/day for replacement produced a significant fall in osteocalcin, indicating bone loss. Lower doses of hydrocortisone (10 mg and 20 mg) produced similar efficacy in terms of quality of life but smaller effects on osteocalcin concentrations and therefore a reduction in bone loss (190). Three studies add evidence of the deleterious effects of oral glucocorticoids and high doses of inhaled glucocorticoids on bone mineral density (191) and the risk of fractures (192,193).

Table 4 Biochemical markers of bone mineral density

Bone formation
Blood
Alkaline phosphatase (bone-specific)
Osteocalcin
Procollagen type I carboxy-terminal propeptide (PICP)
Procollagen type I amino-terminal propeptide (PINP)
Procollagen type III amino-terminal propeptide (PIIINP)
Bone resorption
Blood
Acid phosphatase (acid-resistant)
Type I collagen carboxy-terminal telopeptide (ICTP)
Urine
Calcium
Hydroxyproline
Cross-linked peptides (pyridinium and deoxypyridinoline)

The fluorinated glucocorticoids are said to have relatively more catabolic activity than others and might have a greater effect on the skeleton but such impressions may merely reflect the general potency of some newer glucocorticoids and a tendency to use them in inappropriate doses. A relatively new glucocorticoid, deflazacort, has been proposed to have less effect on bone metabolism, but a double-blind study has failed to show an advantage compared with prednisolone (SEDA-21, 417; 194).

Osteoporosis induced by chronic glucocorticoid therapy has been reviewed in patients with obstructive lung diseases (195) and patients with skin diseases (196).

Presentation

Of the effects of glucocorticoids on the skeleton, osteoporosis is the most important clinically; manifestations can include vertebral compression fractures, scoliosis resulting in respiratory embarrassment, and fractures of the long bones. The risk of vertebral fractures is not different in patients taking or not taking glucocorticoids in whom bone mineral density is similar (197).

Glucocorticoids can even cause osteoporosis when they are used for long-term replacement therapy in the Addison's disease, as has been shown by a study of 91 patients who had taken glucocorticoids for a mean of 10.6 years, in whom bone mineral density was reduced by 32% compared with age-matched controls (SEDA-19, 377; 198). However, these results contrasted with the results of a Spanish study in patients with Addison's disease, in which no direct relation was found between replacement therapy and either bone density or biochemical markers of bone turnover of calcium metabolism (alkaline phosphatase, osteocalcin, procollagen I type, parathormone, and 1,25-dihydroxycholecalciferol) (SEDA-19, 377; 199).

Atraumatic posterior pelvic ring fractures that simulate the form of presentation of metastatic diseases can be produced by glucocorticoid administration (SEDA-19, 377; 200).

Accelerated bone loss, with an increased risk of first hip fracture, occurred in elderly women taking oral glucocorticoids (201). At baseline, 122 (1.5%) women were taking inhaled glucocorticoids only (median dose equivalent to inhaled beclomethasone 168 micrograms/day), 228 (2.8%) were taking oral glucocorticoids (median dose equivalent to prednisone 5 mg/day) with or without inhaled glucocorticoids, and 7718 were not taking any glucocorticoids. The women who were taking oral glucocorticoids had lower mean bone mineral density at 3.6 years than nonusers, with an interim fall that was twice as fast. First hip fracture occurred in 4.8% of the women who were taking oral glucocorticoids and in 2.8% of the women who were not (RR = 2.1; CI = 1.0, 4.4). The researchers said that the power of the study was not sufficient to determine the relative risk of hip fracture in women taking inhaled glucocorticoids.

A reduction in bone mineral density has been described in 23 patients (19 men) with chronic fatigue syndrome taking low-dose glucocorticoids in a double-blind, randomized, placebo-controlled study (202). The patients took hydrocortisone 25–35 mg/day or matched placebo for 3 months. Mean bone mineral density in the spine fell by 2% with hydrocortisone and increased by 1% with placebo.

A group of 367 patients with lung disease taking oral glucocorticoids (177 women, mean age 68 years, 190 men, mean age 70 years) and 734 matched controls completed a questionnaire about lifestyle, fractures, and other possible adverse effects of glucocorticoids (203). The cumulative incidence of fractures from the time of diagnosis was 23% in patients taking oral glucocorticoids and 15% in the controls (OR = 1.8; 95% CI = 1.3, 2.6). Fractures of the vertebrae were more likely (OR = 10; 95% CI = 2.9, 35). The adverse effects were dose-related, with a higher risk of all fractures (OR = 2.22; 95% CI = 1.04, 4.8) and vertebral fractures (OR = 9.2; 95% CI = 2.4, 36) in those who took the highest compared with the lowest cumulative doses (61 versus 5 g).

Systemic glucocorticoids are often prescribed for rheumatoid arthritis. Even in low doses they can have clinical benefits and can inhibit joint damage, but they can cause osteoporotic fractures. In a 2-year double-blind, randomized, placebo-controlled trial in 81 patients (29 men, mean age 62 years) with early active rheumatoid arthritis who had not been treated with disease-modifying antirheumatic drugs, 41 were assigned to oral prednisone 10 mg/day and 40 to placebo. NSAIDs were allowed in both groups and after 6 months, sulfasalazine (2 g/day) could be prescribed as rescue medication. Those who took prednisone had more clinical improvement with less use of concomitant drugs. After month 6, radiological scores had progressed significantly less in those who took prednisone. After 24 months, seven patients had new vertebral fractures, five in the prednisone group and two in the placebo group (204).

Mechanisms

There have been reviews of the mechanisms and adverse effects of glucocorticoids in rheumatoid arthritis (205) and the pathogenesis, diagnosis, and treatment of glucocorticoid-induced osteoporosis in patients with pulmonary diseases (206). Several mechanisms underlie the effect of glucocorticoids on bone, both biochemical and cellular. Effects on calcium are:

(a) increased excretion of calcium into the bowel and inhibition of its absorption;

(b) inhibition of the tubular re-absorption of calcium in the kidney;

(c) increased mobilization of calcium from the skeleton.

When calcium homeostasis cannot be maintained, the resulting hypocalcemia can have serious consequences (SEDA-18, 388) (207,208). This so-called "glucocorticoid hyperparathyroidism" was the explanation traditionally most prominently advanced for glucocorticoid osteoporosis, but it is not the only one and may not be the most central. Other biochemical effects include:

(a) a catabolic effect on protein metabolism, causing a reduction in the bone matrix;

(b) altered vitamin D metabolism, with reduced concentrations of vitamin D metabolites (209);

(c) a dose-dependent reduction of serum osteocalcin, a bone matrix protein that appears to correlate with bone formation.

Measurement of serum osteocalcin is a useful marker for glucocorticoid-induced osteoporosis, and can be used alongside other measures noted below.

Various cellular mechanisms are involved in the production of glucocorticoid-induced osteoporosis (SEDA-20, 375) (210). The major change is a reduction in osteoblast activity that results in a reduced working rate (mean appositional rate), and a reduced active life-span of osteoblasts. The cellular mechanism seems to be related to diminished production of cytokines and other locally acting factors. Increased bone resorption and reduced calcium absorption have also been described. A sophisticated mathematical model has been used to describe changes in calcium kinetics in patients treated with glucocorticoids (SEDA-20, 375) (211). Plasma calcium concentrations were higher than in controls, with a marked reduction in calcium flow into the irreversible stable bone compartment in glucocorticoid-treated patients. The authors concluded that prednisone has direct effects on osteoblast function.

Osteoprotegerin (osteoclastogenesis inhibitory factor, OCIF) has been identified as a novelly secreted cytokine receptor that plays an important role in the negative regulation of osteoclastic bone resorption. There are reports that suggest that glucocorticoids promote osteoclastogenesis by inhibiting osteoprotegerin production in vitro, thereby enhancing bone resorption. However, there are only a few clinical reports in which the regulatory functions of osteoprotegerin have been explored. In order to clarify the potential role of osteoprotegerin in the pathogenesis of glucocorticoid-induced osteoporosis, Japanese investigators have measured serum osteoprotegerin and other markers of bone metabolism before and after glucocorticoid therapy in patients with various renal diseases (212). The findings suggested that short-term administration of glucocorticoids significantly suppresses serum osteoprotegerin and osteocalcin. This might be relevant to the development of glucocorticoid-induced osteoporosis via enhancement of bone resorption and suppression of bone formation. Further long-term studies are needed to elucidate the mechanism of the glucocorticoid-induced reduction in circulating osteoprotegerin and its participation in the pathogenesis of osteoporosis.

Although glucocorticoids can cause changes in trabecular microarchitecture, loss of bone (reduced bone density) seems to be the major determinant of osteoporosis (213). Bone resorption seems to involve the receptor of the activator of the nucleus factor KB ligand (RANK-L) and osteoprotegerin. RANK-L binds to a specific receptor in osteoclasts, and in the presence of the macrophage colony stimulating factor (M-CSF) it induces osteoclastogenesis (the development of mature osteoclasts) and suppression of normal osteoclast apoptosis. Osteoprotegerin is a soluble decoy receptor that binds to and neutralizes RANK-L and so reduces osteoclastogenesis. Glucocorticoids increase the expression of RANK-L and M-CSF and reduce osteoprotegerin production by osteoblasts. The net result is enhanced osteoclastic activity. Other inflammatory mediators, such as tumor necrosis factor-alfa and interleukin-6, have similar biological actions to glucocorticoids. Glucocorticoids reduce osteoblast numbers and function by reducing the replication and differentiation of osteoblasts and by increasing apoptosis in mature osteoblasts. Glucocorticoids inhibit osteoblastic synthesis of type I collagen, the major component of bone extracellular matrix. They can induce apoptosis of osteocytes, and this could be the mechanism of osteonecrosis. Two other factors are involved in bone loss: firstly, glucocorticoids increase renal calcium elimination and reduce intestinal calcium absorption, leading to a negative calcium balance, which can lead to secondary hyperparathyroidism; secondly, glucocorticoids reduce the production of gonadal hormones. The histological effects of glucocorticoids are a reduced rate of bone formation, reduced trabecular wall thickness, and apoptosis of bone cells. These effects lead to osteoporosis and fractures.

Although glucocorticoid use seems to be an important factor for low mineral density, sex hormones have also been suggested as an important determinant of bone mineral content. Bone mineral density and sex hormone status have been studied in 99 men with rheumatoid arthritis and 68 age-matched controls (SEDA-20, 375) (214). There were significant reductions in lumbar and femoral density, and salivary testosterone, androstenedione, and dehydroepiandrosterone in the patients. Salivary testosterone correlated with femoral density. By multiple regression analysis, weight, serum testosterone concentrations, and cumulative dose of glucocorticoid were significant predictors of lumbar bone density. Weight, age, androstenedione concentrations, and cumulative dose of glucocorticoids were significant predictors of femoral bone density.

Dose relation

Dose is an important factor, but these adverse effects have been described after low doses. The risk of hip fracture associated with glucocorticoid use has been studied in Denmark in a population-based case-control study in 6660 subjects with hip fractures and 33 272 age-matched population controls (215). Data on prescriptions for glucocorticoid within the last 5 years before the index date were retrieved from a population-based prescription database. Doses were recalculated to prednisolone

equivalents. Cases and controls were grouped according to cumulative glucocorticoid dose:

1. not used;
2. under 130 mg (equivalent to prednisolone 30 mg/day for 4 days given for an acute exacerbation of asthma);
3. 130–499 mg (equivalent to a short course of prednisolone of 450 mg) for acute asthma;
4. 500–1499 mg (equivalent to prednisolone 7.5 mg/day for 6 months or 800 micrograms/day of inhaled budesonide for 1 year);
5. 1500 mg or more (equivalent to more than 4.1 mg day for 1 year, a long-term high dose).

A conditional logistic regression was used and adjusted for potential confounders including sex, redeemed prescriptions for hormone replacement therapy, antiosteoporotic, anxiolytic, antipsychotic, and antidepressant drugs. Compared with never users, there was an increased risk of hip fracture in glucocorticoid users, with increasing cumulative doses of any type of drug used during the preceding 5 years. For doses of prednisolone under 130 mg, the adjusted risk (OR) was 0.96 (95% CI = 0.89, 1.04); for 130-499 mg the OR was 1.17 (1.01, 1.35); for 500-1499 mg the OR was 1.36 (1.19, 1.56); and for 1500 mg or more the OR was 1.65 (1.43, 1.92). There was an also increased risk when the study population was stratified according to sex, age, and type of glucocorticoid (systemic or topical). This study showed that even a limited daily dose of glucocorticoids (more than an average dose of prednisolone of about 71 micrograms/day) was associated with an increased risk of hip fracture.

Doses of prednisone of 7.5 mg/day can cause premature or exaggerated osteoporosis. However, it is unclear whether a dose of 5 mg/day has the same effect. In a double-blind, randomized, placebo-controlled, 8-week trial 50 healthy postmenopausal women (mean age 57 years) were randomly assigned to prednisone 5 mg/day or matching placebo for 6 weeks, followed by a 2-week recovery phase (216). Prednisone rapidly and significantly decreased serum concentrations of propeptide of type I N-terminal procollagen, propeptide of type I C-terminal procollagen, and osteocalcin, and free urinary deoxypyridinoline compared with placebo. These changes were largely reversed during the recovery period. In conclusion, low-dose prednisone significantly reduced indices of bone formation and bone resorption in postmenopausal women.

Lumbar spine bone mineral density has been assessed in 76 prepubertal asthmatics (mean age 7.7 years, 26 girls) using glucocorticoids (217). After stratification for dose and route of administration, the children who used over 800 micrograms/day of inhaled glucocorticoids, with or without intermittent oral glucocorticoids, had a significant lower weight-adjusted bone density than children who used 400–800 micrograms/day of inhaled glucocorticoids (mean difference –0.05 g/cm^2; 95% CI = –0.02, –0.09). Bone mass was similar in children who did not use inhaled glucocorticoids and those who used 400–800 micrograms/day.

In kidney transplant recipients, lumbar bone loss was significantly higher in 20 patients who took daily prednisone (5.9%, mean dosage 0.19 mg/kg/day) than in 27 patients who used alternate-day prednisone (1.1%, mean dosage 0.15 mg/kg/day) (218).

Time course

The loss of bone mineral after organ and tissue transplant associated with immunosuppressive therapy follows a delayed time course. The long-term effects of immuno-suppressive therapy on bone density have been determined in 25 cardiac transplant patients (SEDA-20, 375) (219). As expected, there was bone loss in the spine during the first year, but this was not maintained during the second and third years after transplantation, despite continuing maintenance immunosuppression with prednisolone. Only four patients, all of whom were hypogonadal, continued to lose bone.

Susceptibility factors

The overall effect of glucocorticoids on bone mineral content differs between patients on comparable treatments, which suggests that some patients are more predisposed than others (SEDA-3, 306), and probably also that the standards of evaluation used in different clinics are not comparable. This variability and the wide range of products and dosage schemes used mean that one does not have a clear impression of what constitutes a safe regimen as far as the skeleton is concerned (SEDA-20, 374), or whether any regimen is safe in this respect. Certainly, in a series of men with rheumatoid arthritis, even a very low dose of glucocorticoids (for example 10 mg or less of prednisolone daily) has proved to have a significant effect on bone mineral density (220); other work has provided similar results (SEDA-20, 374; 221). In another published study, patients who took 1–4 mg/day had the same density as those who were not taking glucocorticoids. Patients who took 5–9 mg/day and those who took more than 10 mg/day had significantly lower bone density (84 and 81% of control values respectively) (SEDA-20, 374; 222).

Glucocorticoid-related complications have been described in 748 adult kidney transplant recipients, followed for at least 1 year. For bone/joint complications, the multivariate analysis showed that the only significant variable was the cumulative duration of glucocorticoid therapy. For avascular necrosis, no variables were significant (SEDA-19, 377; 223).

In a similar study of 65 renal transplant patients treated with immunosuppressive drugs for at least 6 months, multivariate analysis showed that cumulative glucocorticoid dose and female sex were the major predictors of low vertebral bone density (SEDA-19, 377; 224).

In another study, the loss of bone density correlated with the cumulative dose of prednisolone (21 g total dose at 11.4 mg/day) and renal function (SEDA-21, 417; 225).

In a review of renal transplantation during 1974–94, 166 patients were classified into those with osteonecrosis of the femoral head (22 patients) and those without (47 patients) (SEDA-21, 417; 226). The total dose of methyl-prednisolone was higher in those with osteonecrosis. All

five patients who had received intravenous pulse doses over 2000 mg had osteonecrosis.

The risk of vertebral deformity is increased by the combination of an oral glucocorticoid and advanced age, according to the findings in 229 patients (69% women) taking long-term oral glucocorticoids (prednisone equivalents of 5 mg/day or more) and 286 untreated controls (227). The duration of treatment was 0.5–37 (median 4.8) years. More than 60% of the treatment group were aged over 60 years, and most (62%) had been treated for rheumatoid arthritis. Bone mineral density data were analysed in 194 patients. The researchers identified at least one vertebral deformity (defined as a more than 20% reduction in anterior, middle, or posterior vertebral height) in 65 (28%) of the patients in the treatment group, and two or more fractures were identified in 25 (11%). In the treatment group, vertebral deformities were significantly more common in men than in women, and the prevalence of deformities increased with age. Compared with patients aged under 60 years, glucocorticoid-treated patients aged 70–79 years had a five-fold increased risk of vertebral deformity (OR = 5.1; 95% CI = 2.0, 13). The prevalence of vertebral deformities increased significantly with age in the glucocorticoid group. While the mean spine and femoral bone mineral density scores were lower in the glucocorticoid group, logistic regression analysis showed that bone mineral density was only a modest predictor of deformity. Age is an important independent risk factor, with very high prevalence rates in those over 70 years. Increasing duration of glucocorticoid use may increase the risk of fracture.

Osteoporosis is common in Crohn's disease, often because of glucocorticoids. Budesonide as controlled-release capsules is a locally acting glucocorticoid with low systemic availability. In a randomized study in 272 patients with Crohn's disease involving the ileum and/or ascending colon, budesonide and prednisolone were compared for 2 years in doses adapted to disease activity (228). There was active disease in 181, of whom 98 were glucocorticoid-naive; 90 had quiescent disease and were corticosteroid-dependent. Efficacy was similar in the two groups, but treatment-related adverse effects were less frequent with budesonide. The glucocorticoid-naive patients who took budesonide had smaller reductions in bone mineral density than those who took prednisolone (mean −1.04% versus −3.84%).

Comparisons of glucocorticoids

Bone loss induced by glucocorticoids has been assessed in three different populations. A group of 374 subjects (mean age 35 years, 55% women) with mild asthma taking beta-adrenoceptor agonists only, were randomized to inhaled glucocorticoids (budesonide or beclomethasone) or non-glucocorticoid treatment for 2 years (229). Bone mineral density was measured blind after 6, 12, and 24 months. Mean doses of budesonide and beclomethasone were 389 micrograms/day and 499 micrograms/day, respectively. At the end of follow-up, the subjects who had used glucocorticoids had better asthma control. The mean changes in bone density over 2 years in the budesonide, beclomethasone, and control groups were 0.1%, −0.4%, and 0.4% for the lumbar spine and −0.9%, −0.9%, and −0.4% for the neck of the femur. The daily dose of inhaled glucocorticoid was related to the reduction in bone mineral density only at the lumbar spine. Low to moderate doses of inhaled glucocorticoids caused little change in bone mineral density over 2 years and provided better asthma control.

Diagnosis

Several techniques are used to measure bone density. Cortical bone can be assessed in peripheral sites by single-photon absorptiometry and a combination of cortical and trabecular bone in central sites by dual X-ray absorptiometry. Trabecular bone can be assessed by quantitative computer tomography scanning of the lumbar spine. Since single-photon absorptiometry and dual X-ray absorptiometry give a negligible dose of radiation, they are useful for population screening. However, these two techniques are not sensitive enough to show subtle changes in bone density over short periods of time. Quantitative computed tomography gives a significant dose of radiation (of the order of one-tenth of a lateral X-ray of the spine) but can focus on trabecular bone, which has a tenfold greater turnover, compared with cortical bone. Quantitative computed tomography is more sensitive to changing bone density over time.

Other methods, such as the fasting urinary hydroxyproline/creatinine ratio, alkaline phosphatase activity, dual-absorption photometry of the hip, and serum osteocalcin measurements, can also be used, depending on an individual clinic's equipment and experience (SEDA-17, 447).

Management

The prevention and treatment of glucocorticoid bone loss in patients with skin diseases have been reviewed (196). Strategies for the management of this problem have been discussed (SEDA-22, 213) and the clinical implications of trials in the management of glucocorticoid-induced osteoporosis have been reviewed (230). Provided no fractures have occurred, loss of bone mineral density seems to be reversible when treatment is withdrawn (SEDA-18, 389). The management of glucocorticoid-induced osteoporosis has been revised by the UK Consensus Group Meeting on Osteoporosis (SEDA-20, 376; 212) and by the American College of Rheumatology (SEDA-21, 417; 231).

Guidelines for the prevention and treatment of glucocorticoid-induced osteoporosis have been published (232). Although there are several consensus statements and recommendations for prophylactic measures against glucocorticoid-induced osteoporosis in patients with rheumatoid arthritis, prophylaxis is commonly underprescribed. In two recent studies of 191 and 92 patients taking long-term glucocorticoids, relatively few were taking primary prevention, although some were taking vitamin D and calcium tablets. Around 65–68% of all those who qualified for prophylaxis for glucocorticoid-induced osteoporosis did not receive therapy, and only 9% of

those in one study and 21% in the other were taking bisphosphonates (233,234).

Low availability compounds

Bone loss in patients taking oral budesonide has been evaluated in a longitudinal study in which bone mineral density was measured annually for 2 years in 138 patients (67 men, mean age 36 years old) with quiescent Crohn's disease (235). They took budesonide (8.5 mg/day; $n = 48$), prednisone (10.5 mg/day, $n = 45$), or non-steroidal drugs ($n = 45$). After 1 year, the bone mineral density in the lumbar spine fell by 2.36% in those who took budesonide, by 0.61% in those who took prednisone, and by 0.09% in those who took non-steroidal drugs. In the second year, the largest fall occurred in those who took budesonide (1.97%), but the differences between the groups were not significant. After 2 years, bone mineral density in the femoral neck fell by 2.94% with budesonide, 0.36% with prednisone, and 1.05% with the non-steroidal drugs. These results suggest that budesonide can cause bone loss, but the non-randomized design of the study limits conclusions about the comparison between budesonide and prednisone.

Pulse administration

The administration of glucocorticoids in sporadic pulses has been shown not to reduce bone density in patients with multiple sclerosis. In a prospective study, 30 patients were given 1000 mg/day of methylprednisolone intravenously for 3 days, followed by oral prednisone in tapering dosage for 2 weeks. Bone density was determined in the lumbar spine and femoral neck before and at 2, 4, and 6 months after therapy. At baseline, the patients had a reduced bone mass compared with controls; this reduction did not correlate with previous exposure to glucocorticoids. Ambulant patients during follow-up after glucocorticoid pulse therapy had an increase in lumbar bone density (+1.7% at 6 months). Average femoral density did not change; however, in patients who required a walking stick or other aid, femoral density fell (−1.6%), while in those with better ambulation it increased (+2.9%). These results suggest that inactivity is the main factor causing bone loss in patients treated with sporadic pulses of glucocorticoids (SEDA-21, 417; 236).

Calcium and vitamin D analogues

Infusion of ionic calcium has sometimes been used to counteract the malabsorption of calcium in patients taking long-term glucocorticoids, particularly in patients who develop secondary hypoparathyroidism (SEDA-3, 306). There is also evidence that in amenorrheic or menopausal women requiring glucocorticoids, the adverse effects on the vertebrae can be countered by hormonal replacement therapy with estrogen and progesterone (237); progestogens similarly seem to have a promising effect in men, and while they cause a fall in serum testosterone they apparently do not undermine the desired effects of glucocorticoids (SEDA-16, 449).

The administration of calcium and vitamin D3 can prevent bone loss induced by glucocorticoids, and trials have confirmed its efficacy when given for 2 years. Patients taking prednisone and placebo lost bone density in the lumbar spine at a rate of 2% per year. Those taking prednisone and calcium plus vitamin D3 gained bone mineral density at a rate of 0.72% per year. Calcium plus vitamin D3 did not improve bone mineral density in patients who were not taking prednisone (SEDA-21, 417; 238).

In a similar randomized double-blind study, the effects of vitamin D (50 000 units/week) and calcium (1000 mg/day) were evaluated in 62 patients with different rheumatic diseases treated with prednisone (10–100 mg/day) (SEDA-21, 418; 239). The primary outcome was bone mineral density in the lumbar spine at 36 months. Patients taking placebo had reductions of 4.1, 3.8, and 1.5% at 12, 24, and 36 months respectively. Patients taking calcium and vitamin D had reductions of 2.6, 3.7, and 2.2% respectively. The results suggested that preventive therapy could be beneficial early in the prevention of glucocorticoid-induced bone loss, but there was no evidence of long-term beneficial effects. In kidney transplant patients, the preventive administration of 25-hydroxycolecalciferol and calcium reduced bone loss in the spine and femoral neck and the number of new vertebral crush fractures (SEDA-21, 418; 240). In children with rheumatic diseases taking glucocorticoids, calcium and vitamin D supplementation improved spinal bone density, although osteocalcin concentrations remained low (SEDA-19, 378; 241).

A meta-analysis has shown that alfacalcidol and calcitriol prevent bone loss induced by glucocorticoid (effect size = 0.43) but not fractures (242).

Alfacalcidol and vitamin D3 have been compared in patients with established glucocorticoid-induced osteoporosis with or without vertebral fractures (243). Patients taking long-term glucocorticoids were included as matched pairs to receive randomly either alfacalcidol 1 microgram/day plus calcium 500 mg/day (n = 103) or vitamin D3 1000 IU/day plus calcium 500 mg/day (n = 101). The two groups were well matched in terms of mean age, sex ratio, mean height and weight, daily dosage and duration of glucocorticoid therapy, and the percentages of the three underlying diseases (chronic obstructive pulmonary disease, rheumatoid arthritis, and polymyalgia rheumatica). The baseline mean bone mineral density values (expressed as T scores, the number of standard deviations from the mean of the healthy population) at the lumbar spine were −3.26 (alfacalcidol) and −3.25 (vitamin D3) and at the femoral neck −2.81 and −2.84 respectively. The prevalence rates of vertebral and non-vertebral fractures did not differ. During the 3-year study, the median percentage bone mineral density increased at the lumbar spine by 2.4% with alfacalcidol and decreased by 0.8% with vitamin D3. There also was a significantly larger median increase at the femoral neck with alfacalcidol (1.2%) than with vitamin D3 (0.8%). The 3-year rates of patients with at least one new vertebral fracture were 9.7% with alfacalcidol and 25% with vitamin D3

(RR = 0.61; 95% CI = 0.24, 0.81). The 3-year rates of patients with at least one new non-vertebral fracture were 15% with alfacalcidol and 25% with vitamin D3 (RR = 0.41; 95% CI = 0.06, 0.68). The 3-year rates of patients with at least one new fracture of any kind were 19% with alfacalcidol and 41% with vitamin D3 (RR = 0.52; 95% CI = 0.25, 0.71). Those who took alfacalcidol had a substantially larger reduction in back pain than those who took vitamin D3. Generally, adverse effects in both groups were mild, and only three patients taking alfacalcidol and two taking vitamin D3 had moderate hypercalcemia. The authors concluded that alfacalcidol plus calcium is greatly superior to vitamin D3 plus calcium in the treatment of established glucocorticoid-induced osteoporosis.

Calcitonin
Less clear are the results observed after the administration of salmon calcitonin. The usefulness of intranasally administered salmon calcitonin for 2 years has been evaluated in 44 glucocorticoid-dependent asthmatics (SEDA-19, 378; 244). All were taking calcium supplements (1000 mg/day), but one group also took calcitonin (100 IU every other day). Calcitonin increased spinal bone mass during first year of treatment, and maintained bone mass in a steady state during the second year. However, the rate of vertebral fractures was similar in the two groups. The addition of salmon calcitonin did not increase the efficacy of calcium plus vitamin D in the prevention of bone loss in 48 newly diagnosed patients taking glucocorticoids for temporal arteritis and polymyalgia rheumatica in a double-blind, randomized, placebo-controlled trial (SEDA-21, 418; 245). However, salmon calcitonin nasal spray prevented bone loss in the lumbar spine of 31 patients treated with prednisone for polymyalgia rheumatica (SEDA-22, 448; 246). They were randomized to salmon calcitonin nasal spray (200 IU/day) or matched placebo for 1 year. Both groups were treated with calcium supplements if their dietary intake was below 800 mg/day. With calcitonin, the mean bone mineral density in the lumbar spine fell by 1.3% and with placebo by 5% after 1 year. There were no differences in the hip, including the femoral neck and trochanter, or in total body bone density.

Bisphosphonates
There have been several studies of the use of bisphosphonates in preventing glucocorticoid-induced osteoporosis.

Intermittent cyclical etidronate prevented bone loss induced by prednisone in 10 postmenopausal women with temporal arteritis (SEDA-19, 378; 247). Cyclical etidronate (400 mg/day for 2 weeks every 3 months) plus ergocalciferol (0.5 mg/week) was given to 15 postmenopausal women (mean age 63 years) starting glucocorticoid therapy (prednisone 5–20 mg/day). A control group of 11 postmenopausal women (mean age 60 years) with glucocorticoid-induced osteoporosis were treated with calcium supplements only (1 g/day). During the first year, the cyclical regimen significantly increased lumbar and femoral neck bone density compared with placebo (7 and 2.5% for spine and femur respectively). After the second year of cyclical therapy, femoral neck bone density continued to increase while lumbar spine density remained stable (SEDA-20, 376; 248). The effect of intermittent cyclical therapy with etidronate has been investigated in the prevention of bone loss in 117 patients taking high-dose glucocorticoid therapy (a mean daily dose of at least 7.5 mg for 90 days followed by at least 2.5 mg/day for at least 12 months) (249). The patients were randomized to oral etidronate 400 mg/day or placebo for 14 days, followed by 76 days of oral calcium carbonate (500 mg elemental calcium), cycled over 12 months. The mean lumbar spine bone density changed 0.30% and −2.79% in the etidronate and placebo groups respectively. The mean difference between the groups after 1 year (3.0%) was significant. The changes in the femoral neck and greater trochanter were not different between the groups. There was a reduction in pyridinium cross-links, significant from baseline at both 6 and 12 months, in the etidronate group. Osteocalcin increased in the placebo group, and the differences between the groups at 6 and 12 months were −25% and −35% respectively. There was no significant difference between the groups in the number of adverse events, including gastrointestinal disorders. In a placebo-controlled study of the effects of 104 weeks of intermittent cyclical etidronate therapy in 49 patients, the same dose and cycles were used as in the previous study, but calcium (97 mg/day) was given with vitamin D (400 IU) (250). Intermittent cyclical etidronate therapy with vitamin D supplementation significantly increased lumbar spine bone mineral density by 4.5 in patients with osteoporosis resulting from long-term treatment with glucocorticoids.

Intermittent etidronate has been evaluated in a randomized controlled trial in 102 Japanese patients who had taken over 7.5 mg/day of prednisolone for at least 90 days (251). They were randomized to etidronate disodium 200 mg/day for 2 weeks plus calcium lactate 3.0 g/day and alfacalcidol 0.75 micrograms/day) or control (calcium lactate 3.0 g and alfacalcidol 0.75 micrograms/day). Bone mineral density in the lumbar spine and the rate of new vertebral fractures at 48 and 144 weeks were evaluated. With etidronate the mean lumbar spine bone mineral density increased by 3.7% and 4.8% at 48 and 144 weeks respectively. In the control group, the mean lumbar spine bone mineral density increased by 1.5% and 0.4% at 48 and 144 weeks respectively. Of three subgroups, men, premenopausal women, and postmenopausal women, the postmenopausal women had the greatest benefit. Two control patients had new vertebral fractures, whereas there were no fractures with etidronate.

Clodronate 100 mg by intramuscular route once a week was effective in the prevention of glucocorticoid-induced bone loss and fractures in patients with arthritis compared with calcium 1000 mg/day and vitamin D 800 mg/day (252).

Ibandronate can be given intravenously every 3 months. Its efficacy has been demonstrated in men and women with established glucocorticoid-induced osteoporosis in 115 subjects who were randomly assigned to daily calcium supplements (500 mg) plus either ibandronate injections 2 mg every 3 months or daily oral alfacalcidol 1 microgram for up to 3 years (253,254). After 3 years, intermittent intravenous ibandronate produced significantly greater increases than daily oral alfacalcidol in mean bone mineral density in the lumbar spine (13% versus 2.6%), and femoral neck (5.2% versus 1.9%). However, there were no differences between the groups with respect to fractures.

Pamidronate disodium has been compared with calcium supplementation in an open trial of primary prevention of glucocorticoid-induced osteoporosis in 27 patients with different rheumatic conditions, randomly assigned to pamidronate (90 mg intravenously every 3 months) plus calcium (800 mg calcium carbonate) or calcium only for 1 year (SEDA-22, 448; 255). The glucocorticoids were given in a starting dosage of 10–80 mg/day. With pamidronate there was a significant increase in bone density (3.6% lumbar, 2.2% femoral neck), but there was a significant reduction with calcium (−5.3% in both spine and femoral neck).

The effects of risedronate on bone density and vertebral fracture have been studied in 518 patients (mean age 59 years, 40% with rheumatoid arthritis, 56% men, 64% of the women postmenopausal) taking moderate to high doses of oral glucocorticoids (equivalent to prednisone 7.5 mg/day or more) (256). The patients were randomized double-blind to placebo, or risedronate 2.5 or 5 mg/day for 1 year. All took elemental calcium 1000 mg/day and vitamin D 400 IU/day. The mean density of the lumbar spine fell by 1% in the placebo group and increased by 1.3% and 1.9% with risedronate 2.5 and 5 mg respectively. There was a significant reduction of 70% in the risk of vertebral fracture with risedronate 5 mg compared with placebo. There were similar incidences of adverse effects in all the groups.

Similar results have been reported in a clinical trial in 290 patients (38% men, 55% of the women postmenopausal) taking high-dose glucocorticoid therapy (prednisone over 7.5 mg/day or equivalent) (257). The subjects were randomized to receive placebo or risedronate 2.5 or 5 mg/day for 1 year. All took elemental calcium 1000 mg/day and vitamin D 400 IU/day. Risedronate 5 mg increased bone mineral density at 1 year by a mean of 2.9% in the lumbar spine, 1.8% in the femoral neck, and 2.4% in the trochanter. The values for placebo were 0.4%, −0.3%, and 1.0% respectively. The results for risedronate 2.5 mg were positive but not significant compared with placebo. The incidence of spinal fractures was reduced by 70% in the combined risedronate treatment groups compared with placebo. Risedronate and placebo caused similar adverse effects.

In a 1-year extension of a previous double-blind, randomized, placebo-controlled study, two doses of alendronate (5 and 10 mg/day) were compared in 66 men and 142 women taking glucocorticoids (at least 7.5 mg/day of prednisone or equivalent) (258). The extension was also double-blind, but those who had taken alendronate 2.5 mg/day in the previous study were given 10 mg/day.

All the patients took supplementary calcium and vitamin D. The primary end-point was the mean percentage change in lumbar spine bone mineral density from baseline to 2 years. In those who took alendronate 5, 10, and 2.5/10 mg/day, bone mineral density increased significantly by 2.8, 3.9, and 3.7% respectively, and fell by –0.8% with placebo. There were significantly fewer patients with new vertebral fractures in the alendronate group compared with placebo (0.7 versus 6.8%). Adverse events were similar across the groups.

No data are available about the effects on bone mineral density of withdrawing bisphosphonates. Of 183 patients who participated in a randomized, placebo-controlled trial of the efficacy of alendronate 5 and 10 mg/day on the prevention and treatment of glucocorticoid-induced osteoporosis during 1 year 90 participated in a follow-up study for 3.3-4.6 years (259). In the subgroup that continued to take a glucocorticoid (more than 6 mg/day of prednisone or equivalent for more than 1 year) and took alendronate for less than 90 days ($n = 11$), there was bone loss after the end of the trial (–5.1% at the lumbar spine to –9.2% at the femoral neck). In the subgroup that continued to take glucocorticoids and alendronate for more than 300 days ($n = 31$), there was a small gain in the lumbar spine (+0.1%) and no significant loss in the femoral neck (–0.1%). Although the study had limitations, particularly loss to follow-up of a considerable number of patients, the results suggested that sustained treatment with alendronate maintains bone mineral density, and that patients who discontinue alendronate and continue to take glucocorticoids lose bone mass in the femoral neck and lumbar spine.

Parathyroid hormone
Parathyroid hormone (parathormone) is an anabolic osteotrophic agent. Randomized controlled trials have shown the efficacy of human parathormone, hPTH (1-34), in improving bone mass and reducing the risk of fractures in postmenopausal osteoporosis. In 51 women who had been postmenopausal for at least 3 years and who had taken both glucocorticoids (mean dose of prednisone 5-20 mg/day or equivalent for at least 1 year) and hormone replacement therapy (HRT; Premarin 0.625 mg/day or equivalent) were randomized to either HRT + parathormone 40 micrograms/day for 1 year or HRT only (260). Vertebral cross-sectional area increased by 4.8%, and 1 year after treatment was withdrawn it was still 2.6% higher than at baseline. In the control group there was no change. In addition, estimated vertebral compressive strength increased by more than 200% over baseline with parathormone and there was no change in the control group.

Fluoride
Fluoride is a potent stimulator of trabecular bone formation. Sodium monofluorophosphate was given to 48 patients with osteoporosis due to glucocorticoids (more than 10 mg of prednisone equivalents/day). Patients were randomly allocated to 1 g of calcium carbonate (control) or 200 mg of sodium monofluorophosphate plus 1 g of

calcium carbonate for 18 months. At the end of the study lumbar spine bone density had increased by 7.8% in the fluoride group versus 3.3% in the controls. There were no changes in femoral neck density (SEDA-20, 376; 261).

Growth hormone
Growth hormone is a potent anabolic agent that stimulates protein synthesis, cell growth, and osteoblast activity. Recombinant human growth hormone has been used in patients taking long-term glucocorticoid treatment with suppressed endogenous growth hormone responses to GH-releasing hormone (SEDA-20, 376; 262). A single daily dose of 0.1 IU/kg of human growth hormone was given subcutaneously to nine nonobese patients. There was a significant increase in nitrogen balance, osteocalcin, carboxy-terminal propeptide of type I procollagen, and carboxy-terminal telopeptide of type I collagen. Growth hormone also lowered total high density lipoprotein, and low density lipoprotein cholesterol. These preliminary data suggest that growth hormone could ameliorate some adverse effects induced by long-term glucocorticoids.

Others
Other agents are effective in special populations. Vitamin K prevented bone loss in 20 patients with chronic glomerulonephritis treated with prednisolone (263) and ciclosporin 4.8 mg/kg/day prevented glucocorticoid-induced osteopenia in 52 patients taking prednisone 10 mg/day after kidney transplantation (264).

Avascular necrosis
Avascular aseptic necrosis of bone (SEDA-19, 377) (265,266) is a well-recognized adverse effect related to high-dose glucocorticoid therapy (equivalent to more than 4000 mg of prednisone) for extended periods (3 months or longer) but can occur after short-term glucocorticoid therapy. It occurs in a wide range of patients with many different disorders and is particularly likely to involve the femoral and humeral heads. The first lesions are often localized small osteolytic areas in the subchondral bone, where they can be diagnosed early by X-radiography. Magnetic resonance imaging (MRI) is one of the more sensitive techniques to diagnose avascular necrosis of the femoral head. The development and changes in avascular necrosis of the femoral head had been studied by MRI in patients with systemic lupus erythematosus treated with long-term prednisolone administration (SEDA-19, 377; SEDA-19, 164). MRI abnormalities could be detected soon after the start of glucocorticoid therapy or were associated with increased dosages for treating exacerbation of the disease. Normal hips are rarely involved in avascular osteonecrosis. However, aseptic osteonecrosis of the femoral head is often seen in young patients; the lunate, capitate, and patella are their locations. Usually only one joint is involved, although lesions can be multiple. Whether intra-articular injections of glucocorticoids can cause necrosis of bone is still uncertain.

Femoral head necrosis in kidney transplant recipients who receive postoperative immunosuppression with prednisone can be prevented, at least to some extent, by minimizing the dosage of prednisone whenever feasible (267). Of 750 patients (445 men and 305 women) who had undergone kidney transplantation in 1968–95, 374 had received an average of 12.5 g of prednisone during the first year after surgery (high-dose prednisone group) and 276 had received an average of 6.5 g during this time (low-dose prednisone group) plus ciclosporin. Femoral head necrosis occurred in 42/374 patients (11%) in the high-dose prednisone group, an average of 26 months after transplantation. In contrast, femoral head necrosis occurred in only 19/376 patients (5.1%) in the low-dose group an average of 21 months after transplantation. The difference between the high- and low-dose groups was highly significant.

The risk of avascular necrosis has been assessed in a nested case-control study using computer records (268). There were 31 cases during 720 000 person-years Avascular necrosis was strongly associated with glucocorticoid exposure (RR = 16). When total prednisone exposure over 35 months was stratified into three levels (under 440 mg, 440–1290 mg, and over 1290 mg), there was no excess risk for cumulative doses of up to 440 mg (RR = 0; 95% CI = 0, 5). The relative risk was increased for doses between 440 and 1290 mg (RR = 6; CI = 1, 43) and indeterminately increased at doses over 1290 mg (CI = 26, infinity).

In 15 men with osteonecrosis of the femoral head after short-term therapy the mean duration of therapy was 21 (range 7–39) days and the mean dose in milligram equivalents of prednisone was 850 (range 290–3300) mg (269). The time from administration of glucocorticoids to hip pain was 17 (range 6–33) months. A new case of bilateral avascular necrosis of the femoral heads after high-dose short-term dexamethasone therapy as an antiemetic in cancer chemotherapy has been reported (270).

Myopathy

The presence of physiological amounts of glucocorticoids is necessary for the normal functioning of muscle. Excessive glucocorticoid concentrations, in contrast, result in protein catabolism and a reduced rate of muscle protein synthesis (271), and hence in muscle atrophy and fibrosis. The molecular and biochemical basis of myopathy has been widely studied, and the mechanism has been attributed to impairment of glycogen synthesis. Muscle glycogen synthase protein content and activity was measured in samples from 14 patients taking glucocorticoids after kidney transplantation and from 20 healthy subjects (SEDA-21, 418; 272). The patients had impaired activation of glycogen synthase and reduced enzyme activity. Muscular weakness can of course also result from glucocorticoid-induced hypokalemia. In spontaneous Cushing's syndrome, there is muscle involvement in some 50% of cases (273).

Among reports of myopathy in patients taking glucocorticoids, involvement of the respiratory muscles is often mentioned (274,275), possibly because this is particularly

likely to have clinical consequences. Patients on mechanically assisted ventilation may be particularly at risk of myopathy (SEDA-18, 390). However, any muscle can be affected; one often sees weakness and atrophy of the hip muscles and (in about half the cases) the shoulder muscles and the proximal muscles of the limbs.

The myopathy usually develops gradually, without pain, and symmetrically. However, a single epidural injection of a glucocorticoid for lumbar radicular pain has caused Cushing's syndrome and myopathy (SEDA-20, 370; 97).

There is a suggestion that the incidence of myopathy is greatest during treatment with compounds that are fluorinated at the 9-alpha position, such as triamcinolone, but this may simply reflect its general potency. In children, the risk of effects on muscles is relatively high.

Biopsy is not justified as a routine, but it is useful as a diagnostic tool in distinguishing suspected corticoid myopathy from diseases of the muscles or vascular system with inflammation that may have been the indication for giving glucocorticoids in the first place; electromyographic measurements cannot confirm the diagnosis.

After termination of treatment the myopathy normally improves over a period of several months.

Damage to tendons and fascia

Tendons can be injured by glucocorticoids and can rupture (276). Ten cases of Achilles tendon rupture were seen in a single clinic over a 10-year period (SEDA-17, 448). The risk seems to be greater if local (for example intra-articular) injections are used.

Rupture of the plantar fascia induced by glucocorticoids has usually been reported in athletes. However, a case of spontaneous degenerative rupture has been reported in a 72-year-old man who had received four glucocorticoid injections over 1 year for plantar fasciitis (SEDA-21, 418) (277).

- A 69-year-old man with newly diagnosed giant cell arteritis was given prednisone 30 mg bd, and 2 weeks later developed severe pain along his Achilles tendons bilaterally; 1 week later the left tendon ruptured (278). Despite immobilization his pain worsened. The prednisone was gradually tapered and the symptoms abated, with complete recovery.

In the previous literature this adverse reaction was described in patients taking glucocorticoids for from 4 months to several years.

Joints

Among the adverse effects of pulse glucocorticoid therapy, joint manifestations are rare. A woman with systemic lupus erythematosus and nephritis developed transient bilateral knee effusions during pulse therapy with high doses of glucocorticoids (279).

- A 62-year old woman was admitted to hospital with lupus nephritis. A kidney biopsy showed a mesangioproliferative glomerulonephritis (WHO class III). After 4 months of inadequate response to traditional treatment, she started monthly pulse glucocorticoid therapy (methylprednisolone 1 g for 3 days) before immunosuppressive drugs. After 2 days of pulse glucocorticoid therapy she complained of pain and flexion discomfort in both knees, which were swollen. At arthrocentesis synovial fluid was aspirated (5 ml from the right knee and 6 ml from the left). The fluid was colorless, with a high viscosity and excellent mucin clot formation. There was only 1 mononuclear cell/mm^3 in the right knee synovial fluid and no cells in the left. There were no crystals. Inflammatory laboratory measurements carried out simultaneously were unchanged. X-rays of the affected joints were normal. The effusion resolved with arthrocentesis and did not recur.

The author proposed that raised arterial pressure, which is an adverse effect of high dose glucocorticoid treatment, and low oncotic pressure due to a low protein plasma concentration in a patient with nephrotic syndrome, could have increased trans-synovial fluid flow at a lower arterial pressure than normal.

Growth in children

The possibility that inhaled glucocorticoids may impair growth in children is of concern, but difficult to assess, as severe chronic asthma can impair growth. If not adequately controlled, asthma modifies the prepubertal growth spurt, the pubertal growth spurt, and the catch-up phase, which allows the child to attain adult height. There is a wide range of individual responses and some children have adverse effects with relatively small doses of glucocorticoids. It is still not clear whether this is a transient phenomenon, causing a slowing of growth and maturational delay with no adverse effect on adult height, or whether growth can be permanently impaired. Ideally studies should establish the effect of asthma treatments on final adult height (compared with predicted values for sex and parental height). Such studies pose considerable logistic problems. For this reason most studies have measured growth over shorter time spans. Outcome measures have been expressed as the height velocity or growth rate, that is changes in height over a defined time. Alternatively height is measured and compared with that of age- and sex-matched controls. Such relatively short-term studies do not necessarily predict the effects of treatment on eventual adult height.

The growth-inhibiting effects of glucocorticoids in children are related not only to inhibition of growth hormone secretion, but also to the sensitivity of the peripheral tissues to the effects of growth hormone. By means of overnight profile analysis it was shown that glucocorticoid treatment reduces the amplitude but not the number of pulses of the physiological growth hormone secretion (SEDA-14, 335; 280).

Effects on growth occur early in treatment: with sensitive testing methods they can be detected in growing children within a few weeks of starting therapy. The effects can be produced by any route of administration, including even inhalation therapy (at least with dexamethasone) (SEDA-18, 391). Comparisons of attained heights with expected heights in children who have used inhaled or oral glucocorticoids have been summarized in a meta-analysis (SEDA-19, 375; 281). There was a significant but small tendency for glucocorticoid therapy in general to be associated with reduced final height. However, this effect varied according to the route of administration. As expected, there was significant impairment of growth with prednisone and other oral glucocorticoids. On the other hand, inhaled beclomethasone dipropionate was associated with normal stature, even when it was used in higher dosages, for longer durations, or in patients with more severe asthma. In another study in 94 children aged 7–9 years, beclomethasone in a dosage taken by many children with mild asthma (400 micrograms/day) significantly reduced growth (SEDA-20, 369; 282). In children with growth suppression during therapy with inhaled beclomethasone or budesonide (200–400 micrograms/day) there was catch-up growth when they switched to equipotent dosages of inhaled fluticasone (100–200 micrograms/day) (SEDA-21, 414; 283). However, in six children with severe asthma, treatment with inhaled high-dosage fluticasone 1000 micrograms/day was associated with growth retardation and adrenal insufficiency (SEDA-21, 414; 284). In one child, growth rate and adrenal function normalized 9 months after the fluticasone dosage was reduced to 500 micrograms/day.

It is generally agreed that the use of single doses of prednisone on alternate mornings minimizes growth retardation but does not avoid it; in children it has been shown that biochemical markers of growth are lower in patients receiving daily glucocorticoid therapy than in patients treated with an alternate-day regimen or not receiving glucocorticoids (SED-12, 988; 285).

It has long been thought by some physicians that the impairment of growth caused by glucocorticoids can be lessened by switching to corticotropin, but this is uncertain. Compensatory treatment with anabolic hormones is definitely not recommended today, since they do not stimulate growth but actually impede it by promoting closure of the epiphyses. Recombinant growth hormone (rGH) treatment of poorly growing children with glucocorticoid-dependent renal disease has often been observed to improve linear growth. However, the dosage of prednisone has been reported to be a critical factor in determining the efficacy of rGH therapy in glucocorticoid-dependent children (SEDA-19, 375; 286). When the dose of prednisone was greater than 0.35 mg/kg/day, rGH did not increase the linear growth rate. At lower doses, the response was inversely related to the amount of prednisone.

Provided glucocorticoid treatment is terminated before the end of puberty, total growth may catch up with the physiological norm (SEDA-17, 448). Concern has been expressed that fear of growth retardation can result in unjustifiable denial of glucocorticoid therapy. It does, however, seem highly advisable to keep doses as low as possible and to switch to a therapeutic regimen that excludes glucocorticoids as children approach the expected onset of puberty (SEDA-14, 335).

Serum osteocalcin determinations appear to be a helpful marker to evaluate the effects of glucocorticoids on growth in children.

One unanswered question is whether the growth suppression that occurs in children during glucocorticoid treatment persists after treatment is withdrawn and affects final adult height. In an attempt to answer this question, growth 6–7 years after withdrawal of alternate-day prednisone has been evaluated in children (aged 6–14 years) with cystic fibrosis who had participated in a multi-center trial from 1986 to 1991 (287). Of 224 children, 161 had been randomized to prednisone (1 or 2 mg/kg) and 73 to placebo. At the time of the study, 68% were aged 18 years or more. Height fell during prednisone therapy, but catch-up growth began 2 years after withdrawal. However, the heights of the boys treated with prednisone remained significantly lower by 4 cm than those who took placebo. In contrast, in the girls there were no differences in height at 2–3 years after prednisone withdrawal.

Reproductive system

Reduced sperm count and motility and inhibition of the secretory function of the testicles during glucocorticoid treatment have been reported and discussed in relation to the suppression of adrenal androgen production. These reports still await confirmation.

Since amenorrhea is a symptom of Cushing's syndrome, disorders of menstruation are common in fertile women taking higher doses of glucocorticoids (SEDA-3, 305). On the other hand, plasma cortisol concentrations in normally menstruating women have marked circadian variation, the extent of which can reach 200% or more (288), with the peak of the cortisol plasma concentrations at mid-cycle and near its end. Inhibition of ovulation by triamcinolone 25 mg has been reported when the drug is given on day 1 or 2 of the cycle. How glucocorticoids interfere with the hormonal control of the menstrual cycle is still unknown (289).

Women should be warned about the possibility of menstrual disorders after local triamcinolone injections (290). When premenopausal women received their first injection of triamcinolone intra-articularly ($n = 46$), injected into soft tissue ($n = 24$), or epidurally ($n = 7$) they were specifically asked to report flushing or menstrual irregularities during a mean follow-up period of 6 weeks. Of the 77 women in the study, 39 reported menstrual disorders. The onset of menstruation was later than expected in ten women and earlier in 16 women. There was reduced loss of blood and/or a shorter duration of menstruation in four women and increased loss of blood and/or a longer duration of menstruation in 18. Also, 22 women had flushing. Menstrual disorders occurred significantly less often in women who were taking oral contraceptives.

Immunologic

Since the glucocorticoids have immunosuppressive and anti-inflammatory properties, one would not expect allergic reactions to be a problem, except when excipients act as allergens. Nevertheless, allergic reactions to glucocorticoids themselves have been reported (SEDA-21, 419; 291). Immunological reactions to glucocorticoids have been reviewed (292). Reactions can be of types I, III, or IV. Immediate reactions usually occur in patients with asthma and in those who have to use glucocorticoids repeatedly. Other susceptibility factors include female sex and hypersensitivity to acetylsalicylic acid. Often excipients are implicated (succinates, sulfites, and carboxymethylcellulose). Cross-reactivity does not necessarily occur; patients with immediate reactions to hydrocortisone and methylprednisolone can often tolerate prednisone and prednisolone and second-generation compounds, such as dexamethasone and betamethasone. Urticaria after glucocorticoid treatment has been explained as a reaction of the mesenchyme. Also, an increase in eosinophilic leukocytes (which normally are diminished by glucocorticoids) has been reported as a first reaction to treatment with glucocorticoids.

Class I reactions

To date, there have been about 100 published reports of immediate hypersensitivity reactions after oral and parenteral administration of glucocorticoids. Although there is evidence that glucocorticoids themselves can cause these reactions, there is debate about the mechanism. Anaphylactic shock has been described after intranasal hydrocortisone acetate, intramuscular methylprednisolone (SEDA-21, 419; 293), intravenous methylprednisolone (SEDA-22, 448; 294), intramuscular dexamethasone (SEDA-22, 448; 295), and intra-articular methylprednisolone (SEDA-22, 449; 296). A life-threatening anaphylactic-like reaction to intravenous hydrocortisone has been described in patients with asthma (297). Acute laryngeal obstruction has been described after the intravenous administration of hydrocortisone (SEDA-22, 449; 298). There is some reason to believe that sodium succinate esters are more likely to cause hypersensitivity reactions (SEDA-17, 449), but unconjugated glucocorticoids can definitely produce allergy in some cases (SEDA-16, 452).

- A 64-year-old woman with a history of bronchial asthma developed increasing shortness of breath after an upper respiratory tract infection (299). Her medication included inhaled salbutamol as necessary, theophylline 300 mg bd, and aspirin 325 mg/day. She was given nebulized salbutamol and ipratropium and hydrocortisone 200 mg intravenously. Within 30 minutes, she developed a generalized rash, fever (38.3°C), and respiratory distress. She was promptly intubated and mechanical ventilation was started. No further doses of glucocorticoid were given. Skin testing with various parenteral formulations of glucocorticoids produced a 5 mm wheal at the site of hydrocortisone and methylprednisolone injections. She was subsequently given a challenge dose of triamcinolone using a metered-dose inhaler with no reaction, and was therefore continued on this medication.

- An anaphylactoid reaction (angioedema, generalized urticaria, worsening bronchospasm, and marked hypotension) occurred in a 35-year-old man with multiple sclerosis who became allergic to methylprednisolone (dose not stated) after starting treatment with interferon beta-1b (300). He had previously been treated with different courses of methylprednisolone. Clinicians should be aware that the complexity of the effects of interferon beta-1b on the immune system can lead to unexpected outcomes. It is uncertain whether the sequence of events here was due to an effect of interferon beta-1b or to coincidence.

- A 17-year-old boy, with an 11-year history of asthma, had anaphylaxis with respiratory distress shortly after he received intravenous methylprednisolone for an exacerbation of asthma while taking a tapering course of oral prednisone 15 mg/day (301). He had been glucocorticoid-dependent for at least 1 year. He reported having received intravenous glucocorticoids previously. He was treated with inhaled salbutamol and then intravenous methylprednisolone 125 mg over 15–30 seconds, and 3–4 minutes later became flushed and dyspneic, and developed diffuse urticarial lesions on his trunk and face and an undetectable blood pressure. He was treated with adrenaline, but required intubation. Sinus bradycardia developed and then asystole. He was successfully resuscitated and a 10–15 seconds period of generalized tonic-clonic activity was treated with diazepam. He remained unresponsive to stimulation for 30 minutes. However, he awoke 1 hour after his respiratory arrest and was extubated and discharged the following day taking a tapering dosage of prednisone.

- An anaphylactoid reaction occurred in a 68-year-old woman after treatment with intravenous methylprednisolone for asthma. She had developed urticaria with methylprednisolone 1 year earlier, but the reaction had been thought to be related to the solvent in the formulation (302).

- Forty minutes after a first dose of prednisone 25 mg, a 17-year-old girl with a history of aspirin intolerance had generalized flushing, hives, hypogastric pain, and abdominal cramps, followed by vomiting and diarrhea (303). She lost consciousness and developed arterial hypotension. She responded to intravenous diphenhydramine and hydrocortisone. Intradermal skin tests were positive for prednisone and negative for methylprednisolone and hydrocortisone. An oral challenge test with prednisone led to flushing, nausea, dizziness, tachycardia, and hypotension and responded to intravenous diphenhydramine and hydrocortisone. Challenge tests with intravenous methylprednisolone and hydrocortisone were negative.

- A 75-year-old man developed triamcinolone-induced anaphylaxis and dose-related positive prick skin tests to triamcinolone, suggesting that an IgE-mediated hypersensitivity mechanism may have played a part (304).

- A 30-year-old man with recurrent atopic eczema of the head and neck, generalized xerosis, keratosis pilaris of the arms, and a history of dyshidrosis was initially treated with prednisolone-21-acetate ointment (305). His skin eruption became worse. He was given oral prednisolone 25 mg, and 5 hours after the first dose developed intense generalized pruritus with erythema and swelling of the face. After 24 hours there was generalized erythema with disseminated partly follicular papules. There was an eosinophilia (1.1×10^9/l). Total IgE was not raised. Patch tests showed delayed reactions to hydrocortisone 1%, prednisolone 1%, prednisolone-21-acetate ointment, and prednisolone 2.5%. Prick and intradermal tests with methylprednisolone succinate, hydrocortisone succinate, betamethasone, and triamcinolone acetonide in concentrations up to 1 : 10 were negative at 15 minutes. However, 4 hours after intradermal testing, generalized pruritus developed and 24 hours later there was a disseminated partly follicular eczematous reaction with involvement of the flexural areas. Biopsy of the eruptions caused by prednisolone and of the positive skin reaction to methylprednisolone succinate showed superficial dermatitis with a perivascular infiltration consisting predominantly of CD4+ cells and some eosinophils. Immunofluorescence showed increased expression of HLA-DR molecules on the CD4+ and CD8+ cells. During the exanthema caused by prednisolone, interleukin-5 (14 pg/ml), interleukin-6 (38 pg/ml), and interleukin-10 (26 pg/ml) were detected in the blood; 2 months after recovery these cytokines were not detectable.

The authors of the last report commented that generalized delayed type hypersensitivity to systemic administration of a glucocorticoid is rare. Despite the potent immunosuppressive effect of glucocorticoids on immunocompetent cells, the clinical features, the skin biopsy specimen, and the positive delayed skin test reactions strongly suggested an immunological mechanism: T cells were clearly involved and the high concentrations of interleukins 5, 6, and 10 were consistent with a T helper type 2 reaction. The raised concentrations of interleukin-5 were probably responsible for the blood and tissue eosinophilia.

Skin prick tests and intradermal tests to hydrocortisone and methylprednisolone, intradermal tests to betamethasone and dexamethasone, and oral challenge tests to betamethasone and deflazacort were performed in 10 patients with adverse reactions to systemic hemisuccinate esters of hydrocortisone and methylprednisolone (306). The skin prick tests and intradermal tests results suggested the possibility of an IgE-mediated mechanism for allergic reactions to hydrocortisone and methylprednisolone. The authors hypothesized that this mechanism is probably due, at least in part, to a glucocorticoid-glyoxal compound, a degradation product of cortisol, which in aqueous solution may be responsible for presenting steroid carbon rings to the immune system. They suggested that betamethasone and deflazacort could be reserved for emergency use in patients with adverse reactions to other glucocorticoids.

Budesonide has been marketed in oral form for intestinal inflammatory disease. An non-IgE-mediated anaphylactic reaction has been associated with oral budesonide (307).

- A 32-year-old woman with Crohn's disease, who had taken prednisone 20 mg/day and azathioprine 150 mg/day, switched to budesonide 9 mg/day because of weight gain, and 5 minutes after the first capsule her tongue and throat swelled, accompanied by wheeziness and diarrhea. She was given clemastine and recovered after 4 ays. Intracutaneous tests with diluted budesonide suggested a non-IgE-mediated reaction. She had a previous history of a similar reaction to mesalazine. One year later her tongue and throat swelled after intravenous dexamethasone.

Urticaria with angioedema has been described in a patient taking deflazacort (308).

- A 64-year-old woman with allergic alveolitis caused by parakeet feathers improved with intravenous methylprednisolone, and was given oral deflazacort 60 mg/day, to be reduced progressively. After 30 days she developed generalized itchy blotches and lip edema. At that time she was mistakenly taking deflazacort in a dose of 120 mg/day. She was given an antihistamine, without any improvement. Deflazacort was then replaced by prednisolone and her symptoms disappeared immediately. Skin tests (a prick test and an epicutaneous test) were positive with deflazacort. Oral provocation with deflazacort 30 mg was positive, with the immediate appearance of the same symptoms as in the initial episode.

Class III reactions

Allergy to topical glucocorticoids in inflammatory bowel disease has been reported (309).

- A 57-year old Caucasian man with inflammatory bowel disease was given prednisolone metasulfobenzoate sodium enemas twice daily and oral mesalazine 800 mg tds for about 5 months, without improvement. He stopped using the prednisolone enemas but continued to take mesalazine. Within 48 hours of stopping prednisolone his symptoms resolved completely. The theoretical possibility of contact allergy was entertained. Patch tests with a standard battery of contact allergens, including tixocortol pivalate and budesonide, were ++ positive with budesonide. At follow up 3 months later he was symptom free.

The authors advised that allergy to topical glucocorticoids should be considered in patients using rectal steroids whose condition unexpectedly fails to improve or in whom there is unexpected deterioration.

Vasculitis
Exacerbation of giant cell arteritis, with clinical signs of an evolving vertebrobasilar stroke, has been attributed to prednisolone (310).

- A 64-year-old man with giant cell arteritis was given prednisolone 60 mg/day. Within 5 days he developed double vision and agitation and became drowsy and confused. A cranial MRI scan showed recent cerebral lesions and a Doppler scan showed high-resistant blood flow in both vertebral arteries. He had an episode of complete loss of vision and was given dexamethasone

and intravenous heparin followed by warfarin. He gradually improved over the next few weeks but was left with cognitive and memory deficits.

Immunosuppression
Glucocorticoids inhibit the formation of antibodies. Of 111 consecutive heart transplant recipients taking oral prednisone (mean 13.8 months), 57% developed hypogammaglobulinemia (IgG below 7 g/l) (311). Those with severe hypogammaglobulinemia (IgG below 3.5 g/l) were at increassed risk of opportunistic infections compared with those with IgG concentrations over 3.5 g/l (55 versus 5%, OR = 23). Parenteral glucocorticoid pulse therapy was associated with a significantly increased risk of severe hypogammaglobulinemia (OR = 15).

With long-term treatment, IgG subclass deficiencies can become marked (312). There is suppression of the antigen–antibody reaction, and since this reaction itself normally results in liberation of kinins, the latter is also suppressed. Failure of kinin liberation leads in turn to inhibition of invasion of sensitized leukocytes and reduced production and maturation of phagocytes. Undoubtedly, it is true that using minimal effective doses will avoid the most serious consequences, but the problem cannot be fully circumvented, since the anti-inflammatory effects themselves involve some inhibition of the migration of leukocytes and phagocytosis.

Dexamethasone significantly affected the antibody response of preterm infants with chronic lung disease to immunization against *Haemophilus influenzae* (313). Serum samples were obtained before and after immunization from an unselected cohort of 59 preterm infants (30 boys; gestational age 175–208 days). *Haemophilus influenzae* antibodies were measured using ELISA. IgG antibody concentrations in 16 infants who received no dexamethasone were 0.16 and 4.63 microgram/ml before and after immunization respectively. The corresponding values for those who received dexamethasone were 0.10 and 0.51 microgram/ml.

Infection risk

The consequence of this interference with immune responses can be multiplication of bacteria and an increased risk of bacterial intoxication when infection does occur; hence, the frequency and severity of clinical infections tend to increase during glucocorticoid therapy. Aggravation of existing tuberculosis and reactivation of completely quiescent cases of this infection are classic consequences demanding prophylactic measures; atypical mycobacteria have also caused tissue infections (SEDA-17, 449). Other bacterial infections, some severe and proceeding to sepsis, have followed glucocorticoid treatment. There is little evidence that glucocorticoids, even in high dosages and early in the course of infection, significantly alter the ultimate outcome (314). Use of glucocorticoids in the treatment of septic shock is not recommended in the absence of adrenal suppression.

It has been suggested that there are some differences between drugs. The use of fluticasone nasal spray to control polyp recurrence after functional endoscopic sphenoethmoidectomy should be viewed with caution, as it has been said to be associated with a high incidence of severe postoperative infection compared with beclomethasone (SEDA-21, 375; 315).

Acute generalized exanthematous pustulosis due to a glucocorticoid has been reported (SEDA-21, 416; 316).

In a retrospective study, postoperative infectious complications were evaluated in 159 patients with inflammatory bowel disease undergoing elective surgery (317). Immunosuppression consisted of glucocorticoid monotherapy ($n = 56$), a glucocorticoid + azathioprine or mercaptopurine ($n = 52$), and neither a glucocorticoid nor azathioprine or mercaptopurine ($n = 51$). The adjusted odds ratios for any infection and major infections in patients who took glucocorticoid were 3.69 and 5.54 respectively, and in patients who took azathioprine or mercaptopurine 1.68 and 1.20. Thus, preoperative use of glucocorticoid in patients with inflammatory bowel disease increased the risk of postoperative infectious complications.

Bacterial infections

Infections with *Clostridium difficile*, *Pseudomonas aeruginosa*, and *Listeria monocytogenes* (SEDA-22, 450; 318) have occasionally been precipitated or aggravated by glucocorticoids, as has tuberculous peritonitis (SEDA-20, 377; 319).

The cumulative and mean daily dosages of glucocorticoids in patients with systemic lupus erythematosus, inflammatory myopathy, overlap syndrome, or mixed connective tissue disease were the most important risk factors for the development of tuberculosis, according to a study conducted in Korea (320). Records were analysed from 269 patients who had been hospitalized during a 5-year period. In 21 patients active tuberculosis developed after a mean duration of 27 months from diagnosis of their rheumatic disease, an incidence rate of 20 cases per 1000 patient-years. The mean cumulative and daily dosages of prednisolone during the follow-up period were 31 594 and 25 mg respectively in patients who developed tuberculosis, compared with 17 043 and 18 mg in patients who did not. Glucocorticoid pulse therapy was a risk factor for the development of tuberculosis.

- A 43-year-old woman developed cavitary lung tuberculosis after she received methotrexate and glucocorticoid pulse therapy for rheumatoid arthritis (321).

The authors commented that the onset of the lung infection appeared to be closely related to methotrexate and glucocorticoid pulse therapy, because of the interval between drug administration and the onset of tuberculosis, and the lack of other risk factors for opportunistic infections.

In a retrospective study, the use of glucocorticoids during *Pneumocystis jiroveci* pneumonia (mean total dose methylprednisolone 420 mg, mean treatment duration 12 days) did not increase the risk of development or relapse of tuberculosis or other AIDS-related diseases (SEDA-20, 377; 322). The study included 129 patients (72 who took glucocorticoids and 57 who did not) who were

followed up at 6, 12, 18, and 24 months of glucocorticoid therapy. The rates of infections were similar in both groups, and the cumulative rate of tuberculosis at 2 years was 12–13%.

Mycobacterium avium septic arthritis has been reported in two patients with pre-existing rheumatic disease (scleroderma and polymyositis) who were taking prednisolone and azathioprine; the infection was in the left shoulder in one patient and in the knee in the other (323).

The use of glucocorticoids in patients with hematological diseases is a factor that facilitates the occurrence of *Legionella pneumophila* pneumonia, and 10 episodes of this infection were possibly related to glucocorticoids in a series of 67 cases of Legionnaires' disease diagnosed in a single institution during 2.5 years (324).

Viral infections

Infections such as chickenpox can have serious consequences, including death, in patients taking systemic glucocorticoids (SEDA-19, 378; SEDA-20, 377; 325,326). It has been suggested that *Varicella zoster* immunoglobulin should be given to patients in contact with chickenpox if they have taken glucocorticoids in dosages over 0.5 mg/kg/day during the preceding 3 months, in the context of near-fatal chickenpox in a child receiving prednisolone (SEDA-20, 377; 327). Smallpox vaccination has in the past resulted in vaccinia gangrenosum in patients taking glucocorticoids, and the current type of *Varicella* vaccine is much more likely to produce rashes in children who are already taking glucocorticoids than in controls (SEDA-16, 452).

Herpes simplex virus encephalitis after myxedema coma has been described in an 81-year-old man treated with hydrocortisone (100 mg 8-hourly) and levothyroxine (328). In renal transplantation, two cases of death from *Herpes simplex* as a result of glucocorticoid treatment are on record (SED-8, 827; SEDA-17, 449).

Fungal and yeast infections

Fungal and yeast infections (including cases of fulminant fungal pericarditis, mucormycosis, *Aspergillus fumigatus* infection, and cutaneous alternariosis) can be precipitated or aggravated by glucocorticoid treatment (SEDA-17, 449; SEDA-18, 390; SEDA-20, 377; SEDA-21, 418; SEDA-22, 449; 329–332).

Primary esophageal histoplasmosis must be considered in patients who have a history of gastroesophageal reflux disease and are immunosuppressed by long-term glucocorticoids (SEDA-22, 450; 333). Oropharyngeal candidiasis is a well-described adverse effect of inhaled glucocorticoids. However, few cases of esophageal candidiasis have been reported (SEDA-22, 179).

Invasive pulmonary aspergillosis with cerebromeningeal involvement has been described after short-term intravenous administration of methylprednisolone (SEDA-22, 449; 334). Of 473 HIV-infected children, 7 (1.5%) developed invasive aspergillosis during the study period (1987–95) (SEDA-22, 449; 335). Sustained neutropenia or glucocorticoid therapy as predisposing factors for invasive aspergillosis were found in only two patients.

- Fatal pulmonary infection with *Aspergillus fumigatus* and *Nocardia asteroides* has been described in a patient who took prednisone 1 mg/kg/day for 1 month for bronchiolitis obliterans (336).
- Fatal *Aspergillus* myocarditis, probably related to short-term administration of glucocorticoids, has been described in a 58-year-old man, who had an acute exacerbation of his chronic obstructive pulmonary disease and received oxygen, bronchodilators, omeprazole, co-amoxiclav, and intravenous methylprednisolone 40 mg 8-hourly; he died 5 days later and postmortem examination showed a fungal myocarditis (337).
- Fatal aspergillosis with a thyroid gland abscess occurred in a 74-year-old man after treatment with prednisolone for polymyalgia rheumatica (338).
- *Cryptoccocus neoformans* meningitis occurred in a 15-year old child with acute lymphoblastic leukemia (339). The clinical signs, headache, and a sixth nerve palsy on the right side, occurred at the end of the maintenance therapy when complete remission had been obtained (after 100 weeks of maintenance therapy, including multiple intermittent doses of dexamethasone). Culture of the cerebrospinal fluid confirmed cryptococcal meningitis, and antifungal therapy produced a complete clinical response.
- *Scedosporium apiospermum* infection occurred in the left forearm of an 81-year-old man who was taking chronic oral prednisone (increased to 40 mg/day 1 month before presentation) for lung fibrosis (340).

Cutaneous alternariosis (infection with *Alternaria alternata*) has been described in a 78-year-old farmer with idiopathic pulmonary fibrosis taking oral prednisone 20 mg/day (341).

The effect of dexamethasone has been assessed in a retrospective chart review study in neonates weighing less than 1200 g, both with (*n* = 65) and without (*n* = 269) *Candida* sepsis; dexamethasone therapy and prolonged antibiotic therapy were associated with *Candida* infection (342).

In a retrospective study that included 163 consecutive recipients of allogenic hemopoietic stem cell transplants with invasive fungal infections, the possible role of glucocorticoid therapy was evaluated. The administration of high-dose glucocorticoids (2 mg/kg/day or more) was associated with an increased risk of mold infection (HR = 4.0, 95% CI = 1.7, 9.6) and an increased risk of mold infection-related death (1 year survival 11% compared with 44% when patients took doses less than 2 mg/kg/day) (343).

Fatal cerebral involvement in systemic aspergillosis has been described in a 25-year old woman with severe thrombocytopenia (platelet count 10×10^9/l) and mild intermittent leukopenia (granulocytes $0.375-3 \times 10^9$/l) who was taking prednisone 1–1.5 mg/kg/day and azathioprine 100–200 mg/day (344).

Helminth infections
Strongyloidiasis (SEDA-20, 377; SEDA-21, 419; SEDA-22, 449; 345–347) has been precipitated or aggravated by glucocorticoids.

Protozoal infections
Toxoplasmosis has been precipitated by glucocorticoids (348,349).

Pneumocystis jiroveci pneumonia has been precipitated or aggravated by glucocorticoids (SEDA-20, 377; SEDA-22, 450; 272,350,351). There is some concern about the use of glucocorticoids as adjunctive therapy in patients with AIDS who develop *Pneumocystis jiroveci* pneumonia. The immunosuppressant properties of glucocorticoids have been reported to enhance the risk of tuberculosis and other AIDS-related diseases (for example Kaposi's sarcoma or cytomegalovirus infection).

Amebic dysentery has been precipitated by glucocorticoids (352).

Death

Mortality associated with glucocorticoid has been retrospectively studied in 556 patients with chronic obstructive pulmonary disease admitted to a rehabilitation center (353). Median survival was 38 months and 280 patients died during follow-up. On multivariate analysis, oral glucocorticoid use at a prednisone equivalent of 10 mg/day without inhaled glucocorticoid was associated with an increased risk of death (RR = 2.34; 95% CI = 1.24, 4.44), and 15 mg/day increased the risk further (RR = 4.03; 95% CI = 1.99, 8.15). The risk of death was not increased in those using 5 mg/day or when patients used any oral dose in combination with inhaled glucocorticoids.

Long-Term Effects

Drug withdrawal

Suppression of adrenocortical function is one of the consequences of repeated administration of glucocorticoids; after termination of treatment a withdrawal syndrome can occur. In many cases this is unpleasant rather than acutely dangerous; in such instances the patients may have headache, nausea, dizziness, anorexia, weakness, emotional changes, lethargy, and perhaps fever; in some cases severe mental disorders occur and there are repeated reports of benign intracranial hypertension (354). The glucocorticoid withdrawal syndrome also seems to underlie the "glucocorticoid pseudorheumatism" that can occur when the drugs are withdrawn in rheumatic patients.

Withdrawal symptoms disappear if the glucocorticoid is resumed, but as a rule they will in any case vanish spontaneously within a few days. More serious consequences can ensue, however, in certain types of cases and if adrenal cortical atrophy is severe. In patients treated with corticoids for the nephrotic syndrome and apparently cured, the syndrome is particularly likely to relapse on withdrawal of therapy if the adrenal cortex is atrophic (SEDA-3, 305). In some cases, acute adrenocortical insufficiency after glucocorticoid treatment has actually proved fatal. It is advisable to withdraw long-term glucocorticoid therapy gradually so that the cortex has sufficient opportunity to recover. Table 5 lists methods of

Table 5 Suggested methods of withdrawing prednisolone

Circumstances	*Change in daily dose*
The problem has resolved and treatment has been given for only a few weeks	Reduce by 2.5 mg every 3 or 4 days down to 7.5 mg/day; then reduce more slowly, for example by 2.5 mg every week, fortnight, or month
There is uncertainty about disease resolution and/or therapy has been given for many weeks	Reduce by 2.5 mg every fortnight or month down to 7.5 mg/day then reduce by 1 mg every month
Symptoms of the disease are likely to recur on withdrawal (for example rheumatoid arthritis)	Reduce by 1 mg every month

withdrawing prednisolone after long-term therapy in different circumstances (355).

Anorexia nervosa has been precipitated by withdrawal of oral prednisolone for asthma (SEDA-21, 414; 356).

A case of papilledema as a manifestation of raised intracranial pressure has been reported following withdrawal of topical glucocorticoids (SEDA-3, 305).

Panniculitis, which causes erythematous, firm, warm subcutaneous nodules, can occur within 2 weeks of withdrawal of large doses of glucocorticoids, but case reports confirm that resolution without scarring is the rule and that reintroduction of glucocorticoids is not necessary for improvement (357).

Churg–Strauss syndrome has come into prominence with the introduction of the leukotriene receptor antagonists, because they allow glucocorticoid-dependent asthmatics to discontinue their oral prednisolone. Five patients developed Churg–Strauss syndrome when their oral glucocorticoids were withdrawn (358). The duration of oral glucocorticoid therapy was 3–216 months and the dosage of prednisolone was 2.5–25.5 mg/day. The diagnosis of Churg–Strauss syndrome was made from 6 to 83 months after withdrawal of the oral glucocorticoids. These case reports support the hypothesis that it is the withdrawal of glucocorticoids that unmasks the underlying systemic vasculitis in these patients with asthma, rather than an effect of the new therapeutic agents that permits the reduction (and withdrawal) of prednisolone. Case-control studies are needed to determine the respective roles of the new therapeutic agents, prednisolone withdrawal, or other factors in the emergence of Churg–Strauss syndrome in these asthmatic patients

Tumorigenicity

Direct tumor-inducing effects of the glucocorticoids are not known, but the particular risk that malignancies in patients undergoing immunosuppression with these or other drugs will spread more rapidly is a well-recognized problem.

- Progressive endometrial carcinoma associated with azathioprine and prednisone therapy has been reported (359).
- Rapid progression of Kaposi's sarcoma 10 weeks after combined treatment with glucocorticoids and cyclophosphamide has been described; marked improvement of the skin lesions was noted after discontinuation of prednisone therapy (360).

Patients (mean age 39 years, $n = 1862$) who underwent 1924 renal transplantations from March 1995 to May 1997 were followed for 3–150 months. They received one of the following regimens: prednisolone plus azathioprine (group 1; $n = 100$); prednisolone plus azathioprine plus ciclosporin (group 2; $n = 1464$); and the same therapy as group 2 plus either muromonab-CD3 or antithymocyte globulin as induction or antirejection therapy (group 3; $n = 298$). The mean time to appearance of neoplasia after renal transplantation was 48 months. Malignancies developed earlier in group 3 patients (mean time to appearance 31 months) than in group 2 (39 months) and in group 1 (90 months). Seven of the patients who developed malignancies had also received pulse methylprednisolone for acute rejection. The authors concluded that the treatment of acute rejection with pulsed methylprednisolone and the use of muromonab-CD3 and antithymocyte globulin may lead to an increased incidence of malignancies after renal transplantation. They recommended that strategies be implemented for the early detection of malignancy (361)

In seven patients, accelerated growth of Kaposi's sarcoma lesions during glucocorticoid therapy suggested that glucocorticoids can alter the biological behavior of this malignant disease (362). Hydrocortisone accelerates the growth of cell lines derived from Kaposi's sarcoma cells cultured in vitro and this may partially explain these findings. Reports continue to point to the reversibility of the condition when glucocorticoids are withdrawn (363).

Kaposi's sarcoma has been associated with prednisolone therapy in two elderly women (364).

- An 84-year-old woman with polymyalgia rheumatica and a 79-year-old woman with undifferentiated connective tissue disease and leukocytoclastic vasculitis were given prednisolone 20 mg/day with subsequent dosage reductions. The first patient developed a raised purpuric rash and lymphedema of the left leg within 5 months and the second developed large purple nodules on the soles of her feet and the backs of her hands accompanied by periorbital and peripheral edema. Skin biopsies showed Kaposi's sarcoma, and both patients had raised IgG antibody titers to human herpesvirus-8.

Prior infection with herpesvirus-8 is a requisite for the development of Kaposi's sarcoma. The question arises as to how glucocorticoid treatment alone can lead to the emergence of this malignancy. In vitro evidence supports the hypothesis that glucocorticoids have a direct role in stimulating tumor development and the activation of herpesvirus-8.

A possible relation between systemic glucocorticoid use and a risk of esophageal cancer has been described in a population-based study in Denmark, in which the prescriptions database and the Danish cancer registry were linked (365). There was an increase in the number of cases observed ($n = 36$) compared with the number expected ($n = 19$), with a standardized incidence ratio of 1.92 (95% CI = 1.34, 2.65).

Second-Generation Effects

Pregnancy

A single course of a glucocorticoid given to women at risk of preterm delivery promotes fetal lung maturation, reduces the incidence of respiratory distress syndrome, and reduces neonatal morbidity and mortality. In a retrospective analysis of 306 infants of gestational age under 34 weeks, there was an association between glucocorticoid use and gastroesophageal reflux (366). In this series, 71% of the neonates (216/306) received antenatal glucocorticoids. More babies who received antenatal glucocorticoids had clinical evidence of gastroesophageal reflux (27% versus 12%). There was a significant increase in the incidence of gastroesophageal reflux with increasing courses of antenatal steroids: no course 12%, one course 25%, and two or more courses 32%.

However, there is still controversy about the use of single or repeat courses. It seems that betamethasone is more active in reducing neonatal deaths and produces fewer adverse effects than dexamethasone (367).

In a statement, the American Academy of Pediatrics and the Canadian Paediatric Society did not recommend the routine use of systemic dexamethasone for the prevention or treatment of chronic lung disease in infants with very low birthweights, because it does not reduce overall mortality and is associated with impaired growth and neurodevelopment delay (368,369).

In an analysis of 595 preterm infants born at 26–32 weeks gestation during a randomized controlled trial for the prevention of lung disease, glucocorticoids given to women at risk of preterm delivery promoted fetal lung maturation, reduced the incidence of respiratory distress syndrome, and reduced neonatal morbidity and mortality (370). Dexamethasone was given as either two doses of 12 mg 24 hours apart or four doses of 6 mg every 6 hours. Mortality was 9.2% after three or more courses, compared with 4.8% after one or two courses. This association was not explained by other factors (maternal or other common preterm morbidities).

The effects of glucocorticoids on uterine activity and preterm labor in high-order multiple gestations have been retrospectively reviewed (SEDA-20, 377; 371). In 15 women with triplet or quadruplet pregnancies, 17 out of 57 courses of betamethasone were associated with episodes of significant contractions requiring tocolytic intervention; 11 of these episodes were associated with cervical change and four resulted in premature delivery. The authors did not recommend the use of glucocorticoids if patients have more than 3.5 contractions per hour.

Prenatal glucocorticoid therapy to enhance fetal lung maturation reduces neonatal morbidity and mortality. However, adverse effects of serial courses of betamethasone on mother and fetus can occur.

For example, single versus multiple courses of antenatal glucocorticoids have been compared retrospectively in 704 pregnancies that resulted in pre-term births at 24–32 weeks. There three groups: 294 neonates whose mothers had not received glucocorticoids, 257 who had received a single dose, and 153 who had received multiple doses. Multiple doses compared with a single dose was associated with increased positive maternal cultures (44% versus 31%), small for gestational age infants (35% versus 21%), and intraventricular haemorrhage (45% versus 34%) (372).

In a retrospective study of the use of betamethasone every 12 hours versus 24 hours for anticipated preterm delivery in 909 pregnancies, three groups were identified: those who had not received antenatal glucocorticoids, those who had received betamethasone 12 hours apart, and those who received 24-hour dosing (373). There was significantly more maternal antibiotic use (90% versus 84%) and more neonatal surfactant use (40% versus 26%) in the 12-hour group compared with the 24-hour group. For all other outcomes there was no clinically significant difference.

Endocrine

Maternal hyperadrenalism occurred after five courses of betamethasone to enhance fetal lung maturation (374).

- A 26-year-old woman was given intravenous salbutamol 0.3 mg/hour for preterm labor, and intramuscular betamethasone 12 mg/day for 2 days. Daily oral tocolysis (salbutamol 2 mg every 6 hours plus nicardipine 50 mg every 12 hours) and betamethasone every week were continued at home for 3 weeks. The mother developed amyotrophy, acne on the face and trunk, moon face, hirsutism with whiskers, and thin skin. Free urinary cortisol was less than 5 micrograms/day (reference range 25–90), plasma cortisol was less than 10 ng/ml (100–200), and the salivary cortisol was less than 0.6 ng/ml (2.3–4.7). One hour after intramuscular tetracosactide 250 micrograms, her plasma cortisol was 102 ng/ml (reference range over 210) and the salivary cortisol was 3.1 ng/ml (13–25), indicating no adrenocortical response. She was given hydrocortisone 20 mg/day, and 2 months later adrenocortical insufficiency persisted, with a plasma cortisol of 152 ng/ml after corticotropin stimulation. One year later, she still required hydrocortisone 10 mg/day.

Hyperadrenalism has never otherwise been reported after the sequential use of glucocorticoids for fetal lung maturation.

A study in 10 women has been conducted to determine whether betamethasone administered at risk of preterm delivery causes adrenal suppression (375). After adrenal stimulation with corticotropin 1 microgram at 24–25 weeks, each woman received two intramuscular doses of betamethasone 12 mg 24 hours apart; 1 week later, another corticotropin test was followed by another two doses of betamethasone; a third corticotropin stimulation test was carried out 1 week later. All the women had normal baseline and stimulated cortisol concentrations during the first corticotropin stimulation test. Mean baseline serum cortisol concentrations fell with each corticotropin stimulation test (from 700 nmol/l (254 micrograms/l) before betamethasone to 120 nmol/l (43 micrograms/l) 1 week after the second course of betamethasone). The mean stimulated cortisol concentrations also fell significantly, from 910 nmol/l (330 micrograms/l) to 326 nmol/l (118 micrograms/l). There was evidence of adrenal suppression in four patients after the first course of betamethasone and in seven patients after the second course. There was no evidence of Addisonian crisis antepartum or intrapartum.

Musculoskeletal

Osteonecrosis of the femoral head can occur with glucocorticoids in nonpregnant individuals, but has not previously been reported in pregnancy (376).

- A 37-year-old white woman was given betamethasone, two doses of 12 mg over a day, at 24 weeks of a twin pregnancy, because of a history of growth restriction in her first pregnancy. At 25 weeks Doppler of the umbilical vessels suggested a reduction in end-diastolic flow in one twin. Betamethasone was prescribed again and was repeated weekly to a total of six courses because of the high risk of preterm delivery. At 30 weeks she complained of pain in the right hip exacerbated by weight bearing, which increased over the following 7 days until standing was impossible. An MRI scan showed avascular necrosis of the femoral head.

Infection risk

The use of betamethasone for the treatment of premature rupture of membranes during pregnancy is associated with an increased prevalence of maternal and neonatal infections. Two reports have described the risk of infections associated with the use of glucocorticoids during pregnancy. Of 374 patients with preterm premature rupture of membranes, 99 received a single course of glucocorticoids, 72 received multiple courses, and 203 were not treated with glucocorticoids (377). Only multiple courses of betamethasone increased the incidence of early-onset neonatal sepsis, chorioamnionitis, and endometritis in mothers. A single course of glucocorticoid was not significantly associated with any maternal or neonatal infectious complications. The incidence of maternal infections in 37 patients who received three or more courses of betamethasone (median 6, range 3–10) because of the risk of preterm delivery has been evaluated, with 70 healthy pregnant women as controls (378). Of those treated with betamethasone, 65% developed infectious diseases compared with 18% of controls. Symptomatic lower urinary tract infections (35 versus 2.7%) and serious bacterial infections (24 versus 0%) were more frequent in treated mothers. Eight of nine serious infections occurred in patients exposed to five or more courses of glucocorticoids.

Singleton pregnancies delivered at 24–34 weeks after antenatal betamethasone exposure have been prospectively analysed, in order to study the incidence of perinatal infection (379). There were 453 patients, 267 of whom took a single course of betamethasone (two doses of 12 mg in 24 hours), and 186 of whom took a multiple course (more than two doses in the 24 hours after the initial course). Multiple courses were significantly associated with early-onset neonatal sepsis (OR = 5.0; 95% CI = 1.0, 23), neonatal death (OR = 2.9; CI = 1.3, 6.9), chorioamnionitis (OR = 10; CI = 2.1, 65), and endometritis (OR = 3.6; CI = 1.7, 8.1). Respiratory distress and intraventricular hemorrhage were similar in the two groups. Although the study was non-randomized the results suggest an increased risk of neonatal infection and death after multiple courses of dexamethasone during pregnancy.

In a retrospective study in 609 mothers and their 713 infants who were treated with 1–12 courses of antenatal glucocorticoids, data from 369 singleton preterm infants born at 34 weeks or later, 210 multiple gestations, and 134 infants delivered at 35 weeks or later were analysed (380). The incidence of respiratory distress syndrome was 45% for single courses and 35% for multiple courses of glucocorticoids (OR = 0.44; 95% CI = 0.25, 0.79). The multiple-course group also had significantly less cases of patent ductus arteriosus (20 versus 13%). The incidences of death before discharge and other neonatal morbidities were similar. The multiple-course group had a significant reduction of 0.46 cm in head circumference at birth when adjusted for gestational age and pre-eclampsia. The two groups had similar birthweights. Infants born at more than 35 weeks, multiple-gestation infants, and infants who were born more than 7 days after the last dose of glucocorticoid had similar outcomes, regardless of the number of courses they had received. Mothers treated with multiple courses compared with a single course had a significantly higher incidence of postpartum endometritis, even though they had a lower incidence of prolonged rupture of membranes (24 versus 33%) and similar cesarean delivery rates. In conclusion, antenatal exposure to multiple courses of glucocorticoids compared with a single course resulted in a significant reduction in the incidence of respiratory distress syndrome in singleton preterm infants delivered within a week of the last glucocorticoid dose. This was associated with a reduction in head circumference at birth and an increased incidence of maternal endometritis. Whether the potential benefits of repeated therapy outweigh the risks will ultimately be determined in randomized controlled trials.

In a retrospective study of the benefits and risks of multiple courses of glucocorticoids in patients with preterm premature rupture of membranes, 170 preterm singleton infants were evaluated (381). They were divided into three groups: non-use ($n = 50$), single courses ($n = 76$), and multiple courses ($n = 44$). There was a higher incidence of chorioamnionitis those who had received multiple courses.

Teratogenicity

Teratogenic effects of glucocorticoids, which have been demonstrated in animal experiments since 1950, have not generally been confirmed in man. The question whether a disease that has had to be treated with glucocorticoids in pregnancy or the glucocorticoid treatment itself may have caused congenital anomalies reported anecdotally usually cannot be answered in any individual case. Dexamethasone, for instance, given in a suppressive dosage, seems to have been therapeutically effective in endocrine abnormal pregnancy with congenital adreno-genital syndrome (382); how is one to distinguish cause and effect here? Cleft lip and palate, seen in animal studies, have not been encountered more often in the offspring of glucocorticoid-treated women than in those of untreated women. In several small series of patients in whom glucocorticoids were used before and during pregnancy, no congenital abnormalities were seen on follow-up, but material on which to base a firm judgement is lacking. Certainly, the evidence to date does not suggest that on teratological grounds one should hesitate to administer glucocorticoids for therapeutic reasons during pregnancy (SEDA-3, 306).

However, first trimester in utero exposure to a gluco-corticoid was associated with a small risk of major neona-tal malformations, according to the results of a Canadian meta-analysis (383). Six cohort studies and one case-con-trol study were analysed, and the results showed that women who had taken long-term glucocorticoid therapy during pregnancy were more likely to have a baby with a major malformation than women who had not (OR = 2.46; 95% CI = 1.41, 4.29).

Glucocorticoids have been used in cases of hyperemesis gravidarum when standard antiemetics are ineffective. In an observational comparison of women with complicated hyperemesis gravidarum and weight loss, over 5% of pre-pregnant weight treated with (n = 30) or without (n = 25) glucocorticoids, gestational evolution and singleton birth-weights were not different in the two groups (384).

A hydatidiform mole during pregnancy may have been due to the glucocorticoids used in an immunosuppressive regimen (385).

- A 33-year-old woman took immunosuppressive ther-apy after renal transplantation: ciclosporin (dosage adjusted to achieve blood concentrations of 120–160 ng/ml), azathioprine 1 mg/kg (frequency of admin-istration not stated), and methylprednisolone 40 mg/day from day 1 after transplantation, tapered weekly by 4–8 mg/day. Because of rejection symptoms at weeks 1, 4, and 7, she received three cycles of intrave-nous methylprednisolone 250 mg/day, each cycle last-ing 5–7 days; she also received a bolus dose of methylprednisolone 500 mg on day 0. Pregnancy was diagnosed on day 12 after transplantation (9 weeks after conception). At week 6 after transplantation she had a missed abortion. Curettage was performed and a partial hydatidiform mole was detected. She was dis-charged at week 10 and immunosuppressive therapy was tapered.

The teratogenic effects of prednisone have been evalu-ated in a placebo-controlled study in 372 women and a meta-analysis (386). There was no statistical difference in the rate of major anomalies between the glucocorticoid-

exposed women and the controls. The meta-analysis included 10 studies (six cohort and four case-control stu-dies), with data from 535 exposed and 50 845 nonexposed women. The odds ratios for major malformations were 1.5 (95% CI = 0.8, 2.6) for the cohort studies and 3.4 (CI = 2.0, 5.7) for the case-control studies. The results suggest that although prednisone does not represent a major teratogenic risk in humans in therapeutic doses, it does increase the risk of oral cleft defects by an order of 3.4-fold.

Fetotoxicity

The effect of prolonged antenatal betamethasone (three or more weekly administrations) has been studied in 414 fetuses (387). Multidose betamethasone was not associated with higher risks of antenatal maternal fever, chorioamnionitis, reduced birthweight, neonatal adrenal suppression, neonatal sepsis, or neonatal death.

The effects of antenatal dexamethasone on birthweight have been studied in 961 infants and matched controls (388). Dexamethasone-treated infants had significantly lower birthweights (after adjustment for week of gesta-tion). The average differences from controls were 12 g at 24–26 weeks, 63 g at 27–29 weeks, 161 g at 30–32 weeks, and 80 g at 33–34 weeks. In the case of preterm rupture of membranes, the data were not conclusive.

Betamethasone, two doses of 12 mg a day apart, in 40 pregnant women (27–34 weeks) caused important changes in fetal physiology (389). Fetal breathing (the number of breathing episodes and the total breathing time in 30 minutes) fell by 83% and fetal limb and trunk movements fell by 53% and 49% respectively. These changes were transient and returned to the range of nor-mality 96 hours after administration. There were no changes in Doppler velocimetry of the umbilical and mid-dle cerebral arteries. Awareness of these effects may pre-vent unnecessary iatrogenic delivery of preterm infants who present abnormal biophysical profile scores 2 days after glucocorticoid exposure.

Retardation of intrauterine growth by glucocorticoids has been reported not only in animals but also in man. In a 1990 case from France, dwarfism (as well as Cushing's syndrome) was recorded in a child whose mother had received high-dose glucocorticoids during pregnancy.

It has been suggested that the risk of stillbirth may be increased by glucocorticoid treatment; the figures are suggestive, but the possibility that the disorder that led to the use of the glucocorticoid was itself responsible for the less favorable outcome cannot be excluded (390).

Prevention of the respiratory distress syndrome in antici-pated prematurity has become a widely accepted (though not uncontroversial) indication for glucocorticoids in late pregnancy, the compound most often used being dexa-methasone. The timing of such treatment in late pregnancy seems to be of crucial importance (SEDA-3, 306); the pos-sible adverse effects on the mother and child are still being discussed. The issue has been extensively reviewed (SEDA-17, 445). A meta-analysis of 15 trials, involving 1780 patients treated with glucocorticoids and 1780 controls, has shown a lower risk of the syndrome, and a substantial reduction in neonatal mortality (OR = 0.60; 95% CI = 0.48, 0.76), without a higher risk of infection in the mother or maternal pulmonary edema (SEDA-20, 377; 391). In the mother, labor can be delayed by such glucocorticoid therapy (SEDA-3, 306); the combination of this treatment with sympathomimetic drugs may put the mother at risk of fluid retention with pulmonary edema (SED-12, 990), although it is not clear whether this problem only occurs when both drugs are used.

As far as the child is concerned, there may be only moderate adrenal suppression (392), although in some cases substitution treatment with glucocorticoids can be necessary in such babies; short-term treatment with betamethasone shortly before birth generally does not inhibit the infant's adrenal capacity to react to corticotropin (393). A single case of a leukemoid reaction in a preterm infant has been observed, after the mother was given betamethasone shortly before delivery (SEDA-3, 306).

On the other hand, there are many reports of hypertension (394), and electrocardiographic and other studies have often confirmed the presence of a disproportionately serious and bilateral hypertrophic obstructive cardiomyopathy, which unless it proves fatal is, in general, reversible once the glucocorticoids are withdrawn (SEDA-18, 386). Although the issue is confounded by the possibility that infants with bronchopulmonary dysplasia may be innately hypertensive, there seems no doubt as to the effect.

Most babies treated with glucocorticoids for lung dysplasia also show an appreciable rise in blood urea nitrogen, due almost entirely to an increase in structural protein catabolism (395). Serious gastrointestinal complications can occur. In one typical series of premature neonates treated in this way there were three such instances (perforated duodenal ulcer, perforated gastric ulcer, and upper gastrointestinal hemorrhage, the last two proving fatal) (396); the symptoms are apparently not masked by the glucocorticoid, as one would expect in adults. Treated infants also tend to have a low pH, which is unusual in premature babies (SEDA-18, 445).

In 534 individuals aged 30 years, whose mothers had participated in a double-blind, randomized, placebo-controlled trial of antenatal betamethasone (two intramuscular doses 24 hours apart) for the prevention of neonatal respiratory distress syndrome, there were no differences between those exposed to betamethasone and placebo in body size, blood lipids, blood pressure, plasma cortisol, prevalence of diabetes, or history of cardiovascular disease (397). After the oral glucose tolerance test, those who had been exposed to betamethasone had higher plasma insulin concentrations at 30 minutes (61 versus 52 mIU/l) and lower glucose concentrations at 120 minutes (4.8 versus 5.1 mmol/l) than did those exposed to placebo. Antenatal exposure to betamethasone might result in insulin resistance in adult offspring, but has no effect on cardiovascular risk factors at 30 years of age.

In an Italian prospective study, 201 preterm singleton infants received one or more antenatal courses of a glucocorticoid (398). Neurodevelopment was evaluated at 2 years; 138 subjects received at least one complete course of betamethasone (37 multiple) and 63 patients received dexamethasone (33 multiple). The prevalence of infant leukomalacia was 26% after a complete course of glucocorticoid, 40% after one additional course, 42% after two additional courses, and 44% after more than two additional courses. The corresponding prevalences of 2-year infant neurodevelopmental abnormalities, considering the same categories of glucocorticoid exposure, were 18%, 21%, 29%, and 35% respectively. However, most of the risk was related to dexamethasone administration. Compared with betamethasone, exposure to multiple doses of dexamethasone was associated with an increased risk of leukomalacia (OR = 3.21; 95% CI = 1.07, 9.77) and overall 2-year infant neurodevelopmental abnormalities (OR = 3.63; 95% CI = 1.03, 14).

In an Australian cohort study, 541 very preterm infants were followed for physical, cognitive, and psychological assessment up to 6 years after administration of glucocorticoids during pregnancy (399). Although increasing numbers of antenatal glucocorticoid courses (two intramuscular doses of betamethasone 11.4 mg) were associated with a reduction in the rate of cerebral palsy, three or more courses were also associated with increased rates of aggressive/destructive, distractible, and hyperkinetic behavior, and these effects were present at ages 3 and 6 years. Intelligence quotients were unaffected by antenatal use of a glucocorticoid.

In 192 adult offspring (mean age 31 years) of mothers who had taken part in a randomized controlled trial of antenatal betamethasone for the prevention of neonatal respiratory distress syndrome (87 exposed to betamethasone two doses 24 hours apart, and 105 exposed to placebo) there were no alterations in cognitive functioning, working memory and attention, psychiatric morbidity, handedness, or health-related quality-of-life in adulthood (400).

The effects of a single antenatal dose of a glucocorticoid on prostanoids have been evaluated in 43 singleton pregnancies in women who were taking betamethasone or not (401). Betamethasone (dose not described) reduced maternal PGE_2 concentrations, with concomitant increases in the fetoplacental compartment. Umbilical cord thromboxane B_2 concentrations in the treated group were significantly lower than the non-treated group, resulting in a higher ratio of $6\text{-ketoPGF}_{1\alpha}$ to thromboxane B2. Considering the regulatory role of PGE_2 and PGI_2 in fetal lung development and neonatal transition homeostasis, these results suggest a mechanism, at least in part, for the beneficial effects of antenatal glucocorticoids on fetal lung maturation and neonatal cardiopulmonary homeostasis at birth.

Clearly, the duration of such treatment after delivery should be as brief as possible, but there is no reason for such concern as would lead to withholding therapy; one Dutch study with a 10-year follow-up detected no problems with exposed children's intellectual, motor, or social functioning compared with controls (135).

A meta-analysis, including 15 controlled trials and involving more than 1400 women, has shown that antenatal glucocorticoids in women with ruptured membranes may be beneficial in reducing the risks of neonatal death (RR = 0.68; 95% CI = 0.43, 1.07) and respiratory distress syndrome (RR = 0.56; CI = 0.46, 0.70), with no increase in the risk of infection in either the mother (RR = 0.88; CI = 0.61, 1.20) or baby (RR = 1.05; CI = 0.66, 1.68) (402).

A reduction in fetal response to vibroacoustic stimulation (vibroacoustic startle reflex) has been reported during 48 hours after the administration to pregnant women of two doses of betamethasone (12 mg 2 days apart) (403). The authors recommended that this test should not be used to evaluate well-being in fetuses exposed to glucocorticoids.

Susceptibility Factors

Genetic factors

Significant differences in the pharmacokinetics of methylprednisolone have been described in black and white renal transplant patients. Black patients had a slower clearance rate and a lower apparent volume of distribution. They had higher cortisol concentrations throughout the day, with higher nadir concentrations. Some of them had glucocorticoid-associated diabetes, and no white patients did. Further studies are needed to define the differences between the races (SEDA-20, 377; 404).

Age

Children
Inhaled glucocorticoids are recommended as first-line therapy for persistent asthma in children, to reduce both asthma symptoms and inflammatory markers. Treatment should be begun early in the course of the disease, because inhaled glucocorticoids can preserve airway function and prevent airway remodelling and subsequent irreversible airway obstruction (405). Because asthma is a chronic disease requiring long-term treatment, it is very important to balance the safety and efficacy of inhaled glucocorticoids to achieve optimal long-term results. Major safety concerns in children are the potential adverse effects on growth, adrenal function, and bone mass. Overall, the benefits of inhaled glucocorticoids clearly outweigh their potential adverse effects and the risks of poor asthma control. However, high doses of inhaled glucocorticoids in children are still of concern (406). It is of utmost importance to use the lowest effective dose, to limit systemic availability by selecting drugs with high first-pass hepatic inactivation, and to instruct patients on proper inhalation technique. Moreover, the use of adjuvant asthma medications acting by different mechanisms can help to reduce inhaled glucocorticoid dosages (405,406). These add-on therapies include leukotriene modifiers, long-acting beta$_2$-agonists, cromoglicate and nedocromil, and in selected cases theophylline. These agents should be added to, but should not in any case replace, inhaled glucocorticoid therapy (405,406).

The use of postnatal glucocorticoids in very premature infants is controversial; although dexamethasone reduces bronchopulmonary dysplasia, it has been associated with severe adverse effects (407). In 220 infants with a birthweight of 501–1000 g randomized to placebo or dexamethasone (0.15 mg/kg/day for 3 days and tapering over a period of 7 days) the relative risk of death or chronic lung disease

compared with controls was 0.9 (95% CI = 0.8–1.1) at 36 weeks of gestational age (353). Infants treated with dexamethasone were less likely to need supplementary oxygen. Dexamethasone was associated with increased risks of hypertension (RR = 7.4; 95% CI = 2.7, 20.2), hyperglycemia (RR = 2.0; 95% CI = 1.1, 3.6), spontaneous gastrointestinal perforation (13 versus 4%), lower weight, and a smaller head circumference.

Elderly people
Prolonged use of glucocorticoids in elderly people can exacerbate diabetes, hypertension, congestive heart failure, and osteoporosis, or cause depression. In a retrospective, controlled study, the risks of high-dose intravenous or oral glucocorticoid therapy were assessed in 55 patients with Crohn's disease who were over the age of 50 years (408). They had a higher risk of developing hypertension, hypokalemia, and changes in mental state.

Hepatic disease

In patients with acute hepatitis and active hepatitis, protein binding of the glucocorticoids will be reduced and peak concentrations of administered glucocorticoids increased. Conversion of prednisone to prednisolone has been reported to be impaired in chronic active liver disease (409). However, although plasma prednisolone concentrations were more predictable after the administration of prednisolone than of prednisone to a group of healthy subjects (410), there was no difference in patients with chronic active hepatitis. There was also impaired elimination of prednisolone in these patients. In a review of the pharmacokinetics of prednisone and prednisolone it was concluded that fear of inadequate conversion of prednisone into prednisolone was not justified (411). Patients with hepatic disease suffer adrenal suppression more readily (111).

Other features of the patient

Menopause
Significant differences in the pharmacokinetics of prednisolone amongst menopausal women have been described (SEDA-21, 419; 412). The postmenopausal women had reduced unbound clearance (30%), reduced total clearance, and an increased half-life. Similar results are seen in the postmenopausal women who took estrogen or estrogen–progestogen therapy.

Protein binding
The association between low serum albumin concentrations and complications of prednisone has been long recognized, and it is an elementary pharmacokinetic principle that concentrations of unbound drug in plasma (the fraction that can reach the tissues) will be increased when binding of a drug to serum albumin is reduced (413).

Systemic lupus erythematosus
In 539 patients with systemic lupus erythematosus, organ damage was associated with glucocorticoid therapy compared with controls (414). Oral prednisone 10 mg/day for

10 years (cumulative dose 36.6 g) was significantly associated with osteoporotic fractures (RR = 2.5; 95% CI = 1.7, 3.7), symptomatic coronary artery disease (RR = 1.7; CI = 1.1, 2.5), and cataracts (RR = 1.7; CI = 1.4, 2.5). Avascular necrosis was associated with high-dose prednisone (at least 60 mg/day for at least 2 months; RR = 1.2; CI = 1.1, 1.4). Intravenous pulses of methylprednisolone (1000 mg for 1–3 days) were associated with a small increase in the risk of osteoporotic fractures (RR = 1.3; CI = 1.0, 1.8).

Drug Administration

Drug formulations

The development of adverse effects has been evaluated after switching from conventional glucocorticoids to a pH-modified release formulation, Eudragit L-coated budesonide, in 178 patients with Crohn's disease who had taken 5–30 mg/day of prednisolone equivalents for at least 2 weeks (415). The percentage of patients with glucocorticoid-related adverse effects fell from 65% at entry to 43% at the end of the study. The total number of glucocorticoid-related adverse effects fell significantly from 269 to 90. In conclusion, switching from conventional glucocorticoids to budesonide leads to a significant reduction in glucocorticoid-related adverse effects in patients with Crohn's disease without causing rapid deterioration of the disease.

Drug contamination

Unregulated Chinese herbal products adulterated with glucocorticoids have been detected (416). Dexamethasone was present in eight of 11 Chinese herbal creams analysed by UK dermatologists. The creams contained dexamethasone in concentrations inappropriate for use on the face or in children (64–1500 micrograms/g). The cream with the highest concentration of dexamethasone was prescribed to treat facial eczema in a 4-month-old baby. In all cases, it had been assumed that the creams did not contain glucocorticoids. The authors were concerned that these patients received both unlabelled and unlicensed topical glucocorticoids. They wrote that "greater regulation and restriction needs to be imposed on herbalists, and continuous monitoring of side effects of these medications is necessary."

Drug dosage regimens

Daily or alternate-day administration
The unwanted effects of the glucocorticoids can be reduced to some extent by altering the dosage routine, for example by giving them on alternate days or giving the total daily dose every morning.

Because of circadian variation in endogenous glucocorticoid secretion, the pituitary–adrenal axis is suppressed more easily in the night than during the day (417). Thus, administration of the total dose as a single dose in the morning is preferable to twice daily dosing or administration in the evening alone.

Alternate-day therapy (giving twice the daily dose on alternate days) can in some cases maintain the therapeutic efficacy of oral glucocorticoids, while reducing their adverse effects (418–420).

Use in fixed combinations
Fixed combinations of oral glucocorticoids with nonsteroidal anti-inflammatory analgesics or broncholytic drugs that have to be given repeatedly during the day are undesirable, since their pattern of administration is determined in part by the demands of the other components; the glucocorticoid is thus likely to be given in such a way that it alters the circadian rhythm of endogenous glucocorticoids.

Pulse or megadose therapy
Extremely large intravenous doses of glucocorticoids given at longer intervals can sometimes be effective when a patient does not respond to conventional high doses. Systemic lupus erythematosus, various rheumatic diseases, and the treatment of renal graft rejection are indications for this type of use (SEDA-6, 331). High doses of glucocorticoids also have an antiemetic effect in patients with cancers.

No adverse effects are to be expected after a single injection of a high dose of a glucocorticoid, but some serious complications have been observed with repeated use, including both infections and the known direct adverse effects of glucocorticoids. Cases of ventricular dysrhythmias and atrial fibrillation have been reported (SEDA-18, 391). With pulse therapy, the nature of the injected glucocorticoid seems to be important; for example, hydrocortisone, which is more rapidly metabolized, seems to be better tolerated than dexamethasone (SEDA-6, 331).

Pulsed glucocorticoid therapy for moderately severe ulcerative colitis, given on an out-patient basis, can induce remission more quickly than conventional oral glucocorticoid therapy (421). There were no serious adverse effects in 11 patients given pulsed glucocorticoids or in eight treated conventionally. The two regimens were equally efficacious.

Drug administration route

Most knowledge of the adverse effects of glucocorticoids has been acquired in connection with their use as oral products. However, various other routes of administration have been developed, sometimes specifically in the hope of securing a local therapeutic effect while avoiding systemic adverse reactions. Although experience has shown that the latter cannot be eliminated in this way, they can be diminished in some cases. In other cases, new problems arise. Administration by inhalation is covered in the monograph on inhaled glucocorticoids.

Topical administration to the skin
For a list of the local effects of topical glucocorticoids see separate monograph. The percutaneous absorption of high-potency topical glucocorticoids has been documented, but hypothalamic–pituitary–adrenal axis suppression, leading

to clinically significant adrenal insufficiency or Cushing's syndrome, is infrequent. In most cases in which systemic adverse effects occur, misuse of a product can be blamed. For example, a 4-month old boy developed iatrogenic Cushing's syndrome, which occurred when his mother used excessive amounts of clobetasol 17-propionate and hydrocortisone 17-butyrate cream for 2 months to treat a diaper rash (422). Two patients developed adrenal suppression after the unregulated use of betamethasone dipropionate 0.05% ointment (about 80 g/week) or clobetasol 0.05% ointment (up to 100 g/week), obtained without prescription to treat psoriasis (423).

Although glucocorticoids are used to treat eczema, they can sometimes cause or exacerbate it.

- A 74-year-old man developed worsening eczema 24 hours after he applied clobetasol (Decloban) to treat chronic eczema of his external ear (424). Twelve years earlier he had noted exacerbation of a cutaneous lesion after he had applied a topical glucocorticoid. He had also had generalized erythema after an intra-articular injection of paramethasone. Patch tests to a series of glucocorticoids were positive for all drugs except flupametasone, fluocortine, and tixocortol. In addition, intradermal tests were positive to hydrocortisone and prednisolone, despite negative patch tests.

The authors commented that most glucocorticoid-sensitized patients react to several of the same group and less frequently of different groups. No case of hypersensitivity to glucocorticoids of all four classes has previously been reported.

- Chronic lichenified eczema has been attributed to prolonged use of topical methylprednisolone aceponate and budesonide (strength and duration of therapy not stated) in a 26-year-old woman (425). Patch tests were positive for methylprednisolone aceponate and budesonide cream, but negative for all other topical glucocorticoids.
- An 18-year-old woman presented with a pruritic eczematous eruption that developed after topically applying an ointment containing hydrocortisone acetate, neomycin sulfate, and *Centella asiatica* (426). She was positive to all three ingredients of the ointment.

Two patients developed central serous chorioretinopathy after prolonged treatment with glucocorticoids applied locally to the skin (427).

- A 32-year-old man complained of reduced vision and metamorphopsia in the right eye. Best-corrected visual acuity was 20/25 in right eye and 20/20 in left eye. The left fundus was normal but in the right eye there was a well-circumscribed, shallow, serous detachment of the sensory retina. The clinical appearance was consistent with central serous chorioretinopathy, and the diagnosis was confirmed by fluorescein angiography, which showed a leakage point at the superior macula, spreading slowly in an inkblot configuration into the subretinal space. He had seborrheic dermatitis involving the central face, eyebrows, eyelids, and scalp for 2 years treated with topical hydrocortisone acetate cream 1%. After the initial prescription, he used the cream without further medical consultation when his symptoms got worse and used it for 4 weeks, 3–4 times a day before developing central serous chorioretinopathy.
- A 37-year-old man developed blurred vision in the left eye. He had central serous chorioretinopathy in the contralateral eye 5 years before, for which he had been treated with laser photocoagulation. Best-corrected visual acuity was 20/20 in each eye. There were scars from previous laser photocoagulation at the superior macula in the right eye. In the left eye there was a well-delineated area of serous detachment temporal to the fovea and small yellowish precipitates at the posterior aspect of the detached retina. Fluorescein angiography showed a leakage point at the upper pole of the detachment. He had pityriasis versicolor, for which he had used local diflucortolone valerate cream 0.1% in combination with isoconazole nitrate 1%. He had used the cream occasionally but had used it for 3 weeks before the onset of symptoms. He also used diflucortolone valerate cream 0.1% during the first episode of central serous chorioretinopathy.

The effects of exposure to topical glucocorticoids during pregnancy have been evaluated in a population-based follow-up study in 363 primigravida exposed to topical glucocorticoids during pregnancy and 9263 controls who received no prescriptions at all (428). The prevalence of malformations was 2.9% among 170 infants exposed to glucocorticoids during the first trimester and 3.6% among the controls. There were no increases in the risks of low birthweight, malformations, or preterm delivery in the offspring of women who were exposed to topical glucocorticoids during pregnancy.

Topical administration to the eye
Glucocorticoids that have been used for local ophthalmic treatment include medrysone, fluorometholone, tetrahydroxytriamcinolone, and clobetasone. Loteprednol etabonate 0.5% increases intraocular pressure less than dexamethasone. Studies on animal models of uveitis and two randomized double-masked trials showed that loteprednol etabonate 0.5% was less potent than dexamethasone, prednisolone acetate 1%, or fluorometholone, which may partly explain the improved toxicity profile of loteprednol etabonate (429).

Clinicians should not prescribe glucocorticoid-containing eye-drops unless they have performed a slit-lamp examination with tonometry, have assurance of appropriate follow-up, and understand the differential diagnosis, evaluation, and treatment. Unless clearly indicated, prescribing volumes larger than 5 ml or providing refillable prescriptions should be avoided. It should be stressed that excessive use of glucocorticoids can result in corneal Herpes infection and mycosis.

Since glucocorticoids reduce the immunological defences of the body to most types of infection, their use in the eyes should be monitored carefully. When long-term use is necessary, even with oral or inhalation therapy, eye examination should be performed every 6 months. The ophthalmological follow-up of patients using topical glucocorticoids should include tonometry at least twice a year, careful slit-lamp examination for early signs of herpetic or fungal keratitis and for changes in the equatorial and posterior subcapsular portions of the lens, examination of pupillary size and lid position, and staining of the cornea to detect possible punctate keratitis. Blood glucose concentrations should be checked if there are symptoms that suggest hyperglycemia.

Sensory systems

Ocular adverse effects of local or systemic administration of glucocorticoids include cataracts, glaucoma, papilledema, pseudotumor cerebri, activation of corneal infections, superficial keratitis, ptosis, pupillary dilatation, conjunctival palpebral petechiae, uveitis, and scleromalacia. Topical ocular application and facial application can cause high glucocorticoid concentrations in the anterior compartment of the eye. Serious visual loss can occur owing to the development of cataract in patients using glucocorticoid creams.

Glucocorticoid creams applied topically to the skin are routinely used in the treatment of many skin disorders, and their use on the face in severe atopic eczema is relatively common. Three patients developed advanced glaucoma while using topical facial glucocorticoids. Two other patients developed ocular hypertension secondary to topical facial glucocorticoids (430).

The use of a combination of a glucocorticoid with an antimicrobial drug is illogical and should generally be avoided because of the possibility of the emergence of resistant bacterial strains. It would be highly preferable if prescriptions for these drugs were issued by ophthalmologists only, at least in those parts of the world where adequate medical services are available.

Three vision-threatening complications have been described due to the indiscriminate use of glucocorticoid-containing eyedrops (431).

- A 31-year-old man noted a blind spot in his right eye. He had worn contact lenses for 10 years to correct his myopia. He had applied Tobradex ointment (tobramycin 0.3% and dexamethasone 0.1%) to each eye every evening for the past 4 years because of irritation due to contact lenses, and continuous refills of this prescription were obtained through an acquaintance who was employed in a pharmacy. With spectacle correction his visual acuity was 20/25 in each eye. The intraocular pressure was 52 mmHg in his right eye and 37 mmHg in his left eye. The optic discs showed glaucomatous cupping in each eye. Automated visual field testing showed superior and inferior arcuate defects typical of glaucoma in both eyes. Slit-lamp biomicroscopy showed mild papillary conjunctivitis bilaterally due to contact lenses. The antibiotic + glucocorticoid ointment was withdrawn and his bilateral glucocorticoid-induced open-angle glaucoma was treated with antiglaucomatous drugs.
- A 15-year-old boy felt a foreign body sensation in his right eye after he had been raking hay. His local physician prescribed a suspension of tobramycin 0.3% + dexamethasone 0.1% tds, but 6 days later referred him for evaluation of a suspected fungal keratitis. He had a corneal epithelial defect with an underlying dense inflammatory infiltrate. Corneal scrapings contained fungal hyphae and *Fusarium* species was identified. Natamycin 5% was administered topically every hour, the infection resolved, and his visual acuity returned to 20/20 despite a dense corneal scar.
- A 56-year-old woman had bilateral primary open-angle glaucoma without visual field loss, which was well controlled with a long-term topical beta-blocker in each eye. She underwent a left dacryocystorhinostomy for nasolacrimal duct obstruction, but developed persistent tearing and irritation of the left eye several months postoperatively. A suspension of tobramycin 0.3% + dexamethasone 0.1% was prescribed, which she continued to use as needed for 6 months. Pain and reduced vision persisted in her left eye. Corrected visual acuity was 20/20 in her right eye and 20/60 in her left eye. The intraocular pressures were 18 mmHg in her right eye and 68 mmHg in her left eye. Automated visual field testing showed a normal field in her right eye, but only a central island and a crescent of temporal visual field in her left eye. External examination showed persistent nasolacrimal duct obstruction on the left side with mild conjunctival injection. The diagnosis was primary open-angle glaucoma in both eyes, which was exacerbated by topically applied glucocorticoids in her left eye. The antibiotic + glucocorticoid suspension was withdrawn, and a topical ocular hypotensive therapeutic regimen was initiated in her left eye.

Susceptibility factors

Local and systemic adverse effects of ophthalmic glucocorticoids occur in children more often, more severely, and more rapidly than in adults, for unknown reasons. It could be that children have relatively immature chamber angles, giving rise to a rapidly increasing intraocular pressure (432).

Glaucoma has been reported after the use of a glucocorticoid ointment in a young boy (432).

- A 6-year-old boy underwent a resection of levator palpebrae superioris for congenital blepharoptosis. Postoperatively, an ointment containing 0.1% dexamethasone and neomycin (Maxitrol) was applied to the operated eyelid three times a day to reduce lid edema. Four days later the surgical correction was satisfactory and there were no symptoms, but the intraocular pressure was raised to 44 mmHg in the operated eye, although normal in the other eye. The glucocorticoid was withdrawn and topical ocular hypotensive agents were prescribed. The intraocular pressure returned to normal the next day, and the antiglaucoma treatments were maintained for 1 week and tapered over the next 2 weeks. Subsequent follow-up confirmed normal intraocular pressure and no glaucomatous damage.

The ocular hypertensive response in this case could have been due to systemic absorption of glucocorticoid through the skin of the eyelid, especially when there was a surgical wound. Alternatively, a sufficient amount of ointment could have seeped over the eyelid margins, causing the rise in intraocular pressure, similar to the application of eye-drops, as has been reported in another child, who also had Cushing's syndrome, a rare result of ophthalmic glucocorticoids (433).

- An 11-year-old boy with iridocyclitis developed Cushing's syndrome, a posterior subcapsular cataract, and increased intraocular pressure in both eyes after the topical administration of prednisolone acetate 1% eye-drops bilaterally for 6 months. The Cushing's syndrome was aggravated when periocular methylprednisolone acetate was started while bilateral posterior subtenon injections of 80 mg of suspension were continued every 6 weeks for 6 months. He had not used systemic glucocorticoids before.

Topical administration to the nose

The safety of nasal glucocorticoids in the treatment of allergic rhinitis has been reviewed (434,435). The local application of glucocorticoids for seasonal or perennial rhinitis often results in systemic adverse effects. The use of nasal sprays containing a glucocorticoid that has specific topical activity (such as beclomethasone dipropionate or flunisolide) seems to reduce the systemic adverse effects, but they can nevertheless occur, even to the extent of suppression of basal adrenal function in children (436). Local adverse effects include *Candida* infection, nasal stinging, epistaxis, throat irritation (437), and, exceptionally, anosmia (438).

Nervous system

Benign intracranial hypertension with nasal glucocorticoids has been reported (439).

- A 13-year-old boy with Crohn's disease in remission, who had taken fluticasone aqueous nasal spray 50 micrograms to each nostril od regularly for 5 days, gave a 10-day history of head and back pain. He had a right sixth nerve palsy with bilateral swelling of his optic discs. An unenhanced computer tomogram was normal and magnetic resonance imaging excluded cavernous sinus thrombosis. The cerebrospinal fluid was clear with no cells, and protein and glucose concentrations were normal.

Although there was no clear temporal relation between the onset of the symptoms and the regular use of fluticasone, the authors proposed that the fluticasone was responsible, because the symptoms resolved after drug withdrawal. The association remains unproven but it does highlight the possibility of an association.

Sensory systems

Nasal budesonide or beclomethasone 100 micrograms bd for 3–9 months had no effect on the eyes in 26 patients who had undergone endoscopic sinus surgery (440). Ophthalmologic examination, tonometry, visual field testing, and biomicroscopic studies showed no evidence of ocular hypertension or posterior subcapsular cataract.

Ear, nose, and throat

The use of intranasal glucocorticoids in the treatment of allergic and vasomotor rhinitis in Sweden has doubled

over a period of 5 years, and the number of reported cases of nasal septum perforation increased over the same time (441). The most common risk factor in 32 patients with nasal septum perforation (21 women, 11 men) was glucocorticoid treatment. Information from the Swedish Drug Agency showed that 38 cases of glucocorticoid-induced perforation had been reported over 10 years. The number of adverse effects per million Defined Daily Doses averaged 0.21. The risk of perforation was greatest during the first 12 months of treatment and most cases were in young women.

Endocrine

Aqueous nasal triamcinolone spray 220 or 440 micrograms od for the treatment of allergic rhinitis reportedly had no measurable adverse effects on adrenocortical function in 80 children (aged 6–12 years) in a placebo-controlled, double-blind study (442). Plasma triamcinolone concentrations measured over 6 hours fell rapidly and there was little or no accumulation during 6 weeks.

There have been reports of Cushing's syndrome after prolonged use of intranasal betamethasone 0.1% for chronic catarrh in two boys (443) and from an interaction of nasal fluticasone with ritonavir (444).

- A 30-year-old man who was using an intranasal formulation of fluticasone (therapeutic indication not stated), developed Cushing's syndrome about 5 months after starting ritonavir 600 mg bd, zidovudine, and lamivudine for HIV infection. His plasma cortisol concentrations were undetectable, his corticotrophin was low (under 2 pmol/l), and his 24-hours urinary cortisol excretion was under 30 nmol/l. Further investigations were consistent with secondary adrenal failure or with glucocorticoid use. He admitted to having used a topical glucocorticoid cream for 2 months. However, 6 weeks after he stopped using this cream, his plasma cortisol concentrations were still undetectable. It was then established that he had used nasal fluticasone propionate 200 micrograms/day for about 1 year before starting ritonavir. Ritonavir was replaced by nevirapine, and he continued to use fluticasone nasal spray. Three weeks later, his plasma cortisol concentration had increased to 290 nmol/l. Ritonavir was then added and his plasma cortisol concentration fell rapidly. Ritonavir was stopped again and his cortisol concentration normalized and his Cushingoid facies improved.

The authors thought it likely that inhibition of cytochrome P-450 by ritonavir increased the systemic availability of fluticasone and thus caused Cushing's syndrome in this patient.

Musculoskeletal

Osteonecrosis of the femoral head after the use of a glucocorticoid nasal spray has been reported (445).

- A 48-year-old man taking losartan, low-dose amitriptyline, and triamcinolone acetonide nasal spray developed pain in the abdomen and hips. Radiography and magnetic resonance imaging showed rapidly progressive bilateral osteonecrosis of the femoral heads. He had used excessive amounts of nasal glucocorticoids, and during the previous 12 months had used triamcinolone acetonide 110 micrograms qds in each nostril.

Intralesional injection

Intralesional triamcinolone acetonide has been used extensively for the treatment of hypertrophic and keloid scars. Complications are few, usually being local skin color changes, prominent vascular markings, or subcutaneous atrophy. Cushing's syndrome after intralesional administration of triamcinolone acetate has been described in two adults and two children (aged 10 years and 21 months) after treatment of hypertrophic burn scars with intralesional triamcinolone acetonide (SEDA-21, 419) (408). These two children may have had a form of hypersensitivity to triamcinolone acetonide, as Cushing's syndrome was not the result of overdosage.

- Acute anaphylaxis occurred in an 18-year-old man after the third course of intradermal injections of triamcinolone suspension ("Kenalog" 10 mg per treatment) for alopecia areata (446). Subsequent rechallenge with intradermal triamcinolone 1 ml resulted in the same anaphylactic reaction as before and his serum IgE concentration was increased.

Immediate hypersensitivity reactions to paramethasone acetate, causing widespread eruptions, have been described in at least four cases. Delayed allergic reactions are less common.

- A woman had received intralesional paramethasone and other topical glucocorticoids several times for alopecia between the ages of 7 and 18 years (447). When she was 30 she was again treated with intralesional paramethasone for a relapse of alopecia. She developed pruritus after the first intralesional injection and erythema, edema, and vesicles 6–8 hours later. A biopsy showed spongiform lymphocytic folliculitis with spongiosis and exocytosis in the sweat gland ducts and in the pilosebaceous unit. She was treated with triamcinolone cream and her skin lesions resolved. Patch tests were positive for paramethasone, with cross-reactivity to tixocortol pivalate, hydrocortisone, and hydrocortisone butyrate.

Intraspinal injection
Intrathecal
The effects of intrathecal administration, both wanted and unwanted, are still much debated (448). The question as to whether oral glucocorticoid therapy should be preferred to intrathecal injections is raised by the harmful effects that have sometimes occurred after the latter, although some of these may have been caused by irritative substances in the injection fluid (SEDA-6, 331). The same local glucocorticoid concentrations can probably be attained with fewer problems with oral administration. Epidural injection of glucocorticoids seems to be safer than intrathecal injection, but injection of high doses can cause the same systemic adverse effects as seen with oral treatment. Facial flushing and erythema after lumbar

epidural glucocorticoid administration have been reported (SEDA-20, 378; 449).

Glucocorticoids given intrathecally can cause a rise in cerebrospinal fluid protein and carry the risk of arachnoiditis (SED-8, 820). Chemical meningitis has been reported after two intrathecal injections of methylprednisolone acetate (450) and after lumbar facet joint block (SEDA-17, 450). Intraspinal injections of hydrocortisone for multiple sclerosis apparently led in one case to a cauda equina syndrome, with subsequent ulceromutilating acropathy (SEDA-17, 450). Intra-discal injections of triamcinolone acetonide in a number of French cases led to disk or epidural calcification, sometimes symptomless (SEDA-17, 450).

Postlumbar puncture syndrome with abducent nerve palsy followed the use of intrathecal prednisolone for the treatment of low back pain and sciatica (451).

- A 38-year-old woman received intrathecal prednisolone 3 ml (strength not stated) and 1 day later developed a postural headache, nausea, and dizziness. She was treated with intravenous fluids and analgesics. Eight days later she suddenly developed a complete palsy of the right abducent nerve. An MRI brain scan showed contrast meningeal enhancement typical of postlumbar puncture syndrome. She was treated with oral glucocorticoids and blood patching was performed. Her headache began to resolve a week later. Four months later she had almost completely recovered function of her abducent nerve and a repeat MRI scan was normal.

Epidural
The indications, rationale, techniques, alternatives, contraindications, complications, and efficacy of lumbar and caudal epidural glucocorticoid injections have been reviewed (SEDA-21, 420; 452).

Bilateral posterior subcapsular cataracts have been reported after treatment with epidural methylprednisolone for low back pain secondary to degenerative joint disease and disk protrusion (453).

- A 42-year-old man had received 15 epidural injections of methylprednisolone 80 mg over 10 years. About 6 weeks after his last injection, he developed progressively worsening cloudy vision. He had bilateral posterior subcapsular cataracts and subsequently underwent bilateral cataract removal.

The authors commented that it is possible that multiple epidural glucocorticoid injections had contributed to cataract formation. The patient also had several other risk factors for cataracts (cigarette smoking, alcohol consumption, exposure to ultraviolet radiation, low socioeconomic class, and low intake of antioxidant vitamins). However, the role of these other risk factors was speculative.

Symptoms consistent with complex regional pain syndrome have been reported after a cervical epidural glucocorticoid injection (SEDA-22, 451; 454).

Spinal epidural lipomatosis secondary to exogenous administration of glucocorticoids is a rare condition that has been reported almost exclusively in association with systemic treatment. However, local epidural administration has also been implicated (455).

One case of *Staphylococcus aureus* meningitis, a rare complication of epidural analgesia, has been published. The same patient developed a cauda equina syndrome of uncertain etiology, although neural ischemia as a result of meningitis secondary to immunosuppression was possible (SEDA-21, 420; 456). A unique case of transient profound paralysis after epidural glucocorticoid injection (acute paraplegia) has now been reported (SEDA-22, 451; 457). Diplopia associated with the peridural or intrathecal infiltration of prednisolone have not been previously reported (SEDA-22, 451; 458).

Of 31 patients who received 1 ml (40 mg) of methylprednisolone epidurally at the end of microdiscectomy, three developed epidural abscesses (459). These results were compared with a historical series of 400 patients not taking glucocorticoids, who had no deep infection. Although the data were limited, epidural glucocorticoids after discectomy should not be recommended.

Cervical epidural glucocorticoid injection is often used for the treatment of cervical radiculopathy. Subjective patient satisfaction has been reported, but controlled trials have not yet delineated the effectiveness of this procedure. Three cases of severe pain consistent with nerve injury have been reported immediately after cervical epidural glucocorticoid injection, bringing into question the benefit–harm balance of this technique (460).

Intra-articular and periarticular administration
Local injections of glucocorticoids into and around the joints can have a dramatic therapeutic effect, but the catabolic effect can have serious consequences, including adverse effects on joint structure (461) and on local tendons, subcutaneous atrophy, and possibly osteonecrosis. Provided the state of the joint is carefully inspected before any new injection is given, and the interval between the injections is not less than 4 weeks, the risk seems to be small enough to justify treatment in invalidating cases (SEDA-3, 307).

Respiratory
Hiccups have been reported after intra-articular administration (462).

- A 38-year-old man had an intra-articular injection of betamethasone dipropionate (dose not stated) into his right ankle, and the day after had hiccups that lasted for 24 hours and then resolved without treatment. Some months later, because of persistent arthritis, he received a further injection of betamethasone dipropionate into his right ankle. Once again, he had hiccups the following day. On this occasion, the hiccups resolved after 2 weeks, following treatment with levomepromazine.

Psychiatric
Neuropsychiatric effects of glucocorticoids, like hallucinations, can result from intra-articular administration (SEDA-22, 444) (463).

Endocrine
An acute adrenal crisis occurred in a woman who received an intra-articular glucocorticoid for pseudogout of the knee (464).

- An 87-year-old woman received intra-articular betamethasone (Diprophos) 7 mg on three occasions for painful knee joints over 6 months. Six weeks after the last injection she developed diffuse pain and contractures in the legs, fatigue, nausea, abdominal pain, and weight loss of 6 kg. Both knee joints were tender but there was no effusion. Her serum sodium concentration was 123 mmol/l, serum osmolality 254 mosmol/kg, urine sodium 136 mmol/l, and urinary osmolality 373 mosmol/kg. The syndrome of inappropriate antidiuretic hormone secretion was diagnosed, but despite treatment she remained drowsy and hyponatremic. About a week later, she developed hypotension and symptoms of an acute abdomen. Further investigations showed that her basal cortisol concentration was low (36 nmol/l) but it increased to 481 nmol/l after a short tetracosactide test, consistent with acute adrenal crisis. She recovered rapidly after treatment with oral hydrocortisone, but still required glucocorticoid substitution several months later.

Shin
An erythema multiforme-like eruption has been reported after intra-articular triamcinolone in the right knee, with cross-sensitivity to budesonide (465).

- A 70-year-old man had received three intra-articular injections of triamcinolone (dose not stated) into the same knee over 3 months without any allergic reactions. However, 12–24 hours after the last injection he developed pruritus and erythema at the injection site. This eruption was treated with topical budesonide, but within the next few hours, acute eczema developed. The lesions spread to his legs and abdomen, and were erythematous, edematous, and resembled erythema multiforme. He was treated with boric acid solution dressings, emollients, and oral antihistamines. His lesions gradually resolved and did not recur during 8 months of follow-up. A month after the lesions had resolved, he underwent patch testing, which was positive to triamcinolone 1% and budesonide 1% in petrolatum, but negative to other glucocorticoids.

Musculoskeletal
An arthropathy induced by glucocorticoid crystals has been reported (466).

- A 65-year-old man with bilateral osteoarthritis of the knees developed an effusion in the left knee. The swollen joint was treated with an intra-articular injection of triamcinolone hexacetonide 40 mg. The next day, he developed acute arthritis in the injected knee; the joint was swollen and tender and he was unable to walk. Examination of the joint fluid showed 35 ml of a thick, turbid, yellowish synovial fluid with a leukocyte count of $13 \times 10^6/l$ (95% neutrophils). Gram and acridine orange stains were negative. Wet preparations of the specimen with polarizing compensated microscopy showed numerous birefringent, pleomorphic intra- and extracellular crystals of glucocorticoid. He underwent joint lavage with 1 l of isotonic saline and recovered, completely within one day.

The conclusive diagnosis in this case was triamcinolone hexacetonide crystal-induced arthropathy.

Osteomyelitis after three glucocorticoid injections for tennis elbow has been reported; the second injection was given 3 months after the first and the third 2 days later (467). This case illustrates the need for vigilance, even after common procedures, and that exacerbation of symptoms after local glucocorticoid injections should prompt the doctor to review the diagnosis and consider the need for further investigation.

Anaphylaxis occurred in two women after intra-articular administration of paramethasone plus mepivacaine 2% (468).

- A 44-year-old woman developed generalized pruritus 10 minutes after intra-articular paramethasone and mepivacaine and 30 minutes later developed generalized urticaria, tachycardia, and dyspnea. She received emergency treatment and her condition initially improved. However, her symptoms recurred after 6 hours and she was treated again and then discharged taking oral dexchlorpheniramine. She had a history of allergic contact dermatitis due to nickel sulfate sensitization, and 7 years before had had generalized urticaria and dyspnea after intra-articular administration of a glucocorticoid.
- A 31-year-old woman developed generalized pruritus and urticaria, facial edema, and dyspnea 2 hours after the intra-articular administration of paramethasone and mepivacaine. She was treated with an intramuscular glucocorticoid and antihistamines, with worsening of her symptoms. She received intravenous fluids and dexchlorpheniramine, but her symptoms recurred after 1 hour, when she was given subcutaneous adrenaline, intravenous fluids and dexchlorpheniramine. She was later discharged taking oral diphenhydramine. She had a history of a systemic reaction after the administration of a glucocorticoid and a local anesthetic.

Skin prick tests were positive for isolated paramethasone in both patients, but negative for mepivacaine. There has only been one previous report of anaphylaxis in association with paramethasone.

Immunologic

Inadvertent intra-arterial injection
Particularly when injecting glucocorticoids locally, for example to relieve arthritis of the wrist, accidental injection into an artery is possible. Severe local ischemia can result (SEDA-17, 450).

Intracapsular injection
The use of implants for augmentation of the breast can lead to capsular contracture. Patients with intractable capsular contracture are treated with intracapsular injection of triamcinolone. Major complications included three

cases of major atrophy requiring surgical correction. This problem appeared to have been eliminated by reduction of the dose of triamcinolone from 50 to 25 mg. There was one implant puncture (SEDA-19, 379; 469).

Rectal administration
Systemic absorption of glucocorticoids can occur after rectal administration.

- A 48-year-old woman developed avascular necrosis 9 months after she had completed a 3-month course of hydrocortisone 100 mg retention enemas once or twice daily for ulcerative proctitis (470). An MRI scan showed multiple bony infarcts in her distal femora, proximal tibiae, and posterior proximal right fibular head, extending from the diaphysis to the epiphysis, consistent with avascular necrosis.
- Cushing's syndrome occurred in a 65-year-old woman with ulcerative colitis who received a daily betamethasone enema (471).

The authors of the second report reported the pharmacokinetics of betamethasone after rectal dosing, with plasma concentrations of betamethasone high enough to cause Cushing's syndrome. Suppression of the hypothalamic–pituitary–adrenal axis disappeared after the dosage schedule was changed from daily to three times a week. These findings suggest that a considerable amount of betamethasone is absorbed after rectal dosing.

Occupational exposure
Occupational exposure to glucocorticoids can cause adverse effects. Facial plethora has been found in workers manufacturing synthetic glucocorticoids, some of them having grossly abnormal responses to tetracosactide.

- A 58-year-old woman, who had been involved in the manufacturing of glucocorticoid creams and ointments for over 10 years, developed occupational contact sensitization to topical glucocorticoids (472). Patch tests were positive to hydrocortisone, hydrocortisone butyrate, and tixocortol pivalate. Intradermal tests were positive to hydrocortisone succinate, methylprednisolone, and prednisolone. An oral challenge with betamethasone 0.75 mg, 2.5 mg, and 8 mg on three consecutive days resulted in no adverse reactions.

It has been recommended that all workers manufacturing potent glucocorticoids should be screened regularly for glucocorticoid overdosage and should be moved regularly to units processing other drugs (473).

Drug overdose

High doses of glucocorticoids in patients with cancers can increase the risk of metastases, for example in breast cancer; this has been attributed in some cases to immunosuppression (474). These hormones should therefore only be used in patients with those types of tumors for which they are known to improve the efficacy of the cancer treatment.

A curious reaction to intravenous high-dose dexamethasone, used as an antiemetic agent in cancer chemotherapy or for other purposes, is sudden severe itching, burning, and constrictive pain in the perineal region, which has been described in several published reports (SEDA-11, 336; 475).

Drug–Drug Interactions

Albendazole

Dexamethasone reduced the clearance of albendazole and increased its half-life; plasma concentrations almost doubled (SEDA-22, 450; 476).

Amiodarone

Budesonide for collagenous colitis caused Cushing's syndrome in a patient with chronic renal insufficiency taking amiodarone for paroxysmal atrial fibrillation (477).

- An 81-year-old man with persistent diarrhea was given oral budesonide 9 mg/day, following unsuccessful treatment with mesalazine and prednisone. He was also taking amiodarone 100 mg/day. His diarrhea resolved within 6 weeks, and attempts to reduce the dosage of bzudesonide resulted in recurrent diarrhea. After 11 months he developed Cushing's syndrome, which persisted despite a reduction in dosage to 3 mg/day. His mild diarrhea recurred and the dosage of budesonide was increased to 6 mg/day with worsening of Cushing's syndrome; the dosage was reduced to 3 mg/day. Four weeks later amiodarone was withdrawn. The symptoms of Cushing's syndrome resolved within 4 weeks.

The authors suggested that the development of Cushing's syndrome and its persistence at a low dosage of budesonide was caused by inhibition of the metabolism of budesonide by amiodarone.

Anticoagulants

Intravenous methylprednisolone (1 g/day for 3 days) has been reported to inhibit the metabolism of oral anticoagulants (acenocoumarol and fluindione) in 10 patients, increasing the INR by 8 (range 5–20) (478).

Glucocorticoids can also alter the response to anticoagulants. A raised tolerance to heparin has been reported and a fall in fibrinolytic activity has been seen during glucocorticoid treatment (SED-8, 816). The entire clotting mechanism and particularly the prothrombin time should therefore be checked periodically in patients taking glucocorticoids concomitantly with anticoagulants, particularly if the glucocorticoid dose is changed. In addition there is an increased risk of gastric bleeding in patients taking both glucocorticoids and anticoagulants.

Antifungal azoles

Itraconazole 200 mg/day markedly increased plasma methylprednisolone concentrations and reduced morning plasma cortisol concentrations by over 80% in 10 healthy volunteers (479). The C_{max}, AUC, and half-life of methylprednisolone were increased 1.9, 3.9, and 2.4 times respectively.

Itraconazole 200 mg/day orally for 4 days markedly reduced the clearance and increased the half-life of intravenous methylprednisolone from 2.1 to 4.8 hours in a double-blind, randomized, two-phase, crossover study in nine healthy volunteers (SEDA-23, 430; 480). The volume of distribution was not affected. The mean morning plasma cortisol concentration during the itraconazole phase, measured 24 hours after methylprednisolone, was only 9% of that during the placebo phase (11 versus 117 ng/ml).

The authors of these two reports recommended that care be taken when methylprednisolone is prescribed in combination with itraconazole or other potent inhibitors of CYP3A4.

Itraconazole, given orally increased oral prednisolone concentrations by only 24% (481) but increased intravenous dexamethasone concentrations 3.3-fold and oral dexamethasone 3.7-fold (482).

In another study, ketoconazole was given orally as 200 mg od for 4 days, following a single oral dose of budesonide 3 mg either at the same time as ketoconazole or 12 hours before (483). Ketoconazole increased budesonide concentrations (C_{max} and AUC) 6.8- to 7.6-fold when the two drugs were co-administered; with a 12-hour separation, budesonide concentrations increased only 1.7- to 2.1-fold.

Aprepitant

Aprepitant is a neurokinin-1 receptor antagonist that, in combination with a glucocorticoid and a $5HT_3$ receptor antagonist, is very effective in preventing chemotherapy-induced nausea and vomiting. At therapeutic doses it is also a moderate inhibitor of CYP3A4. Coadministration of aprepitant with dexamethasone or methylprednisolone resulted in increased plasma glucocorticoid concentrations (484). These findings suggest that the dose of these glucocorticoids should be adjusted when aprepitant is given.

Calcium channel blockers

Methylprednisolone concentrations increased with the co-administration of diltiazem (2.6-fold) and mibefradil (3.8-fold) (485).

Ciclosporin

Glucocorticoids cause additive immunosuppression when they are given with other immunosuppressants, such as ciclosporin (SEDA-22, 451; 486).

The AUC of plasma prednisolone has been studied in patients with stable renal transplants (487). The prednisolone AUC was significantly higher in women and in those who took ciclosporin. The highest AUC was in women taking estrogen supplements and ciclosporin. A significantly higher proportion of patients taking ciclosporin + azathioprine + prednisolone had glucocorticoid adverse effects compared with those taking azathioprine + prednisolone. Furthermore, more women than men had adverse effects and the prednisone AUC was greater in those with adverse effects than without. Ciclosporin was thought to have increased the systemic availability of prednisolone, most probably by inhibiting P glycoprotein. Because the major contributor to AUC is the maximum post-dose concentration, it may be possible to use single-point monitoring (2 hours after the dose) for routine clinical studies.

Clarithromycin

Clarithromycin inhibits CYP3A4, which is responsible for the metabolic clearance of prednisolone, the biologically active metabolite of prednisone. Clarithromycin (500 mg bd for 2 days) reduced the clearance of methylprednisolone by 65% and significantly increased its plasma concentrations; clarithromycin did not influence the clearance or plasma concentrations of prednisone (488). Acute mania has been reported to be related to inhibition of the metabolic clearance of prednisone by clarithromycin (SEDA-22, 444; 489).

Cyclophosphamide

The effect of prednisone 1 mg/kg on the pharmacokinetics of cyclophosphamide and its initial metabolites 4-hydroxycyclophosphamide and aldophosphamide (the acyclic tautomer of 4-hydroxycyclophosphamide) has been studied between the first and sixth cycles in seven patients (two men) with systemic vasculitis receiving intravenous cyclophosphamide 0.6 g/m^2 as a 1-hour intravenous infusion every 3 weeks for six cycles (490). Prednisone reduced the clearance of cyclophosphamide from 5.8 to 4.0 l/hour, reducing the amount of initial metabolites formed. Although the clinical significance of this interaction is unclear, 4-hydroxycyclophosphamide and aldophosphamide are probably responsible for the cytotoxic activity of cyclophosphamide, and increased cyclophosphamide dosages should be considered in patients taking prednisone.

Diuretics

Glucocorticoids with mineralocorticoid activity potentiate potassium loss when they are given with potassium-wasting diuretics (491).

Globulin

A case report with a review of 27 cases of thromboembolic events after the administration of intravenous globulin with or without glucocorticoids has been published (492). The authors suggested that this combined therapy should be administered with caution because of its potential synergistic thrombotic risk.

Grapefruit juice

Methylprednisolone concentrations increased with the co-administration of grapefruit juice (1.75-fold) (493).

Leukotriene receptor antagonists

In a probable pharmacodynamic interaction, severe peripheral edema followed treatment with montelukast and prednisone for asthma (494).

- A 23-year-old man, with a history of asthma, house dust mite allergy, and rhinoconjunctivitis, presented with acute respiratory symptoms. He was given oral cetirizine, inhaled salmeterol, and fluticasone propionate, and oral prednisone 40 mg/day for 1 week and 20 mg/day for 1 week. His asthma recurred when prednisone was withdrawn and he took oral prednisone 60 mg/day for 1 week and 40 mg/day for 1 week. He also took montelukast 10 mg/day. He then developed severe peripheral edema with a gain in weight of 13 kg. Prednisone was withdrawn and his edema resolved. Montelukast was continued.

The author commented that the patient had tolerated prednisone without montelukast and montelukast without prednisone. However, he had severe edema when both drugs were used together. Montelukast may have potentiated glucocorticoid-induced renal tubular sodium and fluid retention. Both have been associated with edema.

Oral contraceptives

Oral contraceptives increased budesonide concentrations by only 22%, but prednisolone concentrations increased by 131%, suggesting a clinically important interaction (495).

Phenobarbital

Phenobarbital increases the metabolism of glucocorticoids, reducing the half-life by some 50% (496).

Phenytoin

Phenytoin increases the metabolism of glucocorticoids, reducing the half-life by some 50% (496).

Rifampicin

Rifampicin and other drugs that induce liver enzymes increase the metabolism of glucocorticoids (497), sufficient to reduce their therapeutic effects, for example in asthma (498).

Salicylates

Glucocorticoids reduce the plasma concentrations of salicylates (499). If they are given with aspirin or other anti-inflammatory drugs, there may be an additive effect on the gastric wall, leading to an increased risk of bleeding and ulceration (500–502).

Diagnosis of adverse drug reactions

The short Synacthen (tetracosactide) test is the most commonly used test for assessing adrenal suppression. The potential of a simpler and more cost-effective procedure, the morning salivary cortisol concentration, as an out-patient screening tool to detect adrenal suppression in patients using topical intranasal glucocorticoids for rhinosinusitis has been investigated in 48 patients who were using topical glucocorticoids (503). The morning salivary cortisol measurement was a useful screening tool for adrenal suppression in this setting.

Osteoporosis and osteopenia are usually evaluated by measuring bone density using dual-energy X-ray absorptiometry (DXA). However, there is increased interest in measuring not only bone density but also some structural properties of the bone, such as elasticity and trabecular stiffness and connectivity, which are more closely related to bone strength. Quantitative ultrasound could theoretically provide information on bone structure, as has been suggested by a prospective study in patients with glucocorticoid-induced osteoporosis (504), but further studies are needed to define the role of quantitative ultrasonography in the prediction of fracture and in the clinical management of glucocorticoid-induced osteoporosis.

Management of adverse drug reactions

Mood stabilizers, such as lithium, lamotrigine, and carbamazepine, may be effective in treating glucocorticoid-induced mood symptoms. In an open trial, 12 patients with glucocorticoid-induced manic or mixed symptoms were treated with olanzapine 2.5 mg/day initially, increasing to a maximum of 20 mg/day; 11 of the 12 patients had significant improvement (505).

References

1. Kaiser H. Cortisone derivate in Klinik und PraxisStuttgart-New York: Thieme;. 1987.
2. Labhart A. Adrenal cortex. In: Labhart A, editor. Clinical Endocrinology. Berlin-Heidelberg-New York: Springer, 1985:373.
3. Medici TC, Ruegsegger P. Does alternate-day cloprednol therapy prevent bone loss? A longitudinal double-blind, controlled clinical study. Clin Pharmacol Ther 1990;48(4):455–66.
4. Iwasaki E, Baba M. [Pharmacokinetics and pharmacodynamics of hydrocortisone in asthmatic children.]Arerugi 1993;42(10):1555–62.
5. Bone RC, Fisher CJ Jr, Clemmer TP, Slotman GJ, Metz CA, Balk RA. A controlled clinical trial of high-dose methylprednisolone in the treatment of severe sepsis and septic shock. N Engl J Med 1987;317(11):653–8.
6. The Veterans Administration Systemic Sepsis Cooperative Study Group. Effect of high-dose glucocorticoid therapy on mortality in patients with clinical signs of systemic sepsis. N Engl J Med 1987;317(11):659–65.
7. Iuchi T, Akaike M, Mitsui T, Ohshima Y, Shintani Y, Azuma H, Matsumoto T. Glucocorticoid excess induces superoxide production in vascular endothelial cells and elicits vascular endothelial dysfunction. Circ Res 2003; 92: 81–7.
8. Romagnoli C, Zecca E, Vento G, De Carolis MP, Papacci P, Tortorolo G. Early postnatal dexamethasone for the prevention of chronic lung disease in high-risk preterm infants. Intensive Care Med 1999;25(7):717–21.
9. Confalonieri M, Urbino R, Potena A, Piattella M, Parigi P, Puccio G, Della Porta R, Giorgio C, Blasi F, Umberger R, Meduri GU. Hydrocortisone infusion for severe community-acquired pneumonia: a preliminary randomized study. Am J Respir Crit Care Med 2005;171(3):242–8.
10. Garland JS, Alex CP, Pauly TH, Whitehead VL, Brand J, Winston JF, Samuels DP, McAuliffe TL. A three-day course of dexamethasone therapy to prevent chronic lung disease in ventilated neonates: a randomized trial. Pediatrics 1999;104(1 Part 1):91–9.
11. Romagnoli C, Zecca E, Vento G, Maggio L, Papacci P, Tortorolo G. Effect on growth of two different dexamethasone courses for preterm infants at risk of chronic lung disease. A randomized trial. Pharmacology 1999;59(5):266–74.
12. Tarnow-Mordi W, Mitra A. Postnatal dexamethasone in preterm infants is potentially lifesaving, but follow up studies are urgently needed. BMJ 1999;319(7222):1385–6.
13. van de Beek D, de Gans J, McIntyre P, Prasad K. Steroids in adults with acute bacterial meningitis: a systematic review. Lancet Infect Dis 2004; 4: 139–43.
14. Arias-Camison JM, Lau J, Cole CH, Frantz ID 3rd. Meta-analysis of dexamethasone therapy started in the first 15 days of life for prevention of chronic lung disease in premature infants. Pediatr Pulmonol 1999;28(3):167–74.
15. Klein-Gitelman MS, Pachman LM. Intravenous corticosteroids: adverse reactions are more variable than expected in children. J Rheumatol 1998;25(10):1995–2002.
16. Feldweg AM, Leddy JP. Drug interactions affecting the efficacy of corticosteroid therapy. A brief review with an illustrative case. J Clin Rheumatol 1999;5:143–50.
17. Maxwell SR, Moots RJ, Kendall MJ. Corticosteroids: do they damage the cardiovascular system? Postgrad Med J 1994;70(830):863–70.
18. Ellis SG, Semenec T, Lander K, Franco I, Raymond R, Whitlow PL. Effects of long-term prednisone (> = 5 mg) use on outcomes and complications of percutaneous coronary intervention. Am J Cardiol 2004; 93: 1389–90.
19. Sato A, Funder JW, Okubo M, Kubota E, Saruta T. Glucocorticoid-induced hypertension in the elderly. Relation to serum calcium and family history of essential hypertension. Am J Hypertens 1995;8(8):823–8.
20. Thedenat B, Leaute-Labreze C, Boralevi F, Roul S, Labbe L, Marliere V, Taieb A. Surveillance tensionnelle des nourrissons traites par corticotherapie generale pour un hemangiome. [Blood pressure monitoring in infants with hemangiomas treated with corticosteroids.] Ann Dermatol Venereol 2002;129(2):183–5.
21. Stewart IM, Marks JSECG. Abnormalities in steroid-treated rheumatoid patients. Lancet 1977;2(8050):1237–8.
22. Baty V, Blain H, Saadi L, Jeandel C, Canton P. Fatal myocardial infarction in an elderly woman with severe ulcerative colitis. what is the role of steroids? Am J Gastroenterol 1998;93(10):2000–1.
23. Machiels JP, Jacques JM, de Meester A. Coronary artery spasm during anaphylaxis. Ann Emerg Med 1996;27(5):674–5.
24. Sato O, Takagi A, Miyata T, Takayama Y. Aortic aneurysms in patients with autoimmune disorders treated with corticosteroids. Eur J Vasc Endovasc Surg 1995;10(3):366–9.
25. Kotha P, McGreevy MJ, Kotha A, Look M, Weisman MH. Early deaths with thrombolytic therapy for acute myocardial infarction in corticosteroid-dependent rheumatoid arthritis. Clin Cardiol 1998;21(11):853–6.
26. Yunis KA, Bitar FF, Hayek P, Mroueh SM, Mikati M. Transient hypertrophic cardiomyopathy in the newborn following multiple doses of antenatal corticosteroids. Am J Perinatol 1999;16(1):17–21.

27. Gill AW, Warner G, Bull L. Iatrogenic neonatal hypertrophic cardiomyopathy. Pediatr Cardiol 1996;17(5):335–9.

28. Pokorny JJ, Roth F, Balfour I, Rinehart G. An unusual complication of the treatment of a hemangioma. Ann Plast Surg 2002;48(1):83–7.

29. Kothari SN, Kisken WA. Dexamethasone-induced congestive heart failure in a patient with dilated cardiomyopathy caused by occult pheochromocytoma. Surgery 1998;123(1):102–5.

30. Balys R, Manoukian J, Zalai C. Left ventricular hypertrophy with outflow tract obstruction-a complication of dexamethasone treatment for subglottic stenosis. Int J Pediatr Otorhinolaryngol 2005;69(2):271–3.

31. Kucukosmanoglu O, Karabay A, Ozbarlas N, Noyan A, Anarat A. Marked bradycardia due to pulsed and oral methylprednisolone therapy in a patient with rapidly progressive glomerulonephritis. Nephron 1998;80(4):484.

32. Schult M, Lohmann D, Knitsch W, Kuse ER, Nashan B. Recurrent cardiocirculatory arrest after kidney transplantation related to intravenous methylprednisolone bolus therapy. Transplantation 1999;67(11):1497–8.

33. Brumund MR, Truemper EJ, Lutin WA, Pearson-Shaver AL. Disseminated varicella and staphylococcal pericarditis after topical steroids. J Pediatr 1997;131(1 Part 1):162–3.

34. Kaiser H. Cortisonderivate in Klink und Praxis. 7th edn.. Stuttgart: G.Thieme;. 1977.

35. Williamson IJ, Matusiewicz SP, Brown PH, Greening AP, Crompton GK. Frequency of voice problems and cough in patients using pressurized aerosol inhaled steroid preparations. Eur Respir J 1995;8(4):590–2.

36. Lim BS, Choi WY, Choi JW. A case of steroid-induced intractable hiccup. Tuberc Respir Dis 1991;38:304–7.

37. Cersosimo RJ, Brophy MT. Hiccups with high dose dexamethasone administration: a case report. Cancer 1998;82(2):412–4.

38. Ross J, Eledrisi M, Casner P. Persistent hiccups induced by dexamethasone. West J Med 1999;170(1):51–2.

39. Poynter D. Beclomethasone dipropionate aerosol and nasal mucosa. Br J Clin Pharmacol 1977;4(Suppl 3):S295–301.

40. Albucher JF, Vuillemin-Azais C, Manelfe C, Clanet M, Guiraud-Chaumeil B, Chollet F. Cerebral thrombophlebitis in three patients with probable multiple sclerosis. Role of lumbar puncture or intravenous corticosteroid treatment. Cerebrovasc Dis 1999;9(5):298–303.

41. Shinwell ES, Karplus M, Reich D, Weintraub Z, Blazer S, Bader D, Yurman S, Dolfin T, Kogan A, Dollberg S, Arbel E, Goldberg M, Gur I, Naor N, Sirota L, Mogilner S, Zaritsky A, Barak M, Gottfried E. Early postnatal dexamethasone treatment and increased incidence of cerebral palsy. Arch Dis Child Fetal Neonatal Ed 2000;83(3):F177–81.

42. Halliday HL. Postnatal steroids and chronic lung disease in the newborn. Paediatr Respir Rev 2004; 5 Suppl A: S245–8.

43. Yeh TF, Lin YJ, Lin HC, Huang CC, Hsieh WS, Lin CH, Tsai CH. Outcomes at school age after postnatal dexamethasone therapy for lung disease of prematurity. N Engl J Med 2004;350:1304–13.

44. Bentson J, Reza M, Winter J, Wilson G. Steroids and apparent cerebral atrophy on computed tomography scans. J Comput Assist Tomogr 1978;2(1):16–23.

45. Vaughn BV, Ali II, Olivier KN, Lackner RP, Robertson KR, Messenheimer JA, Paradowski LJ, Egan TM. Seizures in lung transplant recipients. Epilepsia 1996;37(12):1175–9.

46. Lorrot M, Bader-Meunier B, Sebire G, Dommergues JP. Hypertension intracranienne benigne: une complication meconnue de la corticotherapie. [Benign intracranial hypertension: an unrecognized complication of corticosteroid therapy.] Arch Pediatr 1999;6(1):40–2.

47. Kalapurakal JA, Silverman CL, Akhtar N, Laske DW, Braitman LE, Boyko OB, Thomas PR. Intracranial meningiomas: factors that influence the development of cerebral edema after stereotactic radiosurgery and radiation therapy. Radiology 1997;204(2):461–5.

48. Laroche F, Chemouilli R, Carlier P. Efficacy of conservative treatment in a patient with spinal cord compression due to corticosteroid-induced epidural lipomatosis. Rev Rheum (English Edn) 1993;30:729–31.

49. Roy-Camille R, Mazel C, Husson JL, Saillant G. Symptomatic spinal epidural lipomatosis induced by a long-term steroid treatment. Review of the literature and report of two additional cases. Spine 1991;16(12):1365–71.

50. Andress HJ, Schurmann M, Heuck A, Schmand J, Lob G. A rare case of osteoporotic spine fracture associated with epidural lipomatosis causing paraplegia following long-term cortisone therapy. Arch Orthop Trauma Surg 2000;120(7–8):484–6.

51. Pinsker MO, Kinzel D, Lumenta CB. Epidural thoracic lipomatosis induced by long-term steroid treatment case illustration. Acta Neurochir (Wien) 1998;140(9):991–2.

52. Parker CT, Jarek MJ, Finger DR. Corticosteroid-associated epidural lipomatosis. J Clin Rheumatol 1999;5:141–2.

53. Kano K, Kyo K, Ito S, Nishikura K, Ando T, Yamada Y, Arisaka O. Spinal epidural lipomatosis in children with renal diseases receiving steroid therapy. Pediatr Nephrol 2005;20(2):184–9.

54. Donaghy M, Mills KR, Boniface SJ, Simmons J, Wright I, Gregson N, Jacobs J. Pure motor demyelinating neuropathy: deterioration after steroid treatment and improvement with intravenous immunoglobulin. J Neurol Neurosurg Psychiatry 1994;57(7):778–83.

55. Urban RC Jr, Cotlier E. Corticosteroid-induced cataracts. Surv Ophthalmol 1986;31(2):102–10.

56. Kaye LD, Kalenak JW, Price RL, Cunningham R. Ocular implications of long-term prednisone therapy in children. J Pediatr Ophthalmol Strabismus 1993;30(3):142–4.

57. Cumming RG, Mitchell P, Leeder SR. Use of inhaled corticosteroids and the risk of cataracts. N Engl J Med 1997;337(1):8–14.

58. Abramson HA. May corticosteroid cataracts be reversible. J Asthma Res 1977;14(3):vii–viii.

59. Lubkin VL. Steroid cataract – a review and a conclusion. J Asthma Res 1977;14(2):55–9.

60. Forman AR, Loreto JA, Tina LU. Reversibility of corticosteroid-associated cataracts in children with the nephrotic syndrome. Am J Ophthalmol 1977;84(1):75–8.

61. Wingate RJ, Beaumont PE. Intravitreal triamcinolone and elevated intraocular pressure. Aust NZ J Ophthalmol 1999;27(6):431–2.

62. Garbe E, LeLorier J, Boivin JF, Suissa S. Risk of ocular hypertension or open-angle glaucoma in elderly patients on oral glucocorticoids. Lancet 1997;350(9083):979–82.

63. Garbe E, LeLorier J, Boivin JF, Suissa S. Inhaled and nasal glucocorticoids and the risks of ocular hypertension or open-angle glaucoma. JAMA 1997;277(9):722–7.

64. Novack GD. Ocular toxicology. Curr Opin Ophthalmol 1994;5(6):110–4.

65. Opatowsky I, Feldman RM, Gross R, Feldman ST. Intraocular pressure elevation associated with inhalation and nasal corticosteroids. Ophthalmology 1995;102(2):177–9.

66. Kwok AK, Lam DS, Ng JS, Fan DS, Chew SJ, Tso MO. Ocular-hypertensive response to topical steroids in children. Ophthalmology 1997;104(12):2112–6.

67. Tham CCY, Ng JSK, Li RTH, Chik KW, Lam DSC. Intraocular pressure profile of a child on a systemic corticosteroid. Am J Ophthalmol 2004;137:198–201.

68. Gass JD, Little H. Bilateral bullous exudative retinal detachment complicating idiopathic central serous chorioretinopathy during systemic corticosteroid therapy. Ophthalmology 1995;102(5):737–47.

69. Karadimas P, Bouzas EA. Glucocorticoid use represents a risk factor for central serous chorioretinopathy: a prospective, case-control study. Graefe's Arch Clin Exp Ophthalmol 2004;242:800–2.

70. Baumal CR, Martidis A, Truong SN. Central serous chorioretinopathy associated with periocular corticosteroid injection treatment for HLA-B27-associated iritis. Arch Ophthalmol 2004;122:926–8.

71. Roth DB, Chieh J, Spirn MJ, Green SN, Yarian DL, Chaudhry NA. Noninfectious endophthalmitis associated with intravitreal triamcinolone injection. Arch Ophthalmol 2003;121:1279–82.

72. Roth DB, Chieh J, Spirn MJ, Green SN, Yarian DL, Chaudhry NA. Noninfectious endophthalmitis associated with intravitreal triamcinolone injection. Arch Ophthalmol 2003;121:1279–82.

73. Chen SDM, Lochhead J, McDonald B, Patel CK. Pseudohypopyon after intravitreal triamcinolone injection for the treatment of pseudophakic cystoid macular oedema. Br J Ophthalmol 2004;88:843–4.

74. Apel A, Campbell I, Rootman DS. Infectious crystalline keratopathy following trabeculectomy and low-dose topical steroids. Cornea 1995;14(3):321–3.

75. Rao GP, O'Brien C, Hicky-Dwyer M, Patterson A. Rapid onset bilateral calcific band keratopathy associated with phosphate-containing steroid eye drops. Eur J Implant Refractive Surg 1995;7:251–2.

76. Ramanathan R, Siassi B, deLemos RA. Severe retinopathy of prematurity in extremely low birth weight infants after short-term dexamethasone therapy. J Perinatol 1995;15(3):178–82.

77. Kushner FH, Olson JC. Retinal hemorrhage as a consequence of epidural steroid injection. Arch Ophthalmol 1995;113(3):309–13.

78. Byers B. Blindness secondary to steroid injections into the nasal turbinates. Arch Ophthalmol 1979;97(1):79–80.

79. Van Dalen JT, Sherman MD. Corticosteroid-induced exophthalmos. Doc Ophthalmol 1989;72(3–4):273–7.

80. Klein JF. Adverse psychiatric effects of systemic glucocorticoid therapy. Am Fam Physician 1992;46(5):1469–74.

81. Doherty M, Garstin I, McClelland RJ, Rowlands BJ, Collins BJ. A steroid stupor in a surgical ward. Br J Psychiatry 1991;158:125–7.

82. Satel SL. Mental status changes in children receiving glucocorticoids. Review of the literature. Clin Pediatr (Phila) 1990;29(7):383–8.

83. Alpert E, Seigerman C. Steroid withdrawal psychosis in a patient with closed head injury. Arch Phys Med Rehabil 1986;67(10):766–9.

84. Hassanyeh F, Murray RB, Rodgers H. Adrenocortical suppression presenting with agitated depression, morbid jealousy, and a dementia-like state. Br J Psychiatry 1991;159:870–2.

85. Nahon S, Pisanté L, Delas N. A successful switch from prednisone to budesonide for neuropsychiatric adverse effects in a patient with ileal Crohn's disease. Am J Gastroenterol 2001;96(1):1953–4.

86. Brown ES, J Woolston D, Frol A, Bobadilla L, Khan DA, Hanczyc M, Rush AJ, Fleckenstein J, Babcock E, Cullum CM. Hippocampal volume, spectroscopy, cognition, and mood in patients receiving corticosteroid therapy. Biol Psychiatry 2004;55:538–45.

87. O'Shea TM, Kothadia JM, Klinepeter KL, Goldstein DJ, Jackson BG, Weaver RG III, Dillard RG. Randomized placebo-controlled trial of a 42-day tapering course of dexamethasone to reduce the duration of ventilator dependency in very low birth weight infants: outcome of study participants at 1-year adjusted age. Pediatrics 1999;104(1 Part 1):15–21.

88. Soliday E, Grey S, Lande MB. Behavioral effects of corticosteroids in steroid–sensitive nephrotic syndrome. Pediatrics 1999;104(4):e51.

89. Kaiser H. Psychische Storungen nach Beclomethasondipropionat-Inhalation?. [Mental disorders following beclomethasone dipropionate inhalation?.] Med Klin 1978;73(38):1334.

90. Keenan PA, Jacobson MW, Soleymani RM, Mayes MD, Stress ME, Yaldoo DT. The effect on memory of chronic prednisone treatment in patients with systemic disease. Neurology 1996;47(6):1396–402.

91. Oliveri RL, Sibilia G, Valentino P, Russo C, Romeo N, Quattrone A. Pulsed methylprednisolone induces a reversible impairment of memory in patients with relapsing-remitting multiple sclerosis. Acta Neurol Scand 1998;97(6):366–9.

92. Newcomer JW, Selke G, Melson AK, Hershey I, Craft S, Richards K, Alderson AL. Decreased memory performance in healthy humans induced by stress-level cortisol treatment. Arch Gen Psychiatry 1999;56(6):527–533.

93. Aisen PS, Davis KL, Berg JD, Schafer K, Campbell K, Thomas RG, Weiner MF, Farlow MR, Sano M, Grundman M, Thal LJ. A randomized controlled trial of prednisone in Alzheimer's disease. Alzheimer's Dis Cooperative Study. Neurology 2000;54(3):588–93.

94. de Quervain DJ, Roozendaal B, Nitsch RM, McGaugh JL, Hock C. Acute cortisone administration impairs retrieval of long-term declarative memory in humans. Nat Neurosci 2000;3(4):313–4.

95. Bermond B, Surachno S, Lok A, ten Berge IJ, Plasmans B, Kox C, Schuller E, Schellekens PT, Hamel R. Memory functions in prednisone-treated kidney transplant patients. Clin Transplant 2005;19(4):512–7.

96. Brown ES, Stuard G, Liggin JD, Hukovic N, Frol A, Dhanani N, Khan DA, Jeffress J, Larkin GL, McEwen BS, Rosenblatt R, Mageto Y, Hanczyc M, Cullum CM. Effect of phenytoin on mood and declarative memory during prescription corticosteroid therapy. Biol Psychiatry 2005;57(5):543–8.

97. Moser NJ, Phillips BA, Guthrie G, Barnett G. Effects of dexamethasone on sleep. Pharmacol Toxicol 1996;79(2):100–2.

98. Chau SY, Mok CC. Factors predictive of corticosteroid psychosis in patients with systemic lupus erythematosus. Neurology 2003;61:104–7.

99. Bolanos SH, Khan DA, Hanczyc M, Bauer MS, Dhanani N, Brown ES. Assessment of mood states in patients receiving long-term corticosteroid therapy and in controls with patient-rated and clinician-rated scales. Ann Allergy Asthma Immunol 2004;92:500–5.

100. Preda A, Fazeli A, McKay BG, Bowers MB Jr, Mazure CM. Lamotrigine as prophylaxis against steroid-induced mania. J Clin Psychiatry 1999;60(10):708–9.

101. Preda A, Fazeli A, McKay BG, Bowers MB Jr, Mazure CM. Lamotrigine of prophylaxis against steroid-induced mania. J. Clin Psychiatry 1999;60(10):708–9.

102. Brown ES, Suppes T, Khan DA, Carmody TJ 3rd. Mood changes during prednisone bursts in outpatients with asthma. J Clin Psychopharmacol 2002;22(1):55–61.

103. Wada K, Suzuki H, Taira T, Akiyama K, Kuroda S. Successful use of intravenous clomipramine in depressive–catatonic state associated with corticosteroid treatment. Int J Psych Clin Pract 2004;8:131–3.

104. Ilbeigi MS, Davidson ML, Yarmush JM. An unexpected arousal effect of etomidate in a patient on high-dose steroids. Anesthesiology 1998;89(6):1587–9.

105. Kramer TM, Cottingham EM. Risperidone in the treatment of steroid-induced psychosis. J Child Adolesc Psychopharmacol 1999;9(4):315–6.

106. Scheschonka A, Bleich S, Buchwald AB, Ruther E, Wiltfang J. Development of obsessive-compulsive behaviour following cortisone treatment. Pharmacopsychiatry 2002;35(2):72–4.

107. Kamoda T, Nakahara C, Matsui A. A case of empty sella after steroid pulse therapy for nephrotic syndrome. J Rheumatol 1998;25(4):822–3.

108. Rabhan NB. Pituitary-adrenal suppression and Cushing's syndrome after intermittent dexamethasone therapy. Ann Intern Med 1968;69(6):1141–8.

109. Zwaan CM, Odink RJ, Delemarre-van de Waal HA, Dankert-Roelse JE, Bokma JA. Acute adrenal insufficiency after discontinuation of inhaled corticosteroid therapy. Lancet 1992;340(8830):1289–90.

110. Clark DJ, Grove A, Cargill RI, Lipworth BJ. Comparative adrenal suppression with inhaled budesonide and fluticasone propionate in adult asthmatic patients. Thorax 1996;51(3):262–6.

111. Marazzi MG, Agnese G, Gremmo M, Cotellessa M, Garibaldi L. Problemi relativi alla funzionalita surrenalica in corso di terapia cortisonica protratta in soggetti con epatite cronica: nota preliminare. [Problems concerning adrenal function during prolonged corticoid treatment in patients with chronic hepatitis. Preliminary note.] Minerva Pediatr 1978;30(11):937–44.

112. Dutau G, Rochiccioli P. Exploration corticotrope au cours des traitements prolongés par le dipropionate de béclométhasone chez l'enfant. [Corticotropic testing during long-term beclomethasone dipropionate treatment asthmatic children.] Poumon Coeur 1978;34(4):247–53.

113. Sumboonnanonda A, Vongjirad A, Suntornpoch V, Petrarat S. Adrenal function after prednisolone treatment in childhood nephrotic syndrome. J Med Assoc Thai 1994;77(3):126–9.

114. Felner EI, Thompson MT, Ratliff AF, White PC, Dickson BA. Time course of recovery of adrenal function in children treated for leukemia. J Pediatr 2000;137(1):21–4.

115. Reiner M, Galeazzi RL, Studer H. Cushing-Syndrom und Nebennierenrinden-Suppression durch intranasale Anwendung von Dexamethasonpraparaten. [Cushing's syndrome and adrenal suppression by means of intranasal use of dexamethasone preparations.] Schweiz Med Wochenschr 1977;107(49):1836–7.

116. Kay J, Findling JW, Raff H. Epidural triamcinolone suppresses the pituitary–adrenal axis in human subjects. Anesth Analg 1994;79(3):501–5.

117. Boonen S, Van Distel G, Westhovens R, Dequeker J. Steroid myopathy induced by epidural triamcinolone injection. Br J Rheumatol 1995;34(4):385–6.

118. Kobayashi S, Warabi H, Hashimoto H. Hypopituitarism with empty sella after steroid pulse therapy. J Rheumatol 1997;24(1):236–8.

119. Grabner W. Zur induzierten NNR-Insuffizienz bei chirurgischen Eingriffen. [Problems of corticosteroid-induced adrenal insufficiency in surgery.] Fortschr Med 1977;95(30):1866–8.

120. Iglesias P, González J, Díez JJ. Acute and persistent iatrogenic Cushing's syndrome after a single dose of triamcinolone acetonide. J Endocrinol Invest 2005;28(11):1019–23.

121. Mukai T. [Antagonism between parathyroid hormone and glucocorticoids in calcium and phosphorus metabolism.]Nippon Naibunpi Gakkai Zasshi 1965;41(8):950–9.

122. Kahn A, Snapper I, Drucker A. Corticosteroid-induced tetany in latent hypoparathyroidism. Arch Intern Med 1964;114:434–8.

123. Fisher JE, Smith RS, Lagrandeur R, Lorenz RP. Gestational diabetes mellitus in women receiving beta-adrenergics and corticosteroids for threatened preterm delivery. Obstet Gynecol 1997;90(6):880–3.

124. Kim YS, Kim MS, Kim SI, Lim SK, Lee HY, Han DS, Park K. Post-transplantation diabetes is better controlled after conversion from prednisone to deflazacort: a prospective trial in renal transplants. Transpl Int 1997;10(3):197–201.

125. Gurwitz JH, Bohn RL, Glynn RJ, Monane M, Mogun H, Avorn J. Glucocorticoids and the risk for initiation of hypoglycemic therapy. Arch Intern Med 1994;154(1):97–101.

126. Bagdade JD, Porte D Jr, Bierman EL. Steroid-induced lipemia. A complication of high-dosage corticosteroid therapy. Arch Intern Med 1970;125(1):129–34.

127. Ettinger WH Jr, Hazzard WR. Elevated apolipoprotein-B levels in corticosteroid-treated patients with systemic lupus erythematosus. J Clin Endocrinol Metab 1988;67(3):425–8.

128. Amin SB, Sinkin RA, McDermott MP, Kendig JW. Lipid intolerance in neonates receiving dexamethasone for bronchopulmonary dysplasia. Arch Pediatr Adolesc Med 1999;153(8):795–800.

129. Tiley C, Grimwade D, Findlay M, Treleaven J, Height S, Catalano J, Powles R. Tumour lysis following hydrocortisone prior to a blood product transfusion in T-cell acute lymphoblastic leukaemia. Leuk Lymphoma 1992;8(1–2):143–6.

130. Lerza R, Botta M, Barsotti B, Schenone E, Mencoboni M, Bogliolo G, Pannacciulli I, Arboscello E. Dexamethasone-induced acute tumor lysis syndrome in a T-cell malignant lymphoma. Leuk Lymphoma 2002;43(5):1129–32.

131. Balli F, Benatti C. Terapia corticosteroidea protratta e metabolismo fosfo-calcico. II. Modificazioni del metabolismo fosfo-calcico in soggetti nefrosici sattoposti a terapia carticosteroidea protratta. [Prolonged corticosteroid therapy and phospho-calcic metabolism. II. Changes of phospho-calcic metabolism in nephrotic subjects subjected to prolonged corticoid therapy.] Minerva Pediatr 1968;20(45):2315–25.

132. Handa R, Wali JP, Singh RI, Aggarwal P. Corticosteroids precipitating hypocalcemic encephalopathy in hypoparathyroidism. Ann Emerg Med 1995;26(2):241–2.

133. Ravina A, Slezak L, Mirsky N, Bryden NA, Anderson RA. Reversal of corticosteroid-induced diabetes mellitus with supplemental chromium. Diabet Med 1999;16(2):164–7.

134. Schneider J, Burmeister H, Ruiz-Torres A. Langzeitstudien uber die Wirksamkeit der Dauertherapie bei hyperergisch-allergischen Erkrankungen mit Prednisolon. [Longitudinal study about the efficacy of long term prednisolone therapy in hyperergic-allergic diseases.] Verh Dtsch Ges Inn Med 1977;83:1785–8.

135. Schmand B, Neuvel J, Smolders-de Haas H, Hoeks J, Treffers PE, Koppe JG. Psychological development of children who were treated antenatally with corticosteroids to prevent respiratory distress syndrome. Pediatrics 1990;86(1):58–64.

136. Bielawski D, Hiatt IM, Hegyi T. Betamethasone-induced leukaemoid reaction in pre-term infant. Lancet 1978;1(8057):218–9.

137. Craddock CG. Corticosteroid-induced lymphopenia, immunosuppression, and body defense. Ann Intern Med 1978;88(4):564–6.

138. Saxon A, Stevens RH, Ramer SJ, Clements PJ, Yu DT. Glucocorticoids administered in vivo inhibit human suppressor T lymphocyte function and diminish B lymphocyte responsiveness in in vitro immunoglobulin synthesis. J Clin Invest 1978;61(4):922–30.

139. Maeshima E, Yamada Y, Yukawa S. Fever and leucopenia with steroids. Lancet 2000;355(9199):198.

140. Patrassi GM, Sartori MT, Livi U, Casonato A, Danesin C, Vettore S, Girolami A. Impairment of fibrinolytic potential in long-term steroid treatment after heart transplantation. Transplantation 1997;64(11):1610–4.

141. The British Thoracic and Tuberculosis Association. Inhaled corticosteroids compared with oral prednisone in patients starting long-term corticosteroid therapy for asthma. Lancet 1975;2(7933):469–73.

142. Salzman GA, Pyszczynski DR. Oropharyngeal candidiasis in patients treated with beclomethasone dipropionate delivered by metered-dose inhaler alone and with Aerochamber. J Allergy Clin Immunol 1988;81(2):424–8.

143. Linder N, Kuint J, German B, Lubin D, Loewenthal R. Hypertrophy of the tongue associated with inhaled corticosteroid therapy in premature infants. J Pediatr 1995;127(4):651–3.

144. Spiro HM. Is the steroid ulcer a myth? N Engl J Med 1983;309(1):45–7.

145. Messer J, Reitman D, Sacks HS, Smith H Jr, Chalmers TC. Association of adrenocorticosteroid therapy and peptic-ulcer disease. N Engl J Med 1983;309(1):21–4.

146. Conn HO, Poynard T. Corticosteroids and peptic ulcer: meta-analysis of adverse events during steroid therapy. J Intern Med 1994;236(6):619–32.

147. Henry DA, Johnston N, Dobson A, Duggan J. Fatal peptic ulcer complications and the use of non-steroidal antiinflammatory drugs, aspirin, and corticosteroids. BMJ (Clin Res Ed) 1987;295:1227.

148. Suazo-Barahona J, Gallegos J, Carmona-Sanchez R, Martinez R, Robles-Diaz G. Nonsteroidal anti-inflammatory drugs and gastrocolic fistula. J Clin Gastroenterol 1998;26(4):343–5.

149. Shimizu T, Yamashiro Y, Yabuta K. Impaired increase of prostaglandin E2 in gastric juice during steroid therapy in children. J Paediatr Child Health 1994;30(2):169–72.

150. Yamanishi Y, Yamana S, Ishioka S, Yamakido M. Development of ischemic colitis and scleroderma renal crisis following methylprednisolone pulse therapy for progressive systemic sclerosis. Intern Med 1996;35(7):583–6.

151. Dwarakanath AD, Nash J, Rhodes JM. "Conversion" from ulcerative colitis to Crohn's disease associated with corticosteroid treatment. Gut 1994;35(8):1141–4.

152. Sharma R, Gupta KL, Ammon RH, Gambert SR. Atypical presentation of colon perforation related to corticosteroid use. Geriatrics 1997;52(5):88–90.

153. Candelas G, Jover JA, Fernandez B, Rodriguez-Olaverri JC, Calatayud J. Perforation of the sigmoid colon in a rheumatoid arthritis patient treated with methylprednisolone pulses. Scand J Rheumatol 1998;27(2):152–3.

154. Mpofu S, Mpofu CMA, Hutchinson D, Maier AE, Dodd SR, Moots RJ. Steroids, non-steroidal anti-inflammatory drugs, and sigmoid diverticular abscess perforation in rheumatic conditions. Ann Rheum Dis 2004;63:588–90.

155. Weissel M, Hauff W. Fatal liver failure after high-dose glucocorticoid pulse therapy in a patient with severe thyroid eye disease. Thyroid 2000;10(6):521.

156. Nanki T, Koike R, Miyasaka N. Subacute severe steatohepatitis during prednisolone therapy for systemic lupus erythematosis. Am J Gastroenterol 1999;94(11):3379.

157. Dourakis SP, Sevastianos VA, Kaliopi P. Acute severe steatohepatitis related to prednisolone therapy. Am J Gastroenterol 2002;97(4):1074–5.

158. Verrips A, Rotteveel JJ, Lippens R. Dexamethasone-induced hepatomegaly in three children. Pediatr Neurol 1998;19(5):388–91.

159. Marinò M, Morabito E, Brunetto MR, Bartalena L, Pinchera A, Marocci C. Acute and severe liver damage associated with intravenous glucocorticoid pulse therapy in patients with Graves' ophthalmopathy. Thyroid 2004;14:403–6.

160. Hamed I, Lindeman RD, Czerwinski AW. Case report: acute pancreatitis following corticosteroid and azathioprine therapy. Am J Med Sci 1978;276(2):211–9.

161. Di Fazano CS, Messica O, Quennesson S, Quennesson ER, Inaoui R, Vergne P, Bonnet C, Bertin P, Treves R. Two new cases of glucocorticoid-induced pancreatitis. Rev Rhum Engl Ed 1999;66(4):235.

162. Khanna S, Kumar A. Acute pancreatitis due to hydrocortisone in a patient with ulcerative colitis. J Gastroenterol Hepatol 2003;18:1010–1.

163. Reichert LJ, Koene RA, Wetzels JF. Acute haemodynamic and proteinuric effects of prednisolone in patients with a nephrotic syndrome. Nephrol Dial Transplant 1999;14(1):91–7.

164. Charpin J, Arnaud A, Boutin C, Aubert J, Murisasco A, Gotte G. Long-term corticosteroid therapy and its effect on the kidney. Acta Allergol 1969;24(1):49–56.

165. Gray D, Shepherd H, Daar A, Oliver DO, Morris PJ. Oral versus intravenous high-dose steroid treatment of renal allograft rejection. The big shot or not? Lancet 1978;1(8056):117–8.

166. Toftegaard M, Knudsen F. Massive vasopressin-resistant polyuria induced by dexamethasone. Intensive Care Med 1995;21(3):238–40.

167. Editorial. Nocturia during steroid therapy. BMJ 1970;4(729):193–4.

168. Wendt H. Klinisch-pharmakologische Untersuchungen zur akneinduzierenden Wirkung von Fluorcortinbutylester. [Clinico-pharmacological studies on the acne-inducing action of fluocortin butylester.] Arzneimittelforschung 1977;27(11a):2245–6.

169. Bioulac P, Beylot C. Etude ultrastructurale d'une leucodermie secondaire à une injection intraarticulaire de corticoides. [Ultrastructural study of a leukoderma secondary to an intra-articular injection of corticoides.] Ann Dermatol Venereol 1977;104(12):883–5.

170. Bondy PhK. Disorders of the adrenal cortex. In: Wilson JD, Foster DW, editors. Williams' Textbook of Endocrinology. 7th edn.. Philadelphia: Saunders, 1985:816.

171. Reinhold K, Schneider L, Hunzelmann N, Krieg T, Scharffetter-Kochanek K. Delayed-type allergy to systemic corticosteroids. Allergy 2000;55(11):1095–6.

172. Shuster S, Raffle EJ, Bottoms E. Skin collagen in rheumatoid arthritis and the effect of corticosteroids. Lancet 1967;2:525.

173. Mathov E, Grad P, Scaglia H. Provocación de hemorragias uterinas anormales y hematomas subcutáneos por el uso de la acetonida de la triamcinoona en pacientes alérgicas. [Provocation of uterine hemorrhages and subcutaneous hematomas by the use of triamcinolone acetonide in allergic patients.] Prensa Med Argent 1971;58(16):826–9.

174. Roy A, Leblanc C, Paquette L, Ghezzo H, Cote J, Cartier A, Malo JL. Skin bruising in asthmatic subjects treated with high doses of inhaled steroids: frequency and association with adrenal function. Eur Respir J 1996;9(2):226–31.

175. Korting HC, Unholzer A, Schafer-Korting M, Tausch I, Gassmueller J, Nietsch KH. Different skin thinning potential of equipotent medium-strength glucocorticoids. Skin Pharmacol Appl Skin Physiol 2002;15(2):85–91.

176. Sener O, Caliskaner Z, Yazicioglu K, Karaayvaz M, Ozanguc N. Nonpigmenting solitary fixed drug eruption after skin testing and intra-articular injection of triamcinolone acetonide. Ann Allergy Asthma Immunol 2001;86(3):335–6.

177. Weber F, Barbaud A, Reichert-Penetrat S, Danchin A, Schmutz JL. Unusual clinical presentation in a case of contact dermatitis due to corticosteroids diagnosed by ROAT. Contact Dermatitis 2001;44(2):105–6.

178. Sener O, Caliskaner Z, Yazicioglu K, Karaayvaz M, Ozanguc N. Nonpigmenting solitary fixed drug eruption after skin testing and intra-articular injection of triamcinolone acetonide. Ann Allergy Asthma Immunol 2001;86(3):335–6.

179. Dooms-Goossens A, Andersen KE, Brandao FM, Bruynzeel D, Burrows D, Camarasa J, Ducombs G, Frosch P, Hannuksela M, Lachapelle JM, Lahti A, Menne T, Wahlberg JE, Wilkinson JD. Corticosteroid contact allergy: an EECDRG multicentre study. Contact Dermatitis 1996;35(1):40–4.

180. Quintiliani R. Hypersensitivity and adverse reactions associated with the use of newer intranasal corticosteroids for allergic rhinitis. Curr Ther Res Clin Exp 1996;57:478–88.

181. Isaksson M, Bruze M, Goossens A, Lepoittevin JP. Patch testing with budesonide in serial dilutions. the significance of dose, occlusion time and reading time. Contact Dermatitis 1999;40(1):24–31.

182. Murata T, Tanaka M, Dekio I, Tanikawa A, Nishikawa T. Allergic contact dermatitis due to clobetasone butyrate. Contact Dermatitis 2000;42(5):305.

183. O'Hagan AH, Corbett JR. Contact allergy to budesonide in a breath-actuated inhaler. Contact Dermatitis 1999;41(1):53.

184. Lew DB, Higgins GC, Skinner RB, Snider MD, Myers LK. Adverse reaction to prednisone in a patient with systemic lupus erythematosus. Pediatr Dermatol 1999;16(2):146–50.

185. Garcia-Bravo B, Repiso JB, Camacho F. Systemic contact dermatitis due to deflazacort. Contact Dermatitis 2000;43(6):359–60.

186. Stingeni L, Caraffini S, Assalve D, Lapomarda V, Lisi P. Erythema-multiforme-like contact dermatitis from budesonide. Contact Dermatitis 1996;34(2):154–5.

187. Roujeau JC, Kelly JP, Naldi L, Rzany B, Stern RS, Anderson T, Auquier A, Bastuji-Garin S, Correia O, Locati F, Mockenhaupt M, Paoletti C, Shapiro S, Shear N, Schüpf E, Kaufman DW. Medication use and the risk of Stevens–Johnson syndrome or toxic epidermal necrolysis. N Engl J Med 1995;333(24):1600–7.

188. Ingber A, Trattner A, David M. Hypersensitivity to an oestrogen–progesterone preparation and possible relationship to autoimmune progesterone dermatitis and corticosteroid hypersensitivity. J Dermatol Treat 1999;10:139–40.

189. Picado C, Luengo M. Corticosteroid-induced bone loss. Prevention and management. Drug Saf 1996;15(5):347–59.

190. Wichers M, Springer W, Bidlingmaier F, Klingmuller D. The influence of hydrocortisone substitution on the quality of life and parameters of bone metabolism in patients with secondary hypocortisolism. Clin Endocrinol (Oxf) 1999;50(6):759–65.

191. Langhammer A, Norjavaara E, de Verdier MG, Johnsen R, Bjermer L. Use of inhaled corticosteroids and bone mineral density in a population based study: the Nord–Trondelag Health Study (the HUNT Study). Pharmacoepidemiol Drug Saf 2004;13:569–79.

192. Suissa S, Baltzan M, Kremer R, Ernst P. Inhaled and nasal corticosteroid use and the risk of fracture. Am J Respir Crit Care Med 2004;169:83–8.

193. Steinbuch M, Youket TE, Cohen S. Oral glucocorticoid use is associated with an increased risk of fracture. Osteoporos Int 2004;15:323–8.

194. Krogsgaard MR, Thamsborg G, Lund B. Changes in bone mass during low dose corticosteroid treatment in patients with polymyalgia rheumatica. a double blind, prospective comparison between prednisolone and deflazacort. Ann Rheum Dis 1996;55(2):143–6.

195. Goldstein MF, Fallon JJ Jr, Harning R. Chronic glucocorticoid therapy-induced osteoporosis in patients with obstructive lung disease. Chest 1999;116(6):1733–49.

196. Yosipovitch G, Hoon TS, Leok GC. Suggested rationale for prevention and treatment of glucocorticoid-induced bone loss in dermatologic patients. Arch Dermatol 2001;137(4):477–81.

197. Selby PL, Halsey JP, Adams KR, Klimiuk P, Knight SM, Pal B, Stewart IM, Swinson DR. Corticosteroids do not alter the threshold for vertebral fracture. J Bone Miner Res 2000;15(5):952–6.

198. Zelissen PM, Croughs RJ, van Rijk PP, Raymakers JA. Effect of glucocorticoid replacement therapy on bone mineral density in patients with Addison disease. Ann Intern Med 1994;120(3):207–10.

199. Valero MA, Leon M, Ruiz Valdepenas MP, Larrodera L, Lopez MB, Papapietro K, Jara A, Hawkins F. Bone density and turnover in Addison's disease: effect of glucocorticoid treatment. Bone Miner 1994;26(1):9–17.

200. Heiner JP, Joyce MJ, Carter JR, Makley JT. Atraumatic posterior pelvic ring fractures simulating metastatic disease in patients with metabolic bone disease. Orthopedics 1994;17(3):285–9.

201. Baltzan MA, Suissa S, Bauer DC, Cummings SR. Hip fractures attributable to corticosteroid use. Study Osteoporotic Fractures Group. Lancet 1999;353(9161):1327.

202. McKenzie R, Reynolds JC, O'Fallon A, Dale J, Deloria M, Blackwelder W, Straus SE. Decreased bone mineral

density during low dose glucocorticoid administration in a randomized, placebo controlled trial. J Rheumatol 2000;27(9):2222–6.

203. Walsh LJ, Wong CA, Oborne J, Cooper S, Lewis SA, Pringle M, Hubbard R, Tattersfield AE. Adverse effects of oral corticosteroids in relation to dose in patients with lung disease. Thorax 2001;56(4):279–84.

204. van Everdingen AA, Jacobs JW, Siewertsz Van Reesema DR, Bijlsma JW. Low-dose prednisone therapy for patients with early active rheumatoid arthritis: clinical efficacy, disease-modifying properties, and side effects: a randomized, double-blind, placebo-controlled clinical trial. Ann Intern Med 2002;136(1):1–12.

205. Townsend HB, Saag KG. Glucocorticoid use in rheumatoid arthritis: benefits, mechanisms, and risks. Clin Exp Rheumatol 2004;22(Suppl 35):S77–82.

206. Gluck O, Colice G. Recognizing and treating glucocorticoid-induced osteoporosis in patients with pulmonary diseases. Chest 2004;125:1859–76.

207. Lukert BP, Adams JS. Calcium and phosphorus homeostasis in man. Effect Corticosteroids. Arch Intern Med 1976;136(11):1249–53.

208. Hahn TJ. Corticosteroid-induced osteopenia. Arch Intern Med 1978;138(Spec No):882–5.

209. Chesney RW, Mazess RB, Hamstra AJ, DeLuca HF, O'Reagan S. Reduction of serum-1, 25-dihydroxyvitamin-D3 in children receiving glucocorticoids. Lancet 1978;2(8100):1123–5.

210. Eastell R. Management of corticosteroid-induced osteoporosis. UK Consensus Group Meeting on Osteoporosis. J Intern Med 1995;237(5):439–47.

211. Goans RE, Weiss GH, Abrams SA, Perez MD, Yergey AL. Calcium tracer kinetics show decreased irreversible flow to bone in glucocorticoid treated patients. Calcif Tissue Int 1995;56(6):533–5.

212. Sasaki N, Kusano E, Ando Y, Yano K, Tsuda E, Asano Y. Glucocorticoid decreases circulating osteoprotegerin (OPG): possible mechanism for glucocorticoid induced osteoporosis. Nephrol Dial Transplant 2001;16(3):479–82.

213. Lespessailles E, Siroux V, Poupon S, Andriambelosoa N, Pothuaud L, Harba R, Benhamou CL. Long-term corticosteroid therapy induces mild changes in trabecular bone texture. J Bone Miner Res 2000;15(4):747–53.

214. Mateo L, Nolla JM, Bonnin MR, Navarro MA, Roig-Escofet D. Sex hormone status and bone mineral density in men with rheumatoid arthritis. J Rheumatol 1995;22(8):1455–60.

215. Vestergaard P, Olsen ML, Paaske Johnsen S, Rejnmark L, Sorensen HT, Mosekilde L. Corticosteroid use and risk of hip fracture: a population-based case-control study in Denmark. J Intern Med 2003;254:486–93.

216. Ton FN, Gunawardene SC, Lee H, Neer RM. J. Effects of low-dose prednisone on bone metabolism. Bone Miner Res 2005;20(3):464–70.

217. Harris M, Hauser S, Nguyen TV, Kelly PJ, Rodda C, Morton J, Freezer N, Strauss BJ, Eisman JA, Walker JL. Bone mineral density in prepubertal asthmatics receiving corticosteroid treatment. J Paediatr Child Health 2001;37(1):67–71.

218. Lane NE. An update on glucocorticoid-induced osteoporosis. Rheum Dis Clin North Am 2001;27(1):235–53.

219. Henderson NK, Sambrook PN, Kelly PJ, Macdonald P, Keogh AM, Spratt P, Eisman JA. Bone mineral loss and recovery after cardiac transplantation. Lancet 1995;346(8979):905.

220. Garton MJ, Reid DM. Bone mineral density of the hip and of the anteroposterior and lateral dimensions of the spine in men with rheumatoid arthritis. Effects of low-dose corticosteroids. Arthritis Rheum 1993;36(2):222–8.

221. Saito JK, Davis JW, Wasnich RD, Ross PD. Users of low-dose glucocorticoids have increased bone loss rates: a longitudinal study. Calcif Tissue Int 1995;57(2):115–9.

222. Buckley LM, Leib ES, Cartularo KS, Vacek PM, Cooper SM. Effects of low dose corticosteroids on the bone mineral density of patients with rheumatoid arthritis. J Rheumatol 1995;22(6):1055–9.

223. Fryer JP, Granger DK, Leventhal JR, Gillingham K, Najarian JS, Matas AJ. Steroid-related complications in the cyclosporine era. Clin Transplant 1994;8(3 Part 1):224–9.

224. Wolpaw T, Deal CL, Fleming-Brooks S, Bartucci MR, Schulak JA, Hricik DE. Factors influencing vertebral bone density after renal transplantation. Transplantation 1994;58(11):1186–9.

225. Yun YS, Kim BJ, Hong SP, Lee TW, Lim CG, Kim MJ. Changes of bone metabolism indices in patients receiving immunosuppressive therapy including low doses of steroids after renal transplantation. Transplant Proc 1996;28(3):1561–4.

226. Saisu T, Sakamoto K, Yamada K, Kashiwabara H, Yokoyama T, Iida S, Harada Y, Ikenoue S, Sakamoto M, Moriya H. High incidence of osteonecrosis of femoral head in patients receiving more than 2 g of intravenous methylprednisolone after renal transplantation Transplant Proc 1996;28(3):1559–60.

227. Naganathan V, Jones G, Nash P, Nicholson G, Eisman J, Sambrook PN. Vertebral fracture risk with long-term corticosteroid therapy: prevalence and relation to age, bone density, and corticosteroid use. Arch Intern Med 2000;160(19):2917–22.

228. Schoon EJ, Bollani S, Mills PR, Israeli E, Felsenberg D, Ljunghall S, Persson T, Haptén-White L, Graffner H, Bianchi Porro G, Vatn M, Stockbrügger RW; Matrix Study Group. Bone mineral density in relation to efficacy and side effects of budesonide and prednisolone in Crohn's disease. Clin Gastroenterol Hepatol 2005;3(2):113–21.

229. Tattersfield AE, Town GI, Johnell O, Picado C, Aubier M, Braillon P, Karlstrom R. Bone mineral density in subjects with mild asthma randomized to treatment with inhaled corticosteroids or non-corticosteroid treatment for two years. Thorax 2001;56(4):272–8.

230. Sambrook PN. Corticosteroid osteoporosis: practical implications of recent trials. J Bone Miner Res 2000;15(9):1645–9.

231. American College of Rheumatology Task Force on Osteoporosis Guidelines. Recommendations for the prevention and treatment of glucocorticoid-induced osteoporosis. Arthritis Rheum 1996;39(11):1791–801.

232. Bone and Tooth Society. National Osteoporosis Society, Royal College of Physicians. Glucocorticoid-induced Osteoporosis Guidelines for Prevention and TreatmentLondon: Royal College of Physicians;. 2002.

233. Hart SR, Green B. Osteoporosis prophylaxis during corticosteroid treatment: failure to prescribe. Postgrad Med J 2002;78(918):242–3.

234. Gudbjornsson B, Juliusson UI, Gudjonsson FV. Prevalence of long term steroid treatment and the frequency of decision making to prevent steroid induced osteoporosis in daily clinical practice. Ann Rheum Dis 2002;61(1):32–6.

235. Cino M, Greenberg GR. Bone mineral density in Crohn's disease: a longitudinal study of budesonide, prednisone, and nonsteroid therapy. Am J Gastroenterol 2002;97(4):915–21.

236. Schwid SR, Goodman AD, Puzas JE, McDermott MP, Mattson DH. Sporadic corticosteroid pulses and osteoporosis in multiple sclerosis. Arch Neurol 1996;53(8):753–7.

237. Lukert BP, Johnson BE, Robinson RG. Estrogen and progesterone replacement therapy reduces glucocorticoid-induced bone loss. J Bone Miner Res 1992;7(9):1063–9.

238. Buckley LM, Leib ES, Cartularo KS, Vacek PM, Cooper SM. Calcium and vitamin D3 supplementation prevents bone loss in the spine secondary to low-dose corticosteroids in patients with rheumatoid arthritis. A randomized, double-blind, placebo-controlled trial. Ann Intern Med 1996;125(12):961–8.

239. Adachi JD, Bensen WG, Bianchi F, Cividino A, Pillersdorf S, Sebaldt RJ, Tugwell P, Gordon M, Steele M, Webber C, Goldsmith CH. Vitamin D and calcium in the prevention of corticosteroid induced osteoporosis: a 3 year followup. J Rheumatol 1996;23(6):995–1000.

240. Talalaj M, Gradowska L, Marcinowska-Suchowierska E, Durlik M, Gaciong Z, Lao M. Efficiency of preventive treatment of glucocorticoid-induced osteoporosis with 25-hydroxyvitamin D3 and calcium in kidney transplant patients. Transplant Proc 1996;28(6):3485–7.

241. Warady BD, Lindsley CB, Robinson FG, Lukert BP. Effects of nutritional supplementation on bone mineral status of children with rheumatic diseases receiving corticosteroid therapy. J Rheumatol 1994;21(3):530–5.

242. Richy F, Ethgen O, Bruyere O, Reginster JY. Efficacy of alphacalcidol and calcitriol in primary and corticosteroid-induced osteoporosis: a meta-analysis of their effects on bone mineral density and fracture rate. Osteoporos Int 2004;15:301–10.

243. Ringe JD, Dorst A, Faber H, Schacht E, Rahlfs VW. Superiority of alfacalcidol over plain vitamin D in the treatment of glucocorticoid-induced osteoporosis. Rheumatol Int 2004;24:63–70.

244. Luengo M, Pons F, Martinez de Osaba MJ, Picado C. Prevention of further bone mass loss by nasal calcitonin in patients on long term glucocorticoid therapy for asthma: a two year follow up study. Thorax 1994;49(11):1099–102.

245. Healey JH, Paget SA, Williams-Russo P, Szatrowski TP, Schneider R, Spiera H, Mitnick H, Ales K, Schwartzberg P. A randomized controlled trial of salmon calcitonin to prevent bone loss in corticosteroid-treated temporal arteritis and polymyalgia rheumatica. Calcif Tissue Int 1996;58(2):73–80.

246. Adachi JD, Bensen WG, Bell MJ, Bianchi FA, Cividino AA, Craig GL, Sturtridge WC, Sebaldt RJ, Steele M, Gordon M, Themeles E, Tugwell P, Roberts R, Gent M. Salmon calcitonin nasal spray in the prevention of corticosteroid-induced osteoporosis. Br J Rheumatol 1997;36(2):255–9.

247. Mulder H, Struys A. Intermittent cyclical etidronate in the prevention of corticosteroid-induced bone loss. Br J Rheumatol 1994;33(4):348–50.

248. Diamond T, McGuigan L, Barbagallo S, Bryant C. Cyclical etidronate plus ergocalciferol prevents glucocorticoid-induced bone loss in postmenopausal women. Am J Med 1995;98(5):459–63.

249. Roux C, Oriente P, Laan R, Hughes RA, Ittner J, Goemaere S, Di Munno O, Pouilles JM, Horlait S, Cortet B. Randomized trial of effect of cyclical etidronate in the prevention of corticosteroid-induced bone loss. Ciblos Study Group. J Clin Endocrinol Metab 1998;83(4):1128–33.

250. Pitt P, Li F, Todd P, Webber D, Pack S, Moniz C. A double blind placebo controlled study to determine the effects of intermittent cyclical etidronate on bone mineral density in patients on long-term oral corticosteroid treatment. Thorax 1998;53(5):351–6.

251. Sato S, Ohosone Y, Suwa A, Yasuoka H, Nojima T, Fujii T, Kuwana M, Nakamura K, Mimori T, Hirakata M. Effect of intermittent cyclical etidronate therapy on corticosteroid induced osteoporosis in Japanese patients with connective tissue disease: 3 year follow up. J Rheumatol 2003;30: 2673–9.

252. Frediani B, Falsetti P, Baldi F, Acciai C, Filippou G, Marcolongo R. Effects of 4-year treatment with once-weekly clodronate on prevention of corticosteroid-induced bone loss and fractures in patients with arthritis: evaluation with dual-energy X-ray absorptiometry and quantitative ultrasound. Bone 2003;33:575–81.

253. Ringe JD, Dorst A, Faber H, Ibach K, Preuss J. Three-monthly ibandronate bolus injection offers favorable tolerability and sustained efficacy advantage over two years in established corticosteroid-induced osteoporosis. Rheumatol (Oxf) 2003;42:743–9.

254. Ringe JD, Dorst A, Faber H, Ibach K, Sorenson F. Intermittent intravenous ibandronate injections reduce vertebral fracture risk in corticosteroid-induced osteoporosis: results from a long-term comparative study. Osteoporos Int 2003;14:801–7.

255. Boutsen Y, Jamart J, Esselinckx W, Stoffel M, Devogelaer JP. Primary prevention of glucocorticoid-induced osteoporosis with intermittent intravenous pamidronate: a randomized trial. Calcif Tissue Int 1997;61(4):266–71.

256. Wallach S, Cohen S, Reid DM, Hughes RA, Hosking DJ, Laan RF, Doherty SM, Maricic M, Rosen C, Brown J, Barton I, Chines AA. Effects of risedronate treatment on bone density and vertebral fracture in patients on corticosteroid therapy. Calcif Tissue Int 2000;67(4):277–85.

257. Reid DM, Hughes RA, Laan RF, Sacco-Gibson NA, Wenderoth DH, Adami S, Eusebio RA, Devogelaer JP. Efficacy and safety of daily risedronate in the treatment of corticosteroid-induced osteoporosis in men and women: a randomized trial. European Corticosteroid-Induced Osteoporosis Treatment Study. J Bone Miner Res 2000;15(6):1006–13.

258. Adachi JD, Saag KG, Delmas PD, Liberman UA, Emkey RD, Seeman E, Lane NE, Kaufman JM, Poubelle PE, Hawkins F, Correa-Rotter R, Menkes CJ, Rodriguez-Portales JA, Schnitzer TJ, Block JA, Wing J, McIlwain HH, Westhovens R, Brown J, Melo-Gomes JA, Gruber BL, Yanover MJ, Leite MO, Siminoski KG, Nevitt MC, Sharp JT, Malice MP, Dumortier T, Czachur M, Carofano W, Daifotis A. Two-year effects of alendronate on bone mineral density and vertebral fracture in patients receiving glucocorticoids: a randomized,

double-blind, placebo-controlled extension trial. Arthritis Rheum 2001;44(1):202–11.

259. Emkey R, Delmas PD, Goemaere S, Liberman UA, Poubelle PE, Daifotis AG, Verbruggen N, Lombardi A, Czachur M. Changes in bone mineral density following discontinuation or continuation of alendronate therapy in glucocorticoid-treated patients: a retrospective, observational study. Arthritis Rheum 2003;48:1102–8.

260. Rehman Q, Lang TF, Arnaud CD, Modin GW, Lane NE. Daily treatment with parathyroid hormone is associated with an increase in vertebral cross-sectional area in postmenopausal women with glucocorticoid-induced osteoporosis. Osteoporos Int 2003;14:77–81.

261. Rizzoli R, Chevalley T, Slosman DO, Bonjour JP. Sodium monofluorophosphate increases vertebral bone mineral density in patients with corticosteroid-induced osteoporosis. Osteoporos Int 1995;5(1):39–46.

262. Giustina A, Bussi AR, Jacobello C, Wehrenberg WB. Effects of recombinant human growth hormone (GH) on bone and intermediary metabolism in patients receiving chronic glucocorticoid treatment with suppressed endogenous GH response to GH-releasing hormone. J Clin Endocrinol Metab 1995;80(1):122–9.

263. Yonemura K, Kimura M, Miyaji T, Hishida A. Short-term effect of vitamin K administration on prednisolone-induced loss of bone mineral density in patients with chronic glomerulonephritis. Calcif Tissue Int 2000;66(2):123–8.

264. Westeel FP, Mazouz H, Ezaitouni F, Hottelart C, Ivan C, Fardellone P, Brazier M, El Esper I, Petit J, Achard JM, Pruna A, Fournier A. Cyclosporine bone remodeling effect prevents steroid osteopenia after kidney transplantation. Kidney Int 2000;58(4):1788–96.

265. Abe H, Sako H, Okino K, Nakane Y, Kodama M, Park KI, Inoue H, Kim CJ, Tomoyoshi T. Clinical study of aseptic necrosis of bone after renal transplantation. Transplant Proc 1994;26(4):1987.

266. Alarcon GS, Mikhail I, Jaffe KA, Bradley LA, Bailey WC. Hip osteonecrosis secondary to the administration of corticosteroids for feigned bronchial asthma. The clinical spectrum of the factitious disorders. Arthritis Rheum 1994;37(1):139–41.

267. Lausten GS, Lemser T, Jensen PK, Egfjord M. Necrosis of the femoral head after kidney transplantation. Clin Transplant 1998;12(6):572–4.

268. Bauer M, Thabault P, Estok D, Chrinstiansen C, Platt R. Low-dose corticosteroids and avascular necrosis of the hip and knee. Pharmacoepidemiol Drug Saf 2000;9:187–91.

269. McKee MD, Waddell JP, Kudo PA, Schemitsch EH, Richards RR. Osteonecrosis of the femoral head in men following short-course corticosteroid therapy: a report of 15 cases. CMAJ 2001;164(2):205–6.

270. Virik K, Karapetis C, Droufakou S, Harper P. Avascular necrosis of bone: the hidden risk of glucocorticoids used as antiemetics in cancer chemotherapy. Int J Clin Pract 2001;55(5):344–5.

271. Gibson JN, Poyser NL, Morrison WL, Scrimgeour CM, Rennie MJ. Muscle protein synthesis in patients with rheumatoid arthritis: effect of chronic corticosteroid therapy on prostaglandin F2 alpha availability. Eur J Clin Invest 1991;21(4):406–12.

272. Ekstrand A, Schalin-Jantti C, Lofman M, Parkkonen M, Widen E, Franssila-Kallunki A, Saloranta C, Koivisto V, Groop L. The effect of (steroid) immunosuppression on skeletal muscle glycogen metabolism in patients after kidney transplantation. Transplantation 1996;61(6):889–93.

273. Anonymous. Corticosteroid myopathy. Lancet 1970;2:1118.

274. Janssens S, Decramer M. Corticosteroid-induced myopathy and the respiratory muscles. Report of two cases. Chest 1989;95(5):1160–2.

275. Weiner P, Azgad Y, Weiner M. The effect of corticosteroids on inspiratory muscle performance in humans. Chest 1993;104(6):1788–91.

276. Halpern AA, Horowitz BG, Nagel DA. Tendon ruptures associated with corticosteroid therapy. West J Med 1977;127(5):378–82.

277. Pai VS. Rupture of the plantar fascia. J Foot Ankle Surg 1996;35(1):39–40.

278. Bunch TJ, Welsh GA, Miller DV, Swaroop VS. Acute spontaneous Achilles tendon rupture in a patient with giant cell arteritis. Ann Clin Lab Sci 2003;33:326–8.

279. Schiavon F. Transient joint effusion: a forgotten side effect of high dose corticosteroid treatment. Ann Rheum Dis 2003;62:491–2.

280. Motson RW, Glass DN, Smith DA, Daly JR. The effect of short- and long-term corticosteroid treatment on sleep-associated growth hormone secretion. Clin Endocrinol (Oxf) 1978;8(4):315–26.

281. Allen DB, Mullen M, Mullen B. A meta-analysis of the effect of oral and inhaled corticosteroids on growth. J Allergy Clin Immunol 1994;93(6):967–76.

282. Doull IJ, Freezer NJ, Holgate ST. Growth of prepubertal children with mild asthma treated with inhaled beclomethasone dipropionate. Am J Respir Crit Care Med 1995;151(6):1715–9.

283. Whitaker K, Webb J, Barnes J, Barnes ND. Effect of fluticasone on growth in children with asthma. Lancet 1996;348(9019):63–4.

284. Todd G, Dunlop K, McNaboe J, Ryan MF, Carson D, Shields MD. Growth and adrenal suppression in asthmatic children treated with high-dose fluticasone propionate. Lancet 1996;348(9019):27–9.

285. Travis LB, Chesney R, McEnery P, Moel D, Pennisi A, Potter D, Talwalkar YB, Wolff E. Growth and glucocorticoids in children with kidney disease. Kidney Int 1978;14(4):365–8.

286. Rivkees SA, Danon M, Herrin J. Prednisone dose limitation of growth hormone treatment of steroid-induced growth failure. J Pediatr 1994;125(2):322–5.

287. Lai HC, FitzSimmons SC, Allen DB, Kosorok MR, Rosenstein BJ, Campbell PW, Farrell PM. Risk of persistent growth impairment after alternate-day prednisone treatment in children with cystic fibrosis. N Engl J Med 2000;342(12):851–9.

288. Diczfalusy E, Landgren BM. Hormonal changes in the menstrual cycle. In: Diczfalusy D, editor. Regulation of Human Fertility. Copenhagen: Scriptor, 1977:21.

289. Cunningham GR, Goldzieher JW, de la Pena A, Oliver M. The mechanism of ovulation inhibition by triamcinolone acetonide. J Clin Endocrinol Metab 1978;46(1):8–14.

290. Mens JM, Nico de Wolf A, Berkhout DJ, Stam HJ. Disturbance of the menstrual pattern after local injection with triamcinolone acetonide. Ann Rheum Dis 1998;57(11):700.

291. Lopez-Serrano MC, Moreno-Ancillo A, Contreras J, Ortega N, Cabanas R, Barranco P, Munoz-Pereira M. Two cases of specific adverse reactions to systemic corticosteroids. J Invest Allergol Clin Immunol 1996;6(5):324–7.

292. Ventura MT, Muratore L, Calogiuri GF, Dagnello M, Buquicchio R, Nicoletti A, Altamura M, Sabba C, Tursi A.

Allergic and pseudoallergic reactions induced by gluco-corticosteroids: a review. Curr Pharm Des 2003;9:1956–64.

293. Moreno-Ancillo A, Martin-Munoz F, Martin-Barroso JA, Diaz-Pena JM, Ojeda JA. Anaphylaxis to 6-alpha-methyl-prednisolone in an eight-year-old child. J Allergy Clin Immunol 1996;97(5):1169–71.

294. van den Berg JS, van Eikema Hommes OR, Wuis EW, Stapel S, van der Valk PG. Anaphylactoid reaction to intravenous methylprednisolone in a patient with multiple sclerosis. J Neurol Neurosurg Psychiatry 1997;63(6):813–4.

295. Figueredo E, Cuesta-Herranz JI, De Las Heras M, Lluch-Bernal M, Umpierrez A, Sastre J. Anaphylaxis to dexa-methasone. Allergy 1997;52(8):877.

296. Mace S, Vadas P, Pruzanski W. Anaphylactic shock induced by intraarticular injection of methylprednisolone acetate. J Rheumatol 1997;24(6):1191–4.

297. Hayhurst M, Braude A, Benatar SR. Anaphylactic-like reaction to hydrocortisone. S Afr Med J 1978;53(7):259–60.

298. Srinivasan V, Lanham PR. Acute laryngeal obstruction – reaction to intravenous hydrocortisone? Eur J Anaesthesiol 1997;14(3):342.

299. Vaghjimal A, Rosenstreich D, Hudes G. Fever, rash and worsening of asthma in response to intravenous hydrocor-tisone. Int J Clin Pract 1999;53(7):567–8.

300. Clear D. Anaphylactoid reaction to methyl prednisolone developing after starting treatment with interferon beta-1b. J Neurol Neurosurg Psychiatry 1999;66(5):690.

301. Schonwald S. Methylprednisolone anaphylaxis. Am J Emerg Med 1999;17(6):583–5.

302. Vanpee D, Gillet JB. Allergic reaction to intravenous methylprednisolone in a woman with asthma. Ann Emerg Med 1998;32(6):754.

303. Polosa R, Prosperini G, Pintaldi L, Rey JP, Colombrita R. Anaphylaxis after prednisone. Allergy 1998;53(3):330–1.

304. Karsh J, Yang WH. An anaphylactic reaction to intra-articular triamcinolone: a case report and review of the literature. Ann Allergy Asthma Immunol 2003;90:254–8.

305. Yawalkar N, Hari Y, Helbing A, von Greyerz S, Kappeler A, Baathen LR, Pichler WJ. Elevated serum levels of interleukins 5, 6, and 10 in a patient with drug-induced exanthem caused by systemic corticosteroids. J Am Acad Dermatol 1998;39(5 Part 1):790–3.

306. Ventura MT, Calogiuri GF, Matino MG, Dagnello M, Buquicchio R, Foti C, Di Corato R. Alternative glucocor-ticoids for use in cases of adverse reaction to systemic glucocorticoids: a study on 10 patients. Br J Dematol 2003;148:139–41.

307. Heeringa M, Zweers P, de Man RA, de Groot H. Drug Points: Anaphylactic-like reaction associated with oral budesonide. BMJ 2000;321(7266):927.

308. Gomez CM, Higuero NC, Moral de Gregorio A, Quiles MH, Nunez Aceves AB, Lara MJ, Sanchez CS. Urticaria–angioedema by deflazacort. Allergy 2002;57(4):370–1.

309. Monk BE, Skipper D. Allergy to topical corticosteroids in inflammatory bowel disease. Gut 2003;52:597.

310. Staunton H, Stafford F, Leader M, O'Riordain D. Deterioration of giant cell arteritis with corticosteroid therapy. Arch Neurol 2000;57(4):581–4.

311. Schols AM, Wesseling G, Kester AD, de Vries G, Mostert R, Slangen J, Wouters EF. Dose dependent increased mortality risk in COPD patients treated with oral glucocorticoids. Eur Respir J 2001;17(3):337–42.

312. Klaustermeyer WB, Gianos ME, Kurohara ML, Dao HT, Heiner DC. IgG subclass deficiency associated with

corticosteroids in obstructive lung disease. Chest 1992;102(4):1137–42.

313. Robinson MJ, Campbell F, Powell P, Sims D, Thornton C. Antibody response to accelerated Hib immunisation in pre-term infants receiving dexamethasone for chronic lung dis-ease. Arch Dis Child Fetal Neonatal Ed 1999;80(1):F69–71.

314. Sprung CL, Caralis PV, Marcial EH, Pierce M, Gelbard MA, Long WM, Duncan RC, Tendler MD, Karpf M. The effects of high-dose corticosteroids in patients with septic shock. A prospective, controlled study. N Engl J Med 1984;311(18):1137–43.

315. Mostafa BE. Fluticasone propionate is associated with severe infection after endoscopic polypectomy. Arch Otolaryngol Head Neck Surg 1996;122(7):729–31.

316. Demitsu T, Kosuge A, Yamada T, Usui K, Katayama H, Yaoita H. Acute generalized exanthematous pustulosis induced by dexamethasone injection. Dermatology 1996;193(1):56–8.

317. Aberra FN, Lewis JD, Hass D, Rombeau JL, Osborne B, Lichtenstein GR. Corticosteroids and immunomodulators: postoperative infectious complication risk in inflammatory bowel disease patients. Gastroenterology 2003;125:320–7.

318. Hedderwick SA, Bonilla HF, Bradley SF, Kauffman CA. Opportunistic infections in patients with temporal arteritis treated with corticosteroids. J Am Geriatr Soc 1997;45(3):334–7.

319. Korula J. Tuberculous peritonitis complicating corticoster-oid therapy for acute alcoholic hepatitis. Dig Dis Sci 1995;40(10):2119–20.

320. Kim HA, Yoo CD, Baek HJ, Lee EB, Ahn C, Han JS, Kim S, Lee JS, Choe KW, Song YW. *Mycobacterium tuberculosis* infection in a corticosteroid-treated rheumatic disease patient population. Clin Exp Rheumatol 1998;16(1):9–13.

321. di Girolamo C, Pappone N, Melillo E, Rengo C, Giuliano F, Melillo G. Cavitary lung tuberculosis in a rheumatoid arthritis patient treated with low-dose metho-trexate and steroid pulse therapy. Br J Rheumatol 1998;37(10):1136–7.

322. Martos A, Podzamczer D, Martinez-Lacasa J, Rufi G, Santin M, Gudiol F. Steroids do not enhance the risk of developing tuberculosis or other AIDS-related diseases in HIV-infected patients treated for *Pneumocystis carinii* pneumonia. AIDS 1995;9(9):1037–41.

323. Bridges MJ, McGarry F. Two cases of *Mycobacterium avium* septic arthritis. Ann Rheum Dis 2002;61(2):186–7.

324. Fernandez-Aviles F, Batlle M, Ribera JM, Matas L, Sabria M, Feliu E. *Legionella* sp pneumonia in patients with hematologic diseases. A study of 10 episodes from a series of 67 cases of pneumonia. Haematologica 1999;84(5):474–5.

325. Rice P, Simmons K, Carr R, Banatvala J. Near fatal chick-enpox during prednisolone treatment. BMJ 1994;309(6961):1069–70.

326. Choong K, Zwaigenbaum L, Onyett H. Severe varicella after low dose inhaled corticosteroids. Pediatr Infect Dis J 1995;14(9):809–11.

327. Burnett I. Severe chickenpox during treatment with corticos-teroids. Immunoglobulin should be given if steroid dosage was > or = 0.5 mg/kg/day in preceding three months BMJ 1995;310(6975):327Erratum in BMJ 1995;310(6978):534.

328. Doherty MJ, Baxter AB, Longstreth WT Jr. Herpes sim-plex virus encephalitis complicating myxedema coma trea-ted with corticosteroids. Neurology 2001;56(8):1114–5.

329. Pingleton WW, Bone RC, Kerby GR, Ruth WE. Oropharyngeal candidiasis in patients treated with triamcinolone acetonide aerosol. J Allergy Clin Immunol 1977;60(4):254–8.

330. Nenoff P, Horn LC, Mierzwa M, Leonhardt R, Weidenbach H, Lehmann I, Haustein UF. Peracute disseminated fatal Aspergillus fumigatus sepsis as a complication of corticoid-treated systemic lupus erythematosus. Mycoses 1995;38(11–12):467–71.

331. Wald A, Leisenring W, van Burik JA, Bowden RA. Epidemiology of Aspergillus infections in a large cohort of patients undergoing bone marrow transplantation. J Infect Dis 1997;175(6):1459–66.

332. Machet L, Jan V, Machet MC, Vaillant L, Lorette G. Cutaneous alternariosis: role of corticosteroid-induced cutaneous fragility. Dermatology 1996;193(4):342–4.

333. Fucci JC, Nightengale ML. Primary esophageal histoplasmosis. Am J Gastroenterol 1997;92(3):530–1.

334. Monlun E, de Blay F, Berton C, Gasser B, Jaeger A, Pauli G. Invasive pulmonary aspergillosis with cerebromeningeal involvement after short-term intravenous corticosteroid therapy in a patient with asthma. Respir Med 1997;91(7):435–7.

335. Shetty D, Giri N, Gonzalez CE, Pizzo PA, Walsh TJ. Invasive aspergillosis in human immunodeficiency virus-infected children. Pediatr Infect Dis J 1997;16(2):216–21.

336. Fernandez JM, Sanchez E, Polo FJ, Saez L. Infección pulmonar por Aspergillus fumigatus y Nocardia asteroides como complicación del tratamiento con glucocorticoides. Med Clin (Barc) 2000;114:358.

337. Carrascosa Porras M, Herreras Martinez R, Corral Mones J, Ares Ares M, Zabaleta Murguiondo M, Ruchel R. Fatal Aspergillus myocarditis following short-term corticosteroid therapy for chronic obstructive pulmonary disease. Scand J Infect Dis 2002;34(3):224–7.

338. Vogeser M, Haas A, Ruckdeschel G, von Scheidt W. Steroid-induced invasive aspergillosis with thyroid gland abscess and positive blood cultures. Eur J Clin Microbiol Infect Dis 1998;17(3):215–6.

339. Mavinkurve-Groothuis AMC, Bokkerink JPM, Verweij PE, Veerman AJP, Hoogerbrugge PM. Cryptococcal meningitis in a child with acute lymphoblastic leukemia. Pediatr Infect Dis J 2003;22:576.

340. Bower CP, Oxley JD, Campbell CK, Archer CB. Cutaneous Scedosporium apiospermum infection in an immunocompromised patient. J Clin Pathol 1999;52(11):846–8.

341. Ioannidou DJ, Stefanidou MP, Maraki SG, Panayiotides JG, Tosca AD. Cutaneous alternariosis in a patient with idiopathic pulmonary fibrosis. Int J Dermatol 2000;39(4):293–5.

342. Pera A, Byun A, Gribar S, Schwartz R, Kumar D, Parimi P. Dexamethasone therapy and Candida sepsis in neonates less than 1250 grams. J Perinatol 2002;22(3):204–8.

343. Fukuda T, Boeckh M, Carter RA, Sandmaier BM, Maris MB, Maloney DG, Martin PJ, Storb RF, Marr KA. Risks and outcomes of invasive fungal infections in recipients of allogenic hematopoietic stem cell transplants after nonmyeloablative conditioning. Blood 2003;102:827–33.

344. Buchheidt D, Hummel M, Diehl S, Hehlmann R. Fatal cerebral involvement in systemic aspergillosis: a rare complication of steroid-treated autoimmune bicytopenia. Eur J Haematol 2004;72:375–6.

345. Sen P, Gil C, Estrellas B, Middleton JR. Corticosteroid-induced asthma: a manifestation of limited hyperinfection syndrome due to Strongyloides stercoralis. South Med J 1995;88(9):923–7.

346. Mariotta S, Pallone G, Li Bianchi E, Gilardi G, Bisetti A. Strongyloides stercoralis hyperinfection in a case of idiopathic pulmonary fibrosis. Panminerva Med 1996;38(1):45–7.

347. Leung VK, Liew CT, Sung JJ. Fatal strongyloidiasis in a patient with ulcerative colitis after corticosteroid therapy. Am J Gastroenterol 1997;92(8):1383–4.

348. Schipperijn AJM. Flare-up of toxoplasmosis due to corticosteroid therapy in pulmonary sarcoidosis. Ned T Geneesk 1970;114:1710.

349. Cohen SN. Toxoplasmosis in patients receiving immunosuppressive therapy. JAMA 1970;211(4):657–60.

350. Sy ML, Chin TW, Nussbaum E. Pneumocystis carinii pneumonia associated with inhaled corticosteroids in an immunocompetent child with asthma. J Pediatr 1995;127(6):1000–2.

351. Bachelez H, Schremmer B, Cadranel J, Mouly F, Sarfati C, Agbalika F, Schlemmer B, Mayaud CM, Dubertret L. Fulminant Pneumocystis carinii pneumonia in 4 patients with dermatomyositis. Arch Intern Med 1997;157(13):1501–3.

352. Kanani SR, Knight R. Amoebic dysentery precipitated by corticosteroids. BMJ 1969;3(662):114.

353. Stark AR, Carlo WA, Tyson JE, Papile LA, Wright LL, Shankaran S, Donovan EF, Oh W, Bauer CR, Saha S, Poole WK, Stoll BJ. National Institute of Child Health and Human Development Neonatal Research Network. Adverse effects of early dexamethasone in extremely-low-birth-weight infants. National Institute of Child Health and Human Development Neonatal Research Network. N Engl J Med 2001;344(2):95–101.

354. Lucas A, Coll J, Salinas I, Sanmarti A. Hipertensión intracraneal benigna tras suspensión de corticoterapia en una paciente previaments intervenida por enfermedad de Cushing. [Benign intracranial hypertension following the suspension of corticotherapy in a female patient previously operated on for Cushing's disease.] Med Clin (Barc) 1991;97(12):473.

355. Richards D, Aronson J. The Oxford Handbook of Practical Drug TherapyOxford: Oxford University Press;. 2004.

356. Morgan J, Lacey JH. Anorexia nervosa and steroid withdrawal. Int J Eat Disord 1996;19(2):213–5.

357. Silverman RA, Newman AJ, LeVine MJ, Kaplan B. Poststeroid panniculitis: a case report. Pediatr Dermatol 1988;5(2):92–3.

358. Le Gall C, Pham S, Vignes S, Garcia G, Nunes H, Fichet D, Simonneau G, Duroux P, Humbert M. Inhaled corticosteroids and Churg–Strauss syndrome: a report of five cases. Eur Respir J 2000;15(5):978–81.

359. Hodgkinson DJ, Williams TJ. Endometrial carcinoma associated with azathioprine and cortisone therapy. A case report. Gynecol Oncol 1977;5(3):308–12.

360. Erban SB, Sokas RK. Kaposi's sarcoma in an elderly man with Wegener's granulomatosis treated with cyclophosphamide and corticosteroids. Arch Intern Med 1988;148(5):1201–3.

361. Thiagarajan CM, Divakar D, Thomas SJ. Malignancies in renal transplant recipients. Transplant Proc 1998;30(7):3154–5.

362. Gill PS, Loureiro C, Bernstein-Singer M, Rarick MU, Sattler F, Levine AM. Clinical effect of glucocorticoids on Kaposi sarcoma related to the acquired immunodeficiency syndrome (AIDS). Ann Intern Med 1989;110(11):937–40.

363. Tebbe B, Mayer-da-Silva A, Garbe C, von Keyserlingk HJ, Orfanos CE. Genetically determined coincidence of Kaposi sarcoma and psoriasis in an HIV-negative patient after prednisolone treatment. Spontaneous regression 8 months after discontinuing therapy. Int J Dermatol 1991;30(2):114–20.

364. Vincent T, Moss K, Colaco B, Venables PJ. Kaposi's sarcoma in two patients following low-dose corticosteroid treatment for rheumatological disease. Rheumatology (Oxford) 2000;39(11):1294–6.

365. Sorensen HT, Mellemkjaer L, Friis S, Olsen JH. Use of systemic corticosteroids and risk of esophageal cancer. Epidemiology 2002;13(2):240–1.

366. Chin S-OS, Brodsky NL, Bhandari V. Antenatal steroid use is associated with increased gastroesophageal reflux in neonates. Am J Perinatol 2003;20:205–13.

367. Jobe AH, Soll RF. Choice and dose of corticosteroid for antenatal treatments. Am J Obstet Gynecol 2004;190: 878–81.

368. Committee on Fetus and Newborn. Postnatal corticosteroids to treat or prevent chronic lung disease in preterm infants. Pediatrics 2002;109(2):330–8.

369. Canadian Paediatric Society and American Academy of Pediatrics. Postnatal corticosteroids to treat or prevent chronic lung disease in preterm infants. Pediatr Child Health 2002;7:20–8.

370. Banks BA, Macones G, Cnaan A, Merrill JD, Ballard PL, Ballard RA. North American TRH Study Group. Multiple courses of antenatal corticosteroids are associated with early severe lung disease in preterm neonates. J Perinatol 2002;22(2):101–7.

371. Elliott JP, Radin TG. The effect of corticosteroid administration on uterine activity and preterm labor in high-order multiple gestations. Obstet Gynecol 1995;85(2):250–4.

372. Ogunyemi D. A comparison of the effectiveness of single-dose vs multi-dose antenatal corticosteroids in pre-term neonates. Obstet Gynaecol 2005;25(8):756–60.

373. Haas DM, McCullough W, Olsen CH, Shiau DT, Richard J, Fry EA, McNamara MF. Neonatal outcomes with different betamethasone dosing regimens: a comparison. J Reprod Med 2005;50(12):915–22.

374. Schmitz T, Goffinet F, Barrande G, Cabrol D. Maternal hypercorticism from serial courses of betamethasone. Obstet Gynecol 1999;94(5 Part 2):849.

375. Helal KJ, Gordon MC, Lightner CR, Barth WH Jr. Adrenal suppression induced by betamethasone in women at risk for premature delivery. Obstet Gynecol 2000;96(2):287–90.

376. Spencer C, Smith P, Rafla N, Weatherell R. Corticosteroids in pregnancy and osteonecrosis of the femoral head. Obstet Gynecol 1999;94(5 Part 2):848.

377. Vermillion ST, Soper DE, Chasedunn-Roark J. Neonatal sepsis after betamethasone administration to patients with preterm premature rupture of membranes. Am J Obstet Gynecol 1999;181(2):320–7.

378. Rotmensch S, Vishne TH, Celentano C, Dan M, Ben Rafael Z. Maternal infectious morbidity following multiple courses of betamethasone. J Infect 1999;39(1):49–54.

379. Vermillion ST, Soper DE, Newman RB. Neonatal sepsis and death after multiple courses of antenatal betamethasone therapy. Am J Obstet Gynecol 2000;183(4):810–4.

380. Abbasi S, Hirsch D, Davis J, Tolosa J, Stouffer N, Debbs R, Gerdes JS. Effect of single versus multiple courses of antenatal corticosteroids on maternal and neonatal outcome. Am J Obstet Gynecol 2000;182(5):1243–9.

381. Yang SH, Choi SJ, Roh CR, Kim JH. Multiple courses of antenatal corticosteroid therapy in patients with preterm premature rupture of membranes. J Perinat Med 2004;32:42–8.

382. Stockli A, Keller M. Kongenitales adrenogenitales Syndrom und Schwangerschaft. [Congenital adrenogenital syndrome and pregnancy.] Schweiz Med Wochenschr 1969;99(4):126–8.

383. Beique LC, Friesen MH, Park LY, Diaz-Citrin O, Koren G, Einarson TR. Major malformations associated with corticosteroid exposure during the first trimester: a meta-analysis. Can J Hosp Pharm 1998;51:83.

384. Moran P, Taylor R. Management of hyperemesis gravidarum: the importance of weight loss as a criterion for steroid therapy. QJM 2002;95(3):153–8.

385. Markert UR, Klemm A, Flossmann E, Werner W, Sperschneider H, Funfstuck R. Renal transplantation in early pregnancy with acute graft rejection and development of a hydatidiform mole. Clin Nephrol 1998;49(6):391–2.

386. Park-Wyllie L, Mazzotta P, Pastuszak A, Moretti ME, Beique L, Hunnisett L, Friesen MH, Jacobson S, Kasapinovic S, Chang D, Diav-Citrin O, Chitayat D, Nulman I, Einarson TR, Koren G. Birth defects after maternal exposure to corticosteroids: prospective cohort study and meta-analysis of epidemiological studies. Teratology 2000;62(6):385–92.

387. Harding JE, Pang J, Knight DB, Liggins GC. Do antenatal corticosteroids help in the setting of preterm rupture of membranes? Am J Obstet Gynecol 2001;184(2):131–9.

388. Bloom SL, Sheffield JS, McIntire DD, Leveno KJ. Antenatal dexamethasone and decreased birth weight. Obstet Gynecol 2001;97(4):485–90.

389. Rotmensch S, Liberati M, Celentano C, Efrat Z, Bar-Hava I, Kovo M, Golan A, Moravski G, Ben-Rafael Z. The effect of betamethasone on fetal biophysical activities and Doppler velocimetry of umbilical and middle cerebral arteries. Acta Obstet Gynecol Scand 1999;78(9):768–73.

390. Warrell DW, Taylor R. Outcome for the foetus of mothers receiving prednisolone during pregnancy. Lancet 1968;1(7534):117–8.

391. Crowley PA. Antenatal corticosteroid therapy: a meta-analysis of the randomized trials, 1972–94. Am J Obstet Gynecol 1995;173(1):322–35.

392. Kairalla AB. Hypothalamic–pituitary–adrenal axis function in premature neonates after extensive prenatal treatment with betamethasone: a case history. Am J Perinatol 1992;9(5–6):428–30.

393. Ohrlander S, Gennser G, Nilsson KO, Eneroth P. ACTH test to neonates after administration of corticosteroids during gestation. Obstet Gynecol 1977;49(6):691–4.

394. Ohlsson A, Calvert SA, Hosking M, Shennan AT. Randomized controlled trial of dexamethasone treatment in very-low-birth-weight infants with ventilator-dependent chronic lung disease. Acta Paediatr 1992;81(10):751–6.

395. Brownlee KG, Ng PC, Henderson MJ, Smith M, Green JH, Dear PR. Catabolic effect of dexamethasone in the preterm baby. Arch Dis Child 1992;67(1 Spec No):1–4.

396. O'Neil EA, Chwals WJ, O'Shea MD, Turner CS. Dexamethasone treatment during ventilator dependency: possible life threatening gastrointestinal complications. Arch Dis Child 1992;67(1 Spec No):10–1.

397. Dalziel SR, Walker NK, Parag V, Mantell C, Rea HH, Rodgers A, Harding JE. Cardiovascular risk factors after

antenatal exposure to betamethasone: 30-year follow-up of a randomised controlled trial. Lancet 2005;365(9474):1856–62.

398. Spinillo A, Viazzo F, Colleoni R, Chiara A, Maria Cerbo R, Fazzi E. Two-year infant neurodevelopmental outcome after single or multiple antenatal courses of corticosteroids to prevent complications of prematurity. Am J Obstet Gynecol 2004;191:217–24.

399. French NP, Hagan R, Evans SF, Mullan A, Newnham JP. Repeated antenatal corticosteroids: effects on cerebral palsy and childhood behavior. Am J Obstet Gynecol 2004; 190: 588–95.

400. Dalziel SR, Lim VK, Lambert A, McCarthy D, Parag V, Rodgers A, Harding JE. Antenatal exposure to beta-methasone: psychological functioning and health related quality of life 31 years after inclusion in randomised controlled trial. BMJ 2005;331(7518):665.

401. Cho S, Beharry KD, Valencia AM, Guajardo L, Nageotte MP, Modanlou HD. Maternal and feto-placental prostanoid responses to a single course of antenatal betamethasone. Prostaglandins Other Lipid Mediat 2005;78(1-4):139–59.

402. Harding JE, Pang J, Knight DB, Liggins GC. Do antenatal corticosteroids help in the setting of preterm rupture of membranes? Am J Obstet Gynecol 2001;184(2):131–9.

403. Rotmensch S, Celentano C, Liberati M, Sadan O, Glezerman M. The effect of antenatal steroid administration on the fetal response to vibroacoustic stimulation. Acta Obstet Gynecol Scand 1999;78(10):847–51.

404. Tornatore KM, Biocevich DM, Reed K, Tousley K, Singh JP, Venuto RC. Methylprednisolone pharmacokinetics, cortisol response, and adverse effects in black and white renal transplant recipients. Transplantation 1995;59(5):729–36.

405. Skoner DP. Balancing safety and efficacy in pediatric asthma management. Pediatrics 2002;109(Suppl 2):381–92.

406. Allen DB. Safety of inhaled corticosteroids in children. Pediatr Pulmonol 2002;33(3):208–20.

407. Thebaud B, Lacaze-Masmonteil T, Watterberg K. Postnatal glucocorticoids in very preterm infants: "the good, the bad, and the ugly"? Pediatrics 2001;107(2):413–5.

408. Akerkar GA, Peppercorn MA, Hamel MB, Parker RA. Corticosteroid-associated complications in elderly Crohn's disease patients. Am J Gastroenterol 1997;92(3):461–4.

409. Powell LW, Axelsen E. Corticosteroids in liver disease: studies on the biological conversion of prednisone to prednisolone and plasma protein binding. Gut 1972;13(9):690–6.

410. Davis M, Williams R, Chakraborty J, English J, Marks V, Ideo G, Tempini S. Prednisone or prednisolone for the treatment of chronic active hepatitis? A comparison of plasma availability. Br J Clin Pharmacol 1978;5(6):501–5.

411. Frey BM, Frey FJ. Clinical pharmacokinetics of prednisone and prednisolone. Clin Pharmacokinet 1990;19(2):126–46.

412. Harris RZ, Tsunoda SM, Mroczkowski P, Wong H, Benet LZ. The effects of menopause and hormone replacement therapies on prednisolone and erythromycin pharmacokinetics. Clin Pharmacol Ther 1996;59(4):429–35.

413. Lewis GP, Jusko WJ, Graves L, Burke CW. Prednisone side-effects and serum-protein levels. A collaborative study. Lancet 1971;2(7728):778–80.

414. Zonana-Nacach A, Barr SG, Magder LS, Petri M. Damage in systemic lupus erythematosus and its association with corticosteroids. Arthritis Rheum 2000;43(8):1801–8.

415. Andus T, Gross V, Caesar I, Schulz HJ, Lochs H, Strohm WD, Gierend M, Weber A, Ewe K, Scholmerich J; German/Austrian Budesonide Study Group. Replacement of conventional glucocorticoids by oral pH-modified release budesonide in active and inactive Crohn's disease: results of an open, prospective, multicenter trial. Dig Dis Sci 2003;48:373–8.

416. Keane FM, Munn SE, du Vivier AW, Taylor NF, Higgins EM. Analysis of Chinese herbal creams prescribed for dermatological conditions. BMJ 1999;318(7183):563–4.

417. Reinberg AE. Chronopharmacology of corticosteroids and ACTH. In: Lammer B, editor. Chronopharmacology. Cellular and Biochemical Interactions. New York and Basel: Marcel Dekker Inc, 1989:137–67.

418. Kimura Y, Fieldston E, Devries-Vandervlugt B, Li S, Imundo L. High dose, alternate day corticosteroids for systemic onset juvenile rheumatoid arthritis. J Rheumatol 2000;27(8):2018–24.

419. Kaiser BA, Polinsky MS, Palmer JA, Dunn S, Mochon M, Flynn JT, Baluarte HJ. Growth after conversion to alternate-day corticosteroids in children with renal transplants: a single-center study. Pediatr Nephrol 1994;8(3):320–5.

420. Blair GP, Light RW. Treatment of chronic obstructive pulmonary disease with corticosteroids. Comparison of daily vs alternate-day therapy. Chest 1984;86(4):524–8.

421. Oshitani N, Kamata N, Ooiso R, Kawashima D, Inagawa M, Sogawa M, Iimuro M, Jinno Y, Watanabe K, Higuchi K, Matsumoto T, Arakawa T. Outpatient treatment of moderately severe active ulcerative colitis with pulsed steroid therapy and conventional steroid therapy. Dig Dis Sci 2003;4:1002–5.

422. Ermis B, Ors R, Tastekin A, Ozkan B. Cushing's syndrome secondary to topical corticosteroids abuse. Clin Endocrinol 2003;58:795–7.

423. Gilbertson EO, Spellman MC, Piacquadio DJ, Mulford MI. Super potent topical corticosteroid use associated with adrenal suppression: clinical considerations. J Am Acad Dermatol 1998;38(2 Part 2):318–21.

424. Marcos C, Allegue F, Luna I, Gonzalez R. An unusual case of allergic contact dermatitis from corticosteroids. Contact Dermatitis 1999;41(4):237–8.

425. Corazza M, Virgili A. Allergic contact dermatitis from 6alpha-methylprednisolone aceponate and budesonide. Contact Dermatitis 1998;38(6):356–7.

426. Oh C, Lee J. Contact allergy to various ingredients of topical medicaments. Contact Dermatitis 2003;49:49–50.

427. Karadimas P, Kapetanios A, Bouzas EA. Central serous chorioretinopathy after local application of glucocorticoids for skin disorders. Arch Ophthalmol 2004; 122: 784–6.

428. Mygind H, Thulstrup AM, Pedersen L, Larsen H. Risk of intrauterine growth retardation, malformations and other birth outcomes in children after topical use of corticosteroid in pregnancy. Acta Obstet Gynecol Scand 2002;81(3):234–9.

429. Whitcup SM, Ferris FL 3rd. New corticosteroids for the treatment of ocular inflammation. Am J Ophthalmol 1999;127(5):597–9.

430. Aggarwal RK, Potamitis T, Chong NH, Guarro M, Shah P, Kheterpal S. Extensive visual loss with topical facial steroids. Eye 1993;7(5):664–6.

431. Baratz KH, Hattenhauer MG. Indiscriminate use of corticosteroid-containing eyedrops. Mayo Clin Proc 1999;74(4):362–6.

432. Chua JK, Fan DS, Leung AT, Lam DS. Accelerated ocular hypertensive response after application of corticosteroid ointment to a child's eyelid. Mayo Clin Proc 2000;75(5):539.

433. Ozerdem U, Levi L, Cheng L, Song MK, Scher C, Freeman WR. Systemic toxicity of topical and periocular corticosteroid therapy in an 11-year-old male with posterior uveitis. Am J Ophthalmol 2000;130(2):240–1.

434. Mehle ME. Are nasal steroids safe? Curr Opin Otolaryngol Head Neck Surg 2003;11:201–5.

435. Salib RJ, Howarth PH. Safety and tolerability profiles of intranasal antihistamines and intranasal corticosteroids in the treatment of allergic rhinitis. Drug Saf 2003;26:863–93.

436. Priftis K, Everard ML, Milner AD. Unexpected side-effects of inhaled steroids: a case report. Eur J Pediatr 1991;150(6):448–9.

437. Stead RJ, Cooke NJ. Adverse effects of inhaled corticosteroids. BMJ 1989;298(6671):403–4.

438. Whittet HB, Shinkwin C, Freeland AP. Anosmia due to nasal administration of corticosteroid. BMJ 1991;303(6803):651.

439. Bond DW, Charlton CP, Gregson RM. Benign intracranial hypertension secondary to nasal fluticasone propionate. BMJ 2001;322(7291):897.

440. Ozturk F, Yuceturk AV, Kurt E, Unlu HH, Ilker SS. Evaluation of intraocular pressure and cataract formation following the long-term use of nasal corticosteroids. Ear Nose Throat J 1998;77(10):846–51.

441. Cervin A, Andersson M. Intranasal steroids and septum perforation – an overlooked complication? A description of the course of events and a discussion of the causes. Rhinology 1998;36(3):128–32.

442. Nayak AS, Ellis MH, Gross GN, Mendelson LM, Schenkel EJ, Lanier BQ, Simpson B, Mullin ME, Smith JA. The effects of triamcinolone acetonide aqueous nasal spray on adrenocortical function in children with allergic rhinitis. J Allergy Clin Immunol 1998;101(2 Part 1):157–62.

443. Findlay CA, Macdonald JF, Wallace AM, Geddes N, Donaldson MD. Childhood Cushing's syndrome induced by betamethasone nose drops, and repeat prescriptions. BMJ 1998;317(7160):739–40.

444. Hillebrand-Haverkort ME, Prummel MF, ten Veen JH. Ritonavir-induced Cushing's syndrome in a patient treated with nasal fluticasone. AIDS 1999;13(13):1803.

445. Mistlin A, Gibson T. Osteonecrosis of the femoral head resulting from excessive corticosteroid nasal spray use. J Clin Rheumatol 2004;10:45–6.

446. Downs AM, Lear JT, Kennedy CT. Anaphylaxis to intradermal triamcinolone acetonide. Arch Dermatol 1998;134(9):1163–4.

447. Miranda-Romero A, Bajo-del Pozo C, Sanchez-Sambucety P, Martinez-Fernandez M, Garcia-Munoz M. Delayed local allergic reaction to intralesional paramethasone acetate. Contact Dermatitis 1998;39(1):31–2.

448. Wilkinson HA. Intrathecal Depo-Medrol: a literature review. Clin J Pain 1992;8(1):49–56.

449. DeSio JM, Kahn CH, Warfield CA. Facial flushing and/or generalized erythema after epidural steroid injection. Anesth Analg 1995;80(3):617–9.

450. Plumb VJ, Dismukes WE. Chemical meningitis related to intrathecal corticosteroid therapy. South Med J 1977;70(10):1241–3.

451. Dumont D, Hariz H, Meynieu P, Salama J, Dreyfus P, Boissier MC. Abducens palsy after an intrathecal glucocorticoid injection. Evidence for a role of intracranial hypotension. Rev Rhum Engl Ed 1998;65(5):352–4.

452. Spaccarelli KC. Lumbar and caudal epidural corticosteroid injections. Mayo Clin Proc 1996;71(2):169–78.

453. Chen YC, Gajraj NM, Clavo A, Joshi GP. Posterior subcapsular cataract formation associated with multiple lumbar epidural corticosteroid injections. Anesth Analg 1998;86(5):1054–5.

454. Siegfried RN. Development of complex regional pain syndrome after a cervical epidural steroid injection. Anesthesiology 1997;86(6):1394–6.

455. Sandberg DI, Lavyne MH. Symptomatic spinal epidural lipomatosis after local epidural corticosteroid injections: case report. Neurosurgery 1999;45(1):162–5.

456. Cooper AB, Sharpe MD. Bacterial meningitis and cauda equina syndrome after epidural steroid injections. Can J Anaesth 1996;43(5 Part 1):471–4.

457. McLain RF, Fry M, Hecht ST. Transient paralysis associated with epidural steroid injection. J Spinal Disord 1997;10(5):441–4.

458. Brocq O, Breuil V, Grisot C, Flory P, Ziegler G, Euller-Ziegler L. Diplopie après infiltrations peridurale et intradurale de prédnisolone. Deux observations. [Diplopia after peridural and intradural infiltrations of prednisolone. 2 cases.] Presse Méd 1997;26(6):271.

459. Lowell TD, Errico TJ, Eskenazi MS. Use of epidural steroids after discectomy may predispose to infection. Spine 2000;25(4):516–9.

460. Field J, Rathmell JP, Stephenson JH, Katz NP. Neuropathic pain following cervical epidural steroid injection. Anesthesiology 2000;93(3):885–8.

461. Sparling M, Malleson P, Wood B, Petty R. Radiographic followup of joints injected with triamcinolone hexacetonide for the management of childhood arthritis. Arthritis Rheum 1990;33(6):821–6.

462. Gutierrez-Urena S, Ramos-Remus C. Persistent hiccups associated with intraarticular corticosteroid injection. J Rheumatol 1999;26(3):760.

463. Daragon A, Vittecoq O, Le Loet X. Visual hallucinations induced by intraarticular injection of steroids. J Rheumatol 1997;24(2):411.

464. Wicki J, Droz M, Cirafici L, Vallotton MB. Acute adrenal crisis in a patient treated with intraarticular steroid therapy. J Rheumatol 2000;27(2):510–1.

465. Valsecchi R, Reseghetti A, Leghissa P, Cologni L, Cortinovis R. Erythema-multiforme-like lesions from triamcinolone acetonide. Contact Dermatitis 1998;38(6):362–3.

466. Selvi E, De Stefano R, Lorenzini S, Marcolongo R. Arthritis induced by corticosteroid crystals. J Rheumatol 2004;31:622.

467. Jawed S, Allard SA. Osteomyelitis of the humerus following steroid injections for tennis elbow. Rheumatology (Oxford) 2000;39(8):923–4.

468. Montoro J, Valero A, Serra-Baldrich E, Amat P, Lluch M, Malet A. Anaphylaxis to paramethasone with tolerance to other corticosteroids. Allergy 2000;55(2):197–8.

469. Caffee HH. Intracapsular injection of triamcinolone for intractable capsule contracture. Plast Reconstr Surg 1994;94(6):824–8.

470. Braverman DL, Lachmann EA, Nagler W. Avascular necrosis of bilateral knees secondary to corticosteroid enemas. Arch Phys Med Rehabil 1998;79(4):449–52.

471. Tsuruoka S, Sugimoto K, Fujimura A. Drug-induced Cushing syndrome in a patient with ulcerative colitis after betamethasone enema: evaluation of plasma drug concentration. Ther Drug Monit 1998;20(4):387–9.

472. Lauerma AI. Occupational contact sensitization to corticosteroids. Contact Dermatitis 1998;39(6):328–9.

473. Newton RW, Browning MC, Iqbal J, Piercy N, Adamson DG. Adrenocortical suppression in workers manufacturing synthetic glucocorticoids. BMJ 1978;1(6105):73–4.

474. Nixon DW, Shlaer SM. Fulminant lung metastases from cancer of the breast. Med Pediatr Oncol 1981;9(4):381–5.

475. Klygis LM. Dexamethasone-induced perineal irritation in head injury. Am J Emerg Med 1992;10(3):268.

476. Takayanagui OM, Lanchote VL, Marques MP, Bonato PS. Therapy for neurocysticercosis: pharmacokinetic interaction of albendazole sulfoxide with dexamethasone. Ther Drug Monit 1997;19(1):51–5.

477. Ahle GB, Blum AL, Martinek J, Oneta CM, Dorta G. Cushing's syndrome in an 81-year-old patient treated with budesonide and amiodarone. Eur J Gastroenterol Hepatol 2000;12(9):1041–2.

478. Costedoat-Chalumeau N, Amoura Z, Aymard G, Sevin O, Wechsler B, Du Cacoub PLT, Diquet B, Ankri A, Piette JC. Potentiation of vitamin K antagonists by high-dose intravenous methylprednisolone. Ann Intern Med 2000;132(8):631–5.

479. Varis T, Kaukonen KM, Kivisto KT, Neuvonen PJ. Plasma concentrations and effects of oral methylprednisolone are considerably increased by itraconazole. Clin Pharmacol Ther 1998;64(4):363–8.

480. Varis T, Kivisto KT, Backman JT, Neuvonen PJ. Itraconazole decreases the clearance and enhances the effects of intravenously administered methylprednisolone in healthy volunteers. Pharmacol Toxicol 1999;85(1):29–32.

481. Varis T, Kivisto KT, Neuvonen PJ. The effect of itraconazole on the pharmacokinetics and pharmacodynamics of oral prednisolone. Eur J Clin Pharmacol 2000;56(1):57–60.

482. Varis T, Kivisto KT, Backman JT, Neuvonen PJ. The cytochrome P450 3A4 inhibitor itraconazole markedly increases the plasma concentrations of dexamethasone and enhances its adrenal-suppressant effect. Clin Pharmacol Ther 2000;68(5):487–94.

483. Seidegard J. Reduction of the inhibitory effect of ketoconazole on budesonide pharmacokinetics by separation of their time of administration. Clin Pharmacol Ther 2000;68(1):13–7.

484. McCrea JB, Majumdar AK, Goldberg MR, Iwamoto M, Gargano C, Panebianco DL, Hesney M, Lines CR, Petty KJ, Deutsch PJ, Murphy MG, Gottesdiener KM, Goldwater DR, Blum RA. Effects of the neurokinin1 receptor antagonist aprepitant on the pharmacokinetics of dexamethasone and methylprednisolone. Clin Pharmacol Ther 2003;74:17–24.

485. Varis T, Backman JT, Kivisto KT, Neuvonen PJ. Diltiazem and mibefradil increase the plasma concentrations and greatly enhance the adrenal-suppressant effect of oral methylprednisolone. Clin Pharmacol Ther 2000;67(3):215–21.

486. Quan VA, Saunders BP, Hicks BH, Sladen GE. Cyclosporin treatment for ulcerative colitis complicated by fatal *Pneumocystis carinii* pneumonia. BMJ 1997;314(7077):363–4.

487. Potter JM, McWhinney BC, Sampson L, Hickman PE. Area-under-the-curve monitoring of prednisolone for dose optimization in a stable renal transplant population. Ther Drug Monit 2004;26:408–14.

488. Fost DA, Leung DY, Martin RJ, Brown EE, Szefler SJ, Spahn JD. Inhibition of methylprednisolone elimination in the presence of clarithromycin therapy. J Allergy Clin Immunol 1999;103(6):1031–5.

489. Finkenbine R, Gill HS. Case of mania due to prednisone–clarithromycin interaction. Can J Psychiatry 1997;42(7):778.

490. Belfayol-Pisante L, Guillevin L, Tod M, Fauvelle F. Possible influence of prednisone on the pharmacokinetics of cyclophosphamide in systemic vasculitis. Clin Drug Invest 1999;18:225–31.

491. Manchon ND, Bercoff E, Lemarchand P, Chassagne P, Senant J, Bourreille J. Frequence et gravité des interactions médicamenteuses dans une population agée: étude prospective concernant 639 malades. [Incidence and severity of drug interactions in the elderly. a prospective study of 639 patients.] Rev Med Interne 1989;10(6):521–5.

492. Feuillet L, Guedj E, Laksiri N, Philip E, Habib G, Pelletier J, Cherif AA. Deep vein thrombosis after intravenous immunoglobulins associated with methylprednisolone. Thromb Haemost 2004;92:662–5.

493. Varis T, Kivisto KT, Neuvonen PJ. Grapefruit juice can increase the plasma concentrations of oral methylprednisolone. Eur J Clin Pharmacol 2000;56(6–7):489–93.

494. Geller M. Marked peripheral edema associated with montelukast and prednisone. Ann Intern Med 2000;132(11):924.

495. Seidegard J, Simonsson M, Edsbacker S. Effect of an oral contraceptive on the plasma levels of budesonide and prednisolone and the influence on plasma cortisol. Clin Pharmacol Ther 2000;67(4):373–81.

496. Schönhofer PS. Interaktionen antirheumatisch wirksamer Substanzen. [Interactions of antirheumatic agents.] Internist (Berl) 1979;20(9):433–8.

497. Strayhorn VA, Baciewicz AM, Self TH. Update on rifampin drug interactions III. Arch Intern Med 1997;157(21):2453–8.

498. Dhanoa J, Natu M, Massey S. Worsening of steroid depending bronchial asthma following rifampicin administration. J Assoc Physicians India 1998;46(2):242.

499. Edelman J, Potter JM, Hackett LP. The effect of intra-articular steroids on plasma salicylate concentrations. Br J Clin Pharmacol 1986;21(3):301–7.

500. Nielsen GL, Sorensen HT, Mellemkjoer L, Blot WJ, McLaughlin JK, Tage-Jensen U, Olsen JH. Risk of hospitalization resulting from upper gastrointestinal bleeding among patients taking corticosteroids: a register-based cohort study. Am J Med 2001;111(7):541–5.

501. Garcia Rodriguez LA, Hernandez-Diaz S. The risk of upper gastrointestinal complications associated with non-steroidal anti-inflammatory drugs, glucocorticoids, acetaminophen, and combinations of these agents. Arthritis Res 2001;3(2):98–101.

502. Weil J, Langman MJ, Wainwright P, Lawson DH, Rawlins M, Logan RF, Brown TP, Vessey MP, Murphy M, Colin-Jones DG. Peptic ulcer bleeding: accessory risk factors and interactions with nonsteroidal anti-inflammatory drugs. Gut 2000;46(1):27–31.

503. Patel RS, Shaw SR, McIntyre HE, McGarry GW, Wallace AM. Morning salivary cortisol versus short Synacthen test as a test of adrenal suppression. Ann Clin Biochem 2004;41:408–10.

504. Cepollaro C, Gonnelli S, Rottoli P, Montagnani A, Caffarelli C, Bruni D, Nikiforakis N, Fossi A, Rossi S, Nuti R. Bone ultrasonography in glucocorticoid-induced osteoporosis. Osteoporos Int 2005;16(8):743–8.

505. Brown ES, Chamberlain W, Dhanani N, Paranjpe P, Carmody TJ, Sargeant M. An open-label trial of olanzapine for corticosteroid-induced mood symptoms. J Affect Disord 2004;83(2–3):277–81.

Corticosteroids—glucocorticoids, inhaled

General Information

Treatment with inhaled glucocorticoids reduces the need for oral glucocorticoids in the treatment of severe asthma. The compounds used for inhalation have high local activity and low systemic availability when delivered to the lung. However, if sufficient amounts of glucocorticoids reach the bronchioles be absorbed, systemic effects will occur. Furthermore, a proportion of the dose intended for inhalation is actually swallowed and is absorbed from the gastrointestinal tract. The consequence is that if sufficiently high doses are used, enough drug will be absorbed from the respiratory and gastrointestinal surfaces to result in systemic effects.

Systemic availability of inhaled glucocorticoids can be reduced in two ways. First, by using esters that reduced local absorption; in the case of beclomethasone the dipropionate is used. Secondly, by using glucocorticoids that are extensively metabolized in the liver after absorption from the gut, such as fluticasone and budesonide. These strategies can be combined: fluticasone is given as the ester fluticasone propionate.

When a patient switches from oral or parenteral therapy to inhalation therapy, the systemic effect is reduced, just as if the dose of systemic glucocorticoid is reduced, and precautions should be taken to avoid withdrawal symptoms.

Systemic availability of inhaled glucocorticoids

The systemic availability of an inhaled glucocorticoid represents the additive and complex combination of pulmonary and gastrointestinal drug absorption. Absorption is influenced by many factors, including delivery device, the use of a spacer, the particle size of the inhaled drug, and the absorption and metabolism of the swallowed drug (1).

In healthy volunteers, high doses of both budesonide and fluticasone were readily absorbed after inhalation from a metered-dose aerosol (2). Fluticasone is extensively metabolized by the liver, so measurable concentrations of parent drug in the systemic circulation reflect efficient absorption across the lung. Lower doses of these inhaled glucocorticoids also result in some systemic absorption, reflected in effects on the hypothalamic–pituitary–adrenal axis (3).

The extent of absorption of inhaled glucocorticoids tends to be less in asthmatic subjects than in healthy volunteers. In a study of fluticasone (500 micrograms via a dry powder device) in asthmatic patients with a wide range of severity, there was a highly significant linear correlation between lung function (expressed as percentage predicted FEV_1) and the absolute magnitude of adrenal suppression (4). In 11 patients with moderately severe asthma (mean FEV_1 54% predicted), who took fluticasone 1000 micrograms/day via a metered-dose inhaler with a spacer, the systemic availability of fluticasone was significantly less (10%) than in 13 healthy controls (21%). The plasma fluticasone concentrations (expressed as AUC) correlated positively with gas transfer (5). In contrast, there was no difference in plasma concentrations of fluticasone and budesonide between 15 mild asthmatics (mean FEV_1 81% predicted) and healthy volunteers after inhalation of 1000 micrograms of either drug with single or repeated dosing (6). Taken together, these studies suggest that patients with severe asthma are protected from the systemic adverse effects of high doses of inhaled glucocorticoids, owing to airways obstruction and reduced lung availability. However, as their lung function improves with continued use of the inhaled glucocorticoids, it is likely that the lung availability of inhaled glucocorticoid will increase. This likely outcome is a compelling argument for reducing the dose of inhaled glucocorticoids to a lowest dose that maintains optimal control of asthma and optimal lung function.

Plasma concentrations have been measured in 13 healthy subjects and eight patients with mild asthma using inhaled fluticasone propionate 1000 micrograms bd via Diskus or pressurized metered-dose inhaler and of budesonide 1000 micrograms bd daily via Turbuhaler for 7 days. Twenty-four-hour plasma cortisol concentrations were determined to assess the systemic activity of fluticasone propionate and budesonide. At steady state, the systemic availability of budesonide via Turbuhaler (39%) was significantly higher than that of fluticasone propionate via Diskus (13%) or inhaler (21%). Fluticasone propionate had a larger distribution volume and slower rates of absorption and clearance. Despite a significantly higher pulmonary availability of budesonide via Turbuhaler, plasma cortisol suppression was less than that of fluticasone propionate via inhaler and similar to that of fluticasone propionate via Diskus. There were no differences between healthy subjects and patients with mild asthma in subgroup analyses. However, this study had some limitations as the doses of fluticasone propionate and budesonide were not equipotent, fluticasone being twice as potent as budesonide (7).

The effects of fluticasone 1500 micrograms/day and budesonide 1600 micrograms/day, both by dry powder inhalation, on three systemic markers (urinary concentrations of total cortisol metabolites, morning serum cortisol, and osteocalcin concentrations) have been investigated in 46 healthy and 31 asthmatic subjects (8). Urinary total cortisol metabolite concentrations represented the most sensitive marker of the systemic effects of inhaled glucocorticoids, and were lower in healthy subjects treated with fluticasone than in asthmatic patients, suggesting greater systemic availability of fluticasone in healthy subjects. A similar correlation was not found for budesonide. Fluticasone impaired the hypothalamic–pituitary–adrenal axis more than budesonide, while budesonide significantly lowered serum osteocalcin concentrations, which reflect osteoblastic activity. The authors suggested that different inhaled glucocorticoids have different effects on the hypothalamic–pituitary–adrenal axis and bone metabolism. This study also had its limitations given that the fluticasone and budesonide doses were not equipotent (9).

The safety and efficacy of fluticasone, beclomethasone dipropionate, and budesonide have been compared in a randomized trial in 133 patients with chronic severe asthma who required at least 1750 micrograms/day of beclomethasone/budesonide (10). The patients were randomized to their regular beclomethasone/budesonide or to fluticasone at about half the dose for 6 months. The patients who used fluticasone had a better safety profile, especially with regard to adrenocortical function and bone turnover, while maintaining asthma control. There were significant increases in morning serum cortisol concentrations, the urine cortisol:creatinine ratio, serum osteocalcin, and the serum (deoxy)-pyridinoline:creatinine ratio only with fluticasone, suggesting less suppression of the hypothalamic–pituitary–adrenal axis. The 2:1 potency ratio for clinical efficacy of fluticasone and budesonide/beclomethasone seems to be maintained even at doses of 2000 micrograms/day or higher.

Since many patients with allergic asthma also have rhinitis, they may be taking both inhaled glucocorticoids for their asthma and intranasal formulations for their hay fever. The total systemic availability of glucocorticoids has been studied after the addition of intranasal therapy in patients already taking inhaled glucocorticoids (11) in 12 moderately severe asthmatic subjects (mean FEV_1 84% predicted), who were randomized in a placebo-controlled, two-way, crossover comparison of inhaled fluticasone (880 micrograms bd) plus intranasal fluticasone (200 micrograms od), inhaled triamcinolone (800 micrograms bd) plus intranasal triamcinolone (220 micrograms od), and respective placebos. Both the inhaled glucocorticoids caused significant suppression of adrenocorticoid activity, although the addition of intranasal formulations did not produce further significant suppression. There were more individual subjects with abnormally low cortisol values when intranasal fluticasone was added. These findings suggest that the dose of intranasal glucocorticoids should be taken into account (particularly if used in the long term) when considering the systemic availability of glucocorticoids used in the treatment of asthma and hay fever.

The concept of the L:T ratio in inhalation therapy is a useful one, where L represents the local or lung availability of an inhaled drug and T the total systemic availability. This ratio will be affected by differences in first-pass metabolism. Another important variable that determines the L:T ratio is the inhalation device. The L:T ratio for budesonide is 0.66–0.85, depending on the method of inhalation (12).

Another way of describing the L:T ratio concept is that of "pulmonary targeting." Drug properties that improve pulmonary targeting include slow absorption from the lungs, low oral systemic availability, and rapid systemic clearance.

budesonide = beclomethasone dipropionate > triamcinolone acetonide = flunisolide. Potency differences can be overcome by giving a larger dose of the less potent

drug. However, comparisons between glucocorticoids must measure the systemic effects as well as the lung effect of each dose (13).

Inhalation devices

The importance of the inhalation device has been shown in studies of beclomethasone. Pressurized metered-dose inhalers containing chlorofluorocarbons produce relatively large particles that deposit less than 10% of the delivered dose in the lungs, primarily in the large airways, more than 90% being deposited in the oropharynx. A hydrofluoroalkane beclomethasone multidose aerosol (Qvar 3M Pharmaceuticals) delivers a smaller particle size. More than 50% is deposited in the lungs in animal and mechanical models. This has been confirmed using radiolabelled Qvar in patients with asthma and in healthy volunteers. In these subjects, 50–60% of the dose is deposited throughout the airways and about 30% in the oropharynx. The breath-activated Autohaler provides lung deposition equivalent to an optimally used Qvar inhaler, by automatically delivering drug early in the inhalation. Neither of these devices is improved by the addition of a spacer (14).

Both inhaled and swallowed fractions cause significant systemic activity, the degree of which depends on the inhaler device used. In one study, systemic activity was greater using a dry power inhaler (52%) than a pressurized metered-dose inhaler with a large volume spacer (28%) (15). It was recommended that when high-dose beclomethasone is used, a pressurized metered-dose inhaler with a large volume spacer would help in limiting potential adverse effects.

The systemic availability of inhaled budesonide has been measured in 15 healthy volunteers, using an open crossover design. Each subject was given three treatments, intravenous budesonide 0.5 mg, inhaled budesonide (from a metered-dose inhaler with a Nebuhaler) 1 mg (200 micrograms × 5) plus oral charcoal, and inhaled budesonide 1 mg without oral charcoal. The treatment order was randomized. The mean systemic availability of inhaled budesonide compared with intravenous budesonide was 36% with charcoal and 35% without charcoal, indicating that the absorption of budesonide from the gastrointestinal tract did not contribute to its systemic availability. Pulmonary deposition was 36% with charcoal and 34% without. When the inhaler was used incorrectly, that is, the canister was shaken only before the first of the five inhalations, systemic availability fell by 50%. This shows that the performance of each inhaler is very dependent on proper use (16).

The available studies suggest that fluticasone is more effective than beclomethasone, triamcinolone, or budesonide. However, budesonide delivered by Turbuhaler has equivalent efficacy to fluticasone delivered by metered-dose inhaler or Diskhaler, and is more effective than beclomethasone. When comparative safety is considered, budesonide and triamcinolone delivered by metered-dose inhaler have less systemic activity than fluticasone. Beclomethasone and fluticasone delivered by metered-dose inhaler are equivalent. Budesonide delivered by

Turbuhaler has less systemic activity than fluticasone delivered by Diskhaler (17).

The equivalence of inhaled glucocorticoids based on equipotent (cortisol suppression) effects has been studied by the Asthma Clinical Research Network (ACRN). Six different inhaled glucocorticoids and matched placebos (beclomethasone chlorofluorocarbon, budesonide dry powder inhaler, fluticasone dry powder inhaler, fluticasone chlorofluorocarbon metered-dose inhaler, flunisolide chlorofluorocarbon, and triamcinolone chlorofluorocarbon) were compared by measuring their systemic effects (18). Glucocorticoid-naïve patients with asthma ($n = 156$) were enrolled at six centers and a one-week doubling dose design was used for each of the six inhaled glucocorticoids and matched placebos to a total of four doses. The best outcome variable for the reliable assessment of a systemic effect was the 12-hour AUC of the hourly overnight plasma cortisol measurements from 8 p.m. to 8 a.m. Microgram comparisons of the glucocorticoids could only be performed at 10% cortisol suppression, because fluticasone did not cause higher suppression. The following equipotent doses (that is, doses producing equal systemic cortisol suppression) were found: flunisolide 936 micrograms; triamcinolone 787 micrograms; beclomethasone 548 micrograms; fluticasone dry powder: 445 micrograms; budesonide 268 micrograms; and fluticasone metered-dose inhaler 111 micrograms. The ranking of systemic effects was very similar to that found earlier in a large meta-analysis (19).

Dry powder inhaler and pressurized metered-dose inhaler for administration of low-dose budesonide (400 micrograms/day) have been compared (20). Only the dry powder caused suppression of the hypothalamic–pituitary–adrenal axis. As effective inhaled glucocorticoid therapy is expected to cause detectable reductions in the physiological secretion of cortisol (1), low-dose budesonide by pressurized metered-dose inhaler is probably not effective. In another study, budesonide inhalation suspension, developed for nebulization to meet the specific needs of infants and young children, did not cause significant suppression of hypothalamic–pituitary–adrenal axis function (basal plasma cortisol concentrations and corticotropin test) in doses from 0.25 to 1.0 mg (21). However, inhaled fluticasone propionate by pressurized metered-dose inhaler with a spacer in 62 children resulted in abnormal morning cortisol concentrations in 36% (17 using a low dose of 176 micrograms/day; 43 using a high dose, over 880 micrograms/day) (22).

In a randomized, double-blind study, adult asthmatic patients took budesonide 800 micrograms/day over 12 weeks either by Easyhaler ($n = 103$) or by Turbuhaler ($n = 58$) dry powder inhaler. The Easyhaler was equivalent to the Turbuhaler with regard to safety and efficacy, but was more acceptable to the patients (23).

Therapeutic studies

Budesonide

Inhaled budesonide has been studied in the management of moderately severe, acute asthma in children (24). After treatment with nebulized terbutaline, 11 children were randomly allocated to receive one dose of either budesonide 1600 micrograms by Turbuhaler or prednisolone 2 mg/kg. There was no significant difference in the improvement of the pulmonary index score or peak expiratory flow rate. Children treated with budesonide had an earlier clinical response than those given prednisolone. Prednisolone caused a fall in serum cortisol concentration. The authors concluded that children with moderately severe asthma attacks could be effectively treated with a short-term course of inhaled budesonide, starting with a high dose and reducing over the following week.

In 81 patients with acute asthma, mean age 38 years, inhaled budesonide 1600 micrograms bd via Turbuhaler was compared with oral prednisolone (40 mg on day 1, reducing to 5 mg by day 7) in a randomized, double-blind, parallel-group design (25). The mean increase in FEV_1 from baseline to day 7 was 17% with budesonide and 18% with prednisolone. Mean values of morning peak expiratory flow rate increased from day 1 to day 7 by 67 l/second with budesonide and by 57 l/second with prednisolone. There were no statistically significant differences between the groups in either symptoms or the number of doses of rescue medication. The authors concluded that high-dose inhaled budesonide may be a substitute for oral therapy in the treatment of an acute attack of asthma.

The effect of supplementary inhaled budesonide in acute asthma has been evaluated in a randomized, double-blind comparison with standard treatment in 44 children aged 6 months to 18 years with a moderate to severe exacerbation of asthma (26). Prednisone 1 mg/kg orally and nebulized salbutamol (0.15 mg/kg) every 30 minutes for three doses and then every hour for 4 hours were given to all children. In addition, each child was given 2 mg of nebulized budesonide or nebulized isotonic saline. There was a more rapid discharge rate in the budesonide group. There were no adverse effects. The authors concluded that nebulized budesonide may be an effective adjunct to oral prednisone in the management of moderate to severe exacerbations of asthma.

Fluticasone

Inhaled fluticasone 500 micrograms bd from a pressurized metered-dose inhaler for 6 months has been compared with placebo in a randomized, double-blind trial in 280 patients with COPD, aged 50–75 years (27). There was no significant difference in the number of patients who suffered one or more exacerbations. Moderate or severe exacerbations occurred significantly more often with placebo than with fluticasone. Diary-card scores, morning peak expiratory flow rate, clinic FEV_1, FVC, and midexpiratory flow all improved significantly with fluticasone. Scores for median daily cough and sputum volume were significantly lower with fluticasone than with placebo. At the end of treatment, patients using fluticasone had increased their 6-minute walking distance significantly more than those using placebo. Fluticasone propionate was tolerated, as well as placebo, with few adverse effects and no clinically important effect on mean serum cortisol concentration. The authors suggested that inhaled glucocorticoids may have an important place in the long-term management of patients with COPD.

Local adverse effects

The local adverse effects of inhaled glucocorticoids have been studied in a prospective, cross-sectional, cohort study in 639 asthmatic children using beclomethasone (721 micrograms/day) or budesonide (835 micrograms/day) for at least one month (28). The local adverse effects included cough (40%), thirst (22%), hoarseness (14%), dysphonia (11%), oral candidiasis (11%), perioral dermatitis (2.9%), and tongue hypertrophy (0.1%). A spacer doubled the incidence of coughing.

Potent glucocorticoids in high local doses increase the risk of local infection and even promote atrophy of the bronchial mucosa. The latter effect has not proved clinically important, but there is an increased incidence of oropharyngeal candidiasis. The incidence varies depending on the population studied and the criteria used to make the diagnosis; candidiasis can affect 13–71% of patients, the highest incidence being seen with doses up to 0.8 mg. Candidiasis rarely requires treatment or withdrawal of the drug. Local measures, such as gargling immediately after inhalation of the aerosol, and the use of a large-volume spacer are effective in reducing the incidence of this complication. However, candidiasis can result in dysphonia.

A local myopathy caused by inhaled glucocorticoids can also cause dysphonia. However, patients with asthma have more dysphonia and vocal fold pathology than healthy controls and inhaled glucocorticoids can improve the voice in some patients (SEDA-21, 188).

In some patients, the propellant used in certain aerosols can cause acute bronchoconstriction (SEDA-6, 332).

Organs and Systems

Sensory systems

Cataract

In a population-based cross-sectional study of vision and common eye diseases in 3654 people, 49–97 years of age, inhaled glucocorticoid use was reported by 370 subjects, of whom 164 reported current use and 206 previous use. Subjects who reported using inhaled glucocorticoids had a higher prevalence of nuclear cataracts (OR = 1.5; CI = 1.2, 1.9) and posterior subcapsular cataracts (OR = 1.9; CI = 1.3, 2.8). The highest prevalence (27%) was in patients whose lifetime dose was more than 2000 mg (relative prevalence 5.5) (SEDA-22, 187).

In 3677 patients undergoing cataract extraction over 2 years compared with a matched control group of 21 868 people, the patients were more likely to undergo cataract extraction if they had used inhaled glucocorticoids for more than 3 years (OR = 3.06; CI = 1.53, 6.13). This risk was not significant in patients who used low to medium doses (1000 micrograms/day or less) when the OR was 1.63 (CI = 0.85, 3.13) after 2 years. The OR was higher in

patients using average daily doses of beclomethasone dipropionate or budesonide (over 1000 micrograms) (OR = 3.40; CI = 1.49, 7.76) after more than 2 years of treatment (29).

In a nested case-control analysis based on a retrospective, observational, cohort study, 103 289 asthmatic patients using inhaled glucocorticoids were identified from the UK General Practice Database and were compared with 98 527 asthmatic patients with no history of glucocorticoid use (30). There was a slightly increased risk of cataract in those who used inhaled glucocorticoids (RR = 1.3; 95% CI = 1.1, 1.5). The relative risk of cataract was 2.0 in oral glucocorticoid users relative to glucocorticoid non-users (95% CI = 1.5, 2.2). The risk ratio increased with extensive use of inhaled glucocorticoids, but not with moderate use. The association of extensive use with cataract was most pronounced in those aged 70 years and over, and there was no effect in those aged under 40. The increased risk of cataract in patients aged 70 years and over persisted after controlling for cataract risk factors, such as smoking, diabetes mellitus, hypertension, and sex.

In another study, treatment for 2 years with fluticasone propionate (500 micrograms bd) had no significant effect on ophthalmic parameters (glaucoma and posterior subcapsular cataracts) (31). Slit lamp examinations were carried out in 157 asthmatic children treated with inhaled budesonide at a mean daily dose of 504 (range 189–1322) micrograms for 3–6 years (mean 4.4 years). Posterior subcapsular cataract due to budesonide was not detected (32).

Glaucoma

A case-control study compared 9793 patients with open-angle glaucoma or ocular hypertension to 38 325 randomly selected controls (33). There was no association between the use of inhaled or intranasal glucocorticoids and the risk of open-angle glaucoma or ocular hypertension. In patients who were currently using high doses, there was a small but significant increase in risk (OR = 1.44; CI = 1.01, 2.06).

Psychological

High doses of oral glucocorticoids can cause adverse psychiatric effects, including mild euphoria, emotional lability, panic attacks, psychosis, and delirium. There have been sporadic case reports of similar reactions in patients using inhaled glucocorticoids. Of 60 preschool children with a recent diagnosis of asthma taking inhaled budesonide 100–200 micrograms/day, nine had suspected psychological adverse events after 18 months, according to their parents (34). The symptoms reported were irritability, depression, aggressiveness, excitability, and hyperactivity. These adverse events disappeared when the medication was terminated or reduced and recurred when budesonide was restarted at higher doses. Most of the symptoms occurred within 2 days from starting the high dose (200 micrograms 2–4 times a day).

Endocrine

Hypothalamic–pituitary–adrenal axis function provides one of the most sensitive markers of the systemic activity of inhaled glucocorticoids (35), and suppression can be used as a surrogate marker for adverse effects of inhaled glucocorticoids in other tissues.

The different methods of assessing hypothalamic–pituitary–adrenal axis activity in patients using inhaled glucocorticoids have been compared (36). The AUC of serum cortisol concentrations was the most reliable method. There were significant positive correlations between AUC and the 8 a.m. serum and salivary cortisol concentrations. The authors favored the non-invasive method of salivary concentration measurement. However, 24-hour urine collection is not recommended, as it correlated only moderately well. This finding is consistent with the results of other studies. Urinary free-cortisol estimation based on immunoassay after inhaled glucocorticoids may be an unreliable surrogate marker of adrenal suppression, and studies using this method should be interpreted with caution (37).

A review of the literature from 1 January 1966 to 31 July 1998 identified 27 studies in which the effects of inhaled glucocorticoids on adrenal function were measured. A meta-regression of adrenal suppression in these 27 studies showed that adrenal suppression occurred with high doses of inhaled glucocorticoids (above 1500 micrograms/day; 750 micrograms/day for fluticasone propionate). However, there is a considerable degree of interindividual susceptibility. Meta-analysis showed significantly greater potency for dose-related adrenal suppression with fluticasone propionate compared with beclomethasone dipropionate, budesonide, or triamcinolone acetonide. Prednisolone and fluticasone propionate were approximately equivalent in a dose ratio of 10:1 (19).

Beclomethasone

Adrenal function has been assessed by low-dose adrenocorticotropin (ACTH) stimulation in 12 adult asthmatic patients using inhaled beclomethasone (200–900 micrograms/day) before and after switching to inhaled fluticasone (200–600 micrograms/day) (38). Switching from beclomethasone to fluticasone led to a 40% reduction in corticosteroid dosage, improved lung function, and caused a significant rise in the adrenal gland response to ACTH. The reduced risk of adrenal gland suppression associated with fluticasone was most notably due to a lower overall dose of inhaled glucocorticoids.

Budesonide

The effects of budesonide aqueous nasal spray (64 micrograms/day) on adrenal function were studied in a 6-week double-blind, placebo-controlled study in 78 patients with allergic rhinitis aged 2–5 years (39). Adrenal function, evaluated by the mean change in morning plasma cortisol concentration after cosyntropin stimulation, was not suppressed. This dose of budesonide by nasal spray is unlikely to have significant systemic activity.

Ciclesonide

The effect of inhaled ciclesonide on adrenal function has been analysed in 164 asthmatic adults in a double-blind, randomized, placebo-controlled study (40). The patients used ciclesonide 320 micrograms once daily, ciclesonide 320 micrograms twice daily, or fluticasone propionate 440 micrograms twice daily for 12 weeks. Adrenal function was significantly suppressed by fluticasone propionate but not by ciclesonide. Oral candidiasis was reported in 2.4% of patients on ciclesonide versus 22% of patients on fluticasone propionate. Even high daily doses of ciclesonide up to 1280 micrograms did not suppress adrenal function, as measured by 24-hour urinary cortisol excretion (41). This is in accordance with other studies in asthmatic subjects, in which serum or 24-hour urinary cortisol concentrations were unchanged by ciclesonide (42–48).

A pharmacokinetic–pharmacodynamic modelling analysis pooled data from 635 adults and children using ciclesonide in daily doses of 40–2880 micrograms to study the effect of ciclesonide on endogenous cortisol release (49). Using an E_{max} model, less than 1% of all observed desisobutyrylciclesonide concentrations were higher than the EC_{50} for cortisol suppression, indicating negligible changes in cortisol concentrations at therapeutically relevant doses. Systemic availability was estimated to be about 50% in patients with impaired liver function, compared with healthy individuals, but this was unlikely to be clinically significant.

In general, ciclesonide in daily doses of up to 640 micrograms can be considered to be safe with respect to adrenal function. Its long-term safety profile is similarly advantageous, and administration in daily doses up to 1280 micrograms over 52 weeks was not associated with systemic or local adverse effects in patients with persistent asthma (50).

Fluticasone

While suppression of adrenal gland function is associated with daily doses of fluticasone above 750 micrograms, the impact of concurrent moderate-dose fluticasone and oral steroids on adrenal response is unknown. Adult patients using intranasal steroids, low-dose fluticasone (440 micrograms/day), or high-dose fluticasone (880 micrograms/day) underwent a low-dose co-syntropin stimulation test to assess adrenal response before and 2 days after oral prednisone 60 mg/day (51). One of 31 control patients and one of 13 patients using moderate-dose fluticasone had suppressed adrenal gland function on the second day of oral prednisone, which normalized by the second week of treatment. However, 14 of 19 patients using high-dose fluticasone had suppressed adrenal gland function on day 2 with recovery in 10 of the 19 patients within 4 weeks. In conclusion, concurrent standard-dose oral prednisone burst and moderate-dose fluticasone transiently suppress adrenal gland function, while concurrent high-dose fluticasone leads to prolonged impairment. Patients using high-dose fluticasone should be closely monitored.

Six patients with pre-existing HIV-lipodystrophy developed symptomatic Cushing's syndrome when treated with inhaled fluticasone at varying doses for asthma while concurrently taking low-dose ritonavir-boosted protease inhibitor antiretroviral regimens for HIV infection (52). Stimulation studies showed evidence of adrenal suppression in all patients. After withdrawal of inhaled fluticasone, four patients developed symptomatic hypoadrenalism, and three required oral glucocorticoid support for several months. Other complications included evidence of osteoporosis (n = 3), crush fractures (n = 1), and exacerbation of pre-existing type 2 diabetes mellitus (n = 1).

In a randomized, placebo-controlled study, the activity of the hypothalamic–pituitary–adrenal axis was assessed at baseline and after 21 days by determining 22-hour time-integrated serum cortisol concentrations, 24-hour urinary cortisol (corrected for creatinine), and morning salivary cortisol concentrations in 153 patients with mild to moderate asthma, randomly assigned to either inhaled flunisolide (500 or 1000 micrograms bd), inhaled fluticasone (110, 220, 330, or 440 micrograms bd), oral prednisone (7.5 mg/day), or placebo (19). Flunisolide and fluticasone caused dose-dependent suppression of the hypothalamic–pituitary–adrenal axis, and fluticasone was significantly more potent. However, the lowest fluticasone dose (110 micrograms/day) had no effect. These findings are consistent with those of a previous meta-analysis, which showed that fluticasone caused a greater dose-related suppression of the hypothalamic–pituitary–adrenal axis than other inhaled glucocorticoids (53). Fluticasone is more lipophilic than flunisolide and therefore has a larger volume of distribution and a longer half-life (35), but it is not clear how this might be associated with the larger effect described here.

The effect of fluticasone aqueous nasal spray on the hypothalamic–pituitary–adrenal axis has been compared with that of oral prednisone and placebo, using a 6-hour tetracosactide infusion test in a 4-week, randomized, double-blind, placebo-controlled study in 105 adults with allergic rhinitis randomly assigned to receive fluticasone 200 micrograms od, fluticasone 400 micrograms bd, oral prednisone 7.5 mg od, oral prednisone 15 mg od, or placebo (54). Fluticasone 400 micrograms bd and both doses of prednisone caused a significant reduction in the morning plasma cortisol concentration. The two fluticasone treatments produced no significant change in the hypothalamic–pituitary–adrenal axis response to co-syntropin. This contrasted with oral prednisone 7.5 or 15 mg od, which significantly reduced both plasma cortisol concentrations after co-syntropin and 24-hour urinary cortisol excretion.

Mometasone

The effect of increasing doses of mometasone furoate and fluticasone propionate by dry powder inhaler on adrenal function was studied by using overnight urinary cortisol in 21 patients with asthma (55). Patients were randomized in a crossover fashion to receive 2-weekly consecutive doubling doses of either fluticasone propionate (500, 1000, and 2000 micrograms/day) or mometasone furoate (400, 800, and 1600 micrograms/day). Both treatments were associated with significant suppression of adrenal function at high and medium doses.

Adrenal suppression with DPI formulations of mometasone furoate and fluticasone propionate has been studied in 21 asthmatic patients in a randomized crossover study (56). Every 2 weeks the patients used consecutive doubling incremental doses of either mometasone furoate via Twisthaler™ (400, 800, and 1600 micrograms/day) or fluticasone propionate via Accuhaler™ (500, 1000, and 2000 micrograms/day). There was significant suppression of adrenal function with both mometasone furoate and fluticasone propionate at high and medium doses.

Triamcinolone

The effect of inhaled triamcinolone on adrenal response has been assessed in 221 patients with chronic obstructive airway disease in a randomized placebo-controlled trial (57). The patients received either inhaled triamcinolone 1200 micrograms/day or placebo for 3 years. Basal cortisol concentrations were significantly lower with triamcinolone than placebo after 1 and 3 years. Cortisol concentrations were not suppressed at 30 minutes and 60 minutes after co-syntropin injection. The authors concluded that triamcinolone is safe in chronic obstructive airway disease patients at the tested dose with respect to adrenal gland response.

Adrenal suppression by inhaled glucocorticoids in children

Inhaled glucocorticoids are being prescribed more and more in younger children at an earlier stage of their disease and for longer periods; children with severe asthma are also treated with larger doses than licensed. Therefore, considerations of their systemic effects are of importance. Symptomatic adrenal insufficiency has been reported in children after various regimens of inhaled glucocorticoids.

- Four boys 4–8 years old with symptomatic adrenal insufficiency had all used consistent high doses of fluticasone propionate 1000–1500 micrograms/day over extended periods (16 months to 5 years) (58). They presented with acute hypoglycemia secondary to iatrogenic adrenal suppression, with abnormal corticotropin tests, although none had Cushingoid features.
- A 33-year-old man and three children (two girls, one boy, 7–9 years) presented with symptomatic adrenal insufficiency (59). All three children had seizures because of hypoglycemia, and the man had a low blood pressure, nausea, and fatigue. In all cases, corticotropin tests were abnormal, showing adrenal insufficiency. The children had used fluticasone propionate 500–2000 micrograms/day and the man had recently switched from fluticasone propionate 1000–2000 micrograms/day to budesonide dry powder inhaler 800 micrograms/day. Only one of the children had used oral glucocorticoids in the previous year.
- A 21-month-old boy had a hypoglycemia-induced seizure in the setting of adrenal suppression (60). He had been given increasing doses of budesonide up to

2000 micrograms qds and oral glucocorticoids until the age of 15 months.

- A 32-month-old girl developed hypoglycemic seizures (61). She had been given fluticasone propionate 440–880 micrograms/day and up to 5 months before the incident oral glucocorticoids.

- Two girls aged 11 and 16 years, one boy aged 12 years, and one woman aged 54 years developed hypothalamic–pituitary–adrenal axis suppression during treatment with inhaled fluticasone propionate 220–880 micrograms bd for long-term control of asthma; however, two of the patients also took oral prednisone or prednisolone (62). Because of poor growth, an 8-year-old girl's asthma medication was changed from budesonide to fluticasone propionate 250 micrograms/day (63). However, 5 months later she had developed a round face. Her early morning cortisol concentration was less than 30 nmol/l (reference range 140–720) and her growth had been no more than 0.5 cm during the past 5 months. Fluticasone propionate was discontinued. After 1 month, her Cushingoid features had resolved and her fasting morning cortisol concentration was 310 nmol/l.

- A 32-year-old woman's asthma regimen was changed from budesonide to fluticasone propionate 500 micrograms/day and salmeterol (44). Eight months later, she was evaluated because of excessive bodyweight gain; her serum cortisol concentration was 16 nmol/l. Fluticasone propionate was replaced with nedocromil and 1 month later her serum cortisol concentration had normalized.

In addition to these case reports, there has been a survey of symptomatic adrenal suppression associated with inhaled glucocorticoids in the UK (64). Only 24% of the questionnaires were returned (709 responses), and there were 28 cases of symptomatic adrenal suppression reported in children and five in adults (including the 10 cases discussed above). The children presented mostly with hypoglycemia and coma, whereas the adults mainly had lethargy and nausea. No obvious precipitating cause was found in 65% of the cases. In four children, diagnosis was delayed by 3 months to 2 years. All but three patients had been treated with fluticasone propionate alone, but at high daily doses (children 500–2000 micrograms, adults 1000–2000 micrograms). One child had used both fluticasone propionate and budesonide, and one adult and one child used beclomethasone dipropionate.

A series of cases has illustrated the unexpected occurrence of symptomatic adrenal insufficiency in eight asthmatic children using inhaled glucocorticoids (65). The authors concluded that therapeutic doses of inhaled glucocorticoids can provoke paradoxical symptoms of adrenal insufficiency. Very high doses (calculated according to body surface area) may partly explain marked suppression of the hypothalamic–pituitary–adrenal axis. The need to taper inhaled glucocorticoid doses and to recognize the possibility of life-threatening acute adrenal insufficiency is of utmost importance.

In a double-blind, randomized pilot study of the efficacy and adverse effects of inhaled fluticasone in 25 newborn preterm infants who required mechanical ventilation for treatment of respiratory distress syndrome, the infants were randomized to receive inhaled fluticasone 1000 micrograms/day or placebo (66). The hypothalamic–pituitary–adrenal axis was assessed by the response to corticotropin-releasing factor. All basal and post-stimulation plasma corticotropin and serum cortisol concentrations were significantly less with inhaled fluticasone than placebo. Cumulative high-dose inhaled glucocorticoids caused moderately severe suppression of both the pituitary and the adrenal glands. This systemic activity is probably associated with pulmonary vascular absorption that avoids hepatic first-pass metabolism.

Chronic inhalation of beclomethasone dipropionate (up to 1000 micrograms/day) can produce adrenal suppression in some children. This effect is reduced by the attachment of a large volume spacer to the aerosol (SEDA-21, 188). Budesonide inhaled from the Turbuhaler, at doses of 800 or 1600 micrograms/day), did not produce any statistically significant suppression of the hypothalamic–pituitary–adrenal axis compared with placebo. The reduction was significant only after 3200 micrograms/day of budesonide when suppression equivalent to 10 mg/day oral prednisone was seen (67). Fluticasone propionate powder, 500 micrograms bd, given using a Diskhaler, for 104 weeks caused only minimal changes in the hypothalamic–pituitary–adrenal axis (31). Inhaled fluticasone propionate 400 micrograms/day for 8 weeks did not cause adrenal suppression in asthmatic children. In children, the benefit/risk ratio generally decreases at doses above 400 micrograms/day of fluticasone propionate (68). Hypothalamic–pituitary–adrenal axis suppression has been reported with inhaled fluticasone propionate at doses in excess of 1000 micrograms/day (SEDA-21, 188).

Endocrine effects of budesonide have been assessed in 29 asthmatic children aged 6 months to 3 years by measuring fasting plasma cortisol concentrations and performing an ACTH stimulation test in a double-blind, randomized, placebo-controlled study (69). The patients received budesonide either 2 mg followed by a stepwise reduction of 25% every second day or 0.5 mg/day or placebo for 8 days. Neither fasting nor 1-hour post-stimulation plasma cortisol concentrations differed in any group.

Adrenal function was suppressed by high-dose inhaled budesonide (400–900 micrograms/m^2/day) in a dose-related manner in 19 children aged 5–12 years (70). Baseline assessments showed significantly less adrenal suppression with budesonide than beclomethasone at comparable doses. In a subsequent randomized, double-blind, placebo-controlled study in 404 asthmatic children aged 6–18 years, inhaled budesonide at a daily dose of up to 800 micrograms for 12 weeks was associated with adrenal suppression in 12%, but adrenal suppression was not clinically apparent in any of the children (71). In a case-control study, 21% of asthmatic children using therapeutic doses of budesonide had signs and symptoms of adrenal suppression (72), but these were not clinically important. Current data suggest individual idiosyncratic sensitivity of some children to inhaled glucocorticoids: eight cases of symptomatic adrenal insufficiency have been identified with therapeutic doses of budesonide (73).

The long-term effects of budesonide on adrenal function have been assessed in 63 asthmatic children using budesonide 400 micrograms/day, nedocromil 16 mg/day, or placebo over 3 years (74). There were no differences in serum cortisol concentrations after ACTH stimulation between the three treatment groups, regardless of the time after ACTH administration or months of follow-up. Cumulative inhaled glucocorticoid exposure did not affect the serum cortisol response to ACTH or urinary free cortisol excretion at 3 years.

Short-term lower-leg growth rate and adrenal function was assessed in 24 children aged 6–12 years using increasing doses of ciclesonide (40, 80, and 160 micrograms) in a randomized, double-blind, placebo-controlled, crossover study (75). Ciclesonide had no effect on lower-leg growth rate or adrenal function.

In a cross-sectional study, adrenal function was assessed in 50 asthmatic children and adolescents using high-dose inhaled fluticasone, by measuring early morning serum cortisol and tetracosactrin stimulation (76). The mean fluticasone daily dose was 925 micrograms for a mean duration of 2 years. In 36 patients with morning serum cortisol concentration less than 400 nmol/l a tetracosactrin stimulation test showed that six had a pathological response. Biochemical evidence of impaired adrenal gland function was thus found in 12% of the patients, suggesting that high-dose fluticasone can be associated with dose-dependent adrenocortical suppression.

Different inhaled glucocorticoids have been compared for their suppressing effects on the hypothalamic–pituitary–adrenal axis (18). In a large meta-analysis, budesonide or beclomethasone dipropionate in doses of over 1500 micrograms/day was associated with adrenal suppression in adults (19). In children, fluticasone propionate 200 micrograms/day or budesonide 400 micrograms/day caused detectable adrenal gland suppression (77). For interpretation of the different studies, it is very important to distinguish between detectable indicators for systemic drug action (that is, reduced morning cortisol) and true suppression of the hypothalamic–pituitary–adrenal axis, as determined by adrenal function tests (standard-dose or low-dose corticotropin test), which are more predictive of possible systemic adverse effects (1).

The fact that fluticasone propionate is involved in the vast majority of the published cases should be discussed further. The systemic concentration of an inhaled glucocorticoid depends on the absorbed fraction of the drug in the gut and in the lung. Swallowed fluticasone propionate is almost completely metabolized in the liver by CYP3A4 (first-pass effect over 99.9%) before reaching the systemic circulation; however, its metabolic clearance can be altered in patients with low CYP3A4 expression and activity (78). Pulmonary absorbed fluticasone propionate is very potent; because of its pronounced lipophilicity, it binds with higher affinity to glucocorticoid receptors and has a larger distribution volume and a longer half-life than other inhaled glucocorticoids (79). These characteristics give it the potential of accumulating with multiple doses.

Other factors that determine the absorbed fraction of inhaled glucocorticoids include the age of the child, as lung deposition of inhaled drugs increases with age (80). Therefore, the minimum effective dose may fall as the child becomes older. Moreover, it is reasonable to hypothesize that systemic absorption will increase once asthma control is established (81). Furthermore, patient adherence and inhaler technique are two factors that can have a large influence on the amount of glucocorticoid inhaled and absorbed.

However, the most important factor is the dose. The safety and efficacy of fluticasone propionate in children in daily doses of 100–200 micrograms have been demonstrated in many studies (82). The doses in the case reports of symptomatic adrenal suppression have to be considered as being excessively high. These reports reflect excessive dosing of inhaled glucocorticoids, and in some cases a residual effect of previous oral glucocorticoid treatment cannot be excluded. The use of excessive doses is empirical and not supported by the literature. All inhaled glucocorticoids have a flat dose–response curve (83). Extensive clinical experience with inhaled glucocorticoids over the past 20 years has suggested that the risk of adrenal insufficiency with inhaled glucocorticoids alone is very low when recommended doses are used (84). To avoid symptomatic adrenal suppression, the lowest effective dose should always be used. Before automatically increasing the dose in refractory patients, the diagnosis should be reconsidered. Furthermore, a reduction in the dosage of inhaled glucocorticoid can also be achieved with the addition of adjuvant therapies, such as leukotriene receptor antagonists and long-acting β_2-adrenoceptor agonists (85).

Monitoring children using inhaled glucocorticoids has been discussed (1). Children using low to moderate doses of inhaled glucocorticoids (up to 200 micrograms of fluticasone propionate or budesonide) do not require routine hypothalamic–pituitary–adrenal axis measurement. In children using consistently higher doses (up to 400 micrograms of fluticasone propionate or budesonide) or using glucocorticoids by other routes, morning plasma cortisol should be monitored periodically because of the increased risk of clinically significant adrenal suppression. If cortisol concentrations are below 276 µmol/l (100 ng/ml), functional testing of the hypothalamic–pituitary–adrenal axis should be considered.

Metabolism

Impaired diabetic control has been reported with high doses of inhaled glucocorticoids.

- A 67-year-old man with asthma and non-insulin-dependent diabetes mellitus, taking glibenclamide 5 mg/day and metformin 1700 mg/day, had glycated hemoglobin concentrations of 7.0–7.3% (86). For asthma, he used nebulized ipratropium bromide 0.5 mg and salbutamol 5 mg qds. He was given inhaled fluticasone propionate 2000 micrograms/day by metered-dose inhaler through a Volumatic spacer device, with beneficial effect. In the third week he developed persistent glycosuria and the dose of fluticasone was reduced stepwise to 500 micrograms/day. He was then rechallenged by increasing his daily dose of fluticasone from 500 to 1000 micrograms. Within a week he had glycosuria, which again resolved on reduction of the dose of fluticasone. His glycated hemoglobin concentration rose to 7.8% after 1000 micrograms/day and to 8.2% after 2000 micrograms/day.

- Deterioration in glucose control occurred in a 64-year-old man with non-insulin-dependent diabetes mellitus (87). High doses of both fluticasone (2000 micrograms/day) and budesonide (2000 micrograms/day) had produced glycosuria despite treatment with glibenclamide and metformin 1700 mg/day. On reducing the dose of budesonide, there was a commensurate fall in glycosylated hemoglobin and glycosuria. There was no glycosuria at a daily maintenance dose of 800 micrograms and the glycosylated hemoglobin fell from 8.2 to 7.2%.

The association between inhaled glucocorticoids and the risk of diabetes mellitus in elderly people (over 65 years) has been investigated in two Canadian studies. In a nested case-control study of the association between current use of inhaled glucocorticoids and the risk of using antidiabetic drugs among 21 645 subjects the risk of diabetes was not statistically significant (88). Moreover, there was no statistically significant increase in risk among users of high-dose beclomethasone compared with non-users. In a retrospective population-based cohort study using administrative databases, the association between oral and inhaled glucocorticoid use and the onset of diabetes mellitus in the elderly was quantified (89). Users of proton pump inhibitors ($n = 53\ 845$) were the controls. Relative to controls, oral glucocorticoid users ($n = 31\ 864$) were more likely to develop diabetes mellitus, but there was no association between the use of inhaled glucocorticoids ($n = 38\ 441$) and diabetes mellitus. These results suggest that the use of inhaled glucocorticoids in elderly people does not significantly increase the risk of diabetes mellitus.

Skin

Reduced skin thickness
Skin thickness (measured with ultrasound) was not significantly different from controls in patients taking low-dose beclomethasone dipropionate (200–800 micrograms/day). There was a reduction in skin thickness of 15–19% in patients using high dose beclomethasone dipropionate (1000–2500 micrograms/day), and 28–33% in patients using long-term oral prednisolone (5–20 mg/day). Bruising occurred in 12% of controls, 33% of patients using low-dose beclomethasone dipropionate, 48% of patients using high-dose beclomethasone dipropionate, and 80% of patients using oral prednisolone (90). Other workers have concluded that patients using beclomethasone dipropionate who report bruising are older (61 versus 52 years), take higher daily doses (1388 versus 1067 micrograms), and have been on treatment longer (55 versus 43 months) (91). The number of bruises

seems to be inversely related to the concentration of urinary cortisol (SEDA-21, 188). In children using budesonide (189–1322 micrograms/day) for 3–6 years, there was no increase in bruising (32).

The effect of long-term inhaled glucocorticoids (800–1000 micrograms/day of either budesonide or beclomethasone) on skin collagen synthesis and thickness has been prospectively investigated in 27 consecutive new asthmatic patients (92). Asthma was treated with a moderate dosage of inhaled glucocorticoids. Skin thickness was measured before treatment and at 3 and 6 months using ultrasound on the abdomen and the upper right arm. Suction blisters were induced on the abdominal skin using a disposable suction blister device. Blister fluid was collected and kept frozen for radioimmunoassay of PINP and PIIINP. Skin punch biopsies were taken from the abdominal wall for the determination of skin hydroxyproline. After 1–2 years, 20 subjects attended for a further measurement of skin thickness. Control data were obtained in 14 healthy women who were followed for 6 months. PINP and PIIINP concentrations in blister fluid were followed in eight male volunteers for 1 year. There was no significant change in abdominal skin thickness after 6 months of inhaled glucocorticoids. In the upper arm there was a small, significant reduction from 1.64 to 1.50 mm after 6 months. After 1–2 years the skin thickness in the abdomen and upper arm was unchanged in 14 subjects who had used only inhaled glucocorticoids, but in six patients who had taken supplementary oral glucocorticoids for one to several weeks there was thinning of the skin in the upper arm but not the abdomen. The procollagen propeptides were markedly reduced in blister fluid at 3 and 6 months. There was no significant change in skin collagen expressed as hydroxyproline. Thus, despite evidence of a reduction in collagen synthesis, skin thickness and collagen did not change, possibly because the degradation and turnover of collagen slowed down. However, in the six patients who subsequently used oral glucocorticoids, skin thickness decreased.

Bruising
Since the original observation of the association between high-dose glucocorticoids and purpura and dermal thinning, easy bruising of the skin has become recognized as a systemic adverse effect of inhaled glucocorticoids (90). In a double-blind crossover study 69 asthmatic subjects received either the usual dose of beclomethasone dipropionate or fluticasone (at half the dose of beclomethasone) both for 4 months (93). The frequency and severity of skin bruising were assessed by questionnaire, and the numbers of bruises were assessed by direct examination. The dose of fluticasone was selected on the basis of previous studies that showed that it had comparable efficacy when given in half the dose of beclomethasone. This dose of fluticasone had comparable efficacy with respect to the control of asthma, but there was no skin bruising. These findings suggest that the systemic availability of equieffective doses of fluticasone is less than that of beclomethasone.

Contact allergy

Nasal glucocorticoids and inhaled glucocorticoids can have adverse effects on the nose and mouth, including pruritus, burning, dryness, erythema, edema, dry cough, and odynophagia; less commonly, they can cause eczema and urticaria, particularly on the face. Contact dermatitis to glucocorticoids can be facilitated by impaired epithelial barriers, and has been found in 4.7% of patients receiving topical hydrocortisone (94). Inhaled glucocorticoids can cause hypersensitivity reactions, especially in patients with chronic eczema who have been sensitized to local glucocorticoids.

Tixocortol pivalate is a marker for glucocorticoid contact allergy, as a positive patch test suggests established contact allergy to hydrocortisone, prednisolone, and their derivatives (95). A literature search via Medline from 1966 to May 2000 revealed only one patient hypersensitive to tixocortol pivalate and budesonide in a pilot study in 34 patients (10 with asthma, 13 with rhinitis, 11 with both) (96). From case reports, the prevalence of glucocorticoid-induced contact allergy has been estimated at 2.9–5%.

Based on these observations it has been concluded that patients who use inhaled glucocorticoids and develop unprecedented skin reactions during therapy should be tested for glucocorticoid-related contact allergy (97). Switching from one of the four main glucocorticoid groups to another might prove successful in these cases.

Two cases of perioral dermatitis have been associated with the use of inhaled glucocorticoids (98).

- A 38-year-old woman who had used inhaled beclomethasone daily (dosage not stated) during the winter for the past 5 years for mild asthma, developed a perioral rash with numerous small pustules and papules. She stopped using beclomethasone and was treated with oral erythromycin and topical tretinoin. Her rash resolved within 4 weeks. One year later, she restarted beclomethasone and her rash reappeared after 2 weeks. There was no recurrence of her perioral dermatitis during subsequent treatment with monthly intramuscular injections of betamethasone.
- A 46-year-old woman, who had used inhaled budesonide (dosage not stated) for 8 years for vasomotor rhinitis, developed a recurrent perioral rash, which responded to treatment with oral erythromycin 1 g/day for 6 weeks. One year later, she had a recurrence, which resolved with oral erythromycin. She continued to use inhaled budesonide.

As cross-reactivity within glucocorticoid groups may be clinically relevant, skin patch testing has been proposed in cases of suspected glucocorticoid allergy, to identify the substances that can be safely administered (99). The prevalence of glucocorticoid allergy has been studied by skin patch testing in 30 patients using inhaled or intranasal glucocorticoids (100). Four patients had a positive patch test (three allergic reactions and one irritant reaction). Eight different glucocorticoids were used, but allergic reactions occurred only with budesonide. The authors therefore suggested that budesonide is more likely to cause contact hypersensitivity, but also referred to the possible relevance of allergic or irritant reactions to preservatives.

Contact allergy to glucocorticoids is not rare in patients with atopic dermatitis. In patients with known contact allergy to budesonide, allergic skin reactions can also occur when inhaled forms of the drug are used, as shown by a randomized, double-blind, placebo-controlled study in 15 non-asthmatic patients with budesonide hypersensitivity on patch testing (101). In four of seven patients who used inhaled budesonide, there was reactivation of the 6-week-old patch test sites and they had new distant skin lesions. No flare-up reactions were observed in the other 11 patients (three had used inhaled budesonide and eight placebo for 1 week). None of the patients developed respiratory symptoms; spirometry and peak expiratory flow rates remained normal.

Musculoskeletal

Bone

Studies of the effects of inhaled glucocorticoids have used biochemical markers of bone function and imaging techniques to assess bone mineral density. Some of the biochemical markers are summarized in Table 1. Initial, short-term studies caused concern about the effect of inhaled glucocorticoids on bone metabolism. Beclomethasone dipropionate 2000 micrograms/day reduced serum osteocalcin concentrations at 1 and 2 weeks, and they returned to normal at 1 and 2 weeks after withdrawal. Nebulized budesonide (2000 micrograms bd) produced a similar increase in FEV_1 to oral prednisolone 30 mg/day given over 5 days. Serum osteocalcin was significantly higher: 2.3 (0.9–3.7) ng/ml with budesonide compared with 0.6 (0–1.2) ng/ml with prednisolone. The 24-hour urinary calcium to creatinine ratio was significantly lower in patients treated with nebulized budesonide (SEDA-22, 183). After 4 weeks on beclomethasone dipropionate or budesonide 800 micrograms/day, there were significant but paradoxical changes in osteocalcin and PICP (both markers of bone formation). Osteocalcin concentrations fell, but PICP concentrations rose. Patients on beclomethasone dipropionate 800 micrograms/day followed for 30 months showed no change in markers of resorption (ICTP) or formation (PICP) (SEDA-22, 183).

While biochemical markers of bone metabolism may be sensitive to the effects of glucocorticoids in the short term, the relation between changes in these markers and intermediate measures, such as bone mineral density, and the more important clinical outcomes of fractures, is unknown. In a random stratified sample of 3222 women in the perimenopausal age range (47–56 years), including 119 women with asthma, bone mineral density was measured to determine whether asthma was a risk factor of osteoporosis and to investigate the effect of inhaled glucocorticoids (102). The subjects had predominantly adult-onset asthma, as the age at diagnosis was over 40 years. There were 26 patients who were treated mainly with

Table 1   Biochemical markers of bone mineral density

Bone formation	Bone resorption
Blood	*Blood*
Alkaline phosphatase (bone-specific)	Acid phosphatase (acid-resistant)
Osteocalcin	Type I collagen carboxy-terminal telopeptide (ICTP)
Procollagen type I carboxy-terminal propeptide (PICP)	*Urine*
Procollagen type I amino-terminal propeptide (PINP)	Calcium
Procollagen type III amino-terminal propeptide (PIIINP)	Hydroxyproline Cross-linked peptides (pyridinium and deoxypyridinoline)

inhaled glucocorticoids (average daily dose 1000 micrograms). The asthmatic women in this general perimenopausal population had slightly reduced spinal and femoral neck bone mineral density compared with non-asthmatic women. These differences were more prominent in women who were not taking hormone replacement therapy. The reduction in bone mineral density may be due to glucocorticoids, and hormone replacement therapy appears to be protective against bone loss in asthmatics as well as healthy subjects. Cross-sectional studies such as this provide information about association but do not imply causality, for which longitudinal studies are required. Studies of the effects of inhaled glucocorticoids on markers of bone mineral density have provided conflicting data (103).

Effects on bone mineral density

Bone mineral density has been measured in a 3-year prospective study in 109 premenopausal asthmatic women, aged 18–45 years, all of whom used inhaled triamcinolone acetonide (104). They were grouped according to their inhaled glucocorticoid use at base line (no glucocorticoids and triamcinolone less than 800 micrograms/day or more than 800 micrograms/day). Therapy with triamcinolone was associated with a dose-related fall in bone mineral density at the hip overall and the trochanter. There was no effect at the femoral neck or the spine. None of the measured serum or urinary markers of bone turnover predicted the degree of bone loss. The dose-related loss of bone mineral density was suggested to be clinically related to prolonged treatment with inhaled glucocorticoids, and periodic bone mineral density assessment in patients taking high-dose inhaled glucocorticoids was proposed.

The effect of beclomethasone on bone mineral density has been examined over 1 year in 36 premenopausal and early postmenopausal women with asthma using inhaled glucocorticoids (beclomethasone at a mean dose of 542 micrograms/day) compared with 45 healthy matched controls (105). In early postmenopausal asthmatic women using beclomethasone, bone mineral density was significantly lower than in the controls, but not in premenopausal asthmatic women using inhaled beclomethasone. Serum osteocalcin concentrations were lower in the early postmenopausal asthmatic women using inhaled glucocorticoids than in the healthy controls, suggesting reduced bone formation, which leads to more pronounced bone loss. Ovarian hormones were suggested to offset the bone-depleting effects of inhaled beclomethasone in premenopausal women by maintaining or stimulating osteoblastic function.

There were significant reductions in bone mineral density in the lumbar spine and femur in 32 asthmatic women taking long-term inhaled beclomethasone (750–1500 micrograms/day) compared with 26 healthy controls (106). Control subjects and asthmatic patients were matched for age, sex, menopausal status, body-mass index, calcium intake, and physical activity. Loss of bone mass was more pronounced in the postmenopausal women. The authors identified several risk factors for accelerated bone loss in the lumbar spine, including postmenopausal status, low body-mass index, long duration of disease, long-term inhaled glucocorticoid therapy, and higher average daily and cumulative inhaled glucocorticoid doses.

The effects of inhaled budesonide 800 micrograms/day and fluticasone 400 micrograms/day on bone metabolism, morning cortisol concentrations, and clinical parameters have been studied in eight asthmatic patients (107). There were no changes in serum and bone alkaline phosphatase, osteocalcin, carboxyterminal propeptide of type 1 procollagen, and urinary calcium and deoxypyridinoline concentrations over 6 months. The authors concluded that fluticasone is as effective as twice the dose of budesonide in controlling asthmatic symptoms, without adverse effects on bone metabolism.

In a prospective comparison of the changes in bone mineral density in adults with mild asthma, 374 subjects with mild asthma (mean FEV_1 86% predicted; mean age 35 years; 55% women) were randomized to receive inhaled budesonide, inhaled beclomethasone, or non-glucocorticoid treatment (the control group) for 2 years (108). Bone mineral density was measured blind after 6, 12, and 24 months. The median daily doses of budesonide (87 subjects) and beclomethasone (74 subjects) were 389 and 499 micrograms respectively. The mean changes in bone density over 2 years in the budesonide, beclomethasone, and control groups were 0.1, −0.4, and 0.4% in the lumbar spine and −0.9, −0.9, and −0.4% in the neck of the femur. The mean daily dose of inhaled glucocorticoid was related to the reduction in bone mineral density only in the lumbar spine. Low to moderate doses of inhaled glucocorticoids caused little change in bone mineral density over 2 years and provided better asthma control.

In a retrospective cohort comparison of patients using inhaled glucocorticoids or bronchodilators with controls, there was an increased risk of fractures, particularly at the hip and spine, in those using inhaled glucocorticoids.

There were no differences in relative fracture risks with different drugs, for example fluticasone, budesonide, beclomethasone (109). In an earlier retrospective study, there was a dose-dependent increase in bone fracture risk with oral glucocorticoids (110).

The effects of inhaled glucocorticoids on bone mineral density (measured using dual X-ray absorptiometry of the spine and hip) and biochemical parameters were followed over 18 months. Mean serum osteocalcin concentrations were significantly lower in patients taking beclomethasone dipropionate or budesonide at doses of 800 micrograms/day and more. However, bone mineral density of the lumbar spine and hip was not affected. The normal advancement of bone mineral density expected in growing children was not affected by inhaled glucocorticoids taken for 7–16 months (SEDA-22, 184).

Treatment with beclomethasone dipropionate 1500 micrograms/day for 6 weeks significantly reduced markers of bone formation (osteocalcin and PICP), whereas fluticasone propionate 750 micrograms/day had no effect. Neither drug affected biochemical markers of bone resorption. There was no significant change in bone density (SEDA-22, 183).

Effects on bone mineral density in children

A cross-sectional study in children (111) showed no significant difference in total and anteroposterior spine bone mineral density between children with asthma treated with long-term budesonide (200–800 micrograms for at least 6 months; $n = 52$) and asthmatic children who had never used inhaled glucocorticoids ($n = 22$). These results are in agreement with those of a larger cross-sectional study of the effects of long-term treatment (3–6 years, mean 4.5 years) with inhaled budesonide on total bone mineral density in children with asthma ($n = 157$). The results provided evidence that long-term treatment with inhaled glucocorticoids in moderate dosages is unlikely to affect bone mineral density adversely in children with asthma (112). However, a study of the association of clinical risk factors and bone density with fractures in 324 prepubertal children, of whom 32 had a fracture, suggested that for total fracture risk bone mineral density may be less important than clinical risk factors (113). In a multivariate model incorporating age, weight, height, breast-feeding history, sports participation, and the use of inhaled glucocorticoids, these factors accounted for 10% of the variability in the risk of fracture. Surprisingly, bone mineral density in the lumbar spine, femoral neck, and total body bone did not differ between those with and without fractures.

In a small cross-sectional study, bone mineral density was studied in 20 prepubertal asthmatic patients treated with moderate to high doses of inhaled glucocorticoids (under 400 micrograms/day beclomethasone or budesonide or over 200 micrograms/day fluticasone) (114). Volumetric trabecular bone mineral density of the lumbar spine and distal radius were measured using dual energy X-ray absorptiometry and were within the reference ranges.

Bone mineral density (measured by dual X-ray absorptiometry) did not change significantly in asthmatic children treated for 3–6 years with a mean daily dose of 504 micrograms (189–1322 micrograms) budesonide (112).

In 23 children, randomized to either fluticasone 100 micrograms bd or beclomethasone 200 micrograms bd for 20 months, there was a significant increase in bone mineral density in the lumbar spine with time, following the normal growth pattern (115).

Comparisons with placebo

More data on the effect of inhaled glucocorticoids on bone mineral density in adults have been generated by the large randomized, multicenter, double-blind, placebo-controlled EUROSCOPE (European Respiratory Society Study on Chronic Obstructive Pulmonary Disease) study of 912 patients with chronic obstructive pulmonary disease randomly assigned to treatment for 3 years with budesonide 800 micrograms/day or placebo (116). There were no significant differences in bone mineral density at L2–4 vertebrae, the femoral neck, trochanter, or Ward's triangle; nor did the fracture rate between budesonide-treated and placebo-treated patients differ. These findings are in contrast to recent data from the Lung Health Study, which showed that triamcinolone 1200 micrograms/day for 4 years was associated with a statistically significant 2% reduction in bone mineral density in the femoral neck compared with placebo (117).

Comparisons of glucocorticoids

In a 12-month, multicenter comparison of fluticasone propionate 250–500 micrograms/day with beclomethasone dipropionate 500–1000 micrograms/day, the two drugs had an equal therapeutic effect. Fluticasone propionate treatment resulted in a higher bone mineral density (assessed at the hip) and higher serum osteocalcin concentrations.

In a prospective randomized comparison of the effects of fluticasone propionate 1000 micrograms/day and budesonide 1600 micrograms/day, over 1 year, bone mineral density measured in the spine was normal at the start of the study and increased slightly with time in both groups, as did serum osteocalcin concentration.

Fluticasone propionate 1000 micrograms/day or beclomethasone dipropionate 2000 micrograms/day taken for 2 years caused no change in biochemical markers of bone metabolism. Bone mineral density, measured by dual X-ray absorptiometry or single-photon absorptiometry, showed no consistent change. However, when bone mineral density was measured using quantitative computed tomography of the lumbar spine, beclomethasone dipropionate was associated with a small fall in bone mineral density, which stabilized by 24 months. It is doubtful that a small fall in bone density seen only on quantitative computed tomography is clinically relevant (SEDA-22, 184).

The efficacy and safety of fluticasone 750 micrograms/day and beclomethasone 1500 micrograms/day delivered by a spacer device have been compared in 30 asthmatic children in a 12-week, randomized, double-blind, cross-over study (118). All of the children had persistent asthma requiring 1000–2000 micrograms/day of inhaled glucocorticoids before the trial. There was no significant difference in efficacy, as judged by daytime and nighttime symptom scores and PEFR. There was a minimal reduction in serum cortisol in both groups. Both groups had identical height gain velocities. At the doses used in this trial, the authors were unable to show a safety advantage of fluticasone over beclomethasone, as assessed by cortisol concentrations.

In a 1-year prospective, randomized, open comparison of inhaled fluticasone 500 micrograms bd with budesonide 800 micrograms bd delivered by metered-dose inhaler and large volume spacer, bone mineral density was measured in 29 patients in the lumbar spine and femoral neck (119). Bone mineral density in the spine increased slightly in both groups over the 12 months. Serum osteocalcin concentrations increased from baseline in both treatment groups (fluticasone +17%, budesonide +14%). The percentage change from baseline in bone mineral density of the spine correlated with the increase in serum osteocalcin. Mean serum cortisol concentrations remained in the reference range after both inhaled glucocorticoids.

It can be hypothesized that different glucocorticoids have different systemic effects, and therefore different effects on bone metabolism. An alternative hypothesis is that these effects are dose dependent (85), support for which comes from a population-based case-control study of 16 341 older patients with hip fractures (mean age 79 years) and 29 889 controls; recent use of an inhaled glucocorticoid was associated with a small dose-dependent increase in the risk of hip fracture (120).

Comparisons with other drugs

Bone mineral density was measured after 7.4 months in 49 asthmatic children, 38 of whom took inhaled beclomethasone, average daily dose 276 micrograms, and 11 sodium cromoglicate, average daily dose 30 mg (121). Children who had used beclomethasone had grown as much as those who used sodium cromoglicate. Trabecular and cortical bone mineral density in the proximal forearm and lumbar spine increased to the same extent in both groups.

The effects of fluticasone 50 micrograms bd or sodium cromoglicate 20 mg qds on growth over 12 months have been studied in 122 asthmatic children aged 4–10 years (122). The mean height velocity was 6 cm/year with fluticasone and 6.5 cm/year with sodium cromoglicate. There was no significant treatment difference in the mean 24-hour urinary-free cortisol concentrations at 6 or 12 months. Mean predicted peak expiratory flow rate improved over 1 year in both groups, but to a greater extent with fluticasone. The authors concluded that growth was normal in mildly asthmatic children using fluticasone (50 micrograms bd) for 1 year. Fluticasone was more effective than sodium cromoglicate, with fewer withdrawals and greater improvement in lung function.

Dose relation

Current evidence suggests that the changes in bone mineral density in asthmatic patients who take inhaled glucocorticoids occur within the high therapeutic range of doses. In patients with mild asthma who are well maintained on low doses of inhaled glucocorticoids, the benefits derived from good control of the asthma appear to outweigh any concerns about minor changes in bone mineral density. The picture is less clear in patients with other risk factors, such as estrogen deficiency and advancing years.

No adverse effect on bone has been shown with beclomethasone dipropionate or budesonide at doses less than 1000 micrograms/day or fluticasone propionate less than 500 micrograms/day. Most patients obtain a good therapeutic response at these doses. Higher doses may be required in some patients. Aerosols delivering doses of beclomethasone dipropionate 250 and 500 micrograms, budesonide 400 micrograms and fluticasone propionate 250 and 500 micrograms should be reserved for patients in whom the requirement for a high dose has been demonstrated in an adequate trial of therapy.

In an uncontrolled study, 56 women with asthma taking long-term inhaled glucocorticoids had bone mineral density measurements of the lumbar spine and hip (123). Women who had taken more than three short courses of systemic glucocorticoids per year over the preceding 3 years were excluded. Data on duration of use and dose of inhaled glucocorticoids were obtained from the patients' medical records. Doses of inhaled glucocorticoids were arbitrarily classified as low (under 500 micrograms/day), medium (500–1000 micrograms/day), and high (over 1000 micrograms/day). More than half the women (61%) had reduced bone mineral density at either the hip or lumbar spine. Amongst the postmenopausal women in the study, 17% of those aged under 65 years had osteoporosis compared with 43% of those aged over 65 years. These figures exceeded those from a national sample of estrogen-deficient women, in which 5.7% under the age of 65 and 29% over the age of 65 years had osteoporosis. Bone mineral density loss increased with higher doses of inhaled glucocorticoids, from 5% in the low-dose group to 50% in the high-dose group. Whilst this is a potentially important finding in women at risk of osteoporosis because of the menopause, there are some aspects of the design of the study that limit the applicability of the findings. There was no appropriate age- and ethnicity-matched control group, and the contribution of nasal glucocorticoids was not accurately assessed.

In a large cross-sectional study, patients aged 20–40 years with asthma who had taken inhaled glucocorticoids for a median of 6 years were studied (124). Patients were excluded if they had taken a course of oral or parenteral glucocorticoids in the past 6 months or more than two courses ever, or if they had had more than 10 inhalers of nasal glucocorticoids or more than 10 prescriptions of a dermal glucocorticoid. Computerized records of general practices were used to identify patients for the study. Bone mineral density was measured at the lumbar spine (L2–L4) and the left femur (neck, Ward's triangle, trochanter). The cumulative dose of inhaled glucocorticoid was expressed as a product of the mean daily dose and time (mg days). This information was obtained from a patient questionnaire and validated against general practice computer and paper records. More than half of the patients (119/196) were women and the median cumulative dose of inhaled glucocorticoid was 876 mg (range 88–4380 mg). There was a significant inverse relation between the cumulative dose of inhaled glucocorticoid and bone mineral density at the spine and hip in both men and women. A doubling of cumulative dose was associated with a 0.16 times SD reduction in bone mineral density. Extrapolation from cross-sectional data such as these requires confirmation in longitudinal studies, since bone loss with oral glucocorticoids is more rapid in the first 12–24 months of therapy.

Bone mineral density has been measured at 3-year intervals in 51 patients taking inhaled glucocorticoids for asthma (125). The patients were divided into a high-dose group taking over 800 micrograms/day of beclomethasone or budesonide ($n = 28$, mean dose 983 micrograms/day) and a control group taking no inhaled glucocorticoid or less than 500 micrograms/day ($n = 23$, mean dose 309 micrograms/day). Whilst there were statistically significant reductions in bone markers, such as serum calcium and phosphorus and osteocalcin, over the 3-year period in each group, there was no significant reduction in bone mineral density in either group of asthmatic patients. Although the change in bone mineral density in the high-dose group was small over the 3-year period and not statistically significant, there was a correlation between bone loss and the daily dose of inhaled glucocorticoids. There was no significant correlation between the changes in bone density and either the initial bone density or biomarkers of bone turnover for the level of physical activity. This longitudinal study has shown the unreliability of biomarkers of bone turnover in predicting changes in bone density (and presumably relevant clinical outcomes, such as risk of fracture) and shows the need for measurement of bone mineral density in asthmatic patients who are deemed to be at risk of bone loss. Such patients include those taking oral glucocorticoids, perimenopausal women not taking hormone replacement therapy, and patients who need high doses of inhaled glucocorticoids. Whilst patients in this study did not have significant changes in bone mineral density over 3 years, the effects of higher doses remain uncertain, so it would be prudent to measure bone mineral density in patients who need higher doses.

Time course

The time course of changes in bone mineral density with inhaled glucocorticoids has yet to be determined. Longitudinal studies will be required to determine whether bone loss is most rapid in the first 12–24 months after initiating inhaled glucocorticoid therapy, as is the case with oral glucocorticoids (126) and whether the risk of fracture falls towards baseline after withdrawal of treatment, as was suggested by the GPRD (General Practice Research Database) study (114).

In older women with asthma, who have an increased risk of osteoporosis, there was no significant change in bone mineral density after 1 year of treatment with beclomethasone dipropionate 1000 micrograms/day (127).

Bone mineral density, bone turnover markers, and adrenal glucocorticoid hormones have been measured in 53 patients (34 women, 19 men) with chronic bronchial asthma who took either inhaled beclomethasone or budesonide in doses of at least 1500 micrograms/day for at least 12 months (128). The patients were divided into those who had taken oral glucocorticoids for more than 1 month and those who had not. Bone mineral density was measured at the lumbar spine and the proximal femur. The values were about one standard deviation lower in men and women taking oral glucocorticoids or very high doses of inhaled glucocorticoids. The reduction in bone mineral density was enough to a double the risk of fracture at these sites. There was suppression of both endogenous glucocorticoid and adrenal androgen production in all subjects. Adrenal androgen suppression may increase the susceptibility of postmenopausal women treated with an oral glucocorticoid to bone loss.

Risk of fracture

Although studies in which biochemical markers of bone turnover are measured for periods of 1–2 months do not predict the development of bone thinning, osteoporosis, or fracture, they can be useful in comparing the potential effects on bone of different glucocorticoids. Studies of bone mineral density over longer time periods relate more directly to osteoporosis and fracture risk.

Whilst there have been several studies of the effects of inhaled glucocorticoids on bone mineral density, there are few data on the effects of inhaled glucocorticoids on the risk of fracture. In a retrospective cohort study the risk of fracture was established by examining the General Practice Research Database (GPRD), which is run by the Medicines Control Agency in the UK (114). Users of inhaled glucocorticoids were defined as permanently registered patients aged 18 years or more who received one or more prescriptions for inhaled glucocorticoids during the time from enrolment in the GPRD until the end of data collection. Patients who received a prescription for oral glucocorticoids for a period of 6 months before to 91 days after the last prescription for an inhaled glucocorticoid were excluded. There were two comparison groups: a bronchodilator group, which included adults who received prescriptions for non-systemic glucocorticoids and bronchodilators, and a second control group who received non-systemic glucocorticoids but never inhaled systemic glucocorticoids or bronchodilators. The database included over 440 000 patients and all patients who had fractures were identified from their medical records during the follow-up period, which was 91 days after the last prescription for an inhaled glucocorticoid. The relative rates of non-vertebral, hip, and vertebral fractures during inhaled glucocorticoid treatment compared with controls were 1.15 (95% CI = 1.10, 1.20), 1.22 (CI = 1.04, 1.43), and 1.51 (CI = 1.22, 1.85) respectively. There were no differences between inhaled glucocorticoids and bronchodilators (non-vertebral fracture relative rate = 1). The authors concluded that users of inhaled glucocorticoids may have an increased risk of fracture, particularly at the hip and spine, but that this excess risk may be related more to the underlying respiratory disease than to the inhaled glucocorticoids.

There were no major differences between the three groups in baseline fracture history. About 1% in each cohort recorded a history of non-vertebral fractures in the year before baseline. During the follow-up, the incidence of non-vertebral fractures was 1.4 fractures per 100 persons with inhaled glucocorticoids, 1.4 with bronchodilators, and 1.1 in the control group. Comparing inhaled glucocorticoid users with a control group, there was a dose response for hip and vertebral fractures. For a standardized daily dose of under 300 micrograms/day of budesonide, hip fracture was 0.95, rising to 1.06 at doses of 300–700 micrograms/day and 1.77 at doses of 700 micrograms/day or more. There was no consistent trend in the rate of fractures amongst users of inhaled glucocorticoid compared with bronchodilators.

This is a noteworthy study because it has examined the most important clinical outcome of change in bone mineral density: the risk of fracture. The results point to an increased risk of fracture, especially at the hip and the vertebral bodies, amongst patients who use inhaled glucocorticoids as well as those using bronchodilators, when compared with patients not using these drugs. Fracture risk tended to fall after withdrawal of inhaled glucocorticoids or bronchodilators. These findings suggest that low-dose inhaled glucocorticoids are not associated with an increased risk of fracture and that patients with chronic respiratory disease who use any inhaled therapy are at risk compared with a control population. There were no differences in fracture risk between the various types of bronchodilators, suggesting that the underlying lung disease itself was the basis of risk rather than any particular type of bronchodilator. The authors noted that 1.9% of patients were using doses of budesonide equivalents of over 1500 micrograms/day and that the possibility of a more pronounced increased fracture risk at these high doses cannot be excluded. The age- and sex-specific incidence of fracture in the control group was similar to that of the general population in the GPRD.

Estimates of the important outcome of bone fracture have shown a small increased risk with inhaled glucocorticoids, but this may well be a feature of the disease rather than the therapy, because comparisons with treatment with bronchodilator drugs show no difference between risk factors in patients taking glucocorticoids or bronchodilators.

Prevention of osteoporosis with bisphosphonates
The effect of high-dose inhaled glucocorticoids and antiresorptive therapy with sodium etidronate has been studied for 18 months in 38 Chinese patients (24 men and 14 premenopausal women aged 30–50 years), of whom 28 were asthmatics who had already been treated for at least 12 months with high-dose inhaled glucocorticoids (beclomethasone or budesonide over 1.5 mg/day), and 10 healthy controls (129). The patients were randomly allocated to (1) no supplement, (2) a calcium supplement 1000 mg/day, or (3) cyclical sodium etidronate 400 mg/day for 14 days followed by calcium 1000 mg/day for 76 days. All three groups continued to take inhaled glucocorticoids. Bone mineral density was measured at the lumbar spine and hip. Bone mineral density in the group one patients fell by about 1% over 18 months and rose by about 1.5% in the healthy controls, neither change being significant. In groups 2 and 3 bone mineral density rose significantly at 12 and 18 months by 2 and 3% respectively. Serum osteocalcin concentrations fell significantly in all three groups of asthmatic patients but not in the controls. There were no significant changes in serum alkaline phosphatase or parathyroid hormone. In the patients taking calcium, with or without etidronate, mean serum calcium increased. The authors suggested that calcium supplementation and cyclical etidronate work by reducing bone resorption, and hence reduced bone turnover, rather than by increasing bone formation. This is consistent with the fall in serum osteocalcin.

The efficacy of clodronate in treating glucocorticoid-induced bone loss in asthmatic subjects has been evaluated in a double-blind study in 74 adults (41 women and 33 men, mean age 57 years) with a long history (mean 8.1 years) of oral and inhaled glucocorticoid use, randomized to clodronate 800, 1600, or 2400 mg/day or placebo (130). There was no increase in bone mineral density with placebo or clodronate 800 mg/day, but a significant dose-related increase with clodronate 1600 and 2400 mg/day. The most common adverse effect was gastric irritation in the patients who took the highest dose of clodronate.

Growth
Oral glucocorticoids inhibit growth by blunting pulsatile growth hormone secretion, by decreasing insulin-like growth factor-1 activity, and by directly inhibiting collagen synthesis (131). Although inhalation reduces systemic exposure, concerns have been raised regarding the potential effects on growth and final height in children, especially when inhaled glucocorticoids are used for long periods.

Uninterrupted administration of moderate-dose inhaled glucocorticoids (for example 400 micrograms/day of budesonide equivalents) has been associated with a suppressed growth rate in some children with asthma. Budesonide reduced the growth by 1 and 1.4 cm over 7 and 12 months, respectively (132). Consequently, in the USA, a class label warning for inhaled glucocorticoids about growth retardation in children was introduced in 1998, when the FDA decided to alter the class labeling for all inhaled and nasal glucocorticoids in children, to indicate that the use of recommended doses might be associated with a reduction in growth velocity (19). However, the available studies suggest that in children, the major advantages of adequate asthma control with inhaled glucocorticoids outweigh any potential adverse effects on growth.

However, results from trials in asthmatic children can be flawed by confounding variables. Severe asthma can itself have a negative effect on growth and adversely affect adult height, as with any chronic disease. Even in well-controlled asthma, children typically show retardation in pubertal growth spurt and attain normal adult height later. As growth in children is non-linear over time, trials over short periods are likely to capture short-term effects of inhaled glucocorticoids rather than the long-term outcome. Furthermore, the growth-retarding effect of inhaled glucocorticoids is more pronounced at the start of treatment.

Long-term studies have suggested that a temporary short-term or medium-term reduction in growth velocity is normally compensated for later on, and individuals attain normal adult height (133,134). The effects of inhaled glucocorticoids on growth rate over weeks and months are dose-dependent, and dose-response curves of pulmonary and adverse systemic effects differ widely, so that individual titration of the inhaled glucocorticoid dose according to the severity of the disease is strongly recommended, and the lowest dose of inhaled glucocorticoids that controls the disease should always be preferred. In conclusion, accumulating evidence shows that children with asthma, even when treated with inhaled glucocorticoids for years, attain normal adult height. However, close growth monitoring during inhaled glucocorticoid therapy is recommended, as idiosyncratic responses can occur, probably owing to individual glucocorticoid receptor polymorphism (135).

A two-part review was published in 2002, addressing the difficulties of assessing the effects of asthma therapy on childhood growth and reviewing the published literature based on the authors' recommendations (136,137). In the first part (136), a simple classification system for growth studies was developed:

- comparisons with placebo (type 1 studies);
- comparisons with non-steroidal asthma therapy (type 2 studies);
- comparisons with another inhaled glucocorticoid (type 3 studies);
- comparisons with "real life" asthma therapy (type 4 studies).

In the context of these different study types, the authors also discussed the choice of end-point, key trial design issues, the selection and numbers of subjects in the active and control groups, the duration of assessments, and methods for measuring height and data analysis. They also elaborated specific recommendations regarding study duration, age/sexual maturity of the patients, exclusion criteria for height and growth velocity, permitted therapy during the study, the protocol for height measurement, the numbers of patients for adequate statistical power, and methods for statistical analysis (136).

In the second part, they selected 18 growth studies that included minimal criteria, such as selected control group, measured height by stadiometry, and at least a 12-month duration; they compared the design attributes of these studies with the described recommendations (137). Of the 18 selected studies, 17 were susceptible to one or more important confounding factors; nevertheless, the outcomes of all 18 studies were considered to be

consistent. In summary, impaired growth velocity was found with budesonide and beclomethasone dipropionate compared with placebo, non-steroidal treatment, and fluticasone propionate during 1–2 years of therapy, but none of the inhaled glucocorticoids appeared to affect final height (137). Growth in children treated with low-dose fluticasone propionate (up to 200 micrograms/day) for 1 year is similar to growth in those treated with placebo or non-steroidal therapy. Standard pediatric doses of inhaled glucocorticoids (less than 800 micrograms of budesonide and less than 400 micrograms of budesonide or fluticasone) are considered not to affect growth adversely (84,138). The risk of growth suppression depends on the dose, the administration regimen, and the delivery device.

An important confounding factor is the influence of non-adherence to inhaled glucocorticoid treatment (139). Sensitive and reliable measures of adherence should be applied when evaluating long-term effects on height.

The time of dosing can influence the effect of inhaled glucocorticoids on growth suppression in the prepubertal child, since growth hormone secretion is generally confined to nighttime. Therefore, once-daily morning dosing could be advantageous (140).

For clinical practice, the lowest effective dose should be achieved, and all children using inhaled glucocorticoids should have their growth measured every 6 months, as this is a sensitive method of detecting significant systemic effects (84,140).

These results apply to children over 4 years of age; for younger children only assumptions can be entertained and age-specific studies are needed (140).

Dose relation

Lumbar spine bone mineral density has been assessed in 76 prepubertal asthmatics (mean age 7.7 years, 26 girls) using glucocorticoids (141). After stratification for dose and route of administration, the children who used over 800 micrograms/day of inhaled glucocorticoids, with or without intermittent oral glucocorticoids, had a significant lower weight-adjusted bone density than children who used 400–800 micrograms/day of inhaled glucocorticoids (mean difference –0.05 g/cm^2; 95% CI = –0.02, –0.09). Bone mass was similar in children who did not use inhaled glucocorticoids and those who used 400–800 micrograms/day.

The authors of a review concluded, from short-term and intermediate-term growth studies, that there are no clinically significant adverse effects on growth with inhaled glucocorticoids at normal pediatric doses (100–200 micrograms/day budesonide equivalents), but that growth retardation can occur with all inhaled glucocorticoids at higher doses (142). Individual idiosyncratic adverse reactions are rare. Long-term studies and studies that have examined the effect on final adult height have been consistent in showing significantly reduced growth rates during the first months and up to 2 years of treatment with inhaled glucocorticoids. However, children treated with inhaled glucocorticoids attain their predicted adult height to the same extent as their healthy peers. It is important to note that changes in growth rate during the first year of inhaled glucocorticoid treatment cannot be used to predict final adult height.

Growth velocity measured over a 12-month period in prepubertal children with asthma was reduced by prior treatment with inhaled glucocorticoids for an average of 2.7 years. However, measurement of biochemical markers (Table 1) gave conflicting results. Osteocalcin concentrations were reduced, but alkaline phosphatase did not change. PINP and PIIINP were reduced, but PICP increased. ICTP, a marker for collagen I degradation, fell.

Comparisons of glucocorticoids

Fluticasone propionate 400 micrograms/day or budesonide 800 micrograms/day were administered for 20 weeks to children with moderate to severe asthma aged 4–12 years. Fluticasone propionate was superior to budesonide in improving peak expiratory flow and comparable in controlling symptoms. Growth was reduced with budesonide treatment compared with fluticasone propionate treatment mean difference, 6.2 mm (CI = 2.9, 9.6). There was no difference in serum cortisol suppression (143).

Comparisons with other drugs

Beclomethasone dipropionate 400 micrograms/day and salmeterol 50 micrograms bd were compared in asthmatic children treated for 12 months. Beclomethasone dipropionate treatment resulted in better overall asthma control. Over 12 months, linear growth was 3.96 cm/year in the children using beclomethasone dipropionate, compared with 5.40 cm/year in those who used salmeterol and 5.04 cm/year in a placebo group (SEDA-22, 186).

The long-term effects of inhaled glucocorticoids on growth in children have been recently assessed. In the so-called CaAMP Study (144), children aged 5–12 years with mild to moderate asthma were randomized to budesonide 200 micrograms bd (n = 311), nedocromil 8 mg bd (n = 312), or placebo (n = 418). At the end of the 4–6 year treatment period, the mean increase in height in the budesonide group was 1.1 cm less than in the placebo group. The difference between budesonide and placebo in the rate of growth was evident primarily within the first year but did not increase thereafter, and all the groups had similar growth velocity by the end of the treatment period.

Comparisons with oral glucocorticoids

A meta-analysis of 21 studies in which 810 asthmatic children were treated with oral prednisolone (8 trials) and/or beclomethasone dipropionate, dosage range 200–900 micrograms/day (12 trials) has been reported. Significant suppression of growth occurred with oral glucocorticoids but not with beclomethasone dipropionate (145).

Reversibility

Growth data obtained in 50 children who used beclomethasone dipropionate over 7 months suggested that any growth suppression is temporary and that growth velocity recovers during continuing treatment. Growth velocity fell most in the first 6 weeks of treatment, from 0.140 to 0.073 mm/week (0.067 mm/week; 95%

CI = 0.015, 0.120). There were similar reductions at 12 and 18 weeks. After this, growth velocity increased to rates seen before treatment began: 0.138 mm/week at 24 weeks and 0.120 mm/week at 30 weeks (146).

Long-term use of beclomethasone dipropionate 400–600 micrograms/day was reported to delay the onset of puberty. However, subsequent catch-up growth was unaffected and subjects reached their normal predicted adult height (147).

Children taking budesonide (mean daily dose 412 micrograms, range 110–877 micrograms) for periods of 3–13 years have been followed to adulthood to determine their final height (134). These 142 budesonide-treated children were compared with 18 control patients with asthma who had never taken inhaled glucocorticoids and 51 healthy siblings of the patients in the budesonide group. These children, who had taken long-term inhaled glucocorticoids, attained normal adult height. There was no evidence of a dose–response relation between the mean daily dose of budesonide, the cumulative dose, or the duration of treatment with budesonide and the difference between the measured and target adult heights.

These studies are important, because several previous reports of growth during a period of 1 year after beginning treatment with inhaled glucocorticoids (in daily doses of about 400 micrograms of budesonide) identified growth retardation of about 1.5 cm. The mechanism for the termination after 1 year of the effects on growth is uncertain.

Immunologic

Hypersensitivity to inhaled glucocorticoids is rare.

- An asthmatic patient using inhaled budesonide and salbutamol developed an acute asthma attack. Despite emergency treatment the patient deteriorated, requiring endotracheal intubation and assisted ventilation, and there was no improvement until the glucocorticoid was withdrawn, after which there was steady improvement. Skin prick tests with prednisolone, sodium hemisuccinate, and 6-methylprednisolone-sodium hemisuccinate were positive. Thirty minutes after intradermal 6-methylprednisolone-sodium hemisuccinate 4 mg, the patient developed a dry cough, dyspnea, and wheezing and a 17% fall in FEV_1.
- A 37-year-old woman who was pregnant developed Churg–Strauss syndrome after withdrawal of her usual high-dose inhaled glucocorticoid therapy (drug not stated) that she had used for 3 years for bronchial asthma (148).

The authors of the second report commented that activated eosinophils and their cytotoxic products, such as eosinophil catatonic protein, may play a part in the pathogenesis of Churg–Strauss syndrome. Measuring serum concentrations of eosinophil catatonic protein may be useful in monitoring disease activity, since concentrations were increased before treatment and normalized afterwards.

Infection risk

Inhaled or topical immunosuppressive and anti-inflammatory glucocorticoids increase the risk of oral candidiasis (149). Patients who harbor oral *Candida* before they use inhaled glucocorticoids may have an increased risk. The location and degree of oral candidiasis seems to be related to dosage, administration frequency, and inhalation technique. Preventive measures include using a spacer, lowering the dosage, and rinsing the mouth after use.

The frequency of oral candidiasis has been studied in 143 asthmatic patients using inhaled glucocorticoids (96 fluticasone and 47 beclomethasone dipropionate), 11 asthmatic patients not using inhaled glucocorticoids, and 86 healthy volunteers (150). Quantitative fungal cultures were performed by aseptically obtaining a retropharyngeal wall swab. The growth of *Candida* species was significantly greater in asthmatic patients taking inhaled glucocorticoids. The presence of *Candida* was also significantly greater in patients with oral symptoms than in asymptomatic patients, and in patients using fluticasone (26%) compared with those using beclomethasone (11%). The presence of *Candida* correlated with the dose of fluticasone but not with the inhaled dose of beclomethasone. *Candida* species were rarely found in asthmatic patients not using glucocorticoids or in healthy volunteers. Gargling with Invasive aspergillosis occurred after high-dose inhaled fluticasone (440 micrograms qds) and zafirlukast 20 mg/day in a 44-year old man with moderately severe asthma; this is the first report of invasive pulmonary aspergillosis associated with an inhaled glucocorticoid (151).

Second-Generation Effects

Teratogenicity

Congenital malformations that may be associated with inhaled budesonide in pregnancy have been evaluated using the Swedish Medical Birth Registry (152). Of 2014 infants whose mothers started to use inhaled budesonide in early pregnancy, 75 (3.7%) had a congenital malformation; the corresponding rate among all infants born in 1995–97 was 3.5%. Five infants had chromosomal anomalies that were unlikely to have been caused by drugs. This study did not identify teratogenic properties of inhaled budesonide.

Drug–Drug Interactions

HIV protease inhibitors

Cushing's syndrome can be caused by the co-administration of a glucocorticoid and inhibitors of CYP3A4, such as HIV protease inhibitors, resulting in increased plasma glucocorticoid concentrations.

- Cushing's syndrome occurred in a 44-year-old HIV-positive patient who used inhaled fluticasone (500 micrograms qds) for severe asthma for 2 years (153). Stavudine and nevirapine were replaced by abacavir and ritonavir + lopinavir and 2 months later he developed the typical features of Cushing syndrome.

In this case an interaction of ritonavir + lopinavir with fluticasone was suspected, because fluticasone is metabolized by CYP3A4, which ritonavir inhibits.

Itraconazole

Interactions with other drugs can increase plasma concentrations of inhaled glucocorticoids. Itraconazole, a potent inhibitor of CYP3A4, markedly increased plasma concentrations of inhaled budesonide (154).

Cushing's syndrome of rapid onset occurred during combined treatment with inhaled budesonide and itraconazole (155).

- A 4-year old boy with cystic fibrosis developed persistent bronchospasm. Allergic bronchopulmonary aspergillosis was suspected and he was given oral itraconazole 100 mg bd, inhaled formoterol 12 micrograms/day, and inhaled budesonide 200 micrograms bd. After 2 weeks his respiratory symptoms had improved but he had a moon face and swollen abdomen, his blood pressure was 121/75 mmHg, and his weight had increased by 1.5 kg. A morning sample showed low cortisol concentrations (under 3 ng/ml) and a reduced plasma ACTH (12 pg/ml). Itraconazole was withdrawn and budesonide was reduced and withdrawn after 2 weeks. He was given hydrocortisone to prevent acute adrenal insufficiency. He recovered over the next 3 months.

This adverse effect could have been due to inhibition of the metabolism of budesonide by itraconazole.

Cushing's syndrome has been attributed to the combination of itraconazole and inhaled budesonide (156).

- A 70-year-old white woman taking inhaled budesonide 400 micrograms tds developed multiple, small, purple, non-tender nodules in the subcutaneous tissues of her left leg. Biopsy of a nodule showed fungal hyphae, and *Scedosporium apiospermum* was isolated. She was treated with itraconazole suspension 200 mg bd, with complete clinical resolution after 4 weeks. Within 8 weeks after starting itraconazole, she developed swollen ankles, shortness of breath, fatigue, lethargy, and progressive severe leg weakness. Her doctor attributed her increased breathlessness to worsening asthma and increased the dose of inhaled budesonide to 800 micrograms bd. She had a Cushingoid appearance, her skin was thin, with multiple bruises over her body, her blood pressure was 170/90 mmHg, and she had proximal muscle weakness in the legs. The plasma cortisol concentration was below 2 (reference range 50–250) µg/l and tetracosactide 250 micrograms produced a rise to 11 µg/l after 60 minutes. The adrenocorticotropic hormone (ACTH) concentration was below 6.8 (9–52) ng/l and the 24-hour urine free cortisol was below 73 (350–1100) µg/l. Itraconazole and inhaled budesonide were withdrawn, and the secondary adrenal insufficiency was treated with hydrocortisone replacement. Inhaled beclomethasone 250 micrograms bd was given by metered-dose inhaler and 4 weeks later she developed a local recurrence of the *S. apiospermum* infection, which was treated with voriconazole 200 mg bd for 3 months, with complete resolution.

Voriconazole is predominantly metabolized by CYP2C19, and although it is an inhibitor of CYP3A4 its inhibitory effects are much less than those of itraconazole, as shown in this case, in which it appeared not to interact with beclomethasone, while itraconazole did.

Ritonavir

Ritonavir is a potent inhibitor of CYP3A4. In healthy volunteers a low dose of ritonavir increases the plasma concentrations of fluticasone and reduces cortisol concentrations, probably due to increased systemic availability of fluticasone. Ritonavir has also caused Cushing's syndrome in a patient using fluticasone propionate 1000 micrograms/day (157). Five cases of iatrogenic Cushing's syndrome with osteoporosis and secondary adrenal failure have been described in patients with HIV taking oral ritonavir and inhaled glucocorticoids (four fluticasone and one budesonide) (158).

References

1. Allen DB. Sense and sensitivity: assessing inhaled corticosteroid effects on the hypothalamic–pituitary–adrenal axis. Ann Allergy Asthma Immunol 2002;89(6):537–9.
2. Minto C, Li B, Tattam B, Brown K, Seale JP, Donnelly R. Pharmacokinetics of epimeric budesonide and fluticasone propionate after repeat dose inhalation—intersubject variability in systemic absorption from the lung. Br J Clin Pharmacol 2000;50(2):116–24.
3. Donnelly R, Williams KM, Baker AB, Badcock CA, Day RO, Seale JP. Effects of budesonide and fluticasone on 24-hour plasma cortisol. A dose-response study. Am J Respir Crit Care Med 1997;156(6):1746–51.
4. Weiner P, Berar-Yanay N, Davidovich A, Magadle R. Nocturnal cortisol secretion in asthmatic patients after inhalation of fluticasone propionate. Chest 1999;116(4):931–4.
5. Brutsche MH, Brutsche IC, Munawar M, Langley SJ, Masterson CM, Daley-Yates PT, Brown R, Custovic A, Woodcock A. Comparison of pharmacokinetics and systemic effects of inhaled fluticasone propionate in patients with asthma and healthy volunteers: a randomised crossover study. Lancet 2000;356(9229):556–61.
6. Lofdahl CG, Thorsson L. No difference between asthmatic patients and healthy subjects in lung uptake of fluticasone propionate. Eur Respir J 1999;14:466S.
7. Harrison TW, Wisniewski A, Honour J, Tattersfield AE. Comparison of the systemic effects of fluticasone propionate and budesonide given by dry powder inhaler in healthy and asthmatic subjects. Thorax 2001;56(3):186–91.
8. Fabbri L, Melara R. Systemic effects of inhaled corticosteroids are milder in asthmatic patients than in normal subjects. Thorax 2001;56(3):165–6.
9. Berend N, Kellett B, Kent N, Sly PD, Bowler S, Burdon J, Dennis C, Gibson P, James A, Jenkins C. Collaborative Study Group of the Australian Lung Foundation. Improved safety with equivalent asthma control in adults with chronic severe asthma on high-dose fluticasone propionate. Respirology 2001;6(3):237–46.
10. Dubus JC, Marguet C, Deschildre A, Mely L, Le Roux P, Brouard J, Huiart L. Reseau de Recherche Clinique en Pneumonologie Pédiatrique. Local side-effects of inhaled corticosteroids in asthmatic children: influence of drug, dose, age, and device. Allergy 2001;56(10):944–8.
11. Wilson AM, Lipworth BJ. 24 hour and fractionated profiles of adrenocortical activity in asthmatic patients receiving inhaled and intranasal corticosteroids. Thorax 1999;54(1):20–6.
12. Borgstrom L. Local versus total systemic bioavailability as a means to compare different inhaled formulations of the same substance. J Aerosol Med 1998;11(1):55–63.
13. Kelly HW. Establishing a therapeutic index for the inhaled corticosteroids. Part I. Pharmacokinetic/pharmacodynamic comparison of the inhaled corticosteroids. J Allergy Clin Immunol 1998;102(4 Pt 2):S36–51.
14. Leach C. Targeting inhaled steroids. Int J Clin Pract Suppl 1998;96:23–7.
15. Trescoli C, Ward MJ. Systemic activity of inhaled and swallowed beclomethasone dipropionate and the effect of different inhaler devices. Postgrad Med J 1998;74(877):675–7.
16. Thorsson L, Edsbacker S. Lung deposition of budesonide from a pressurized metered-dose inhaler attached to a spacer. Eur Respir J 1998;12(6):1340–5.
17. O'Byrne PM, Pedersen S. Measuring efficacy and safety of different inhaled corticosteroid preparations. J Allergy Clin Immunol 1998;102(6 Pt 1):879–86.
18. Martin RJ, Szefler SJ, Chinchilli VM, Kraft M, Dolovich M, Boushey HA, Cherniack RM, Craig TJ, Drazen JM, Fagan JK, Fahy JV, Fish JE, Ford JG, Israel E, Kunselman SJ, Lazarus SC, Lemanske RF Jr, Peters SP, Sorkness CA. Systemic effect comparisons of six inhaled corticosteroid preparations. Am J Respir Crit Care Med 2002;165(10):1377–83.
19. Lipworth BJ. Systemic adverse effects of inhaled corticosteroid therapy: A systematic review and meta-analysis. Arch Intern Med 1999;159(9):941–55.
20. Goldberg S, Einot T, Algur N, Schwartz S, Greenberg AC, Picard E, Virgilis D, Kerem E. Adrenal suppression in asthmatic children receiving low-dose inhaled budesonide: comparison between dry powder inhaler and pressurized metered-dose inhaler attached to a spacer. Ann Allergy Asthma Immunol 2002;89(6):566–71.
21. Irani AM, Cruz-Rivera M, Fitzpatrick S, Hoag J, Smith JA. Effects of budesonide inhalation suspension on hypothalamic–pituitary–adrenal-axis function in infants and young children with persistent asthma. Ann Allergy Asthma Immunol 2002;88(3):306–12.
22. Eid N, Morton R, Olds B, Clark P, Sheikh S, Looney S. Decreased morning serum cortisol levels in children with asthma treated with inhaled fluticasone propionate. Pediatrics 2002;109(2):217–21.
23. Tukiainen H, Rytila P, Hamalainen KM, Silvasti MS, Keski-Karhu J. Finnish Study Group. Safety, tolerability and acceptability of two dry powder inhalers in the administration of budesonide in steroid-treated asthmatic patients. Respir Med 2002;96(4):221–9.
24. Volovitz B, Bentur L, Finkelstein Y, Mansour Y, Shalitin S, Nussinovitch M, Varsano I. Effectiveness and safety of inhaled corticosteroids in controlling acute asthma attacks in children who were treated in the emergency department: a controlled comparative study with oral prednisolone. J Allergy Clin Immunol 1998;102(4 Pt 1):605–9.

25. Nana A, Youngchaiyud P, Charoenratanakul S, Boe J, Lofdahl CG, Selroos O, Stahl E. High-dose inhaled budesonide may substitute for oral therapy after an acute asthma attack. J Asthma 1998;35(8):647–55.

26. Sung L, Osmond MH, Klassen TP. Randomized, controlled trial of inhaled budesonide as an adjunct to oral prednisone in acute asthma. Acad Emerg Med 1998;5(3):209–13.

27. Paggiaro PL, Dahle R, Bakran I, Frith L, Hollingworth K, Efthimiou J. Multicentre randomised placebo-controlled trial of inhaled fluticasone propionate in patients with chronic obstructive pulmonary disease. International COPD Study Group. Lancet 1998;351(9105):773–80Erratum in: Lancet 1998;351(9120):1968.

28. Jick SS, Vasilakis-Scaramozza C, Maier WC. The risk of cataract among users of inhaled steroids. Epidemiology 2001;12(2):229–34.

29. Garbe E, Suissa S, LeLorier J. Association of inhaled corticosteroid use with cataract extraction in elderly patients. JAMA 1998;280(6):539–43Erratum in: JAMA 1998;280(21):1830.

30. Kennedy L, Rusch VW, Strange C, Ginsberg RJ, Sahn SA. Pleurodesis using talc slurry. Chest 1994;106(2):342–6.

31. Li JT, Ford LB, Chervinsky P, Weisberg SC, Kellerman DJ, Faulkner KG, Herje NE, Hamedani A, Harding SM, Shah T. Fluticasone propionate powder and lack of clinically significant effects on hypothalamic–pituitary–adrenal axis and bone mineral density over 2 years in adults with mild asthma. J Allergy Clin Immunol 1999;103(6):1062–8.

32. Agertoft L, Larsen FE, Pedersen S. Posterior subcapsular cataracts, bruises and hoarseness in children with asthma receiving long-term treatment with inhaled budesonide. Eur Respir J 1998;12(1):130–5.

33. Garbe E, LeLorier J, Boivin JF, Suissa S. Inhaled and nasal glucocorticoids and the risks of ocular hypertension or open-angle glaucoma. JAMA 1997;277(9):722–7.

34. Hederos CA. Neuropsychologic changes and inhaled corticosteroids. J Allergy Clin Immunol 2004;114:451–2.

35. Casale TB, Nelson HS, Stricker WE, Raff H, Newman KB. Suppression of hypothalamic–pituitary–adrenal axis activity with inhaled flunisolide and fluticasone propionate in adult asthma patients. Ann Allergy Asthma Immunol 2001;87(5):379–85.

36. Nelson HS, Stricker W, Casale TB, Raff H, Fourre JA, Aron DC, Newman KB. A comparison of methods for assessing hypothalamic–pituitary–adrenal HPA axis activity in asthma patients treated with inhaled corticosteroids. J Clin Pharmacol 2002;42(3):319–26.

37. Fink RS, Pierre LN, Daley-Yates PT, Richards DH, Gibson A, Honour JW. Hypothalamic–pituitary–adrenal axis function after inhaled corticosteroids: unreliability of urinary free cortisol estimation. J Clin Endocrinol Metab 2002;87(10):4541–6.

38. Niitsuma T, Okita M, Sakurai K, Morita S, Tsuyuguchi M, Matsumura Y, Hayashi T, Koshishi T, Oka K, Homma M. Adrenal function as assessed by low-dose adrenocorticotropin hormone test before and after switching from inhaled beclomethasone dipropionate to inhaled fluticasone propionate. J Asthma 2003;40:515–22.

39. Kim KT, Rabinovitch N, Uryniak T, Simpson B, O'Dowd L, Casty F. Effect of budesonide aqueous nasal spray on hypothalamic–pituitary–adrenal axis function in children with allergic rhinitis. Ann Allergy Asthma Immunol 2004;93:61–7.

40. Lipworth BJ, Kaliner MA, LaForce CF, Baker JW, Kaiser HB, Amin D, Kundu S, Williams JE, Engelstaetter R, Banerji DD. Effect of ciclesonide and fluticasone on hypothalamic–pituitary–adrenal axis function in adults with mild-to-moderate persistent asthma. Ann Allergy Asthma Immunol 2005;94:465–72.

41. Szefler SJ, Rohatagi S, Williams JE, Lloyd M, Kundu S, Banerji D. Ciclesonide, a novel inhaled steroid, does not affect hypothalamic–pituitary–adrenal axis function in patients with moderate-to-severe persistent asthma. Chest 2005;128(3):1104–14.

42. Derom E, Van DV, V, Marissens S, Engelstatter R, Vincken W, Pauwels R. Effects of inhaled ciclesonide and fluticasone propionate on cortisol secretion and airway responsiveness to adenosine 5'monophosphate in asthmatic patients. Pulm Pharmacol Ther 2005;18:328–36.

43. Langdon CG, Adler M, Mehra S, Alexander M, Drollmann A. Once-daily ciclesonide 80 or 320 microg for 12 weeks is safe and effective in patients with persistent asthma. Respir Med 2005;99:1275–85.

44. Pearlman DS, Berger WE, Kerwin E, LaForce C, Kundu S, Banerji D. Once-daily ciclesonide improves lung function and is well tolerated by patients with mild-to-moderate persistent asthma. J Allergy Clin Immunol 2005;116:1206–12.

45. Postma DS, Sevette C, Martinat Y, Schlosser N, Aumann J, Kafe H. Treatment of asthma by the inhaled corticosteroid ciclesonide given either in the morning or evening. Eur Respir J 2001;17:1083–8.

46. Szefler S, Rohatagi S, Williams J, Lloyd M, Kundu S, Banerji D. Ciclesonide, a novel inhaled steroid, does not affect hypothalamic–pituitary–adrenal axis function in patients with moderate-to-severe persistent asthma. Chest 2005;128:1104–14.

47. Weinbrenner A, Huneke D, Zschiesche M, Engel G, Timmer W, Steinijans VW, Bethke T, Wurst W, Drollmann A, Kaatz HJ, Siegmund W. Circadian rhythm of serum cortisol after repeated inhalation of the new topical steroid ciclesonide. J Clin Endocrinol Metab 2002;87:2160–3.

48. Lee DK, Fardon TC, Bates CE, Haggart K, McFarlane LC, Lipworth BJ. Airway and systemic effects of hydrofluoroalkane formulations of high-dose ciclesonide and fluticasone in moderate persistent asthma. Chest 2005;127:851–60.

49. Rohatagi S, Krishnaswami S, Pfister M, Sahasranaman S. Model-based covariate pharmacokinetic analysis and lack of cortisol suppression by the new inhaled corticosteroid ciclesonide using a novel cortisol release model. Am J Ther 2005;12:385–97.

50. Chapman KR, Boulet LP, D'Urzo AD. Long-term administration of ciclesonide is safe and well tolerated in patients with persistent asthma. 4th Triennial World Asthma Meeting (WAM). February 16–19, Bangkok, Thailand, 2004:61.

51. Nguyen KL, Lauver D, Kim I, Aresery M. The effect of a steroid "burst" and long-term, inhaled fluticasone propionate on adrenal reserve. Ann Allergy Asthma Immunol 2003;91:38–43.

52. Samaras K, Pett S, Gowers A, McMurchie M, Cooper DA. Iatrogenic Cushing's syndrome with osteoporosis and secondary adrenal failure in human immunodeficiency virus-infected patients receiving inhaled corticosteroids and ritonavir-boosted protease inhibitors: six cases. J Clin Endocrinol Metab 2005;90(7):4394–8.

53. Patel L, Wales JK, Kibirige MS, Massarano AA, Couriel JM, Clayton PE. Symptomatic adrenal insufficiency during inhaled corticosteroid treatment. Arch Dis Child 2001;85(4):330–4.

54. Vargas R, Dockhorn RJ, Findlay SR, Korenblat PE, Field EA, Kral KM. Effect of fluticasone propionate aqueous nasal spray versus oral prednisone on the hypothalamic–pituitary–adrenal axis. J Allergy Clin Immunol 1998;102(2):191–7.

55. Fardon TC, Lee DK, Haggart K, McFarlane LC, Lipworth BJ. Adrenal suppression with dry powder formulations of fluticasone propionate and mometasone furoate. Am J Respir Crit Care Med 2004;170:960–6.

56. Fardon TC, Lee DK, Haggart K, McFarlane LC, Lipworth BJ. Adrenal suppression with dry powder formulations of fluticasone propionate and mometasone furoate. Am J Respir Crit Care Med 2004;170:960–6.

57. Eichenhorn MS, Wise RA, Madhok TC, Gerald LB, Bailey WC, Tashkin DP, Scanlon PD. Lack of long-term adverse adrenal effects from inhaled triamcinolone. Lung Health Study II. Chest 2003;124:57–62.

58. Drake AJ, Howells RJ, Shield JP, Prendiville A, Ward PS, Crowne EC. Symptomatic adrenal insufficiency presenting with hypoglycaemia in children with asthma receiving high dose inhaled fluticasone propionate. BMJ 2002;324(7345):1081–2.

59. Todd GR, Acerini CL, Buck JJ, Murphy NP, Ross-Russell R, Warner JT, McCance DR. Acute adrenal crisis in asthmatics treated with high-dose fluticasone propionate. Eur Respir J 2002;19(6):1207–9.

60. Dunlop KA, Carson DJ, Shields MD. Hypoglycemia due to adrenal suppression secondary to high-dose nebulized corticosteroid. Pediatr Pulmonol 2002;34(1):85–6.

61. Kennedy MJ, Carpenter JM, Lozano RA, Castile RG. Impaired recovery of hypothalamic–pituitary–adrenal axis function and hypoglycemic seizures after high-dose inhaled corticosteroid therapy in a toddler. Ann Allergy Asthma Immunol 2002;88(5):523–6.

62. Duplantier JE, Nelson RP Jr, Morelli AR, Good RA, Kornfeld SJ. Hypothalamic–pituitary–adrenal axis suppression associated with the use of inhaled fluticasone propionate. J Allergy Clin Immunol 1998;102(4 Pt 1):699–700.

63. Zimmerman B, Gold M, Wherrett D, Hanna AK. Adrenal suppression in two patients with asthma treated with low doses of the inhaled steroid fluticasone propionate. J Allergy Clin Immunol 1998;101(3):425–6.

64. Todd GR, Acerini CL, Ross-Russell R, Zahra S, Warner JT, McCance D. Survey of adrenal crisis associated with inhaled corticosteroids in the United Kingdom. Arch Dis Child 2002;87(6):457–61.

65. Wilkinson SM, Cartwright PH, English JS. Hydrocortisone: an important cutaneous allergen. Lancet 1991;337(8744):761–2.

66. Ng PC, Fok TF, Wong GW, Lam CW, Lee CH, Wong MY, Lam K, Ma KC. Pituitary–adrenal suppression in preterm, very low birth weight infants after inhaled fluticasone propionate treatment. J Clin Endocrinol Metab 1998;83(7):2390–3.

67. Aaronson D, Kaiser H, Dockhorn R, Findlay S, Korenblat P, Thorsson L, Kallen A. Effects of budesonide by means of the Turbuhaler on the hypothalmic–pituitary–adrenal axis in asthmatic subjects: a dose-response study. J Allergy Clin Immunol 1998;101(3):312–9.

68. Lipworth BJ. Airway and systemic effects of inhaled corticosteroids in asthma: dose response relationship. Pulm Pharmacol 1996;9(1):19–27.

69. Volovitz B, Nussinovitch M. Effect of high starting dose of budesonide inhalation suspension on serum cortisol concentration in young children with recurrent wheezing episodes. J Asthma 2003;40:625–9.

70. Yiallouros PK, Milner AD, Conway E, Honour JW. Adrenal function and high dose inhaled corticosteroids for asthma. Arch Dis Child 1997;76:405–10.

71. Shapiro G, Bronsky EA, LaForce CF, Mendelson L, Pearlman D, Schwartz RH, Szefler SJ. Dose-related efficacy of budesonide administered via a dry powder inhaler in the treatment of children with moderate to severe persistent asthma. J Pediatr 1998;132:976–82.

72. Priftis KN, Papadimitriou A, Gatsopoulou E, Yiallouros PK, Fretzayas A, Nicolaidou P. The effect of inhaled budesonide on adrenal and growth suppression in asthmatic children. Eur Respir J 2006;27:316–20.

73. Patel L, Wales JK, Kibirige MS, Massarano AA, Couriel JM, Clayton PE. Symptomatic adrenal insufficiency during inhaled corticosteroid treatment. Arch Dis Child 2001;85:330–4.

74. Bacharier LB, Raissy HH, Wilson L, McWilliams B, Strunk RC, Kelly HW. Long-term effect of budesonide on hypothalamic–pituitary–adrenal axis function in children with mild to moderate asthma. Pediatrics 2004;113:1693–9.

75. Agertoft L, Pedersen S. Short-term lower-leg growth rate and urine cortisol excretion in children treated with ciclesonide. J Allergy Clin Immunol 2005;115:940–5.

76. Sim D, Griffiths A, Armstrong D, Clarke C, Rodda C, Freezer N. Adrenal suppression from high-dose inhaled fluticasone propionate in children with asthma. Eur Respir J 2003;21:633–6.

77. Kannisto S, Korppi M, Remes K, Voutilainen R. Adrenal suppression, evaluated by a low dose adrenocorticotropin test, and growth in asthmatic children treated with inhaled steroids. J Clin Endocrinol Metab 2000;85(2):652–7.

78. Shimada T, Yamazaki H, Mimura M, Inui Y, Guengerich FP. Interindividual variations in human liver cytochrome P-450 enzymes involved in the oxidation of drugs, carcinogens and toxic chemicals: studies with liver microsomes of 30 Japanese and 30 Caucasians. J Pharmacol Exp Ther 1994;270(1):414–23.

79. Derendorf H, Hochhaus G, Meibohm B, Mollmann H, Barth J. Pharmacokinetics and pharmacodynamics of inhaled corticosteroids. J Allergy Clin Immunol 1998;101(4 Pt 2):S440–6.

80. Onhoj J, Thorsson L, Bisgaard H. Lung deposition of inhaled drugs increases with age. Am J Respir Crit Care Med 2000;162(5):1819–22.

81. Russell G. Inhaled corticosteroids and adrenal insufficiency. Arch Dis Child 2002;87(6):455–6.

82. Russell G. Fluticasone propionate in children. Respir Med 1994;88(Suppl A):25–9.

83. Bousquet J, Ben-Joseph R, Messonnier M, Alemao E, Gould AL. A meta-analysis of the dose-response relationship of inhaled corticosteroids in adolescents and adults with mild to moderate persistent asthma. Clin Ther 2002;24(1):1–20.

84. Sizonenko PC. Effects of inhaled or nasal glucocorticosteroids on adrenal function and growth. J Pediatr Endocrinol Metab 2002;15(1):5–26.

85. Allen DB. Safety of inhaled corticosteroids in children. Pediatr Pulmonol 2002;33(3):208–20.

86. Faul JL, Tormey W, Tormey V, Burke C. High dose inhaled corticosteroids and dose dependent loss of diabetic control. BMJ 1998;317(7171):1491.

87. Faul JL, Cormican LJ, Tormey VJ, Tormey WP, Burke CM. Deteriorating diabetic control associated with high-dose inhaled budesonide. Eur Respir J 1999;14(1):242–3.

88. Dendukuri N, Blais L, LeLorier J. Inhaled corticosteroids and the risk of diabetes among the elderly. Br J Clin Pharmacol 2002;54(1):59–64.

89. Blackburn D, Hux J, Mamdani M. Quantification of the risk of corticosteroid-induced diabetes mellitus among the elderly. J Gen Intern Med 2002;17(9):717–20.

90. Capewell S, Reynolds S, Shuttleworth D, Edwards C, Finlay AY. Purpura and dermal thinning associated with high dose inhaled corticosteroids. BMJ 1990;300(6739):1548–51.

91. Mak VH, Melchor R, Spiro SG. Easy bruising as a side-effect of inhaled corticosteroids. Eur Respir J 1992;5(9):1068–74.

92. Haapasaari K, Rossi O, Risteli J, Oikarinen A. Effects of long-term inhaled corticosteroids on skin collagen synthesis and thickness in asthmatic patients. Eur Respir J 1998;11(1):139–43.

93. Malo JL, Cartier A, Ghezzo H, Mark S, Brown J, Laviolette M, Boulet LP. Skin bruising, adrenal function and markers of bone metabolism in asthmatics using inhaled beclomethasone and fluticasone. Eur Respir J 1999;13(5):993–8.

94. Dooms-Goossens A. Allergy to inhaled corticosteroids: a review. Am J Contact Dermatitis 1995;6:1–3.

95. Isaksson M, Bruze M, Hornblad Y, Svenonius E, Wihl JA. Contact allergy to corticosteroids in asthma/rhinitis patients. Contact Dermatitis 1999;40(6):327–8.

96. Isaksson M. Skin reactions to inhaled corticosteroids. Drug Saf 2001;24(5):369–73.

97. Israel E, Banerjee TR, Garrett MPH, Fitzmaurice GM, Kotlov TV, LaHive K, LeBoff MS. Effects of inhaled glucocorticoids on bone density in premenopausal women. N Engl J Med 2001;345(13):941–7.

98. Shiri J, Amichai B. Perioral dermatitis induced by inhaled corticosteroids. J Dermatol Treat 1998;9:259–60.

99. Ellepola AN, Samaranayake LP. Inhalational and topical steroids, and oral candidosis: a mini review. Oral Dis 2001;7(4):211–6.

100. National Asthma Education Program, National Institutes of Health. Guidelines for the Diagnosis and Management of Asthma. Publication No 91–3042 Bethesda: United States Department of Health and Human Services;. 1991.

101. Isaksson M, Bruze M. Allergic contact dermatitis in response to budesonide reactivated by inhalation of the allergen. J Am Acad Dermatol 2002;46(6):880–5.

102. Laatikainen AK, Kroger HP, Tukiainen HO, Honkanen RJ, Saarikoski SV. Bone mineral density in perimenopausal women with asthma: a population-based cross-sectional study. Am J Respir Crit Care Med 1999;159(4 Pt 1):1179–85.

103. Wong CA, Subakumar G, Casey PM. Effects of asthma and asthma therapies on bone mineral density. Curr Opin Pulm Med 2002;8(1):39–44.

104. Fujita K, Kasayama S, Hashimoto J, Nagasaka Y, Nakano N, Morimoto Y, Barnes PJ, Miyatake A. Inhaled corticosteroids reduce bone mineral density in early postmenopausal but not premenopausal asthmatic women. J Bone Miner Res 2001;16(4):782–7.

105. Sivri A, Coplu L. Effect of the long-term use of inhaled corticosteroids on bone mineral density in asthmatic women. Respirology 2001;6(2):131–4.

106. Harmanci E, Colak O, Metintas M, Alatas O, Yurdasiper A. Fluticasone propionate and budesonide do not influence bone metabolism in the long term treatment of asthma. Allergol Immunopathol (Madr) 2001;29(1):22–7.

107. Reilly SM, Hambleton G, Adams JE, Mughal MZ. Bone density in asthmatic children treated with inhaled corticosteroids. Arch Dis Child 2001;84(2):183–4.

108. Tattersfield AE, Town GI, Johnell O, Picado C, Aubier M, Braillon P, Karlstrom R. Bone mineral density in subjects with mild asthma randomised to treatment with inhaled corticosteroids or non-corticosteroid treatment for two years. Thorax 2001;56(4):272–8.

109. Poon E, Fewings JM. Generalized eczematous reaction to budesonide in a nasal spray with cross-reactivity to triamcinolone. Australas J Dermatol 2001;42(1):36–7.

110. Bennett ML, Fountain JM, McCarty MA, Sherertz EF. Contact allergy to corticosteroids in patients using inhaled or intranasal corticosteroids for allergic rhinitis or asthma. Am J Contact Dermat 2001;12(4):193–6.

111. Bahceciler NN, Sezgin G, Nursoy MA, Barlan IB, Basaran MM. Inhaled corticosteroids and bone density of children with asthma. J Asthma 2002;39(2):151–7.

112. Agertoft L, Pedersen S. Bone mineral density in children with asthma receiving long-term treatment with inhaled budesonide. Am J Respir Crit Care Med 1998;157(1):178–83.

113. Ma DQ, Jones G. Clinical risk factors but not bone density are associated with prevalent fractures in prepubertal children. J Paediatr Child Health 2002;38(5):497–500.

114. van Staa TP, Leufkens HG, Cooper C. Use of inhaled corticosteroids and risk of fractures. J Bone Miner Res 2001;16(3):581–8.

115. Gregson RK, Rao R, Murrills AJ, Taylor PA, Warner JO. Effect of inhaled corticosteroids on bone mineral density in childhood asthma: comparison of fluticasone propionate with beclomethasone dipropionate. Osteoporos Int 1998;8(5):418–22.

116. Johnell O, Pauwels R, Lofdahl CG, Laitinen LA, Postma DS, Pride NB, Ohlsson SV. Bone mineral density in patients with chronic obstructive pulmonary disease treated with budesonide Turbuhaler. Eur Respir J 2002;19(6):1058–63.

117. Lung Health Study Research Group. Effect of inhaled triamcinolone on the decline in pulmonary function in chronic obstructive pulmonary disease. N Engl J Med 2000;343(26):1902–9.

118. Fitzgerald D, Van Asperen P, Mellis C, Honner M, Smith L, Ambler G. Fluticasone propionate 750 micrograms/day versus beclomethasone dipropionate 1500 micrograms/day: comparison of efficacy and adrenal function in paediatric asthma. Thorax 1998;53(8):656–61.

119. Hughes JA, Conry BG, Male SM, Eastell R. One year prospective open study of the effect of high dose inhaled steroids, fluticasone propionate, and budesonide on bone markers and bone mineral density. Thorax 1999;54(3):223–9.

120. Hubbard RB, Smith CJ, Smeeth L, Harrison TW, Tattersfield AE. Inhaled corticosteroids and hip fracture: a population based case control study. Am J Respir Crit Care Med 2002;166(12 Pt 1):1563–6.

121. Martinati LC, Bertoldo F, Gasperi E, Fortunati P, Lo Cascio V, Boner AL. Longitudinal evaluation of bone mass in asthmatic children treated with inhaled beclomethasone dipropionate or cromolyn sodium. Allergy 1998;53(7):705–8.

122. Price JF, Russell G, Hindmarsh PC, Weller P, Heaf DP, Williams J. Growth during one year of treatment with fluticasone propionate or sodium cromoglycate in children with asthma. Pediatr Pulmonol 1997;24(3):178–86.

123. Bonala SB, Reddy BM, Silverman BA, Bassett CW, Rao YA, Amara S, Schneider AT. Bone mineral density in women with asthma on long-term inhaled corticosteroid therapy. Ann Allergy Asthma Immunol 2000;85(6 Pt 1): 495–500.

124. Wong CA, Walsh LJ, Smith CJ, Wisniewski AF, Lewis SA, Hubbard R, Cawte S, Green DJ, Pringle M, Tattersfield AE. Inhaled corticosteroid use and bone-mineral density in patients with asthma. Lancet 2000;355(9213):1399–403.

125. Boulet LP, Milot J, Gagnon L, Poubelle PE, Brown J. Long-term influence of inhaled corticosteroids on bone metabolism and density. Are biological markers predictors of bone loss? Am J Respir Crit Care Med 1999;159(3):838–44.

126. Sambrook P, Birmingham J, Kempler S, Kelly P, Eberl S, Pocock N, Yeates M, Eisman J. Corticosteroid effects on proximal femur bone loss. J Bone Miner Res 1990;5(12):1211–6.

127. Herrala J, Puolijoki H, Impivaara O, Liippo K, Tala E, Nieminen MM. Bone mineral density in asthmatic women on high-dose inhaled beclomethasone dipropionate. Bone 1994;15(6):621–3.

128. Ebeling PR, Erbas B, Hopper JL, Wark JD, Rubinfeld AR. Bone mineral density and bone turnover in asthmatics treated with long-term inhaled or oral glucocorticoids. J Bone Miner Res 1998;13(8):1283–9.

129. Wang WQ, Ip MS, Tsang KW, Lam KS. Antiresorptive therapy in asthmatic patients receiving high-dose inhaled steroids: a prospective study for 18 months. J Allergy Clin Immunol 1998;101(4 Pt 1):445–50.

130. Herrala J, Puolijoki H, Liippo K, Raitio M, Impivaara O, Tala E, Nieminen MM. Clodronate is effective in preventing corticosteroid-induced bone loss among asthmatic patients. Bone 1998;22(5):577–82.

131. Lo Cascio V, Bonucci E, Imbimbo B, Ballanti P, Adami S, Milani S, Tartarotti D, DellaRocca C. Bone loss in response to long-term glucocorticoid therapy. Bone Miner 1990;8(1):39–51.

132. Allen DB. Influence of inhaled corticosteroids on growth: a pediatric endocrinologist's perspective. Acta Paediatr 1998;87(2):123–9.

133. Norjavaara E, Gerhardsson De Verdier M, Lindmark B. Reduced height in swedish men with asthma at the age of conscription for military service. J Pediatr 2000;137(1): 25–29.

134. Agertoft L, Pedersen S. Effect of long-term treatment with inhaled budesonide on adult height in children with asthma. N Engl J Med 2000;343(15):1064–9.

135. Brand PL. Inhaled corticosteroids reduce growth. Or do they? Eur Respir J 2001;17(2):287–94.

136. Price J, Hindmarsh P, Hughes S, Effthimiou J. Evaluating the effects of asthma therapy on childhood growth: principles of study design. Eur Respir J 2002;19(6):1167–78.

137. Price J, Hindmarsh P, Hughes S, Efthimiou J. Evaluating the effects of asthma therapy on childhood growth: what can be learnt from the published literature? Eur Respir J 2002;19(6):1179–93.

138. Wolthers OD. Growth problems in children with asthma. Horm Res 2002;57(Suppl 2):83–7.

139. Wolthers OD, Allen DB. Inhaled corticosteroids, growth, and compliance. N Engl J Med 2002;347(15):1210–1.

140. Allen DB. Inhaled corticosteroid therapy for asthma in preschool children: growth issues. Pediatrics 2002;109(Suppl 2):373–80.

141. Pedersen S. Do inhaled corticosteroids inhibit growth in children? Am J Respir Crit Care Med 2001;164(4):521–35.

142. Thorsson L, Edsbacker S, Kallen A, Lofdahl CG. Pharmacokinetics and systemic activity of fluticasone via Diskus and pMDI, and of budesonide via Turbuhaler. Br J Clin Pharmacol 2001;52(5):529–38.

143. Ferguson AC, Spier S, Manjra A, Versteegh FG, Mark S, Zhang P. Efficacy and safety of high-dose inhaled steroids in children with asthma: a comparison of fluticasone propionate with budesonide. J Pediatr 1999;134(4):422–7.

144. The Childhood Asthma Management Program Research Group. Long-term effects of budesonide or nedocromil in children with asthma. N Engl J Med 2000;343(15):1054–63.

145. Allen DB, Mullen M, Mullen B. A meta-analysis of the effect of oral and inhaled corticosteroids on growth. J Allergy Clin Immunol 1994;93(6):967–76.

146. Doull IJ, Campbell MJ, Holgate ST. Duration of growth suppressive effects of regular inhaled corticosteroids. Arch Dis Child 1998;78(2):172–3.

147. Balfour-Lynn L. Growth and childhood asthma. Arch Dis Child 1986;61(11):1049–55.

148. Priori R, Tomassini M, Magrini L, Conti F, Valesini G. Churg–Strauss syndrome during pregnancy after steroid withdrawal. Lancet 1998;352(9140):1599–600.

149. Sears MR, Taylor DR. The beta 2-agonist controversy. Observations, explanations and relationship to asthma epidemiology. Drug Saf 1994;11(4):259–83.

150. Fukushima C, Matsuse H, Tomari S, Obase Y, Miyazaki Y, Shimoda T, Kohno S. Oral candidiasis associated with inhaled corticosteroid use: comparison of fluticasone and beclomethasone. Ann Allergy Asthma Immunol 2003;90:646–51.

151. Leav BA, Fanburg B, Hadley S. Invasive pulmonary aspergillosis associated with high-dose inhaled fluticasone. N Engl J Med 2000;343(8):586.

152. Kallen B, Rydhstroem H, Aberg A. Congenital malformations after the use of inhaled budesonide in early pregnancy. Obstet Gynecol 1999;93(3):392–5.

153. Rouanet I, Peyriere H, Mauboussin JM, Vincent D. Cushing's syndrome in a patient treated by ritonavir/lopinavir and inhaled fluticasone. HIV Med 2003;4:149–50.

154. Raaska K, Niemi M, Neuvonen M, Neuvonen PJ, Kivisto KT. Plasma concentrations of inhaled budesonide and its effects on plasma cortisol are increased by the cytochrome P4503A4 inhibitor itraconazole. Clin Pharmacol Ther 2002;72(4):362–9.

155. De Wachter E, Vanbesien J, De Schutter I, Malfroot A, De Schepper J. Rapidly developing Cushing syndrome in a 4-year-old patient during combined treatment with itraconazole and inhaled budesonide. Eur J Pediatr 2003;162:488–9.

156. Bolland MJ, Bagg W, Thomas MG, Lucas JA, Ticehurst R, Black PN. Cushing's syndrome due to interaction between inhaled corticosteroids and itraconazole. Ann Pharmacother 2004;38:46–9.

157. Clevenbergh P, Corcostegui M, Gerard D, Hieronimus S, Mondain V, Chichmanian RM, Sadoul JL, Dellamonica P. Iatrogenic Cushing's syndrome in an HIV-infected patient treated with inhaled corticosteroids (fluticasone propionate) and low dose ritonavir enhanced PI containing regimen. J Infect 2002;44(3):194–5.

158. Samaras K, Pett S, Gowers A, McMurchie M, Cooper DA. Iatrogenic Cushing's syndrome with osteoporosis and secondary adrenal failure in human immunodeficiency virus-

infected patients receiving inhaled corticosteroids and ritonavir-boosted protease inhibitors: six cases. J Clin Endocrinol Metab 2005;90(7):4394–8.

Corticosteroids—glucocorticoids, topical

The local adverse effects of topical glucocorticoids (1,2) are listed in Table 1. They include transient local

Table 1 Local adverse effects of topical glucocorticoids

Effects on the pilosebaceous unit
  Perioral dermatitis (SEDA-5, 151)
  Steroid rosacea or rosacea-like dermatitis; cannot be differentiated from perioral dermatitis and can be identical
  Steroid acne
  Exacerbation of pre-existing rosacea
  Hypertrichosis of the face
Atrophic changes
  Cigarette-paper wrinkling of the skin
  Telangiectasia (SEDA-6, 153)
  Petechiae, ecchymoses
  Striae rubrae distensae, mainly in the inguinal and axillary regions (occlusion effect)
  Susceptibility of the skin to minor trauma
  Fragile skin in surgery
  Delayed wound healing
  Worsening of existing ulceration
  Photosensitivity of atrophic skin
Effects on the immune system
  Aggravation of pre-existing folliculitis
  Development of extensive, but unrecognized dermatophytic infections ("tinea incognito")
  Perpetuation of masked infections with *Candida albicans*
  Conversion of scabies into the Norwegian type
  Widespread lesions of molluscum contagiosum
  "Galloping" impetigo
  (Possibly) exacerbation or dissemination of viral skin infections
  Generalized pustular psoriasis
  Generalized urticaria
  Spreading of malignant skin lesions
  Suppression of pruritus
  Allergic contact dermatitis* (SEDA-15, 139)
Ocular effects
  Ocular hypertension
  Open-angle glaucoma (9)
  Uveitis
  Posterior subcapsular cataracts (9)
Nasal effects
  Nasal septal perforation (steroid aerosols)
Skin lesions
  Acne
  Hirsutism
  Ecchymoses
  Milia
  Granuloma gluteale infantum
  Pseudocicatrices stellaires spontanées
  Eczema craquelatum after withdrawal

Elastoidosis cutanée nodulaire à cystes et à comedones
Favre-Raacouchot
Erythrosis interfollicularis colli
Cutis punctata linearis colli or "stippled skin"
Effects on skin color
  Hypopigmentation
  Hyperpigmentation
  Striae
Miscellaneous effects
  Tachyphylaxis to the vasoconstrictor effect of topical glucocorticoids
Systemic adverse effects of topical administration
  Cushing's syndrome
  Suppression of the hypothalamic–pituitary–adrenal axis
  Growth retardation (SEDA-6, 151)
  Hyperglycemia
  Benign intracranial hypertension after withdrawal
  Subcapsular cataract
  Pancreatitis
  Bony avascular necrosis (9)
  Psychiatric symptoms
  Fluid retention
  Hypertension (SEDA-7, 167)

erythema, calcinosis cutis, cramps (due to injection of crystals into a vessel), amaurosis (a dubious report), depigmentation, skin atrophy, and skin necrosis (3,4). The systemic adverse effects of topical glucocorticoids (5–8), which are those to be expected from systemic use, are also listed in Table 1.

References

1. De Groot AC, Weyland JW, Nater JP. Unwanted Effects of Cosmetics and Drugs used in Dermatology. 3rd ed.. Amsterdam: Elsevier;. 1994.
2. Miller JA, Munro DD. Topical corticosteroids: clinical pharmacology and therapeutic use. Drugs 1980;19(2):119–34.
3. Rimbaud P, Meynadier J, Guilhou JJ, Meynadier J. Complications dermatologiques locales secondaires aux injections cortisonées. [Local dermatological complications secondary to corticosteroid injections.] Nouv Presse Méd 1974;3(11):665–8.
4. Davy A, Guillerot E, Boyer C. A propos d'un accident iatrogène consecutif à une injection de corticoïdes au cou de pied. [An iatrogenic complication subsequent to an injection of corticoids into the instep.] Phlebologie 1986;39(3):527–37.
5. Walsh P, Aeling JL, Huff L, Weston WL. Hypothalamus–pituitary–adrenal axis suppression by superpotent topical steroids. J Am Acad Dermatol 1993;29(3):501–3.
6. Dhein S. Cushing-Syndrom nach externer Glukokortikoid-Applikation bei psoriasis. [Cushing syndrome following external glucocorticoid administration in psoriasis.] Z Hautkr 1986;61(3):161–6.
7. Lawlor F, Ramabala K. Iatrogenic Cushing's syndrome—a cautionary tale. Clin Exp Dermatol 1984;9(3):286–9.
8. Olsen EA, Cornell RC. Topical clobetasol-17-propionate: review of its clinical efficacy and safety. J Am Acad Dermatol 1986;15(2 Pt 1):246–55.
9. McLean CJ, Lobo RF, Brazier DJ. Cataracts, glaucoma, and femoral avascular necrosis caused by topical corticosteroid ointment. Lancet 1995;345(8945):330.
10. Isaksson M, Dooms-Goossens AN. Contact allergens—what's new? Corticosteroids. Clin Dermatol 1997;15(4):527–31.

11. Dooms-Goossens A. Allergy to inhaled corticosteroids: a review. Am J Contact Dermatitis 1995;6:1–3.
12. Whitmore SE. Delayed systemic allergic reactions to corticosteroids. Contact Dermatitis 1995;32(4):193–8.

Corticosteroids— mineralocorticoids

General Information

Aldosterone is the principal physiological salt-retaining mineralocorticoid, but it is unsuitable for routine medical use since it is rapidly inactivated when given orally. Desoxycorticosterone (DCA, DOCA, desoxycortone) was used for a long time, but it had to be taken sublingually (or implanted or injected) to avoid inactivation during passage through the liver. Overdosage of desoxycorticosterone, leading to hypertensive encephalopathy and permanent brain damage, has been described (SED-8, 820).

The approximate potency of various mineralocorticoids relative to cortisone is shown in Table 1.

Fludrocortisone is the compound that is most often used at present for long-term mineralocorticoid treatment. The dose of fludrocortisone needed in chronic adrenocortical insufficiency varies very widely, from 0.05 to 1.0 mg/day. In salt-losing forms of the congenital adrenogenital syndrome up to 0.2 mg/day may be needed. In doses appropriate to the individual's needs, adverse reactions to the glucocorticoid effects of fludrocortisone rarely prove problematic; the main problem is to adjust the dosage (as well as salt intake) to these needs, since the adverse effects that can be experienced mainly reflect relative overdosage; if high doses are to be used, meticulous monitoring is required.

Table 1 Approximate potency of various mineralocorticoids relative to cortisone

Compound	Route of administration	Mineralo-corticoid effect	Gluco-corticoid effect
Cortisone	Oral	1	1
Desoxy-corticosterone	Sublingual	50	Negligible
Fludrocortisone	Oral	150	10–20
Aldosterone	Injected	500	None

Organs and Systems

Cardiovascular

Edema, hypertension, and cardiac hypertrophy can occur with fludrocortisone (1). Hypertension is the most common reason for reducing the dosage.

Fluid retention due to mineralocorticoid effects can cause cardiac failure (1).

- Congestive heart failure occurred in a 47-year-old woman after she had taken fludrocortisone 100 micrograms/day for 2 weeks for Addison's disease (2). Ten months later, fludrocortisone 25 micrograms/day was restarted, and the dosage was increased to 100 micrograms/day over 2 months. At follow-up after 4 months she was well, without fluid retention or electrolyte abnormalities.

Electrolyte balance

Hypokalemia due to fludrocortisone can cause muscle weakness (3).

Drug–Drug Interactions

Phenytoin

In two patients with adrenal insufficiency, phenytoin increased fludrocortisone dosage requirements (4).

Potassium-sparing diuretics

Potassium-sparing diuretics, such as prorenoate and spironolactone, can prevent the potassium-losing effects of fludrocortisone (5).

References

1. Hussain RM, McIntosh SJ, Lawson J, Kenny RA. Fludrocortisone in the treatment of hypotensive disorders in the elderly. Heart 1996;76(6):507–9.
2. Bhattacharyya A, Tymms DJ. Heart failure with fludrocortisone in Addison's disease. J R Soc Med 1998;91(8):433–4.
3. Rivera VM. Fludrocortisone acetate and muscular weakness. JAMA 1973;225:993.
4. Keilholz U, Guthrie GP Jr. Adverse effect of phenytoin on mineralocorticoid replacement with fludrocortisone in adrenal insufficiency. Am J Med Sci 1986;291(4):280–3.
5. Ramsay LE, Shelton JR, Tidd MJ. The pharmacodynamics of single doses of prorenoate potasssium and spironolactone in fludrocortisone treated normal subjects. Br J Clin Pharmacol 1976;3(3):475–82.

Corticotrophins (corticotropin and tetracosactide)

General Information

The adrenocorticotrophic hormone ACTH (corticotropin) stimulates the adrenal cortex to secrete the glucocorticoids hydrocortisone (cortisol) and corticosterone, the mineralocorticoid aldosterone, and a number of weakly androgenic substances, as well as a small amount of testosterone. Aldosterone synthesis is also regulated by renin and angiotensin.

This monograph should be read in conjunction with the monograph on glucocorticoids. It is not always clear which adverse effects are specific to corticotrophins and which simply result from the secretion of the glucocorticoids that they induce; conversely, almost any adverse effect associated with glucocorticoids can in principle also occur with corticotrophins.

Structures and nomenclature

Natural ACTH (corticotropin) is a polypeptide consisting of 39 amino acids. Its hormonal activity is related to the first 24 amino acids in a sequence that is found in both animal and human pituitary glands. The differing sequences of the remaining 15 amino acids in animals can lead to antibody formation and hence to allergic reactions when animal hormones are injected into humans. From 1970 onwards, therefore, even highly purified corticotropin preparations of animal origin were largely displaced by the so-called "synthetic ACTH" or "synthetic corticotropin," better known by its generic name of tetracosactide (rINN), which contains only the first 24 amino acids, hence avoiding much of the antigenicity of the complete molecule. Collectively, corticotropin and tetracosactide are known as the corticotrophins.

Since the development of tetracosactide, other modifications to the corticotropin molecule have been made, and some clinical work has been done with products containing fewer than 24 amino acids, for example 1–18. However, none has proved more usable than tetracosactide. The replacement of some naturally occurring amino acids by others may intensify or prolong the effect of the polypeptide.

Production and elimination

Fluctuations in the rates of secretion of glucocorticoids from the adrenal cortex are determined by variations in the rate of release of corticotropin from the anterior pituitary, and this in turn is controlled by the hypothalamic corticotropin-releasing hormone (CRH). Since release of CRH is affected by circulating glucocorticoid concentrations, a negative-feedback control operates to keep the system in balance. It follows from this that if glucocorticoids are administered exogenously they will operate through this feedback to suppress adrenal function.

The mode of inactivation and excretion of corticotropin is still almost completely unknown; its biological half-life has been variously assessed as several minutes or several hours.

Uses

Corticotrophins can be used diagnostically to investigate adrenocortical insufficiency. Corticotropin has also been used therapeutically in most of the conditions for which systemic glucocorticoids are indicated, although such use is now fairly limited. However, corticotropin is used in certain neurological disorders, such as infantile spasms and multiple sclerosis. The main indications for corticotropin and tetracosactide are thus diagnostic rather than therapeutic; for the latter purpose they are being increasingly replaced by CRH.

General adverse effects

Corticotrophins share all the adverse effects of glucocorticoids, including impaired immunity, but they do not depress adrenocortical function. In addition, the melanocyte-stimulating hormone (MSH) sequence in the corticotropin molecule can result in hyperpigmentation, and induction of androgen secretion can lead to virilization. Corticotrophins also have additional unwanted effects of their own, such as myoclonic encephalopathy and adrenal hemorrhage. Hypersensitivity reactions occur occasionally, but have become less frequent since older preparations of animal origin were phased out. Tumor-inducing effects have not been observed.

Organs and Systems

Cardiovascular

Corticotropin has been reported to cause enlargement of cardiac tumors in tuberous sclerosis (1).

- A female infant with tuberous sclerosis had multiple large cardiac tumors in the left and right ventricles. Corticotropin was given (dose not stated; once a day for 2 weeks, tapering over 3 months) at 4 months for infantile spasms. At 6 months a heart murmur was detected. Echocardiography showed pronounced enlargement of the tumors in both ventricles and a small tumor extending from the upper portion of the interventricular septum into the left ventricular outflow tract. An electrocardiogram showed 2–3 mm ST segment depression in leads I, aVL, and V4-6. Gated single photon emission CT showed low perfusion at the lateral and inferior regions of the left ventricle, indicating myocardial ischemia. Corticotropin was withdrawn and 3 months later the patient was asymptomatic. An echocardiogram showed that the tumors had reduced in size, and there was concomitant improvement in the electrocardiogram.

There is a risk of myocardial hypertrophy in children on prolonged treatment with ACTH (2), an effect that could reflect increased androgen secretion and thus be more likely to occur than with glucocorticoids.

Hypertension, with or without simultaneous hypertrophic myopathy, is a common feature of adrenal stimulation that seems to be common with depot tetracosactide but not simple tetracosactide (3). During treatment for infantile spasms, hypertension occurred more often in those treated with high doses (SEDA-19, 374) (4), and changes in cardiac function, such as left ventricular shortening fraction, can occur early and sometimes before systolic hypertension (SEDA-19, 374) (5).

Respiratory

Corticotropin and to a lesser extent tetracosactide can cause asthma in sensitive subjects (6). The question as to whether tetracosactide or glucocorticoids should be preferred for the treatment of chronic asthmatic bronchitis has been discussed mainly with respect to adverse effects, particularly adverse endocrine effects and effects on growth. An earlier belief that corticotropin might be more effective in children has not been confirmed.

Nervous system

In 138 Japanese patients with West syndrome treated with low-dose tetracosactide, the initial effects on seizures and long-term outcome were not related to dose (daily dose 0.005–0.032 mg/kg, 0.2–1.28 IU/kg; total dose 0.1–0.87 mg/kg, 4–35 IU/kg) (7). There were moderate or severe adverse effects in 30% of the patients. There was slight loss of brain volume on CT/MRI scans in 64% of the patients, moderate loss in 23%, and severe loss in 4%. The severity of adverse effects correlated with the total dose of corticotropin, and the severity of brain volume loss due to corticotropin correlated well with the daily and total doses. The authors recommended a reduction in the dose of corticotropin in order to avoid serious adverse effects.

Brain shrinkage has been described as a possible adverse effect of corticotropin treatment of infantile spasms, and this has been confirmed using magnetic resonance imaging (SEDA-20, 368) (8,9). Changes in midline structures (volume reductions in the pons, corpus callosum, and cerebellum) seem to show that the beneficial effect of corticotropin in infantile spasms could be due to a direct effect on the brainstem. Cerebral shrinkage and subdural hematoma occurred after the administration of high doses of corticotropin for West syndrome (total dose 4.5–6.75 mg) and subdural hematoma occurred in two children (aged 2 and 5 months) during the administration of low doses of tetracosactide (0.01 mg/kg/day; total dose 0.24–0.26 mg) (10).

Drowsiness, hypotonia, and irritability were observed in 37% of infants given corticotropin in a randomized comparison of corticotropin with vigabatrin in the treatment of infantile spasms (SEDA-22, 442; 11).

Myoclonic encephalopathy appears to be a specific, if rare, complication of corticotropin, not seen with the glucocorticoids (12).

Sensory systems

Bilateral subcapsular cataracts and glaucoma have been reported as possible risks (13), but they presumably reflect glucocorticoid effects.

Bilateral macular degeneration has been described with tetracosactide (13), but presumably reflects glucocorticoid effects.

Central serous retinopathy has been linked to the therapeutic use of corticotrophins or glucocorticoids or to endogenous corticotropin hypersecretion. Bilateral central serous retinopathy has been reported in a woman treated with tetracosactide intramuscularly (SEDA-22, 442) (14).

Psychological, psychiatric

Mood changes continue to be reported in association with corticotropin (15). Emotional instability or psychotic tendencies can be aggravated, while euphoria, insomnia, and personality changes such as hypomania and depression can be precipitated, sometimes even with psychotic manifestations. Although it seems reasonable to assume that one is dealing here mainly with an effect of the glucocorticoids secreted in response to corticotropin, it should be recalled that segments of the corticotropin molecule themselves have effects on brain function and could conceivably play a role.

Endocrine

Corticotropin can promote the development of a more or less pronounced Cushingoid state. Corticotropin also increases the metabolic clearance rate of cortisol, aldosterone, and desoxycorticosterone (SEDA-1, 282).

Prolonged stimulation by corticotropin leads to adrenocortical cell hyperplasia and an increase in the size and weight of the adrenal glands; massive enlargement can be demonstrated by computerized tomography as well as clinical examination (16).

Acute adrenal hemorrhage, either unilateral (17) or bilateral (18), has been observed repeatedly after corticotropin administration, and causes an acute abdominal crisis. Although it is usually seen in children, hemorrhage can also occur in adults (SEDA-17, 451).

Even a single dose of corticotropin can cause inhibition of thyrotrophic hormone secretion (19), although the effect is brief. Conversely, thyroid hormones increase the sensitivity of adrenocortical cells in vitro to corticotropin (20) and hyperthyroidism increases sensitivity to corticotropin (21,22).

Corticotropin suppresses the growth hormone response to hypoglycemia (23).

Androgen secretion due to corticotropin can cause virilization in women (24).

Fluid balance

Corticotropin affects mineral and fluid balance in varying degrees, as would be expected from its effect on mineralocorticoid secretion.

Hematologic

Marked leukocytosis has been described, despite the absence of infection, in a patient treated with tetracosactide (SED-12, 980); the effect may well have been due to glucocorticoid secretion rather than to tetracosactide itself.

Gastrointestinal

A relative indication for corticotropin is the occasional gastrointestinal intolerance that occurs with oral glucocorticoids. In these cases, however, only the local effects of the glucocorticoids can be avoided, and not their systemic effects on the gastrointestinal tract (25).

Urinary tract

Renal calcinosis can develop as a result of hypercalciuria and is a major concern in the treatment of infantile spasms with corticotropin. In 16 infants, corticotropin, often associated with anticonvulsants, results in increased urinary excretion of calcium and phosphate, with increased parathormone serum concentrations and in some cases generalized aminoaciduria (26). This makes it imperative that the dose of corticotropin and the duration of treatment be kept to the minimum required to ensure efficacy. In one case in which calcified stones were removed surgically, recurrence was apparently prevented, despite the presence of a Cushingoid state, by long-term chlorothiazide (27).

Skin

Allergic skin reactions, for example urticaria, can occur. Since the first 13 amino acids in the corticotropin peptide are the same as in MSH, treatment with corticotropin can occasionally cause hyperpigmentation. The shorter peptide chain in tetracosactide can even cause rather more pronounced melanocyte-stimulatory effects. Long-term treatment with depot tetracosactide has itself caused melanoderma (SED-12, 980) and, in one series of 41 patients, there was hyperpigmentation in 3 of them (SEDA-1, 281).

Immunologic

Although the incidence of severe allergic reactions to natural corticotropin of animal origin fell as progressively purer products were introduced, the problem remained for a small minority of patients. Exact figures are difficult to cite, but hypersensitivity reactions have sometimes even been described in patients with no history of corticotropin treatment, presumably sensitized by other animal material. Hypersensitivity to corticotropin generally causes only dizziness, nausea and vomiting, or cutaneous hypersensitivity reactions, but in several instances shock with circulatory failure has been observed (28). In a number of patients who were allergic to porcine corticotropin, no such problems were observed when tetracosactide was given. This suggests that the absence of most of the antigenic part of the original molecule reduces the risk of hypersensitivity reactions. However, the smaller synthetic molecule can still stimulate the formation of antibodies in some individuals (SEDA-12, 979) (29).

However, allergic reactions and anaphylactic shock have been observed during treatment with tetracosactide and have even proved fatal. Local reactions have even been seen after the administration of small doses for intracutaneous testing. In the early years of tetracosactide use, the frequency of local and general reactions to a long-acting acetylated tetracosactide was estimated at as little as one in 30 000 (SED-12, 979), but it is doubtful whether this figure can be supported today, unless one interprets it as referring only to major calamities. Indeed, subclinical immune reactions to both natural and tetracosactide appear to be fairly common during long-term treatment of patients with asthma, with an incidence of intradermal reactions of about 50%, a prevalence of IgE antibodies that is significantly higher than in controls, and a high incidence of low-titer agglutinating antibodies to corticotropin. The antibodies can result in a gradual loss of effect.

Infection risk

Pneumonia due to *Pneumocystis jiroveci* (formerly *Pneumocystis carinii*) has been attributed to high-dose corticotropin (30).

- An infant girl was given corticotropin 80 U/day for infantile spasms. After 5 weeks she became increasingly lethargic, with reduced oral intake, cough, an increased respiratory rate (50 breaths/minute), and a fever of 38.6°C. Investigations were consistent with pneumonia and she was given intravenous ceftriaxone. She initially improved, but 36 hours later her respiratory distress worsened and she required intubation and mechanical ventilation. The diagnosis of *P. jiroveci* pneumonia was confirmed and she was given intravenous co-trimoxazole and glucocorticoids. Her respiratory distress resolved and she was extubated 10 days later. Immunological testing after the withdrawal of corticotropin did not show any abnormalities that could have predisposed her to *P. jiroveci* pneumonia.

The authors commented that a transient immunodeficiency related to corticotrophin may have predisposed to the development of *P. jiroveci* pneumonia.

Long-Term Effects

Drug withdrawal

Relative adrenocortical insufficiency can follow withdrawal of corticotropin treatment (presumably because the cortex has adapted itself to a constant high level of stimulation) and can persist for some months. Glucocorticoid substitution has to be provided during this period. The risk of this effect can be reduced by keeping the dose of corticotropin as low as possible.

Second-Generation Effects

Pregnancy

There are no firm data on the use of corticotropin in pregnancy; both glucocorticoid and androgenic effects might be expected to affect the fetus.

Susceptibility Factors

Age

Although it has been stated in reviews that treatment with corticotropin inhibits growth much less than glucocorticoid treatment does, the growth hormone response to stimuli is reduced, and since growth hormone secretion is impaired during corticotropin treatment, claims for the greater safety of this therapy in children with asthma must be treated with reservations.

Other features of the patient

Susceptibility factors for adverse effects are as for glucocorticoids. In addition, patients with a known allergic tendency should preferably not receive these substances, unless sufficient supervision is possible to cope with unexpected allergic reactions, at least until tolerance has been demonstrated.

Drug–Drug Interactions

Coumarin anticoagulants

In 10 of 14 patients taking dicoumarol or phenindione who also took corticotropin for 4–9 days, there was a small increase in the effects of the anticoagulants (31). One patient taking ethyl biscoumacetate developed bleeding after taking corticotropin 20 mg/day for 3 days (32). However, in contrast, reduced efficacy of ethyl biscoumacetate has been described (33).

References

1. Hiraishi S, Iwanami N, Ogawa N. Images in cardiology. Enlargement of cardiac rhabdomyoma and myocardial ischaemia during corticotropin treatment for infantile spasm. Heart 2000;84(2):170.
2. Lang D, Muhler E, Kupferschmid C, Tacke E, von Bernuth G. Cardiac hypertrophy secondary to ACTH treatment in children. Eur J Pediatr 1984;142(2):121–5.
3. Kusse MC, van Nieuwenhuizen O, van Huffelen AC, van der Mey W, Thijssen JH, van Ree JM. The effect of non-depot ACTH(1–24) on infantile spasms. Dev Med Child Neurol 1993;35(12):1067–73.
4. Hrachovy RA, Frost JD Jr, Glaze DG. High-dose, long-duration versus low-dose, short-duration corticotropin therapy for infantile spasms. J Pediatr 1994;124(5 Pt 1):803–6.
5. Starc TJ, Bierman FZ, Pavlakis SG, Challenger ME, De Vivo DC, Gersony WM. Cardiac size and function during adrenocorticotropic hormone-induced systolic systemic hypertension in infants. Am J Cardiol 1994;73(1):57–64.
6. Grabner W. Zur induzierten NNR-Insuffizienz. (Problems of corticosteroid-induced adrenal insufficiency in surgery.) Fortschr Med 1977;95(30):1866–8.
7. Ito M, Aiba H, Hashimoto K, Kuroki S, Tomiwa K, Okuno T, Hattori H, Go T, Sejima H, Dejima S, Ikeda H, Yoshioka M, Kanazawa O, Kawamitsu T, Ochi J, Miki N, Noma H, Oguro K, Ozaki N, Tamamoto A, Matsubara T, Miyajima T, Fujii T, Konishi Y, Okuno T, Hojo H. Low-dose ACTH therapy for West syndrome: initial effects and long-term outcome. Neurology 2002;58(1):110–4.
8. Konishi Y, Yasujima M, Kuriyama M, Konishi K, Hayakawa K, Fujii Y, Ishii Y, Sudo M. Magnetic resonance imaging in infantile spasms: effects of hormonal therapy. Epilepsia 1992;33(2):304–9.
9. Konishi Y, Hayakawa K, Kuriyama M, Saito M, Fujii Y, Sudo M. Effects of ACTH on brain midline structures in infants with infantile spasms. Pediatr Neurol 1995;13(2):134–6.
10. Ito M, Miyajima T, Fujii T, Okuno T. Subdural hematoma during low-dose ACTH therapy in patients with West syndrome. Neurology 2000;54(12):2346–7.
11. Vigevano F, Cilio MR. Vigabatrin versus ACTH as first-line treatment for infantile spasms: a randomized, prospective study. Epilepsia 1997;38(12):1270–4.
12. Rutgers AW, Links TP, le Coultre R, Begeer JH. Behavioural disturbances after effective ACTH-treatment of the dancing-eyes syndrome. Dev Med Child Neurol 1988;30(3):408–9.
13. Williamson J, Dalakos TG. Posterior subcapsular cataracts and macular lesions after long-term corticotrophin therapy. Br J Ophthalmol 1967;51(12):839–42.
14. Zamir E. Central serous retinopathy associated with adrenocorticotrophic hormone therapy. A case report and a hypothesis. Graefes Arch Clin Exp Ophthalmol 1997;235(6):339–44.
15. Minden SL, Orav J, Schildkraut JJ. Hypomanic reactions to ACTH and prednisone treatment for multiple sclerosis. Neurology 1988;38(10):1631–4.
16. Liebling MS, Starc TJ, McAlister WH, Ruzal-Shapiro CB, Abramson SJ, Berdon WE. ACTH induced adrenal enlargement in infants treated for infantile spasms and acute cerebellar encephalopathy. Pediatr Radiol 1993;23(6):454–6.
17. Levin TL, Morton E. Adrenal hemorrhage complicating ACTH therapy in Crohn's disease. Pediatr Radiol 1993;23(6):457–8.
18. Dunlap SK, Meiselman MS, Breuer RI, Panella JS, Ficho TW, Reid SE Jr. Bilateral adrenal hemorrhage as a complication of intravenous ACTH infusion in two patients with inflammatory bowel disease. Am J Gastroenterol 1989;84(10):1310–2.
19. Prummel MF, Brokken LJ, Wiersinga WM. Ultra short-loop feedback control of thyrotropin secretion. Thyroid 2004;14(10):825–9.
20. Simonian MH. ACTH and thyroid hormone regulation of 3 beta-hydroxysteroid dehydrogenase activity in human fetal adrenocortical cells. J Steroid Biochem 1986;25(6):1001–6.
21. Jasani MK. Anti-inflammatory steroids: mode of action in rheumatoid arthritis and homograft reaction. In: Born GVR, Farah A, Herken H, Welch AD, editors. Handbook of Experimental Pharmacology. Berlin–Heidelberg–New York: Springer-Verlag, 1979:589.
22. Labhart A, Martz G. Fundamentals of hormone treatment of nonendocrine disorders. In: Labhart A, editor. Clinical Endocrinology. Berlin–Heidelberg–New York: Springer-Verlag, 1986:1067.
23. McGregor VP, Banarer S, Cryer PE. Elevated endogenous cortisol reduces autonomic neuroendocrine and symptom responses to subsequent hypoglycemia. Am J Physiol Endocrinol Metab 2002;282(4):E770–7.
24. Garren LD, Gill GN, Masui H, Walton GM. On the mechanism of action of ACTH. Recent Prog Horm Res 1971;27:433–78.

25. Mathies H. Probleme der symptomatischen Therapie rheumatischer Erkrankungen mit Glukokortikoiden und nichtsteroidalen Antirheumatika. [Problems in symptomatic therapy of rheumatic diseases with glucocorticoids and nonsteroidal antirheumatic agents.] Internist (Berl) 1979;20(9):414–25.

26. Riikonen R, Simell O, Jaaskelainen J, Rapola J, Perheentupa J. Disturbed calcium and phosphate homeostasis during treatment with ACTH of infantile spasms. Arch Dis Child 1986;61(7):671–6.

27. Katzir Z, Shvil Y, Landau EH, Popovtzer MM. Thiazide therapy for ACTH-induced hypercalciuria and nephrolithiasis. Acta Paediatr 1992;81(3):277–9.

28. Riikonen R, Simell O, Dunkel L, Santavuori P, Perheentupa J. Hormonal background of the hypertension and fluid derangements associated with adrenocorticotrophic hormone treatment of infants. Eur J Pediatr 1989;148(8):737–41.

29. Glass D, Nuki G, Daly JR. Development of antibodies during long-term therapy with corticotrophin in rheumatoid arthritis. II. Zinc tetracosactrin (Depot Synacthen). Ann Rheum Dis 1971;30(6):593–6.

30. Dunagan DP, Rubin BK, Fasano MB. *Pneumocystis carinii* pneumonia in a child receiving ACTH for infantile spasms. Pediatr Pulmonol 1999;27(4):286–9.

31. Hellem AJ, Solem JH. The influence of ACTH on prothrombin–proconvertin values in blood during treatment with dicumarol and phenylindanedione. Acta Med Scand 1954;150(5):389–93.

32. Van Cauwenberge H, Jaques LB. Haemorrhagic effect of ACTH with anticoagulants. Can Med Assoc J 1958;79(7):536–40.

33. Chatterjea JB, Salomon L. Antagonistic effect of A.C.T.H. and cortisone on the anticoagulant activity of ethyl biscoumacetate BMJ 1954;4891:790–2.

PROSTAGLANDINS

General Information

Eicosanoids are the oxygenated metabolites of 20-carbon unsaturated fatty acids found in the phospholipids of cell membranes (Greek eikosi = 20). The eicosanoids include the prostaglandins, thromboxanes, and leukotrienes. Precursor fatty acids include arachidonic acid $C20:4n–6$ (for 2-series prostaglandins and thromboxane and 4-series leukotrienes), dihomogammalinolenic acid $C20:3n–6$ (for PGE_1), and eicosapentaenoic acid $C20:5n–3$ (for 3-series prostaglandins and 5-series leukotrienes). Naturally occurring eicosanoids are predominantly metabolites of arachidonic acid, reflecting the dominance of $n–6$ fatty acids in the terrestrial food chain.

The principal biologically active, naturally occurring prostaglandins are prostaglandin E_1 (PGE_1), prostaglandin E_2 (PGE_2), prostaglandin $F_{2\alpha}$ ($PGF_{2\alpha}$), prostacyclin (PGI_2), and thromboxane (TXA_2). These agents have various, sometimes opposed, biological actions (1). Their half-lives are short, owing to their rapid breakdown (a few minutes for PGE_2 and $PGF_{2\alpha}$, a few seconds for PGI_2) (2). Prostaglandins thus have principally local biological actions. Analogues (mostly methyl derivatives) have been synthesized and are more slowly inactivated. The adverse reactions encountered when prostaglandins are used therapeutically will depend on the indications (see Table 1), since these will determine the dose and route of administration and hence the type of reaction likely to occur. Many of the problems experienced are attributable to their main pharmacological effects (Table 2).

Nomenclature

The names of prostaglandins are generally abbreviated to a three-letter abbreviation with a subscripted number.

Table 1 Indications for prostaglandin therapy

In obstetrics
  First- and second-trimester abortion
  Cervical reopening
  Induction of labor
  Augmentation of labor
  Postpartum hemorrhage
  Ectopic pregnancy
  Lactation suppression
In gastrointestinal disease
  Peptic ulceration
  Liver transplantation
  Chemotherapy-induced mucosal lesions
In cardiovascular disease
  Congenital cardiac malformations
  Raynaud's syndrome
  Chronic obstructive pulmonary disease
  Adult respiratory distress syndrome
  Pulmonary hypertension
  Arterial occlusive disease
  Extracorporeal circulation
In urology
  Erectile dysfunction
  Cystitis after radiation or chemotherapy
In ophthalmology
  Glaucoma

The first two letters are always PG; the third is E, F, or I. The recommended International Non-proprietary Names (rINNs) of various prostaglandins are given in Table 3. The convention is that, for example, PGE_1 is the name given to the endogenous prostaglandin and alprostadil is the name given to the same compound available for exogenous administration.

Synthetic analogues of PGE_1, PGE_2, PGF_1, $PGF_{2\alpha}$, and PGI_2

Synthetic analogues of prostaglandins are listed in Table 4. Their use allows reduction of dosages and adverse effects. In general, they cause fewer adverse effects than their naturally occurring counterparts, although this depends on the method of administration. Newer analogues (3) and oral forms (4) are in development.

General adverse effects

The most prominent and frequent adverse effects of prostaglandins are those on the gastrointestinal tract. However, the most dangerous are likely to be the cardiovascular effects, which in predisposed patients can sometimes cause life-threatening collapse and heart failure. Hyperthermia and headache are frequent nervous system effects. Epileptiform convulsions occur rarely. When used for termination of pregnancy, uterine hyperstimulation and, less often, uterine rupture can occur (5). Hypersensitivity to prostaglandins can cause skin reactions, bronchospasm (also seen as a direct pharmacological effect), and occasionally anaphylaxis. Tumor-inducing effects have not been reported. There have been a few reports of infants with limb deformities with and without Möbius sequence after exposure to misoprostol (a PGE_1 analogue) in the first trimester.

Prostaglandins in cardiovascular disease

Maintenance of the ductus arteriosus
PGE_1 and PGE_2 are effective in maintaining the patency of the ductus arteriosus in the initial management of congenital cardiac malformations (6,7). The most frequent adverse effects during prolonged treatment are diarrhea, necrotizing enterocolitis, cortical hyperostosis (8–10), fever, respiratory depression and apnea, and seizure-like activity (11). The frequency of adverse effects is not necessarily reduced with low-dose intravenous or oral administration (12). Maternal/fetal hyperglycemia due to reduced insulin secretion is rare, except in the infants of diabetic mothers (13). Less common adverse effects include gastric outlet obstruction due to antral hyperplasia (14).

Raynaud's phenomenon and digital ischemia
Studies of PGE_1 infusion for treatment of Raynaud's syndrome have shown variable changes in frequency of attacks and of healing ischemic digital ulcers (15–18). Prostacyclin infusion (using PGI_2 or its synthetic analogue iloprost) appears to have beneficial effects, both in reducing the severity and frequency of attacks and healing ischemic digital ulcers. Adverse effects are common and

Table 2 Actions of prostaglandins

Prostaglandin E series
  Increased hormone secretion
    Growth hormone, corticotropin, thyrotropin, luteinizing hormone, thyroid hormone, insulin, glucocorticoids, progesterone, erythropoietin, renin
  Increased body temperature
  Sensitization of pain-mediating nerve fibers
  Increased force of myocardial contraction
  Increased blood flow in gastric mucosa, liver, kidney, and placenta
  Increased renal secretion of sodium, potassium, and water
  Antagonistic action against antidiuretic hormone
  Increased intraocular pressure
  Increased permeability of blood capillaries
  Increased gastrointestinal motility
  Reduced gastrointestinal secretions
  Reduced blood pressure
  Bronchodilatation
  Inhibition of bronchial secretions
  Sedation
  Contraction of the non-pregnant uterus
  Induction of abortion and labor
Prostaglandin F series
  Bronchial constriction, especially in patients with asthma
  Reduced pulmonary blood flow and increased pulmonary blood pressure
  Increased erythropoietin secretion
  Increased neurotransmission at sympathetic nerve endings
  Increased gastrointestinal motility
  Reduced blood pressure
  Sedation (effects on the central nervous system)
  Luteolytic effects in mammalian species (except man)
  Induction of abortion and labor
Prostaglandin I series
  Reduced platelet aggregation
  Reduced mean arterial pressure
  Reduced total peripheral and pulmonary resistances
  Increased heart rate
  Increased renal secretion of sodium (tubular effect)

Table 3 Recommended International Non-proprietary Names (rINNs) and chemical names of the major prostaglandins

Prostaglandin	rINN	Chemical name (omitting stereochemical information)
PGE_1	Alprostadil	11,15-dihydroxy-9-oxoprosta-13-en-1-oic acid
PGE_2	Dinoprostone	11,15-dihydroxy-9-oxoprosta-5,13-dien-1-oic acid
$PGF_{2\alpha}$	Dinoprost	9,11,15-trihydroxyprosta-5,13-dien-1-oic acid
PGI_2 (PGX, prostacyclin)	Epoprostenol	6,9-epoxy-11,15-dihydroxyprosta-5,13-dien-1-oic acid

include headache, flushing, jaw pain, nausea, vomiting, diarrhea, and inflammation and pain at the injection site (19,20). Iloprost has also been used effectively in the treatment of local gangrene secondary to chemotherapy (21). Application of a PGE_2 analogue to the skin produced both subjective and objective improvement in patients with Raynaud's syndrome and produced only minor self-limiting adverse effects (headache, flushing, and diarrhea) (22).

Peripheral vascular disease
Synthetic PGI_2 has been used in arterial occlusive disease as an anti-aggregatory drug (23–28). Adverse effects are common (85%). Headache, fever, nausea, anorexia,

diarrhea, pain at the infusion site, and arthralgia are the most prominent. A single study has suggested an increased risk of thromboembolism after the use of iloprost in peripheral vascular disease (29).

Beraprost, an epoprostenol (PGI_2) analogue, has been studied in intermittent claudication. Adverse events include gastrointestinal disorders, headaches, skin disorders, and fever (30).

Primary pulmonary hypertension
Initial studies of continuous intravenous prostacyclin infusion in patients with primary pulmonary hypertension have shown sustained improvement in pulmonary artery pressure, exercise capacity, and survival compared with

Table 4 Synthetic analogues of prostaglandins
(rINNs except where stated)

PGE₁ analogues
  Enisoprost
  Limaprost
  Mexiprostil
  Misoprostol
  Ornoprostil
  Rioprostil
  Rosaprostol
PGE₂ analogues
  Arbaprostil
  Enprostil
  Gemeprost
  Meteneprost
  Nocloprost
  Sulprostone
  Trimoprostil
  Viprostol
PGF₁ analogues
  Prostalene (pINN)
PGF₂ₐ analogues
  Alfaprostol
  Bimatoprost
  Carboprost
  Cloprostenol
  Fenprostalene
  Fluprostenol
  Latanoprost
  Luprostiol
  Tiaprost
  Travoprost
  Unoprostone
PGI₂ analogues
  Beraprost
  Cicaprost
  Ciprostene
  Iloprost

historical controls (31,32). Minor complications (diarrhea, jaw pain, flushing, photosensitivity, and headache) were dose-related. Serious complications were related to problems with the drug delivery system, including catheter thrombosis, sepsis, and temporary interruption of the infusion, resulting in abrupt deterioration (31).

Regulation of pulmonary vascular perfusion in advanced respiratory disease
PGE_1 significantly reduces right ventricular pulmonary after-load in patients with pulmonary hypertension due to chronic obstructive airways disease (33). PGE_1 can also be useful in the treatment of adult respiratory distress syndrome (34). Preliminary studies using aerosolized prostacyclin showed a reduction in pulmonary artery pressure and improved arterial oxygenation with reduction in intrapulmonary shunt in ventilated patients with adult respiratory distress syndrome (35) and severe community-acquired pneumonia (36). However, ventilated patients with severe community-acquired pneumonia and pre-existing fibrosis required much higher doses, with a reduction in systemic vascular resistance and an increase in intrapulmonary shunting (36). A single report described improved oxygenation, mainly due to reduction of intrapulmonary shunting, in two neonates with pulmonary hypertension treated with aerosolized prostacyclin (37).

Other uses
PGI_2 has been used to reduce the re-stenosis rate during transluminal coronary angioplasty (38).

Prostacyclin infusion (using PGI_2 or its synthetic analogue, iloprost) has been used during extracorporeal circulation to prevent blood clotting in the dialyser coil (39). The risk of severe hypotension can be avoided by carefully controlling the infusion rate.

Prostaglandins in gastrointestinal disease

Peptic ulceration and NSAID-induced gastropathy
Prostaglandins of the E series (misoprostol, enprostil) have antiulcer activity in the upper gastrointestinal tract (40). They inhibit gastric acid secretion at modest doses and provide mucosal protection against noxious agents, including non-steroidal anti-inflammatory drugs, smoking, alcohol, and chemotherapy. They have been used to prevent NSAID-induced gastroduodenal lesions (41,42). They may also be effective in preventing NSAID-induced renal impairment (43).

The cure rate for gastric and duodenal ulcers is comparable to the results with H_2-receptor antagonists (44–46). Relapses appear to be fewer with prostaglandin therapy (44,45). Healing of duodenal ulcers refractory to H_2-receptor antagonists has been described.

Diarrhea (4–38%), abdominal pain or cramp, flatulence, and nausea or vomiting account for most of the adverse effects reported. No biochemical or hematological adverse effects have been noted.

These agents are contraindicated in women of childbearing age, unless they are using adequate contraceptive measures, because of uncertain abortifacient effects. They have been used as illegal abortifacients in some countries (47).

Prostaglandins in liver disease

Liver failure and transplant dysfunction
Prostaglandins of the E series (both intravenous and oral formulations) have been used to treat fulminant hepatic failure, primary non-function following orthotopic liver transplantation, and recurrent hepatitis B infection after orthotopic liver transplantation in open trials (48–50). Adverse effects are almost universal. They include gastrointestinal symptoms (abdominal pain and cramping, watery diarrhea), which affect 33–100% and are more common with oral formulations and possibly amongst those with raised blood glucose concentrations. Cardiovascular effects, which affect about 33%, include migraine, hypotension, peripheral edema, and myocardial infarction (in those with pre-existing risk factors). Painful clubbing and cortical hyperostosis (92–100%) developed 10–60 days after the start of intravenous or oral therapy. Arthritis/arthralgia developed in 8% of those receiving intravenous and 92% of those taking oral PGE_1 or PGE_2.

All adverse reactions appear to be dose-related and resolve with reductions in dose. Two patients developed calcium oxalate stones after 1 year of oral therapy (51).

Prostaglandins in urology

Prostacyclin infusion in men with persistent pain associated with Peyronie's disease was of little value but produced marked adverse effects (bradycardia, hypotension, nausea, flushing) (52).

A single dose of PGE_1 into the corpus cavernosum is highly effective in inducing artificial penile erection in cases of erectile dysfunction. The reported adverse effects include pain and a burning sensation, prolonged penile erection, and local fibrosis. The incidence of pain was high (75%) in older studies (53), while later data improved to 13–44% (54–57). Pain is cited as a prominent factor in non-adherence to therapy and in the dropout rate of patients from self-injection programs, although the incidence may fall with time (57). An alprostadil sterile powder formulation had a lower incidence of pain after penile injection (6.6%), attributed to lower doses and the lack of alcohol in the formulation (58). Burning and pain can be reduced by using a lower initial dose, with incremental increases until a satisfactory erection is produced (59).

Although the incidence of priapism varies in different studies, depending on its definition (erection lasting anywhere from 2 to 11 hours), an analysis of 48 studies in 8090 patients showed an overall incidence of 1% (55).

Prolonged erections induced by PGE_1 usually require drainage and phenylephrine irrigation, although a small percentage can be managed with oral terbutaline or oral pseudoephedrine if treated within 3 hours of PGE_1 injection (56). Local fibrosis is infrequent, occurring in 2% at 6 months and in 8% at 18 months (60). A single case of Peyronie's-like plaque and penile curvature deformity has been reported after repeated PGE_1 use (61).

Complications of alprostadil injections include hematoma and ecchymoses (8%) and systemic effects (6%), which mostly occur in the urogenital system (testicular pain and swelling, scrotal pain and edema, changes in urinary frequency, hematuria, and pelvic pain) (62). In 1% there were symptoms related to hypotension.

Massive diffuse hemorrhage due to cyclophosphamide-induced or radiation cystitis has been treated successfully with intravesicular PGE_1, PGE_2, and carboprost. Febrile reactions and severe bladder spasm are dose-dependent (63–65).

Prostaglandins in ophthalmology

Topical PGE_2 and $PGF_{2\alpha}$ significantly reduce intraocular pressure for at least 24 hours and are used in the treatment of glaucoma. Derivatives of the isopropyl ester of $PGF_{2\alpha}$ appear to be the most effective. Transient ocular adverse effects include conjunctival hyperemia, local irritation, intermittent photophobia, and pain in the eye (66–68). Newer derivatives, such as latanoprost, travoprost, and bimatoprost, appear to be better tolerated, with less severe and less frequent adverse effects (69). They reduce intraocular pressure by increasing uveoscleral outflow.

The ocular pressure-lowering effect of latanoprost appears to be additive with timolol, with mild transient hyperemia in 50% of those treated with latanoprost alone (70).

Latanoprost, travoprost, and bimatoprost cause increased pigmentation of the iris in some patients after prolonged treatment (3.0–4.5 months) (71). Most data have been obtained with latanoprost, and it appears that there is a predisposition to iris pigmentation in patients with eyes of hazel or heterochromic color. As latanoprost and travoprost are selective agonists at $PGF_{2\alpha}$ receptors, it is likely that the phenomenon is mediated by these receptors. Latanoprost stimulates melanogenesis in iris melanocytes, and transcription of the tyrosinase gene is upregulated. No evidence of harmful consequences of this adverse effect has been found, and the only disadvantage appears to be potential heterochromia between the eyes in unilaterally treated patients: the heterochromia is likely to be permanent, or very slowly reversible (72–74).

The adverse effects of travoprost include gradual darkening of the color of the iris and the eyelid skin, increased thickness, number, and darkness of the eyelashes, conjunctival hyperemia, and ocular pruritus (75).

Cystoid macular edema, iritis, *Herpes simplex* keratitis, periocular skin darkening, and headaches have been described in patients treated with prostaglandin analogues. These adverse effects occur rarely, and cystoid macular edema, iritis and *H. simplex* keratitis occur in eyes with risk factors. Repeated rechallenge with masked controls is required to establish a causal relation. However, even without firm establishment of a causal relation, caution is advised with the use of prostaglandin analogues in the eyes of patients with risk factors for macular edema, iritis, and *H. simplex* keratitis (76).

The ocular adverse effects of latanoprost include conjunctival hyperemia, iris pigmentation, periocular skin color changes, anterior uveitis, and cystoid macular edema in pseudophakic patients (77,78). *H. simplex* dendritic keratitis has been reported after treatment with latanoprost (79). In patients with uveitic glaucoma, latanoprost can cause increased intraocular pressure and recurrence of inflammation (80).

Exacerbation of angina pectoris has been described in association with latanoprost (81). $PGF_{2\alpha}$ is a vasoconstrictor, and systemic absorption of topical latanoprost can cause vasoconstriction in coronary arteries.

Three patients had new-onset migraine after using latanoprost, perhaps through activation of the trigeminal vascular system (82).

Prostaglandins in obstetrics

Prostaglandins of the E and F series are widely used in obstetrics for ripening the uterine cervix and stimulating uterine contraction at any stage of pregnancy. They are used in first- and second-trimester abortions, cervical priming, the induction and augmentation of labor, and postpartum hemorrhage (83–89). The route of administration can be vaginal, cervical, extra-amniotic, intra-amniotic, oral, intramuscular, or intravenous, and varies according to indication. Mifepristone (RU 486), a synthetic 19-norsteroid and progesterone antagonist, has been used in combination with synthetic prostaglandins in the induction of abortion.

A less well-established use involves intratubal injection of $PGF_{2\alpha}$ for ectopic pregnancy (90,91). Oral PGE_2 can be used to suppress lactation, for which it is as effective as bromocriptine, and causes less breast tenderness (92).

Organs and Systems

Cardiovascular

Both PGE_2 and $PGF_{2\alpha}$ commonly cause a fall in blood pressure and a degree of bradycardia (1,93). PGE_2 can cause vasodilatation of small vessels and $PGF_{2\alpha}$ can cause vasoconstriction (94). These changes are common but often mild. However, angina pectoris and myocardial infarction have been reported with prostaglandins of all types, particularly after inadvertent intramyometrial injection (95–98). A single case of pulmonary edema after the infusion of PGE_1 has been reported (99). In patients with pre-existing cardiovascular disease, the risk of serious aggravation is very real, and both pre-existing hypertension and states of shock can be worsened. A severe rise in maternal blood pressure occurred in a few cases in which fetal death was associated with unresolved pre-eclampsia.

Respiratory

People with asthma are more sensitive than healthy subjects to bronchoconstriction induced by $PGF_{2\alpha}$ (100,101).

Nervous system

Increased body temperature, pyrexia (both intra- and postpartum), and chills are thought to result from central stimulation of temperature regulatory centers by prostaglandins (102,103). Headache and migraine are the most common adverse effects on the central nervous system (5,104).

Prostaglandin therapy can cause electroencephalographic abnormalities (105). Convulsions, which occur occasionally, are a particular risk in epileptic patients (5,104,105). The combination of prostaglandins and oxytocin can be complicated by tonic-clonic seizures (106).

Enhancement of the pain sensation may reflect a direct effect on nerve fibers. The presence of pain correlates well with the effect on the uterus.

Sensory systems

Increased intraocular pressure and miosis have been reported (5,104).

Mouth and teeth

Gingivitis has been associated with obstetric prostaglandins (5).

Gastrointestinal

Nausea, vomiting, diarrhea, and abdominal pain (107) occur in about 90% of all patients given prostaglandins

systemically. The frequency and duration of these adverse effects depend on the mode of application, the dosage, and the molecule used, and are very variable (108).

Reproductive system

Uterine hypertonia and hyperstimulation are well-recognized adverse effects of induction of abortion and labor with prostaglandins. Cervical rupture and uterine rupture have been reported with every prostaglandin and analogue, even in previously unscarred uteri (5,109–116). The risks can be minimized by using lower doses (0.5 mg intracervically or 3 mg intravaginally), by allowing longer intervals between re-applications, and by avoiding combination with oxytocin, which has a potentiating effect. However, there is a single case report of uterine rupture in a multiparous woman with unscarred uterus following low-dose (1.5 mg) intravaginal PGE_2 (117). In the event of uterine hyperstimulation, beta$_2$-adrenoceptor agonists may reduce uterine contractility. Intensive monitoring of uterine activity and fetal condition is mandatory, since the rate of absorption of PGE_2 after intravaginal or cervical administration is unpredictable.

Second-Generation Effects

Teratogenicity

Seven Brazilian infants were born with limb deficiencies both with and without Möbius sequence after exposure to misoprostol in the first trimester during unsuccessful abortion attempts (118).

Fetotoxicity

Like oxytocin, prostaglandins have been responsible rarely for fetal distress and even fetal death (119,120). The risk of fetal death underlines the importance of cardiotocography during prostaglandin (pre)induction. Prostaglandins should be used with extreme caution if there is a risk of placental insufficiency (120).

The incidence of neonatal jaundice was not increased after induction of labor with prostaglandins (47).

Susceptibility Factors

When PGE_2 and $PGF_{2\alpha}$ are used for induction of labor and abortion, the following contraindications must be respected and (until proven otherwise) also apply to the methyl analogues of these two prostaglandins:

- previous cesarean section or hysterotomy (because of the risk of rupture) (110);
- previous major abdominal surgery;
- prior abnormal delivery;
- a history of severe abdominal inflammation and/or infection;
- a predisposition to uterine cramps or tetanus uteri.

However, uneventful vaginal deliveries have been reported in patients with two previous cesarean sections in whom labor was induced with vaginal PGE_2 (121).

Women with a history of six or more deliveries and anomalies of the fetus (for example hydrocephalus causing cephalopelvic disproportion) must also be excluded.

Predispositions to glaucoma, epilepsy, pre-eclampsia, hypertension, asthma, and ischemic heart disease are relative contraindications.

Drug Administration

Drug administration route

Intrauterine infusion
Intrauterine infusion (intra-amniotic or extra-amniotic) has been reported to be associated with fewer gastrointestinal symptoms and less fever than parenteral or intravaginal administration (122). In intra-amniotic use, the puncture must be guided by ultrasonography, and before injection a control aspiration of some amniotic fluid is required in order to avoid intrauterine or intravascular injection. Uterine rupture has been described with intra-amniotic treatment.

Intramuscular or intradermal injection
Inflammation and pain are common at the site of injection when prostaglandins are given intramuscularly or intradermally (123,124).

Intravenous injection
Prostaglandins have been used intravenously, both for induction of mid-trimester abortion and for induction of labor in cases of intrauterine death. The same adverse effects as described above occur, and are usually very pronounced. Routine premedication with an antiemetic and an antidiarrheal agent significantly reduces gastrointestinal adverse effects.

Inhalation
Intravenous epoprostenol increases exercise tolerance, improves pulmonary hemodynamics, and improves survival in patients with primary pulmonary hypertension. However, there are limitations to intravenous administration, and a significant proportion of patients develop catheter-related problems, such as thrombosis, pump failure, and catheter-related sepsis. In an attempt to improve delivery, several trials of aerosolized prostacyclin have been undertaken, primarily in patients with primary pulmonary hypertension.

There has been a sequential comparison of inhaled nitric oxide 40 ppm with aerosolized iloprost 14–17 micrograms in 35 adults with primary pulmonary hypertension (125). Five of the patients had minor headache and facial flushing during inhalation of iloprost, but these symptoms were short-lived and abated a few minutes after the inhalation ended. One patient had mild jaw pain after aerosolized iloprost, but again this was short-lived. There was an unexpected increase in pulmonary artery pressure in 10 patients and vascular resistance in six patients who received nitric oxide. The authors were uncertain of the cause of this increase, as nitric oxide generally behaves as a vasodilator, but they noted that

nitric oxide is a vasoconstrictor in certain conditions, such as the presence of hemolysate (126).

There has been a trial of aerosolized iloprost in 24 patients with primary pulmonary hypertension and New York Heart Association class III or IV disability, who were refractory to conventional medical treatment (127). They were given aerosolized iloprost in a total daily dose of 100–150 micrograms (in 6–8 divided doses, given every 2–3 hours while awake) over 12 months. The treatment was generally well tolerated, except for coughing during inhalation, which was common initially but resolved spontaneously in all patients within the first 4 weeks. Five patients reported symptoms of flushing, headache, and jaw pain at the end of inhalation, but all rated the symptoms as mild and none discontinued treatment because of adverse effects. There was an asymptomatic but significant fall in systemic arterial pressure (from 98 to 90 mmHg) and vascular resistance at 3 and 12 months compared with baseline.

The effects of aerosolized iloprost have been reported in three patients with severe pulmonary hypertension (mean pulmonary artery pressure 50 mmHg or more) who were already being treated with intravenous epoprostenol (10–16 micrograms/kg/minute) (128). The aim of the study was to replace continuous intravenous epoprostenol with intermittent aerosolized iloprost (150–300 micrograms/day in 6–18 divided doses). All three patients had gradual weaning of intravenous epoprostenol (1 micrograms/kg/minute every 3–10 hours) under close supervision and hemodynamic monitoring in intensive care. All three had initial falls in pulmonary arterial pressure and improved right ventricular function with inhaled iloprost. The first could not be fully weaned from epoprostenol, because of right ventricular failure with dyspnea and hypoxemia, accompanied by a three-fold increase in serum bilirubin and lactate dehydrogenase and echocardiographically demonstrated right ventricular failure. The second and third patients both tolerated complete withdrawal of epoprostenol. However, one developed right ventricular failure within 2 hours of withdrawal. The third was successfully discharged from hospital taking aerosolized therapy, but presented 2 weeks later with severe right ventricular failure. Thus, caution should be taken in patients who have been previously maintained on intravenous prostacyclin when trying to convert to aerosolized therapy, as there appears to be a high chance of treatment failure, which can occur abruptly.

Platelet function after inhaled prostacyclin has been measured in a randomized, double-blind study in 28 patients undergoing elective cardiothoracic surgery (129). They were given aerosolized prostacyclin (5 or 10 micrograms) for 6 hours postoperatively. All the patients, regardless of dose, had a lower rate of platelet aggregation in response to adenosine diphosphate (ADP) than controls. There were no differences in clinically significant indices, such as chest tube drainage or bleeding time. This study has shown that prostacyclin, given as an aerosol, can cause measurable alterations in platelet function, with a possibly higher risk of bleeding.

References

1. Dusting GJ, Moncada S, Vane JR. Prostaglandins, their intermediates and precursors: cardiovascular actions and regulatory roles in normal and abnormal circulatory systems. Prog Cardiovasc Dis 1979;21(6):405–30.

2. Nakano J. General pharmacology of prostaglandins. In: Cuthbert MF, editor. The Prostaglandins: Pharmacological and Therapeutic Advances. Philadelphia: JB Lippincott, 1973:23–124.

3. Hattori R, Yui Y, Shirotani M, Kawai C. A stable prostacyclin analogue, 9B methylcarbacyclin (U-61, 431F). Cardiovasc Drug Rev 1992;10:233–42.

4. Hildebrand M, Pfeffer M, Mahler M, Staks T, Windt-Hanke F, Schutt A. Oral iloprost in healthy volunteers. Eicosanoids 1991;4(3):149–54.

5. Karim SMM. Prostaglandin—physiological basis of practical applications. In: Proceedings 6th Asia and Oceania Congress in Endocrinology 1978;.

6. Momma K, Takao A, Sone K, Tashiro M. Prostaglandin E1 treatment of ductus-dependent infants with congenital heart disease. Int Angiol 1984;3:33.

7. van der Sijp JR, Rohmer J. Prostaglandinetherapie bij pasgeborenen met een ductus Botalli-afhankeliijke circulatie. [Prostaglandin therapy in newborn infants with a Botalli duct-dependent circulation.] Tijdschr Kindergeneeskd 1985;53(1):20–5.

8. Woo K, Emery J, Peabody J. Cortical hyperostosis: a complication of prolonged prostaglandin infusion in infants awaiting cardiac transplantation. Pediatrics 1994;93(3):417–20.

9. Letts M, Pang E, Simons J. Prostaglandin-induced neonatal periostitis. J Pediatr Orthop 1994;14(6):809–13.

10. Kaufman MB, El-Chaar GM. Bone and tissue changes following prostaglandin therapy in neonates. Ann Pharmacother 1996;30(3):269–77.

11. Lewis AB, Freed MD, Heymann MA, Roehl SL, Kensey RC. Side effects of therapy with prostaglandin E1 in infants with critical congenital heart disease. Circulation 1981;64(5):893–8.

12. Singh GK, Fong LV, Salmon AP, Keeton BR. Study of low dosage prostaglandin—usages and complications. Eur Heart J 1994;15(3):377–81.

13. Cohen MH, Nihill MR. Postoperative ketotic hyperglycemia during prostaglandin E1 infusion in infancy. Pediatrics 1983;71(5):842–4.

14. Peled N, Dagan O, Babyn P, Silver MM, Barker G, Hellmann J, Scolnik D, Koren G. Gastric-outlet obstruction induced by prostaglandin therapy in neonates. N Engl J Med 1992;327(8):505–10.

15. Gryglewski RJ. Prostacyclin: pharmacology and clinical trials. Int Angiol 1984;3:89.

16. Katoh K, Kawai T, Narita M, Uemura J, Tani K, Okubo T. Use of prostaglandin E1 (lipo-PGE1) to treat Raynaud's phenomenon associated with connective tissue disease: thermographic and subjective assessment. J Pharm Pharmacol 1992;44(5):442–4.

17. Langevitz P, Buskila D, Lee P, Urowitz MB. Treatment of refractory ischemic skin ulcers in patients with Raynaud's phenomenon with PGE1 infusions. J Rheumatol 1989;16(11):1433–5.

18. Mohrland JS, Porter JM, Smith EA, Belch J, Simms MH. A multiclinic, placebo-controlled, double-blind study of prostaglandin E1 in Raynaud's syndrome. Ann Rheum Dis 1985;44(11):754–60.

19. Wigley FM, Wise RA, Seibold JR, McCloskey DA, Kujala G, Medsger TA Jr, Steen VD, Varga J, Jimenez S, Mayes M, Clements PJ, Weiner SR, Porter J, Ellman M, Wise C, Kaufman LD, Williams J, Dole W. Intravenous iloprost infusion in patients with Raynaud phenomenon secondary to systemic sclerosis. A multicenter, placebo-controlled, double-blind study. Ann Intern Med 1994;120(3):199–206.

20. Belch JJ, Newman P, Drury JK, McKenzie F, Capell H, Leiberman P, Forbes CD, Prentice CR. Intermittent epoprostenol (prostacyclin) infusion in patients with Raynaud's syndrome. A double-blind controlled trial. Lancet 1983;1(8320):313–5.

21. Vowden P, Wilkinson D, Kester RC. Treatment of digital ischaemia associated with chemotherapy using the prostacyclin analogue iloprost. Eur J Vasc Surg 1991;5(5):593–5.

22. Belch JJ, Madhok R, Shaw B, Leiberman P, Sturrock RD, Forbes CD. Double-blind trial of CL115,347, a transdermally absorbed prostaglandin E2 analogue, in treatment of Raynaud's phenomenon. Lancet 1985;1(8439):1180–3.

23. Gruss JD, Vargas-Montano H, Bartels D, et al. Use of prostaglandins in arterial occlusion diseases. Int Angiol 1984;3:7.

24. Shionoya S. Clinical experience with prostaglandin E1 in occlusive arterial disease. Int Angiol 1984;3:99.

25. Tanabe T, Mishima Y, Shionoya Y, Katsumara T, Kusaba A. Effect of intravenous drip infusion of prostaglandin E1 on peripheral vascular reconstruction. Int Angiol 1984;3(Suppl):63.

26. Nizankowski R, Krolikowski W, Bielatowicz J, Szczeklik A. Prostacyclin for ischemic ulcers in peripheral arterial disease. A random assignment, placebo controlled study. Thromb Res 1985;37(1):21–8.

27. Telles GS, Campbell WB, Wood RF, Collin J, Baird RN, Morris PJ. Prostaglandin E1 in severe lower limb ischaemia: a double-blind controlled trial. Br J Surg 1984;71(7):506–8.

28. Staben P, Albring M. Treatment of patients with peripheral arterial occlusive disease Fontaine stage III and IV with intravenous iloprost: an open study in 900 patients. Prostaglandins Leukot Essent Fatty Acids 1996;54(5):327–33.

29. Kovacs IB, Mayou SC, Kirby JD. Infusion of a stable prostacyclin analogue, iloprost, to patients with peripheral vascular disease: lack of antiplatelet effect but risk of thromboembolism. Am J Med 1991;90(1):41–6.

30. Lievre M, Azoulay S, Lion L, Morand S, Girre JP, Boissel JP. A dose-effect study of beraprost sodium in intermittent claudication. J Cardiovasc Pharmacol 1996;27(6):788–93.

31. Barst RJ, Rubin LJ, McGoon MD, Caldwell EJ, Long WA, Levy PS. Survival in primary pulmonary hypertension with long-term continuous intravenous prostacyclin. Ann Intern Med 1994;121(6):409–15.

32. Higenbottam TW, Spiegelhalter D, Scott JP, Fuster V, Dinh-Xuan AT, Caine N, Wallwork J. Prostacyclin (epoprostenol) and heart-lung transplantation as treatments for severe pulmonary hypertension. Br Heart J 1993;70(4):366–70.

33. Gassner A, Sommer G, Fridrich L, Magometschnigg D, Priol A. Der Einfluss von Prostaglandin E1 (Alprostadil) auf die pulmonale Hypertonie bei Patienten mit chronisch obstructiven Atemwegserkrankungen (COPD). [Effect of prostaglandin El (alprostadil) on pulmonary hypertension in patients with chronic obstructive respiratory tract diseases (COPD).] Prax Klin Pneumol 1988;42(7):521–4.

34. Sinzinger H, Fitscha P. Leberfunktionsparameter und Fibrinogen bei i.a. und i.v. PGE1-infusion. [Liver function

parameters and fibrinogen in intra-arterial and intravenous PGE1 infusion.] Wien Klin Wochenschr 1988;100(14):488–90.

35. Walmrath D, Schneider T, Pilch J, Grimminger F, Seeger W. Aerosolised prostacyclin in adult respiratory distress syndrome. Lancet 1993;342(8877):961–2.

36. Walmrath D, Schneider T, Pilch J, Schermuly R, Grimminger F, Seeger W. Effects of aerosolized prostacyclin in severe pneumonia. Impact of fibrosis. Am J Respir Crit Care Med 1995;151(3 Pt 1):724–30.

37. Bindl L, Fahnenstich H, Peukert U. Aerosolised prostacyclin for pulmonary hypertension in neonates. Arch Dis Child Fetal Neonatal Ed 1994;71(3):F214–6.

38. Darius H, Nixdorff U, Zander J, Rupprecht HJ, Erbel R, Meyer J. Effects of ciprostene on restenosis rate during therapeutic transluminal coronary angioplasty. Agents Actions Suppl 1992;37:305–11.

39. Zusman RM, Rubin RH, Cato AE, Cocchetto DM, Crow JW, Tolkoff-Rubin N. Hemodialysis using prostacyclin instead of heparin as the sole antithrombotic agent. N Engl J Med 1981;304(16):934–9.

40. O'Keefe SJ, Spitaels JM, Mannion G, Naiker N. Misoprostol, a synthetic prostaglandin E1 analogue, in the treatment of duodenal ulcers. A double-blind, cimetidine-controlled trial. S Afr Med J 1985;67(9):321–4.

41. Graham DY, White RH, Moreland LW, Schubert TT, Katz R, Jaszewski R, Tindall E, Triadafilopoulos G, Stromatt SC, Teoh LS. Duodenal and gastric ulcer prevention with misoprostol in arthritis patients taking NSAIDs. Misoprostol Study Group. Ann Intern Med 1993;119(4):257–62.

42. Grazioli I, Avossa M, Bogliolo A, Broggini M, Carcassi A, Carcassi U, Cecconami L, Ligniere GC, Colombo B, Consoli G, et al. Multicenter study of the safety/efficacy of misoprostol in the prevention and treatment of NSAID-induced gastroduodenal lesions. Clin Exp Rheumatol 1993;11(3):289–94.

43. Wilkie ME, Davies GR, Marsh FP, Rampton DS. Effects of indomethacin and misoprostol on renal function in healthy volunteers. Clin Nephrol 1992;38(6):334–7.

44. Goldin E, Fich A, Eliakim R, Zimmerman J, Ligumsky M, Rachmilewitz D. Comparison of misoprostol and ranitidine in the treatment of duodenal ulcer. Isr J Med Sci 1988;24(6):282–5.

45. Wilson DE. Misoprostol and gastroduodenal mucosal protection (cytoprotection). Postgrad Med J 1988;64(Suppl 1):7–11.

46. Watkinson G, Hopkins A, Akbar FA. The therapeutic efficacy of misoprostol in peptic ulcer disease. Postgrad Med J 1988;64(Suppl 1):60–77.

47. Lange AP, Secher NJ, Westergaard JG, Skovgard I. Neonatal jaundice after labour induced or stimulated by prostaglandin E2 or oxytocin. Lancet 1982;1(8279):991–4.

48. Greig PD, Woolf GM, Sinclair SB, Abecassis M, Strasberg SM, Taylor BR, Blendis LM, Superina RA, Glynn MF, Langer B, Levy GA. Treatment of primary liver graft nonfunction with prostaglandin E1. Transplantation 1989;48(3):447–53.

49. Flowers M, Sherker A, Sinclair SB, Greig PD, Cameron R, Phillips MJ, Blendis L, Chung SW, Levy GA. Prostaglandin E in the treatment of recurrent hepatitis B infection after orthotopic liver transplantation. Transplantation 1994;58(2):183–92.

50. Tancharoen S, Jones RM, Angus PW, Michell ID, McNicol L, Hardy KJ. Prostaglandin E1 therapy in orthotopic liver transplantation recipients: indications and outcome. Transplant Proc 1992;24(5):2248–9.

51. Cattral MS, Altraif I, Greig PD, Blendis L, Levy GA. Toxic effects of intravenous and oral prostaglandin E therapy in patients with liver disease. Am J Med 1994;97(4):369–73.

52. Strachan JR, Pryor JP. Prostacyclin in the treatment of painful Peyronie's disease. Br J Urol 1988;61(6):516–7.

53. Waldhauser M, Schramek P. Efficiency and side effects of prostaglandin E1 in the treatment of erectile dysfunction. J Urol 1988;140(3):525–7.

54. Derouet H, Weirauch A, Bewermeier H. Prostaglandin E1 (PGE1) in der Diagnostik und Langzeittherapie der erektilen Dysfunktion. [Prostaglandin E1 (PGE1) in diagnosis and long-term therapy of erectile dysfunction.] Urologe A 1996;35(1):62–7.

55. Lea AP, Bryson HM, Balfour JA. Intracavernous alprostadil. A review of its pharmacodynamic and pharmacokinetic properties and therapeutic potential in erectile dysfunction. Drugs Aging 1996;8(1):56–74.

56. Canale D, Giorgi PM, Lencioni R, Morelli G, Gasperi M, Macchia E. Long-term intracavernous self-injection with prostaglandin E1 for the treatment of erectile dysfunction. Int J Androl 1996;19(1):28–32.

57. The European Alprostadil Study Group. The long-term safety of alprostadil (prostaglandin-E1) in patients with erectile dysfunction. Br J Urol 1998;82(4):538–43.

58. Colli E, Calabro A, Gentile V, Mirone V, Soli M. Alprostadil sterile powder formulation for intracavernous treatment of erectile dysfunction. Eur Urol 1996;29(1):59–62.

59. Chen J, Godschalk M, Katz PG, Mulligan T. The lowest effective dose of prostaglandin E1 as treatment for erectile dysfunction. J Urol 1995;153(1):80–1.

60. Lowe FC, Jarow JP. Placebo-controlled study of oral terbutaline and pseudoephedrine in management of prostaglandin E1-induced prolonged erections. Urology 1993;42(1):51–4.

61. Chen J, Godschalk M, Katz PG, Mulligan T. Peyronie's-like plaque after penile injection of prostaglandin E1. J Urol 1994;152(3):961–2.

62. Linet OI, Ogrinc FG. Efficacy and safety of intracavernosal alprostadil in men with erectile dysfunction. The Alprostadil Study Group. N Engl J Med 1996;334(14):873–7.

63. Hemal AK, Vaidyanathan S, Sankaranarayanan A, Ayyagari S, Sharma PL. Control of massive vesical hemorrhage due to radiation cystitis with intravesical instillation of 15 (s) 15-methyl prostaglandin F2-alpha. Int J Clin Pharmacol Ther Toxicol 1988;26(10):477–8.

64. Levine LA, Jarrard DF. Treatment of cyclophosphamide-induced hemorrhagic cystitis with intravesical carboprost tromethamine. J Urol 1993;149(4):719–23.

65. Trigg ME, O'Reilly J, Rumelhart S, Morgan D, Holida M, de Alarcon P. Prostaglandin E1 bladder instillations to control severe hemorrhagic cystitis. J Urol 1990;143(1):92–4.

66. Flach AJ, Eliason JA. Topical prostaglandin E2 effects on normal human intraocular pressure. J Ocul Pharmacol 1988;4(1):13–8.

67. Lee PY, Shao H, Xu LA, Qu CK. The effect of prostaglandin F2 alpha on intraocular pressure in normotensive human subjects. Invest Ophthalmol Vis Sci 1988;29(10):1474–7.

68. Patel SS, Spencer CM. Latanoprost. A review of its pharmacological properties, clinical efficacy and tolerability in the management of primary open-angle glaucoma and ocular hypertension. Drugs Aging 1996;9(5):363–78.

69. Serle JB. Pharmacological advances in the treatment of glaucoma. Drugs Aging 1994;5(3):156–70.

70. Rulo AH, Greve EL, Hoyng PF. Additive effect of latanoprost, a prostaglandin F2 alpha analogue, and timolol in patients with elevated intraocular pressure. Br J Ophthalmol 1994;78(12):899–902.

71. Stjernschantz JW, Albert DM, Hu DN, Drago F, Wistrand PJ. Mechanism and clinical significance of prostaglandin-induced iris pigmentation. Surv Ophthalmol 2002;47(Suppl 1):S162–75.

72. Fristrom B. A 6-month, randomized, double-masked comparison of latanoprost with timolol in patients with open angle glaucoma or ocular hypertension. Acta Ophthalmol Scand 1996;74(2):140–4.

73. Watson P, Stjernschantz J. A six-month, randomized, double-masked study comparing latanoprost with timolol in open-angle glaucoma and ocular hypertension. The Latanoprost Study Group. Ophthalmology 1996;103(1):126–37.

74. Camras CB. Comparison of latanoprost and timolol in patients with ocular hypertension and glaucoma: a six-month masked, multicenter trial in the United States. The United States Latanoprost Study Group. Ophthalmology 1996;103(1):138–47.

75. Chernin T. The eyes have it. FDA clears several ophthalmic drops for glaucoma in a row. Drug Topics 2001;145:20.

76. Schumer RA, Camras CB, Mandahl AK. Putative side effects of prostaglandin analogues. Surv Ophthalmol 2002;47(Suppl 1):S219.

77. Linden C. Therapeutic potential of prostaglandin analogues in glaucoma. Expert Opin Investig Drugs 2001;10(4):679–94.

78. Wand M, Ritch R, Isbey EK Jr, Zimmerman TJ. Latanoprost and periocular skin color changes. Arch Ophthalmol 2001;119(4):614–5.

79. Ekatomatis P. *Herpes simplex* dendritic keratitis after treatment with latanoprost for primary open angle glaucoma. Br J Ophthalmol 2001;85(8):1008–9.

80. Sacca S, Pascotto A, Siniscalchi C, Rolando M. Ocular complications of latanoprost in uveitic glaucoma: three case reports. J Ocul Pharmacol Ther 2001;17(2):107–13.

81. Mitra M, Chang B, James T. Drug points. Exacerbation of angina associated with latanoprost. BMJ 2001;323(7316):783.

82. Weston BC. Migraine headache associated with latanoprost. Arch Ophthalmol 2001;119(2):300–1.

83. Hayashi RH, Castillo MS, Noah ML. Management of severe postpartum hemorrhage due to uterine atony using an analogue of prostaglandin F2 alpha. Obstet Gynecol 1981;58(4):426–9.

84. Pulkkinen MO, Kajanoja P, Kivikoski A, Saastamoinen J, Selander K, Tuimala R. Abortion with sulprostone, a prostaglandin E2 derivative. Int J Gynaecol Obstet 1980;18(1):40–3.

85. Robins J, Surrago EJ. Alternatives in midtrimester abortion induction. Obstet Gynecol 1980;56(6):716–22.

86. Thong KJ, Robertson AJ, Baird DT. A retrospective study of 932 second trimester terminations using gemeprost (16,16 dimethyl-trans delta 2 PGE1 methyl ester). Prostaglandins 1992;44(1):65–74.

87. Hill NCW, Selinger M, Ferguson J, MacKenzie IZ. Management of intra-uterine fetal death with vaginal administration of gemeprost or prostaglandin E2: a random allocation controlled trial. J Obstet Gynaecol 1991;11:422–6.

88. Poulsen HK, Moller LK, Westergaard JG, Thomsen SG, Giersson RT, Arngrimsson R. Open randomized comparison of prostaglandin E2 given by intracervical gel or vagitory for preinduction cervical ripening and induction of labor. Acta Obstet Gynecol Scand 1991;70(7–8):549–53.

89. Jaschevatzky OE, Dascalu S, Noy Y, Rosenberg RP, Anderman S, Ballas S. Intrauterine PGF2 alpha infusion for termination of pregnancies with second-trimester rupture of membranes. Obstet Gynecol 1992;79(1):32–4.

90. Egarter C, Husslein P. Treatment of tubal pregnancy by prostaglandins. Lancet 1988;1(8594):1104–5.

91. Eckford S, Fox R. Intratubal injection of prostaglandin in ectopic pregnancy. Lancet 1993;342(8874):803.

92. England MJ, Tjallinks A, Hofmeyr J, Harber J. Suppression of lactation. A comparison of bromocriptine and prostaglandin E2. J Reprod Med 1988;33(7):630–2.

93. Lee JB. Cardiovascular–renal effects of prostaglandins: the antihypertensive, natriuretic renal "endocrine" function. Arch Intern Med 1974;133(1):56–76.

94. Olsson AG, Carlson LA. Clinical, hemodynamic and metabolic effects of intraarterial infusions of prostaglandin E1 in patients with peripheral vascular disease. Adv Prostaglandin Thromboxane Res 1976;1:429–32.

95. Bugiardini R, Galvani M, Ferrini D, Gridelli C, Tollemeto D, Mari L, Puddu P, Lenzi S. Myocardial ischemia induced by prostacyclin and iloprost. Clin Pharmacol Ther 1985;38(1):101–8.

96. Fliers E, Duren DR, van Zwieten PA. A prostaglandin analogue as a probable cause of myocardial infarction in a young woman. BMJ 1991;302(6773):416.

97. Lennox CE, Martin J. Cardiac arrest following intramyometrial prostaglandin E2. J Obstet Gynaecol 1991;11:263–4.

98. Meyer WJ, Benton SL, Hoon TJ, Gauthier DW, Whiteman VE. Acute myocardial infarction associated with prostaglandin E2. Am J Obstet Gynecol 1991;165(2):359–60.

99. White JL, Fleming NW, Burke TA, Katz NM, Moront MG, Kim YD. Pulmonary edema after PGE1 infusion. J Cardiothorac Anesth 1990;4(6):744–7.

100. Smith AP, Cuthbert MF. The response of normal and asthmatic subjects to prostaglandins E2 and F2alpha by different routes, and their significance in asthma. Adv Prostaglandin Thromboxane Res 1976;1:449–59.

101. Fishburne JI Jr, Brenner WE, Braaksma JT, Hendricks CH. Bronchospasm complicating intravenous prostaglandin F 2a for therapeutic abortion. Obstet Gynecol 1972;39(6):892–6.

102. Milton AS. Modern views on the pathogenesis of fever and the mode of action of antipyretic drugs. J Pharm Pharmacol 1976;28(Suppl 4):393–9.

103. Callen PJ, de Louvois J, Hurley R, Trudinger BJ. Intrapartum and postpartum pyrexia and infection after induction with extra-amniotic prostaglandin E2 in tylose. Br J Obstet Gynaecol 1980;87(6):513–8.

104. Haller U, Kubli R. Klinische Nebenwirkungen und Komplikationen der Prostaglandine bei Abortinduktion. Gynekologie 1978;11:39.

105. Lyneham RC, Low PA, McLeod JC, Shearman RP, Smith ID, Korda AR. Convulsions and electroencephalogram abnormalities after intra-amniotic prostaglandin F2a. Lancet 1973;2(7836):1003–5.

106. Sederberg-Olsen J, Olsen CE. Prostaglandin–oxytocin induction of mid-trimester abortion complicated by grand mal-like seizures. Acta Obstet Gynecol Scand 1983;62(1):79–81.

107. Rachmilewitz D. Prostaglandins and diarrhea. Dig Dis Sci 1980;25(12):897–9.

108. Kirton KT, Kimball FA, Porteus SE. Reproductive physiology: prostaglandin-associated events. Adv Prostaglandin Thromboxane Res 1976;2:621–5.

109. Cederqvist LL, Birnbaum SJ. Rupture of the uterus after midtrimester prostaglandin abortion. J Reprod Med 1980;25(3):136–8.

110. Bromham DR, Anderson RS. Uterine scar rupture in labour induced with vaginal prostaglandin E2. Lancet 1980;2(8192):485–6.

111. El-Etriby EK, Daw E. Rupture of the cervix during prostaglandin termination of pregnancy. Postgrad Med J 1981;57(666):265–6.

112. Sawyer MM, Lipshitz J, Anderson GD, Dilts PV Jr. Third-trimester uterine rupture associated with vaginal prostaglandin E2. Am J Obstet Gynecol 1981;140(6):710–1.

113. Geirsson RT. Uterine rupture following induction of labour with prostaglandin E2 pessaries, an oxytocin infusion and epidural analgesia. J Obstet Gynecol 1981;2:76.

114. Thavarasah AS, Achanna KS. Uterine rupture with the use of Cervagem (prostaglandin E1) for induction of labour on account of intrauterine death. Singapore Med J 1988;29(4):351–2.

115. Maymon R, Shulman A, Pomeranz M, Holtzinger M, Haimovich L, Bahary C. Uterine rupture at term pregnancy with the use of intracervical prostaglandin E2 gel for induction of labor. Am J Obstet Gynecol 1991;165(2):368–70.

116. Maymon R, Haimovich L, Shulman A, Pomeranz M, Holtzinger M, Bahary C. Third-trimester uterine rupture after prostaglandin E2 use for labor induction. J Reprod Med 1992;37(5):449–52.

117. Azem F, Jaffa A, Lessing JB, Peyser MR. Uterine rupture with the use of a low-dose vaginal PGE2 tablet. Acta Obstet Gynecol Scand 1993;72(4):316–7.

118. Gonzalez CH, Vargas FR, Perez AB, Kim CA, Brunoni D, Marques-Dias MJ, Leone CR, Correa Neto J, Llerena Junior JC, de Almeida JC. Limb deficiency with or without Mobius sequence in seven Brazilian children associated with misoprostol use in the first trimester of pregnancy. Am J Med Genet 1993;47(1):59–64.

119. Quinn MA, Murphy AJ. Fetal death following extra-amniotic prostaglandin gel. Report of two cases. Br J Obstet Gynaecol 1981;88(6):650–1.

120. Beck I, Clayton JK. Hazards of prostaglandin pessaries in postmaturity. Lancet 1982;2(8290):161.

121. Chattopadhyay SK, Sherbeeni MM, Anokute CC. Planned vaginal delivery after two previous caesarean sections. Br J Obstet Gynaecol 1994;101(6):498–500.

122. Quinn MA, Shekleton PA, Wein R, Kloss M. Single dose extra-amniotic prostaglandin gel for midtrimester termination of pregnancy. Aust NZ J Obstet Gynaecol 1980;20(2):77–9.

123. Moncada S, Ferreira SH, Vane JR. Sensitization of pain receptors of dog knee joint by prostaglandins. In: Robinson HJ, Vane JR, editors. Prostaglandin Synthetase Inhibitors. New York: Raven Press, 1974:189.

124. Ferreira SH, Moncada S, Vane JR. Prostaglandins and signs and symptoms of inflammation. In: Robinson HJ, Vane JR, editors. Prostaglandin Synthetase Inhibitors. New York: Raven Press, 1974:175.

125. Hoeper MM, Olschewski H, Ghofrani HA, Wilkens H, Winkler J, Borst MM, Niedermeyer J, Fabel H, Seeger W, Grimminger F, et al. A comparison of the acute hemodynamic effects of inhaled nitric oxide and aerosolized iloprost in primary pulmonary hypertension. German PPH study group. J Am Coll Cardiol 2000;35(1):176–82.

126. Voelkel NF, Lobel K, Westcott JY, Burke TJ. Nitric oxide-related vasoconstriction in lungs perfused with red cell lysate. FASEB J 1995;9(5):379–86.

127. Hoeper MM, Schwarze M, Ehlerding S, Adler-Schuermeyer A, Spiekerkoetter E, Niedermeyer J, Hamm M, Fabel H. Long-term treatment of primary pulmonary hypertension with aerosolized iloprost, a prostacyclin analogue. N Engl J Med 2000;342(25):1866–70.

128. Schenk P, Petkov V, Madl C, Kramer L, Kneussl M, Ziesche R, Lang I. Aerosolized iloprost therapy could not replace long-term IV epoprostenol (prostacyclin) administration in severe pulmonary hypertension. Chest 2001;119(1):296–300.

129. Haraldsson A, Kieler-Jensen N, Wadenvik H, Ricksten SE. Inhaled prostacyclin and platelet function after cardiac surgery and cardiopulmonary bypass. Intensive Care Med 2000;26(2):188–94.

Alprostadil

General Information

Alprostadil is PGE_1 available for exogenous administration. Alprostadil is widely used in neonates with cyanotic congenital heart disease to maintain the patency of the ductus arteriosus. Reported adverse effects include fever, apnea, flushing, bradycardia, and hyperostosis. Continuous chronic infusion of alprostadil via a portable pump and neuromuscular electrical stimulation help to improve the quality of life in patients with severe chronic heart failure waiting for a donor heart, as both treatments can be performed at home.

Of 15 neonates with hypoplastic left heart syndrome (nine boys and six girls; median weight 3123 g) included in a cardiac transplant program between January 1993 and August 1996, who received continuous perfusion of alprostadil from the time of diagnosis of the cardiomyopathy, 13 received transplants and 6 died in the operating room (1). All had short-term adverse effects from the continuous perfusion of alprostadil, including slight fever and irritability. However, none had apneic pauses. Cortical hyperostosis occurred in 13 and antral hyperplasia in 12, but in all transplanted cases regression of the antral hyperplasia was seen after 6 months and regression of the cortical hyperostosis was seen after 12 months.

Organs and Systems

Cardiovascular

Moderate or severe phlebitis can occur at the site of venepuncture in some patients who receive alprostadil by infusion. It is sometimes severe enough to necessitate withdrawal of therapy. The frequency and severity of phlebitis has been investigated in 18 men, mean age 63 (range 47–78) years, with peripheral vascular disease who received a 2-hour infusion twice daily (2). Although it is usual to dissolve 60 micrograms of alprostadil in 500 ml of fluid to avoid phlebitis, in this study 200 ml was used to prevent volume overload. The solution was neutralized to pH 7.4 with 4 ml of 7% sodium bicarbonate. Two patients had grade 0, four grade 1, 11 grade 2, and one grade 3 phlebitis (by Dinley's criteria (3)). Age correlated negatively with the severity of phlebitis. Usually, alprostadil infusion therapy is stopped when phlebitis reaches grade 4 or more, but there were no such cases in this study.

Respiratory

Bilateral pleural effusions have been associated with alprostadil (4).

- After surgery to re-attach an amputated hand, a 75-year-old man was given urokinase 240 000 U/day and heparin 20 000 U/day, each for 6 days, and alprostadil 120 micrograms/day for 12 days. From day 7 he started to have respiratory distress, which progressed gradually. A chest X-ray and CT on day 12 showed bilateral pleural effusions and a pericardial effusion. There was mild peripheral edema. The total protein was 52 g/l, albumin 22 g/l, and hemoglobin 7.6 g/dl. Analysis of the pleural fluid showed that it was an exudate, with a positive Rivalta reaction, carcinoembryonic antigen 1.7 ng/ml, glucose 6.3 mmol/l; total protein 29 g/l, lactate dehydrogenase 129 U/l, total cholesterol 0.8 mmol/l, and no acid-fast bacilli. Alprostadil was withdrawn, and after 8 days the pleural effusion disappeared and the respiratory distress improved.

The mechanism of pleural effusion in the present case was suspected to be increased capillary permeability due to alprostadil; hypoalbuminemia probably also contributed.

Hematologic

Investigators from the Department of Pediatrics in Johns Hopkins Hospital, after seeing a neonate who had marked leukocytosis temporally related to alprostadil, conducted a retrospective study of neonatal leukocytosis induced by alprostadil in 45 neonates (5). They concluded that alprostadil infusion is a predictable cause of leukocytosis in neonates with congenital heart disease. Alprostadil-induced leukocytosis was especially prominent in three patients with splenic disorders associated with the heterotaxy syndrome. Many of the other adverse effects of alprostadil, including respiratory depression, hypotension, fever, and lethargy, were also associated with sepsis. The authors considered that it is reasonable to look for sepsis in infants receiving alprostadil, but that it is equally reasonable to withdraw empirical therapy once infection has been ruled out. Leukocytosis associated with alprostadil infusion has not been previously reported and is not listed in the alprostadil package insert.

Skin

Penile shaft lichen sclerosus has been reported in a 63-year-old man in association with alprostadil

intracavernous injection for erectile dysfunction (6). The authors suggested that the lichen sclerosus had been caused by (1) an isomorphic response to the trauma of repeated needle injection; (2) a local cutaneous response to alprostadil-induced collagen synthesis or alprostadil-induced fibroblast production of IL-6, with secondary paracrine/autocrine-induced collagen synthesis by improper skin exposure by direct injection to the skin or by retrograde flow of alprostadil through the needle puncture tract; or (3) a random occurrence of separate events.

A neonate with transposition of the great vessels developed urticaria during treatment with alprostadil (7). While flushing and peripheral edema are well recognized, urticaria has not been described before.

Allergic contact dermatitis has been attributed to latanoprost (8).

- An 85-year-old man with glaucoma developed tearing, red eyes, and pruritic, edematous, eczematous eyelids. Treatment for presumed ocular rosacea and seborrhea with oral tetracyclines, topical glucocorticoids, and metronidazole gel was unhelpful. He was using topical carboxymethylcellulose sodium 1%, propylmethylcellulose 0.3%, polyvinyl alcohol 1.4%, latanoprost, and levobunolol. Patch-testing with a standard 64-antigen patch elicited a strong reaction only to balsam of Peru. However, repeated open application of levobunolol and latanoprost for 4 days elicited a strong positive reaction to latanoprost.

The harlequin color change is an unusual cutaneous phenomenon observed in neonates as transient benign episodes of sharply demarcated erythema on half of the infant, with simultaneous contralateral blanching. This self-resolving phenomenon usually occurs in the setting of hypoxia, as seen in prematurity or congenital heart disease. Two neonates with congenital heart anomalies demonstrated the harlequin color change (9). In one the skin showed a course related to the dose of systemic prostaglandin E_1, suggesting a possible association.

- A full-term girl with transposition of the great vessels and an intact intraventricular septum developed a migratory macular erythema on the tenth day of life. The color change was blanchable, with no surface changes, and distributed mostly on the head and neck, with a few patches on the trunk and midline demarcation. There was no correlation between the color change and the position of the child. The event lasted several hours and resolved spontaneously with no skin sequelae. Intravenous diphenhydramine had no effect. At the time of this episode, the child was clinically stable and mechanically ventilated, with normal vital signs and acid-base balance. Medications consisted of PGE_1 by continuous infusion, furosemide, midazolam, morphine, and pancuronium (doses not stated). One day later, arterial switch surgery was performed and PGE_1 was withdrawn. No further color change or rash occurred after withdrawal of PGE_1.
- A full-term girl with pulmonary atresia and an intact intraventricular septum had balloon dilatation of the pulmonary valve performed on the third day of life.

Eight days later she developed a macular blanchable erythema involving several areas of the head and neck and on one-half of the trunk with sharp demarcation along the midline. The color change did not respond to intravenous diphenhydramine. The episode lasted 30 minutes and resolved spontaneously. Medications at the time were PGE_1 by continuous infusion, furosemide, propranolol, midazolam, morphine, and pancuronium (doses not stated). On the same day as the initial episode of color change, she developed cardiovascular instability with low oxygen saturation. After she had been intubated and ventilated, a bolus of PGE_1 was administered (dose not stated). The color change recurred, showing prominent macular erythema in a migratory pattern over the face and neck, and on either side of the truncal midline. The erythema was brighter and more extensive than in the previous episode, and was not affected by position. The colour change was not responsive to intravenous diphenhydramine or topical hydrocortisone. This second episode recurred intermittently over the next 8 days, becoming significantly less prominent as PGE_1 was gradually weaned. After the withdrawal of PGE_1, no further color change was noted.

As this adverse effect is not serious, PGE_1 should be continued until surgical correction is performed. Recognition of the association between systemic PGE_1 infusion and the harlequin color change may assist the clinician to manage neonates with cyanotic heart disease and to avoid unnecessary exposure to pharmacological agents given to treat the rash.

Musculoskeletal

Alprostadil infusion can produce bone cortical hyperostosis. Periosteal changes have been described in 15 neonates after the administration of alprostadil for more than 1 week (10). Serum alkaline phosphatase activity was significantly raised. The long bones and clavicles were most commonly involved and symmetrically affected. The scapula was involved in two cases and the ribs in seven. The involvement of clavicles has not been previously reported.

Hypertrophic osteoarthropathy has been reported in a woman with severe chronic heart failure who was referred for cardiac rehabilitation (11).

- A 56-year-old woman with muscle weakness and severe chronic heart failure (NYHA Class III) caused by aortic coarctation received an intravenous infusion of alprostadil 5 nanograms/kg/minute. Although her hemodynamics improved, her muscle weakness and exercise intolerance persisted. Neuromuscular electrical stimulation of both thigh muscles was begun. However, during simultaneous continuous intravenous infusion of alprostadil, she developed pain in her knees and elbows. The overlying skin was warm and dusky red and the subcutaneous tissues were swollen. The discomfort was aggravated by motion. There were signs of non-inflammatory synovial effusions and X-rays showed symmetric bilateral periosteal bone deposition in the distal humerus and synovial effusions

in both knees. The bone scintigram showed increased bilateral symmetrical tracer uptake in both knees, ankles, wrists, and carpal bones, and increased radionuclide uptake in periarticular regions. Secondary hypertrophic osteoarthropathy caused by continuous intravenous infusion of alprostadil was diagnosed. The dosage of alprostadil was reduced to 2.5 nanograms/kg/minute, and the signs of osteoarthropathy disappeared within 5 days.

Sexual function

Intracavernosal alprostadil was effective and well tolerated in the treatment of erectile dysfunction, according to the results of a 6-month study (funded by Pharmacia & Upjohn) in 848 men (mean age 52 years) with at least a 4-month history of erectile dysfunction (12). This is provided that the individual dose is established by titration and patients receive training in injection techniques and periodic supervision during treatment. An initial dose was established for each patient and the patients then administered the alprostadil themselves at home. Of 727 evaluable patients, 682 (94%) had at least one erectile response after the injection of alprostadil, and 88% of injections lead to a satisfactory sexual response. The most commonly reported adverse event was penile pain, reported by 44% of patients, but only after 8% of injections. In just over half of the patients who had penile pain, the condition was reported as mild. Prolonged erection, penile fibrosis, and priapism occurred in 8, 4, and 0.9% of patients respectively. Treatment was withdrawn because of medical events in 4% of patients, and drug-related events accounted for treatment withdrawal in 2% of patients.

There is a high dropout rate from self-injection therapy for erectile dysfunction. Of 86 patients aged 36–76 years who had been using home treatment for at least 3 months, 17 had discontinued treatment (13). The patients were evaluated by interview and clinical examination. Patients still in the program used one injection every 2 weeks, and those who had given up treatment had used one injection in 3 weeks. They were in the program for 39 and 16 months respectively, and had used a mean of 50 versus 12 injections respectively. There was no difference in the number of injections that produced unsatisfactory penile rigidity, prolonged erections, hematomas at the injection site, corporeal fibrosis, secondary penile deviation, or mean estimated duration of a drug-induced erection. Patient satisfaction, estimated partner satisfaction, increase in self-esteem, and negligible effort in performing injections were all significantly better for those still in the program. The authors commented that the reasons for dropout from self-injection therapy were not based on objective adverse effects and discomfort. Patients who leave the program are less motivated, less satisfied with the quality of drug-induced sexuality, consider the effort of giving the injections to be substantial, and have not achieved improved self-esteem.

There has been a report of a long-term follow-up program for treatment of erectile dysfunction in 32 patients who used alprostadil for a minimum of 5 years under standardized protocol conditions (14). All the patients had organic erectile dysfunction, and their mean age was 59 years. The period of observation was on average 75 months, and the mean dose of alprostadil was 14 μg. In all, 6799 injections were registered. The average number of injections was 213 per patient, 2.8 injections per month per patient. As regards adverse effects, hematomas occurred in 1.9% of the patients and there were five cases of prolonged erection (0.07%) caused by unauthorized redosing. Three patients developed reversible penile nodules. In 10 patients, the initial dosage had to be increased. Five patients dropped out after 5 years, none of them because of treatment complications.

The impact of treatment with transurethral alprostadil for erectile dysfunction on the quality of life of 249 men and their partners has been evaluated (15). The men had organic erectile dysfunction of more than 3 months' duration and self-administered transurethral alprostadil in an open, dose-escalating, outpatient study. Patients with a sufficient response (n = 159) were randomly assigned double-blind to either active medication or placebo for 3 months at home. Drug-related urogenital pain was reported by 12% of patients during outpatient dosing. However, this pain was usually mild, and only five patients (2%) discontinued treatment. One patient reported minor urethral bleeding/spotting. The transurethral administration of alprostadil was associated with minimal or no discomfort in 83–88% of patients. In the outpatient study, dizziness occurred in one patient and hypotension in one patient. During home treatment, drug-related urogenital pain was reported by 11 patients (14%), minor urethral bleeding/spotting by one (1.3%), and dizziness by 2 (2.6%). One patient reported prolonged erections on two occasions during home treatment, each lasting less than 5 hours.

The incidence of priapism after intracorporeal administration of alprostadil is 1%. Priapism after medicated urethral system for erection (MUSE) has been reported (16).

- A 57-year-old man with erectile impotence, who had previously been treated with intracorporeal injections of papaverine and alprostadil, resulting in recurrent episodes of priapism necessitating aspiration, decided to try intraurethral alprostadil (MUSE). The dose needed to achieve a full erection in the clinic was titrated to 1 μg, but after 5 months this was found to be inadequate unless supplemented by a hot bath before MUSE administration. The patient stated that with MUSE alone the erection lasted for 5–10 minutes but on the two previous occasions when he had had a hot bath for 20 minutes and then used MUSE, the erection had lasted 3–4 hours. However, on the third occasion, priapism lasted 20 hours and necessitated corporeal aspiration for detumescence.

Immunologic

When latanoprost was applied for 4 months to the eyes in 14 patients, there was an increase in HLA-DR expression (17). Since HLA-DR is a marker of ocular surface inflammation, these results suggested a subclinical inflammatory reaction to latanoprost. However, the clinical significance of HLA-DR expression is not clear.

References

1. Caballero S, Torre I, Arias B, Blanco D, Zabala JI, Sanchez Luna M. Efectos secundarios de la prostaglandina E1 en el manejo del sindrome de corazon izquierdo hipoplastico en espera de trasplante cardiaco. [Secondary effects of prostaglandin E1 on the management of hypoplastic left heart syndrome while waiting for heart transplantation.] An Esp Pediatr 1998;48(5):505–9.
2. Fujita M, Hatori N, Shimizu M, Yoshizu H, Segawa D, Kimura T, Iizuka Y, Tanaka S. Neutralization of prostaglandin E1 intravenous solution reduces infusion phlebitis. Angiology 2000;51(9):719–23.
3. Lewis GB, Hecker JF. Infusion thrombophlebitis. Br J Anaesth 1985;57(2):220–33.
4. Watanabe H, Anayama S, Horiuchi T, Sato E, Hamada Y, Ishihara H. Pleural effusion caused by prostaglandin E1 preparation. Chest 2003; 123: 952–3.
5. Arav-Boger R, Baggett HC, Spevak PJ, Willoughby RE. Leukocytosis caused by prostaglandin E1 in neonates. J Pediatr 2001;138(2):263–5.
6. English JC 3rd, King DH, Foley JP. Penile shaft hypopigmentation: lichen sclerosus occurring after the initiation of alprostadil intracavernous injections for erectile dysfunction. J Am Acad Dermatol 1998;39(5 Pt 1):801–3.
7. Carter EL, Garzon MC. Neonatal urticaria due to prostaglandin E1. Pediatr Dermatol 2000;17(1):58–61.
8. Jerstad KM, Warshaw E. Allergic contact dermatitis to latanoprost. Am J Contact Dermat 2002;13(1):39–41.
9. Rao J, Campbell ME, Krol A. The harlequin color change and association with prostaglandin E1. Pediatr Dermatol 2004; 21: 573–6.
10. Nadroo AM, Shringari S, Garg M, al-Sowailem AM. Prostaglandin induced cortical hyperostosis in neonates with cyanotic heart disease. J Perinat Med 2000;28(6):447–52.
11. Crevenna R, Quittan M, Hulsmann M, Wiesinger GF, Keilani MY, Kainberger F, Leitha T, Fialka-Moser V, Pacher R. Hypertrophic osteoarthropathy caused by PGE1 in a patient with congestive heart failure during cardiac rehabilitation. Wien Klin Wochenschr 2002;114(3):115–8.
12. Alvarez E, Andrianne R, Arvis G, Boezaart F, Buvat J, Czyzyk A, et al. The long-term safety of alprostadil (prostaglandin-E1) in patients with erectile dysfunction. The European Alprostadil Study Group. Br J Urol 1998;82(4):538–43.
13. Lehmann K, Casella R, Blochlinger A, Gasser TC. Reasons for discontinuing intracavernous injection therapy with prostaglandin E1 (alprostadil). Urology 1999;53(2):397–400.
14. Hauck EW, Altinkilic BM, Schroeder-Printzen I, Rudnick J, Weidner W. Prostaglandin E1 long-term self-injection programme for treatment of erectile dysfunction—a follow-up of at least 5 years. Andrologia 1999;31(Suppl 1):99–103.
15. Williams G, Abbou CC, Amar ET, Desvaux P, Flam TA, Lycklama a Nijeholt GA, Lynch SF, Morgan RJ, Muller SC, Porst H, Pryor JP, Ryan P, Witzsch UK, Hall MM, Place VA, Spivack AP, Todd LK, Gesundheit N. The effect of transurethral alprostadil on the quality of life of men with erectile dysfunction, and their partners. MUSE Study Group. Br J Urol 1998;82(6):847–54.

16. Bettocchi C, Ashford L, Pryor JP, Ralph DJ. Priapism after transurethral alprostadil. Br J Urol 1998;81(6):926.
17. Guglielminetti E, Barabino S, Monaco M, Mantero S, Rolando M. HLA-DR expression in conjunctival cells after latanoprost. J Ocul Pharmacol Ther 2002;18(1):1–9.

Beraprost

General Information

Beraprost is a stable, orally active analogue of PGI_2. It has been tested in patients with intermittent claudication in a randomized, placebo-controlled trial (1). Beraprost improved walking distance more often than placebo. It also reduced the incidence of critical cardiovascular events, but the trial was not powered for statistical validation of this effect. As with iloprost, headache and flushing were the most common adverse effects.

Reference

1. Lievre M, Morand S, Besse B, Fiessinger JN, Boissel JP. Oral Beraprost sodium, a prostaglandin I(2) analogue, for intermittent claudication: a double-blind, randomized, multicenter controlled trial. Beraprost et Claudication Intermittente (BERCI) Research Group. Circulation 2000;102(4):426–31.

Bimatoprost

General Information

Bimatoprost is an analogue of $PGF_{2\alpha}$, used to treat glaucoma. It is believed to lower intraocular pressure by increasing the outflow of aqueous humor through both the trabecular meshwork and uveoscleral routes.

Organs and Systems

Sensory systems

Bimatoprost can cause gradual darkening of the color of the eyes and the eyelid skin, increased thickness, numbers and darkness of eyelashes, conjunctival hyperemia, and ocular pruritus (1). Darkening of the iris occurs in 1.1% of patients (2).

Hair

Eyelash growth was reported in 36–48% of patients after 6 months of using bimatoprost (2).

References

1. Cantor LB. Bimatoprost: a member of a new class of agents, the prostamides, for glaucoma management. Expert Opin Investig Drugs 2001;10(4):721–31.
2. Sherwood M, Brandt J. Bimatoprost Study Groups 1 and 2. Six-month comparison of bimatoprost once-daily and twice-daily with timolol twice-daily in patients with elevated intraocular pressure. Surv Ophthalmol 2001;45(Suppl 4):S361–8.

Carboprost

General Information

Carboprost is a 15-methylated analogue of $PGF_{2\alpha}$. It is used in termination of pregnancy, in the management of labor, and to treat postpartum hemorrhage and uterine atony.

Organs and Systems

Respiratory

Pulmonary edema has been attributed to carboprost (1).

- An 18-year-old woman at 37 weeks gestation was given prostaglandin E_2 gel for cervical ripening followed by oxytocin. After delivery by cesarean section uterine atony, which did not respond to oxytocin and methylergometrine maleate, was treated with intramyometrial 15-methyl-prostaglandin $F_{2\alpha}$ 0.25 mg. After 5 minutes, her SpO_2 fell to 89 and she had dyspnea and sinus tachycardia due to acute pulmonary edema.

Gastrointestinal

Vomiting is a common adverse effect of $PGF_{2\alpha}$ (2).

Reproductive system

Uterine rupture has been reported after intramuscular injection of carboprost to terminate a mid-trimester pregnancy (3).

Drug Administration

Drug overdose

A neonate was accidentally given a large dose of carboprost and recovered (4).

- A full-term neonate was accidentally given carboprost 250 µg intramuscularly in an error for hepatitis vaccine. Within 15 minutes, he became tachypneic and hypertensive and then developed bronchospasm and dystonic movements and/or seizure activity in the arms. He was hyperthermic and had diarrhea. He recovered within 18 hours.

References

1. Rodriguez de la Torre MR, Gallego Alonso JI, Gil Fernandez M. Edema pulmonar en una cesarea relacionado con la administracion de 15-metil prostaglandina F2 alpha. [Pulmonary edema related to administration of 15-methyl-prostaglandin F2 alpha during a cesarean section.] Rev Esp Anestesiol Reanim 2004;51(2):104–7.
2. Biswas A, Roy S. A comparative study of the efficacy and safety of synthetic prostaglandin E2 derivative and 15-methyl prostaglandin F2 alpha in the termination of midtrimester pregnancy. J Indian Med Assoc 1996;94(8):292–3.
3. Tripathy SN. Uterine rupture following intramuscular injection of carboprost in midtrimester pregnancy termination. J Indian Med Assoc 1985;83(9):328.
4. Mrvos R, Kerr FJ, Krenzelok EP. Carboprost exposure in a newborn with recovery. J Toxicol Clin Toxicol 1999;37(7):865–7.

Dinoprostone

General Information

Dinoprostone is PGE_2 available for exogenous administration.

Organs and Systems

Reproductive system

Uterine rupture occurred after labor had been induced with dinoprostone at 10 days after term; the baby was born dead (1).

- A 26-year-old woman, whose first child had been delivered by elective cesarean section at 38 weeks of gestation because of a breech presentation, was given two doses of dinoprostone vaginal gel 1 mg 6 hours apart; 8 hours after the second dose her cervix was soft, fully effaced, and dilated to 3 cm. Since her uterine contractions were only mild and irregular, she underwent amniotomy and an infusion of oxytocin was begun. Fetal tachycardia occurred 4 hours later, with recurrent decelerations. Prolonged deceleration of the fetal heart then occurred and there was fresh vaginal bleeding. Uterine rupture was suspected and the neonate was delivered by emergency cesarean section, but could not be resuscitated. The mother required a blood transfusion, but subsequently made a good recovery.

The authors commented that induction with prostaglandins in women with a previous lower segment cesarean scar is associated with a risk of symptomatic scar rupture no greater than 0.6%, and the vaginal delivery rate is about 75%, that is similar to rates quoted for spontaneous labor in women with a cesarean scar. At present, faced with the lack of comparative evidence, clinicians can only provide women with the best estimate of risk based on uncontrolled observational data.

Reference

1. Vause S, Macintosh M. Evidence based case report: use of prostaglandins to induce labour in women with a caesarean section scar. BMJ 1999;318(7190):1056–8.

Enprostil

General Information

Enprostil is a synthetic analogue of PGE_2.

Organs and Systems

Gastrointestinal

Even in doses insufficient to control ulcer symptoms, enprostil has a higher incidence of adverse effects than the H_2-receptor antagonists. In a randomized, double-blind, endoscopically controlled study, 98 patients with gastric ulcers were treated with either enprostil 70 micrograms bd or ranitidine 150 mg bd (1). The healing rates at 4, 8, and 12 weeks were similar. After ulcer healing, half the patients were followed for 1 year without treatment and the others were given enprostil 70 micrograms/day. Diarrhea was a common adverse effect of enprostil, and seven patients withdrew because of diarrhea or abdominal pain.

Reference

1. Morgan AG, Pacsoo C, Taylor P, McAdam WA. A comparison between enprostil and ranitidine in the management of gastric ulceration. Aliment Pharmacol Ther 1990;4(6):635–641.

Epoprostenol

General Information

Epoprostenol is PGI_2 available for exogenous administration. It has become the preferred long-term treatment for patients with primary pulmonary hypertension who continue to have symptoms in spite of conventional therapy. However, tolerance, which always occurs, has made dosing uncertain. The effectiveness of epoprostenol given according to an aggressive dosing strategy for longer than 1 year has been investigated in these patients (1). The dose of epoprostenol was increased by

2.4 nanograms/kg/minute each month to the maximum tolerated dose. Adverse effects were common and included diarrhea, jaw pain, headaches, and flushing in all patients.

Organs and Systems

Respiratory

Pulmonary veno-occlusive disease is a rare form of pulmonary hypertension associated with fibrotic occlusion of the smaller pulmonary veins. Although vasodilator therapy is effective in many patients with primary pulmonary hypertension, the role of vasodilators in veno-occlusive disease is unclear, because of concerns about precipitating pulmonary edema. There have been reports of successful therapy with oral vasodilators or intravenous prostacyclin. In contrast, there has been a description of a patient who developed acute pulmonary edema and respiratory failure 15 minutes after the start of a low-dose prostacyclin infusion 2 nanograms/kg/minute, leading to death an hour later (2). This case has several important implications for the management of patients with pulmonary hypertension. Although previous reports suggested that prostacyclin may be safe in patients with pulmonary veno-occlusive disease, the experience reported here suggests that even in very low doses prostacyclin can produce acute decompensation. Thus, consideration must be given to the diagnosis of pulmonary veno-occlusive disease in all patients with suspected primary pulmonary hypertension.

Further cases of pulmonary edema have been reported during continuous intravenous epoprostenol in patients with severe pulmonary hypertension and pulmonary capillary hemangiomatosis, a rare condition characterized by proliferation of thin-walled microvessels in the alveolar walls (3). This report suggests that epoprostenol should not be used in such patients.

- A 66-year-old woman with scleroderma and severe pulmonary hypertension was given continuous intravenous epoprostenol 2 and then 4 nanograms/kg/minute (total duration 48 hours) (4). Two weeks later her dyspnea had improved, but her leg was swollen and her oxygen saturation had fallen. Her dosage of epoprostenol was increased to 5 nanograms/kg/minute. One month later she developed increasing dyspnea, a non-productive cough, severe edema of her legs, and severe hypoxemia. She had gained 5 kg in weight and there were new bibasal lung crackles. A chest X-ray showed bilateral air-space opacities and bilateral effusions. Her PaO_2 was 5.7 kPa, $PaCO_2$ 3.9 kPa, and the arterial pH 7.51. Pulmonary veno-occlusive disease was diagnosed and the infusion of epoprostenol was gradually tapered over the next 48 hours. She died 6 days later withsided heart failure. At autopsy, histological examination showed thickening of the alveolar septa by proliferation of dilated capillaries on both sides of the alveolar walls, consistent with pulmonary capillary hemangiomatosis.

- A 61-year-old woman developed pulmonary edema during treatment with epoprostenol for severe pulmonary hypertension associated with limited scleroderma (5). She received an infusion of epoprostenol 1 nanogram/kg/minute, and the dosage was increased by 1–2 nanograms/kg/minute every 15 minutes. At a dosage of 6 nanograms/kg/minute, her pulmonary vascular resistance had fallen by 60% and her cardiac output had increased by 55%. However, at this dosage, she became acutely dyspneic. Epoprostenol was withdrawn, she was treated with furosemide and high-flow oxygen, and her symptoms resolved. Because no other therapy was available, she agreed to restart epoprostenol therapy the next day, 1 nanogram/kg/minute, increasing by 1 nanogram/kg/minute every 24 hours to 3 nanograms/kg/minute at discharge. Over the next 6 months, the dosage of epoprostenol was gradually increased to 20 nanograms/kg/minute. She had a significant improvement in her exercise tolerance and there was no evidence of pulmonary edema. However, after about 7 months of marked clinical improvement, she developed right ventricular decompensation. Increased doses of epoprostenol were ineffective and she died. Autopsy showed severe obliterative and plexogenic pulmonary arteriopathy.

This is the first case in which epoprostenol has been successfully restarted. The authors commented that pulmonary edema during acute infusion of epoprostenol is considered a contraindication to its further use. They theorized that the pulmonary edema could have occurred secondary to the dramatic increase in pulmonary perfusion at 6 nanograms/kg/minute of epoprostenol and subsequent rapid shifts in vascular hydrostatic pressure. The slow increase in dosage during reinstitution may have averted the dramatic increase in pulmonary perfusion.

Interstitial pneumonia has been reported in a patient taking epoprostenol for primary pulmonary hypertension (6).
{Case report starts}

- A 25-year-old woman with primary pulmonary hypertension, dyspnea, and exacerbation of edema was given an infusion of epoprostenol 0.5 ng/kg/minute with incremental increases of 0.5 ng/kg/minute every 12 hours. After 5 days she was receiving 4.5 ng/kg/minute. Her chest X-ray showed rapid changes in bilateral infiltrates and her respiration gradually deteriorated so that she required tracheal intubation and inhaled nitric oxide 10–20 ppm. Despite intensive antibiotic therapy, her oxygenation did not improve. The flow rate of nitric oxide was increased and she was given methylprednisolone 500 mg/day for 3 days and then weaned to oral prednisolone 40 mg/day. Her oxygenation improved and the dose of prednisolone was reduced to 20 mg/day. Ten days after intubation, she had massive bleeding from a gastric ulcer, which required a blood transfusion and endoscopic hemostasis. Prednisolone was withdrawn. One week later, her chest X-ray began to show bilateral infiltrates and a CT scan showed diffuse nodular interstitial changes, consistent with interstitial pneumonia. She was given methylprednisolone 500 mg/day for 3 days followed by prednisolone 40 mg/day, which resulted in significant improvement. Because the cause of her respiratory failure was unknown a lymphocyte stimulation test was conducted with epoprostenol and was positive (273% compared with control). She was given prostaglandin E_1 (PGE_1) instead of epoprostenol, after which her oxygenation, chest X-ray, and CT scan became stable.

Hematologic

Patients with end-stage liver failure, portal hypertension, and associated pulmonary artery hypertension (portopulmonary hypertension) have a high mortality when undergoing liver transplantation. Successful transplantation in these patients may depend on efforts to reduce pulmonary artery pressure. To this end, some centers are using a continuous intravenous infusion of epoprostenol, which has been shown to improve symptoms, extend life span, and reduce pulmonary artery pressure in patients with primary pulmonary hypertension. There have been four cases in which treatment of portopulmonary hypertension with continuous intravenous epoprostenol was followed by the development of progressive splenomegaly, with worsening thrombocytopenia and leukopenia (7). This finding may limit the usefulness of epoprostenol in portopulmonary hypertension and influence the timing of transplantation in such patients.

Skin

Common dose-limiting adverse effects of epoprostenol (including flushing) are attributed to vasodilatation. However, patients can develop a persistent rash distinct from the flushing associated with epoprostenol. The clinical and pathological findings have been described in 12 patients who developed a persistent rash while receiving long-term epoprostenol for pulmonary arterial hypertension (8).

Drug-drug interactions

Anticoagulants

Anticoagulants and continuous intravenous infusion of epoprostenol are the standard treatments for primary pulmonary hypertension. However, their combined use increases the likelihood of hemorrhagic complications, as demonstrated in a retrospective study of 31 consecutive patients with primary pulmonary hypertension (mean age, 29 years, 10 men, 21 women), nine of whom had 11 bleeding episodes; nine episodes were cases of alveolar hemorrhage and two patients had severe respiratory distress (9). The mean dose of epoprostenol at the time of the first bleeding episode was 89 ng/kg/minute. More of the patients who had a bleeding episode died (67% versus 41%).

Management of adverse drug reactions

Long-term therapy with epoprostenol, a potent prostacyclin and short-acting vasodilator, improves hemodynamics, exercise capacity, and survival in adults and children with pulmonary hypertension. However, epoprostenol has several inherent drawbacks (SEDA-24, 463). Bosentan, a dual endothelin receptor antagonist, lowers pulmonary artery pressure and resistance and improves exercise tolerance in adults with pulmonary arterial hypertension. Based on a case series that suggested that epoprostenol can be withdrawn from a select group of adults with normal pulmonary pressures, it has been shown that bosentan facilitates the reduction of epoprostenol dosages and the severity of its associated adverse effects, without adversely affecting hemodynamic parameters in selected children (10). Further randomized studies are required to determine if use of bosentan concomitantly with epoprostenol improves hemodynamics and may allow safe weaning or discontinuation of epoprostenol.

In a double-blind, placebo-controlled study, the Bosentan Randomized trial of Endothelin Antagonist Therapy for Pulmonary Arterial Hypertension (BREATHE-2), 33 patients took epoprostenol (2 ng/kg/min initially, increasing to a mean dosage of 14 ng/kg/min at week 16) and were then randomized for 16 weeks in a 2:1 ratio to bosentan (62.5 mg bd for 4 weeks then 125 mg bd) or placebo (11). There was a non-significant trend towards hemodynamic and clinical improvement with to the combination. There were several early and late major complications (four withdrawals with bosentan + epoprostenol: two deaths due to cardiopulmonary failure, one clinical worsening, and one increase in hepatic transaminases; and one withdrawal due to increased hepatic transaminases with placebo + epoprostenol. Power was the major limitation of this study, in which only 33 patients were enrolled, and the results should be interpreted with caution. Additional information is needed to evaluate the benefit to harm balance of combined bosentan + epoprostenol therapy in pulmonary arterial hypertension.

References

1. McLaughlin VV, Genthner DE, Panella MM, Rich S. Reduction in pulmonary vascular resistance with long-term epoprostenol (prostacyclin) therapy in primary pulmonary hypertension. N Engl J Med 1998;338(5):273–7.
2. Palmer SM, Robinson LJ, Wang A, Gossage JR, Bashore T, Tapson VF. Massive pulmonary edema and death after prostacyclin infusion in a patient with pulmonary veno-occlusive disease. Chest 1998;113(1):237–40.
3. Humbert M, Maitre S, Capron F, Rain B, Musset D, Simonneau G. Pulmonary edema complicating continuous intravenous prostacyclin in pulmonary capillary hemangiomatosis. Am J Respir Crit Care Med 1998;157(5 Pt 1):1681–1685.
4. Gugnani MK, Pierson C, Vanderheide R, Girgis RE. Pulmonary edema complicating prostacyclin therapy in pulmonary hypertension associated with scleroderma: a case of pulmonary capillary hemangiomatosis. Arthritis Rheum 2000;43(3):699–703.
5. Farber HW, Graven KK, Kokolski G, Korn JH. Pulmonary edema during acute infusion of epoprostenol in a patient

with pulmonary hypertension and limited scleroderma. J Rheumatol 1999;26(5):1195–6.

6. Morimatsu H, Goto K, Matsusaki T, Katayama H, Matsubara H, Ohe T, Morita K. Rapid development of severe interstitial pneumonia caused by epoprostenol in a patient with primary pulmonary hypertension. Anesth Analg 2004; 99: 1205–7.

7. Findlay JY, Plevak DJ, Krowka MJ, Sack EM, Porayko MK. Progressive splenomegaly after epoprostenol therapy in portopulmonary hypertension. Liver Transpl Surg 1999;5(5):362–5.

8. Myers SA, Ahearn GS, Selim MA, Tapson VF. Cutaneous findings in patients with pulmonary arterial hypertension receiving long-term epoprostenol therapy. J Am Acad Dermatol 2004; 51: 98–102.

9. Ogawa A, Matsubara H, Fujio H, Miyaji K, Nakamura K, Morita H, Saito H, Kusano KF, Emori T, Date H, Ohe T. Risk of alveolar hemorrhage in patients with primary pulmonary hypertension—anticoagulation and epoprostenol therapy. Circ J 2005; 69(2): 216–20.

10. Ivy DD, Doran A, Clausen L, Bingaman D, Yetman A. Weaning and discontinuation of epoprostenol in children with idiopathic pulmonary arterial hypertension receiving concomitant bosentan. Am J Cardiol 2004; 93: 943–6.

11. Humbert M, Barst RJ, Robbins IM, Channick RN, Galie N, Boonstra A, Rubin LJ, Horn EM, Manes A, Simonneau G. Combination of bosentan with epoprostenol in pulmonary arterial hypertension: BREATHE-2. Eur Respir J 2004; 24: 353–9.

Gemeprost

General Information

Gemeprost is an analogue of PGE_2. Vaginal gemeprost is effective in inducing first and second trimester abortion and in cervical priming before vacuum aspiration. Pyrexia, vomiting, and diarrhea were experienced in 20% of patients (1).

In a double-blind, randomized, controlled trial, 896 healthy women requesting a medical abortion (57–63 days gestation, mean age 25 years) were randomized to a single oral dose of mifepristone 200 or 600 mg, both followed in 48 hours by gemeprost 1 mg vaginally (2). The complete abortion rates were similar with the lower and higher doses of mifepristone (92 versus 92%). The incidences of adverse effects were similar, with the exception of nausea at 1 week, which was less frequent in the low-dose group (3.6 versus 7.6%).

Organs and Systems

Cardiovascular

Two women developed myocardial ischemia during treatment with gemeprost for termination of pregnancy (3).

- A 29-year-old woman, a smoker with a history of renal insufficiency, obesity, hypertension, hypercholesterolemia, and cardiac dysrhythmias, underwent termination

of pregnancy at 10 weeks with a pessary of gemeprost 1 mg and 5 hours later dilatation and evacuation, followed by tubal ligation. After surgery, her blood pressure became unmeasurable, her heart rate dropped to 40/minute, and she developed ventricular fibrillation. She was given streptokinase and intravenous heparin for suspected pulmonary embolism; her blood pressure rose and was maintained with adrenaline and noradrenaline. Angiography showed an 80% stenosis of her right coronary artery and complete occlusion of the anterior interventricular branch. Blood flow was re-established by coronary angioplasty.

- A 32-year-old woman, a smoker, had an evacuation after the death of her fetus at 18 weeks. Two pessaries of gemeprost 1 mg were inserted 7.25 hours apart, and about 90 minutes later she became unconscious, apneic, and cyanotic, and had dilated pupils and no detectable blood pressure or pulse. She was given 100% oxygen, intravenous adrenaline and dobutamine, and a crystalloid infusion. Her systolic pressure rose to 100 mmHg. Coronary angiography showed left and circumflex coronary artery spasm.

The author commented that the myocardial ischemia experienced by both of these patients was thought to be due to prostaglandin-induced coronary spasm. It would be prudent to monitor every woman treated with gemeprost during the course of an abortion.

Skin

Toxic epidermal necrolysis has been attributed to mifepristone/gemeprost (4).

References

1. Thong KJ, Robertson AJ, Baird DT. A retrospective study of 932 second trimester terminations using gemeprost (16,16 dimethyl-trans delta 2 PGE1 methyl ester). Prostaglandins 1992;44(1):65–74.

2. Weston BC. Migraine headache associated with latanoprost. Arch Ophthalmol 2001;119(2):300–1.

3. Schulte-Sasse U. Life threatening myocardial ischaemia associated with the use of prostaglandin E1 to induce abortion. BJOG 2000;107(5):700–2.

4. Lecorvaisier-Pieto C, Joly P, Thomine E, Tanasescu S, Noblet C, Lauret P. Toxic epidermal necrolysis after mifepristone/gemeprost-induced abortion. J Am Acad Dermatol 1996;35(1):112.

Iloprost

General Information

Iloprost is an analogue of prostacyclin (PGI_2), the pharmacodynamic properties of which it mimics, namely inhibition of platelet aggregation, vasodilatation, and cytoprotection (as yet ill-defined). Iloprost has greater chemical stability than prostacyclin, which facilitates its clinical use (1).

Iloprost is mainly used in patients with chronic critical leg ischemia due to atherosclerosis or Buerger's disease. Episodic digital ischemia in patients with systemic sclerosis or related disorders is another use. The most frequently observed adverse effects, facial flushing and headache, are caused by profound vasodilatation.

Most clinical experience with iloprost has been gained in patients with critical leg ischemia. An intermittent intravenous infusion of up to 2 nanograms/kg/minute for 2–4 weeks reduced rest pain and improved ulcer healing in roughly half of the patients with critical leg ischemia, including diabetics. Compared with placebo, the improvement obtained with iloprost was significant in most but not all individual clinical trials. In addition, a meta-analysis showed a 15% reduction in major amputation rate compared with placebo (2).

Observational studies

The use of iloprost has been proposed in patients with systemic sclerosis, a disease that is often characterized by pulmonary hypertension and Raynaud's phenomenon. Three patients with systemic sclerosis who were treated with iloprost developed acute thrombotic events (3). In one case, intestinal infarction occurred 1 day after infusion of iloprost. In another patient the left kidney was not perfused 22 days after the last infusion of iloprost because of thrombosis of the left renal artery. The last patient, 9 months after the start of treatment with iloprost, and 5 days after the last infusion, had an anterolateral myocardial infarction. The authors commented that their observations did not allow them to conclude that there is a direct relation between infusion of iloprost and thrombotic events. However, they said that this possibility should be considered, and they suggested that risk factors for thromboembolism should be carefully evaluated in each patient with systemic sclerosis who is receiving iloprost.

Inhalation of aerosolized iloprost is being tested in patients with severe primary or secondary pulmonary hypertension refractory to conventional therapy. The aim is to produce predominantly pulmonary vasodilatation without significant systemic effects. In an uncontrolled series of 19 patients, the most common adverse effects of inhaled iloprost were coughing, nausea, edema, and thoracic pain (4). In most patients, these effects were transient and rarely required a change in therapy.

Comparative studies

In a randomized, controlled study of cyclic iloprost or nifedipine in 46 patients with systemic sclerosis, the predictable adverse effects of iloprost (headache, nausea and vomiting, and diarrhea) were common but quickly resolved after the end of the infusion (5). They rarely required a temporary dose reduction. Hypotension occurred less often than with nifedipine.

The effects of PGE_1 and iloprost on microcirculation have been investigated in a randomized crossover study in 36 patients with peripheral arterial occlusive disease stage III and IV according to Fontaine (6). They received PGE_1 and iloprost by single 3-hour intravenous infusions on two different days at doses recommended by the manufacturers or as have been used in previous studies (PGE_1: first hour 20 micrograms, next 2 hours 30 micrograms each; iloprost: first hour 0.5 ng/kg/minute, next 2 hours 1.0 ng/kg/minute). Adverse effects occurred in 19% (PGE_1) and 31% (iloprost). Dosage reduction was required in three patients receiving iloprost (hypotension, nausea, irritation of the infused vein), and in none in those receiving PGE_1.

Placebo-controlled studies

A multicenter, randomized, parallel-group comparison of two different doses of oral iloprost and placebo has been conducted, to identify the optimal dose of oral iloprost on the basis of efficacy and tolerability in patients with Raynaud's phenomenon secondary to systemic sclerosis (7). A total of 103 patients were given total daily doses of iloprost of 100 micrograms ($n = 33$) or 200 micrograms ($n = 35$) or placebo ($n = 35$) for 6 weeks. The mean percentage reductions in the frequency, total daily duration, and severity of attacks of Raynaud's phenomenon were greater in the iloprost groups at the end of treatment and at the end of follow-up. Adverse effects were reported by 80% of patients taking placebo, 85% taking oral iloprost 100 micrograms/day, and 97% taking oral iloprost 100 micrograms/day. There were significant differences in the frequency of five types of adverse events. Headache, flushing, nausea, and trismus were all more common with increasing iloprost dose, while flu-like illnesses were most commonly reported in the placebo group. Treatment was prematurely discontinued in 9, 30, and 51% respectively, and discontinuation was precipitated by adverse events in 6, 27, and 51%.

General adverse effects

The adverse effects of iloprost occur within or above the usual dosage range and are predictable from its pharmacological effects. Minor vascular reactions during infusion (characterized by facial flushing and headache) are so common as to make double-blind trials impossible. Gastrointestinal effects become more prevalent at higher dosages, and include nausea, vomiting, abdominal cramps, and diarrhea. Less common adverse effects include restlessness, sweating, local erythema along the infusion line, wheals, fatigue, and muscle pain. Clinically significant hypotension is rare with the doses tested. The untoward effects resolve rapidly after the infusion is discontinued.

Therapy with iloprost is usually started with a dosage of 0.5 nanogram/kg/minute and increased in increments until either minor vascular reactions occur or a dosage of 2 nanograms/kg/minute has been reached. The optimal total dose remains to be established.

Organs and Systems

Cardiovascular

Myocardial ischemia is unusual during infusion of iloprost. It mainly occurs in patients with pre-existing coronary disease, when it is ascribed to a steal phenomenon detrimental to the subendocardial tissue. As a rule it is transient and exceptionally proceeds to infarction. However, such an event has now been reported in a patient with systemic sclerosis (8).

- A 57-year-old man with a 1-year history of systemic sclerosis and ischemia of several digits received a first infusion of iloprost using the recommended stepwise increasing dosage scheme; he developed sudden chest pain, with inferior ST segment elevation. Emergency coronary angiography showed an occlusion of the circumflex coronary artery, for which a stent was inserted. At angiography 3 years earlier his coronary arteries had been normal. He died 5 months later from cardiogenic pulmonary edema.

Musculoskeletal

Four women with CREST syndrome or systemic sclerosis had pain and eventually contracture of the masseter muscles during infusion of iloprost for severe attacks of Raynaud's phenomenon (9). The adverse effect was quickly reversed by reducing the infusion rate. There were no electrocardiographic or cardiac enzyme changes. The mechanism of this effect is obscure.

Drug Administration

Drug administration route

An oral formulation has been investigated in patients with Raynaud's phenomenon secondary to systemic sclerosis and in patients with severe ischemia due to Buerger's disease or to atherosclerosis. The first reports were not particularly encouraging in terms of efficacy. Tolerance is acceptable: 6% of patients discontinued iloprost compared with 2% with placebo (10,11).

References

1. England MJ, Tjallinks A, Hofmeyr J, Harber J. Suppression of lactation. A comparison of bromocriptine and prostaglandin E2. J Reprod Med 1988;33(7):630–2.
2. Lee JB. Cardiovascular-renal effects of prostaglandins: the antihypertensive, natriuretic renal "endocrine" function. Arch Intern Med 1974;133(1):56–76.
3. Tedeschi A, Meroni PL, Del Papa N, Salmaso C, Boschetti C, Miadonna A. Thrombotic events in patients with systemic sclerosis treated with iloprost. Arthritis Rheum 1998;41(3):559–60.
4. Olschewski H, Ghofrani HA, Schmehl T, Winkler J, Wilkens H, Hoper MM, Behr J, Kleber FX, Seeger W. Inhaled iloprost to treat severe pulmonary hypertension. An uncontrolled trial. German PPH Study Group. Ann Intern Med 2000;132(6):435–43.
5. Pfeiffer N, Grierson I, Goldsmith H, Hochgesand D, Winkgen-Bohres A, Appleton P. Histological effects in the iris after 3 months of latanoprost therapy: the Mainz 1 study. Arch Ophthalmol 2001;119(2):191–6.
6. Schellong S, Altmann E, Von Bilderling P, Rudofsky G, Waldhausen P, Rogatti W. Microcirculation and tolerability following i.v. infusion of PGE1 and iloprost: a randomized

cross-over study in patients with critical limb ischemia. Prostaglandins Leukot Essent Fatty Acids 2004; 70: 503–9.
7. Black CM, Halkier-Sorensen L, Belch JJ, Ullman S, Madhok R, Smit AJ, Banga JD, Watson HR. Oral iloprost in Raynaud's phenomenon secondary to systemic sclerosis: a multicentre, placebo-controlled, dose-comparison study. Br J Rheumatol 1998;37(9):952–60.
8. Marroun I, Fialip J, Deleveaux I, Andre M, Lamaison D, Cabane J, Piette JC, Eschalier A, Aumaitre O. Infarctus du myocarde sous iloprost chez un patient atteint de sclérodermie. [Myocardial infarction and iloprost in a patient with scleroderma.] Therapie 2001;56(5):630–2.
9. Boubakri C, Bouchou K, Guy C, Roy M, Cathebras P. Douleurs masseterines: un effet indésirable méconnu de l'iloprost. [Masseter pain: aé little known, undesirable effect of iloprost.] Presse Méd 2000;29(35):1935–6.
10. Olsson AG, Carlson LA. Clinical, hemodynamic and metabolic effects of intraarterial infusions of prostaglandin E1 in patients with peripheral vascular disease. Adv Prostaglandin Thromboxane Res 1976;1:429–32.
11. Bugiardini R, Galvani M, Ferrini D, Gridelli C, Tollemeto D, Mari L, Puddu P, Lenzi S. Myocardial ischemia induced by prostacyclin and iloprost. Clin Pharmacol Ther 1985;38(1):101–8.

Latanoprost

General Information

Latanoprost is an analogue of $PGF_{2\alpha}$, used to treat glaucoma. The use of latanoprost and unoprostone in the treatment of open-angle glaucoma and ocular hypertension has been reviewed (1). More data on safety are needed to calculate its benefit-to-harm balance.

Latanoprost caused reduced intraocular pressure by 20–40% in adults with open-angle glaucoma or ocular hypertension, but its efficacy and safety in children have not been widely reported. Most children reported so far gained little benefit on intraocular pressure from latanoprost, but older children and those with juvenile-onset open-angle glaucoma do gain a significant ocular hypotensive effect. Systemic and ocular adverse effects in children using latanoprost are infrequent (2).

Organs and Systems

Cardiovascular

Two patients in their seventies developed hypertension during treatment with topical latanoprost (dosage not stated) for open-angle glaucoma; both were also taking tocopherol (vitamin E) supplements. Neither had a previous history of hypertension (3). The authors commented that it is likely that systemic absorption of topical latanoprost could cause hypertension. Self-medication with vitamin E has been reported to aggravate or precipitate hypertension.

Coronary spasm has been attributed to latanoprost (4).

- A 58-year-old man with stable angina pectoris started to use latanoprost eye drops and over the next few days his angina worsened and occurred at rest. After 15 days, he had syncope during physical exercise. Angiography showed coronary spasm.

Respiratory

Latanoprost rarely causes systemic effects. However, it aggravated respiratory symptoms in a patient with chronic bronchitis and emphysema, with improvement after latanoprost was withdrawn (5).

Nervous system

Three cases of headache after latanoprost have been described (6).

- A 65-year-old man with primary open-angle glaucoma intolerant of dipivefrin and beta-blockers used latanoprost in both eyes at bedtime. He had no prior history of migraine, but he began to have headaches, the frequency and severity of which increased until they were occurring daily. The pain was not relieved by over-the-counter or narcotic analgesics, and he was virtually incapacitated. Latanoprost was discontinued and he had almost immediate relief, with only one migraine during the following week, and he was headache-free for the next 10 months. He then agreed to rechallenge. After the second night of latanoprost therapy his headache recurred, and therapy was withdrawn 2 days later when he had incapacitating pain. Headache did not recur within 4 months of follow-up.
- A 65-year-old man with primary open-angle glaucoma, using levobunolol hydrochloride 0.5%, was given a nighttime dose of latanoprost. The next morning he awoke with a severe bifrontal throbbing headache, photophobia, and slight blurring of vision. The headache intensified, and 4 days later a CT scan was normal. On the sixth day he stopped using latanoprost. His headache disappeared within 24 hours and did not recur during follow-up for 1 year.
- A 54-year-old woman with primary open-angle glaucoma, using betaxolol hydrochloride 0.5%, had mild progression of visual field loss in her left eye. Latanoprost was added nightly to her left eye. A few hours after the first dose she was awakened by a severe unilateral pounding headache extending from the left eye and brow to the left cranium. There were no associated neurological symptoms. The headache resolved spontaneously the next day, but recurred on three nights after instillation of latanoprost. On the fourth night the headache did not occur. She continued to use latanoprost, and the headache did not return.

Sensory systems

Corneal damage

Four patients treated with latanoprost developed dendritiform epitheliopathy, a sign of corneal toxicity; the lesions reversed in 1–4 weeks after latanoprost withdrawal (7).

Three cases of *Herpes simplex* keratitis developed during latanoprost therapy (8).

- One patient, with a history of *H. simplex* keratitis, had recurrence with latanoprost (4 months); the infection resolved on withdrawal but recurred on rechallenge.
- The second patient, with a history of *H. simplex* keratitis, had bilateral recurrence with latanoprost (1 month); antiviral therapy did not eradicate the infection until latanoprost was withdrawn.
- The third patient developed the infection after 1 month; the keratitis cleared on withdrawal of latanoprost and antiviral therapy; reinstitution of latanoprost with prophylactic antiviral medication (valaciclovir) kept the cornea clear, but as soon as the antiviral drug was discontinued, *H. simplex* virus keratitis reappeared.

Although the mechanism is unclear, it is known that inhibitors of prostaglandin synthesis reduce recurrence of epithelial *H. simplex* infections and prostaglandins may stimulate their occurrence.

Iris pigmentation

Latanoprost can produce darkening of the iris in 10–25% of patients treated for 0.5–2 years. The incidence of iris pigmentation differs between eyes with differently colored irises: green–brown, yellow–brown, and blue–brown eyes, in that order, have the highest incidences, whereas eyes with uniformly blue, grey, or green irises are much less affected, even after 2 years of treatment. About 60% of eyes with an initial green–brown iris will have increased pigmentation within 1 year. The corresponding figure for initially blue–brown eyes is about 20%. All patients who have developed increased pigmentation of the iris have been withdrawn from studies, and during follow-up for up to almost 3 years the change in iris pigmentation has been stable without signs of reversibility or further increase. Nevi and freckles have not changed color or size. Apart from the change in color the iris looks normal and pigmentation dispersion has not been observed. No cell proliferation is involved and the change in color is due to melanogenesis. It has been concluded that the change in iris pigmentation is unlikely to cause any long-term consequence besides the cosmetic one. The possibility of late loss of pigment and induction of a pigmentary glaucoma also seems unlikely; melanocytes in the iris are continent and do not release melanin (9). In an observational cohort study of 43 patients, 30 had a definite acquired iris anisochromia (10).

The time of onset of the changes in iris pigmentation can be as early as 3 months. The earliest reported change in iris color occurred in a 78-year-old woman, whose iris color changed from blue–green to brown–green within 4 weeks (11). The pigmentation is irreversible. In a 50-year-old man with peripheral iris darkening after latanoprost treatment, the darkening did not change appreciably for several years after withdrawal (12).

The fine structure of an iridectomy specimen from a 65-year-old woman treated with latanoprost has been reported (13). She received latanoprost for 13.5 months and the drug was withdrawn because of iris color change. She underwent cataract surgery 16 months after stopping the drug and a sector iridectomy was obtained. The authors found some melanocytes with atypical features, including nuclear chromatin margination, prominent nucleoli, and invagination of the nucleoli. These characteristics are also seen in precancerous lesions, in the normal ageing iris, and in patients with glaucoma.

The effects of latanoprost on iris structure were assessed in 17 patients with bilateral primary open-angle glaucoma. In each case an iridectomy was performed in one eye, which served as a control. The other eye was then treated with latanoprost for 6 months followed by iridectomy. Light and electronic microscopy showed no evidence of early ultrastructural changes in the latanoprost-treated eyes (14).

The long-term safety of topical latanoprost in the long-term treatment of open-angle glaucoma has been assessed in two studies. To investigate the possible appearance of trabecular pigmentation, 50 subjects who used latanoprost were evaluated by gonioscopic photography of the inferior quadrant at baseline and every 3 months during the first year and every 6 months during the second and third years (15). In all 41 subjects (79 eyes) completed the 3-year follow-up and none had any increase in the grade of trabecular pigmentation, including 10 subjects (20 eyes) in whom iris pigment increased. The safety of latanoprost after 5 years of treatment has been reported in 380 subjects, of whom 353 were evaluated at 4 years and 344 completed the 5th year (16). In 127 (33%) there was increased iris pigmentation in one or both eyes after 5 years. Of the patients who developed iris pigmentation, 89% had a baseline eye color known to be susceptible to color change (mixed-color irises containing brown areas). Patient with blue-grey eyes and no brown pigment did not develop increased iris pigmentation. In the 127 patients who developed iris pigmentation, it occurred during the first 8 months of the study in 94, during the first 12 months in 103, and during the first 24 months in 103. All developed the condition after 36 months. There was hypertrichosis in 14%.

Seven patients using different topical prostaglandin F_{2a} analogues developed bilateral poliosis, which appeared at 1.5–6 months after the start of therapy (17). Four used latanoprost, two used bimatoprost, and one used travaprost.

The mechanism of iris pigmentation due to latanoprost is unknown. In an in vitro experiment using uveal melanocytes, the addition of latanoprost increased melanin content, melanin production, and tyrosinase activity (18). Alpha-methyl-para-tyrosine, an inhibitor of tyrosinase (the enzyme that transforms tyrosine to levodopa), completely prevented the latanoprost-induced stimulation of melanogenesis.

Of 17 patients requiring filtering surgery for primary open-angle glaucoma randomized to receive latanoprost ($n = 8$) or alternative medications ($n = 9$) for 3 months before surgery, all had peripheral iridectomy specimens,

and there were color changes in one case (19). No morphological changes or cellular proliferation were found in any specimen.

Iris cyst associated with latanoprost has been described in a 76-year-old woman (20). Latanoprost was given for 5 weeks, and during a re-examination a large iris cyst was observed in her right eye. The cyst disappeared 3 weeks after latanoprost withdrawal.

Uveitis

In four patients with complicated open-angle glaucoma, in whom anterior uveitis appeared to be associated with latanoprost, the uveitis was unilateral and occurred only in the eye receiving latanoprost in three patients. In one patient, latanoprost was used in both eyes, and the uveitis was bilateral (21). Four of five eyes had a history of prior inflammation and/or prior incisional surgery. All patients were rechallenged. The uveitis improved after withdrawal and recurred after rechallenge in all eyes. The authors concluded that topical prostaglandin analogues may be relatively contraindicated in patients with a history of uveitis or prior ocular surgery. There may also be a risk in eyes that have not had previous uveitis or incisional surgery.

Optic disc and macular edema

A case of bilateral optic disc edema has been described (22).

- A 64-year-old woman was included in a randomized, double-blind trial of drugs used in the treatment of ocular hypertension. After 3 months, examination of the optic nerve showed bilateral edema. She had been using latanoprost 0.0005% eye-drops at night to both eyes. Latanoprost was withdrawn and the disc edema resolved at 1 week.

Cystoid macular edema developed in two patients treated with topical latanoprost for glaucoma (23). Latanoprost was withdrawn, and the cystoid macular edema was treated with topical corticosteroids and ketorolac, with improvement in visual acuity. The macular edema resolved in both cases.

Cystoid macular edema has been reported in four other patients shortly after they started to use latanoprost (24) and other reports have appeared (25–29). A possible explanation is enhanced disruption of the blood–aqueous barrier induced by latanoprost (28).

A review of the published literature (28 eyes in 25 patients) has shown that in all cases there were other associated risk factors, so that a definitive conclusion about a causal relation cannot be reached (30). Nevertheless, latanoprost should be used with caution in patients with risk factors for cystoid macular edema and special surveillance is necessary.

Choroidal detachment

The use of latanoprost after trabeculectomy can cause choroidal detachment (31).

- A 36-year-old man with juvenile open-angle glaucoma in both eyes and traumatic glaucoma in the left eye had extensive iridodialysis and angle recession of about 180° in the left eye. He was treated with topical timolol 0.5% bd and later daily latanoprost 0.005% to both eyes. Immediately after surgery for cataract extraction and intraocular lens implantation combined with trabeculectomy he had a large fall in intraocular pressure and 2 days later developed severe pain, gross impairment of vision, and intense congestion in the left eye. Indirect ophthalmoscopy showed an inferior choroidal detachment. Topical latanoprost was immediately stopped in the left eye and systemic prednisolone 1.5 mg/kg/day was continued. Within 7 days, the choroidal detachment settled.

The authors suggested that the drastic fall in intraocular pressure after trabeculectomy had resulted from an unusually large increase in uveoscleral outflow because of latanoprost. This was because of the additive effect of two factors: trabeculectomy-associated ciliary body detachment and the pre-existing cleft between the ciliary body stroma and the sclera, evidenced by extensive angle recession. The latter was perhaps responsible for the large fall in intraocular pressure (from 32 to 16 mmHg) when latanoprost was first introduced. Although the patient did not have uveitis, prostaglandin-mediated damage to the blood retinal barrier could also have contributed to choroidal detachment. They cautioned against the use of latanoprost as an adjunctive pressure-lowering agent after glaucoma filtration surgery.

Iris cyst

An iris cyst has been attributed to latanoprost (32).

- A 67-year old woman with advanced chronic angle-closure glaucoma was treated with laser iridotomy on both eyes followed by pilocarpine 2% and a beta-blocker. Later she used latanoprost instead, and intraocular pressures were maintained at 12-15 mmHg. There were no abnormal responses except mild hyperemia of the conjunctivae. After about 9 months she developed an iris pigment epithelial cyst on the posterior iris surface. Latanoprost was withdrawn and dorzolamide and a beta-blocker used instead. The iris cyst gradually shrank and completely disappeared from the pupil margin within 5 months. During follow-up for 4 months there was no recurrence.

Skin

Hyperpigmentation of the eyelids can occur during latanoprost therapy.

- A 62-year old Korean woman treated with latanoprost for 4 months developed eyelid pigmentation in both upper and lower eyelids of both eyes (33). There was no increase in iris pigmentation. The eyelid pigmentation gradually diminished after withdrawal, but minimal brownish coloration remained along the lower eyelid folds in both eyes at 4 months.
- A 75-year-old woman with open-angle glaucoma who had used latanoprost for 15 months reported that the skin around her eyes was much darker than on the rest of her face (34). The darkening had occurred gradually. Latanoprost was withdrawn; 1 month later there was a discernible lightening of the periocular skin and 2 months after withdrawal the skin was significantly lighter.

Hair

Eyelashes

Latanoprost causes growth of lashes and ancillary hairs around the eyelids, with greater thickness and length of lashes, additional rows of lashes, and conversion of vellus to terminal hairs in canthal areas and regions adjacent to lashes. As well as increased growth, there is also increased pigmentation. Vellus hairs on the lower eyelids also undergo increased growth and pigmentation. Latanoprost caused changes in eyelashes in 26% of 194 patients over 12 months; the changes included increased length, thickness, density, and color (19).

Latanoprost therapy for 2–17 days can cause changes comparable to chronic therapy. The increased number and length of visible lashes are consistent with the ability of latanoprost to induce and prolong anagen growth in telogen (resting) follicles while producing hypertrophic changes in the involved follicles. Laboratory studies suggest that the initiation and completion of the effects of latanoprost on hair growth occur very early in the anagen phase and that the likely target is the dermal papilla.

Latanoprost can even reverse alopecia of the eyelashes (35).

- A 53-year-old woman, with glaucoma and loss of the eyelashes secondary to alopecia following an allergic response to ibuprofen was given latanoprost (36). After 3 weeks her eyelashes were noticeable and 2 months later full growth had occurred.
- Quantitative analysis of eyelash lengthening in 17 patients treated with latanoprost showed a significant increase in eyelash length in the treated eyes (37).

Increased pigmentation of the eyelashes has been reported in a patient treated with latanoprost (38).

Sweat glands

Heavy sweating occurred in a 6-year-old boy with aniridia and glaucoma during treatment with latanoprost eye-drops (39). Other combinations of drugs for glaucoma had been ineffective in reducing the intraocular pressure. He was given latanoprost eye-drops (dose not stated) at night in combination with a beta-blocker during the day. However, at night he had very heavy sweating. His pyjamas had to be changed regularly about 1–2 hours after he went to sleep. When latanoprost was withdrawn, the heavy sweating resolved. When it was restarted, the heavy sweating recurred.

The author commented that systemic absorption occurred for the most part through the mucous membranes of the nose and throat, since the sweating was less severe when the boy's lacrymal points were compressed for 10 minutes after the administration of latanoprost.

- A 55-year-old woman with primary chronic angle glaucoma was given latanoprost ophthalmic solution (0.005%, 1 drop/day) (40). After 3 days, 1–2 hours after administration, she reported severe sweating involving the entire body and drenching all her clothes. The excessive sweating disappeared on withdrawal of latanoprost and did not occur when she was given bimatoprost. One month later, latanoprost was restarted and the severe sweating recurred on the first day of therapy. Latanoprost was withdrawn and bimatoprost was started again.

Infection risk

Two cases of *H. simplex* virus dermatitis of the periocular skin have been reported in patients using latanoprost (41). Cases of *H. simplex* keratitis are mentioned above, under sensory systems.

Second-Generation Effects

Teratogenicity

Latanoprost exposure has been reported in 11 pregnancies (42). All the women used latanoprost in the first trimester, and embryo exposure lasted from a minimum of 4 days to a maximum of 70 days. There was complete follow-up in 10 cases: nine women delivered normal fetuses without malformations and one pregnancy was complicated by early spontaneous abortion 2 weeks after treatment was completed in a 46-year-old primigravida. The children were considered normal at follow-up within 2 years.

Drug-drug interactions

Non-steroidal anti-inflammatory drugs

Latanoprost induces the formation of endogenous prostaglandins including prostaglandin E_2 (dinoprostone), which could affect extracellular matrix metabolism in ciliary smooth muscle cells. It has therefore been hypothesized that latanoprost ophthalmic solution may reduce intraocular pressure by either direct signal transduction through prostaglandin $F_{2\alpha}$ receptors and by an indirect action through induced endogenous prostaglandins. Non-steroidal anti-inflammatory drugs (NSAIDs) inhibit the induction of endogenous prostaglandins by suppressing the activity of cyclo-oxygenases. Moreover, recent studies have shown that some NSAIDs also inhibit the formation of latanoprost-induced endogenous prostaglandins. Thus, NSAIDs may oppose intraocular pressure reduction by latanoprost. In a prospective observer masked study of the effects of bromfenac sodium hydrate eye-drops on latanoprost-induced intraocular pressure reduction in 13 volunteers (43). Latanoprost significantly reduced intraocular pressure by about 5.7 mmHg, and this effect was attenuated by about 1.5 mmHg by co-

administration of bromfenac. Bromfenac on its own did not affect intraocular pressure.

References

1. Eisenberg DL, Camras CB. A preliminary risk-benefit assessment of latanoprost and unoprostone in open-angle glaucoma and ocular hypertension. Drug Saf 1999;20(6):505–14.
2. Enyedi LB, Freedman SF. Latanoprost for the treatment of pediatric glaucoma. Surv Ophthalmol 2002;47(Suppl 1):S129–32.
3. Peak AS, Sutton BM. Systemic adverse effects associated with topically applied latanoprost. Ann Pharmacother 1998;32(4):504–5.
4. Marti V, Guindo J, Valles E, Domínguez de Rozas JM. Angina variante asociada con latanoprost. Med Clin (Barc) 2005; 125(6): 238–9.
5. Veyrac G, Chiffoleau A, Cellerin L, Larousse C, Bourin M. Latanoprost (Xalatan) et effect systémique respiratoire? A propos d'un cas. [Latanoprost (Xalatan) and a systemic respiratory effect? Apropos of a case.] Therapie 1999;54(4):494–6.
6. Weston BC. Migraine headache associated with latanoprost. Arch Ophthalmol 2001;119(2):300–1.
7. Sudesh S, Cohen EJ, Rapuano CJ, Wilson RP. Corneal toxicity associated with latanoprost. Arch Ophthalmol 1999;117(4):539–40.
8. Wand M, Gilbert CM, Liesegang TJ. Latanoprost and *Herpes simplex* keratitis. Am J Ophthalmol 1999;127(5):602–4.
9. Alm A. Prostaglandin derivates as ocular hypotensive agents. Prog Retin Eye Res 1998;17(3):291–312.
10. Teus MA, Arranz-Marquez E, Lucea-Suescun P. Incidence of iris colour change in latanoprost treated eyes. Br J Ophthalmol 2002;86(10):1085–8.
11. Pappas RM, Pusin S, Higginbotham EJ. Evidence of early change in iris color with latanoprost use. Arch Ophthalmol 1998;116(8):1115–6.
12. Camras CB, Neely DG, Weiss EL. Latanoprost-induced iris color darkening: a case report with long-term follow-up. J Glaucoma 2000;9(1):95–8.
13. Grierson I, Lee WR, Albert DM. The fine structure of an iridectomy specimen from a patient with latanoprost-induced eye color change. Arch Ophthalmol 1999;117(3):394–6.
14. Pfeiffer N, Grierson I, Goldsmith H, Appleton P, Hochgesand D, Winkgen A. Fine structural evaluation of the iris after unilateral treatment with latanoprost in patients undergoing bilateral trabeculectomy (the Mainz II study). Arch Ophthalmol 2003; 121: 23–31.
15. Nakamura Y, Nakamura Y, Morine-Shinjo S, Sakai H, Sawaguchi S. Assessment of chamber angle pigmentation during longterm latanoprost treatment for open-angle glaucoma. Acta Ophthalmol Scand 2004; 82: 158–60.
16. Alm A, Schoenfelder J, McDermott J. A 5-year, multicenter, open-label, safety study of adjunctive latanoprost therapy for glaucoma. Arch Ophthalmol 2004; 122: 957–65.
17. Chen CS, Wells J, Craig JE. Topical prostaglandin F(2alpha) analog induced poliosis. Am J Ophthalmol 2004; 137: 965–6.
18. Drago F, Marino A, La Manna C. Alpha-methyl-p-tyrosine inhibits latanoprost-induced melanogenesis in vitro. Exp Eye Res 1999;68(1):85–90.
19. Netland PA, Landry T, Sullivan EK, Andrew R, Silver L, Weiner A, Mallick S, Dickerson J, Bergamini MV,

Robertson SM, Davis AA. Travoprost Study Group. Travoprost compared with latanoprost and timolol in patients with open-angle glaucoma or ocular hypertension. Am J Ophthalmol 2001;132(4):472–84.

20. Krohn J, Hove VK. Iris cyst associated with topical administration of latanoprost. Am J Ophthalmol 1999;127(1):91–3.

21. Fechtner RD, Khouri AS, Zimmerman TJ, Bullock J, Feldman R, Kulkarni P, Michael AJ, Realini T, Warwar R. Anterior uveitis associated with latanoprost. Am J Ophthalmol 1998;126(1):37–41.

22. Stewart O, Walsh L, Pande M. Bilateral optic disc oedema associated with latanoprost. Br J Ophthalmol 1999;83(9):1092–3.

23. Callanan D, Fellman RL, Savage JA. Latanoprost-associated cystoid macular edema. Am J Ophthalmol 1998;126(1):134–5.

24. Ayyala RS, Cruz DA, Margo CE, Harman LE, Pautler SE, Misch DM, Mines JA, Richards DW. Cystoid macular edema associated with latanoprost in aphakic and pseudophakic eyes. Am J Ophthalmol 1998;126(4):602–4.

25. Avakian A, Renier SA, Butler PJ. Adverse effects of latanoprost on patients with medically resistant glaucoma. Arch Ophthalmol 1998;116(5):679–80.

26. Gaddie IB, Bennett DW. Cystoid macular edema associated with the use of latanoprost. J Am Optom Assoc 1998;69(2):122–8.

27. Heier JS, Steinert RF, Frederick AR Jr. Cystoid macular edema associated with latanoprost use. Arch Ophthalmol 1998;116(5):680–2.

28. Miyake K, Ota I, Maekubo K, Ichihashi S, Miyake S. Latanoprost accelerates disruption of the blood–aqueous barrier and the incidence of angiographic cystoid macular edema in early postoperative pseudophakias. Arch Ophthalmol 1999;117(1):34–40.

29. Moroi SE, Gottfredsdottir MS, Schteingart MT, Elner SG, Lee CM, Schertzer RM, Abrams GW, Johnson MW. Cystoid macular edema associated with latanoprost therapy in a case series of patients with glaucoma and ocular hypertension. Ophthalmology 1999;106(5):1024–9.

30. Schumer RA, Camras CB, Mandahl AK. Latanoprost and cystoid macular edema: is there a causal relation? Curr Opin Ophthalmol 2000;11(2):94–100.

31. Sodhi PK, Sachdev MS, Gupta A, Verma LK, Ratan SK. Choroidal detachment with topical latanoprost after glaucoma filtration surgery. Ann Pharmacother 2004; 38: 510–1.

32. Lai IC, Kuo MT, Teng IMC. Iris pigment epithelial cyst induced by topical administration of latanoprost. Br J Ophthalmol 2003; 87: 366.

33. Kook MS, Lee K. Increased eyelid pigmentation associated with use of latanoprost. Am J Ophthalmol 2000;129(6):804–6.

34. Wand M, Ritch R, Isbey EK Jr, Zimmerman TJ. Latanoprost and periocular skin color changes. Arch Ophthalmol 2001;119(4):614–5.

35. Johnstone MA, Albert DM. Prostaglandin-induced hair growth. Surv Ophthalmol 2002;47(Suppl 1):S185–202.

36. Mansberger SL, Cioffi GA. Eyelash formation secondary to latanoprost treatment in a patient with alopecia. Arch Ophthalmol 2000;118(5):718–9.

37. Sugimoto M, Sugimoto M, Uji Y. Quantitative analysis of eyelash lengthening following topical latanoprost therapy. Can J Ophthalmol 2002;37(6):342–5.

38. Reynolds A, Murray PI, Colloby PS. Darkening of eyelashes in a patient treated with latanoprost. Eye 1998;12(Pt 4):741–3.

39. Schmidtborn F. Systemische Nebenwirkung von Latanoprost bei einem Kind mit Aniridie und Glaukom. [Systemic side-effects of latanoprost in a child with aniridia and glaucoma.] Ophthalmologe 1998;95(9):633–4.

40. Kumar H, Sony P, Gupta V. Profound sweating episodes and latanoprost. Clin Experiment Ophthalmol 2005; 33(6): 675.

41. Morales J, Shihab ZM, Brown SM, Hodges MR. *Herpes simplex* virus dermatitis in patients using latanoprost. Am J Ophthalmol 2001;132(1):114–6.

42. De Santis M, Lucchese A, Carducci B, Cavaliere AF, De Santis L, Merola A, Straface G, Caruso A. Latanoprost exposure in pregnancy. Am J Ophthalmol 2004; 138: 305–6.

43. Kashiwagi K., Tsukahara S. Effect of non-steroidal anti-inflammatory ophthalmic solution on intraocular pressure reduction by latanoprost. Br J Ophthalmol 2003; 87: 297–301.

Misoprostol

General Information

Misoprostol, an analogue of PGE_1, is licensed for use in the management of gastroduodenal ulceration. It is an effective myometrial stimulant of the pregnant uterus and is used for the induction of labor and as abortifacient, both alone and in combination with other substances (for example mifepristone). It provides an effective alternative to gemeprost, the most widely used prostaglandin pessaries in combination with mifepristone.

Vaginal misoprostol is more effective and better tolerated than oral misoprostol for induction of first and second trimester abortions after the administration of mifepristone (1,2). It is more effective than either gemeprost or sulprostone combined with mifepristone for induction of first trimester abortion, although uterine rupture has been reported (3).

Intramuscular methotrexate 50 mg/m^2 followed by intravaginal misoprostol was effective in the induction of first trimester abortion. Adverse events following the administration of misoprostol included nausea (12%), vomiting (8.1%), diarrhea (7.4%), and fevers/chills (3.4%) (4).

Observational studies

A single intravaginal dose of misoprostol 800 micrograms can obtain an abortion. The success rate has been assessed in 102 pregnant patients with amenorrhea for less than 42 weeks (5). After 1 day and 3 days of administration the abortion rates were 72 and 87% respectively. A second dose 7 days later increased the cumulative rate to 92%. The main complaints were pain (85%), nausea (21%), and headache (18%). Similar results were obtained in 2295 pregnant women (up to 56 days of gestation), who took a single oral dose of mifepristone (200 mg) and were randomized to self-administer misoprostol 800 micrograms/day at home for 1, 2, or 3 days (6). Complete abortion rates were 98, 98, and 96% among those who took misoprostol for 1, 2, and 3 days respectively. There were similar frequencies of adverse effects in all groups (cramping, nausea, fever/chills, dizziness, vomiting, headache, and diarrhea).

Misoprostol has been used to induce abortions in 150 adolescents (age range 12–17 years) at gestations of 63–84 days (7). They received vaginal misoprostol 800 micrograms/day to a maximum of three doses. Complete abortion occurred in 84%. Adverse effects were more frequent in these adolescents than in adult women, and included nausea (31%), vomiting (41%), diarrhea (48%), dizziness (19%), headache (17%), a subjective feeling of fever (26%), flushing (16%), and chills (49%).

The efficacy and tolerability of sublingual misoprostol has been evaluated in an uncontrolled trial in China in 50 women who requested medical abortions at up to 12 weeks of gestation (8). All received three doses of misoprostol 600 micrograms sublingually 3-hourly, and two more doses of 600 micrograms sublingually if an abortion did not occur. The overall complete abortion rate was 86% and the mean number of doses of misoprostol required was four. There was no significant change in hemoglobin concentration and the median duration of vaginal bleeding was 15 days. Lower abdominal pain, fatigue, diarrhea, fever, and chills were the most common adverse effects, and they occurred more often (from 70 to 100%) than in studies in which repeated doses of vaginal misoprostol were used.

In a retrospective study in patients with pre-eclampsia undergoing cervical ripening the complications associated with vaginal misoprostol (n = 95) and dinoprostone (n = 108) vaginal inserts before induction of labor have been reported (9). The incidence of uterine hyperstimulation requiring emergency cesarean section because of fetal heart rate abnormalities was significantly higher among patients who received misoprostol (18% versus 8.3%). The overall incidence of abruptio placenta was also significantly higher among those who received misoprostol (14% versus 1.9%).

Comparative studies

Different prostaglandins

Extra-amniotic dinoprost ($PGF_{2\alpha}$) and intracervical misoprostol have been compared for termination of pregnancy in 40 women at 16–24 weeks of gestation (10). All the women given dinoprost aborted within 28 hours and 16 within 20 hours; termination of pregnancy was complete in 13 cases. With misoprostol, all the women aborted within 20 hours, 18 within 13 hours; termination of pregnancy was complete in 17 cases. The mean time to induction of abortion was 16 hours for extra-amniotic dinoprost and 10 hours for intracervical misoprostol (significantly quicker). The incidence of prostaglandin-associated pyrexia, vomiting, and diarrhea was significantly higher with dinoprost. Abdominal pain was similar in the two groups.

Oxytocin

Misoprostol and oxytocin have been compared in three trials during vaginal and cesarean delivery. The first trial included 663 women (mean age 25 years, mean parity 2)

with uncomplicated vaginal deliveries (11). They were randomized to receive two tablets of misoprostol (total dose 400 micrograms, dissolved in saline 5 ml and given as a micro-enema) or oxytocin (10 IU intramuscularly), with a double-dummy technique. There were no significant differences between the groups in mean hemoglobin and hematocrit, volume of blood loss, or duration of third-stage labor. Shivering (38 versus 15%) and an increased mean temperature were significantly more common among those who received misoprostol.

The second trial included 60 women who were randomized to oral misoprostol (400 micrograms) or intravenous oxytocin (10 IU) during cesarean section (12). Estimated blood loss was 545 ml (95% CI = 476, 614) in those given misoprostol and 533 ml (95% CI = 427, 639) in those given oxytocin. The hemoglobin concentration and hematocrit were similar in the two groups.

The third trial included 2058 patients (mean age 28 years, 53% nulliparous) with a singleton pregnancy, a low risk of postpartum hemorrhage, and vaginal delivery (13). They were randomly assigned to either intramuscular Syntometrine 1 ml (oxytocin 5 units plus ergometrine 0.5 mg) or oral misoprostol 600 micrograms. There were no significant differences between the two groups in mean blood loss, the incidence of postpartum hemorrhage, or the fall in hemoglobin concentration. The need for oxytocic medication was higher with misoprostol, but manual removal of the placenta was required more often. Shivering (30 versus 9.9%) and transient pyrexia (temperature over 38°C, 8.5 versus 1.3%) were more common with misoprostol. Misoprostol could be an alternative to oxytocic drugs in reducing postpartum blood loss.

Placebo-controlled studies

Oral misoprostol 400 micrograms has been compared with placebo in the routine management of the third-stage of labor. In this study shivering was a specific adverse effect of oral misoprostol in the puerperium (19 versus 5%; RR = 3.69; 95% CI = 2.05, 6.64) (14).

The adverse effects of misoprostol have been evaluated in a large double-blind randomized placebo-controlled trial sponsored by the WHO in 15 clinics in 11 countries in 2219 healthy pregnant women requesting medical abortion after up to 63 days of amenorrhea (15). They were given oral mifepristone 200 mg on day 1, followed by 800 micrograms either orally or vaginally on day 3. The oral group and one of the vaginal groups continued taking oral misoprostol 400 micrograms bd for 7 days and the vaginal-only group took oral placebo. Pregnancy-related symptoms abated in all the groups after misoprostol and breast tenderness was reduced by mifepristone. Oral misoprostol was associated with a higher frequency of nausea and vomiting than vaginal administration at 1 hour after administration. With oral misoprostol, diarrhea was more frequent at 1, 2, and 3 hours after administration. Misoprostol caused *fever* during at least 3 hours after administration in up to 6% of the women, the peak being slightly higher and later with vaginal administration. Lower abdominal pain peaked at 1 and 2 hours after oral misoprostol and at 2 and 3 hours after vaginal misoprostol. In the two groups of women who continued to take misoprostol, 27% had diarrhea between the misoprostol visit and the 2-week follow up visit, compared with 9% in the placebo group.

Systematic reviews

A systematic review of the use of misoprostol for induction of labor has been published (16). The meta-analysis included all randomized clinical trials registered in the Cochrane Pregnancy and Childbirth Group. Vaginal misoprostol was associated with increased uterine hyperstimulation, both without fetal heart changes (RR = 1.67; CI = 1.30, 2.14) and with associated fetal heart rate changes (RR = 1.45; CI = 1.04, 2.04). There was also an increase in meconium-stained amniotic fluid (RR = 1.38; CI = 1.06, 1.79).

General adverse effects

The most common adverse effects during misoprostol use in labor include pyrexia (temperature over 38°C), shivering, postpartum hemorrhage, nausea, vomiting, diarrhea, hot flushes, headache, and vertigo. When it is used in the first or second trimesters for pregnancy termination, its adverse effects include fever, chills, vomiting, diarrhea, moderate and severe abdominal pain, profuse bleeding, dysfunctional uterine bleeding, dizziness, and headache.

Organs and Systems

Reproductive system

The effects of vaginal misoprostol for third trimester cervical ripening or induction of labor has been reviewed (17).

Several cases of uterine rupture due to misoprostol after second trimester have been reported. However, unexpectedly, administration of misoprostol for cervical ripening before surgical evacuation of a missed abortion reportedly produced *uterine rupture* in the first trimester (18).

- A 30-year-old woman with amenorrhea for 8 weeks had vaginal bleeding probably secondary to a missed abortion. Transvaginal ultrasonography showed a single fetus of 6 weeks without cardiac activity. She was scheduled for dilatation and evacuation but 1 hour after a single oral dose of misoprostol 400 micrograms she developed severe abdominal pain, hypotension (70/40 mmHg), and abdominal distension and rebound tenderness. The hemoglobin concentration was 6.5 g/l. Emergency laparoscopy showed a 1.5 cm rupture of the left uterine horn.

She had had a previous cesarean section, but it is very unlikely that that contributed, because the uterine rupture occurred at a different site to the caesarean incision (low-flap transverse section).

Infection risk

There were four deaths in previously healthy women due to endometritis and toxic shock syndrome within 1 week after medically induced abortions with oral mifepristone 200 mg and vaginal misoprostol 800 micrograms; in two cases *Clostridium sordellii* was found (19). Another similar case was reported in Canada in 2001. Endometritis and toxic shock syndrome associated with *C. sordellii* are rare. Of 10 cases identified by authors in the previous literature, eight occurred after the delivery of live-born infants, one after a medical abortion, and one was not associated with pregnancy. The cases produced an FDA alert with a "Dear Health Care Provider" letter from the manufacturer and publication of a "Dispatch" in the Morbidity and Mortality Weekly Report (20).

Body temperature

Severe hyperthermia has been reported after misoprostol (21).

- A 31-year primigravida had a missed abortion after 12 weeks of amenorrhea and was admitted for evacuation of the uterus. Preoperative cervical priming was done with intravaginal misoprostol 600 micrograms. Within 30 minutes of insertion of the misoprostol tablets she had chills and rigors, felt unwell, and started to have lower abdominal cramps. She was febrile (39.5°C) and her pulse rate was 90/minute. The undissolved misoprostol tablets were removed digitally and her vagina was douched. Ice sponging lowered her temperature. A rectal suppository of diclofenac 25 mg and an intramuscular injection of promethazine 25 mg were given. Her temperature remained high at 38°C for 3 hours and normalized after 5 hours.

Second-Generation Effects

Pregnancy

Cervical laceration associated with misoprostol has been reported in a 33-year-old woman who received four doses of vaginal misoprostol (total dose 100 micrograms) for labor induction. Uterine rupture has occurred during induction of labor with misoprostol, usually in women who have had a previous cesarean section (22,23). Uterine dehiscence occurred in one and uterine rupture in three of 48 women with prior cesarean sections treated with intravaginal misoprostol 50 micrograms for cervical ripening (24). In comparison, uterine rupture occurred in one of 89 women who had an oxytocin infusion and none of 24 patients who received intravaginal alprostadil.

- Transvaginal misoprostol for induction of labor caused uterine rupture in a 26-year-old woman with a previous low transverse cesarean delivery (25).
- In two cases, disruption of prior uterine incisions occurred after misoprostol (26).
- In two cases, uterine rupture occurred after inappropriate use (27). In one case the dose of 200 micrograms was too high. In the other case oxytocin was started 5

hours after the second misoprostol tablet, while the usual recommendation is to wait at least 12 hours. One patient had also had a previous dilatation and curettage for spontaneous abortion, which is a predisposing factor for uterine rupture in labor.

Seven pregnant women who had uterine rupture after intravaginal administration of misoprostol for induction of labor (SEDA-23, 436) had all undergone cesarean section in previous pregnancies (28).

- The first four women (aged 26–36 years) underwent induction of labor at 37–40 weeks of gestation. They received 1–2 doses of intravaginal misoprostol 25 micrograms; three of the women then received intravenous oxytocin. Soon after the first woman began pushing, there was fetal heart rate deceleration and the fetal head could not be palpated in the vagina. Emergency laparotomy showed that the baby was free in the abdominal cavity and the woman had a bladder defect. The bladder and uterine defects were repaired successfully and the mother received a transfusion of packed erythrocytes.
- In the second case, there was sudden fetal bradycardia. Laparotomy showed a large clot overlying the previous uterine incision. Dissection through the hematoma showed complete separation of the uterine incision. After delivery, the uterine rupture site and a cervical laceration were successfully repaired.
- The third woman had sudden-onset severe abdominal pain and fetal decelerations were detected. Emergency laparotomy showed complete separation of the uterine scar; both the fetus and the placenta were free in the abdominal cavity. The uterine defect was repaired and the woman recovered. However, the baby subsequently died.
- The fourth woman began to have extreme pain and fetal bradycardia then occurred. Uterine rupture from the previous incision was found at emergency cesarean section, with the baby's arm extending through the lacerated area. The uterine defect was successfully repaired.
- Uterine rupture also occurred in another three women (ages not stated) after misoprostol (dosages not stated) was used to induce labor. One underwent cesarean section because labor did not progress. During the procedure, the fetal hand and head were outside the uterine cavity (maternal and fetal outcome not stated).
- The other two women underwent emergency cesarean deliveries because of fetal bradycardia. Both had complete uterine wall separation; one had a stellate laceration involving the previous incision, and the other had a hematoma associated with the scar disruption. Outcomes were good in both cases.

In view of these cases, the authors recommended that there be a moratorium on the use of misoprostol in the setting of a scarred uterus until the relative risks have been thoroughly investigated in appropriately controlled trials.

Uterine rupture has also been associated with misoprostol (200 micrograms vaginally) during second trimester termination of pregnancy. Occasionally, uterine rupture can occur in women who have not had a previous cesarean section, as happened in two women, one of whom had a normal delivery and the other curettage after abortion (29).

Misoprostol is not approved by the FDA for any obstetric indication. In 2000, the manufacturers GD Searle distributed a "Dear Health Care Provider" letter in the USA, emphasizing the fact that misoprostol, by any route of administration, is not intended for the induction of labor or as a cervical ripening agent before termination of pregnancy (30). Searle has become aware of instances in which misoprostol was used for such purposes, in spite of its being specifically contraindicated for use during pregnancy. The following serious adverse events have been reported after such off-label use: maternal or fetal death; uterine hyperstimulation; uterine rupture or perforation requiring surgical repair, hysterectomy, or salpingo-oophorectomy; amniotic fluid embolism; severe vaginal bleeding; retained placenta; shock; fetal bradycardia; and pelvic pain. Searle does not intend to study or support the use of misoprostol for pregnancy termination or labor induction. The company is therefore unable to provide complete risk information for misoprostol when it is used for such purposes. Furthermore, the effects of misoprostol on the later growth, development, and functional maturation of children who are exposed to it during induction of labor have not been established.

Teratogenicity

The common phenotypical effects of exposure of the fetus to misoprostol in utero have been defined in 42 infants who were exposed to misoprostol during the first 3 months of gestation, and then born with congenital abnormalities (31). Equinovarus with cranial nerve defects occurred in 17 infants. Ten children had equinovarus as part of more extensive arthrogryposis. The most distinctive phenotypes were arthrogryposis confined to the legs (five cases) and terminal transverse limb defects (nine cases), with or without Möbius' syndrome. The most common dose of misoprostol was 800 (range 200–16 000) micrograms. Deformities attributed to vascular disruption were found in these children. The authors suggested that the uterine contractions induced by misoprostol cause vascular disruption in the fetus, including brainstem ischemia. Information on the effects of taking misoprostol during pregnancy should be made more widely available, to dissuade women from misusing the drug. Additional information on the risk associated with continuing a pregnancy to term after a failure of mifepristone and prostaglandin has been provided (32).

Data from Brazil, where misoprostol has been used orally and vaginally as an abortifacient, have suggested a relation between the use of misoprostol by women in an unsuccessful attempt to terminate pregnancy and Möbius' syndrome (congenital facial paralysis) in their infants (33). The frequencies of misoprostol use during the first trimester by mothers of infants in whom Möbius' syndrome was diagnosed and mothers of infants with neural-tube defects have been compared. There were 96 infants with Möbius' syndrome and 96 with neural-tube defects. The mean age at the time of the diagnosis of Möbius' syndrome was 16 (range 0.5–78) months and the diagnosis of neural-tube defects was made within 1 week of birth in most cases. Of the mothers of the infants with Möbius' syndrome, 47 had used misoprostol in the first trimester of pregnancy, compared with three of the mothers of the infants with neural-tube defects (OR = 30; 95% CI = 12, 76). Of the mothers of the infants with Möbius' syndrome, 20 had taken misoprostol only orally (OR = 39; CI = 9.5, 159), 20 had taken misoprostol both orally and vaginally, three had taken it vaginally, and four did not report how they had taken it. The authors concluded that attempted abortion with misoprostol is associated with an increased risk of Möbius' syndrome in infants.

In another case-control study in Brazil, 93 cases of prenatal exposure to misoprostol and 279 controls were recruited (34). Vascular disruption defects (transverse terminal limb reductions, Möbius and/or Poland sequences, hypoglossia–hypodactyly sequence, arthrogryposis, intestinal atresia, hemifacial microsomia, microtia, and porencephalic cyst) were identified in 32 exposed infants compared with only 12 controls.

In another case-control study in Brazil, congenital anomalies were compared in 34 misoprostol-exposed children and 4639 unexposed controls (35). Misoprostol exposure significantly increased the risk of arthrogryposis (OR = 8.5; 95% CI = 2, 37), hydrocephalus (OR = 4.2; CI = 1.5, 12), terminal transverse limb reduction (OR = 12; CI = 3.5, 41), and limb constriction ring or skin scars (OR = 40; CI = 11, 153). There were 13 different defects not previously described in the misoprostol-exposed cases, but only holoprosencephaly and bladder exstrophy significantly exceeded the expected number.

Mothers who used misoprostol during pregnancy as an abortifacient had an increased risk of having a baby with congenital anomalies (OR = 2.4; 95% CI = 1.0, 6.2), as reported in a case-control study in Fortaleza, Brazil (36). Multiple malformations have been described associated with the use of misoprostol (37).

- A 23-year-old woman took oral misoprostol 600 micrograms/day twice when she was 7 weeks pregnant to induce an abortion. At 12 weeks she developed a *Varicella* infection. At 15 weeks, ultrasound showed a fetus of 14.5 weeks size with several abnormalities. After amniocentesis at 17 weeks, an elective abortion was performed. The fetus had amputation deformities at the proximal interphalangeal joints of four fingers, with distal fusion of the proximal finger stumps by thin strands of tissue; the index finger was normal. The left leg had an amputation deformity at the mid-tibial/fibular level. There was an omphalocele. Histological examination of the placenta showed an absence of amnion on the chorionic surface, with reactive changes in the superficial chorionic stroma and "vernix granulomas" on the chorionic surface. These findings are diagnostic of early amnion rupture. There were no features of *Varicella* embryopathy.

Möbius' syndrome in association with congenital central alveolar hypoventilation has been described in Brazil (38).

Misoprostol-induced arthrogryposis has been reported in 15 Brazilian patients (39).

Drug Administration

Drug administration route

In a randomized controlled trial, 74 primigravidae who were undergoing surgical abortion were randomly assigned to misoprostol 400 micrograms sublingually or vaginally 2–4 hours before surgery (40). Efficacy was similar in the two groups. Women who took sublingual misoprostol had significantly more *nausea* (63% versus 32%), vomiting (29% versus 6%), diarrhea (6% versus 0%), and unpleasant taste in the mouth (39% versus 3%) compared with the women who used vaginal misoprostol.

In another study, 100 pregnant women who opted for termination of pregnancy at 6–12 weeks gestation were randomly allocated to misoprostol 400 micrograms sublingually or vaginally 2 hours before suction evacuation (41). There was a significant difference between the sublingual and vaginal misoprostol groups with respect to mean cervical dilatation (8.6 mm versus 6.8 mm). However, the durations of the procedures (3.03 versus 3.16 minutes) and the amounts of blood loss (29 versus 31.2 ml) were not different. The women who used sublingual misoprostol had significantly more shivering and preoperative vaginal bleeding (68% versus 56%). Sublingual misoprostol is an effective alternative to vaginal administration for cervical priming before surgical abortion, despite a higher incidence of adverse effects.

The pharmacokinetics of misoprostol 600 mg after oral and rectal administration have been compared in 20 women after delivery (42). After rectal administration there was a higher AUC, but lower C_{max} and a later t_{max}; these findings are consistent with a slower speed but a greater extent of absorption. In 275 women randomized to oral misoprostol 600 micrograms or rectal misoprostol 400 or 600 micrograms after delivery, shivering was reported by 76% of the patients given oral misoprostol and 55% of those given rectal misoprostol. Thus, rectal misoprostol is associated with less toxicity than oral misoprostol.

References

1. el-Refaey H, Rajasekar D, Abdalla M, Calder L, Templeton A. Induction of abortion with mifepristone (RU 486) and oral or vaginal misoprostol. N Engl J Med 1995;332(15):983–7.
2. Jain JK, Mishell DR Jr. A comparison of misoprostol with and without laminaria tents for induction of second-trimester abortion. Am J Obstet Gynecol 1996;175(1):173–7.

3. Phillips K, Berry C, Mathers AM. Uterine rupture during second trimester termination of pregnancy using mifepristone and a prostaglandin. Eur J Obstet Gynecol Reprod Biol 1996;65(2):175–6.

4. Creinin MD, Vittinghoff E, Keder L, Darney PD, Tiller G. Methotrexate and misoprostol for early abortion: a multicenter trial. I. Safety and efficacy. Contraception 1996;53(6):321–7.

5. Bugalho A, Mocumbi S, Faundes A, David E. Termination of pregnancies of <6 weeks gestation with a single dose of 800 microg of vaginal misoprostol. Contraception 2000;61(1):47–50.

6. Schaff EA, Fielding SL, Westhoff C, Ellertson C, Eisinger SH, Stadalius LS, Fuller L. Vaginal misoprostol administered 1, 2, or 3 days after mifepristone for early medical abortion: A randomized trial. JAMA 2000;284(15):1948–53.

7. Acharya G, Al-Sammarai MT, Patel N, Al-Habib A, Kiserud T. A randomized, controlled trial comparing effect of oral misoprostol and intravenous syntocinon on intraoperative blood loss during cesarean section. Acta Obstet Gynecol Scand 2001;80(3):245–50.

8. Tang OS, Miao BY, Lee SW, Ho PC. Pilot study on the use of repeated doses of sublingual misoprostol in termination of pregnancy up to 12 weeks gestation: efficacy and acceptability. Hum Reprod 2002;17(3):654–8.

9. Fontenot MT, Lewis DF, Barton CB, Jones EM, Moore JA, Evans AT. Abruptio placentae associated with misoprostol use in women with preeclampsia. J Reprod Med 2005; 50(9): 653–8.

10. Ghorab MN, El Helw BA. Second-trimester termination of pregnancy by extra-amniotic prostaglandin F2alpha or endocervical misoprostol. A comparative study. Acta Obstet Gynecol Scand 1998;77(4):429–32.

11. Ng PS, Chan AS, Sin WK, Tang LC, Cheung KB, Yuen PM. A multicentre randomized controlled trial of oral misoprostol and i.m. syntometrine in the management of the third stage of labour Hum Reprod 2001;16(1):31–5.

12. Oyelese Y, Landy HJ, Collea JV. Cervical laceration associated with misoprostol induction. Int J Gynaecol Obstet 2001;73(2):161–2.

13. Al-Hussaini TK. Uterine rupture in second trimester abortion in a grand multiparous woman. A complication of misoprostol and oxytocin. Eur J Obstet Gynecol Reprod Biol 2001;96(2):218–9.

14. Hofmeyr GJ, Nikodem VC, de Jager M, Gelbart BR. A randomised placebo controlled trial of oral misoprostol in the third stage of labour. Br J Obstet Gynaecol 1998;105(9):971–5.

15. Honkanen H, Piaggio G, Hertzen H, Bartfai G, Erdenetungalag R, Gemzell-Danielsson K, Gopalan S, Horga M, Jerve F, Mittal S, Thi Nhu Ngoc N, Peregoudov A, Prasad RN, Pretnar-Darovec A, Shah RS, Song S, Tang OS, Wu SC; WHO Research Group on Post-Ovulatory Methods for Fertility Regulation. WHO multinational study of three misoprostol regimens after mifepristone for early medical abortion. BJOG 2004; 111: 715–25.

16. Hofmeyr GJ, Gulmezoglu AM, Alfirevic Z. Misoprostol for induction of labour: a systematic review. Br J Obstet Gynaecol 1999;106(8):798–803.

17. Hofmeyr GJ, Gulmezoglu AM. Vaginal misoprostol for cervical ripening and induction of labour. Cochrane Database Syst Rev 2003; (1): CD000941.

18. Kim JO, Han JY, Choi JS, Ahn HK, Yang JH, Kang IS, Song MJ, Nava-Ocampo AA. Oral misoprostol and uterine rupture in the first trimester of pregnancy: a case report. Reprod Toxicol 2005; 20(4): 575–7.

19. Fischer M, Bhatnagar J, Guarner J, Reagan S, Hacker JK, Van Meter SH, Poukens V, Whiteman DB, Iton A, Cheung M, Dassey DE, Shieh WJ, Zaki SR. Fatal toxic shock syndrome associated with Clostridium sordellii after medical abortion. N Engl J Med 2005; 353(22): 2352–60.

20. Centers for Disease Control and Prevention. Clostridium sordellii toxic shock syndrome after medical abortion with mifepristone and intravaginal misoprostol—United States and Canada, 2001–2005. MMWR Morb Mortal Wkl Rep 2005; 54: 724.

21. Fong YF, Singh K, Prasad RN. Severe hyperthermia following use of vaginal misoprostol for pre-operative cervical priming. Int J Gynaecol Obstet 1999;64(1):73–4.

22. Gherman RB, McBrayer S, Browning J. Uterine rupture associated with vaginal birth after cesarean section: a complication of intravaginal misoprostol? Gynecol Obstet Invest 2000;50(3):212–3.

23. Jwarah E, Greenhalf JO. Rupture of the uterus after 800 micrograms misoprostol given vaginally for termination of pregnancy. BJOG 2000;107(6):807.

24. Hill DA, Chez RA, Quinlan J, Fuentes A, LaCombe J. Uterine rupture and dehiscence associated with intravaginal misoprostol cervical ripening. J Reprod Med 2000;45(10):823–6.

25. Sciscione AC, Nguyen L, Manley JS, Shlossman PA, Colmorgen GH. Uterine rupture during preinduction cervical ripening with misoprostol in a patient with a previous Caesarean delivery. Aust NZ J Obstet Gynaecol 1998;38(1):96–7.

26. Wing DA, Lovett K, Paul RH. Disruption of prior uterine incision following misoprostol for labor induction in women with previous cesarean delivery. Obstet Gynecol 1998;91(5 Pt 2):828–30.

27. Fletcher H, McCaw-Binns A. Rupture of the uterus with misoprostol (prostaglandin El) used for induction of labour. J Obstet Gynaecol 1998;18(2):184–5.

28. Plaut MM, Schwartz ML, Lubarsky SL. Uterine rupture associated with the use of misoprostol in the gravid patient with a previous cesarean section. Am J Obstet Gynecol 1999;180(6 Pt 1):1535–42.

29. Mathews JE, Mathai M, George A. Uterine rupture in a multiparous woman during labor induction with oral misoprostol. Int J Gynaecol Obstet 2000;68(1):43–4.

30. Searle GD. Important drug warning concerning unapproved use of intravaginal or oral misoprostol in pregnant women for induction of labor or abortion. Media Release 23 August 2000.

31. Gonzalez CH, Marques-Dias MJ, Kim CA, Sugayama SM, Da Paz JA, Huson SM, Holmes LB. Congenital abnormalities in Brazilian children associated with misoprostol misuse in first trimester of pregnancy. Lancet 1998;351(9116):1624–7.

32. Sitruk-Ware R, Davey A, Sakiz E. Fetal malformation and failed medical termination of pregnancy. Lancet 1998;352(9124):323.

33. Pastuszak AL, Schuler L, Speck-Martins CE, Coelho KE, Cordello SM, Vargas F, Brunoni D, Schwarz IV, Larrandaburu M, Safattle H, Meloni VF, Koren G. Use of misoprostol during pregnancy and Möbius' syndrome in infants. N Engl J Med 1998;338(26):1881–5.

34. Vargas FR, Schuler-Faccini L, Brunoni D, Kim C, Meloni VF, Sugayama SM, Albano L, Llerena JC Jr, Almeida JC, Duarte A, Cavalcanti DP, Goloni-Bertollo E, Conte A, Koren G, Addis A. Prenatal exposure to misoprostol and vascular disruption defects: a case-control study. Am J Med Genet 2000;95(4):302–6.

35. Orioli IM, Castilla EE. Epidemiological assessment of misoprostol teratogenicity. BJOG 2000;107(4):519–23.

36. Brasil R, Coelho HL, D'Avanzo B, La Vecchia C. Misoprostol and congenital anomalies. Pharmacoepidemiol Drug Saf 2000;9:401–3.

37. Genest DR, Di Salvo D, Rosenblatt MJ, Holmes LB. Terminal transverse limb defects with tethering and omphalocele in a 17 week fetus following first trimester misoprostol exposure. Clin Dysmorphol 1999;8(1):53–8.

38. Nunes ML, Friedrich MA, Loch LF. Association of misoprostol, Moebius syndrome and congenital central alveolar hypoventilation. Case report. Arq Neuropsiquiatr 1999;57(1):88–91.

39. Coelho KE, Sarmento MF, Veiga CM, Speck-Martins CE, Safatle HP, Castro CV, Niikawa N. Misoprostol embryotoxicity: clinical evaluation of fifteen patients with arthrogryposis. Am J Med Genet 2000;95(4):297–301.

40. Hamoda H, Ashok PW, Flett GM, Templeton A. A randomized controlled comparison of sublingual and vaginal administration of misoprostol for cervical priming before first-trimester surgical abortion. Am J Obstet Gynecol 2004; 190: 55–9.

41. Vimala N, Mittal S, Kumar S, Dadhwal V, Sharma Y. A randomized comparison of sublingual and vaginal misoprostol for cervical priming before suction termination of first-trimester pregnancy. Contraception 2004; 70: 117–20.

42. Khan RU, El-Refaey H. Pharmacokinetics and adverse-effect profile of rectally administered misoprostol in the third stage of labor. Obstet Gynecol 2003; 101: 968–74.

Sulprostone

General Information

Sulprostone is a synthetic prostaglandin analogue of PGE_2 used for inducing uterine contraction.

In large series, sulprostone has had good tolerability with a very low complication rate. The most severe complication is myocardial infarction secondary to coronary spasm, with a frequency of one in 20 000, usually in smokers and women over 35 years of age with cardiovascular disease (SEDA-23, 436).

Organs and Systems

Cardiovascular

Several experimental studies have provided support for the hypothesis that coronary spasm plays a major role in the pathophysiology of myocardial infarction during the administration of sulprostone. However, the possibility of myocardial infarction is not mentioned in the product information.

- Two cases of myocardial infarction (one fatal) have been reported in patients receiving sulprostone with mifepristone (1,2).
- Myocardial infarction has been reported in a woman aged 35 years with normal coronary arteries and good left ventricular function (3).

- A 30-year-old woman developed uterine atony and bleeding after induced abortion because of fetal death at 17 weeks of gestation (4). Sulprostone was given intravenously at a rate of 500 micrograms/hour. When additional sulprostone was injected into the uterine cervix, the patient sustained a myocardial infarction, with ventricular fibrillation and cardiocirculatory arrest, most probably due to coronary artery spasm. She was resuscitated and recovered completely.

Sulprostone should be used with care, particularly in patients with cardiac risk factors, and only in settings equipped to manage complications.

Cardiac dysrhythmias have been reported after the administration of misoprostol.

- A 38-year-old woman developed complete heart block, ventricular fibrillation, and subsequent asystole about 7 minutes after intravenous sulprostone 30 micrograms over 5 minutes, after she had previously been given a total dose of intramyometrial sulprostone 500 micrograms at seven different points for postpartum hemorrhage after cesarean section (5).

The time-course suggested that the most likely cause of the arrest was the intravenous sulprostone. Contributory causes may have been hemorrhagic shock, electrolyte abnormalities, and hypothermia (from massive blood transfusion).

- Cardiac arrest occurred in a 39-year-old woman 3.5 hours after the administration of sulprostone 250 micrograms directly into the uterine wall for postpartum hemorrhage after manual removal of the placenta (6). She had specific contraindications to sulprostone, as formulated by the French authorities: age over 35 years, heavy cigarette smoking, and cardiovascular risk factors.

In the Netherlands, sulprostone is registered for intravenous administration only. The authors strongly advised against administration directly into the uterine wall.

Nervous system

Seizures have been described during pregnancy termination induced by sulprostone (7).

Liver

Sulprostone has been associated with minor abnormalities of liver function (8).

Urinary tract

Sulprostone has been associated with minor abnormalities of kidney function (8).

Reproductive system

Sulprostone can cause rupture of the uterine cervix (9).

- A 43-year-old woman, who had previously had a first trimester miscarriage that required evacuation of the uterus and a normal vaginal delivery at term 4 years before, was admitted for an abortion at 16 weeks.

Ripening of the cervix was started with a pessary of gemeprost 1 mg. After 3 hours, when the cervix was 1 cm dilated, an intramuscular injection of sulprostone 500 mg was given. After 30 minutes she developed persistent abdominal pain, which became a continuous cramping and then a shooting pain; a male fetus of 170 g was aborted. There was a 3 cm longitudinal cervical rupture located posteriorly that reached the posterior fornix.

References

1. Anonymous. A death associated with mifeprostone/sulprostone. Lancet 1991;337:969–70.
2. Ulmann A, Silvestre L, Chemama L, Rezvani Y, Renault M, Aguillaume CJ, Baulieu EE. Medical termination of early pregnancy with mifepristone (RU 486) followed by a prostaglandin analogue. Study in 16,369 women. Acta Obstet Gynecol Scand 1992;71(4):278–83.
3. Feenstra J, Borst F, Huige MC, Oei SG, Stricker BH. Acuut myocardinfarct na toediening van sulproston. [Acute myocardial infarct following sulprostone administration.] Ned Tijdschr Geneeskd 1998;142(4):192–5.
4. Kulka PJ, Quent P, Wiebalck A, Jager D, Strumpf M. Myocardial infarction after sulprostone therapy for uterine atony and bleeding: a case report. Geburtshilfe Frauenheilk 1999;59:634–7.
5. Chen FG, Koh KF, Chong YS. Cardiac arrest associated with sulprostone use during caesarean section. Anaesth Intensive Care 1998;26(3):298–301.
6. Beerendonk CC, Massuger LF, Lucassen AM, Lerou JG, van den Berg PP. Circulatiestilstand na gebruik van sulproston bij fluxus post partum. [Circulatory arrest following sulprostone administration in postpartum hemorrhage.] Ned Tijdschr Geneeskd 1998;142(4):195–7.
7. Brandenburg H, Jahoda MG, Wladimiroff JW, Los FJ, Lindhout D. Convulsions in epileptic women after administration of prostaglandin E2 derivative. Lancet 1990;336(8723):1138.
8. Ranjan V, Hingorani V, Kinra G, Agarwal N, Pande Y. Evaluation of sulprostone for second trimester abortions and its effects on liver and kidney function. Contraception 1982;25(2):175–84.
9. Corrado F, D'Anna R, Cannata ML. Rupture of the cervix in a sulprostone induced abortion in the second trimester. Arch Gynecol Obstet 2000;264(3):162–3.

Travoprost

General Information

Travoprost is a derivative of fluprostenol and $PGF_{2\alpha}$ and has intraocular pressure-lowering activity.

Organs and Systems

Sensory systems

Travoprost causes changes in iris pigmentation (3.1–5.0%) and changes in eyelash characteristics, including length, thickness, density, and color (44–57%), similar to those described with latanoprost, after 12 months (1).

Gastrointestinal

Abdominal cramp has been attributed to travoprost (2).

- A 34-year-old woman with primary open-angle glaucoma began topical application of travoprost ophthalmic solution (0.004%, 1 drop/day) and 30 minutes later developed abdominal cramp that lasted for 2 hours. The same symptoms appeared on 3 days after drug administration. The pain disappeared after travoprost withdrawal.

In order to investigate this adverse effect, a series of single-blind trials were carried out with the informed consent of the patient (including rechallenge with travoprost and other prostaglandin analogues and dechallenges). Abdominal cramp did not develop after substitution of travoprost with latanoprost or isotonic saline, but recurred on rechallenge with travoprost.

References

1. Netland PA, Landry T, Sullivan EK, Andrew R, Silver L, Weiner A, Mallick S, Dickerson J, Bergamini MV, Robertson SM, Davis AATravoprost Study Group. Travoprost compared with latanoprost and timolol in patients with open-angle glaucoma or ocular hypertension. Am J Ophthalmol 2001;132(4):472–84.
2. Lee YC. Abdominal cramp as an adverse effect of travoprost. Am J Ophthalmol 2005; 139(1): 202–3.

Unoprostone

General Information

Unoprostone is a synthetic prostaglandin analogue of $PGF_{2\alpha}$ used in the treatment of glaucoma. Its mechanism of action is believed to be by enhancing uveoscleral outflow, like latanoprost.

Organs and Systems

Sensory systems

The use of unoprostone in the treatment of open-angle glaucoma and ocular hypertension has been reviewed (1). Most of the literature is in Japanese. The adverse effects of unoprostone are similar to those of latanoprost: conjunctival hyperemia, iris pigmentation, hypertrichosis and hyperpigmentation of eyelashes, and rarely systemic effects (1).

Reference

1. Eisenberg DL, Camras CB. A preliminary risk-benefit assessment of latanoprost and unoprostone in open-angle glaucoma and ocular hypertension. Drug Saf 1999;20(6):505–14.

SEX HORMONES AND RELATED DRUGS

Androgens and anabolic steroids

See also individual agents and Hormonal
contraceptives—male

General Information

The classic androgen is natural testosterone, which can be
given orally in micronized form, but has much more often
been used as the orally active 17-methyl derivative or an
injectable ester. Androgens are used to some extent in male
hypogonadism, when they can promote libido and potency
and increase the frequency of erections and the volume of
the ejaculate (1). The use of androgens by either sex as
"sexual tonics" is a matter of dispute. Some centers have
used androgens to treat postmenopausal women complaining of weak libido, poor energy, or a feeling of malaise (2);
workers who use this contentious approach have suggested
that they should be given in association with estrogens,
because of the adverse effects of androgens on serum lipids.

While some anabolic steroids are still available in the
legitimate trade, others are manufactured and distributed
illegally, and the contents and potency of these are
unknown; some adverse effects could be due to impurities
or content variation.

From about 1955 onwards, a number of so-called anabolic steroids were developed for which it was claimed, on
the basis of animal experiments, that the virilizing effects
had been reduced compared with testosterone, whereas
the effects on tissue build-up and nitrogen retention had
been maintained. These compounds were therefore promoted for such purposes as the promotion of appetite and
weight increase in children and the advancement of con-
valescence. In fact, it has never been at all clear that these
compounds are anything other than weak and expensive
androgens. Their supposed dissociation of anabolic and
androgenic effects was based on a misleading animal
model and was largely disproved. The benefits that they
were thought to confer in conditions such as aplastic
anemia and uremia were minimal or dubious, and their
adverse effects were pronounced. There are still those
who would argue for the use of anabolic steroids, alongside erythropoietin, in renal anemia (3), but this practice
is now unusual. Yet as they disappeared from pharmacy
shelves, the anabolic steroids began to return anew
through largely surreptitious channels. The western literature on the use and effects of performance-enhancing
drugs as a whole suggests that anabolic-androgenic steroids are currently used in up to 1% of women, 0.5?3% of
high school girls, 1?5% of men, 1?12% of high school
boys, and up to 67% of some groups of elite athletes,
often alongside other agents reputed to enhance physical
development or performance (4). Even in "tonic" doses,
androgens can cause virilization in women and precocious
development of secondary characteristics in children.
In the much higher doses later developed for use in such
conditions as aplastic anemia, mammary carcinoma,
terminal uremia, and even hereditary angioedema (5),
their androgenic effects are very pronounced indeed,

and other serious complications can occur, for example
in the liver (SED-12, 1038) (6–12). One formerly well-
known "anabolic" steroid, metandienone (Dianabol), was
withdrawn as early as 1982, and other withdrawals have
followed.

When androgen therapy is used in postmenopausal
women who complain of poor libido, poor energy, or a
feeling of malaise (2), it should be given in association with
estrogens, because of its adverse effects on serum lipids.

Anabolic steroids are also still used in refractory anemias, although with recombinant human erythropoietin
now widely available they appear to be seen mainly as a
means of increasing the response to erythropoietin in
highly resistant cases; combination treatment with erythropoietin, a glucocorticoid, and nandrolone has also
been recommended for treating myelodysplastic syndromes (13). Again, in such exceptional situations the
risks of anabolic steroids have to be accepted.

Placebo-controlled studies

A well-founded indication for the cautious use of androgens in women is to treat those who have much reduced
sexual desire after a surgical menopause and are troubled
by it. In a 24-week, randomized, double-blind, placebo-
controlled, parallel-group, study, 447 women aged 24–70
years were randomized to receive placebo or transdermal
testosterone patches in dosages of 150, 300,or 450 micrograms twice weekly, and 318 subjects completed the study
(14). There were marginally significant successes in
restoring sexual desire and activity, but only in the two
higher dose groups. There were no serious safety concerns, but adverse effects were not discussed in detail.

Androgen replacement therapy in men

The notion that many men in later life require androgen
supplementation to counter the effects of the "andropause" is more widespread in some countries than others,
both among practitioners and the public, and it is heavily
debated (15,16). Much of the evidence adduced to support the use of so-called "androgen supplementation" in
older men, such as an attempt to demonstrate its use as a
supportive treatment in depression (17), is far from convincing. Proponents of this therapy call for the development of more specific formulations for this purpose, while
others argue that such treatment is rarely justified and
should be strictly limited to a minority of men with severe
and evident hypogonadism. It has, after all, to quote a
sober review, "never been definitively established that the
decline in testosterone seen in most aging men results in
an androgen deficient state with health-related outcomes
that can be improved by androgen therapy" (18). In that
situation it is indefensible to run risks. A thorough review
of the literature has turned up much evidence for the
benefit of short-term testosterone treatment in selected
subjects, provided prostate cancer can be excluded, but
also marked reservations regarding the safety or otherwise of long-term use. Potential risks include erythrocytosis, edema, gynecomastia, and prostate stimulation. The
possibility of significantly increased risks of prostate cancer and cardiovascular disease has been considered (19).

Another thorough review has concluded that there is no place for such treatment in healthy older men (20). It is not clear to what extent the less favorable aspects of ageing are really attributable to androgen decline; nor is it clear that aged tissues remain androgen sensitive, nor that such treatment is necessarily safe. However, certain idiosyncratic adverse effects of androgen treatment, which can include disordered sleep and breathing, as well as polycythemia, are clearly dose related, suggesting that dose escalation to increase efficacy may create or aggravate undesirable adverse effects.

Hormonal contraception in men

The use of intramuscular testosterone + oral desogestrel for hormonal contraception in men is discussed in a separate monograph (Hormonal contraceptives—male).

General adverse reactions

Adverse effects of pharmacological doses of androgens include, as one would expect from male hormones, hirsutism with acne and other signs of virilization, along with adverse lipoprotein profiles, endometrial hyperplasia in women, and an increased risk of cardiovascular disease. Some compounds are particularly likely to cause liver disorders.

Male hormone replacement therapy has been reviewed (21). Hypogonadism can be accompanied by hot flushes, similar to those seen in postmenopausal women, and gynecomastia. The potential risks of testosterone replacement in adult men are precipitation or worsening of sleep apnea, hastened onset of clinical significant prostate disease, benign prostatic hyperplasia, prostatic carcinoma, gynecomastia, fluid retention, polycythemia, exacerbation of hypertension, edema, and an increased risk of cardiovascular disease.

The adverse effects of long-term testosterone therapy in HIV-positive men are irritability, weight gain, fatigue, hair loss, reduced volume of ejaculate, testicular atrophy, truncal acne, breast tenderness, and increased aggression (22).

Supraphysiological concentrations of androgen hormones can cause acne, hirsutism, and deepening of the voice.

Adverse effects of androgens in men

The safety of androgen therapy for cardiovascular and prostatic disease is uncertain. Kraus, after a careful review of the literature from a German perspective, has pointed out that androgen substitution must be approached with caution; even if the hazards are dubious, the need for such treatment is even more doubtful: "···.The lack of clear hazards from testosterone substitution in the aging male does not indicate unrestricted treatment safety. Until all doubts are cleared, each treatment should be carefully documented and monitored" (23).

While opinions are many and varied, only a few groups have made an adequate effort to acquire firm data on relative benefits and harms. In a randomized study using the anabolic androgen oxandrolone, 32 men aged 60–87

took oxandrolone 20 mg/day for 12 weeks or placebo (24). Oxandrolone produced significant increases in lean body mass and muscle strength during treatment, but 12 weeks after the treatment had ended these measures were no long different from baseline; however, there was some improvement in fat mass during the study, which was largely discernible 12 weeks later. These modest short-term effects hardly seem to provide a justification for anabolic treatment of the elderly in view of the risks involved.

Adverse effects of androgens in women

There are clear differences of opinion about the use of androgens in women. An Australian reviewer has argued that women may have symptoms secondary to androgen deficiency and that "prudent" androgen replacement can be effective in relieving both the physical and psychological symptoms of such insufficiency (25). The reviewer suggested that testosterone replacement for women is safe, with the caveat that doses should be restricted to the "therapeutic" window for androgen replacement in women, such that the beneficial effects on well-being and quality of life are achieved without incurring undesirable virilizing effects. The predominant symptom of women with androgen deficiency is claimed to be loss of sexual desire after a premature or natural menopause, while other indications for androgens include premenopausal iatrogenic androgen deficiency states, glucocorticoid-induced bone loss, management of wasting syndromes, and possibly premenopausal bone loss, premenopausal loss of libido, and the treatment of the premenstrual syndrome.

Some reservations about this approach arise when one considers the possible adverse effects and the doubts that have been raised as to whether there is in fact a safe therapeutic window when treating women with androgens. This comes clearly to the fore in a thoughtful paper by another Australian author, a speech therapist (26). For women treated with androgens or related compounds for any reason, virilization of the voice, which soon becomes permanent, is a distressing complication that has not received a great deal of specific study. This review provides some pointers for clinical practice. She reports on four women aged 27–58 years who sought otolaryngological examination because of significant alterations to their voices, the primary concerns being hoarseness, lowering of habitual pitch, difficulty in projecting their speaking voices, and loss of control over their singing voices. Otolaryngological examination with a mirror or flexible laryngoscope showed no apparent abnormality of vocal fold structure or function, and the women were referred for speech pathology with diagnoses of functional dysphonia. Objective acoustic measures using the Kay Visipitch showed significant lowering of the mean fundamental frequency in each woman, and perceptual analysis of the patients' voices during quiet speaking, projected voice use, and comprehensive singing activities showed a constellation of features typically noted in pubescent men. The original diagnosis of functional dysphonia was queried, prompting further exploration of each woman's medical history. In each case the vocal symptoms had started shortly after the beginning of treatment with medications containing virilizing agents, notably danazol, nandrolone decanoate, and testosterone. Although some of the vocal symptoms abated in severity with 6 months of voice therapy and after withdrawal of the drugs, a number of symptoms remained permanent, suggesting that each subject had suffered significant alterations in vocal physiology, including muscle tissue changes, muscle coordination dysfunction, and proprioceptive dysfunction. The study showed that both the projected speaking voice and the singing voice proved highly sensitive to virilizing effects.

It has been known for more than 30 years that some 50% of women have voice changes with anabolic steroids. While it has sometimes been thought that safe doses can be identified, studies of individual patients, including one of the cases documented here, throw doubt on this. The effects can be disastrous for any woman and incapacitating to a singer; clearly the use in women of any product having any androgenic potency must be undertaken with great reticence.

Organs and Systems

Cardiovascular

Particularly when androgens/anabolics are misused to promote extreme muscular development, there is a risk of cardiomegaly and ultimate cardiac failure. Androgen-induced hypertension may be due to a hypertensive shift in the pressure-natriuresis relation, either by an increase in proximal tubular reabsorption or by activation of the renin–angiotensin system (27). This effect is not related to higher doses or longer treatment and can develop after a few months but can also be delayed for many years.

Respiratory

There has been a single published report, which could have been coincidental, of obstructive sleep apnea during use of testosterone (28).

Nervous system

Use of androgenic steroids is likely to produce a sensation of energy and euphoria, but also with a tendency to sleeplessness and irritability (1). More extreme changes in mental state can result in extreme swings in mood, ranging from depression to aggressive elation. An unusual complication in one case was a toxic confusional state and choreiform movements caused by an anabolic steroid (SED-12, 1038) (29), but it may have been due to the non-specific results of endocrine stress in a susceptible individual.

- A 40-year-old Korean woman who had taken oxymetholone for aplastic anemia (doses not stated) developed cerebral venous thrombosis accompanied by a tentorial subdural hematoma (30).

Hiccups have been classified as a neurological reaction that can be triggered by many factors. There have been a few published reports of persistent hiccups associated with oral and intravenous glucocorticoids and one of progesterone-induced hiccups, which were thought to be secondary to the glucocorticoid-like effects of progesterone on the brainstem.

- Anabolic steroid-induced hiccups have been reported in a champion power lifter (31). The hiccups occurred within 12 hours of an increase in the dose of oral methandrostenolone from 50 to 75 mg/day, and persisted for 12 consecutive hours until medical attention was sought. The hiccups abated rapidly after the dose of methandrostenolone was reduced, but he was unwilling to abandon it completely.

Psychological, psychiatric

In the late 1980s various reports seemed to show that the use of anabolic steroids was linked to aggressive behavior and mood changes, even to the extent of inducing or potentiating violent crime (32,33). During the decade that followed, a series of other papers similarly linked high circulating concentrations of testosterone to increased degrees of aggression and related changes in mood. Undoubtedly, some of these findings are well-founded, but one must always be alert to the fallacy that individuals with particular pre-existent personality traits might be more susceptible than others to become bodybuilders, to use anabolic steroids, or to take testosterone. This possibility remains open after the completion of a thorough study of weightlifters at various American academic centers. In 20 male weightlifters, 10 of whom were taking anabolic steroids (metandrostenolone, testosterone, and nandrolone), supranormal testosterone concentrations were associated with increased aggression (34). Users tended to have a greater degree of depression, agitation, psychic or somatic anxiety, hypochondriasis, and hopelessness on the Hamilton Depression Scale; on the Modified Manic State Rating Scale, users showed more talkativeness, restlessness, threatening language, irritability, and sexual preoccupation. However, the results of the Personality Disorder Questionnaire suggested that this finding, while valid, was to some extent confounded by the personality disorder profile of the steroid users. The latter showed "cluster B" personality disorder traits for antisocial, borderline, and histrionic personality disorder, significantly differing in this respect from non-users. Men who use androgenic anabolic steroids to enhance their sporting achievements seem to be more likely to have cyclic depression (35), but young men who have stopped using anabolic steroids can also develop depression and fatigue as withdrawal effects (36).

In a useful review of the entire field there is particular reference to the contested evidence on the behavioral effects of these compounds (37). The authors observed that certain of these complications, in particular hypomania and increased aggressiveness, have been confirmed in some, but not all, randomized controlled studies. Epidemiological attempts to determine whether anabolic steroids trigger violent behavior have failed, primarily because of high rates of non-participation. Studies of the use of anabolic steroids in different populations typically report a prevalence of repeated use of 1–5% among adolescents. The symptoms and signs of the use of anabolic steroids seem to be often overlooked by health-care professionals, and the number of cases of complications is virtually unknown. The authors suggested that future epidemiological research in this area should focus on retrospective case-control studies and perhaps also on prospective cohort studies of populations selected for a high prevalence of anabolic steroid use, rather than large-scale population-based studies.

Androgens can rarely cause psychotic mania.

- A 28-year-old man with AIDS and a history of bipolar disorder was given a testosterone patch to counter progressive weight loss and developed worsening mania with an elevated mood, racing thoughts, grandiose delusions, and auditory hallucinations (38). His condition improved in hospital after removal of the patch and the administration of antipsychotic drugs. No cause for the psychosis, other than the use of testosterone, was found.

Suicide—or attempted suicide—in eight users of anabolic steroids has been described in Germany; the cases were related variously to hypomanic states during use of anabolic steroids or depression after withdrawal (39). Some of the users had committed acts of violence while using the drugs. In all cases, there were risk factors for suicidality and the drugs may simply have triggered the suicidal decision.

Endocrine

While both androgens and anabolic steroids have male hormone effects, resulting in virilization, they suppress endogenous secretion of follicle-stimulating hormone (FSH) and luteinizing hormone (LH); the result is that on withdrawal the system is for a time deprived of sufficient amounts of male hormone (40); this can lead to hypogonadism until endogenous secretions recover. A transdermal product has a particularly marked effect on circulating concentrations of serum dehydrotestosterone, and this may prove to be the case with other forms of administration; the effects of dehydrotestosterone on the prostate and other systems do not appear to have been systematically studied.

Although concerns regarding the risk of anabolic steroids usually relate primarily to their peripheral and organic adverse effects, the fact that serious hypothalamic?pituitary dysfunction can occur, and can be slow to recover, is often overlooked.

- A 37-year-old bodybuilder developed gynecomastia and severe acne, together with headaches and weight gain. Sexual function and desire were much reduced (41). For two periods of 18 weeks in each year he had been taking cocktails containing methylandrostenediol, stanozolol, mesterolone, metenolone enanthate, trebolone acetate, androlone laurate, and drostanolone propionate, surely a record in anabolic steroid polypharmacy. Circulating concentrations of luteinizing hormone and follicle stimulating hormone were undetectable and plasma testosterone was critically low. A hypothalamic function test with LH-RH showed

an inadequate response. He was treated effectively with high doses of LH-RH 200 micrograms/day for 3 days, and normal function progressively returned.

Metabolism

In women androgens alone have unfavorable effects on lipids and are atherogenic (2). However, the simultaneous administration of estrogens appears to have a protective effect on the lipid profile. Androgen implants combined with estrogens cause a fall in total cholesterol and LDL cholesterol, without significant effects on HDL cholesterol or triglycerides. There is a similar reduction in total cholesterol in postmenopausal women treated with estrogen plus methyltestosterone, with a reduction in HDL2 cholesterol and triglycerides but no change in LDL cholesterol. Testosterone replacement therapy should therefore be given to women only if they are concurrently using estrogen replacement therapy.

In men a small reduction in high-density lipoprotein cholesterol tends to be accompanied by a significant reduction in total cholesterol and low-density lipoprotein cholesterol, which is consistent with an absence of added cardiovascular risk (42).

In sufficient doses, androgens can alter regional fat distribution, with a reduction in subcutaneous fat; despite their body-building effects they have therefore been used as part of slimming programs in men (43). In women, testosterone causes an increase in lean body mass with a reduction in total body fat (44).

One residual medical use for oxandrolone in some centers is as a growth-promoting treatment for girls with Turner's syndrome, in which it is regarded by certain workers as an acceptable supplement (in a dose of 0.06 mg/kg/day) to recombinant human growth hormone. A risk of this treatment is altered glucose metabolism, but this effect is usually transient. In a series of 18 patients, one girl developed non-ketotic hyperglycemia 50 months after the end of treatment; in the other 17 girls the effect of treatment on glucose metabolism was reversible (45). There was a moderate, but not significant, rise in fasting blood glucose throughout the course of the longitudinal study. Fasting insulin increased continuously during treatment but fell after the end of treatment; subsequent concentrations were slightly higher than before treatment, but this could have been an effect of age.

Fluid balance

Androgens, particularly oxymetholone, can lead to increased water retention (46), but it is not clear whether this occurs via a mineralocorticoid or an estrogenic effect.

Hematologic

Hemoglobin can increase with high doses of androgens (47). Polycythemia as a complication of androgen treatment seems to be directly related to the intensity and duration of treatment. There is a little evidence that should it occur (for example after treatment with intramuscular androgens) it can be reversed by changing to the use of transdermal testosterone. However it remains unclear whether this is related to the mode of administration or simply to the fact that a lower dose is used (48).

Severe aplastic anemia has been reported.

- A 26-year-old woman developed severe aplastic anemia, complicated by superior sagittal sinus thrombosis, while taking fluoxymesterone 30 mg/day (49).

Anabolic steroids have been reported to be thrombogenic (50–52). Stanozolol, fluomesterone, metandienone, methyltestosterone, oxymesterone, and oxymetholone all reduce the synthesis or increase the degradation of clotting factors; as a rule this effect is not clinically significant, but it can result in an interaction with anticoagulants.

Liver

Particularly because the bulk of oral treatment with androgens has been with a 17-substituted compound (methyltestosterone) there have been considerable problems with liver toxicity (5). Liver dysfunction, first indicated by a rise in alkaline phosphatase and then by increases in other enzymes, transaminases and lactate dehydrogenase, is the earliest and most common sign of dysfunction. Peliosis hepatis (characterized by blood-filled cysts in the liver), hepatomas, and hepatocellular carcinoma can follow with prolonged treatment. Large hepatocellular carcinomas have been described on various occasions (8). The anabolic steroids are as risky in this respect as more traditional androgens; a case of a liver cell adenoma in a child (9) and two cases of nodular hepatocellular carcinoma (10) have been reported in patients who took oxymetholone, metenolone acetate, or other anabolic steroids for 5–15 years. It must be stressed that the complication is not limited to the 17-substituted compounds; other anabolic steroids and androgens, if given in sufficient doses (which are likely to be in excess of physiological amounts), can also damage liver function. Early damage to liver function, for example by methyltestosterone, has been shown to be reversible (6), but longer-term effects are not. The reversibility however depends on the nature of the derangement. Patients with severe cholestasis occurring late with stanozolol recovered biochemically over 3–6 months after drug withdrawal (7).

- A Japanese girl aged 20 years, who had been legitimately treated with oxymetholone (30 mg/day) for 6 years for aplastic anemia, developed a hepatic adenoma (53). In this case, in contrast to some earlier reports, there was a predisposing factor in the form of familial adenomatous polyposis.
- Reversible hepatotoxicity, in the form of abnormal liver function tests, led to the withdrawal of stanozolol in a patient with lipodermatosclerosis (54). Since some dermatologists continue to have faith in anabolic steroids in this condition, the patient was then given oxandrolone, which is reputed to be less hepatotoxic. The hepatic problems did not recur, although several months later the patient developed a cardiomyopathy, which may have been coincidental.

In a double-blind placebo-controlled study in 52 HIV-positive individuals, oxymetholone 50 mg bd or tds for 16 weeks led to improvements in appetite and well-being and weight gain. However, there was marked derangement of liver function tests in 27% of patients taking the lower dose and 35% of those taking the higher dose (55). Liver damage has always been problematic with drugs in this class, and in such patients it might very well prove to outweigh any benefit on general physical state. One should add that any useful effects that may emerge in patients with HIV could just as well be obtained with plain androgens, for example small doses of testosterone (56).

One of the few valid uses remaining for anabolic androgens is temporary relief of Fanconi anemia while awaiting hemopoietic cell transplantation. However, in one case a large adenoma ruptured shortly after transplantation, with a fatal result (57).

Skin

Acne is common in patients taking androgens (58). When the effect of testosterone and anabolic steroids on the size of sebaceous glands was studied in a series of male athletes, high doses of all the products tested were found to enlarge the glands (59).

It has been claimed that testosterone implants are much less likely to cause acne than are injections of testosterone enanthate in equivalent doses; it is not clear why this might be expected and the claim seems dubious.

Multiple halo nevi have been described in a patient who took oxymetholone (SED-12, 1038) (60).

Testosterone gel is effective transdermally, although a report on its use in the form of AA2500 (brand name), which releases 50 or 100 mg/day, points to an unusually high incidence of local sensitivity reactions; it is not clear whether this is due to testosterone itself or to excipients absent from the placebo comparator (61).

Hair

Hirsutism is common in patients taking androgens, and is often irreversible (62,63). In contrast, in women, loss of scalp hair can occur (64). Of 81 female-to-male transsexual subjects, mean age 37 years (range 21–61), treated with testosterone esters ($n = 61$; 250 mg intramuscularly every 2 weeks) or testosterone undecanoate ($n = 20$; 160–240 mg/day orally), 31 developed male-pattern baldness; thinning of the hair was related to the duration of androgen administration and was present in about half of the transsexuals after 13 years (65).

Musculoskeletal

The ability of androgens to counter osteoporosis is the basis of their use as a supplement to estrogens in one version of hormone replacement therapy. Testosterone can increase markers of bone formation (66). However, the early closure of epiphyses, with an arrest of growth, is a risk if children are exposed to these substances; this latter effect may be produced by the estrogen to which testosterone is metabolized. In some patients with excessive growth (such as Klinefelter's syndrome or Marfan syndrome) the effect is exploited therapeutically (SEDA-21, 434). Follow-up in these subjects at the age of 21–30 years showed no abnormalities of testicular function as a consequence of treatment.

A potential adverse effect of oxandrolone is acceleration of puberty and skeletal maturation (67).

- A 9-year-old boy with early puberty took oxandrolone for 22 months because of constitutional delay of growth. His height velocity increased above the 97th percentile and his bone age developed twice as fast as his chronological age. The oxandrolone was withdrawn, but his growth velocity did not decrease and his bone age continued to accelerate.

The authors hypothesized that oxandrolone could have induced early puberty. They concluded that in young children oxandrolone should be used with caution for short periods only.

Sexual function

In men, the (often desired) effects can include an increase in libido. After some time, androgenic treatment in men will lead to a reduction in the volume of the testes and azoospermia or oligospermia because of suppression of gonadotropins. Severe priapism occasionally occurs.

- A 20-year-old man with idiopathic hypogonadotrophic hypogonadism receiving a testosterone ester in a dose of 250 mg intramuscularly every 2 weeks developed priapism (68).

Reproductive system

In women and children, the main effect will be one of virilization in its various forms, ranging from hirsutism and deepening of the voice to enlargement of the female clitoris and male pattern baldness; the effect on the voice rapidly becomes irreversible because of changes in the larynx; laryngeal polyps have also been observed (69). In women, menstrual abnormalities are likely. Short-term treatment can produce increases in estradiol, dihydrotestosterone, testosterone (total and unbound), and the ratio of dihydrotestosterone to testosterone.

When ill-advisedly used to promote growth in boys by administration for some years, oxandrolone caused gynecomastia in a high proportion of subjects treated; 23 of the 33 patients affected subsequently required mastectomy (70,71).

Long-Term Effects

Drug abuse

There is a persistent illegal market in androgenic anabolic steroids, to promote physical strength. A difficulty in determining the ultimate consequences of anabolic steroid abuse for body-building or to advance sporting achievement is that individuals who are susceptible to such abuse may well have taken several different types of substance at the same time or in succession. Indeed, an analysis of the hair of seven body-builders showed what the authors termed a "complete pharmacopeia" of drug residues, ranging from glucocorticoids, anabolic steroids, and androgens to beta-adrenoceptor agonists, antidepressants, diuretics, and human chorionic gonadotropin (72).

The claimed body-building effect of the so-called anabolic compounds reflects their ability to promote muscular development, even beyond physiological limits, and this can bring with it cardiovascular complications. Surreptitious misuse by athletes remains a recurrent problem in professional sport (73); apart from the cardiovascular risks, one observes numerous physiological changes, including effects on plasma levels of enzymes, minerals and vitamins and reduced concentrations of HDL cholesterol (74).

According to an extensive review published in 2004 (75) , the main untoward effects that male athletes most often self-report are an increase in sexual drive, acne vulgaris, increased body hair, and increased aggressive and hostile behavior. Mood disturbances (for example depression, mania and hypomania, and psychotic features) are likely to be dose- and drug-dependent. Anabolic dependence or withdrawal effects (such as depression) seem to occur only in a small number of users. Drug intake will derange endogenous production of testosterone and gonadotropins, and this effect may persist for months after drug withdrawal. Cardiovascular risk factors may undergo deleterious alterations, including raised blood pressure and depression of serum high-density lipoprotein (HDL), HDL2, and HDL3 cholesterol concentrations.

In echocardiographic studies in male athletes, anabolic drugs did not seem to affect cardiac structure and function, although in animal studies they have hazardous effects on heart structure and function, while in other studies they did not damage the liver. Many other adverse effects have been associated with misuse, including disturbance of endocrine and immune function, alterations of the sebaceous system and skin, hemostatic changes, and changes in the urogenital tract.

- Poststeroid balance disorder was diagnosed in a 20-year-old Polish athlete who had been given two courses of metandienone, oxymetholone, and nandrolone phenylpropionate (76). Vertigo occurred twice just after "doping" and persisted in spite of a 1.5-year break in taking anabolic steroids. There was positional nystagmus, the eye-tracking test was abnormal, and there were abnormal responses in caloric tests. In computed dynamic posturography, the incidence and degree of body sway were increased and consequently the field of the outspread area was enlarged. These findings pointed to a permanent poststeroid disorder of the central part of the equilibrium organ.
- A German report of a 22-year-old male body-builder who had taken both testosterone propionate and nandrolone decanoate in rising doses over a period of 4 months detailed the emergence of fulminant acne, a sternoclavicular bone lesion, and loss of libido (77). Severe acne after excessive androgen use has been reported before, and the apparently osteoarthritic complication in this case was probably secondary to the acne.

- A Texas group observed erythrocytosis in a young body-builder taking androgens and followed up this observation by examining hematological measures in nine male competitive body-builders who admitted to using these steroids illicitly (78). Although erythropoietin concentrations were normal (and even tended to be low), six subjects had a raised hematocrit with erythrocytosis.
- Cholestasis and renal insufficiency occurred together in a German body-builder who had been taking two anabolic steroids together over a period of 80 days (79).
- A large hepatic hematoma led to intra-abdominal hemorrhage in a 24-year-old man who for 2 years had taken two anabolic steroids as well as clomiphene and human chorionic gonadotropin (80). The authors obtained information from health clubs that users commonly took some 300 mg of nandrolone weekly, whereas the recommended dose was only 50 mg monthly.

An Australian study of 41 past and present users of anabolic steroids, together with controls from a similar population ("potential users") has vividly portrayed the risks that prolonged use of these products brings (81). Complications included alterations in libido (61%), changes in mood (48%), reduced testicular volume (46%), and acne (43%). The mean systolic and diastolic blood pressures were raised in 29% of current users, 37% of past users, and only 8% of controls, although these differences were not significant. Gynecomastia was found in 10 past users (37%), two current users (12%), and none of the controls, while mean testicular volume was significantly smaller in current users (18 ml). There were abnormal liver function tests in 20 past users (83%), eight present users (62%), and five potential users (71%).

- A partial empty sella syndrome occurred in an elite 39-year-old body-builder with a 17-year history of drug abuse involving growth hormone, anabolic steroids, testosterone, and thyroid hormone (82).

The pituitary is a hormone-responsive gland, but it has not previously been shown to suffer negative feedback in response to any of these substances. Any one of them could in principle have contributed to the effect, or it could have been an indirect consequence of drug abuse, by way of an increase in intracranial pressure, which is a known cause of empty sella syndrome.

The reversibility of the long-term physical effects of these drugs, notably cardiac hypertrophy, has been studied in 32 bodybuilders or powerlifters, including 15 athletes who had not been using anabolic drugs for at least 12 months and 17 current abusers; there was also a control group of 15 weightlifters who were non-users (83). The mean systolic blood pressure was higher in users (mean 140 mmHg) than in ex-users (130 mmHg) or weightlifters (125 mmHg). Left ventricular muscle mass related to fat-free body mass and the ratio of mean left ventricular wall thickness to internal diameter were not significantly higher in users and ex-users than in controls. Left ventricular wall thickness related to fat-free body mass was also lower in non-user weightlifters, but did not differ between users and ex-users. In all groups, systolic left ventricular function was within the reference range. The maximum late transmitral Doppler flow velocity was higher in users than in non-user controls. One has to conclude that several years after discontinuation of anabolic steroid abuse, strength athletes still show slight concentric left ventricular hypertrophy in comparison with anabolic-free strength athletes.

Drug withdrawal

Withdrawal of high doses of androgens or anabolic steroids after the system has become accustomed to them can lead to menopause-like reactions, such as anxiety, chills, tachycardia, anorexia, piloerection, insomnia, sweats, hypertension, myalgia, nausea, vomiting, irritability, and hot flushes. Young men who have used these compounds can experience depression and fatigue for a time after withdrawal.

Tumorigenicity

Danazol is a weak androgen and also has a series of other hormonal and anti-hormonal properties. It inhibits pituitary gonadotropin and has been used in the treatment of endometriosis, fibrocystic disease of the breast, idiopathic thrombocytopenic purpura, and hereditary angioedema. Its hepatotoxic effects include reversible rises in serum transaminases and cholestatic hepatitis; a few cases of hepatocellular tumors have been reported.

- A 34-year-old woman who had taken danazol 400 mg/day for 13 years for hereditary angioedema developed a mass in the right hypochondrium. Her alcohol intake was under 20 g/day. She had a large heterogeneous hepatic tumor, a well-differentiated hepatocellullar carcinoma in a non-cirrhotic liver.

The hypothesis that hepatocellular carcinoma had been caused by danazol was accepted in the absence of other causes (84).

It has been stressed in a recent and very extensive American review that the benefit to harm balance of androgen replacement has still not been adequately examined (85). In an otherwise positive review of this form of treatment, it has been pointed out that androgens are growth factors for pre-existing prostate cancer (86). Before therapy is begun, careful digital rectal examination and determination of the serum concentration of prostate-specific antigen (PSA) should be performed, in order to exclude evident or suspected prostate cancer. The first 3–6 months after starting testosterone therapy is the most critical time for monitoring effects on the prostate. It is therefore important to monitor PSA concentrations every 3 months for the first year of treatment; thereafter, regular monitoring during therapy is mandatory, primarily to ensure prostate safety but also with a view to cardiovascular and hematological safety.

In this connection it may also be noted that, following a joint meeting in 2004, the International Society of Andrology, the International Society for the Study of the Aging Male, and the European Association of Urology revised their earlier recommendations on the definition, diagnosis, and management of late onset hypogonadism (87). While by no means rejecting androgen replacement therapy, the recommendations remain cautious and are explicitly intended to be regarded as provisional until larger-scale, long-term studies are available.

A particular reason for caution is the fact that in this age group there will be a fair proportion of subjects at risk of prostate cancer. It is possible that in these subjects testosterone might further increase the risk or actually precipitate the neoplasm. In a review of the medical records of six urology practices, men undergoing testosterone supplementation for sexual dysfunction or "rejuvenation" who were found to have prostate cancer after initiation of exogenous testosterone supplementation were identified (88). Cases were analysed to determine the clinical and pathological parameters that characterized the presentation of prostate cancer. A total of 20 men were found to have prostate cancer after the start of testosterone therapy. Prostate cancer was detected within 2 years in 11 men (55%) and from 28 months to 8 years in the rest. The tumors were of moderate and high grade, being of Gleason sums 6, 7, and 8–10 in nine men (45%), six men (30%), and five men (25%) respectively. The median serum prostate specific antigen (PSA) concentration at diagnosis tended to be low, at 5.1 (range 1.1–329) ng/ml, and digital rectal examination was generally more sensitive than PSA in detecting the cancer. Patients seen by non-urologist physicians were monitored less often for prostate cancer during use of testosterone than those followed by urologists. The authors therefore concluded that prostate cancer may become clinically apparent within months to a few years after the start of testosterone treatment. In their view, physicians who prescribe testosterone supplements and patients who take them should be cognizant of this risk, and serum PSA testing and digital rectal examination should be performed frequently during treatment.

Second-Generation Effects

Fertility

Not surprisingly, azoospermia is a classic consequence of intensive use of anabolic androgenic steroids, and it can be reflected in sterility. A well-documented case has shown that in at least some cases the condition can be reversed and fertility restored by treatment with gonadotrophins (HMG and HCG) (89).

Susceptibility Factors

Age

In just a few medical situations, the marginal benefits of "anabolic" androgens may still outweigh their risks. The need to treat life-threatening episodes of severe hereditary angioma in children may for example justify use of oxandrolone or other anabolic drugs, but the doses required are likely to cause marked virilization (90). In children, who may be exposed to androgens or anabolic steroids accidentally or in ill-advised therapy (for example to improve appetite), there will be a particular risk of virilization, premature sexual development, and early closure of the epiphyses. Virilization has even been reported after topical androgen administration (91).

The long-term use of oxandrolone has been studied in children with very severe burns (covering 40% or more of the body surface). Under controlled conditions, 84 children (56 girls and 28 boys; mean age 8 years) received treatment for 1 year with placebo or oral oxandrolone 0.1 mg/kg bd (92). At discharge (95% healed) and at 6, 9, and 12 months after the burn, oxandrolone improved lean body mass, bone mineral content, and bone mineral density compared with placebo and there was no adverse effect on hepatic transaminases. The latter finding, and the absence of other adverse effects, suggests that this treatment of very severely burnt children is defensible.

Interest in the use of androgens in elderly men continues, with on the one hand the long-standing hope that potency and libido may be restored, and, on the other hand, the belief that cardiovascular prospects might be improved. The uncertainties that exist in this latter respect have been well reviewed in a paper that merits reading in full; it is best summarized in the author's own conclusion that "··· overall, the androgens are as likely to prevent arterial disease as they are to cause it ···" (93).

The use of oxandrolone has been restudied in a prospective comparative investigation in 61 children with 40% total body surface area burns (94). They were randomized to receive oral oxandrolone 0.1 mg/kg bd (n = 30) or placebo (n = 31) for 12 months after the injury. Oxandrolone significantly improved lean body mass, bone mineral content, and muscle strength. Serum IGF-1, T3 uptake, and free thyroxine index were significantly increased by oxandrolone. There were significant increases in height and weight during and after the end of treatment. A broader view of these problems from burns experts is needed for final assessment. The conclusion regarding effects on height must be regarded with some caution, since androgens can result in early closure of the epiphyses. However, the essential question must be whether recovery was accelerated or rendered more complete.

Sex

In women, as well as men, androgens have effects on sexual function, bone health, muscle mass, body composition, mood, energy, and the sense of well-being. Androgen insufficiency has clearly been demonstrated in women with hypopituitarism, after adrenalectomy and oophorectomy, and in some women who take oral estrogen therapy, which increases sex hormone-binding globulin. The indications for administering androgens to women are not well-defined, nor is it clear which doses can be safely used; both testosterone and dehydroepiandrosterone (DHEA) have been used. The risks of *rash* or poorly dosed androgen treatment are evident, but the literature provides little guidance; further study is clearly needed (95).

The effect of androgens on cardiovascular function and prognosis, breast and endometrial tissues, and mood and anger need careful investigation, and this is still largely lacking (96).

There is still disagreement as to whether the concept of "female sexual dysfunction" is a genuine pathological entity or a concept artificially constructed to promote the sale of particular drugs. In a thorough review published by the Mayo Clinic it was stressed that failure of sexual performance in women can have many causes (for example psychological and marital) and that it demands an individualized therapeutic approach, which is not necessarily medicinal. However, for certain patients androgens may prove useful, especially in strengthening libido. The risks are evident, notably manifestations of virilization of the user and masculinization of a female fetus should pregnancy occur (97).

Transsexuals

When androgens are used to treat female-to-male transsexuals, a minor problem is the tendency for them to develop male pattern baldness, while a greater problem appears to be an increase in the risk of coronary heart disease. It has been suggested that the development of baldness might in these subjects actually serve as an early indicator for the risk of coronary complications, but a retrospective study in 81 transsexuals seems to show that the two effects simply occur coincidentally. Thinning of hair was related to the duration of androgen administration and present in about 50% of Frightward arrowM transsexuals after 13 years. None of the coronary risk factors at follow-up, nor proportional changes, was associated with the degree of baldness, except that there was an unexpected tendency to lower fasting glucose concentrations in balding subjects (98).

HIV infection

One possible use of anabolic agents is in the treatment of the physical wasting associated with HIV infection. Some experience has been gained, but it is still not clear whether such treatment is warranted, bearing in mind the limited benefits that can be expected and the well-documented risks of anabolic drug therapy (99). The effects and adverse effects of testosterone replacement with a non-genital transdermal system, Androderm, have been studied in 41 HIV-positive men with low testosterone concentrations (100). Nine men taking placebo and 11 taking testosterone reported adverse events. Five men taking testosterone had reactions at the site of administration; other adverse events in this group included problems related to resistance mechanisms ($n = 2$), gastrointestinal system ($n = 2$), and skin and appendages ($n = 1$); there was one severe adverse event (a suicidal amitriptyline overdose). There were skin reactions at the site of application of the placebo or testosterone patch in 19% of the participants. One man had blisters on one occasion, related to rupture of the patch. The mean erythrocyte count increased with testosterone and fell with placebo. Hemoglobin concentration increased with testosterone and fell with placebo.

Diabetes mellitus

Older data pointed to some reduction in insulin requirements when patients with diabetes mellitus received androgens, and it is wise to avoid these drugs altogether in patients with diabetes.

Drug Administration

Drug formulations

Testosterone is available as oral testosterone undecanoate, buccal testosterone, intramuscular testosterone esters, testosterone implants, and testosterone transdermal patches and gel. Proponents of transdermal testosterone products, such as gels and scrotal or non-scrotal dermal patches, claim that they have a good safety profile (101). Transdermal testosterone replacement certainly improves bone mass and lean body mass, reduces fat mass, and improves mood and sexual function. There are said to be no harmful effects on the prostate and lipids. Acne, polycythemia, and gynecomastia are stated to be less common with this form of therapy than with the intramuscular esters. To date these claims must be regarded with some reservations; it is not at all clear that in equieffective doses the local or topical forms of administration dissociate wanted and unwanted effects.

After oral administration there is large variability in systemic availability, which makes this route generally unsuitable.

Buccal testosterone tablets provide sustained release of testosterone and also bypass first-pass metabolism in the liver. Small-scale work with a bioadhesive buccal tablet of testosterone has shown that adequate serum concentrations can be obtained and that the buccal tablet (administered twice daily) is well tolerated (102). Other work has confirmed that twice-daily buccal application is optimal to maintain therapeutic serum concentrations of testosterone and its metabolites (103–105); however, it appears that about one patient in six initially has a degree of oral discomfort from the presence of the "mucoadhesive" tablet, although this fades after a few days and does not seriously affect compliance. Common adverse effects of buccal testosterone include gum irritation, pain, and tenderness, and edema (106) and headache (107).

Intramuscular testosterone is given as a deep intramuscular injection of single testosterone esters or a mixture of testosterone propionate, testosterone phenylpropionate, testosterone isocaproate, and testosterone decanoate (Sustanon), every 2–3 weeks. In one series of 551 injections, 162 were associated with pain and bleeding; injection in the gluteal site caused fewer complaints and was less susceptible to bleeding, but was painful more often than injection in the deltoid muscle or thigh (108). There were no serious adverse effects and the only systemic adverse effect was episodes of sudden non-productive cough associated with faintness after eight injections which the authors thought might have been due to pulmonary oil microembolism. Systemic availability of testosterone after intramuscular administration is variable and there can be fluctuations in mood and sexual function

(109). High testosterone concentrations can cause raised lipid concentrations (110).

Topical application of testosterone, as a gel or from transdermal patches, can lead to absorption and systemic effects (SEDA-16, 158). Transdermal absorption of testosterone (usually from treatment of vulvar lichen sclerosus et atrophicus) can lead to increased libido, clitoral hypertrophy, pubic hirsutism, thinning of the scalp hair, facial acne, voice change, hirsutism, and even virilization (111).

The use of transdermal patches for administering testosterone to hypogonadal men ("Andropatch") seems logical and convenient, but a British study in 50 treated patients showed that patient acceptance was surprisingly poor (112). There were adverse effects in 84%, mostly skin problems; 72% requested a return to depot injections, and 5% returned to oral therapy. The reservoir patches, 6 cm in diameter, were, to quote the report literally, judged to be too large, uncomfortable, and visually obtrusive, while the noise they made on bodily movement distracted dogs, wives, and children; they fell off in showers and attracted ribald remarks from sports partners; they could only be removed with difficulty and left bald red marks on the body. The nature of the complaints suggests that they might be accommodated by further technical development of the product.

Of 123 men who used "AndroGel 1%" for periods up to 42 months, 12 had some local skin irritation, but only one discontinued treatment as a result (113).

However, one needs to be cautious when faced with claims that topical hormonal products are better tolerated than those administered orally or by other routes. Topical testosterone has sometimes been used in women as a treatment for different vulvar conditions, and hirsutism and other signs of virilization have been described by several authors. Clearly, close monitoring is needed (114).

One unusual variant involves applying a transdermal preparation to the scrotum (115), a technique that has been claimed to mimic more closely the natural pattern of release of endogenous testosterone. It is not clear that applying it at this site has any special merit, although some work suggests that the scrotal skin is less likely than other skin areas to exhibit local reactions. Certainly topical preparations of testosterone can elicit such reactions, with pruritus and blistering being common, while induration, erythema, and allergic reactions can also occasionally occur.

Testosterone implants, like implants of other substances, can be subject to extrusion, probably in about a tenth of cases treated, and can also give rise to local irritation (116).

Drug–Drug Interactions

Anticoagulants

Many androgens and anabolic steroids reduce the dose of oral anticoagulant that a patient requires, sometimes by as much as 25% (117), and hemorrhage has sometimes resulted from their use. From the results of a study in which stanozolol reduced warfarin requirements, the investigators concluded that stanozolol increased fibrinolysis, reduced the production of vitamin K-dependent clotting factors, and increased the amount of the natural anticoagulant antithrombin III (118).

References

1. Birkhauser MH. Chemistry, physiology and pharmacology of sex steroids. J Cardiovasc Pharmacol 1996;28(Suppl 5):S1–S13.
2. Vermeulen A. Plasma androgens in women. J Reprod Med 1998;43(Suppl 8):725–33.
3. Navarro JF. In the erythropoietin era, can we forget alternative or adjunctive therapies for renal anaemia management? Nephrol Dial Transplant 2003;18:2222–6.
4. Boyce EG. Use and effectiveness of performance-enhancing substances. J Pharm Pract 2003;16:22–36.
5. Cicardi M, Castelli R, Zingale LC, Agostoni A. Side effects of long-term prophylaxis with attenuated androgens in hereditary angioedema: comparison of treated and untreated patients. J Allergy Clin Immunol 1997;99(2):194–6.
6. Pandita R, Quadri MI. Constitutional aplastic anemia. Indian Pediatr 1988;25(5):469–72.
7. Kaunitz AM. The role of androgens in menopausal hormonal replacement. Endocrinol Metab Clin North Am 1997;26(2):391–7.
8. Lowdell CP, Murray-Lyon IM. Reversal of liver damage due to long term methyltestosterone and safety of non-17 alpha-alkylated androgens. BMJ (Clin Res Ed) 1985;291(6496):637.
9. Evely RS, Triger DR, Milnes JP, Low-Beer TS, Williams R. Severe cholestasis associated with stanozolol. BMJ (Clin Res Ed) 1987;294(6572):612–3.
10. McCaughan GW, Bilous MJ, Gallagher ND. Long-term survival with tumor regression in androgen-induced liver tumors. Cancer 1985;56(11):2622–6.
11. Sanchez JMC, Becerra EP, Martin AA, et al. Adenoma hepatico después del tratamiento con oximetolona. Rev Esp Pediatr 1988;44:195.
12. Oda K, Oguma N, Kawano M, Kimura A, Kuramoto A, Tokumo K. Hepatocellular carcinoma associated with long-term anabolic steroid therapy in two patients with aplastic anemia. Nippon Ketsueki Gakkai Zasshi 1987;50(1):29–36.
13. Tsiara SN, Chaidos A, Gouva M, Christou L, Panteli K, Kapsali E, Bourantas KL. Successful treatment of refractory anemia with a combination regimen containing recombinant human erythropoietin, low-dose methylprednisolone and nandrolone. J Exp Clin Cancer Res 2004;23:47–52.
14. Braunstein GD, Sundwall DA, Katz M, Shifren JL, Buster JE, Simon JA, Bachman G, Aguirre OA, Lucas JD, Rodenberg C, Buch A, Watts NB. Safety and efficacy of a testosterone patch for the treatment of hypoactive sexual desire disorder in surgically menopausal women: a randomized, placebo-controlled trial. Arch Intern Med 2005;165:1582–9.
15. Nieschlag E, Behre HM, Bouchard P, Corrales JJ, Jones TH, Stalla GK, Webb SM, Wu FCW. Testosterone replacement therapy: current trends and future directions. Hum Reprod Update 2004;10:409–19.

16. Mudali S, Dobs AS. Effects of testosterone on body composition of the aging male. Mech Ageing Dev 2004;125:297–304.

17. Orengo CA, Fullerton L, Kunik ME. Safety and efficacy of testosterone gel 1% augmentation in depressed men with partial response to antidepressant therapy. J Geriat Psychiatry Neurol 2005;18:20–4.

18. Anonymous. Treatment of androgen deficiency in the aging male. Fertil Steril 2004;81:1437–40.

19. Tan RS, Culberson JW. An integrative review on current evidence of testosterone replacement therapy for the andropause. Maturitas 2003;45:15–27.

20. Liu PY, Swerdloff RS, Veldhuis JD. The rationale, efficacy and safety of androgen therapy in older men: future research and current practice recommendations. J Clin Endocrinol Metab 2004;89:4789–96.

21. Tenover JL. Male hormone replacement therapy including "andropause". Endocrinol Metab Clin North Am 1998;27(4):969–87.

22. Maguen S, Wagner GJ, Rabkin JG. Long-term testosterone therapy in HIV-positive men: side-effects and maintenance of clinical benefit. AIDS 1998;12(3):327–8.

23. Krause W. Testosteronsubstitution beim alternden Mann. Welche fragen sind beantwortet? [Testosterone substitution in aging males. Which questions are answered?] Urologe A 2004;43:1097–100.

24. Schroeder ET, Zheng L, Yarasheski KE, Qian D, Stewart Y, Flores C, Martinez C, Terk M, Sattler FR. Treatment with oxandrolone and the durability of effects in older men. J Appl Physiol 2004;96:1055–62.

25. Davis SR. The therapeutic use of androgens in women. J Steroid Biochem Mol Biol 1999;69(1–6):177–84.

26. Baker J. A report on alterations to the speaking and singing voices of four women following hormonal therapy with virilizing agents. J Voice 1999;13(4):496–507.

27. Reckelhoff JF, Granger JP. Role of androgens in mediating hypertension and renal injury. Clin Exp Pharmacol Physiol 1999;26(2):127–31.

28. Sandblom RE, Matsumoto AM, Schoene RB, Lee KA, Giblin EC, Bremner WJ, Pierson DJ. Obstructive sleep apnea syndrome induced by testosterone administration. N Engl J Med 1983;308(9):508–10.

29. Tilzey A, Heptonstall J, Hamblin T. Toxic confusional state and choreiform movements after treatment with anabolic steroids. BMJ (Clin Res Ed) 1981;283(6287):349–50.

30. Chu K, Kang DW, Kim DE, Roh JK. Cerebral venous thrombosis associated with tentorial subdural hematoma during oxymetholone therapy. J Neurol Sci 2001;185(1):27–30.

31. Dickerman RD, Jaikumar S. The hiccup reflex arc and persistent hiccups with high-dose anabolic steroids: is the brainstem the steroid-responsive locus? Clin Neuropharmacol 2001;24(1):62–4.

32. Pope HG Jr, Katz DL Affective and psychotic symptoms associated with anabolic steroid use. Am J Psychiatry 1988;145:487–90.

33. Conacher GN, Workman DG. Violent crime possibly associated with anabolic steroid use. Am J Psychiatry 1989;146:679.

34. Perry PJ, Kutscher EC, Lund BC, Yates WR, Holman TL, Demers L. Measures of aggression and mood changes in male weightlifters with and without androgenic anabolic steroid use. J Forensic Sci 2003;48:646–51.

35. Copeland J, Peters R, Dillon P. Anabolic–androgenic steroid use disorders among a sample of Australian competitive and recreational users. Drug Alcohol Depend 2000;60(1):91–6.

36. Christiansen K. Behavioural effects of androgen in men and women. J Endocrinol 2001;170(1):39–48.

37. Thiblin I, Petersson A. Pharmacoepidemiology of anabolic androgenic steroids: a review. Fundam Clin Pharmacol 2005;19:27–44.

38. Weiss EL, Bowers MB Jr, Mazure CM. Testosterone-patch-induced psychotic mania. Am J Psychiatry 1999;156(6):969.

39. Thiblin I, Runeson B, Rajs J. Anabolic androgenic steroids and suicide. Ann Clin Psychiatry 1999;11(4):223–31.

40. Anderson SJ, Bolduc SP, Coryllos E, Griesemer B, McLain LAmerican Academy of PediatricsCommittee on Sports Medicine and Fitness. Adolescents and anabolic steroids: a subject review. Pediatrics 1997;99(6):904–8.

41. Van Breda E, Keizer HA, Kuipers H, Wolffenbuttel BHR. Androgenic anabolic steroid use and severe hypothalamic-pituitary dysfunction: a case study. Int J Sports Med 2003;24:195–6.

42. Schleich F, Legros J-J. Effects of androgen substitution on lipid profile in the adult and aging hypogonadal male. Eur J Endocrinol 2004;151:415–24.

43. Lovejoy JC, Bray GA, Greeson CS, Klemperer M, Morris J, Partington C, Tulley R. Oral anabolic steroid treatment, but not parenteral androgen treatment, decreases abdominal fat in obese, older men. Int J Obes Relat Metab Disord 1995;19(9):614–24.

44. Davis SR, Burger HG. Androgens and the postmenopausal woman. J Clin Endocrinol Metab 1996;81(8):2759–63.

45. Joss EE, Zurbrugg RP, Tonz O, Mullis PE. Effect of growth hormone and oxandrolone treatment on glucose metabolism in Turner syndrome. A longitudinal study. Horm Res 2000;53(1):1–8.

46. International Programme on Chemical Safety. Poisons Information Monograph 915.

47. Bebb RA, Anawalt BD, Christensen RB, Paulsen CA, Bremner WJ, Matsumoto AM. Combined administration of levonorgestrel and testosterone induces more rapid and effective suppression of spermatogenesis than testosterone alone: a promising male contraceptive approach. J Clin Endocrinol Metab 1996;81(2):757–62.

48. Siddique H, Smith JC, Corrall RJM. Reversal of polycythaemia induced by intramuscular androgen replacement using transdermal testosterone therapy. Clin Endocrinol 2004;60:143–5.

49. Kaito K, Kobayashi M, Otsubo H, Ogasawara Y, Sekita T, Shimada T, Hosoya T. Superior sagittal sinus thrombosis in a patient with aplastic anemia treated with anabolic steroids. Int J Hematol 1998;68(2):227–9.

50. Ferenchick GS. Are androgenic steroids thrombogenic? N Engl J Med 1990;322(7):476.

51. Lowe GD, Thomson JE, Reavey MM, Forbes CD, Prentice CR. Mesterolone: thrombosis during treatment, and a study of its prothrombotic effects. Br J Clin Pharmacol 1979;7(1):107–9.

52. Toyama M, Watanabe S, Kobayashi T, Iida K, Koseki S, Yamaguchi I, Sugishita Y. Two cases of acute myocardial infarction associated with aplastic anemia during treatment with anabolic steroids. Jpn Heart J 1994;35(3):369–73.

53. Nakao A, Sakagami K, Nakata Y, Komazawa K, Amimoto T, Nakashima K, Isozaki H, Takakura N, Tanaka N. Multiple hepatic adenomas caused by long-term administration of androgenic steroids for aplastic

anemia in association with familial adenomatous polyposis. J Gastroenterol 2000;35(7):557–62.

54. Segal S, Cooper J, Bolognia J. Treatment of lipodermatosclerosis with oxandrolone in a patient with stanozolol-induced hepatotoxicity. J Am Acad Dermatol 2000;43(3):558–9.

55. Hengge UR, Stocks K, Faulkner S, Wiehler H, Lorenz C, Jentzen W, Hengge D, Ringham G. Oxymetholone for the treatment of HIV-wasting: a double-blind, randomized, placebo-controlled phase III trial in eugonadal men and women. AIDS 2003;17:699–710.

56. Dobs A. Role of testosterone in maintaining lean body mass and bone density in HIV-infected patients. Int J Impot Res 2003;15:S21–5.

57. Kumar AR, Wagner JE, Auerbach AD, Coad JE, Dietz CA, Schwarzenberg SJ, MacMillan ML. Fatal hemorrhage from androgen-related hepatic adenoma after hematopoietic cell transplantation. J Pediatr Hematol Oncol 2004;26:16–18.

58. Zouboulis CC, Degitz K. Androgen action on human skin—from basic research to clinical significance. Exp Dermatol 2004;13(Suppl 4):5–10.

59. Kiraly CL, Collan Y, Alen M. Effect of testosterone and anabolic steroids on the size of sebaceous glands in power athletes. Am J Dermatopathol 1987;9(6):515–9.

60. Jhung JW, Edelstein LM, Church A. Multiple halo nevi developing after oxymetholone treatment of "aplastic anemia". Cutis 1973;12:56.

61. Steidle C, Schwartz S, Jacoby K, Sebree T, Smith T, Bachand R. AA2500 testosterone gel normalizes androgen levels in aging males with improvements in body composition and sexual function. J Clin Endocrinol Metab 2003;88:2673–8.

62. Muller SA. Hirsutism. Am J Med 1969;46(5):803–17.

63. Muller OA. Hirsutismus und Androgenexzess: Diagnostische Probleme, therapeutische Schwierigkeiten. [Hirsutism and androgen excess: diagnostic problems, therapeutic difficulties.] Med Monatsschr Pharm 1982;5(11):329–36.

64. Birch MP, Lalla SC, Messenger AG. Female pattern hair loss. Clin Exp Dermatol 2002;27(5):383–8.

62. Giltay EJ, Toorians AW, Sarabdjitsingh AR, de Vries NA, Gooren LJ. Established risk factors for coronary heart disease are unrelated to androgen-induced baldness in female-to-male transsexuals. J Endocrinol 2004;180(1):107–12.

66. Wang C, Eyre DR, Clark R, Kleinberg D, Newman C, Iranmanesh A, Veldhuis J, Dudley RE, Berman N, Davidson T, Barstow TJ, Sinow R, Alexander G, Swerdloff RS. Sublingual testosterone replacement improves muscle mass and strength, decreases bone resorption, and increases bone formation markers in hypogonadal men—a clinical research center study. J Clin Endocrinol Metab 1996;81(10):3654–62.

67. Doeker B, Muller-Michaels J, Andler W. Induction of early puberty in a boy after treatment with oxandrolone? Horm Res 1998;50(1):46–8.

68. Zelissen PM, Stricker BH. Severe priapism as a complication of testosterone substitution therapy. Am J Med 1988;85(2):273–4.

69. Keul J, Deus B, Kindermann W. Anabole Hormone: Schädigung, Leistungsfähigkeit und Stoffwechsel. [Anabolic steroids: damages, effect on performance, and on metabolism.] Med Klin 1976;71(12):497–503.

70. Joss EE, Schmidt HA, Zuppinger KA. Oxandrolone in constitutionally delayed growth, a longitudinal study up to final height. J Clin Endocrinol Metab 1989;69(6):1109–15.

71. Moore DC, Ruvalcaba RHA. Late onset gynecomastia associated with oxandrolone therapy in adolescents with short stature. J Pediatr Endocrinol 1991;4:249.

72. Dumestre-Toulet V, Kintz P, Cirimele V, Gromb S, Ludes BJ. Analyse des cheveux de 7 culturistes: toute une pharmacopée. J Med Leg Droit Med 2001;44:38–44.

73. Perlmutter G, Lowenthal DT. Use of anabolic steroids by athletes. Am Fam Physician 1985;32(4):208–10.

74. Costill DL, Pearson DR, Fink WJ. Anabolic steroids use among athletes: changes in HDL-C levels. Phys Sportsmed 1984;12:113.

75. Hartgens F, Kuipers H. Effects of androgenic–anabolic steroids in athletes. Sports Med 2004;34:513–54.

76. Bochnia M, Medras M, Pospiech L, Jaworska M. Poststeroid balance disorder—a case report in a body builder. Int J Sports Med 1999;20(6):407–9.

77. Assmann T, Arens A, Becker-Wegerich PM, Schuppe HC, Lehmann P. Acne fulminans with sternoclavicular bone lesions and azoospermia after abuse of anabolic steroids. H G Z Hautkr 1999;74:570–2.

78. Dickerman RD, Pertusi R, Miller J, Zachariah NY. Androgen-induced erythrocytosis: is it erythropoietin? Am J Hematol 1999;61(2):154–5.

79. Habscheid W, Abele U, Dahm HH. Schwere Cholestase mit Nierenversagen durch Anabolika bei einem Bodybuilder. [Severe cholestasis with kidney failure from anabolic steroids in a body builder.] Dtsch Med Wochenschr 1999;124(36):1029–32.

80. Schumacher J, Muller G, Klotz KF. Large hepatic hematoma and intraabdominal hemorrhage associated with abuse of anabolic steroids. N Engl J Med 1999;340(14):1123–4.

81. O'Sullivan AJ, Kennedy MC, Casey JH, Day RO, Corrigan B, Wodak AD. Anabolic–androgenic steroids: medical assessment of present, past and potential users. Med J Aust 2000;173(6):323–7.

82. Dickerman RD, Jaikumar S. Secondary partial empty sella syndrome in an elite bodybuilder. Neurol Res 2001;23(4):336–8.

83. Urhausen A, Albers T, Kindermann W. Are the cardiac effects of anabolic steroid abuse in strength athletes reversible? Heart 2004;90:496–501.

84. Crampon D, Barnoud R, Durand M, Ponard D, Jacquot C, Sotto JJ, Letoublon C, Zarski JP. Danazol therapy: an unusual aetiology of hepatocellular carcinoma. J Hepatol 1998;29(6):1035–6.

85. Hijazi RA, Cunningham GR. Andropause: is androgen replacement therapy indicated for the aging male? Ann Rev Med 2005;56:117–37.

86. Ebert T, Jockenhovel F, Morales A, Shabsigh R. The current status of therapy for symptomatic late-onset hypogonadism with transdermal testosterone gel. Eur Urol 2005;47:137–46.

87. Lunenfeld B, Saad F, Hoesl CE. ISA, ISSAM and EAU recommendations for the investigation, treatment and monitoring of late-onset hypogonadism in males: scientific background and rationale. Aging Male 2005;8:59–74.

88. Gaylis FD, Lin DW, Ignatoff JM, Amling CL, Tutrone RF, Cosgrove DJ. Prostate cancer in men using testosterone supplementation. J Urol 2005;174:534–8.

89. Menon DK. Successful treatment of anabolic steroid-induced azoospermia with human chorionic gonadotropin and human menopausal gonadotropin. Fertil Steril 2003;79:1659–61.

90. Church JA. Oxandrolone treatment of childhood hereditary angioedema. Ann Allergy Asthma Immunol 2004;92:377–8.

91. Kunz GJ, Klein KO, Clemons RD, Gottschalk ME, Jones KL. Virilization of young children after topical androgen use by their parents. Pediatrics 2004;114(1):282–4.

92. Murphy KD, Thomas S, Mlcak RP, Chinkes DL, Klein GL, Herndon DN. Effects of long-term oxandrolone administration in severely burned children. Surgery 2004;136:219–24.

93. Crook D. Androgen therapy in the aging male: assessing the effect on heart disease. Aging Male 1999;2:151–6.

94. Przkora R, Jeschke MG, Barrow RE, Suman OE, Meyer WJ, Finnerty CC, Sanford AP, Lee J, Chinkes DL, Mlcak RP, Herndon DN, Pruitt Jr BA, Gamelli RL. Metabolic and hormonal changes of severely burned children receiving long-term oxandrolone treatment. Ann Surg 2005;242:384–91.

95. Cameron DR, Braunstein GD. Androgen replacement therapy in women. Fertil Steril 2004;82:273–89.

96. Basaria S, Dobs AS. Safety and adverse effects of androgens: how to counsel patients. Mayo Clin Proc 2004;79 (4 Suppl):S25-S32.

97. Shifren JL. The role of androgens in female sexual dysfunction. Mayo Clin Proc 2004;79 (4 Suppl):S19-S24.

98. Giltay EJ, Toorians AWFT, Sarabjitsingh AR, de Vries NA, Gooren LJG. Established risk factors for coronary heart disease are unrelated to androgen-induced baldness in female-to-male transsexuals. J Endocrinol 2004;180:107–12.

99. Taiwo BO. HIV-associated wasting: brief review and discussion of the impact of oxandrolone. AIDS Patient Care STDS 2000;14(8):421–5.

100. Bhasin S, Storer TW, Asbel-Sethi N, Kilbourne A, Hays R, Sinha-Hikim I, Shen R, Arver S, Beall G. Effects of testosterone replacement with a nongenital, transdermal system, Androderm, in human immunodeficiency virus-infected men with low testosterone levels. J Clin Endocrinol Metab 1998;83(9):3155–62.

101. Basaria S, Dobs AS. New modalities of transdermal testosterone replacement. Treatments Endocrinol 2003;2:1–9.

102. Ross RJM, Jabbar A, Jones TH, Roberts B, Dunkley K, Hall J, Long A, Levine H, Cullen DR. Pharmacokinetics and tolerability of a bioadhesive buccal testosterone tablet in hypogonadal men. Eur J Endocrinol 2004;150:57–63.

103. Wang C, Swerdloff R, Kipnes M, Matsumoto AM, Dobs AS, Cunningham G, Katznelson L, Weber TJ, Friedman TC, Snyder P, Levine HL. New testosterone buccal system (Striant) delivers physiological testosterone levels: pharmacokinetics study in hypogonadal men. J Clin Endocrinol Metab 2004;89:3821–9.

104. Korbonits M, Slawik M, Cullen D, Ross RJ, Stalla G, Schneider H, Reincke M, Bouloux P.M, Grossman AB. A comparison of a novel testosterone bioadhesive buccal system, Striant, with a testosterone adhesive patch in hypogonadal males. J Clin Endocrinol Metab 2004;89:2039–43.

105. Dobs AS, Matsumoto AM, Wang C, Kipnes MS. Short-term pharmacokinetic comparison of a novel testosterone buccal system and a testosterone gel in testosterone deficient men. Curr Med Res Opin 2004;20:729–38.

106. Wang C, Swerdloff R, Kipnes M, Matsumoto AM, Dobs AS, Cunningham G, Katznelson L, Weber TJ, Friedman TC, Snyder P, Levine HL. New testosterone

107. Ross RJ, Jabbar A, Jones TH, Roberts B, Dunkley K, Hall J, Long A, Levine H, Cullen DR. Pharmacokinetics and tolerability of a bioadhesive buccal testosterone tablet in hypogonadal men. Eur J Endocrinol 2004;150(1):57–63.

108. Mackey MA, Conway AJ, Handelsman DJ. Tolerability of intramuscular injections of testosterone ester in oil vehicle. Hum Reprod 1995;10(4):862–5.

109. Jockenhovel F. Testosterone supplementation: what and how to give. Aging Male 2003;6(3):200–6.

110. Whitsel EA, Boyko EJ, Matsumoto AM, Anawalt BD, Siscovick DS. Intramuscular testosterone esters and plasma lipids in hypogonadal men: a meta-analysis. Am J Med 2001;111(4):261–9.

111. Parker LU, Bergfeld WF. Virilization secondary to topical testosterone. Cleve Clin J Med 1991;58(1):43–6.

112. Parker S, Armitage M. Experience with transdermal testosterone replacement therapy for hypogonadal men. Clin Endocrinol (Oxf) 1999;50(1):57–62.

113. Wang C, Cunningham G, Dobs A, Iranmanesh A, Matsumoto AM, Snyder PJ, Weber T, Berman N, Hull L, Swerdloff RS. Long-term testosterone gel (Androgel) treatment maintains beneficial effects on sexual function and mood, lean and fat mass, and bone mineral density in hypogonadal men. J Clin Endocrinol Metab 2004;89:2085–98.

114. Hernandez-Nunez A, Dauden E, Garcia-Villalta M, Rios-Buceta L, Garcia-Diez A. Hirsutism secondary to topical testosterone: report of two cases and review of the literature. J Eur Acad Dermatol Venereol 2004;18:208–10.

115. Jordan WP Jr. Allergy and topical irritation associated with transdermal testosterone administration: a comparison of scrotal and nonscrotal transdermal systems. Am J Contact Dermat 1997;8(2):108–13.

116. Handelsman DJ, Mackey MA, Howe C, Turner L, Conway AJ. An analysis of testosterone implants for androgen replacement therapy. Clin Endocrinol (Oxf) 1997;47(3):311–6.

117. Weser JK, Sellers E. Drug interactions with coumarin anticoagulants. 2. N Engl J Med 1971;285(10):547–58.

118. Acomb D, Shaw PW. A significant interaction between warfarin and stanozolol. Pharm J 1985;234:73.

Antiandrogens

General Information

Antiandrogens include steroids, such as cyproterone acetate, and non-steroidal agents, such as bicalutamide, flutamide, and nilutamide. They have different endocrine effects and therefore different adverse effects (1). Cyproterone acetate tends to result in a loss of sexual interest and erectile dysfunction, whereas most men experience this only moderately or not at all during non-steroidal treatment. The most common adverse effects of the non-steroidal agents are gynecomastia and breast pain. Although the incidence of these events varies considerably between studies, and it is tempting for a reviewer to revise his preferences as new work appears, there is probably no real difference in the incidence of hormonal adverse effects between the three non-steroidal agents. However, there are important differences between them in other respects. Cyproterone acetate has been linked to adverse changes in serum lipids as well as significant, and in some cases fatal, cardiovascular events; it can also induce hepatotoxic effects. Nilutamide is associated with delayed adaptation to darkness, alcohol intolerance, and interstitial pneumonitis. Flutamide is associated with a greater risk of serious hepatotoxicity than bicalutamide or nilutamide. Diarrhea is also more likely to occur during therapy with flutamide than the other antiandrogens. In contrast, no specific non-pharmacological complications have been linked to bicalutamide, while diarrhea and abnormal liver function occur less often than with flutamide. Bicalutamide is a useful alternative to castration in men with prostatic cancer, especially since it appears somewhat less likely to cause impotence or loss of libido (2,3,4).

Antiandrogens are widely used in treating benign prostatic hyperplasia, but there is a tendency for patients to abandon treatment early. A Dutch group has sought to develop optimal treatment strategies for lower urinary tract symptoms suggestive of benign prostatic hyperplasia (5). Within a large general practice database all men aged 45 years and over with new diagnoses of benign prostatic hyperplasia were followed up; 26% discontinued therapy; discontinuation was not in the first place due to adverse reactions. The probability of early discontinuation was higher if the patients were primarily concerned by symptoms related to voiding, post-micturition, or storage rather than if they experienced a range of symptoms. The risk of early discontinuation was higher if patients had a normal prostate-specific antigen concentration. Older age and a higher chronic disease score protected against early treatment.

Finasteride is a selective inhibitor of 5-alpha-reductase. It thereby reduces prostatic concentrations of dihydrotestosterone and so reduces prostatic size (6,7,8). It is therefore used to treat benign prostatic hyperplasia (9,10,11,12) and in the prevention and treatment of prostate cancer (13). It is poorly effective in patients with prostatic obstruction and small prostate glands (14), but in patients with glands larger than 40 ml it produces significant symptomatic improvement.

The ability of finasteride to block the conversion of testosterone to dihydrotestosterone also makes it useful in both male-pattern baldness (15) and hirsutism related to hyperandrogenism (for example, in polycystic ovary syndrome) in women (16).

In the normal daily dose of 1 mg, which is sufficient to treat male pattern hair loss, finasteride is well tolerated over long periods. There is a very slightly higher incidence of impaired sexual function in users compared with placebo (17). In women too, low doses of finasteride (2.5 mg/day) are well tolerated when used to treat hirsutism (18). However, many of the problems seen with finasteride have undoubtedly been due to its use in unnecessarily high doses. Particularly when it is used for cosmetic purposes there has been doubt as to how far dosages can be reduced while maintaining acceptable effects. Long-term information on its safety in women with hirsutism is sparse, and in principle it might adversely affect an unborn child (16). The dose should certainly be kept as low as possible.

Observational studies

Hirsutism

In women with hirsutism low doses of finasteride (2.5 mg/ day) are generally well tolerated (19). However, in a randomized study in 38 hirsute women finasteride 2.5 mg every 3 days was as effective as 2.5 mg/day and better tolerated (20).

Prostate cancer

The effect of adding finasteride 5 mg/day to high-dose bicalutamide 150 mg/ day has been studied in 41 men with advanced prostate cancer treated over a mean of 3.9 years (21). The serum prostate-specific antigen (PSA) concentration was measured every 2 weeks until disease progression. At the first nadir of PSA, the median fall from baseline was 96.5%; a second nadir occurred in 30 of 41 patients, with a median fall of 98.5% from baseline. The median times to each nadir were 3.7 and 5.8 weeks respectively. The median time to treatment failure was 21 months. Adverse effects were minor, including gynecomastia. Sex drive was normal in 17 of 29 men at baseline and in 12 of 24 men at the second PSA nadir, but one-third of the men had spontaneous erections at both times. The authors concluded that finasteride provided additional intracellular androgen blockade when added to bicalutamide. The duration of control was comparable to that achieved with castration, with preserved sexual function in some patients.

Comparative studies

Androgenetic alopecia

In an open comparative study of androgenetic alopecia in 90 men oral finasteride (1 mg/day for 12 months; n = 65) was compared with 5% topical minoxidil solution twice daily (n = 25) (22). The cure rates were 80% for oral finasteride and 52% for topical minoxidil. The adverse effects were all mild, and did not lead to withdrawal of treatment. Of the 65 men given oral finasteride, six had loss of libido, and one had an increase in body hair at other sites; irritation of the scalp was seen in one of those who used minoxidil. These adverse events disappeared as soon as the treatment was withdrawn. The laboratory data did not show any statistically or clinically significant changes from baseline values to the endpoint, except for the serum total testosterone concentration, which was increased, and free testosterone and serum prostate-specific antigen in the finasteride group which were reduced from baseline values.

Benign prostatic hyperplasia
The benefit of combining an alpha-adrenoceptor antagonist with a 5-alpha-reductase inhibitor has been assessed in men with benign prostatic hyperplasia (23). Modified-release alfuzosin was more effective than finasteride, with no additional benefit in combining the drugs. The adverse effects of alpha-blockade were postural hypotension, hypotension, headache, dizziness, and malaise; the adverse effects of finasteride were ejaculatory disorders and impotence.

The therapeutic and adverse effects of dibenyline, finasteride, and a combination of the two in 190 patients with symptomatic benign prostatic hyperplasia have been evaluated (24). Adverse effects were more common with dibenyline than with finasteride alone or in combination with dibenyline. The drop-out rate was higher with dibenyline (16%) than finasteride alone (7.5%) or the two in combination (4.6%). The reported adverse effects are listed in Table 1.

In short-term studies the herbal preparation saw palmetto (*Serenoa repens*) and finasteride seem to give a similar degree of relief in benign prostatic hyperplasia (25). However, in a prospective 1-year comparative randomized trial in 64 men with category III prostatitis or chronic pelvic pain syndrome, in which finasteride 5 mg/day was compared with saw palmetto 325 mg/day, the mean NIH Chronic Prostatitis Symptom Index score fell from 24 to 18 with finasteride, but scarcely or not at all with saw palmetto (26). Adverse events included headache (n = 3) with saw palmetto and reduced libido (n = 2) with finasteride. Although one might envisage even more prolonged studies, these findings hardly suggest that saw palmetto is a serious replacement for finasteride, even though it is well tolerated.

In a prospective 1-year comparative randomized trial in 64 men with category III prostatitis or chronic pelvic pain syndrome, finasteride was 5 mg/day was compared with saw palmetto 325 mg/day (27). At 1 year the mean NIH Chronic Prostatitis Symptom Index score fell from 24 to 18 in the finasteride group, but scarcely or not at all in the saw palmetto group. Adverse events included headache (n = 3) in the saw palmetto group and reduced libido (n = 2) in the finasteride group. Although one might envisage even more prolonged studies these findings hardly suggest that saw palmetto is a serious replacement for finasteride even though it is well tolerated.

Prostate cancer
Although flutamide is sufficiently well tolerated in prostatic cancer, the much older drug cyproterone acetate continues to show up favorably. In a direct comparison between the two drugs in 310 men the two were equally

Table 1 Adverse effect of finasteride with or without dibenyline in benign prostatic hyperplasia

Adverse effect	Finasteride	Dibenyline	Combination
Light-headedness	1.9%	25%	19%
Nasal stuffiness	–	9.9%	11%
Impotence	9.3%	17%	17%

effective in delaying progression of the cancer and prolonging survival; however, adverse effect profiles were more favorable for cyproterone acetate overall and in particular with respect to gynecomastia, diarrhea, and nausea (28).

Polycystic ovary syndrome
In 44 women with polycystic ovary syndrome treated with finasteride or flutamide for 6 months the adverse effects of flutamide were reduced libido, gastrointestinal disorders, and dry skin (29). Finasteride caused reduced libido, headache, and dry skin. Dry skin was reported in 68% of users of flutamide and in only 27% of users of finasteride.

Placebo-controlled studies

Androgenetic alopecia
In an unusual study, finasteride 1 mg/day was used for 1 year to treat male-pattern baldness in nine subjects; each had an identical twin who received placebo (30). Finasteride significantly improved hair growth. There were no drug-related adverse events, either clinical or biochemical.

Of 1553 men with male-pattern baldness who took finasteride 1 mg/day, all of whom had initially taken part in one of two 1-year placebo-controlled studies, 1215 continued into further controlled studies over another 4 years (31). There was durable improvement in scalp hair over 5 years and no new safety concerns were identified.

Hirsutism
The effects of finasteride for 9 months on hirsutism and serum concentrations of basal gonadotropins, androgens, estrogen, and sex hormone-binding globulin have been studied in 18 women with idiopathic hirsutism (32). Nine took oral finasteride 7.5 mg/day and the other nine took placebo. Hirsutism improved significantly with finasteride after 6 and 9 months; placebo had no significant effect. Adverse effects were headache and modest depression during the first month. Libido did not change. Hirsute patients who took finasteride had a marked fall in dihydrotestosterone from the third month and a significant increase in serum testosterone concentrations from the sixth month of treatment.

Benign prostatic hyperplasia
The effects of finasteride and placebo on quality of life have been evaluated for 12 months in a diverse population of 2342 men with benign prostatic hyperplasia (33). Symptom scores fell significantly at month 3 in those taking finasteride and continued to improve throughout the study. The incidence of drug-related sexual adverse experiences was significantly higher in the finasteride group, but led to withdrawal in only 1.5% of patients.

Prostate cancer
The effects of bicalutamide 150 mg/day, in addition to standard non-medicinal care, have been tested in an internationally co-ordinated series of randomized placebo-controlled studies in more than 8000 patients with

localized or locally advanced prostate cancer (34). At this dosage, sufficient to increase the length of progression-free survival, patients with locally advanced disease gained most benefit from bicalutamide. Overall survival was similar with bicalutamide and placebo. Survival appeared to be improved by bicalutamide in those with locally advanced disease, whereas it was reduced by bicalutamide in those with localized disease. The most common adverse events with bicalutamide were gynecomastia and breast pain.

In 9060 men who had participated in the randomized, placebo-controlled Prostate Cancer Prevention Trial in the USA for 7 years, finasteride 5 mg/day either prevented or delayed the appearance of prostate cancer, with an overall reduction in cancer incidence of 25% (35). However, of the 757 tumors that occurred with finasteride, no less than 37% were classified as relatively malignant (Gleason grades 7, 8, 9, or 10), whereas in the placebo group of 1068 tumors only 22% received this grading. The absolute number of high-grade tumors was also rather higher in the finasteride group (n = 280) than in the placebo group (n = 237). Sexual adverse effects (reduced volume of ejaculate, erectile dysfunction, loss of libido, gynecomastia) were also significantly more common in the treated group than in those taking placebo, but in the finasteride group urinary problems, such as prostatic hyperplasia or problems with micturition, were markedly reduced. The authors suggested that "physicians can use these results to counsel men regarding the use of finasteride" but it is hard to see that it provides a simple choice.

Systematic reviews

In a Spanish systematic review of the world literature there were firm conclusions about the value of finasteride in reducing the symptoms of benign prostatic hyperplasia in doses that are well tolerated in all respects (36).

Organs and Systems

Cardiovascular

The long-term effects and adverse effects of finasteride have been studied in a multicenter study of 3270 men (37). There was a background history of cardiovascular disease in 40% of the patients at baseline, and myocardial infarction was reported in 1.5% of those who took finasteride and 0.5% of those who took placebo, a significant difference.

Respiratory

An 88-year-old man developed interstitial pneumonitis while taking flutamide 375 mg/day for prostatic cancer (38). After 3 weeks he developed dyspnea and bilateral pulmonary interstitial infiltrates; glucocorticoid therapy and withdrawal of flutamide resulted in clinical improvement.

Special senses

Cataract has been associated with finasteride therapy (39).

- A 43-year-old man developed impaired vision in both eyes over 3 months. Anterior subcapsular opacities were found in both eyes, necessitating cataract extraction. He had been taking finasteride 1 mg/day for 3 years to treat the early stage of androgenic alopecia. It was suspected that the drug was responsible and the treatment was therefore withdrawn.

Endocrine

In men finasteride had no affect on serum concentrations of luteinizing hormone, follicle-stimulating hormone, cortisol, or estradiol (40). In women finasteride had no effect on basal and gonadorelin-stimulated gonadotropin secretion, the pulsatility of luteinizing hormone secretion, or the concentrations of estradiol, prolactin, free testosterone, androstenedione, dehydroepiandrosterone sulfate, or sex hormone-binding globulin; there were significant reductions in plasma concentrations of cortisol, dihydrotestosterone, and 3-alpha-androstanediol glucuronide (41).

Thyroid function has been studied in 183 patients with prostate cancer who were being treated with continuous androgen deprivation therapy; 64 were being treated with a luteinizing hormone-releasing hormone (LHRH) agonist alone and 119 others with an LHRH agonist + bicalutamide 50 mg/day (42). Treatment lasted an average of 43 months. Mean concentrations of T3 and free T4 were very similar to those in a control group of post-surgical patients without medicinal treatment or recurrence. However, the mean TSH concentration was 16 (4.4–120) mU/l in the controls and 18 (1.5–66) mU/l in the treated group, and the serum concentration of TSH was higher than 5 mU/l in six treated patients (2.1%). There was also a mild reduction in the free T4 serum concentration in treated patients. It therefore seems that androgen deprivation therapy with bicalutamide alters some thyroid function tests.

Metabolism

A marked rise in blood glucose concentration must be a very rare effect of anti-androgen therapy, but a Japanese group has described two patients with prostate cancer with this complication (43).

- A 61-year-old man with a 7-year history of diabetes, well-controlled with diet and acarbose, developed prostate cancer and was given leuprorelin acetate and flutamide. After the second injection of leuprorelin his fasting glucose and hemoglobin A_{1c} concentrations were markedly raised (23 mmol/l and 11% respectively).
- An 81-year-old man with no history of diabetes developed diabetes mellitus after using leuprorelin for prostate carcinoma for 6 months. His fasting glucose was 19 mmol/l and his HbA_{1c} was 9.9%.

In both cases the blood glucose concentration was successfully corrected with a brief course of insulin and was thereafter maintained in the reference range using pioglitazone. This is encouraging, but the toxicity of pioglitazone must surely be borne in mind (see Chapter 42), especially in this type of elderly patient.

In men finasteride did not affect serum lipids, including total cholesterol, low density lipoproteins, high density lipoproteins, or triglycerides (40).

Hematologic

The use of androgen blockade in the treatment of prostatic cancer is, at least for a period, highly effective, but it commonly causes anemia or aggravates the anemia that is often already present in such patients. The onset and degree of the anemia in such cases has been studied in 42 patients with adenocarcinoma of the prostate, stage C, who underwent combined androgen blockage using LH-RH-A and antiandrogen treatment (leukopride acetate 3.75 mg intramuscularly every month plus oral flutamide 250 mg every 8 hours) (44). Patients who developed severe symptomatic anemia were treated with erythropoietin. Observations continued over 6 months. The mean hemoglobin concentration fell significantly from 14.2 g/dl at the start to 12.7 g/dl at 6 months, but there was severe and clinically evident anemia (less than 11 g/dl) in only six patients (14%). The development of severe anemia did not correlate with testosterone baseline values, age, or clinical stage. Its approach was detectable by the third month. The condition was readily correctable with recombinant erythropoietin.

Gastrointestinal

Gastrointestinal effects are common when flutamide is used to treat advanced cases of prostate cancer. At doses of 250 mg every 8 hours or 500 mg/day, 23 of 106 men had gastrointestinal problems, irrespective of the dosage regimen (45). There was no difference in the incidence of these effects in the 56 men who had previously received external beam radiation and 50 others who had undergone radical prostatectomy. This suggests that the gastrointestinal adverse effects of flutamide are not due to a local toxic effect.

Enterocolic lymphocytic phlebitis has been temporally associated with flutamide treatment (46). Although the association could have been coincidental, the facts suggest that the report should be taken seriously.

- A 53-year-old man developed ileocecal intussusception due to an edematous ischemic cecum, due to enterocolic lymphocytic phlebitis, with numerous associated thrombi. The phlebitis involved not only the ischemic area but also other sites, notably the entire right colon, terminal ileum, and appendix. All layers of the bowel wall were involved. The mesenteric veins were also prominently affected, but the arteries were spared. There was a marked lymphocytic infiltrate involving the epithelium of the entire right colon, ileum, and appendix.

This is the first reported case of enterocolic lymphocytic phlebitis, a rare form of vasculitis, in conjunction with lymphocytic colitis, lymphocytic enteritis, and lymphocytic appendicitis. The fact that the patient was taking flutamide at the same time suggests that this peculiar form of lymphocytic inflammation of the veins and mucosa could represent a drug reaction. It should be recalled that diarrhea is a common complication of flutamide use, and perhaps occurs in severe degree in some 15% of men taking full-dose treatment.

Liver

Flutamide causes hepatotoxicity in some 0.36% of patients, and for this reason alone it should not be used in the absence of a serious indication. Whether bulimia nervosa in women justifies its use is open to doubt, since non-pharmacological methods of treatment are available. Furthermore, bulimia nervosa in women can be associated with raised serum testosterone concentrations. In a small double-blind study of the use of flutamide, citalopram, a combination of the two, or placebo in 31 women over 3 months, all the active treatments reduced the tendency to binge eating (47). However, there was a moderate and reversible increase in serum transaminase activities, leading to withdrawal in two of the 19 subjects who were taking flutamide either alone or in combination.

Pancreas

The incidence of acute pancreatitis as a suspected complication of finasteride treatment has been examined in a case-control study in a Danish regional population of 490 000 over 7 years. Of 302 men aged 60 and older with incident acute pancreatitis, three had been exposed to finasteride; of 2994 controls 37 had been exposed to finasteride. After adjustment for alcohol-related diseases, gallstone disease, hyperlipidemia, hypercalcemia, and hyperparathyroidism, the authors found no evidence of an increased risk of acute pancreatitis in users of finasteride (48).

Skin

Cutaneous adverse effects of flutamide, which as a whole are common, include some cases of photosensitivity.

- A 70-year-old man who had taken flutamide for 4 months for prostatic carcinoma photosensitivity was associated with a positive rechallenge test (49). The authors provided evidence that this might have represented an early form of lupus erythematosus. The theory was supported by histology and by the fact that in the literature there is at least one case of flutamide induced lupus.

Photosensitivity as a complication of flutamide treatment has been described; in one unusually severe case, erythroderma proceeded to extensive vitiligo (50).

Musculoskeletal

Androgen deprivation therapy for prostatic cancer, whether it is carried out surgically or medicinally, carries a substantial risk of osteoporosis and spinal fractures. These risks have been quantified to some extent (51). In 87 elderly men treated in this way over a long period, 38 had radiographic evidence of spinal fractures. They had an initial mean prostate specific antigen of 53 ng/ml and had received androgen deprivation therapy for a mean of 40 months. Mean spinal and femoral neck bone mineral densities were significantly lower than in men without spinal fractures. The duration of androgen deprivation therapy, low serum 25-hydroxycolecalciferol concentrations, and a history of alcohol excess (defined as more than four standard drinks daily) were the main determinants of spinal fractures.

Reversible severe myopathy during treatment with finasteride has been described in a 70-year-old man (52).

Sexual function

Very long-term treatment of prostatic enlargement with finasteride, for example over 10 years, continues to be sufficiently well tolerated, although adverse effects, mostly relating to sexual function, do occur (53,54). The incidence and nature of these adverse effects has been well documented in The Proscar Long-term Efficacy and Safety Study (PLESS), a 4-year, randomized, double-blind, placebo-controlled trial in 3040 men, all of whom took finasteride 5 mg/day (55). At screening, 46% of all the patients reported some history of sexual dysfunction. During the first year of the study, 15% of the finasteride-treated patients and 7% of the placebo-treated patients had sexual adverse events that were considered drug related; during years 2–4, there was no between-group difference in the incidence of new sexual adverse events (7% in each group). Sexual adverse events resolved while continuing therapy in 12% of those taking finasteride and 19% of those taking placebo.

The incidence of erectile dysfunction induced by finasteride is difficult to estimate, since in many users of the drug other causes are present; they include advanced age, heart disease, diabetes, hypertension, smoking, and hypercholesterolemia. Benign prostatic hyperplasia itself can also aggravate or even induce erectile dysfunction. Analysis of a questionnaire study in New Jersey suggested that such pathological factors can have a greater role in inducing erectile dysfunction than drugs such as finasteride and alpha-blockers, although the latter can clearly contribute (56).

At an oral dose of 1 mg/day finasteride has no major adverse effects on measures of semen production or quality (57), although it can cause a slight reduction in the volume of ejaculate (15).

There is a higher incidence of impaired sexual function in men who take finasteride compared with placebo (58,59). The incidence of erectile dysfunction has been estimated at 5% (60), but it is difficult to estimate, since in many users of the drug other causes are present, including advanced age, heart disease, diabetes, hypertension, smoking, and hypercholesterolemia. Benign prostatic hyperplasia itself can also aggravate or even induce erectile dysfunction. A questionnaire study in New Jersey

suggested that such pathological factors have a greater role in inducing erectile dysfunction than drugs such as finasteride and alpha-adrenoceptor antagonists, although the latter can clearly contribute (61).

The long-term efficacy and safety of finasteride have been studied in 102 patients with benign prostatic hyperplasia (62). Adverse experiences due to sexual dysfunction continued throughout the study, but the low continuous dropout rate may have reflected a natural process in this aged population, and not necessarily a drug-related effect.

The incidence and nature of adverse effects of finasteride on sexual function have been documented in The Proscar Long-term Efficacy and Safety Study (PLESS), a 4-year, randomized, double-blind, placebo-controlled trial in 3040 men, all of whom took finasteride 5 mg/day (63). At screening, 46% of all the patients reported some history of sexual dysfunction. During the first year of the study, 15% of the finasteride-treated patients and 7% of the placebo-treated patients had sexual adverse events that were considered to be drug-related; during years 2–4 there was no between-group difference in the incidence of new sexual adverse events (7% in each group). Sexual adverse events resolved during continued therapy in 12% of those taking finasteride and 19% of those taking placebo.

In a long-term multicenter study of finasteride in 3270 men the numbers of serious adverse events and withdrawals because of adverse events were significantly higher with placebo (37). Drug-related adverse effects in 1% or more of patients were reduced libido, ejaculation disorders, and impotence. A total of 273 patients, 165 (10%) taking finasteride and 108 (7%) taking placebo, reported a sexual adverse event during the treatment period, including change in libido, ejaculation disorders, impotence, or orgasmic dysfunction.

The effects of finasteride (n = 545), tamsulosin, or the proprietary herbal remedy Permixon on sexual function have been studied in patients with lower urinary tract symptoms due to benign prostatic hyperplasia (64). At 6 months tamsulosin and finasteride caused slight increases in sexual disorders and Permixon caused a slight improvement. Ejaculation disorders were the most frequently reported adverse effects after tamsulosin or finasteride.

However, an Italian investigation of sexual and erectile function, using questionnaires directed to 186 patients treated at various centers with finasteride 1 mg/day for 4–6 months has challenged the accepted wisdom; the authors concluded that (as judged by the five-item International Index of Erectile Function) there was no adverse effect on erection after this period of time (65).

Reproductive system

Of 65 women with idiopathic hirsutism who took either finasteride 5 mg/day or the long-acting gonadorelin agonist leuprorelin (3.75 mg monthly as an intramuscular depot), none had either menstrual abnormalities or other adverse effects (66). However, adequate doses may not have been used, since the hirsutism score improved in only 36% of the patients who took leuprorelin and 14% of those who took finasteride. Serum concentrations of total testosterone, free testosterone, androstenedione, and dehydroepiandrosterone fell in patients treated with leuprorelin, but only serum total testosterone and free testosterone concentrations fell significantly with finasteride.

Breasts

Reversible painful gynecomastia has been reported as an adverse effect of finasteride in a dose as low as 1 mg/day (67); it can be unilateral (68) or bilateral (69). Some reports of gynecomastia in users of finasteride relate to doses as low as 1 mg/day (70).

- A 23-year-old man who was taking finasteride 1 mg/day for 2 months for androgenetic alopecia developed painful enlargement of his right breast (71). Treatment was withdrawn and resolution occurred after 2 months.

However, breast cancer can be misdiagnosed as benign gynecomastia (see below).

In a series of studies from Italy an attempt was made to determine whether giving anastrozole 1 mg/day and/or tamoxifen 20 mg/day could prevent gynecomastia and breast pain due to bicalutamide 150 mg/day (72). In a 48-week double-blind study tamoxifen reduced the symptoms but anastrozole did not.

It is possible to reduce the incidence of gynecomastia in men taking antiandrogens by prophylactic irradiation of the breast. In a major randomized clinical study of antiandrogen use in Scandinavia, breast irradiation, generally using single-fraction electrons (12 to 15 Gy), was given to 174 (69%) of 253 patients (73). After 1 year physician evaluations suggested some form of gynecomastia in 71% and 28% of the non-irradiated and irradiated patients respectively, some form of breast enlargement in 78% and 44%, and some degree of breast tenderness in 75% and 43%.

Long-Term Effects

Tumorigenicity

Striking evidence of the association of finasteride with male breast cancer comes from the Medical Therapy of Prostatic Symptoms (MTOPS) study, a National Institutes of Health (NIH)-sponsored study of about 3047 men that compared finasteride, doxazosin, and the combination for the treatment of benign prostatic hyperplasia. The rate of breast cancer in this trial for men taking finasteride either alone or with doxazosin was four in 1554, or nearly 200 times that of the general population; one man in the finasteride + doxazosin group and three in the finasteride-alone group developed male breast cancer (74).

- A 53-year-old man developed unilateral gynecomastia following finasteride therapy for alopecia (75). On needle biopsy the mammary mass was diagnosed as

adenocarcinoma on the basis of nuclear atypia and particularly because of cytoplasmic vacuolization, but excision biopsy showed only benign gynecomastia with no evidence of malignant change.

In one case a man taking bicalutamide developed gynecomastia, which proceeded to breast cancer (76).

An elderly man with prostate cancer took long-term flutamide and developed adenocarcinoma of the breast (77). There could have been several reasons for this complication. Unlike LH-releaser-based hormonal therapy for prostatic cancer, antiandrogens cause hyperestrogenemia owing to suppressed negative feedback of androgens on LHRH and LH production, stimulation of testicular androgen production, and transformation to estrogens in peripheral target tissues. It is true that, in this particular individual, there were other susceptibility factors, namely BRCA-1 mutation and chromosome 9 inversion, which has been previously shown to impinge upon testicular function and intracrine balance of androgens versus estrogens. However, the authors stressed that men with prostate cancer who take antiandrogens may be at risk of breast cancer and they advised caution in the use of the treatment in men with risk factors for male breast cancer.

Susceptibility factors

Age

In 3040 men with benign prostatic hyperplasia the effects of finasteride 5 mg/day for 4 years were studied in those over and under 65 years (78). In both groups the drug was effective and there were no significant differences in cardiovascular adverse events between placebo and finasteride. There were significant differences between placebo and finasteride in the overall incidence of typical drug-related adverse events, but there were no specific differences associated with age. The principal events were impotence (8.8%), reduced libido (6.8%), reduced volume of ejaculate (3.5%), other disorders of ejaculation (1.5%), rash (0.6%), breast enlargement (0.5%), and breast tenderness (0.2%).

Drug Administration

Drug dosage regimens

The difficulty in weighing benefit against harm when selecting a regimen for patients with hormone-refractory prostate carcinoma is compounded by the fact that patients differ markedly in their needs and responses. This is underlined by the outcome of a panel study undertaken by the Society of Urologic Oncology (79). However, its only firm recommendation, after considering all the medicinal alternatives, was that "management strategies should be targeted toward the individual patient".

In a phase II study of androgen suppression therapy for prostate cancer, 95 patients with recurrent or metastatic prostate cancer received cyclical 8-month periods of treatment with leuprolide acetate and nilutamide, with intermittent rest periods (80). Recovery periods were progressively lengthened until the treatment failed to achieve normal prostate-specific antigen (PSA) concentrations. The 95 subjects received 245 cycles of treatment. The median duration of rest periods was 8 months and the median time to treatment failure was 47 months. There was testosterone recovery during rest periods in 117 cycles (61%). There was mild anemia in 33%, 44%, and 67% of cycles 1, 2, and 3 respectively. Sexual function recovered during the rest periods in 47% of cycles. There was no significant overall change in body mass index at the end of the treatment period. Osteoporosis was documented in at least one site, evaluated in 41 patients (37%). The results of this study suggest that intermittent use of androgen suppression has the potential to reduce adverse effects, allowing recovery of the hemoglobin concentration, permitting return of sexual function, and avoiding weight gain.

Many of the problems seen with finasteride have undoubtedly been due to its use in unnecessarily high doses. Particularly when used for cosmetic ends there has been doubt as to how far dosage can be reduced while maintaining an acceptable effect. Finasteride continues to be used to treat hirsutism in women and is effective, although long-term information on safety is sparse, and in principle it might adverse affect an unborn child (81). The dose should certainly be kept as low as possible.

In a randomized study in 38 hirsute women finasteride 2.5 mg every 3 days was as effective as the higher daily dose formerly used and better tolerated (82).

Drug-drug interactions

Cyproterone acetate

Sequential administration of flutamide and cyproterone acetate has been associated with toxic hepatitis (83).

Sibutramine

An interaction of finasteride with sibutramine has been described (84).

- A 30-year man who was being successfully treated for obesity with sibutramine started to take finasteride to treat alopecia. Soon afterwards he developed paranoid psychotic behavior. The reaction abated and disappeared when finasteride was withdrawn.

The suggested mechanism of this interaction was that finasteride inhibited the hepatic metabolism of sibutramine, which then displaced finasteride from its plasma protein binding sites; inhibition of 5HT (serotonin) and noradrenaline reuptake by sibutramine then triggering the psychotic event.

Interference with diagnostic routines

Finasteride reduces serum prostate-specific antigen concentrations (60). In participants in the Prostate Cancer Prevention Trial who had an end of study biopsy (928

with cancer and 8620 with a negative biopsy) or an interim diagnosis of prostate cancer (n = 671) those who took finasteride had a median fall in PSA of 2% after year 1, while the controls had an increase of 3% (85). By the end of the study PSA had increased annually by 6% (placebo) and 7% (finasteride). In those with interim diagnoses PSA increased by 11% (placebo) and 15% (finasteride) each year before diagnosis. Cases with high grade disease (Gleason 7 and above) had greater increases in PSA than cases with low grade disease. The authors concluded that in men who have taken finasteride for more than 1 year the PSA concentration will need to be adjusted to determine whether it is in the reference range. In the Prostate Cancer Prevention Trial the adjustment factor required to preserve a median PSA concentration increased from 2 at 24 months to 2.5 at 7 years after the start of finasteride treatment.

References

1. Fourcade R-O, McLeod D. Tolerability of antiandrogens in the treatment of prostate cancer. UroOncol 2004;4:5–13.
2. Fradet Y. Bicalutamide (Casodex) in the treatment of prostate cancer. Exp Rev Anticancer Ther 2004;4:37–48.
3. Ciarra A, Cardi A, Di Silverio F. Antiandrogen monotherapy: recommendations for the treatment of prostate cancer. Urol Int 2004;72:91–8.
4. Schellhammer PF, Davis JW. An evaluation of bicalutamide in the treatment of prostate cancer. Clin Prost Cancer 2004;2:213–9.
5. Verhamme KMC, Dieleman JP, Bleumink GS, Bosch JLHR, Stricker BHCh, Sturkenboom MCJM. Treatment strategies, patterns of drug use and treatment discontinuation in men with LUTS suggestive of benign prostatic hyperplasia: the Triumph Project. Eur Urol 2003;44:539–45.
6. Peters DH, Sorkin EM. Finasteride. A review of its potential in the treatment of benign prostatic hyperplasia. Drugs 1993;46(1):177–208.
7. Steiner JF. Finasteride: a 5 alpha-reductase inhibitor. Clin Pharm 1993;12(1):15–23.
8. Steiner JF. Clinical pharmacokinetics and pharmacodynamics of finasteride. Clin Pharmacokinet 1996;30(1):16–27.
9. Nickel JC, Fradet Y, Boake C, Pommerville PJ, Perreault J-P, Afridi SK, Elhilali MM, Barr RE, Beland GA, Bertrand PE, et al. Efficacy and safety of finasteride therapy for benign prostatic hyperplasia: results of a 2-year randomized controlled trial (the PROSPECT study). Can Med Assoc J 1996;155:1251–9.
10. Nickel JC. Long-term implications of medical therapy on benign prostatic hyperplasia end points. Urology 1998;51 Suppl A:50–7.
11. Edwards JE, Moore RA. Finasteride in the treatment of clinical benign prostatic hyperplasia: a systematic review of randomised trials. BMC Urol 2002;2:14.
12. Jimenez Cruz J.F, Quecedo Gutierrez L, Del Llano Senaris J. Finasterida. Diez anos de uso clinico. Revision sistematica de la literatura. Actas Urol Esp 2003;27:202–15.
13. Reddy GK. Finasteride, a selective 5-alpha-reductase inhibitor, in the prevention and treatment of human prostate cancer. Clin Prostate Cancer 2004;2(4):206–8.
14. Ekman P. A risk-benefit assessment of treatment with finasteride in benign prostatic hyperplasia. Drug Saf 1998;18:161–70.

15. Libecco JF, Bergfeld WF. Finasteride in the treatment of alopecia. Expert Opin Pharmacother 2004;5(4):933–40.

16. Townsend KA, Marlowe KF. Relative safety and efficacy of finasteride for treatment of hirsutism. Ann Pharmacother 2004;38(6):1070–3.

17. Whiting DA, Olsen EA, Savin R, Halper L, Rodgers A, Wang L, Hustad C, Palmisano J. Efficacy and tolerability of finasteride 1 mg in men aged 41 to 60 years with male pattern hair loss. Eur J Dermatol 2003;13:150–60.

18. Bayram F, Muderris I, Guven M, Ozcelik B, Kelestimur F. Low-dose 2.5 mg/day) finasteride treatment in hirsutism. Gynecol Endocrinol 2003;17:419–22.

19. Bayram F, Muderris I, Guven M, Ozcelik B, Kelestimur F. Low-dose 2.5 mg/day) finasteride treatment in hirsutism. Gynecol Endocrinol 2003;17:419–22.

20. Tartagni M, Schonauer MM, Cicinelli E, Petruzzelli F, De Pergola G, De Salvia MA, Loverro G. Intermittent low-dose finasteride is as effective as daily administration for the treatment of hirsute women. Fertil Steril 2004;82:752–5.

21. Tay M-H, Kaufman DS, Regan MM, Leibowitz SB, George DJ, Febbo PG, Manola J, Smith MR, Kaplan ID, Kantoff PW, Oh WK. Finasteride and bicalutamide as primary hormonal therapy in patients with advanced adenocarcinoma of the prostate Ann Oncol 2004;15:974–8.

22. Arca E, Acikgoz G, Tastan HB, Kose O, Kurumlu Z. An open, randomized, comparative study of oral finasteride and 5% topical minoxidil in male androgenetic alopecia. Dermatology 2004;209:117–25.

23. De Bruyne FMJ, Jardin A, Colloi D, Resel L, Witjes WPJ, Delauche-Cavallier MC, McCarthy C, Geffriaud-Ricouard C. Sustained release alfuzosin, finasteride and the combination of both in the treatment of benign prostatic hyperplasia. Eur Urol 1998;34:169–75.

24. Kuo HC. Comparative study for therapeutic effect of dibenyline, finasteride and combination drugs for symptomatic benign prostatic hyperplasia. Urol Int 1998;60:85–91.

25. Carraro JC, Raynaud JP, Koch G, Chisholm GD, Di Silverio F, Teillac P, Da Silva FC, Cauquil J, Chopin DK, Hamdy FC, Hanus M, Hauri D, Kalinteris A, Marencak J, Perier A, Perrin P. Comparison of phytotherapy (Permixon) with finasteride in the treatment of benign prostate hyperplasia: a randomized international study of 1,098 patients. Prostate 1996;29(4):231–40.

26. Kaplan SA, Volpe MA, Te AE. A prospective 1-year trial using saw palmetto versus finasteride in the treatment of category III prostatitis/chronic pelvic pain syndrome. J Urol 2004;171:284–8.

27. Kaplan SA, Volpe MA, Te AE. A prospective 1-year trial using saw palmetto versus finasteride in the treatment of category III prostatitis/chronic pelvic pain syndrome. J Urol 2004;171:284–8.

28. Schroder FH, Whelan P, De Reijke TM., Kurth KH, Pavone-Macaluso M, Mattelaer J, Van Velthoven RF, Debois M, Collette L. Metastatic prostate cancer treated by flutamide versus cyproterone acetate: final analysis of the "European Organization for Research and Treatment of Cancer" (EORTC) protocol 30892. Eur Urol 2004;45:457–64.

29. Falsetti L, De Fusco D, Eleftheriou G, Rosina B. Treatment of hirsutism by finasteride and flutamide in women with polycystic ovary syndrome Gynaecol Endosc 1997;6:251–7.

30. Stough DB, Rao NA, Kaufman KD, Mitchell C. Finasteride improves male pattern hair loss in a randomized study in identical twins. Eur J Dermatol 2003;12:32–7.

31. Kaufman KD. Long-term (5-year) multinational experience with finasteride 1 mg in the treatment of men with androgenetic alopecia. Eur J Dermatol 2002;12:38–49.

32. Ciotta L, Cianci A, Calogero AE, Palumbo MA, Marletta E, Sciuto A, Palumbo G. Clinical and endocrine effects of finasteride, a 5α-reductase inhibitor in women with idiopathic hirsutism. Fertil Steril 1995;64:299–306.

33. Byrnes CA, Morton AS, Liss CL, Lippert MC, Gillenwater JY. Efficacy, tolerability, and effect on health-related quality of life of finasteride versus placebo in men with symptomatic benign prostatic hyperplasia: a community based study. CUSP Investigators. Community based study of Proscar. Clin Ther 1995;17:956–69.

34. Wirth MP, See WA, McLeod DG, Iversen P, Morris T, Carroll K; Casodex Early Prostate Cancer Trialists' Group. Bicalutamide 150 mg in addition to standard care in patients with localized or locally advanced prostate cancer: results from the second analysis of the early prostate cancer program at median followup of 5.4 years. J Urol 2004;172:1865–70.

35. Thompson IM, Goodman PJ, Tangen CM, Lucia MS, Miller GJ, Ford LG, Lieber MM, Cespedes RD, Atkins JN, Lippman SM, Carlin SM, Ryan A, Szczepanek CM, Crowley JJ, Coltman CA Jr. The influence of finasteride on the development of prostate cancer. New Engl J Med 2003;349:215–24.

36. Jimenez Cruz J.F, Quecedo Gutierrez L, Del Llano Senaris J. Finasterida: Diez anos de uso clinico. Revision sistematica de la literatura. Actas Urol Esp 2003;27:202–15.

37. Margerger MJ. Long-term effects of finasteride in patients with benign prostatic hyperplasia: a double-blind, placebo-controlled multicenter study. Urology 1998;51:677–86.

38. Nomura M, Sato H, Fujimoto N, Matsumoto T. Interstitial pneumonitis related to flutamide monotherapy for prostate cancer. Int J Urol 2004;11:798–800.

39. Chou S-Y, Kao S-C, Hsu W-M. Propecia-associated bilateral cataract. Clin Exp Ophthalmol 2004;32:106–8.

40. Gormley GJ, Stoner E, Rittmaster RS, Gregg H, Thompson DL, Lasseter KC, Vlasses PH, Stein EA. Effects of finasteride (MK-906), a 5 alpha-reductase inhibitor, on circulating androgens in male volunteers. J Clin Endocrinol Metab 1990;70(4):1136–41.

41. Fruzzetti F, de Lorenzo D, Parrini D, Ricci C. Effects of finasteride, a 5 alpha-reductase inhibitor, on circulating androgens and gonadotropin secretion in hirsute women. J Clin Endocrinol Metab 1994;79(3):831–5.

42. Morote J, Esquena S, Orsola A, Salvador C, Trilla E, Cecchini L, Raventos CX, Planas J, Catalan R, Reventos J. Effect of androgen deprivation therapy in the thyroid function test of patients with prostate cancer Anti-Cancer Drugs 2005;16:863–6.

43. Inaba M, Otani Y, Nishimura K, Takaha N, Okuyama A, Koga M, Azuma J, Kawase I, Kasayama S. Combination therapy with rofecoxib and finasteride in the treatment of men with lower urinary tract symptoms (LUTS) and benign prostatic hyperplasia. Metab Clin Exp 2005;54:55–9.

44. Bogdanos J, Karamanolakis D, Milathianakis C, Repousis P, Tsintavis A, Koutsilieris M. Combined androgen blockade-induced anemia in prostate cancer patients without bone involvement. Anticancer Res 2003;23:1757–62.

45. Langenstroer P, Porter HJ, McLeod DG, Thrasher JB. Direct gastrointestinal toxicity of flutamide: comparison of irradiated and nonirradiated cases. J Urol 2004;171:684–6.

46. Wright CL, Cacala S. Enterocolic lymphocytic phlebitis with lymphocytic colitis, lymphocytic appendicitis, and lymphocytic enteritis. Am J Surg Pathol 2004;28:542–7.

47. Sundblad C, Landen M, Eriksson T, Bergman L, Eriksson E. Effects of the androgen antagonist flutamide and the serotonin reuptake inhibitor citalopram in bulimia nervosa: a placebo-controlled pilot study. J Clin Psychopharmacol 2005;25:85–8.

48. Floyd A, Pedersen L, Nielsen GL, Thorlacius-Ussing O, Sorensen HT. Risk of acute pancreatitis in users of finasteride: a population-based case-control study. J Clin Gastroenterol 2004;38:276–8.

49. Kaur C, Thami GP. Flutamide-induced photosensitivity: is it a forme fruste of lupus? Br J Dermatol 2003;148:603–4.

50. Rafael JP, Manuel GG, Antonio V, Carlos MJ. Widespread vitiligo after erythroderma caused by photosensitivity to flutamide. Contact Dermatitis 2004;50:98–100.

51. Diamond TH, Bucci J, Kersley JH, Aslan P, Lynch WB, Bryant C. Osteoporosis and spinal fractures in men with prostate cancer: risk factors and effects of androgen deprivation therapy. J Urol 2004;172:529–32.

52. Haan J, Hollander JMR, van Duinen SG, Saxena PR, Wintzen AR. Reversible severe myopathy during treatment with finasteride. Muscle Nerve 1997;20:502–4.

53. Lam JS, Romas NA, Lowe FC. Long-term treatment with finasteride in men with symptomatic benign prostatic hyperplasia: 10-year follow-up. Urology 2003;61:354–8.

54. Lowe FC, McConnell JD, Hudson PB, Romas NA, Boake R, Lieber M, Elhilali M, Geller J, Imperto-McGinely J, Andriole GL, Bruskewitz RC, Walsh PC, Bartsch G, Nacey JN, Shah S, Pappas F, Ko A, Cook T, Stoner E, Waldstreicher J. Long-term 6-year experience with finasteride in patients with benign prostatic hyperplasia. Urology 2003;61:791–6.

55. Wessells H, Roy J, Bannow J, Grayhack J, Matsumoto AM, Tenover L, Herlihy R, Fitch W, Labasky R, Auerbach S, Parra R, Rajfer J, Culbertson J, Lee M, Bach MA, Waldstreicher J. Incidence and severity of sexual adverse experiences in finasteride and placebo-treated men with benign prostatic hyperplasia. Urology 2003;61:579–84.

56. Sadeghi-Nejad H, Sherman N, Lue J. Comparison of finasteride and alpha-blockers as independent risk factors for erectile dysfunction. Int J Clin Pract 2003;57:484–7.

57. McClellan KJ, Markham A. Finasteride. A review of its use in male pattern hair loss. Drugs 1999;57:111–26.

58. Lam JS, Romas NA, Lowe FC. Long-term treatment with finasteride in men with symptomatic benign prostatic hyperplasia: 10-year follow-up. Urology 2003;61:354–8.

59. Lowe FC, McConnell JD, Hudson PB, Romas NA, Boake R, Lieber M, Elhilali M, Geller J, Imperto-McGinely J, Andriole GL, Bruskewitz RC, Walsh PC, Bartsch G, Nacey JN, Shah S, Pappas F, Ko A, Cook T, Stoner E, Waldstreicher J. Long-term 6-year experience with finasteride in patients with benign prostatic hyperplasia. Urology 2003;61:791–6.

60. Neal DE. Drugs in focus: finasteride. Presc J 1995;35:89–95.

61. Sadeghi-Nejad H, Sherman N, Lue J. Comparison of finasteride and alpha-blockers as independent risk factors for erectile dysfunction. Int J Clin Pract 2003;57:484–7.

62. Ekman P. Maximum efficacy of finasteride is obtained within 6 months and maintained over 6 years. Eur Urol 1998;33:312–7.

63. Wessells H, Roy J, Bannow J, Grayhack J, Matsumoto AM, Tenover L, Herlihy R, Fitch W, Labasky R, Auerbach S, Parra R, Rajfer J, Culbertson J, Lee M, Bach MA, Waldstreicher J. Incidence and severity of sexual adverse experiences in finasteride and placebo-treated men with benign prostatic hyperplasia. Urology 2003;61:579–84.

64. Zlotta AR, Teillac P, Raynaud JP, Schulman CC. Evaluation of male sexual function in patients with lower urinary tract symptoms (LUTS) associated with benign prostatic hyperplasia (BPH) treated with a phytotherapeutic agent (Permixon®), tamsulosin or finasteride. Eur Urol 2005;48:269–76.

65. Tosti A, Pazzaglia M, Soli M, Rossi A, Rebora A, Atzori L, Barbareschi M, Benci M, Voudouris S, Vena GA. Evaluation of sexual function with an International Index of Erectile Function in subjects taking finasteride for androgenetic alopecia. Arch Dermatol 2004;140:857–8.

66. Bayhan G, Bahceci M, Demirkol T, Ertem M, Yalinkaya A, Erden AC. A comparative study of a gonadotropin-releasing hormone agonist and finasteride on idiopathic hirsutism. Clin Exp Obstet Gynecol 2000;27:203–6.

67. Wade MS, Sinclair RD. Reversible painful gynaecomastia induced by low dose finasteride (1 mg/day). Australas J Dermatol 2000;41:55.

68. Ferrando J, Grimalt R, Alsina M, Bulla F, Manasievska E. Unilateral gynecomastia induced by treatment with 1 mg of oral finasteride. Arch Dermatol 2002;138:543–4.

69. Kim BJ, Kim YJ, Ro BI. Two cases of reversible bilateral painful gynecomastia induced by 1 mg oral finasteride (Propecia). Korean J Dermatol 2003;41:232–4.

70. Kim BJ, Kim YJ, Ro BI. Two cases of reversible bilateral painful gynecomastia induced by 1 mg oral finasteride (Propecia). Korean J Dermatol 2003;41:232–4.

71. Kim H, Kye K, Seo Y, Suhr K, Lee J, Park J. A case of unilateral idiopathic gynecomastia aggravated by low-dose finasteride. Korean J Dermatol 2004;42:643–5.

72. Boccardo F, Rubagotti A, Battaglia M, Di Tonno P, Selvaggi F.P, Conti G, Comeri G, Bertaccini A, Martorana G, Galassi P, Zattoni F, Macchiarella A, Siragusa A, Muscas G, Durand F, Potenzoni D, Manganelli A, Ferraris V, Montefiore F, Trump DL. Evaluation of tamoxifen and anastrozole in the prevention of gynecomastia and breast pain induced by bicalutamide monotherapy of prostate cancer. Urol Oncol 2005;23:377.

73. Widmark A, Fossa SD, Lundmo P, Damber J-E, Vaage S, Damber L, Wiklund F, Klepp O. Does prophylactic breast irradiation prevent antiandrogen-induced gynecomastia? Evaluation of 253 patients in the randomized Scandinavian trial SPCG-7/SFUO-3. Urology 2003;61:145–51.

74. See SC, Ellis RJ. Male breast cancer during finasteride therapy. J Natl Cancer Inst 2004;96:338–9.

75. Zimmerman RL, Fogt F, Cronin D, Lynch R. Cytologic atypia in a 53-year-old man with finasteride-induced gynecomastia. Arch Pathol Lab Med 2000;124:625–7.

76. Chianakwalam C.I, McCahy P, Griffiths N.J. A case of male breast cancer in association with bicalutamide-induced gynaecomastia. Breast 2005;14:163–4.

77. Karamanakos P, Mitsiades CS, Lembessis P, Kontos M, Trafalis D, Koutsilieris M. Male breast adenocarcinoma in a prostate cancer patient following prolonged anti-androgen monotherapy. Anticancer Res 2004;24:1077–81.

78. Kaplan SA, Holtgrewe HL, Bruskewitz R, Saltzman B, Mobley D, Narayan P, Lund RH, Weiner S, Wells G, Cook TJ, Meehan A, Waldstreicher J. Comparison of the efficacy and safety of finasteride in older versus younger men with benign prostatic hyperplasia. Urology 2001;57:1073–7.

79. Chang SS, Benson MC, Campbell SC, Crook J, Dreicer R, Evans CP, Hall MC, Higano C, Kelly WK, Sartor O, Smith Jr JA. Society of Urologic Oncology position statement. Redefining the management of hormone-refractory prostate carcinoma. Cancer 2005;103:11–21.

80. Malone S, Perry G, Segal R, Dahrouge S, Crook J. Long-term side-effects of intermittent androgen suppression therapy in prostate cancer. Results of a phase II study. BJU Int 2005;96:514–20.
81. Townsend KA, Marlowe KF. Relative safety and efficacy of finasteride for treatment of hirsutism. Ann Pharmacother 2004;38:1070–3.
82. Tartagni M, Schonauer MM, Cicinelli E, Petruzzelli F, De Pergola G, De Salvia MA, Loverro G. Intermittent low-dose finasteride is as effective as daily administration for the treatment of hirsute women. Fertil Steril 2004;82:752–5.
83. Manolakopoulos S, Bethanis S, Armonis A, Economou M, Avgerinos A, Tzourmakliotis D. Toxic hepatitis after sequential administration of flutamide and cyproterone acetate. Dig Dis Sci 2004;49:462–5.
84. Dogol Sucar D, Botelho Sougey E, Brandao Neto J. Psychotic episode induced by potential drug interaction of sibutramine and finasteride. Rev Bras Psiquiatr 2002;24:30–3.
85. Etzioni RD, Howlader N, Shaw PA, Ankerst DP, Penson DF, Goodman PJ, Thompson IM. Long-term effects of finasteride on prostate specific antigen levels: results from the prostate cancer prevention trial. J Urol 2005;174(3):877-81 [erratum 2071].

Aromatase inhibitors

General Information

The development of newer antiestrogens continues in the hope of attaining a better benefit to harm balance, particularly in the adjuvant treatment of early breast cancer after the menopause (1,2). The third-generation aromatase inhibitors inhibit the production of estrogen (3). Anastrozole and letrozole are non-steroids, and exemestane (a steroid with some androgenic activity) is a derivative of the androgen androstenedione, the natural substrate of aromatase. Early findings were positive, as demonstrated by a first analysis of the ATAC ("Arimidex, Tamoxifen Alone or in Combination") trial, with a median follow-up of 33 months and a safety analysis after as many as 37 months of treatment (4). The latest safety analysis seemed to confirm that endometrial cancer vaginal bleeding and discharge, cerebrovascular events, venous thromboembolic events, and hot flushes all occurred less often in the anastrozole group, whereas musculoskeletal disorders and fractures continued to occur less often in the tamoxifen group. However, there is still debate about whether the aromatase inhibitors have significant advantages over tamoxifen (5); proponents argue that they are associated with fewer adverse effects (including endometrial cancer as well as those listed above) than tamoxifen (6). However, although they may cause fewer hot flushes, gynaecological, and thromboembolic adverse effects than tamoxifen, they may cause more musculoskeletal complications and sexual dysfunction. There is also variability in the actions of the different aromatase inhibitors, and they are not interchangeable (7).

Organs and Systems

Cardiovascular

Of 8028 postmenopausal women with receptor-positive early breast cancer who were randomly assigned double-blind to letrozole, tamoxifen, or a sequence of these agents for 5 years, 7963 were included in an analysis of cardiovascular events over a median follow-up time of 30 months (8). There was a similar overall incidence of cardiac adverse events (letrozole 4.8%; tamoxifen 4.7%), but more grade 3–5 events with letrozole (2.4% versus 1.4%), an excess that was only partly attributable to prior hypercholesterolemia. There were more thromboembolic events with tamoxifen (3.9% versus 1.7% overall and 2.3% versus 0.9% for grade 3–5 events). There were no significant differences between tamoxifen and letrozole in the incidence of hypertension or cerebrovascular events.

The risk of venous thromboembolism in women taking anastrozole is lower than that in women taking tamoxifen (1.6% versus 2.4%) (9), but still higher than in the untreated population. Cases of pulmonary embolism have been reported in an 80-year-old woman taking anastrozole (10) and a 72-year-old woman taking letrozole (11).

Sensory systems

Retinal hemorrhages were sought in 35 women taking anastrozole 1 mg/day, 38 taking tamoxifen 20 mg/day, and 53 controls (12). There were retinal hemorrhages within the posterior pole in four of those taking anastrozole and none of the controls or those taking tamoxifen. Two of those taking anastrozole had a flame hemorrhage in the retinal nerve fiber layer and two had a blot hemorrhage deeper in the retina.

Metabolism

In 55 overweight or obese postmenopausal women w ho took tamoxifen (n = 27) or exemestane (n = 28) for 1 year, frat mass fell significantly with exemestane but not tamoxifen. Triglycerides and high-density lipoprotein cholesterol fell significantly and low-density lipoprotein cholesterol rose significantly with exemestane (13).

In 147 postmenopausal women with early breast cancer who took exemestane in a placebo-controlled study, exemestane caused modest reductions in high-density lipoprotein cholesterol and apolipoprotein, but had no major effect on lipid profile, homocysteine concentrations, or coagulation (14).

In 122 postmenopausal patients with metastatic breast cancer who were randomized to exemestane 25 mg/day (n = 62) or tamoxifen 20 mg/day (n = 60), neither exemestane nor tamoxifen had adverse effects at 8, 24 or 48 weeks on concentrations of total cholesterol, HDL cholesterol, apolipoproteins A1 or B, or lipoprotein a (15). Exemestane lowered triglyceride concentrations while tamoxifen increased them.

Hematologic

Reversible thrombocytopenia occurred in a 64-year-old woman with recurrent breast cancer taking letrozole 2.5 mg/day (16).

Liver

Acute hepatitis has been attributed to anastrozole (17).

Urinary tract

Sclerosing glomerulonephritis has been attributed to anastrozole in a 73-year-old postmenopausal woman with breast cancer (18).

Skin

- A 54-year-old Chinese woman developed a rapidly evolving vesicobullous eruption on her face, trunk, and legs, covering 50% of her body surface area, 2 weeks after she had taken letrozole on two separate occasions; histology was consistent with toxic epidermal necrolysis (19).
- Diffuse non-scarring alopecia occurred in a 37-year-old premenopausal woman with relapsed breast cancer 6 months after she had started to take letrozole 2.5 mg/ day and triptorelin 3.75 mg every 28 days; it resolved with topical minoxidil (20).

Musculoskeletal

Myalgia occurred in 12% of patients in a study of letrozole (21). In 12 patients with non-metastatic breast cancer who reported severe musculoskeletal pain while taking letrozole (n = 11) or exemestane (n = 1), the most common reported symptoms were severe early morning stiffness and hand/wrist pain causing impaired ability to completely close/stretch the hand/fingers and to perform daily activities and work-related skills (22). Six had to discontinue treatment owing to severe symptoms. Trigger finger and carpal tunnel syndrome were the most frequently reported clinical signs. Ultrasound examination showed fluid in the tendon sheath surrounding the digital flexor tendons. MRI scans showed enhancement and thickening of the tendon sheath in all 12.

Joint pain, which can be disabling, is common in women taking aromatase inhibitors (5–40%) (23). In 24 women mean age 59 years with joint pain of greater than 5/10 on a visual analogue scale, pain was due to osteoarthritis, shoulder tendinitis, or paraneoplastic aponeurositis in five cases; the other 19 had inflammatory pain of the fingers, wrists, shoulders, forefeet, ankles, or knees, with slight synovial thickening of the proximal interphalangeal joints and metacarpophalangeal joints (24). Nine had antinuclear antibodies and four had rheumatoid factor. Ten had sicca syndrome of the eyes or mouth, seven had probable Sjögren's syndrome according to the San Diego criteria, and one had definite Sjögren's syndrome. One had rheumatoid arthritis, one had Hashimoto thyroiditis, and two had positive hepatitis C serology.

Of 53 postmenopausal women with estrogen receptor-positive breast cancer taking anastrozole, 14 had joint symptoms (13 with digital stiffness and three with arthralgias of wrist and shoulders) (25). Joint symptoms tended to occur in the patients who had previously undergone chemotherapy, but there was no relation between prior hormonal therapy and joint symptoms. Seven patients who stopped taking anastrozole improved. Five who had grade 1 digital stiffness continued taking anastrozole. Two who had with grade 1 stiffness took a Chinese herbal medicine, improved, and continued to take anastrozole.

Aromatase inhibitors increase bone turnover by near complete estrogen depletion, leading to reduced bone mineral density and an increased risk of fractures. Bisphosphonates plus calcium and vitamin D supplementation mitigate this (26). In an open, multicenter, randomized study in 602 women with early-stage breast cancer taking letrozole 2.5 mg/day, zoledronic acid 4 mg every 6 months prevented bone loss (27).

In 70 postmenopausal women with completely resected breast cancers who were disease-free after taking tamoxifen for 2–3 years, a switch to exemestane resulted in increases in serum bone alkaline phosphatase and the carboxy-terminal telopeptide of type I collagen and a fall in parathormone; bone mineral density worsened (28).

In 147 postmenopausal women with early breast cancer who took exemestane in a placebo-controlled study, the mean annual rate of bone mineral density loss was 2.17% versus 1.84% in the lumbar spine and 2.72% versus 1.48% in the femoral neck with exemestane versus placebo. The mean changes in T score after 2 years were −0.21 versus −0.11 in the hip and −0.30 versus −0.21 in the lumbar spine (14).

Carpal tunnel syndrome has been reported in six patients taking aromatase inhibitors (29). Most subsequently experienced relief after withdrawal and/or switching to tamoxifen. In clinical trials of anastrozole and exemestane, carpal tunnel syndrome occurred in about 3% (30,31,32).

Immunologic

Subacute cutaneous lupus erythematosus has been attributed to anastrozole (33).

A 67-year-old woman developed Henoch-Schönlein purpura, with a leukocytoclastic vasculitis and joint pains, after taking anastrozole for 10 months; the symptoms resolved within 2 weeks of withdrawal (34).

Long-Term Effects

Tumorigenicity

In four patients with prostate tumors who were treated with exemestane (two with and two without bicalutamide) there was progression of the tumor after 4 weeks, assessed by measurement of prostate-specific antigen and radiological signs (35). Three of the four had a significant increase in bone pain only a few days after starting treatment and a clear improvement in these symptoms after withdrawal. The study was stopped prematurely and the authors concluded that exemestane has no role to play in the treatment of prostate cancer.

Susceptibility Factors

Renal and hepatic disease

The pharmacokinetics of a single oral dose of exemestane 25 mg have been studied in postmenopausal subjects with normal hepatic function (n = 9), moderately impaired hepatic function (n = 9), severely impaired hepatic function (n = 8), normal renal function (n = 6), moderately impaired renal function (n = 6), and severely impaired renal function (n = 7) (36). Exposure to exemestane was increased two- to three-fold in patients with hepatic impairment; the apparent oral clearance and apparent volume of distribution of exemestane were reduced. Renal impairment was also associated with two- to three-fold increases in exposure due to reduced clearance. However, because exemestane has a relatively large safety margin, the authors considered that these effects were of no clinical significance.

Drug-Drug Interactions

Gefitinib

Liver toxicity attributed to gefitinib in a 63-year-old woman was thought to have been due to inhibition of the metabolism of gefitinib by anastrozole (37).

Tamoxifen

In 34 post-menopausal women with early breast cancer anastrozole 1 mg/day for 28 days had no effect on the pharmacokinetics of tamoxifen 20 mg/day (38).

However, in 12 patients who took letrozole 2.5 mg/day for 6 weeks with and without tamoxifen 20 mg/day plasma concentrations of letrozole were reduced by 38% during combination therapy (39). Tamoxifen did not significantly alter the effect of letrozole in suppressing estradiol, estrone, and estrone sulfate. The authors suggested that sequential therapy might be preferable with these two drugs.

References

1. Powles TJ. Anti-oestrogenic chemoprevention of breast cancer—the need to progress. Eur J Cancer 2003;39:572–9.
2. Miller WR, Jackson J. The therapeutic potential of aromatase inhibitors. Exp Opin Invest Drugs 2003;12:337–51.
3. Smith RE, Good BC. Chemoprevention of breast cancer and the trials of the National Surgical Adjuvant Breast and Bowel Project and others. Endocr Relat Cancer 2003;10:347–57.
4. Baum M, Buzdar A, Cuzick J, Forbes J, Houghton J, Howell A, Sahmoud T; the ATAC (Arimidex, Tamoxifen Alone or in Combination) Trialists' Group. Anastrozole alone or in combination with tamoxifen versus tamoxifen alone for adjuvant treatment of postmenopausal women with early-stage breast cancer: results of the ATAC (Arimidex, Tamoxifen Alone or in Combination) trial efficacy and safety update analyses. Cancer 2003;98:1802–10.
5. Nabholtz JM. Long-term safety of aromatase inhibitors in the treatment of breast cancer. Ther Clin Risk Manag 2008;4(1):189–204.
6. Aapro MS, Forbes JF. Three years' follow-up from the ATAC trial is sufficient to change clinical practice: a debate. Breast Cancer Res Treat 2003;80:S3–11.
7. Miller WR, Bartlett J, Brodie AM, Brueggemeier RW, di Salle E, Lønning PE, Llombart A, Maass N, Maudelonde T, Sasano H, Goss PE. Aromatase inhibitors: are there differences between steroidal and nonsteroidal aromatase inhibitors and do they matter? Oncologist 2008;13(8):829–37.
8. Mouridsen H, Keshaviah A, Coates AS, Rabaglio M, Castiglione-Gertsch M, Sun Z, Thürlimann B, Mauriac L, Forbes JF, Paridaens R, Gelber RD, Colleoni M, Smith I, Price KN, Goldhirsch A. Cardiovascular adverse events during adjuvant endocrine therapy for early breast cancer using letrozole or tamoxifen: safety analysis of BIG 1-98 trial. J Clin Oncol 2007;25(36):5715–22.
9. Howell A, Cuzick J, Baum M, Buzdar A, Dowsett M, Forbes JF, Hoctin-Boes G, Houghton J, Locker GY, Tobias JS. Results of the ATAC (Arimidex, Tamoxifen, Alone or in Combination) trial after completion of 5 years' adjuvant treatment for breast cancer. Lancet 2005;365(9453):60–2.
10. Lycette JL, Luoh SW, Beer TM, Deloughery TG. Acute bilateral pulmonary emboli occurring while on adjuvant aromatase inhibitor therapy with anastrozole: Case report and review of the literature. Breast Cancer Res Treat 2006;99(3):249–55.
11. Oyan B, Altundag K, Ozisik Y. Does letrozole have any place in adjuvant setting in breast cancer patients with documented hypercoagulability? Am J Clin Oncol 2004;27(2):210–1.
12. Eisner A, Falardeau J, Toomey MD, Vetto JT. Retinal hemorrhages in anastrozole users. Optom Vis Sci 2008;85(5):301–8.
13. Francini G, Petrioli R, Montagnani A, Cadirni A, Campagna S, Francini E, Gonnelli S. Exemestane after tamoxifen as adjuvant hormonal therapy in postmenopausal women with breast cancer: effects on body composition and lipids. Br J Cancer 2006;95(2):153–8.
14. Lønning PE, Geisler J, Krag LE, Erikstein B, Bremnes Y, Hagen AI, Schlichting E, Lien EA, Ofjord ES, Paolini J, Polli A, Massimini G. Effects of exemestane administered for 2 years versus placebo on bone mineral density, bone biomarkers, and plasma lipids in patients with surgically resected early breast cancer. J Clin Oncol 2005;23(22):5126–37.
15. Atalay G, Dirix L, Biganzoli L, Beex L, Nooij M, Cameron D, Lohrisch C, Cufer T, Lobelle JP, Mattiaci MR, Piccart M, Paridaens R. The effect of exemestane on serum lipid profile in postmenopausal women with metastatic breast cancer: a companion study to EORTC Trial 10951, 'Randomized phase II study in first line hormonal treatment for metastatic breast cancer with exemestane or tamoxifen in postmenopausal patients'. Ann Oncol 2004;15(2):211–7.
16. Sperone P, Gorzegno G, Berruti A, Familiari U, Dogliotti L. Reversible pancytopenia caused by oral letrozole assumption in a patient with recurrent breast cancer. J Clin Oncol 2002;20(17):3747–8.
17. de la Cruz L, Romero-Vazquez J, Jiménez-Sáenz M, Padron JR, Herrerias-Gutierrez JM. Severe acute hepatitis in a patient treated with anastrozole. Lancet 2007;369(9555):23–4.

18. Kalender ME, Sevinc A, Camci C, Turk HM, Karakok M, Akgul B. Anastrozole-associated sclerosing glomerulone-phritis in a patient with breast cancer. Oncology 2007;73(5-6):415–8.

19. Chia WK, Lim YL, Greaves MW, Ang P. Toxic epidermal necrolysis in patient with breast cancer receiving letrozole. Lancet Oncol 2006;7(2):184–5.

20. Carlini P, Di Cosimo S, Ferretti G, Papaldo P, Fabi A, Ruggeri EM, Milella M, Cognetti F. Alopecia in a preme-nopausal breast cancer woman treated with letrozole and triptorelin. Ann Oncol 2003;14(11):1689–90.

21. Goss PE, Ingle JN, Martino S, Robert NJ, Muss HB, Piccart MJ, Castiglione M, Tu D, Shepherd LE, Pritchard KI, Livingston RB, Davidson NE, Norton L, Perez EA, Abrams JS, Therasse P, Palmer MJ, Pater JL. A rando-mized trial of letrozole in postmenopausal women after five years of tamoxifen therapy for early-stage breast can-cer. N Engl J Med 2003;349(19):1793–802.

22. Morales L, Pans S, Paridaens R, Westhovens R, Timmerman D, Verhaeghe J, Wildiers H, Leunen K, Amant F, Berteloot P, Smeets A, Van Limbergen E, Weltens C, Van den Bogaert W, De Smet L, Vergote I, Christiaens MR, Neven P. Debilitating musculoskeletal pain and stiffness with letrozole and exemestane: associated tenosynovial changes on magnetic resonance imaging. Breast Cancer Res Treat 2007;104(1):87–91.

23. Khanduri S, Dodwell DJ. Aromatase inhibitors and muscu-loskeletal symptoms. Breast 2008;17(1):76–9.

24. Laroche M, Borg S, Lassoued S, De Lafontan B, Roché H. Joint pain with aromatase inhibitors: abnormal frequency of Sjögren's syndrome. J Rheumatol 2007;34(11):2259–63.

25. Ohsako T, Inoue K, Nagamoto N, Yoshida Y, Nakahara O, Sakamoto N. Joint symptoms: a practical problem of ana-strozole. Breast Cancer 2006;13(3):284–8.

26. Coleman RE, Body JJ, Gralow JR, Lipton A. Bone loss in patients with breast cancer receiving aromatase inhibitors and associated treatment strategies. Cancer Treat Rev 2008;34 Suppl 1:S31–42.

27. Brufsky A, Harker WG, Beck JT, Carroll R, Tan-Chiu E, Seidler C, Hohneker J, Lacerna L, Petrone S, Perez EA. Zoledronic acid inhibits adjuvant letrozole-induced bone loss in postmenopausal women with early breast cancer. J Clin Oncol 2007;25(7):829–36.

28. Gonnelli S, Cadirni A, Caffarelli C, Petrioli R, Montagnani A, Franci MB, Lucani B, Francini G, Nuti R. Changes in bone turnover and in bone mass in women with breast cancer switched from tamoxifen to exemestane. Bone 2007;40(1):205–10.

29. Nishihori T, Choi J, DiGiovanna MP, Thomson JG, Kohler PC, McGurn J, Chung GG. Carpal tunnel syndrome asso-ciated with the use of aromatase inhibitors in breast cancer. Clin Breast Cancer 2008;8(4):362–5.

30. ATAC Trialists' Group results of the ATAC (Arimidex, Tamoxifen, Alone or in Combination) trial after completion of 5 years' adjuvant treatment for breast cancer. Lancet 2005;365:60–2.

31. The Arimidex, Tamoxifen, Alone or in Combination (ATAC) Trialists Group. Comprehensive side effect profile of anastrozole and tamoxifen as adjuvant treatment for early stage breast cancer: long term safety analysis of the ATAC trial. Lancet Oncol 2006;7:633–43.

32. Coombes RC, Hall E, Gibson LJ, Paridaens R, Jassem J, Delozier T, Jones SE, Alvarez I, Bertelli G, Ortmann O, Coates AS, Bajetta E, Dodwell D, Coleman RE, Fallowfield LJ, Mickiewicz E, Andersen J, Lønning PE, Cocconi G, Stewart A, Stuart N, Snowdon CF, Carpentieri M, Massimini G, Bliss JM, van de Velde C; Intergroup Exemestane Study. A randomized trial of exemestane after two to three years of tamoxifen therapy in postmeno-pausal women with primary breast cancer. N Engl J Med 2004;350(11):1081–92.

33. Trancart M, Cavailhes A, Balme B, Skowron F. Anastrozole-induced subacute cutaneous lupus erythemato-sus. Br J Dermatol 2008;158(3):628–9.

34. Conti-Beltraminelli M, Pagani O, Ballerini G, Richetti A, Graffeo R, Ruggeri M, Forni V, Pianca S, Schönholzer C, Mainetti C, Cavalli F, Goldhirsch A. Henoch-Schönlein purpura (HSP) during treatment with anastrozole. Ann Oncol 2007;18(1):205–7.

35. Bonomo M, Mingrone W, Brauchli P, Hering F, Goldhirsch A; Swiss Group for Clinical Cancer Cancer Research, a member of the Swiss Institute of Applied Cancer Research. Exemestane seems to stimulate tumour growth in men with prostate carcinoma. Eur J Cancer 2003;39(14):2111–2.

36. Jannuzzo MG, Poggesi I, Spinelli R, Rocchetti M, Cicioni P, Buchan P. The effects of degree of hepatic or renal impair-ment on the pharmacokinetics of exemestane in postmeno-pausal women. Cancer Chemother Pharmacol 2004;53(6):475–81.

37. Carlini P, Papaldo P, Fabi A, Felici A, Ruggeri EM, Milella M, Ciccarese M, Nuzzo C, Cognetti F, Ferretti G. Liver toxicity after treatment with gefitinib and anastrozole: drug-drug interactions through cytochrome P450? J Clin Oncol 2006;24(35):e60–1.

38. Dowsett M, Tobias JS, Howell A, Blackman GM, Welch H, King N, Ponzone R, von Euler M, Baum M. The effect of anastrozole on the pharmacokinetics of tamoxifen in post-menopausal women with early breast cancer. Br J Cancer 1999;79(2):311–5.

39. Dowsett M, Pfister C, Johnston SR, Miles DW, Houston SJ, Verbeek JA, Gundacker H, Sioufi A, Smith IE. Impact of tamoxifen on the pharmacokinetics and endocrine effects of the aromatase inhibitor letrozole in postmenopausal women with breast cancer. Clin Cancer Res 1999;5(9):2338–43.

Chlorotrianisene

General Information

Chlorotrianisene is a non-steroidal triphenylethylene with estrogen and antiestrogen activity. Diethylstilbestrol and other non-steroidal estrogens came into vogue at a time when the cost of producing steroidal estrogens, whether synthetic or of natural origin, was still prohibitive. They have fallen out of favor, in view of the association between diethylstilbestrol in pregnancy and second gen-eration injury. There is no reason for believing that the short-term acute adverse reactions to these non-steroidal compounds differ from those of estrogenic steroids.

Chlorotrianisene does not bind in vitro to the uterine estrogen receptor but has potent estrogenic and antiestro-genic actions in vivo, suggesting that it is a prodrug. Its antiestrogenic activity has been proposed to be due to a reactive intermediate (1).

Organs and Systems

Hematologic

In 50 postpartum women who took chlorotrianisene for lactation suppression in a double-blind, randomized, placebo-controlled study, antithrombin III concentrations were significantly lower on the third day postpartum compared with placebo (2).

References

1. Kupfer D, Bulger WH. Inactivation of the uterine estrogen receptor binding of estradiol during P-450 catalyzed metabolism of chlorotrianisene (TACE). Speculation that TACE antiestrogenic activity involves covalent binding to the estrogen receptor. FEBS Lett 1990;261(1):59–62.
2. Niebyl JR, Bell WR, Schaaf ME, Blake DA, Dubin NH, King TM. The effect of chlorotrianisene as postpartum lactation suppression on blood coagulation factors. Am J Obstet Gynecol 1979;134(5):518–22.

Clomiphene

General Information

Clomiphene is a very weak non-steroidal estrogen; it blocks the feedback effect of endogenous estrogens on the pituitary, promoting the further secretion of gonadotropins. The primary use of clomiphene in women is in the induction of ovulation. In men, it has been used to treat infertility in view of its ability to increase endogenous production of testosterone (1).

General adverse effects

In one large study, some adverse reactions in treated women were due to its ovulatory effects and others were direct reactions to the substance itself (2). The most common problem was ovarian enlargement (14%), followed by hot flushes (11%), abdominal and pelvic discomfort (7.0%), and nausea and vomiting (2.1%). Incidental symptoms were breast discomfort, vaginal changes, psychological symptoms, headache, heavier menses, and increased urinary frequency. Sporadic case-reports on clomiphene in the literature relate to fetal ovarian dysplasia or maternal psychosis (SEDA-7, 391), either of which may have been coincidental. However, it must be borne in mind that the substance is related structurally to triparanol, an obsolete drug that produced a series of disastrous adverse effects some 40 years ago.

In another study, the adverse effects of the antiestrogenic effects of clomiphene citrate were hot flushes (10%), mood swings, depression, headaches (1%), pelvic pain (5.5%), nausea (2%), breast tenderness (2–5%), dryness and loss of hair (0.3%), visual symptoms, halos and streaks around lights (particularly at night), blurring, and scotoma (1.5%) (3).

Organs and Systems

Nervous system

In a multicenter WHO study, two men withdrew because of visual disturbances, dizziness, and headaches (4).

Reproductive system

In some men taking clomiphene in the hope of improving subfertility, a non-bacterial pyospermia developed and could well have had an adverse effect on the outcome; it appeared more commonly in clomiphene users than controls (5).

Long-Term Effects

Tumorigenicity

Mammary cancer in the mother has been suspected as a risk of clomiphene, but specific investigations into the matter have not supported this suspicion (SED-12, 1034) (6).

A case of testicular seminoma in a man receiving both clomiphene and mesterolone for 15 months for oligospermia has been described (7), but it is unlikely that the drug was responsible.

Malignant melanoma
Concern that the drug treatment of female infertility might predispose the user to malignant melanoma was first engendered by a US study published in 1995 (8). Among women who had used clomiphene citrate for infertility, the incidence of melanoma was higher (RR = 1.8; 95% CI = 0.8, 3.5) than among American women in general. However, in a case-cohort study of nearly 4000 infertile women there was a similar increase in the incidence of melanoma among those who had been treated with human chorionic gonadotropin compared with the rest; there was no association with the use of clomiphene.

Quite apart from the inherent discrepancy in these findings, several pieces of evidence have confused the debate. In the first place, the cohort of melanoma cases was small—barely a handful. In the second place, some earlier papers had suggested that infertility in women might of itself have an association with melanoma. The same impression came from various studies, in which the incidences of cancers in infertile women were examined (9–11). If that were true, it could affect the initial findings in either direction: a high spontaneous incidence might mask a real drug effect, or it might provide a predisposition to melanoma, which the drugs might then more readily trigger.

In the meantime, data from Australia have shown no greater incidence of melanoma among women who had used fertility drugs and undergone in vitro fertilization than in the country's general female population (12). Since then there has been one more significant paper, again from Australia, using data from a specialized fertility clinic in Queensland, relating to all women who attended the center over a decade (13). Whenever possible, the women were traced and their subsequent history noted. Originally intended as a retrospective case-cohort study using a subcohort, the approach had to be amended because no cases of melanoma were found in the subcohort. The work therefore proceeded as a matched case-control study; all the data were taken and set against publicly available figures on melanoma in Queensland. After some necessary exclusions, 3186 women were included; care was taken to minimize recall bias. Fourteen women developed melanoma after fertility treatment, eight cases being invasive. The expected incidence in the general population would have been 15.8 cases in the same period. The incidence actually observed was therefore only 0.89 of that anticipated (95% CI = 0.54, 1.48). The numbers of women who had used clomiphene or human menopausal gonadotropin were too small to make more differentiated calculations, but the incidence of melanoma seemed to correspond to that in the general population.

On current evidence there seems no reason to discourage fertility-promoting drug treatments because of any risk of melanoma; they may even reduce it to some extent. However, this does not alter the fact that the data are deficient in various ways. Quite apart from the small numbers of melanoma cases that have been recorded, all the work to date has been performed in relatively sunny parts of the world; it is not known what would happen in other climates. Within countries there are sharp differences in melanoma figures; in the USA, where about 32 000 new cases of skin melanoma were projected for 1994 (14), the highest melanoma rates occur among light-skinned populations in areas of intense sunlight, for example Arizona; the same applies to Queensland, Australia. In the USA as a whole there is a melanoma incidence among whites of 12.4 per 100 000 (15), while mortality rates vary inversely with latitude (16). Furthermore, in whites, there has been a recent increase in the incidence of melanoma, during the precise period that this type of treatment has become popular, but probably for entirely different reasons, which may be associated with lifestyles and holiday habits; the reported incidence in whites rose by no less than 102% from 1973 to 1991 (16). Finally, as the Australian authors themselves stressed, the fact that the Queensland clinic was a private institution specializing in IVF/GIFT therapy means that women with endocrine-associated or ovulation-associated infertility may not have been referred to it so readily.

All this makes it very difficult to find a baseline incidence for melanoma with which cases treated for infertility can be compared. It is to be hoped that data of this type will continue to arrive from other centers, so that a definitive judgement will become possible.

Second-Generation Effects

Teratogenicity

Suspicions that clomiphene might adversely affect a fetus that has developed as a result of successful ovulation induction are difficult to confirm or allay, since the condition for which clomiphene is being used, that is subfertility, might itself be associated with a risk of malformation. The fear originally arose after 18 cases of trisomy had been reported

in the USA; later data on a large series of clomiphene-induced pregnancies (17) indicated that if there was indeed such risk it must be very small; a study of 200 instances of Down's syndrome showed that none of them had been exposed to the drug (SEDA-6, 357). Another report concerned a case of congenital retinopathy (SEDA-7, 391).

Cornel and colleagues concluded in 1989 that there was a relative risk of at least two of an association between disturbed fertility and neural tube defects (18), but others found no evidence for an association between maternal clomiphene use and such defects. The authors of a pooled analysis of all published work concluded that any increase in neural tube defects is likely to be less than two-fold and that there may in fact be no increase at all (1).

One unusual possibility is a change in the sex ratio; in one study the ratio of boys to girls among infants conceived after induction of ovulation with clomiphene was 0.85, significantly different from the normal human sex ratio at birth, which is about 1.06 (19).

An unusual condition that has been tentatively ascribed to clomiphene is persistence of the hyperplastic primary vitreous, that is fetal ophthalmic tissue that normally resolves before birth. If more than a trace of the material persists, ocular complications, including cataract and retinal detachment, can result. In a case reported from Canada, there had been an estimated 3 weeks of exposure to high doses of clomiphene (100 mg/day) after gestation, and the child's vision was severely impaired (20). This is probably not a mere chance association, since several cases of visual defects of various types after exposure to clomiphene have been described before, and in some animal studies the drug does adversely affect ocular development.

A possible link between clomiphene and hypospadias in male offspring has been reported (21). This possible link has been further examined in a case-control study, based on records of 319 cases of hypospadias recorded in four counties of Denmark over 30 years and prescribing records over that time, and a comparable control group (22). There was no evidence of a link between clomiphene and hypospadias.

References

1. Greenland S, Ackerman DL. Clomiphene citrate and neural tube defects: a pooled analysis of controlled epidemiologic studies and recommendations for future studies. Fertil Steril 1995;64(5):936–41.
2. Kistner RW. The use of clomiphene citrate in the treatment of anovulation. Semin Drug Treat 1973;3(2):159–76.
3. Vollenhoven BJ, Healy DL. Short- and long-term effects of ovulation induction. Endocrinol Metab Clin North Am 1998;27(4):903–14.
4. World Health Organization. A double-blind trial of clomiphene citrate for the treatment of idiopathic male infertility. Int J Androl 1992;15(4):299–307.
5. Matthews GJ, Goldstein M, Henry JM, Schlegel PN. Nonbacterial pyospermia: a consequence of clomiphene citrate therapy. Int J Fertil Menopausal Stud 1995;40(4):187–91.
6. Kimbel HK. Inquiry of the 'Arzneimittelkommission der Deutschen Arzteschaft'. Personal communication. 1978.

7. Neoptolemos JP, Locke TJ, Fossard DP. Testicular tumour associated with hormonal treatment for oligospermia. Lancet 1981;2(8249):754.
8. Rossing MA, Daling JR, Weiss NS, Moore DE, Self SG. Risk of cutaneous melanoma in a cohort of infertile women. Melanoma Res 1995;5(2):123–7.
9. Ron E, Lunenfeld B, Menczer J, Blumstein T, Katz L, Oelsner G, Serr D. Cancer incidence in a cohort of infertile women. Am J Epidemiol 1987;125(5):780–90.
10. Brinton LA, Melton LJ 3rd, Malkasian GD Jr, Bond A, Hoover R. Cancer risk after evaluation for infertility. Am J Epidemiol 1989;129(4):712–22.
11. Modan B, Ron E, Lerner-Geva L, Blumstein T, Menczer J, Rabinovici J, Oelsner G, Freedman L, Mashiach S, Lunenfeld B. Cancer incidence in a cohort of infertile women. Am J Epidemiol 1998;147(11):1038–42.
12. Venn A, Watson L, Lumley J, Giles G, King C, Healy D. Breast and ovarian cancer incidence after infertility and in vitro fertilisation. Lancet 1995;346(8981):995–1000.
13. Young P, Purdie D, Jackman L, Molloy D, Green A. A study of infertility treatment and melanoma. Melanoma Res 2001;11(5):535–41.
14. Boring CC, Squires TS, Tong T, Montgomery S. Cancer statistics, 1994. CA Cancer J Clin 1994;44(1):7–26.
15. In: Rees LAG, Eisner MP, Kosary CL, Hankey BF, Miller BA, Clegg L, Edwards BK, editors. SEER Cancer Statistics Review, 1973–1999. Bethesda MD: National Cancer Institute, 2002:23–124 http:/seer.cancer.gov/csr/1973-1999/.
16. Glass AG, Hoover RN. The emerging epidemic of melanoma and squamous cell skin cancer. JAMA 1989;262(15):2097–100.
17. Gysler M, March CM, Mishell DR Jr, Bailey EJ. A decade's experience with an individualized clomiphene treatment regimen including its effect on the postcoital test. Fertil Steril 1982;37(2):161–7.
18. Cornel MC, ten Kate LP, Dukes MN, de Jong-v D, Berg LT, Meyboom RH, Garbis H, Peters PW. Ovulation induction and neural tube defects. Lancet 1989;1(8651):1386.
19. James WH. The sex ratio of infants born after hormonal induction of ovulation. Br J Obstet Gynaecol 1985;92(3):299–301.
20. Bishai R, Arbour L, Lyons C, Koren G. Intrauterine exposure to clomiphene and neonatal persistent hyperplastic primary vitreous. Teratology 1999;60(3):143–5.
21. Wilcox AJ, Baird DD, Weinberg CR, Hornsby PP, Herbst AL. Fertility in men exposed prenatally to diethylstilbestrol. N Engl J Med 1995;332:1411–6.
22. Sorensen HT, Pedersen L, Skriver MV, Norgaard M, Norgard B, Hatch EE. Use of clomifene during early pregnancy and risk of hypospadias: population based case-control study. BMJ 2005;330:126–7.

Cyclofenil

General Information

Cyclofenil is a weak non-steroidal estrogen related to diethylstilbestrol. For a number of years it was used for inducing ovulation, but has lost favor; more recently there have been studies of its possible effects in Raynaud's phenomenon secondary to scleroderma (1).

Up to 2% of patients taking cyclofenil complain of nausea, vomiting, hot flushes, or headache. Mild abdominal pain has been reported in up to 18%, ovarian enlargement without cysts in 3%, and galactorrhea in 4%. There have been a few case reports of hemolytic anemia (SED-12, 1034) (2).

Organs and Systems

Liver

Cyclofenil can cause reversible mild cholestatic jaundice. The authors of a review of 30 patients with hepatic reactions to cyclofenil concluded that liver derangement due to cyclofenil is probably related to metabolic hypersusceptibility rather than to a direct toxic effect (3). There is a surprising lack of such reports from countries where cyclofenil was widely used: in France, at least, the number of cases of hepatitis occurring is known to have been much greater than that reported in print, and the drug was abandoned in that country in 1988.

References

1. Pope J, Fenlon D, Thompson A, Shea B, Furst D, Wells G, Silman A. Cyclofenil for Raynaud's phenomenon in progressive systemic sclerosis. Cochrane Database Syst Rev 2000;(2):CD000955.
2. Wollheim FA, Ljunggren HO, Blom-Bulow B. Hemolytic anemia during cyclofenil treatment of scleroderma. Acta Med Scand 1981;210(5):429–30.
3. Olsson R, Tyllstrom J, Zettergren L. Hepatic reactions to cyclofenil. Gut 1983;24(3):260–3.

Danazol

See also Androgens and anabolic steroids

General Information

Danazol is a weak androgen and can thus exert the adverse effects of androgens, but because it inhibits LH and FSH secretion it can also elicit menopausal-like symptoms. However, from time to time it has other types of adverse effect. It has been used with some success in the management of pelvic pain associated with endometriosis (1), heavy menstrual bleeding (2), and idiopathic thrombocytopenic purpura (3). It is ineffective in unexplained subfertility (4).

Organs and Systems

Cardiovascular

A 42-year-old woman, with no history of smoking, had an acute myocardial infarct 2 months after she had started to take danazol 100 mg/day (5). There have been occasional reports of thrombosis during danazol treatment, possibly because of effects on low-density lipoprotein cholesterol, raised glucose concentrations, or an increase in the platelet count. It would at all events seem wise to avoid danazol in patients at particular risk of coronary artery disease.

Respiratory

A patient developed pulmonary fibrosis after having taken danazol for 2 months for idiopathic thrombocytopenic purpura (6). He developed bilateral pneumothoraces and pneumomediastinum and died. An association between danazol and lung fibrosis has been reported only once before; here it could have been coincidental or a reflection of a pathological process underlying the originally diagnosed disorder.

Liver

Like other anabolic steroids, danazol can cause cholestatic jaundice (7).

In five women with advanced, recurrent, or persistent endometrial cancer not amenable to other means of treatment, danazol 100 mg qds had to be withdrawn because of toxicity, four with hepatic complications (8).

A further case of danazol-induced hepatocellular carcinoma has been reported (9), to add to three described before.

- A 37-year-old woman with refractory idiopathic thrombocytopenic purpura, who had responded dramatically to danazol 600 mg/day after the failure of other forms of treatment, developed a multinodular well-differentiated trabeculovesicular hepatocellular tumor after 5 years. There were no metastases and no invasion of the lymph nodes, and after chemoembolization she received an orthoptic liver transplant. A year later she remained in good condition.

References

1. Selak V, Farquhar C, Prentice A, Singla A. Danazol for pelvic pain associated with endometriosis. Cochrane Database Syst Rev 2007;(4):CD000068.
2. Beaumont H, Augood C, Duckitt K, Lethaby A. Danazol for heavy menstrual bleeding. Cochrane Database Syst Rev 2007;(3):CD001017.
3. Andrès E, Zimmer J, Noel E, Kaltenbach G, Koumarianou A, Maloisel F. Idiopathic thrombocytopenic purpura: a retrospective analysis in 139 patients of the influence of age on the response to corticosteroids, splenectomy and danazol. Drugs Aging 2003;20(11):841–6.
4. Hughes E, Brown J, Tiffin G, Vandekerckhove P. Danazol for unexplained subfertility. Cochrane Database Syst Rev 2007;(1):CD000069.
5. Boos C.J, Dawes M, Jones R, Farrell T. Danazol treatment and acute myocardial infarction. J Obstet Gynecol 2003;23:327–8.
6. Pakhale S, Moltyaner Y, Chamberlain D, Lazar N. Rapidly progressive pulmonary fibrosis in a patient treated with danazol for idiopathic thrombocytopenic purpura. Can Resp J 2004;11:55–7.
7. Malaguarnera M, Santangelo N, Motta M, Pistone G. Danazol induced cholestasis: pathogenetic hypothesis. Panminerva Med 1997;39(3):244–7.
8. Covens A, Brunetto VL, Markman M, Orr JW Jr, Lentz SS, Benda J. Phase II trial of danazol in advanced, recurrent, or persistent endometrial cancer: a Gynecologic Oncology Group study. Gynecol Oncol 2003;89:470–4.
9. Confavreux C, Seve P, Broussolle C, Renaudier P, Ducerf C. Danazol-induced hepatocellular carcinoma. Quart J Med 2003;96:317–8.

Diethylstilbestrol

General Information

For a complete account of the adverse effects of estrogens, readers should consult the following monographs as well as this one:

- Estrogens
- Hormonal contraceptives—emergency contraception
- Hormonal contraceptives—oral
- Hormone replacement therapy—estrogens
- Hormone replacement therapy—estrogens + androgens
- Hormone replacement therapy—estrogens + progestogens.

Diethylstilbestrol and other non-steroidal estrogens came into vogue at a time when the cost of producing steroidal estrogens, whether synthetic or of natural origin, was still prohibitive. They have largely fallen out of favor, in view of the association between the use of diethylstilbestrol in pregnancy and second-generation injury. There seems to be no reason for believing that the short-term acute adverse reactions to these non-steroidal compounds differ from those of estrogenic steroids.

Diethylstilbestrol continues to be recommended in some centers as one of the agents of last resort when prostate cancer proves refractory to steroid hormones or androgen deprivation therapy has done all it can (1). In a Japanese study in which 16 patients were given a daily intravenous injection of diethylstilbestrol diphosphate 250 mg for 28 days, the short-term response was favorable and the drug was well tolerated (2).

Organs and Systems

Cardiovascular

In a randomized study of men treated hormonally for prostatic cancer (3), cardiovascular adverse effects were reported more often in patients treated with diethylstilbestrol than in those treated with cyproterone acetate. The risk was highest during the first 6 months of treatment.

Mineral balance

Profound hypocalcemia occurred in a patient with osteoblastic metastatic carcinoma of the prostate after treatment with diethylstilbestrol 15 mg/day for 7 days (SED-12, 1032) (4).

Hematologic

The risk of thromboembolic complications when diethylstilbestrol is used in treating prostatic cancer is well documented, but there has been some doubt as to the mechanisms involved. Oral diethylstilbestrol diphosphate 300 mg/day has been compared with LR-RH agonist therapy or no treatment in 35 patients with prostatic cancer (5). Diethylstilbestrol reduced the concentrations of protein S to below the lower limit of normal in 24 of the 35 cases. There was also some reduction in antithrombin III concentrations. These results were consistently confirmed in a follow-up group of eight further patients who took diethylstilbestrol. Since these very low concentrations of protein S are virtually the same as those found in congenital deficiency, it seems likely that this plays a role in the development of cardiovascular complications during diethylstilbestrol treatment.

Liver

Liver damage has again been attributed to diethylstilbestrol (6).

- A 65-year-old man started to take diethylstilbestrol 1 mg bd for prostatic cancer (Gleason grade 3). After 11 years of treatment without metastasis he was switched to treatment with an LH-RH analogue, which was regarded as safer, but at this time his liver function tests were found to be seriously deranged. Biopsy showed established cirrhosis with steatohepatitis. He had no history of excessive alcohol intake, and it seemed likely that the diethylstilbestrol was the cause of the liver disorder.

A Japanese paper of 1989 reported six similar cases, but no others appear to be on record.

Immunologic

In 13 women exposed to diethylstilbestrol in utero compared with similar control subjects with respect to the in vitro T cell response to the mitogens phytohemagglutinin, concanavalin A, and interleukin-2, incorporation of tritiated thymidine into T cells from diethylstilbestrol-exposed women was increased three-fold over a range of concentrations in response to concanavalin A, increased by 50% over a range of concentrations in response to phytohemagglutinin, and increased two-fold in response to the endogenous mitogen interleukin-2 (7). This in vitro evidence of a change in T cell-mediated immunity clearly raises questions about the clinical consequences.

Long-Term Effects

Tumorigenicity

Exposure to diethylstilbestrol during pregnancy in 4836 women has been reported to carry a relative risk of 1.27 of breast cancer later in life. However, the authors found no evidence to support the link between diethylstilbestrol exposure and ovarian, endometrial, or other cancers.

In a 25-year follow-up study there were very slightly more breast tumors in women using diethylstilbestrol in pregnancy and significantly more cancer deaths (8).

In one study there was a six-fold risk of endometrial cancer among estrogen users compared with non-users; long-term users (over 5 years) had a 15-fold risk; there were excess risks for both diethylstilbestrol and conjugated estrogens (9).

Diethylstilbestrol can cause hepatic adenomas and carcinomas in experimental animals (10), and hepatocellular carcinoma has been reported in a man who took a total of 668 g over 12 years for suspected carcinoma of the prostate (11).

Second-Generation Effects

Teratogenicity

Diethylstilbestrol was used extensively in pregnancies between 1940 and about 1975, in the belief that it could protect threatened pregnancies and counter the risk of spontaneous abortion. Toward the end of that period, increasingly clear evidence emerged that diethylstilbestrol could have an adverse effect on the second generation that did not become apparent until puberty or adulthood, and perhaps could also appear in the third generation (12). It appears to be the only estrogen with this effect, but it is naturally not excluded that some structurally related non-steroidal estrogens might carry the same risk, although these have never been used in the same way in pregnancy.

The current difficulty in many reports of second-generation complications is to determine whether the mother actually took diethylstilbestrol during her pregnancy. In a case of a very large clear-cell carcinoma of the cervix in a teenager with no known history of maternal use of diethylstilbestrol, in view of the dates it was likely to have been non-drug-related, but the possibility of third-generation effects must also be borne in mind (13).

Clear cell adenocarcinomas of the vagina and cervix induced by prenatal exposure to this drug metastasize to the lungs. The secondaries generally appear within 2–3 years of the initial diagnosis. Unusually, a case has been reported in which pulmonary metastases occurred more than 15 years after presentation of the primary tumor (14). This makes it clear that patients of this type should be followed up in the very long term.

History

Diethylstilbestrol provides several illustrations of how societies cope with the risks of harm from a drug. Under different brand names diethylstilbestrol has been given to a wide range of patients over many years, mostly pregnant women and aging men with prostate cancer. The history of iatrogenic disease as a result of the use of diethylstilbestrol in pregnant women shows that patients can play an important role in securing legitimacy for research and the publication of data on the harmful effects of a drug.

Diethylstilbestrol was given to pregnant women in many countries, mainly in the 1940s to 1970s, in the mistaken belief that it would prevent miscarriage and provide strong healthy babies (15,16). The application to market diethylstilbestrol in the USA was the first new drug application submitted to the FDA shortly after the 1938 Food, Drugs, and Cosmetics Act had been passed; permission was granted, although diethylstilbestrol had already been identified as a carcinogen in animals (17). Diethylstilbestrol was especially popular in some maternity clinics in North America, serving middle-class and upper-middle class women, and in the Netherlands, where the Queen's gynecologist promoted it. In other countries it was dispensed through public health maternity centers.

In the USA, evidence showing that it was ineffective for its intended purpose appeared by the 1950s. However, conclusions based on animal experiments, as well as a major double-blind, controlled clinical trial (18), remained unheeded, partly because prescribing physicians trusted their collegial loyalty more than data that implicitly threw doubt on their practice.

In 1971, a rare form of aggressive cancer in the vagina of young girls was attributed to the girls' exposure to diethylstilbestrol in utero in a report that was based on a case-control study of eight young women, two of whom had died, at the Massachusetts General Hospital (19). It was already clear from this small study that monitoring young women exposed to diethylstilbestrol would save lives. However, months and even years were to pass before the discovery led to any public action, at different times in different countries. Only after 5 months, when the risk of cancer in patients exposed to diethylstilbestrol was featured at hearings in the US Congress, did the FDA react. The FDA's Administrator then announced that diethylstilbestrol products were to be labelled with a warning that diethylstilbestrol was contraindicated in pregnancy and should not be given to pregnant women because of risk of the cancer in the offspring (20).

Drug regulatory agencies in other countries in which diethylstilbestrol had also been commonly used in pregnancy delayed taking action. In the Netherlands, the first change of labelling to include a warning to physicians that diethylstilbestrol given to pregnant women might harm the fetus was implemented in 1972. A similar change in labelling was introduced in France in 1977. In many other countries, the news that some daughters of women who had taken diethylstilbestrol while pregnant were at risk of developing a potentially lethal cancer was passed over in silence.

In Britain, the medical community was alerted to the risks by an editorial in the British Medical Journal in 1971, but it was only in 1973 that the Committee on Safety of Medicines advised against the use of diethylstilbestrol during pregnancy (21). In Britain, drugs were commonly not labelled with information about their contents, nor with warnings of risk until well into the 1990s; thus, patients were kept in ignorance. No measures have yet been taken in Britain to alert the public to the need for medical surveillance of women who have been exposed to diethylstilbestrol in utero.

It is estimated that in the USA, the Netherlands, and France, diethylstilbestrol was given to over 5.3 million pregnant women, and it is known that it has been given to pregnant women in most parts of the world. Single cases of clear-cell vaginal carcinoma from many countries are known, but systematic studies have not been conducted everywhere.

One in a thousand young women exposed to diethylstilbestrol before birth have been estimated to be at risk of developing clear-cell vaginal adenocarcinoma (22). Exposure to diethylstilbestrol in utero also has a range of other effects on exposed women, including malformations of the reproductive organs and difficulties in conception and carrying a pregnancy to term. Some of the men exposed to diethylstilbestrol in utero have urogenital malformations and an increased risk of testicular cancer (23).

Most of the women who suspected that they had taken diethylstilbestrol were to learn of the problems from the media, and they had to guess that their daughters might be at risk of developing cancer. When they tried to discover whether they had been given diethylstilbestrol during pregnancy, many of the women found that their obstetricians were not willing to give them access to their own medical records. In a report from a nationwide US survey intended to locate pregnant women who had been given diethylstilbestrol during 1940–72, the investigators complained that at some clinics they had encountered extreme difficulties in getting access to the records (24). Women who have been exposed to diethylstilbestrol sometimes say that never have so many medical files reportedly been lost through fire and inundation, as when they asked for access to records that might document the use of diethylstilbestrol during pregnancy.

Many doctors did not notice or did not heed warnings in the early 1970s about the risks of giving diethylstilbestrol to pregnant women. As late as 1974, according to one writer, some 11 000 prescriptions for diethylstilbestrol to be used during pregnancy were written in the USA (25). In 1976, it was observed that diethylstilbestrol was given to unsuspecting pregnant women in several Latin-American countries (25). In other countries, prescribing physicians' responses to reports that linked the use of diethylstilbestrol during pregnancy with cancer risks in their daughters were even slower. The latest documented prescription of diethylstilbestrol in Europe was in Spain in 1983 (26).

The first batches of educational material for physicians, with warnings and advice regarding health care for women who had been exposed to diethylstilbestrol, were distributed in the USA in 1971, in the Netherlands in 1974, and in France in 1989. No such material has been distributed in Britain.

Mothers in the USA who had taken diethylstilbestrol formed an organization, DES Action, to inform the public about the risks and to alert exposed mothers that their daughters needed regular medical examinations, so that potential tumor development would be detected early. Through DES Action they also gave each other mutual support during litigation against the manufacturers and acted politically to ensure that health care would be available for their daughters. DES Action groups outside the USA were formed in Australia, Belgium, Canada, France, Great Britain, Italy, Ireland, and the Netherlands. DES Action was still in the 1990s a prime mover in securing resources for research and follow-up of women who had been exposed to diethylstilbestrol, and in promoting educational programs for those women and for medical professionals.

Initiatives by medical researchers, by DES Action, and by the Public Citizen's Health Research Group secured funding in the USA for medical research on the prevalence of cancer and other effects in the young women who had been exposed in utero, and eventually also the men. The US National Institute for Environmental Health Sciences (NIEHS) has been one of the centers for toxicological studies of the effects of diethylstilbestrol. A substantial amount of research on the effects of diethylstilbestrol—animal experiments as well as epidemiological studies—has produced a valuable body of knowledge about how hormones affect the development of the fetus and prime the individual for disease later in life.

As in the case of thalidomide, the emotional engagement evoked by the harm caused by diethylstilbestrol in pregnancy led to committed action. Some physicians have devoted a major part of their careers to finding out why and how diethylstilbestrol produced adverse effects. The anger over the harm caused by diethylstilbestrol inspired patients to a commitment to prevent further harm by engaging in political action and achieving an effective response from legislators and governmental administrators. Despite the abandonment of diethylstilbestrol in pregnancy for habitual or threatened abortion, its late effects continue to be reported. Essentially, the female offspring of these pregnancies tend to develop vaginal changes (adenosis, with cervical ectropion) when reaching adolescence or adulthood and these can subsequently give rise to a clear-cell adenocarcinoma. Whereas carcinomas are a late and infrequent event, even in exposed subjects, cervical vaginal adenosis is common, the incidence probably being some 30% (27). The estimated tumor risk is only 0.14–1.4 per 1000 diethylstilbestrol-exposed subjects, but since up to 6 million fetuses were exposed to diethylstilbestrol between 1940 and 1970 the total number affected in some way may be very high indeed. There is also a high incidence of fertility disturbances among these daughters, and their own pregnancies apparently stand a high chance of not going normally to term (SED-12, 1023) (28). Analogous changes were found in male offspring (29). As in the case of thalidomide, an important element in determining cause and effect was the characteristic nature of the defect: the vaginal pathology does occur spontaneously but is highly unusual. A major problem has been the fact that the defect is as a rule only recognizable so many years after birth, by which time the history of the original treatment may be difficult or impossible to reconstruct. Even today the material is not homogeneous and strict statistical analysis of some of the epidemiological data has been claimed to point to a series of shortcomings. This does not undermine the clear conclusion

that the drug is indeed responsible for the effects described (30).

Epidemiological studies on the complications of the use of diethylstilbestrol in pregnancy will certainly produce new data as time goes on: most of the data will probably continue to come from the USA and the Netherlands, where diethylstilbestrol was much more widely used to treat habitual or threatened abortion than elsewhere. In France 150 000–200 000 pregnancies were involved; in the Netherlands, with a much smaller population, 180 000–380 000 pregnant women were treated with diethylstilbestrol up to 1976.

Vaginal adenosis and adenocarcinoma

Second-generation (and possible third-generation) effects of diethylstilbestrol continue to be reported (31,32). Typical is a 1987 update analysing 519 cases of clear-cell carcinoma of the vagina and cervix identified by the Registry for Research on Hormonal Transplacental Carcinogenesis of the University of Chicago (23); in 60% of all cases the patient's mother could be shown to have used diethylstilbestrol during pregnancy. The median age at diagnosis was 19 years. The authors argued that in view of the relative rarity of the tumors, even in exposed women, one could consider that diethylstilbestrol is not a complete carcinogen and that some other factor is also involved in the pathogenesis of this type of carcinoma. The particular question of third-generation injury has actually been the subject of judicial proceedings in the USA (31,32); on the balance of evidence it seems that it can occur, although the mechanism is not clear.

Evidence has also emerged on long-term survival in young women with a clear-cell adenocarcinoma of the vagina, 20% of whom had been exposed to diethylstilbestrol and 80% had not (33). The probabilities of survival at 5 and 10 years for diethylstilbestrol-associated cases were 84 and 78% respectively, compared with 69 and 60% for those not associated with diethylstilbestrol. These differences were not due to differences in clinical prognostic factors, but suggest differences in tumor behavior for as yet undetermined reasons.

Although it is more than 30 years since the full extent of the injury to offspring by the ill-advised use of diethylstilbestrol during pregnancy became clear, details of that injury are still being filled in as the individuals concerned grow older. The picture will continue to develop as long as this generation of individuals lives, and it is even possible that findings in the third generation will throw light on the persisting injury to the family.

Psychological research among "DES daughters" has shown how traumatic it can be for a woman to learn of her prenatal exposure to diethylstilbestrol, and the extent to which this creates persistent uncertainty about her health; the failure of a physician to provide reliable information and continuing support can severely undermine her faith in health care (34).

Long-term studies of the pregnancy experiences of women exposed to diethylstilbestrol in utero, compared with unexposed women, now include one in the US National Collaborative Diethylstilbestrol Adenosis

Table 1 Outcomes in pregnancies exposed and not exposed to diethylstilbestrol

Outcome	Exposed (%)	Non-exposed (%)
Full-term delivery	64	85
Spontaneous abortion	19	10
Preterm delivery	12	4.1
Ectopic pregnancy	4.2	0.8

cohort and one in the Chicago cohort and their respective non-exposed comparison groups. A review of questionnaire replies from 3373 exposed daughters and from controls has confirmed that diethylstilbestrol-exposed women were less likely than unexposed women to have had full-term live births and more likely to have had premature births, spontaneous pregnancy losses, or ectopic pregnancies (35). The data are shown in Table 1. Second-trimester spontaneous pregnancy losses were much more common in diethylstilbestrol-exposed women.

Pregnancy

The long and tragic tale of the complications resulting from the use of diethylstilbestrol in pregnancy between 1948 and 1975 has still not yet been fully told. The methodological errors made by OW Smith in the 1948 paper that launched this dangerous and ineffective treatment have been reviewed as a striking example of the need for critical clinical studies in any field (36). Although the use of diethylstilbestrol in pregnancy fortunately ended in much of the world more than 30 years ago, cases are still being reported of women who were exposed to the drug during their prenatal life and later developed severe reproductive problems. There have been various cases of rupture of the uterus in mid-pregnancy, and a rupture of a previously unscarred uterus during the first trimester has now also bee reported (37).

- A 28 year-old woman undergoing her first pregnancy developed a uterine rupture in the anterior fundal area of the uterus during the first trimester. Both tubes were normal.

The event presumably reflected thinness of the uterine wall, which has been described before in women who were exposed to diethylstilbestrol before birth.

Other cancers

Long-term data are also accumulating on the actual incidence of genital cancer in women exposed to diethylstilbestrol in utero (38). In the Netherlands, a country in which diethylstilbestrol was used intensively in pregnancy, there is evidence that the risk of cervical cancer in these women is trebled, rather than doubled as was previously supposed (39).

- A diethylstilbestrol-exposed woman developed concurrent primary cancers of both the vagina and the endometrium at the age of 39 (40).

However, it is important to bear in mind that cases occur in which there is no history of the mother's having taken

diethylstilbestrol during pregnancy. In one such case, HIV/AIDS infection was also a predisposing factor for vaginal carcinoma and this could explain a proportion of new cases that are being reported today (41).

A further follow-up and analysis of 3879 women, taken from two earlier US studies, who had been exposed to diethylstilbestrol during pregnancy has been presented (42). The results showed a modest association between diethylstilbestrol exposure and the risk of breast cancer (RR = 1.27; 95% CI = 1.07, 1.52). The increased risk was not further aggravated by a family history of breast cancer, by use of oral contraceptives, or by HRT. There was no evidence that diethylstilbestrol was associated with a raised risk of ovarian, endometrial, or other hormone-associated cancers.

Sensory systems

A study in the USA has produced some evidence that in people with amblyopia, those who were exposed to diethylstilbestrol before birth may be more likely to develop myopia (43).

Menstrual and vaginal disturbances

The effects of in-utero exposure to diethylstilbestrol on the menstrual cycle have been studied prospectively in 198 women and in 162 unexposed controls (44). A major limitation of this study was the exclusion of women with a severe menstrual abnormality. Exposure to diethylstilbestrol was associated with a statistical significantly lower duration of menstrual bleeding but not with dysmenorrhea. For most women exposed to diethylstilbestrol, any effects on reproductive hormonal function are in all probability minor, if present at all.

Even the classic genital manifestations of diethylstilbestrol in women who have been exposed to it in fetal life may be overlooked unless one is alert to them; vaginal discharge with ectropion should cause one to enquire as to possible prenatal diethylstilbestrol exposure (45).

Autoimmune disease

During the last 15 years, various additional aspects of the diethylstilbestrol problem have given rise to concern. One emerged in 1988 from a large multicenter epidemiological cohort study established by the US National Cancer Institute (DESAD Project), in which it was found that women exposed in utero to diethylstilbestrol had a 50% increased incidence of autoimmune disease (46).

Third-generation effects

Even more disconcerting than the second-generation effects in women exposed to diethylstilbestrol during pregnancy is the possibility of third-generation effects. There is no certainty regarding these, but worrying cases have been reported at intervals over the last thirty years or more (SED-14, 1449).

- Ovarian carcinoma occurred in an adolescent girl with a suggestive history. The tumor was a small-cell carcinoma of the ovary, which is excessively rare in childhood and adolescence (47). Her grandmother had taken diethylstilbestrol when she was pregnant with her mother. Her mother had in later life undergone hysterectomy for a cervical dysplasia, another condition that could have been due to exposure to diethylstilbestrol.

A current hypothesis is that in utero exposure to diethylstilbestrol leads to genetic or epigenetic changes in the primordial oocytes that are formed in the first trimester of gestation in the daughter. These changes can then be inherited by grandchildren.

Drug Administration

Drug formulations

The parenteral formulation diethylstilbestrol diphosphate is less commonly used than the oral formulation. In Japan, 24 elderly patients with advanced relapsed prostatic cancer were treated with high doses supplemented with ethinylestradiol (doses unclear); there was some slight therapeutic effect, but there were gastrointestinal symptoms and fluid retention (48). Also in Japan, a few patients with advanced disease were treated using intravenous diethylstilbestrol diphosphate 500 mg/day for 20 consecutive days to a total dose of 10 g; the authors' conclusion was more positive but adverse events were not specified (49).

Drug contamination

Contamination of isoniazid tablets with diethylstilbestrol was the cause of several cases of precocious puberty in a children's tuberculosis ward (50).

References

1. Lonning PE, Taylor PD, Anker G, Iddon J, Wie L, Jorgensen LM, Mella O, Howell A. High-dose estrogen treatment in postmenopausal breast cancer patients heavily exposed to endocrine therapy. Breast Cancer Res Treat 2001;67(2):111–6.
2. Takezawa Y, Nakata S, Kobayashi M, Kosaku N, Fukabori Y, Yamanaka H. Moderate dose diethylstilbestrol diphosphate therapy in hormone refractory prostate cancer. Scand J Urol Nephrol 2001;35(4):283–7.
3. Pavone-Macaluso M, de Voogt HJ, Viggiano G, Barasolo E, Lardennois B, de Pauw M, Sylvester R. Comparison of diethylstilbestrol, cyproterone acetate and medroxyprogesterone acetate in the treatment of advanced prostatic cancer: final analysis of a randomized phase III trial of the European Organization for Research on Treatment of Cancer Urological Group. J Urol 1986;136(3):624–31.
4. Harley HA, Mason R, Phillips PJ. Profound hypocalcaemia associated with oestrogen treatment of carcinoma of the prostate. Med J Aust 1983;2(1):41–2.
5. Hayashi N, Wada T, Ikemoto I, Oishi Y, Suzuki H, Ueda M. Decrease in anticoagulant factors in patients with prostate cancer treated with diethylstilbestrol diphosphate. Nippon Hinyokika Gakkai Zasschi 2003;94:420–7.
6. Cooper L, Palmer M, Oien K. Cirrhosis with steatohepatitis following longterm stilboestrol treatment. J Clin Pathol 2003;56:639.
7. Burke L, Segall-Blank M, Lorenzo C, Dynesius-Trentham R, Trentham D, Mortola JF. Altered immune response in adult women exposed to diethylstilbestrol in utero. Am J Obstet Gynecol 2001;185(1):78–81.
8. Herbst AL, editor. Intrauterine exposure to diethlystilbestrol in the human. Proceedings, "Symposium on DES". Chicago: American College of Obstetricians and Gynecologists, 1977.
9. Antunes CM, Strolley PD, Rosenshein NB, Davies JL, Tonascia JA, Brown C, Burnett L, Rutledge A, Pokempner M, Garcia R. Endometrial cancer and estrogen use. Report of a large case-control study. N Engl J Med 1979;300(1):9–13.
10. Williams GM, Iatropoulos M, Cheung R, Radi L, Wang CX. Diethylstilbestrol liver carcinogenicity and modification of DNA in rats. Cancer Lett 1993;68(2–3):193–8.
11. Rosinus V, Maurer R. [Diättylstilböstrol-induziertes Leberzellkarzinom? Diethylstilbestrol-induced liver cancer?] Schweiz Med Wochenschr 1981;111(30):1139–42.
12. Martino MA, Nevadunsky NS, Magliaro TJ, Goldberg MI. The DES (diethylstilbestrol) years: bridging the past into the future. Prim Care Update Ob Gyns 2002;9:7–12.
13. Ding D-C, Chang F-W, Yu M-H. Huge clear cell carcinoma of the cervix in teenager not associated with diethylstilbestrol: a brief case report. Eur J Obstet Gynecol Reprod Biol 2004;117:115-6.
14. Hall WB, Detterbeck FC, Livasy CA, Fowler WC Jr. Endobronchial clear cell adenocarcinoma occurring in a patient 15 years after treatment for DES-associated vaginal clear cell adenocarcinoma. Gynecol Oncol 2004;93:708–10.
15. Smith OW. Diethylstilbestrol in prevention of complications of pregnancy. Am J Obstet Gynecol 1948;56:821–34.
16. Smith OW, Smith GV. The influence of diethylstilbestrol on the progress and outcome of pregnancy as based on a comparison of treated with untreated primigravidas. Am J Obstet Gynecol 1949;58(5):994–1009.
17. Lacassagne A. Apparition d'adénocarcinomes mammaires chez des souris mâles traités par une substance oestrogène synthétique. Comptes Rend Séances Soc Biol 1938;129:641–3.
18. Dieckmann WJ, Davis ME, Rynkiewicz LM, Pottinger RE. Does the administration of diethylstilbestrol during pregnancy have therapeutic value? Am J Obstet Gynecol 1953;66(5):1062–81.
19. Herbst AL, Ulfelder H, Poskanzer DC. Adenocarcinoma of the vagina. Association of maternal stilbestrol therapy with tumor appearance in young women. N Engl J Med 1971;284(15):878–81.
20. US Department of Health, Education and Welfare, Food and Drug Administration. Certain estrogens for oral or parenteral use. Drugs for human use. Drug efficacy study implementation. Federal Register 1971;36(217):21537–8.
21. Mitchell S, Wait J. Face the Facts. BBC Radio 4 21 February 2000.
22. Melnick S, Cole P, Anderson D, Herbst A. Rates and risks of diethylstilbestrol-related clear-cell adenocarcinoma of the vagina and cervix. An update. N Engl J Med 1987;316(9):514–6.
23. Palmlund I. Exposure to a xenoestrogen before birth: the diethylstilbestrol experience. J Psychosom Obstet Gynaecol 1996;17(2):71–84.
24. Nash S, Tilley BC, Kurland LT, Gundersen J, Barnes AB, Labarthe D, Donohew PS, Kovacs L. Identifying and tracing a population at risk: the DESAD Project experience. Am J Public Health 1983;73(3):253–9.

25. Norwood C. In: At highest risk: environmental hazards to young and unborn children. New York: McGraw-Hill, 1980:141.

26. Direcks A, Figueroa S, Mintzes B, Banta D. DES European Study: DES Action the Netherlands for the European Commission Programme "Europe Against Cancer". Utrecht: DES Action the Netherlands 1991;13:25.

27. Sopena-Bonnet B. L'adénose cervico-vaginale: l'une des conséquences possibles de l'exposition in utero au DES. Contracept Fertil Sex 1989;17:461.

28. Senekjian EK, Potkul RK, Frey K, Herbst AL. Infertility among daughters either exposed or not exposed to diethylstilbestrol. Am J Obstet Gynecol 1988;158(3 Pt 1):493–8.

29. Hembree WC, Nagler HM, Fang JS, Myles EL, Jagiello GM. Infertility in a patient with abnormal spermatogenesis and in utero DES exposure. Int J Fertil 1988;33(3):173–7.

30. Buitendijk S. Diethylstilbestrol and the next generation—a challenge to the evidence? In: Dukes MNG, editor. Side Effects of Drugs, Annual 12. Amsterdam: Elsevier, 1988:346–8.

31. Lynch HT, Quinn T, Severin MJ. Diethylstilbestrol, teratogenesis and carcinogenesis: medical/legal implications of its long-term sequelae, including third-generation effects. Int J Risk Safety Med 1990;1:171.

32. Curran WJ. The DES product liability story in America: the third generation litigation. Int J Risk Safety Med 1992;3:229.

33. Waggoner SE, Mittendorf R, Biney N, Anderson D, Herbst AL. Influence of in utero diethylstilbestrol exposure on the prognosis and biologic behavior of vaginal clear-cell adenocarcinoma. Gynecol Oncol 1994;55(2):238–44.

34. Duke SS, McGraw SA, Avis NE, Sherman A. A focus group study of DES daughters: implications for health care providers. Psychooncology 2000;9(5):439–44.

35. Kaufman RH, Adam E, Hatch EE, Noller K, Herbst AL, Palmer JR, Hoover RN. Continued follow-up of pregnancy outcomes in diethylstilbestrol-exposed offspring. Obstet Gynecol 2000;96(4):483–9.

36. Bamigboye AA, Hofmeyr GJ, Morris J. Diethylstilbestrol—haunting lessons. S Afr Med J 2003;93:346–7.

37. Porcu G, Courbiere B, Sakr R, Carcopino X, Gamerre M. Spontaneous rupture of a first-trimester gravid uterus in a woman exposed to diethylstilbestrol in utero: a case report. J Reprod Med 2003;48:744–6.

38. Herbst AL. Behavior of estrogen-associated female genital tract cancer and its relation to neoplasia following intrauterine exposure to diethylstilbestrol (DES). Gynecol Oncol 2000;76(2):147–56.

39. Verloop J, Rookus MA, van Leeuwen FE. Prevalence of gynecologic cancer in women exposed to diethylstilbestrol in utero. N Engl J Med 2000;342(24):1838–9.

40. Keller C, Nanda R, Shannon RL, Amit A, Kaplan AL. Concurrent primaries of vaginal clear cell adenocarcinoma and endometrial adenocarcinoma in a 39-year old woman with in utero diethylstilbestrol exposure. Int J Gynecol Cancer 2001;11(3):247–50.

41. Izquierdo Mendez N, Herraiz Martinez MA, Furio Bacete V, Cristobal Garcia I, Vidart Aragon JA, Escudero Fernandez M. Adenocarcinoma de celulas claras de cupula vaginal sin relacion con des (dietilestilbestrol): a proposito de un caso y revision de la literatura. Acta Ginecol 2001;58:21–6.

42. Titus-Ernstoff L, Hatch EE, Hoover RN, Palmer J, Greenberg ER, Ricker W, Kaufman R, Noller K, Herbst AL, Colton T, Hartge P. Long-term cancer risk in women given diethylstilbestrol (DES) during pregnancy. Br J Cancer 2001;84(1):126–33.

43. Lempert P. Myopia in diethylstilboestrol exposed amblyopic subjects. Br J Ophthalmol 1999;83(1):126.

44. Hornsby PP, Wilcox AJ, Weinberg CR, Herbst AL. Effects on the menstrual cycle of in utero exposure to diethylstilbestrol. Am J Obstet Gynecol 1994;170(3):709–15.

45. Wingfield M. Not just a cervical ectropion. Three case reports of diethylstilbestrol (DES) exposed women presenting with vaginal discharge and cervical ectropion. J Obstet Gynaecol 1999;19(6):649–51.

46. Noller KL, Blair PB, O'Brien PC, Melton LJ 3rd, Offord JR, Kaufman RH, Colton T. Increased occurrence of autoimmune disease among women exposed in utero to diethylstilbestrol. Fertil Steril 1988;49(6):1080–2.

47. Blatt J, Van Le L, Weiner T, Sailer S. Ovarian carcinoma in an adolescent with transgenerational exposure to diethylstilbestrol. J Pediatr Hematol/Oncol 2003;25:635–6.

48. Hisamatsu H, Sakai H, Kanetake H. High-dose intravenous diethylstilbestrol diphosphate (DES-DP) in the treatment of prostatic cancer during relapse. Nioshinihon J Urol 2002;64:199–202.

49. Michinaga S, Ariyoshi A. High-dose intravenous diethylstilbestrol diphosphate therapy for hormone-refractory prostate cancer. Nishinihon J Urol 2002;64:203–5.

50. Weber WW, Grossman M, Thom JV, Sax J, Chan JJ, Duffy M. Drug contamination with diethylstilbestrol. Outbreak of precocious puberty due to contaminated isonicoeinic acid hydrazide (INH). N Engl J Med 1963;268:411–5.

Estrogens

General Information

For a complete account of the adverse effects of estrogens, readers should consult the following monographs as well as this one:

- Diethylstilbestrol
- Hormonal contraceptives—emergency contraception
- Hormonal contraceptives—oral
- Hormone replacement therapy—estrogens
- Hormone replacement therapy—estrogens + androgens
- Hormone replacement therapy—estrogens + progestogens.

The physiological secretion of endogenous estrogens rises and falls during the monthly cycle; it is much lower before the menarche and after the menopause than during the period of fertility. Any use of estrogens that deviates from this pattern is therefore unphysiological.

Types of estrogen

The primary estrogen in premenopausal women is 17-β-estradiol (E2), which is synthesized by developing ovarian follicles. Estradiol is oxidized to estrone (E1) and then to estriol (E3). Estrone is also produced in peripheral tissues by aromatization of androstenedione, an androgen precursor that is produced by both the ovaries and the adrenal glands; after the menopause, estrone produced in this way becomes the predominant estrogen. All of the estrogens are sulfated and glucuronidated before excretion.

Natural 17-β-estradiol undergoes first-pass metabolism when given by mouth, and other compounds have therefore been preferred for therapeutic purposes. For the estrogen component of the oral contraceptives, mestranol (ethinylestradiol-3-methyl ether) was originally used, but since it was suspected of adverse effects it was by 1969 largely replaced by unesterified ethinylestradiol. 17-α-estradiol has also been synthesized (or extracted from pomegranates) and studied, but it binds much more weakly than the 17-α congener to estrogen receptors. 17-β-estradiol in micronized form, to improve systemic availability, has also been used in various products, especially in Scandinavia.

For estrogen replacement therapy, the less potent estrogens, estrone and estriol, have been widely used, as well as the semi-synthetic compound epimestrol.

In North America, much publicity has for many years been devoted to the supposed merits of "equine estrogens," also known as "conjugated estrogens" (Premarin), described as comprising a natural product extracted from the urine of pregnant mares. However, since pregnant mares were an inadequate source of starting material, these preparations have for a long time apparently been based primarily on synthetic substances (estrone with some equilin), although in some products a small amount of natural material may be present. The Food and Drug Administration in the USA long took the view that sodium estrone sulfate and sodium equilin sulfate were the sole active ingredients of the original product, but this was challenged by the manufacturers, who adduced evidence that dehydroestrone sulfate, and perhaps other components, could play a role. Overall, however, the view seems to be that the effects of Premarin are similar to those of other weak estrogens, whether given singly or in combination.

For injectable formulations used in estrogenic hormone replacement therapy, various esters of beta-estradiol have been most widely used.

Estradiol (E2) (rINN)

As noted above, 17-β-estradiol has hardly been used by the oral route, except in micronized form. The micronized product is also available in the form of an intranasal spray for the treatment of menopausal symptoms; this can give rise to mild irritation, leading to sneezing (1).

Estriol (E3) (rINN) and estrone (E1) (rINN)

Estriol is a very weak estrogen, usually given in oral doses of 1–2 mg/day, which has effects similar to those of ethinylestradiol at about 1/100th of this dosage: that is the vulva and vagina respond, but there is little effect on the endometrium. Similar considerations apply to estrone and to conjugated equine estrogens; most of the activity in the latter is in fact due to the presence of sodium estrone, which appears to be added to most formulations, in view of the limited supply of genuine equine estrogens.

Epimestrol (rINN)

The adverse effects of epimestrol (3-methoxy-17-epiestriol), a very weak estrogen with some ovulation-inducing effects, are largely as one would expect. In one series, hot flushes, insomnia, anorexia, nausea, and vomiting were reported in 1.5%, headache in 3%, and uterine bleeding in 38% (2). Ovarian hyperstimulation is rare but not unknown. As is usual with such treatment, the incidence of the adverse effects reported varies greatly, no doubt reflecting differences in the motivation of the patients and the schemes of administration used.

Ethinylestradiol (rINN)

Ethinylestradiol is discussed under hormonal contraceptives.

Fosfestrol (rINN)

Fosfestrol is an unusual agent used in Japan for the treatment of prostatic carcinoma but not accepted by experts in Europe. Described as an estrogen, in European studies it had a high incidence of complications, including fluid retention (16%), myocardial infarction (10%), and thromboembolism (6.3%). A case of adrenocortical insufficiency has now been documented in Japan, involving a 59-year-old man who had taken the drug for 10 years (3).

Nylestriol (rINN)

Nylestriol is an estriol derivative (cyclopentylethinylestriol), which has been tested in animals in combination with levonorgestrel as a potential agent for the treatment of post-menopausal osteoporosis. In a preliminary placebo-controlled study over 1 year using nylestriol 0.5 mg + levonorgestrel 0.15 mg once weekly in 119 patients, the combination produced no adverse effects on the uterus or breasts and there was no uterine bleeding (4).

Quinestrol (rINN)

Quinestrol is an ether of ethinylestradiol. It is stored in body fat and hence acts for weeks or months after a single oral dose; in the event of adverse reactions, this makes prompt termination of exposure impossible.

Non-steroidal estrogens

The non-steroidal estrogens diethylstilbestrol (rINN) and cyclofenine (rINN) are covered in separate monographs.

Uses

Estrogens are used principally for:

- relief of the symptoms of the menopause
- treatment of postmenopausal vaginal atrophy
- contraception, in combination with a progestogen
- hormone replacement therapy, alone or in combination with a progestogen, an androgen, or both.

Hormone replacement therapy should be distinguished from the short-term therapeutic use of estrogen (or hormonal combinations) around the time of the climacteric for the relief of acute (primarily vasomotor) symptoms; such treatment can generally be limited to some 6–12 months although if it is then withdrawn the symptoms may recur (5). Confusion between these two forms of treatment has led to a series of misunderstandings regarding the adverse effects of true hormone replacement therapy.

Oral contraception and hormone replacement therapy are dealt with specifically in separate monographs. Here the general adverse effects of estrogens for any indication are reviewed.

There is also interest in the possible neuroprotective effects of estrogens on the nervous system, since estrogen may act as an antiapoptotic agent, an antioxidant, or a neurotrophic modulating agent, promoting cross-talk with neurotrophic factors (6). This could in theory prove helpful in the treatment of conditions such as Parkinsonism, but no selective agent with such usefulness, and devoid of unwanted effects on other systems, has so far emerged. In the meantime, tibolone, sometimes described as a "gonadomimetic" agent, because of its ability to stimulate certain estrogen receptors selectively, has been used, although without any clear success, in the hope of potentiating the effects of fluoxetine on major depression (7).

"Equine estrogens" (Premarin)

The controversy regarding the composition of Premarin and what are regarded as its generic equivalents has been outlined above. While still in use for hormone replacement therapy, these products have also been used as a means of reducing unwanted bleeding, for example in uremia (8,9), although their efficacy has been challenged. Estrogens have also been used in the treatment of bleeding in hereditary hemorrhagic telangiectasia (10,11).

General adverse effects

Salt and water retention due to estrogens can cause weight gain and a rise in blood pressure. Changes in liver function tests can occur and jaundice is sometimes seen. Mild gastrointestinal upsets are not unusual. Unwanted endocrine effects include uncomfortable stimulation of the breasts and endometrial bleeding. In men, estrogens produce gynecomastia. Hypersensitivity reactions are rare and include urticaria, edema, and bronchospasm.

Estrogens can be associated with endometrial carcinoma, liver tumors, and breast tumors; they can also promote the further growth of pre-existing estrogen-dependent tumors.

When conjugated estrogens are used to control bleeding they are generally given only in short courses and are therefore well tolerated. As recommendations for control of bleeding involve administration of Premarin on a limited number of occasions (no more than five or seven doses) the usual hormonal problems associated with estrogens will be avoided. Gross hepatic disease is regarded as a contraindication. Headache, flushing, and nausea have been observed after intravenous injections and slow injection is therefore recommended.

Men taking estrogens generally do so in the course of palliative treatment for malignancies (prostatic carcinoma), for which high doses have sometimes been used. Estrogen therapy in men with prostate cancer may be superior to castration in terms of efficacy, but orally administered estrogens are associated with adverse effects: gynecomastia, loss of sexual function, and unacceptable cardiovascular toxicity (12). Low-dose estrogens in combination with anti-androgens or antithrombotic agents may be better tolerated.

Estrogenic effects of non-estrogens

Over the last 50 years, it has been realized that environmental chemicals, such as pesticides and industrial chemicals, can have hormone-like effects in wildlife and humans (13). These chemicals may:

- mimic the effect of endogenous hormones
- antagonize the effect of endogenous hormones
- alter the synthesis and metabolism of endogenous hormones
- alter the synthesis and metabolism of hormone receptors.

There have been reports that aviation crop dusters handling DDT had reduced sperm counts and workers at a plant producing the insecticide kepone had reduced libido, became impotent, and had low sperm counts. Subsequently, animal experiments showed that these pesticides have estrogen-like activity. Man-made compounds used in the manufacture of plastics interfered with experiments on natural estrogens. Some detergents and antioxidants are not themselves estrogenic, but on degradation during sewage treatment can release estrogenic alkyl phenols, such as bisphenol-A, nonylphenol, and phenylphenols. Polycarbonate flasks release bisphenol-A, which can also contaminate the contents of canned food in which polycarbonate coatings are used; bisphenol-A is also used in dental sealants and composites and can leach from teeth into saliva. Polystyrene tubes can release nonylphenol. The surfactant nonoxynol is used as intravaginal spermicide and condom lubricant; in animals it is metabolized to free nonylphenol. Other xeno-estrogens include the plasticizers benzylbutylphthalate and dibutylphthalate, the antioxidant butylhydroxyanisole, the rubber additive *para*-phenylphenol, and the disinfectant *ortho*-phenylphenol.

Organs and Systems

Cardiovascular

Estrogens have both wanted and unwanted effects on the cardiovascular system, depending on the manner in which they are used. Hormone replacement therapy is used in the hope of reducing the risk of ischemic heart disease after the menopause. The reduction in risk may be as much as 50% and is attributed variously to vasodilatation mediated by the endothelial production of prostaglandin I_2 (prostacyclin), effects on coagulation factors and endothelial function, and improvements in serum lipids (increased concentrations of HDL cholesterol and reduced concentrations of LDL and total cholesterol) (14), but variable effects on triglycerides. However, estrogens (especially as used in contraception but also postmenopausally) can have a marked effect on clotting factors and renin substrate, increasing the risk of thromboembolism.

The Coronary Drug Project in men taking different doses of estrogens showed a dose-related increase in myocardial infarction and thromboembolic diseases (15).

A Greek group set out to determine in a randomized, double-blind study the effect of hormonal or antihormonal therapy on serum VE-cadherin in 28 healthy postmenopausal women, who received either 17-beta-estradiol (2 mg/day) with norethisterone acetate (1 mg/day) or alternatively raloxifene HCl alone (60 mg/day) for 6 months (16). Serum VE-cadherin, which was estimated at baseline and at month 6, fell significantly in both groups. These findings suggest that these drugs may preserve interendothelial junction integrity and control vascular permeability. Although this effect may favorably influence the progress of an atheromatous lesion, its clinical impact, for example on coronary artery disease, remains uncertain.

Respiratory

Allergic bronchospasm occurs very rarely with estrogens (17), but has been reported several times in women with an existing allergic tendency or a history of asthma; some asthmatic women have worse symptoms during the luteal phase of the menstrual cycle. In affected cases, the link with estrogens can be demonstrated by rechallenge.

Nervous system

Various types of headache can occur; in patients with migraine, attacks can be precipitated, usually with prominent visual phenomena.

- In a woman with history of chorea in the distant past, a vaginal cream containing estrogens precipitated an attack.

In a randomized, double-blind, placebo-controlled arm of the Women's Health Initiative, 10 739 postmenopausal women, aged 50–79 years, with prior hysterectomies, were randomly assigned to receive either conjugated equine estrogen 0.625 mg/day or placebo. There was an increased risk of stroke (RR = 1.39; 95% CI = 1.10, 1.77).

Sensory systems

Retinal vein occlusion (18–21), retinal artery occlusion (22), and optic neuritis (23,24) have been described in women taking estrogens.

In older women, estrogens cause a slight rise in intraocular pressure (SED-12, 1031) (25).

Psychological, psychiatric

The effects of estrogens on mood tend to be positive, and improved performance in intellectual tests has been described (SEDA-20, 382) (26); this is in parallel with the known effects of endogenous estrogens. During the menopause some women become depressed and irritable, and the ability of estrogens to correct this has been delineated in various studies, including work with estradiol given transdermally (27). Some workers also claim increased vigilance, and have concluded that this is

reflected in encephalographic changes. There is even some evidence of an improvement in mental balance and self-control when estrogens are given to demented and aggressive old people of both sexes (28). However, all of these effects of estrogens on mood or mental performance are only likely to last for as long as the treatment does, and the effects on mood may occur only at the start of treatment; altered mood can follow acute withdrawal.

Endocrine

In postmenopausal women taking long-term mestranol there was a fall in the serum concentration of unbound (free) thyroxine, but it was not associated with hypothyroidism; the serum concentration of thyroid-stimulating hormone was unchanged (29).

Metabolism

Conflicting data concerning the effects of oral contraceptives on carbohydrate metabolism have been presented; the effects are probably clinically insignificant. However, estrogen hormone replacement therapy with a sequential-type product containing mestranol and norethisterone caused significantly impaired glucose tolerance (30).

There is no doubt that with appropriate treatment regimens, altered lipid metabolism due to estrogens can improve (31). In women with familial hypertriglyceridemia or increased triglycerides from other causes, oral estrogens can increase triglyceride concentrations. However, transdermal estrogens can lower triglycerides and generally produce smaller changes in lipoproteins than oral therapy, although it may be that whatever differences are observed merely reflect differing degrees of absorption.

Porphyria can be precipitated by estrogens, and familial porphyria cutanea tarda can become manifest (32).

Metal metabolism

Estrogens increase serum copper concentrations (SED-12, 1030) (33).

Fluid balance

Retention of water and salt and consequent weight gain are common during estrogen therapy. Fluid retention can cause a feeling of abdominal pressure, sensations resembling the premenstrual syndrome, breast tenderness, bloating, and edema. These symptoms can largely be relieved by a mild diuretic, but it is only practicable to use this approach if the estrogen treatment is cyclical and the symptoms thus intermittent, since it is undesirable to give diuretics continuously to healthy women over a long period of time.

Hematologic

There is a risk of thrombosis with estrogens, discussed in detail in the monograph on Hormonal contraception. Both superficial and deep complications can occur in either sex. Effects on clotting factors and renin are involved: in one small study, men taking estrogens had increased concentrations of factor VII, factor VIII, and fibrinogen, pointing to a hypercoagulable state and platelet activation (34).

In hormone replacement therapy, the risk of deep vein thrombosis is increased by a factor of 2–4 (35–37). The absolute increase in the treated population as a whole is low, with about one case of venous thromboembolism in 5000 women-years of use of hormone replacement therapy. However, in the subgroup with pre-existing risk factors, such as obesity, varicose veins, smoking, and a prior history of venous thromboembolism or superficial thrombophlebitis, the increase in risk from hormone replacement therapy can be substantial; among these women are those with a genetic predisposition to thrombosis, generally due to some form of thrombophilia, such as deficiency of the coagulation inhibitors protein S, protein C, or antithrombin III. In any of these subjects thrombosis can occur early in hormone replacement therapy. However, this tendency to early occurrence of deep vein thrombosis also seems to be present in all those who take hormone replacement therapy.

The mechanisms of thrombotic complications are multiple. Fibrinolytic activity falls in postmenopausal women when a high dose (250 micrograms/day) of ethinylestradiol is given for 10 days in preparation for prolapse operation (38). On the other hand, long-term administration of mestranol 80 micrograms/day to postmenopausal women for 1 year or longer increased the concentrations of fibrinogen and l-trypsin inhibitor and reduced plasminogen (SED-12, 1030) (39). There is also evidence that even low doses of oral estrogens increase the amount of thrombin generated in vivo.

It has been suggested, on the basis of a case of multiple systemic arterial thrombi in a patient with a prosthetic heart valve, that if estrogens are needed in such individuals they should be combined with anticoagulants. One would be inclined to extend the warning: any woman with a pre-existing risk of thrombosis should be examined very carefully before deciding to give estrogens at all.

The hypercoagulability that can occur with conjugated estrogens has been reported to be less pronounced than with oral contraceptives, but it is not clear that it is less than that seen with other types of estrogen used in hormone replacement therapy (40). The hematological effects of different estrogens are additive; various reports have demonstrated this for ethinylestradiol and diethylstilbestrol (41), which would mean that nothing would be gained by using several estrogens in parallel at reduced doses.

Some work suggests that when estrogens are given parenterally or transdermally rather than orally, the unwanted effects on the clotting process are reduced (42). The most important pharmacokinetic difference is that first-pass metabolism in the liver is avoided in all forms of non-oral therapy, which in the case of estrogens includes percutaneous gels, implants into the abdominal wall or buttocks, transdermal patches, and vaginal tablets, rings, and creams. It may therefore be prudent to use transdermal estrogens or another form of parenteral therapy when seeking to prevent osteoporosis in women with a tendency to thrombosis or hypertension.

For reasons that are not clear, other facets of the blood system are also affected by estrogens. After 6-months treatment with low doses of conjugated estrogens, hemoglobin concentration and mean erythrocyte counts were significantly reduced (43); on the other hand, the hematocrit was significantly increased by high-dose estrogen + androgen at 6 months, while the mean white blood cell count was significantly increased by low-dose estrogen + androgen at 12 months (43).

Mesenteric venous thrombosis has been reported in men taking estrogen therapy for carcinoma of the prostate (SED-12, 1032) (44).

Gastrointestinal

Estrogens can cause dose-related nausea, which is not reduced by using enteric-coated tablets. It has been claimed that there is a significantly lower incidence of nausea with estrogen + androgen than with conjugated estrogens.

Intestinal ischemia has occasionally been attributed to conjugated estrogens (26,45).

There is some reason to distinguish this from the ischemia that can be caused by oral contraceptives, in that it is restricted to the colon, can have a chronic or remitting course, can present with non-specific abdominal and colonic symptoms, can be reversible despite continued use of estrogen, and does not require surgical treatment. The symptoms of intestinal ischemia resolve within days to weeks after withdrawal of the estrogen. However, oral contraceptives have also been reported to cause ischemic colitis.

- A 19-year-old woman developed abdominal cramps, nausea, vomiting, diarrhea, and rectal bleeding (46). She was taking no medications other than Norinyl-2 (norethindrone 2 mg and mestranol 1 mg), which she had taken for 6 months. Just before the onset of the symptoms she had taken dimenhydrinate 100 mg and two ExLax tablets (90 mg of phenolphthalein) for constipation. Colonic X-rays showed impaired mesenteric circulation and bowel ischemia. Her symptoms subsided within 96 hours of withdrawing the oral contraceptive and giving supportive therapy (including intravenous fluid infusion, nasogastric suction, analgesics, and antiemetics). Further radiology showed that the ischemia had resolved.

Estrogens can cause or aggravate constipation (47), but when it occurs it is more likely to be due to the calcium carbonate that many women take as a daily supplement in postmenopausal treatment.

Liver

Changes in liver function tests can occur during estrogen treatment (48). In one comparative study, ethinylestradiol had an unfavorable effect on liver protein synthesis (SED-12, 1030) (49).

Cholestatic jaundice has often been reported with oral estrogens and is probably related to an effect on the permeability of the canalicular membrane (SEDA-20, 381). Cholestatic jaundice induced by a subcutaneous estrogen implant has also been reported in the absence of any other cause of liver disease (SEDA-20, 381). After removal of the implant the patient's symptoms resolved. The authors' explanation was that fragmentation of the implant had led to release of excessive amounts of estradiol.

The effects of estrogens on liver function differ with the type of estrogen used, problems being particularly associated with 17-substituted steroids. Significant reductions in transaminases, lactate dehydrogenase, and alkaline phosphatase have been found at 6 and 12 months with various forms of estrogen therapy. A reduction in mean bilirubin concentration has been described at 6 months with high-dose conjugated estrogens, and a significant increase in mean bilirubin concentration with low-dose estrogen + androgen at 12 months.

In some studies, women taking estradiol or conjugated estrogens for hormone replacement therapy had no cholestasis or hepatotoxicity, as assessed by rises in serum alkaline phosphatase, bilirubin, or transaminases, whereas these effects did occur with ethinylestradiol.

Pancreas

There is a small but significant risk of acute pancreatitis at 2–78 weeks after the start of hormone replacement therapy; the pain usually abates within 10 days of withdrawal (50).

Urinary tract

In the past, hypernephroma was thought to result from estrogen treatment. However, there is no clear evidence that this is so. There is evidence that older women with an intact uterus become more susceptible to urinary tract infections by taking estrogens (51). This is surprising, since some other studies, admittedly in selected patients, have shown a reduction in such infections when hormone replacement therapy is used. In another study, hormone replacement therapy improved urinary incontinence and nocturia after 6 months in postmenopausal women, without affecting bacteriuria (52).

Skin

Diffuse prickly erythema has been attributed to ethinylestradiol in various oral contraceptive formulations.

- A woman taking an oral contraceptive (Marvelon, ethinylestradiol 30 micrograms + desogestrel 150 micrograms) developed diffuse prickly erythema in an exposed site less than 20 minutes after sun exposure (53). Phototesting showed photosensitivity in the UVB and UVA ranges, but routine patch and photopatch tests with Marvelon were negative. All abnormal findings reversed 4 months after withdrawal of the oral contraceptive, but reappeared when she started using another oral contraceptive (Microgynon 30, ethinylestradiol 30 micrograms + levonorgestrel 150 micrograms). Phototesting was again abnormal. Her symptoms disappeared after withdrawal of the oral contraceptive. Porphyrin production was normal.

Although the estrogen and progestogen were not tested separately in this patient, the photosensitivity was most probably due to the estrogen, because the oral contraceptives that she used contained ethinylestradiol 30 micrograms with different progestogens, and photosensitivity has been described with estrogens (54).

- A 47-year-old postmenopausal woman developed eczematous lesions at the sites of application of an estradiol transdermal system and subsequently at the sites of application of an estradiol gel (55). She was therefore given oral estrogen instead, but this promptly elicited a systemic pruritic rash. The causal link was in all instances confirmed by patch-testing.

Estrogens can cause chloasma (56).

Papillomatous melanocytic nevi can be induced by estrogens (57), and melanocytic lesions can contain large numbers of estrogen and progestogen receptors (58).

When transdermal estrogens are used there can be problems with poor adhesion and skin irritation. The latter occurs more often in hot humid weather and can rarely proceed to edema, induration, a vesicular rash, residual pigmentation, itching, and erythema (59).

Three patients developed erythema nodosum during estrogen replacement therapy (60).

Topical estrogens can reduce skin aging (61), for example with reduced wrinkling and increased firmness in the dermis of perimenopausal women, although it is not clear that the effect is more marked than with oral treatment. Certainly, estrogens augment dermal water content by increasing hyaluronic acid and mucopolysaccharides, improving the structure of elastic fibers, and increase vascularization.

Sexual function

Libido, sexual activity (including masturbation), and orgasm increase in women taking the combination of an estrogen with an androgen, but it is not clear that estrogens alone have any such effect (62,63). Reduced libido and reduced sexual activity are to be expected in men treated with estrogens.

Reproductive system

All estrogens, even less potent ones, can cause endometrial hypertrophy and bleeding in a proportion of users after the menopause; in high doses the complication is common (64). With continuous estrogen therapy, the bleeding is irregular and unpredictable, whereas cyclical use of a combination with a progestogen is likely to produce something resembling normal menstruation, although it generally abates as treatment continues (64).

Estrogens can cause painful tingling and swelling of the breasts, sometimes requiring withdrawal of treatment. Frank gynecomastia can occur in men by exposure to estrogens in a factory environment and has even been described in an elderly man whose wife used an estrogen-containing vaginal lubricant (SEDA-6, 350).

In men, estrogens cause pigmentation of the areola followed by gynecomastia, both during oral treatment and local application (65). Estrogen-induced gynecomastia can be prevented in men with prostatic carcinoma by irradiating the breast region before starting therapy.

Because in some societies excessive height in women is considered a social disadvantage, a minority of physicians have long used estrogens to arrest rapid growth in adolescent girls. The question has always been whether this might adversely affect reproductive function in later life. A retrospective cohort study, based on 371 women who had undergone such treatment (with diethylstilbestrol or ethinylestradiol) and 409 controls, has been published (66). After adjustment for age, the treated women were more likely than the controls to have tried at some time for 12 months or more to become pregnant without success (RR = 1.80), more likely to have seen a doctor because they were having difficulty becoming pregnant (RR = 1.80; CI = 1.39, 2.32), and more likely to have taken fertility drugs at some time (RR = 2.05; CI = 1.39, 3.04). The treated group was 40% less likely to conceive in any given menstrual cycle of unprotected intercourse. These striking findings raise much doubt as to the wisdom of using estrogens to arrest growth in girls.

Immunologic

Estrogens can have adverse immunological effects, which could predispose to infections (67).

The immunological effects of two contraceptive combinations, namely Valette (dienogest 2.0 mg + ethinylestradiol 0.03 mg) and Lovelle (desogestrel 0.15 mg + ethinylestradiol 0.02 mg), have been examined during one treatment cycle (68). Lovelle significantly increased the numbers of lymphocytes, monocytes, and granulocytes. Valette reduced the CD4 lymphocyte count after 10 days and Lovelle did the opposite. Lovelle increased CD19 and CD23 cell counts after 21 days. Phagocytic activity was unaffected by either formulation. After 10 days both contraceptives reduced serum IgA, IgG, and IgM concentrations, which remained low at day 21 with Lovelle but returned to baseline with Valette. Secretory IgA was unaffected by either contraceptive. Neither treatment affected concentrations of interleukins, except for a significant difference between the treatment groups in interleukin-6 after 10 days, which resolved after 21 days. Concentrations of non-immunoglobulin serum components fluctuated; macroglobulin was increased by Valette. However, total protein and albumin concentrations were reduced more by Lovelle than Valette. Complement factors also fluctuated. There was no evidence of sustained immunosuppression with either Valette or Lovelle.

Angioedema and urticaria have often been attributed to food allergy, in the absence of any other explanation. In 26 young women in whom these conditions had been attributed to food allergy there was reason to believe that estrogens in oral contraceptives were in fact responsible (69). All the patients had a deficiency of C1 esterase inhibitor. Withdrawal of oral contraception caused an increase in C1 esterase inhibitor concentrations and activity, associated with recovery or marked improvement in the symptoms that had formerly been attributed to food allergy. The relatively high frequency of women taking cyproterone acetate in this population was striking. Replacement of the initial contraception containing ethinylestradiol by a progestogen-only regimen maintained or even accentuated these good therapeutic results.

A severe anaphylactic reaction occurred in one patient who was given an intravenous formulation of conjugated estrogens (SED-12, 1033) (70). Some formulations of conjugated estrogens contain foreign (equine) material.

Long-Term Effects

Tumorigenicity

For the sake of simplicity the carcinogenic effects of estrogens in all formulations, including the combined oral contraceptives, are included here.

Knowledge of tumor induction by sex steroids is largely based on interpretation of epidemiological data, with careful exclusion of possible confounding elements. Hepatic tumors have given rise to most concerns, but some evidence also indicates an increased incidence of various other malignancies, including carcinomas of the breast, endometrium, and prostate (71).

The overall incidence of reproductive cancers attributable to oral contraceptive use has been estimated in a modeling analysis (72). The authors assumed a 50% reduction in ovarian and endometrial cancers associated with 5 years or more of tablet use, and used two alternative scenarios for breast and cervical cancer effects. If oral contraceptive use produces a 20% increase in breast cancer before age 50 and the same increase in cervical cancer, then for every 100 000 tablet users there would be 44 fewer reproductive cancers and these users would gain one more day free of cancer. If instead the increase in risk of early breast cancer and of cervical cancer is 50%, oral contraceptive users would have 11 fewer cancer-free days.

Liver tumors

In dealing with liver tumors, it is essential to consider all the various types of sex steroids in a single review since they seem to resemble one another closely in their long-term effects on this organ. The nomenclature used in the literature is unfortunately confusing: most reports differentiate between "hepatic adenoma" and "focal nodular hyperplasia," but the latter term is also sometimes used to cover the whole range. Other terms that have been used are "focal cirrhosis," "regenerative hyperplasia," "hamartoma," "mixed adenoma," and "benign hepatoma," while "peliosis" may constitute a precancerous state.

Androgens and anabolic steroids

There is no essential difference between androgens and so-called anabolic steroids. High doses of either, such as can be used in refractory anemias, have been associated with the induction of benign liver tumors and primary hepatocellular carcinoma. The fact that primary hepatoma, liver adenoma, and peliosis are uncommon conditions and that there is a considerable overlap between the patients concerned and the tiny fraction of the population taking high-dose androgens strongly suggests that the association of both events is more than coincidental (73). Some animal studies and in vitro studies have also pointed to a hepatic carcinogenic effect of anabolic steroids. No cases seem to have been described in sportsmen who have used high-dose androgens or in girls suffering from precocious puberty, but the former at least often use these drugs for relatively short periods; furthermore, such use is likely to be surreptitious and thus poorly documented. Most of the widely used compounds in this class, including methyltestosterone, have been reported to induce liver tumors. The apparent exceptions are the nortestosterone derivatives without 17-alpha substitution. Whether these drugs are indeed safer or whether they have merely been used less often in high doses is not known.

The incidence of liver tumors following the use of androgens and anabolic steroids still cannot be calculated. What is clear is that if these products are used in high doses or over long periods of time (and there is now much doubt about whether they are more than marginally effective in such conditions as osteoporosis and aplastic anemia), techniques such as CT scanning and ultrasonography should be used routinely to ensure early detection of liver lesions.

Oral contraceptives, estrogens, and benign liver tumors

The effects of oral contraceptives on the liver include not only benign liver tumors (focal nodular hyperplasia, hepatic adenoma, and hemangioma) (74) and hepatocellular carcinoma, but also peliosis hepatis (75), sinusoid dilatation (76), and such probably unrelated shorter-term complications as jaundice and gallstones.

However, the causal association between oral contraceptives and certain benign liver tumors has been well documented in humans, and the same association arises with conjugated estrogens (77), diethylstilbestrol, and probably antiestrogens. The evidence for the link is based on many case reports, reviewed in SEDA, and on some case-control studies, which first appeared in 1976 and 1981, pointing to a correlation (SED-14, 1450). The relative risk of benign liver tumors in users of conjugated estrogens or oral contraceptives compared with non-users may be about 40:1, although the figure is still low in absolute terms. Animal studies suggest in fact that estrogens, taken alone or in combination with progestogens, can increase the size of pre-existing liver tumors, but do not initiate tumor formation themselves; however, whether these formulations actually induce tumors or promote a latent tendency to tumor development is not of essential importance. Although there is some evidence that liver cell adenomas can regress after oral contraceptives are withdrawn (78), they do not always do so (79).

The impact of female sex hormones on the natural history of liver hemangiomas has been prospectively evaluated over 1–17 years in 94 women with 181 hemangiomas diagnosed by ultrasound (80). There was an increase in the size of the lesions in 5 of 22 patients exposed to hormone therapy compared with 7 of 72 controls. Three variables (ultrasonographic pattern, number of hemangiomas, and hormone therapy) predicted whether or not a given hemangioma would increase in size. Hormone therapy significantly increased the risk of hemangioma enlargement but there was significant enlargement only

in a minority of women. It would seem that in women with existing hepatic hemangiomas who are to receive hormone therapy (oral contraception or HRT) periodic ultrasound examination is advisable to detect any tendency to enlargement. The risk of a de novo hemangioma as a result of exposure to female sex hormone therapy is probably negligible.

It is clear that any woman with "pill"-associated liver lesions should avoid all further use of hormonal contraceptives and related products.

Oral contraceptives and malignant liver cancer

Malignant cancer of the liver is still a very rare disease in young women, but case-control studies are possible. Evidence from both sides of the Atlantic suggested from 1987 onwards that there might be a significant relation between oral contraceptives and hepatocellular carcinoma (81–83). However, even the best of these studies had some limitations, for example incomplete data as regards a history of hepatitis or the extent of contraceptive use. One authoritative attempt to estimate the degree of risk was made by the World Health Organization in 1989, matching 122 newly diagnosed cases of primary liver cancer to 802 controls; the relative risk of liver cancer in women who had at any time used combined oral contraceptives was estimated at 0.71; there was no consistent link with months of use or time since first or last use (84). A major examination of the issue appeared in 1992, when it was concluded that the relative risk for sometime users of oral contraceptives was 1.6, rising to 2.0 in those who used the products for more than 10 years (85).

In a review of the earliest studies of hepatocellular carcinoma, it was concluded that oral contraceptives may not interact with other hepatic carcinogens, and that if they do not interact they may not measurably enhance the risk of liver cancer in parts of the world where hepatitis B virus is endemic and hepatocellular carcinoma is common (86). Others have since suggested a positive association between parity or gravidity and hepatocellular carcinoma, which needs to be further explored (87).

Conjugated estrogens

The same association with benign liver tumors arises with conjugated estrogens (77), diethylstilbestrol (q.v.), and probably antiestrogens. The evidence for the link is based on very numerous case reports from the field, reviewed in the Annuals in this series, but also on some case-control investigations. Studies of the latter type first appeared in 1976 and 1981, and both pointed to a correlation (SED-12, 1024). The relative risk of benign liver tumors in users of conjugated estrogens or oral contraceptives compared with non-users may be about 40:1, although the figure is still low in absolute terms.

Uterine tumors

The extent to which tumors of the reproductive tract are associated with hormonal treatment varies greatly with the type of tumor and the type of treatment involved.

Hormonal replacement therapy and endometrial carcinoma

In untreated women, the main risk factors for endometrial carcinoma are age, obesity, nulliparity, late menopause (and possibly early menarche), the Stein–Leventhal syndrome, exposure to exogenous estrogens, radiation, and certain systemic diseases, including diabetes mellitus, hypertension, hypothyroidism, and arthritis (SED-14, 1451) (88). Certain of these risk factors indicate that an altered endocrine state with increased estrogen stimulation is a predisposing cause, and one might thus in theory expect estrogen treatment (and notably hormonal replacement therapy) to increase the risk (SEDA-22, 466).

In women with an intact uterus, the risk of endometrial hyperplasia and cancer increases with increasing dose and duration of estrogen use. Adding a progestogen to estrogen-only therapy for at least 12 days a month greatly reduces this risk. However, it is not clear why the complication develops only in certain users. The risk of developing endometrial cancer during HRT seems to vary individually, perhaps because of genetic rather than exogenous factors. In women with endometrial cancer, women who reported ever taking HRT were more than twice as likely to develop endometrial cancer as women who had never taken it (OR = 2.24; 95% CI = 1.19, 4.23) and among these women the risk of endometrial cancer was higher for women homozygous for the CYP17 T-allele (OR = 4.10; 95% CI = 1.64, 10.3), but not for women with the C-allele. These preliminary findings suggest that CYP17 or other variants in estrogen biosynthesis or metabolism pathways may be markers of susceptibility to endometrial cancer among users of estrogen replacement therapy (89).

Two epidemiological studies published in 1975 first suggested that the use of estrogens during and after the menopause increased the risk of endometrial cancer, and in 1986 the authors of an authoritative review (90) endorsed these findings, concluding that there was an increase in risk among users, relative to non-users, of 4–9 times; the risk increased with both the strength of the medication and the duration of use. A 1990 review of data up to that time suggested that estrogen replacement therapy, continued for over 2 years without concurrent progesterone therapy, was associated with an approximately three-fold increase in the risk of both localized and extrauterine cancer; this risk increased with duration of use and persisted for over 6 years after withdrawal of therapy (91). These studies have been criticized from a methodological point of view, particularly since there is evidence of a detection bias that arises from the increased diagnostic attention received by women with uterine bleeding after estrogen exposure and perhaps also from a greater tendency of women to bleed from a pre-existing tumor when estrogens are given (92). It could be that the magnitude of the association between estrogens and endometrial cancer has been greatly overestimated for such reasons, and that the real odds ratio is less than estimated, but it seems unlikely that the risk can be disproved. There is, for example, some older evidence that even when the above-mentioned bias has largely been eliminated, there

is still a correlation between the use of estrogens and endometrial carcinoma, the evidence being strongest for the first-generation oral contraceptive products, which contained large amounts of estrogen. One such study still found a six-fold risk among estrogen users compared with non-users (93); long-term users (over 5 years) had a 15-fold risk; there were excess risks for both diethylstilbestrol and conjugated estrogens. Another well-controlled study, from 1986, similarly found increased risks with conjugated estrogens, the greatest increases in risk being associated with a dosage of 0.625 mg/day or greater and duration of use of 10 years or more (94). Although according to this study the risk remained high even among women who had stopped using conjugated estrogens 5 or more years before, one cannot ignore an earlier finding, based on evidence from a large group practice, that a sharp downward trend in the incidence of endometrial cancer occurred in parallel with a substantial reduction in prescriptions for replacement estrogens (95).

Among the many papers that have since then incriminated estrogens, particularly the conjugated estrogens so widely used in North America, some have presented more subtle conclusions. One paper specifically incriminated estrone (96), but this is of course a major component of conjugated estrogens. A case-control study from Buffalo, New York, found that while patients with endometrial cancer and healthy controls had used similar amounts of menopausal estrogens, estrogen users had a significantly higher frequency of low-grade tumors and a correspondingly better survival rate (97). Menopausal estrogens became popular much later in Europe, and relatively little evidence has emerged to complement the US findings. In 1983, however, when Persson in Sweden completed a very large cohort study, he found that while among women treated with estrogens there was no significant increase in endometrial cancer compared with the control population, there was indeed a significantly increased incidence of premalignant lesions among women who had used estrogens alone for more than 3 years (98). A protracted case-control study in a Swiss population pointed in the same direction; the use of HRT for 5 years or more created a mean relative risk of 1.9, and use for 5 years or more a relative risk of 5.1 (CI 2.7, 9.8) (99). This, as well as evidence that progestogens have some protective effect on the endometrium (100), emphasizes the need for prospective studies in different subpopulations taking different types of replacement therapy.

Some helpful evidence comes from related fields. It should be borne in mind, for example, that the question of an increased risk of endometrial hyperplasia and endometrial cancer also arises in patients with estrogen-producing tumors of the ovaries, obesity, and polycystic ovarian syndrome (101) and in patients with breast cancer who are using tamoxifen (102).

During one 3-year study, under 1% of 596 women taking placebo or an estrogen + a progestogen had an abnormal endometrial biopsy. Of women taking an unopposed estrogen, 12% developed typical hyperplasia, 23% complex hyperplasia, and 28% simple hyperplasia. Use of HRT for 15 or more years resulted in a significantly higher relative risk of 1.3 for breast cancer, but was also associated with a significantly lower total mortality (103). The use of combined therapy was not associated with an increased risk of endometrial carcinoma, unless the progestogen was added for less than 10 days each month (104).

Detailed studies may also help to clarify further the risks and the possible interaction of estrogens with other susceptibility factors for endometrial tumors; there is, for example, an impression that the risk is greater in lean than in overweight women, although upper abdominal obesity is thought to reflect a higher risk. Patients who develop endometrial cancer often have an increase in estrogen production, reduced ovulation, and a lower sex hormone binding globulin concentration, resulting in high concentrations of free estrogen. As regards subjects of low susceptibility, the cancer threat may be less in women who have used oral contraceptives earlier.

One can also recognize some correlations between the subtype of tumor and the type of hormonal exposure. Unopposed hyperestrogenism is most likely to be associated with the endometrioid type of endometrial carcinoma, rather than with clear-cell, serous-papillary, and mucinous carcinomas.

Remarkably, the survival curves for women taking estrogens and developing adenocarcinomas are actually better than in women not taking estrogens and not developing adenocarcinomas. In 1822 women with angiographically documented severe coronary artery disease, the mortality among estrogen users was 4% compared with 35% among non-users, suggesting that the benefit of postmenopausal estrogen replacement therapy may be even greater in women with established coronary artery disease than it is in healthy women. A possible explanation is that estrogen replacement therapy in postmenopausal women reduces the risk of coronary heart disease by 5% or more.

Like a history of breast cancer, a history of cancer of the endometrium is commonly regarded as a reason to avoid HRT with estrogens. One study, though limited in duration, provided encouraging evidence that such treatment at least does not adversely affect the rate of recurrence or the survival time (105).

Of 249 women with surgical stage I, II, and III endometrial cancer treated between 1984 and 1998, 130 used estrogen replacement after their primary cancer treatments and half of these used progesterone in addition to estrogen. Among this cohort, 75 matched treatment-control pairs were identified. The hormone users were followed for a mean of 83 months and the non-hormone users for a mean of 69 months. There were two recurrences among the 75 HRT users compared with 11 recurrences in the 75 non-hormone users. Hormone users had a statistically significant longer disease-free interval than untreated women. Whether this is sufficient to conclude that the effect is actually positive is not clear, but no evidence of an increase in risk came to the fore.

In view of the possibility that HRT can trigger malignancy in the endometrium itself, it is not surprising to find that it has also been reported to do so in endometriosis deposits elsewhere. An adenocarcinoma arose after many years of HRT in abdominal areas of endometriosis in a

woman who had undergone hysterectomy and salpingo-oophorectomy 17 years before (106). It is of course known that some 1–2% of endometriosis deposits undergo malignant degeneration, and the link with HRT could therefore have been fortuitous.

The minimum dose of continuously administered norethindrone acetate needed to reduce significantly the incidence of endometrial hyperplasia associated with the use of 17-β-estradiol 1 mg/day has been investigated in a large, controlled, comparative study in 1146 women over 12 months (107). The results suggested that continuous norethindrone acetate at doses as low as 0.1 mg/day is fully effective, at least during the first year of treatment.

The evidence that concurrent use of progestogens reduces the risk of cancer induction needs to be further supplemented; if this beneficial effect of progestogens truly exists, one must still determine how they can best be used. They are widely used, but not consistently, and increase the risk of endometrial cancer both during and after treatment. Some workers have recommended that for partial protection of the endometrium, dosages of medroxyprogesterone acetate of 2.5 mg/day continuously or 5.0 mg/day given for 14 days per cycle are the minimum required to counteract the endometrial effects of continuous therapy with estrogens (108). The added medroxyprogesterone is claimed to have no effect on the efficacy of the estrogen in treating vasomotor symptoms or in preventing osteoporosis. Others have concluded that administration of continuous rather than cyclical estrogen + progestogen therapy is more likely to maintain the beneficial effects of the estrogen and yet protect against the increase in endometrial carcinoma that occurs with estrogen therapy alone (109). However, progestogens have a negative impact on circulating lipids (55); it is possible that this adverse effect is less when using natural progesterone, but this is hardly practicable. The risk of endometrial hyperplasia and endometrial cancer with estrogens given alone must therefore be balanced against this negative impact.

Thus, although our knowledge is still incomplete and needs to be extended, it is highly likely that estrogen replacement therapy given without progestogens considerably increases the risk of endometrial carcinoma. It seems likely that the use of concurrent progestogen treatment reduces the risk, but it is still uncertain how this supplementary treatment can best be administered.

The possibility that the risk of endometrial complications might have been incorrectly estimated and commonly underestimated has been examined with the hypothesis that the method of endometrial examination or sampling is crucial (110). Hysteroscopy was performed in 98 menopausal women with endometrial thickening, and the findings were matched with those of histopathology based on various means of tissue collection, including suction curettage, oriented-streak curettage, hysteroscopically targeted biopsies, or polypectomy and hysterectomy. There was an abnormal endometrium in 35 patients (65% in symptomatic and 22% in asymptomatic women) and there were six carcinomas, 18 polyps, and 11 cases of hyperplasia.

Hysteroscopy had a sensitivity of 89% and a specificity of 98%. With blind sampling, tissue collection was too scant to make diagnosis possible in 29% of patients, while in 81% of patients in whom hysteroscopy showed cystic atrophy the pathologist failed to confirm this condition. Moreover, eight endometrial polyps (36%) detected by hysteroscopy were missed when samples were studied in the laboratory. Hysteroscopy with targeted sampling thus appears to be the most effective method for assessing the endometrial lining and detecting unwanted changes.

The endometrial effects of transdermal sequential combination therapy with estradiol and levonorgestrel in various doses has been examined over 1 year in 468 postmenopausal women, who each month used patches that released estradiol for 1 week followed later in the month by combined patches that released both estradiol and levonorgestrel, again for 1 week (111). The dose of estradiol was 50–100 micrograms/day and that of levonorgestrel 15–20 micrograms/day. Endometrial biopsies, obtained from 399 subjects, generally showed good tolerance for all the various combinations tested. However, there were two cases of endometrial hyperplasia at the highest doses, while the lowest dose was associated with less bleeding than the two higher doses and a somewhat different histological pattern.

Oral contraceptives and endometrial cancer

Suggestive case histories raised at an early phase the notion of a possible correlation of oral contraceptives with endometrial cancer. Among cases of endometrial cancer there seemed to be an excess of users of oral contraceptives, particularly of the early high-dose estrogen type. With the virtual demise of these early products, the situation seems to have reversed: a 1983 study from the Centers for Disease Control (CDC) in Atlanta showed that women who had used fixed combinations for oral contraception at some time in their lives had a relative risk of endometrial cancer of only 0.5 compared with never-users (112). The protective effect occurred only in women who had used oral contraception for at least 12 months, and lasted for at least 10 years after withdrawal. The WHO adopted the same view in 1988 in the light of multinational data (113). As in the case of hormonal replacement therapy, the protective effect seems to be due to the progestogen component.

Many studies have also shown a duration-related protective effect of combined oral contraceptives on endometrial cancer, the risk before age 60 being reduced by 38% after 2 years of use and up to a 70% reduction after 12 years (114). This beneficial effect continued for at least 15 years after the end of use. As with ovarian cancer, the CASH study results suggest that the lower-dose combined oral contraceptives have a protective effect similar to that of the higher-dose tablets (115).

Oral contraceptives, cervical neoplasms, and adenosis

A 1988 statistical analysis of data from the Royal College of General Practitioners study in Britain pointed clearly to an association between oral contraceptive use and cervical neoplasms (116); of 47 000 women followed since 1965, those who had at some time used oral contraceptives had a significantly higher incidence of cervical cancer than never-users after standardization of other variables, including a history of sexually transmitted disease. The incidence increased with duration of use, attaining four-fold control values after 10 years of use. Other studies (117,118) similarly showed an increased risk with increased duration of use but also with the use of formulations that contained a higher proportion of estrogen or in users with a history of genital infections or abnormal Papanicolaou smears. Benign cervical adenosis and adenomatous polyps have been seen in oral contraceptive users and were prominent in some early reports (SED-11, 857). They often (but not always) disappear when medication is stopped.

By the mid-1980s it was fair to conclude that: (a) oral contraceptive use did not appear to increase the subsequent incidence of abnormal cytology among women who had normal smears at the time they began to use the products; (b) extended oral contraceptive use (over 6 years) appeared to increase by several times the rate of conversion of pre-existing cervical dysplasia to carcinoma in situ. Generally speaking, subsequent data have tended to be compatible with those conclusions, for example pointing to an increased incidence of micro-invasive cervical carcinoma and again stressing the changes in cytology and the extent to which the effect differs with the strength and composition of the product. The average risk figures that emerge are generally in line with those found in a Norwegian study, in which, after correcting for other risk factors, relative rates were found of 1.5 for current users and 1.4 for past users as compared with never-users (119). Clearly, confounding factors, such as differences in sexual activity, age at first coitus, and the number of sexual partners, can confuse the issue and make interpretation more complex (120). In addition, any discussion of the issue must today take into account the current view of the human papilloma virus (HPV) as a sexually transmitted agent that is the main cause of cervical cancer (121), and the possible influence of Herpes simplex virus type 2, smoking, and other known or emergent risk factors.

The most authoritative view on cervical cancer at present is that expressed by the WHO in 1992: "Recent studies suggest that use of oral contraceptives for more than 5 years is associated with a modest increase in relative risk (ranging from 1.3 to 1.8). The extent to which this reflects a biological relationship is uncertain, particularly given the absence of reliable information on the role of possible infectious agents, such as the human papilloma viruses ···" (122). In the present state of knowledge, all women taking oral contraceptives over long periods should undergo regular routine screening by cervical cytology to ensure early detection of premalignant and malignant processes.

In 2002 the Chief Medical Officer of the UK Department of Health issued an urgent communication to all Health Professionals that oral contraceptives may contribute to the development of cervical cancer in women with high-risk type HPV, because of an association between an increased risk of cervical cancer and increasing duration of use of oral contraceptives (123). There was a three-fold increase in risk after 5–9 years of oral contraceptive use versus a four-fold increase after 10 or more years in women with HPV, which is sexually transmitted. There are more than 80 HPV, only a few of which are associated with an increased risk of cervical cancer. With the current evidence it is difficult to state what the main precipitating factors for cervical cancer are—the use of oral contraceptives, sexual activity, the type of HPV, or the duration of infection. While cervical screening is not perfect, 80–90% of cervical abnormalities can be detected and treated in women who attend regular screening programmes. The Chief Medical Officer therefore advised that all sexually active women, especially those taking long-term oral contraceptives, should be encouraged to have regular cervical smears.

Oral contraceptives and uterine fibroids

In a long-term, follow-up study in Scandinavia, the risk of fibroids fell consistently with increasing duration of oral contraceptive use (124). A decade earlier, the British Royal College of Physicians study had similarly suggested a protective effect, while an Oxford study had not, but once more the issue is confused by the change in composition of oral contraceptives over the years; more recent papers thus carry the most weight. On the other hand a causal relation between apoplectic leiomyomas and oral contraceptive usage was strongly suggested by Myles and Hart in the light of their study of five histologically distinctive uterine smooth muscle neoplasms with multifocal hemorrhages (125). They thought that effects of hormonal steroids on the blood vessels in pre-existing leiomyomas might be responsible for intimal hyperplasia with or without accompanying thrombi.

Ovarian tumors
Hormone replacement therapy

While the risk that hormone replacement therapy may cause endometrial tumors has been widely discussed, less attention has been given to the possibility that it could increase the risk of epithelial ovarian cancer. Since cancer of the ovary has some risk factors in common with endometrial cancer (notably low parity and obesity), this possible risk needs to be considered, especially in view of the fact that the endometrioid epithelial type of ovarian tumor is histologically so similar to adenocarcinoma of the endometrium.

The issue has been examined in a large Australian case-control study. A total of 793 eligible incident diagnoses of epithelial ovarian cancer in 1990–93 among women living in Queensland, New South Wales, and Victoria were identified. These were compared with 855 eligible female controls selected at random. Standard questionnaires were used to obtain histories. There were no clear associations between the use of hormone replacement therapy overall and the risk of ovarian cancer. However, unopposed estrogen replacement therapy was associated with a significant increase in the risk of endometrioid or clear-cell epithelial ovarian tumors. In addition, the risk associated with estrogen replacement therapy was much larger in women with an intact genital tract than in

those with a history of either hysterectomy or tubal ligation. The authors therefore suggested that postmenopausal estrogen replacement may be a risk factor associated with endometrioid and clear-cell tumors in particular.

The risk of ovarian cancer with various hormonal replacement regimens has been examined in a nationwide study in Sweden in relation to plain estrogen regimens as well as estrogen + sequentially added progestogens or continuously added progestogens (126). Between 1993 and 1995, the investigators enrolled 655 women with histologically verified ovarian cancers and 3899 randomly selected population controls, all aged 50–74. Data on the use of estrogen replacement therapy were collected by postal questionnaires. The risk of ovarian cancer was higher among ever-users than never-users as regards both plain estrogen supplementation (OR = 1.43, 95% CI = 1.02, 2.00) and estrogens with sequentially added progestogens (OR = 1.54, 95% CI = 1.15, 2.05); the increase in risk applied to the serous, mucinous, and endometrioid subtypes. For all cancer types combined, the greatest increases in risk were seen when hormone use exceeded 10 years. The odds ratios after ever use of low-potency estrogens were 1.18 (95% CI = 0.89, 1.55) for oral and 1.33 (95% CI = 1.03, 1.72) for vaginal use. There was no increase in risk among users of continuously added progestogens. In other words, the continuous addition of progestogens appeared to reduce or eliminate the risk.

Oral contraceptives

The results of two major British prospective studies of 1974 and 1976 (127,128) suggested that oral contraceptive treatment was unrelated to the development of benign ovarian tumors; these and other studies also suggested that follicular and lutein cysts are suppressed in women using oral contraceptives. With regard to ovarian cancer, somewhat later data suggested a reduced risk in oral contraceptive users; impressive case-control work from the USA in 1981 seemed to show this protective effect when oral contraceptives had been taken for 4 years or more, the risk of ovarian cancer then being decreased by a mean of some 40%; the effect was even greater when the contraceptives had been used for a longer period (129). Very similarly, in 1988, the results of a multi-country study backed by the WHO suggested that sometime users of combined oral contraceptives had a risk rate that was only 71% of that in non-users, while women who had used oral contraceptives for 5 or more years had about a 50% reduction in risk (113). It should be added, however, that not all reviewers find these trends significant.

A meta-analysis of epidemiological studies of ovarian cancer showed a summary estimated relative risk of 0.64 for ever-use of combined oral contraceptives, implying a 36% reduction in ovarian cancer risk (130). This protective effect increased with increasing duration of oral contraceptive use and continued for at least 10 years after discontinuation. Although most of the oral contraceptives reported in these studies were older, higher-dose formulations, the Cancer and Steroid Hormone (CASH) study included users of tablets containing ethinylestradiol 35 µg or less, and this subgroup of women had a reduced risk of ovarian cancer (115).

With conjugated estrogens, the risk of ovarian cancer was stated in 1977 to increase two- to three-fold (SED-12, 1026), but this conclusion was based primarily on findings in women who had also taken diethylstilbestrol, and it was therefore not generally accepted. A 1982 study in which there was an apparent slight increase in ovarian epithelial carcinoma among American women taking estrogens was similarly open to challenge (SEDA-7, 385) and the link cannot be regarded as having been established (131).

Breast neoplasms
Oral contraceptives
Shortly after the first oral contraceptives were introduced around 1959, the fact that some women noticed acute effects on the breast led to fears that the ultimate consequence might be induction of mammary disorders, particularly tumors; the same concerns were raised about estrogen replacement therapy (132). The debate on this issue has now continued for more than 30 years and it is characterized by contradictions, discrepancies in scientific findings, qualified statements, and controversies and a massive output of data and opinions. The present review will necessarily be confined to some of the highlights of the discussion, presented in Table 1, leading up to a summary of the present situation and the questions that still remain open.

It is clear from the studies reported in Table 1 (133–149) that there is no simple relation between treatment with hormonal oral contraceptives and the incidence of breast cancer. As in the case of other neoplasms, studies are confounded by the influence of many factors, including age, parity, age at first delivery, family history, pre-existent fibrocystic disease, geographical or

Table 1 The possible association of oral contraceptives with breast neoplasms

Type of study	Findings	Source
Review of nine major studies of oral contraceptives	Reduced risk of breast cancer in eight studies; greater effect with higher doses; clinically significant with 2 years of use	(133)
Case-control study	Link between oral contraceptives and breast cancer, but only in those aged 30–34 years; coincidental?	(134)
Prospective epidemiological study	Link between oral contraceptives and breast cancer if used before first full-term pregnancy; high doses associated with a higher risk	(135)
Case-control study	No link between oral contraceptives and breast cancer	(136)
Historical study of breast cancer cases	Four-fold increased risk with injectable estrogens	(137)
Case-control study	No link between oral contraceptives and breast cancer	(138)
Case-control study	Ever-users of oral contraceptives had 1.1 risk compared with never-users; higher doses produce a slightly higher risk; duration of use irrelevant; family history: higher risk; use after age 40: risk increased by 50%	(139)
Editorial	Greater risk if oral contraceptives used long-term in early life?	(140)
Case-control study	Ever-users of oral contraceptives had 0.9 (0.8, 1.2) risk compared with never-users; family history and use of oral contraceptives before first pregnancy irrelevant	(112)
Epidemiological study (extension of Pike, 1981)	Link between oral contraceptives and breast cancer if used before first full-term pregnancy: high doses associated with a higher risk	(135)
Case-control study	Pike's results not confirmed; may be some protective effect of oral contraceptives?	(136)
Case-control study	No link with oral contraceptives	(141)
Case-control study	No link with oral contraceptives, except for a 30% increase if taken before first full pregnancy	(142)
Epidemiological study	No link with oral contraceptives, even in subpopulations	(143)
Epidemiological study	No link with oral contraceptives, even in subpopulations	(144)
Case-control study	Evidence of risk if duration and dosage considered	(145)
International case-control study	Risk doubled by use of oral contraceptives for 12 years; risk increased by duration of use; risk increased by use before first pregnancy; results may only be valid for Swedish women under 40; not seen in older or Norwegian women	(146)
Population-based case control study	No link with oral contraceptives	(144)
Narrative review	No risk	(147)
Systematic review	Greater risk with oral contraceptives in women with a history of fibroadenomas	(148)
Case-control study	Significantly more cases of breast cancer with depot medroxyprogesterone; no link with oral contraceptives	(149)
Population-based, case-control study	12-fold risk increase when young women use oral contraceptives for 12 years or more	(148)
Narrative review	Most studies have found no link with oral contraceptives; no reason for serious concern; possibly slightly higher frequency in industrialized countries	(113)
Narrative review	No increased risk from past use of oral contraceptives in women aged over 45 years; weak link in younger women with long-term use	(122)

environmental influences, the ages at which the menarche and menopause have occurred, and progressive changes in the spectrum of contraceptives in use. Information bias can easily mislead. The possible influence of the long latency likely to be involved in any effect has been heavily debated; breast tumors may have been present for many years by the time they become clinically detectable; many tumors induced by oral contraceptives may therefore so far have been missed, but conversely, oral contraceptives must often have been prescribed to women who unknowingly were already suffering from breast cancer. One must also bear in mind the apparently spontaneous increase in the incidence of breast cancer over the last 40 years. Finally, when cancers are found, there is little or nothing to distinguish them histologically from tumors that arise spontaneously (150).

Four meta-analyses have shown no increased risk of breast cancer in women who have ever taken an estrogen, compared with non-users. However, most studies suggest an increased risk of breast cancer among women who take estrogen for 5–10 years or longer. The summary relative risk estimate based on the findings of these studies is 1.32 (95% C1 = 1.16, 1.51) for women who reported long-term use compared with never-users. The increased risk of breast cancer may not persist after estrogen therapy is withdrawn, suggesting that estrogen acts as a promoter rather than a cause of breast cancer (151). In one publication from the Nurse's Health Study, the estimated risk of breast cancer associated with estrogen alone was 1.36 compared with 1.50 for estrogen + progestogen therapy (152). A later analysis from the same cohort showed that women who took unopposed estrogen had a 5% per year increased risk of breast cancer compared with 9% per year in women taking an estrogen + a progestogen. The most promising marker is the increase in breast density that occurs in 15–50% of women who take replacement estrogen (151).

The lower the dose of the hormonal components the less the risk of this complication, as has been shown in a population based case-control study in the USA in some 3000 women (153); the design of the study was originally described in 1995 (154). Women who had recently used oral contraceptives containing more than 35 micrograms of ethinylestradiol per tablet were at a significantly higher risk of breast cancer than users of lower dose formulations and at both doses the risk was higher than among never-users (respective relative risks of 1.99 and 1.27). The relation was particularly marked among women under 35 years of age, In whom the respective relative risks were 3.62 and 1.91. The authors also found significant trends of increasing breast cancer risk for tablets with higher progestogen and estrogen potencies, and these were again most pronounced among women under 35.

Non-invasive breast carcinoma, i.e. breast carcinoma in sit, has been studied in Connecticut in 2003 by examining data on 875 cases of ductal carcinoma in situ registered between 1994 and 1998, as well as data on 999 controls. The risk of ductal carcinoma in situ was not increased in women who had ever used oral contraceptives compared

with women who had never used them; nor was it significantly increased in any subgroup of ever-users (155).

There are some circumstances in which it is prudent to avoid using oral contraceptives, or in which frequent control of the state of the breasts is essential. These include (a) very long-term use before the first full pregnancy; (b) prolonged use of high-dose formulations; (c) uninterrupted use in women with a family history of breast cancer or with a personal history of fibroadenoma.

Finally, it is clear that the increase in the use of estrogen-containing contraceptives during the last 30 years cannot be held responsible for the current population-wide increase in breast cancer; as the International Committee for Research in Reproduction pointed out in 1989, the overwhelming proportion of the current rise in cases of breast cancer is among women who are too old to have taken oral contraceptives when they were younger. In addition, calculations suggest that even if an adverse effect among younger users of oral contraceptives were proved, it would still only account for a few percent of all breast cancers occurring in Western countries.

Patients with breast cancer who have discontinued estrogens less than 1 year before diagnosis have a significantly higher survival rate (156). Current users of estrogens at breast cancer diagnosis have a survival rate 5 years longer than non-users. However, they also have an increased incidence of breast cancer. This increased survival disappears when corrected for stage at diagnosis, when one can see that estrogen use relates most strongly to early-stage tumors. One might therefore expect that these tumors are less aggressive and that they result in an increased survival after diagnosis. The effect of hormone replacement therapy on breast cancer mortality may even be beneficial (157,158). Indicators of biological aggressiveness are the c-er 6 B2 oncoprotein, ploidy, tumor proliferation rate, and the presence of estrogen receptors (159).

Hormone replacement therapy

As far as hormone replacement therapy is concerned (Table 2) one must provisionally conclude, with the authors of a major Canadian study published in 1992, that long-term past use of estrogens is not related to risk, but that current estrogen use increases the risk of breast cancer to a modest degree, and that the addition of progestogens probably does not remove the increased risk resulting from the use of unopposed estrogen (160). Neither later research nor extensive reviews (171) have further clarified existing knowledge on the ability of HRT to modify the risks of certain malignancies.

The main concern relates to the increased risk of breast cancer. HRT is thought to increase the risk in about 6 per 1000 users aged 50–59 and 12 per 1000 in older women, the risk being further increased when combined estrogen + progestogen regimens are used. The risk of endometrial cancer is unaltered or very slightly reduced; randomized trials examining other important but rarer malignancies, like ovarian, gall-bladder, and urinary bladder cancer, are either non-existent or too small to detect any effect reliably (172).

Table 2 Some studies of the association between hormone replacement therapy and breast neoplasms

Type of study	Findings	Source
Prospective comparative study of users and non-users	Positive link between breast cancer and HRT, provided the menopause was natural	(95)
Cohort study following up long-term users of HRT	Slight increase in breast cancer, possibly accentuated by progestogens; possible methodological problems	(SED-12, 1027) (161)
	Risk increased with HRT by up to 30%	(162)
	Link between HRT and breast cancer uncertain, but Nurse's Health Study suggested a relative risk of 1.36; adding a progestogen reduces the risk	(163)
17 relevant studies of HRT reviewed	Risk increased by 20% with use for over 10 years and 50% with use for over 20 years	(164)
Review	At least 10 acceptable epidemiological papers point to a link between long-term HRT and breast cancer	(165)
Case-control study	No increase in risk among users of combined estrogen + progestogen HRT	(166)
Large case-control study	No increased risk of breast cancer with HRT	(167)
Case-control study	Increased risk among users of any type of HRT for more than 10 years; OR 2.1	(168)
Iowa Women's Health Study	HRT associated most strongly with an increased risk of invasive breast cancer and modest increases in risk of invasive ductal or lobular carcinoma of the breast	(169)
Million Women Study	Current users of HRT more likely than never-users to develop breast cancer	(170)

Breast cancer

There is today no reasonable doubt that hormone replacement therapy increases the risk of breast cancer. As always, however, the devil is in the detail, and argument continues as to nature and extent of the risk and the approaches or dosage schemes that might be relatively safe. The epidemiological figures continue to be interpreted in a manner much influenced by the writer's optimism or pessimism. The most useful estimates are still those from the 1997 analysis of 51 epidemiological studies (a 2% risk for each year of use) and from the Women's Health Initiative (a relative risk of 1.26 when combined therapy is compared with placebo). More subtle approaches are now estimating the risk by histological type. Tumor registry data from three eastern states in the USA, suggested that lobular carcinoma was associated with estrogen therapy within the last 2 years (OR = 1.8) and recent use of combined therapy (OR = 3.6), whereas ductal carcinoma showed no correlation with either type of HRT (173).

A prospective population study in Sweden has looked further into the question of how the incidence of breast cancer during HRT might be influenced by the type of replacement therapy used, i.e. with or without a progestogen (174). From 1995 onwards, data were collected on 6586 women aged 50-64 years in the Lund area of Sweden, with no reported breast cancer on inclusion. Information on their use of HRT during the period from December 1995 to February 2000 was obtained by questionnaire. Between their inclusion in the study and December 2001, 101 developed breast cancer. Only ever-use of the continuous combined estrogen + progestogen formula differed significantly between cases and controls (45% versus 24%). Compared with never-users, exclusive users of combined estrogen + progestogen had

the highest age-adjusted hazard ratio (HR = 3.3; 95% CI = 1.9, 5.6), followed by users of combined estrogen + progestogen in addition to other HRT formulas (HR = 2.8; 95% CI = 1.4, 5.5). There was no significant increase in women who exclusively used other HRT formulas. On this evidence it can be concluded that women who used combined estrogen + progestogen had over three times the risk of breast cancer compared with never-users and twice the risk compared with users of other types of HRT.

In the Iowa Women's Health Study of postmenopausal women for 11 years, during which 1520 specific breast cancers occurred in the at-risk cohort of 37 105 women, it was concluded that exposure to hormone replacement therapy was associated most strongly with an increased risk of invasive breast cancer with a favorable prognosis. There was a more modest increase in the risk of invasive ductal or lobular carcinoma of the breast (169).

Precisely because a careful watch has to be kept for signs of malignant change in the breast in users of HRT, it is important to recognize the possible influence of the hormonal treatment itself on the breast, even in the absence of cancerous change. In the past an increase in parenchymal density, ranging from 11% to 52% has been described. In a new prospective study of this issue in Turkey, 182 menopausal women were given HRT (estrogen alone, sequential use of progestogens + estrogens, continuous use of both types of hormone, or tibolone alone) (175). Breast examinations and mammography were carried out at the outset and repeated after a mean of 11.6 months. The parenchymal density of the breast was increased by an average of some 18% in all cases; the effect was most marked in women who took the combined product continuously (a 25% increase in density) and least in the users of tibolone (a 5.5% increase). The increase in density was particularly striking in obese women and was twice as severe in women with a family history of breast cancer; in the series as a whole, it ran parallel with an increase in breast tenderness. However, there was no atypia, and the changes were therefore not considered to constitute a contraindication to continued HRT.

In a relatively small but meticulously designed study of not only actual breast cancer but all possible forms of breast changes in 300 women aged 30-50 years, of whom 120 had taken HRT and 180 had never been exposed to it, the women were divided into four categories: those with normal breast tissue, those with fibrocystic disease, those with cellular atypia, and those with breast cancer (176). Another group of women were also identified who had breast implants. Changes in breast tissue were determined using breast-enhanced scintigraphy. The breasts were "normal" in 122 (40%), of whom 84 (69%) had not taken HRT. This accounted for 47% of the women not taking hormone therapy (84 of 180), while only 32% of the women taking HRT (38 of 120) had normal breasts. This difference was statistically significant. There was a greater overall incidence of breast abnormality in women taking HRT and a lower incidence in pathology among women not taking HRT when cumulatively analysed for FCD, cellular atypia, and breast cancer. This difference was statistically significant for women with breast cancer, of whom 63% (10 of 16) were taking HRT. This work suggests that the initial empirical observations of a higher incidence of HRT among women with breast cancer may have a relation to underlying changes in breast tissue that are associated with differences in mitochondrial content and activity. Perhaps one should stress that this paper was concerned primarily with defining the entire spectrum of changes that can occur in the breast during HRT; it did not address the question of existing evidence about the association between HRT and breast cancer.

Breast tumors that develop in HRT users have prognostically favorable histological features, but it is unclear if this is the case for both short-term and long-term use. In 2000 women aged over 55 years with invasive breast cancer diagnosed over 7 years short-term users of HRT (5 years or less) were about 50% less likely to develop poorly differentiated breast tumors or node-positive tumors than non-users (177). Longer term users of HRT were also less likely to develop poorly differentiated tumors, but the incidence of node-positive tumors was not reduced compared with controls. Tumor size was not significantly related to the duration of treatment.

Many clinicians continue to withhold estrogen-based replacement therapy from women who have a history of breast cancer because they fear impairing their prognosis; the evidence is not firm, but experts continue to urge caution in the absence of firm data either way (178). A well-designed study from Finland in 131 such women, two-thirds of whom used HRT, showed no increase in the breast cancer recurrence rate after an average of 2.5 years (179). However, the limited size of the study (and the fact that various different forms of HRT were used) make it difficult to exclude the risk on the basis of these data alone.

Because hyperplastic or fibrocystic changes in the breast may be pre-malignant, there has been a study of 42 women who at breast biopsy had atypical hyperplasia, 74 age-matched women with proliferative fibrocystic changes, and 74 with non-proliferative fibrocystic changes (180). The patients were aged 26–77 years, and had taken predominantly HRT (usually conjugated estrogen) but sometimes oral contraceptives. There was a strong association between exogenous hormone use and the presence of atypical hyperplasia. The authors considered that their results were in line with the theory that there is a continuum between hyperplasia and carcinoma and considered that exogenous hormone use may influence the transition from one to the other in a (still undefined) subset of women.

It is difficult to interpret a Japanese report of a woman aged 62 years who developed a benign fibrous tumor of the breast. The mass, which had been noted 1 year before, progressively enlarged. Bearing in mind that such fibrous tumors of the breast are almost always premenopausal, it may be significant that she had been taking estrogens irregularly for the previous 10 years but had taken them intensively during the last year. In addition, there was positive immunohistochemical nuclear staining for estrogen receptor antibodies in stromal cells (181).

By far the largest piece of evidence to emerge on the risk of breast cancer is that from the Million Women Study (170). In all, more than a million women aged 50–64 were recruited into this study between 1996 and 2001 and are being followed up with respect to cancer incidence and deaths. There were 9364 incident invasive breast cancers and 637 breast cancer deaths after an average of 2.6 and 4.1 years of follow-up respectively. Current users of HRT at recruitment were more likely than never-users to develop breast cancer (adjusted RR = 1.66; 95% CI = 1.58, 1.75) and die from it (1.22; 1.00, 1.48). Past users of hormone replacement therapy were not at an increased risk. The risk was significantly increased among current users of formulations containing estrogen only, estrogen + progestogen, and tibolone, but the risk was substantially greater for estrogen + progestogen than for other types of hormone replacement therapy. The risks were significantly increased separately for oral, transdermal, and implanted estrogen-only formulations. In current users of each type of hormone replacement therapy the risk of breast cancer increased with increasing total duration of use. Although the conclusions of this major study are roughly similar to those of the Women's Health Initiative, it has already been challenged on methodological and statistical grounds as presenting an unjustified threat to the continued use of HRT in women who need it (182).

When breast cancers occur in women taking estrogen replacement therapy they are sometimes claimed to be less aggressive than in other women. The effect of the duration or type of replacement therapy on the aggressiveness of such tumors has been studied in 1105 consecutive postmenopausal patients treated for operable breast cancer at the European Institute of Oncology (183). Tumors in women who had been exposed to estrogen replacement therapy were characterized by better stage distribution, a smaller diameter, and less extensive involvement of the axillary lymph nodes; histological grade III tumors were less common. The prognosis was generally better in women who took estrogen replacement therapy for more than 5 years. Tumors with estrogen-positive receptors were more common in the controls, but this tendency was reversed when the comparison was limited to those who had had particularly long exposure. Overall, these findings seem to confirm that prolonged use of estrogen replacement therapy does reduce the degree of aggressiveness of breast cancer, but they still have to be set against the evidence that the incidence of such cancers is increased.

The pathological spectrum of breast cancers that develop in users of HRT is not necessarily the same as that of cancers that develop spontaneously. In a retrospective study of 10 874 postmenopausal Danish Nurses over 10 years, using data retrieved from the National Cancer Registry, there were breast cancers in 244 women, 172 being invasive ductal carcinomas (184). Compared with never users, current users of HRT had an increased risk of a hormone receptor-positive breast cancer, but no increased risk of receptor-negative breast cancer ($RR = 3.29$; $95\%CI = 2.27, 4.77$). The risk of a diagnosis of a "low histological malignancy" grade of cancer was higher than that of high malignancy grade ($RR = 4.13$). For breast cancers with other prognostic characteristics, the risk was increased equally for the favorable and non-favorable types. Current users of HRT had a two- to four-fold increased risk of breast cancer with various prognostic characteristics, both the favorable and non-favorable types. As regards receptor status, the risk with HRT was statistically significantly higher for hormone receptor-positive breast cancer than with receptor-negative breast cancer.

It would be helpful if there were a reliable means of identifying women at an increased risk of breast cancer when taking decisions on HRT. The possibility that the androgen receptor gene might provide a clue, in view of earlier evidence that women with a higher number of CAG repeat lengths on this gene have increased breast cancer rates, has been studied in 404 women with breast cancer (185). Among postmenopausal users of estrogen + progestogen treatment, carriers of the less active AR-CAG had a statistically significantly higher mean percentage breast density (41%) than carriers of the more active AR-CAG. It is thus possible that the number of AR-CAG repeats will ultimately be helpful in predicting the breast cancer risk in women taking HRT.

Another approach to the study of the effects of hormone replacement therapy on the breast is to examine breast density, using mammography and the Wolfe classification. In a randomized study of 166 menopausal women, using this technique, there was increased breast density after 6 months of treatment; eight times more commonly in those who took estradiol and norethisterone acetate than in those who took tibolone (186). The significance of this increased density is not clear, but it should for the present be regarded as undesirable,

perhaps representing the prodromal phase of more serious complications.

Whatever the level of breast cancer risk presented by postmenopausal hormonal cancer therapy, there is little doubt that it varies with the precise regimen. It is true that this does not come clearly to the fore in all the relevant studies, but that may simply be because the question was not specifically examined. In a thoughtful study of data from the E3N-EPIC cohort investigation, the risk of breast cancer associated with HRT was assessed in 54 548 postmenopausal women (mean age at inclusion 53 years) who had not taken any HRT in the year before entering the investigation. There were 948 primary invasive breast cancers during follow-up over an average of 5.8 years, and a modestly increased overall breast cancer risk compared with non-users ($RR = 1.2$) (187). However, while the relative risk was only 1.1 ($CI = 0.8, 1.6$) for estrogens used alone it was 1.3 (1.1, 1.5) when estrogens were used in combination with oral progestogens. The risk was significantly greater with HRT containing synthetic progestins than with HRT containing micronized progesterone, the relative risks being 1.4 (1.2, 1.7) and 0.9 (0.7, 1.2) respectively. When combined with synthetic progestins, both oral estrogen and transdermal/percutaneous estrogen were associated with a significantly increased risk; for transdermal/percutaneous estrogen, this was the case even when exposure was less than 2 years. These findings suggest that when estrogens used for HRT are combined with synthetic progestogens even short-term use may increase the risk of breast cancer. It also seems that micronized progesterone may be preferable to synthetic progestins for short-term HRT. Findings such as these need more follow-up if the safest form of HRT is to be clearly identified.

Meanwhile in Australia an attempt has been made to estimate the national incidence of breast cancer due to hormone replacement therapy and to come to grips with it. The investigators used the attributable fraction technique, with prevalence data derived from the 2001 Australian Health Survey and published rates of breast cancer relative risks from HRT. In Australia 12% of adult women are current HRT users, and 11 783 breast cancers were reported in 2001, of which 1066 (9%) were potentially attributable to HRT (188). Restricting HRT to women under 65 years, withdrawing HRT after 10 years, or limiting combined estrogen and progesterone HRT to 5 years (but otherwise keeping prescription patterns to 2001 levels) were considered to be approaches that could reduce the annual national breast cancer case load by 280 (2.4%), 555 (4.7%), and 674 (5.7%) cases respectively.

Endometrial cancer

It has long been considered that the risk of endometrial carcinoma may be somewhat reduced by HRT, but that the risk is affected by the dose of progestogen used, if any. In a recent population-based case-control study covering 647 cases and 1209 controls, users of estrogen + medroxyprogesterone acetate (MPA) given for 10–24 days monthly in a dose of 100 mg/month or more showed the same risk of endometrial cancer as women not using HRT

(189). However, the relative risk was only 0.8 (95% CI 0.5-1.5) in those who used a lower monthly MPA dose. Among users of a continuous combined hormone regimen, the risk of endometrial cancer was low relative to untreated women, regardless of the MPA dose. These findings hardly suggest that the dose of progestogen has very much effect on the risk of endometrial cancer.

In a critical review of all the relevant evidence on combined estrogen + progestogen HRT about 15% of the endometrial biopsies taken from women on sequential HRT showed proliferative activity, including atypical endometrial hyperplasia in up to 1% of the cases (190). Most biopsies taken from women taking continuous combined HRT show endometrial atrophy. About 2–3% of these women will have proliferative activity, usually without atypical hyperplasia. There was no increased risk of endometrial cancer in the extensive WHI and HERS studies, but various endogenous factors, such as obesity, diabetes mellitus, the distribution of estrogen receptors alpha and beta, and genetic polymorphisms for receptors and enzymes, might alter the endometrial effects of various types of HRT. These authors considered that there should be a liberal indication for endometrial biopsies when HRT is used. Since the incidence of atypical hyperplasia or carcinoma under unopposed estrogen therapy is 2–10%, this type of HRT should not be used in non-hysterectomized women. As far as the risk of endometrial cancer from any kind of HRT is concerned, the different molecular pathways of endometrial carcinogenesis (types 1 and 2 cancers) should be taken into account. These authors noted that tibolone leaves the endometrium unaffected.

Malignant melanoma

Mortality and incidence rates of malignant melanoma and skin cancer have increased in most Western countries during the last 20 years, clearly for reasons unconnected with oral contraception. However, endocrinological factors can affect the melanocytes and the spread of malignant melanoma. Estrogen receptors have been noted in malignant melanoma cells, and estrogens are known to stimulate melanogenesis, an effect that is enhanced by simultaneous administration of progestogens. Oral contraceptives might therefore have an effect; the fact that chloasma has long been known to occur in some oral contraceptive users is perhaps relevant (191).

One large epidemiological study from California showed that women taking oral contraceptives, particularly long-term users, had a relatively high incidence of malignant melanoma (192). In Australia, there was a significant association with melanoma in women who had used oral contraceptives for at least 10 years before diagnosis (193). In a Canadian study, on the other hand, there was no association between the risk of superficially spreading melanoma or nodular melanoma and the use of either oral contraceptives or menopausal estrogens (SED-12, 1029) (194); however, it was suggested that there might be a risk in some subpopulations. One must be alert for confounding factors: for example, among oral contraceptive users there could be a relatively higher

proportion of physically active and sporting women who are more susceptible than the average to expose themselves to sunlight. The results of a case control study in Philadelphia specifically on intraocular malignant melanoma showed that hormonal factors played only a limited role in the causation of this condition (SED-12, 1029) (195).

Pituitary tumors

A 1978 WHO report quoted an unpublished study by March in which pituitary adenomas were found in 26% of women with secondary amenorrhea following the use of oral contraceptives, yet in only 13% of cases who had not used these products (118). The difference was significant, but selection bias might have explained the results.

Non-Hodgkin's lymphoma

Weak evidence from interview studies conducted in the past suggested that the risk of non-Hodgkin's lymphoma might be increased by estrogen treatment. A case-control study in a total population of some 300 000 adults in the Netherlands, using primary discharge diagnoses and pharmacy dispensing records now appears to have discounted this supposed risk (196).

Other cancers

While the incidence of some tumors is increased in HRT users, that of other tumors seems to be reduced, the reduced incidence of colorectal cancer having been documented. The authors of a review brought together data on this issue from a series of case-control studies conducted in Italy between 1983 and 1999 involving a total of 537 cancers occurring in ever-users and 6439 reported in never-users; there was a control group of 6976 women with acute, non-neoplastic conditions (197). In the overall analysis there was an inverse relation between HRT and the occurrence of cancer of the colon (OR = 0.7), rectum (OR = 0.5) and liver (OR = 0.2), There were excess risks for cancers of the gallbladder (OR = 3.2), breast (OR = 1.1), endometrium (OR = 3.0), and urinary bladder (OR = 2.0). There was also a non-significant increase in the risk of ovarian cancer. The very small increase in breast cancer risk in this study is striking when one sets these findings against other work, cited above.

HRT after gynecological malignancies

It is widely considered that women who have already suffered breast cancer and have been treated for it should not receive estrogen therapy, but some workers express doubts as to whether this is indeed risky. The influential results of the Women's Health Initiative study concerning the risks of HRT did not address this specific subgroup of users. A recent review has examined more than 30 studies of the issue, involving in all 1558 breast cancer survivors treated with estrogen or estrogen + progestogen replacement therapy (198). Overall, the recurrence rate accrued from the uncontrolled studies was 7.3% (53 of 728). The average rate culminating from 11 case-controlled studies was 11% (99 of 830) in treated patients versus 20% (739 of 3640) in their untreated counterparts. There was no increase in recurrent disease among treated patients but the study was not conclusive because of deficiencies in some of the studies reviewed.

The possible effects of hormonal therapy on women who have been treated for endometrial or other malignancies have been reviewed (198). Data derived from 537 women involved in four case-control studies showed that early use of estrogens very greatly reduces the incidence of recurrences. The impact of estrogen on other gynecological malignancies is not as clear. Incomplete data in the literature suggest a slight increase in recurrence of ovarian cancer but indicate that there is no effect on most other gynecological malignancies. However, a previous history of cervical adenocarcinoma definitely excludes the use of these hormonal regimens.

Second-Generation Effects

Fertility

In 1993, Sharpe and Skakkebaek published a theory that environmental and other forms of exposure of males to estrogens, particularly during fetal life, might explain the increasing incidence of reduced sperm counts and developmental disorders of the male genital system (199). Such exposure could be in part due, for example, to dietary changes in mothers: a low-fiber diet results in a great reabsorption of endogenous estrogens, and there is an increasing use in the diet of soya, which is a rich source of phytoestrogens. The topic goes beyond the scope of this volume, but it is not impossible that baseline exposure to estrogens in the diet or environment could increase the sensitivity of individuals to estrogens that are administered therapeutically or for purposes of contraception.

Teratogenicity

The best-known second-generation effects of estrogens are the genital complications that result from the formerly widespread use in pregnancy of diethylstilbestrol (q.v.), mainly between 1940 and 1975. Although it is difficult to reconstruct medical histories dating back to this period, evidence continues to emerge. The evidence is covered in the monograph on Oral contraceptives.

Hormone replacement therapy is generally given at a time when pregnancy can be excluded, but in principle some of the risks discussed in connection with oral contraceptives would arise if a women taking hormone replacement therapy were to become pregnant. In 1980, an authoritative Scientific Group of the World Health Organization (WHO) surveyed the entire question of the effects of female sex hormones on fetal development and infant health (200), and after 25 years one can conclude that later reports in the literature have almost entirely supported its conclusions.

Congenital abnormalities
Records available in Finland have been used to seek correlations between hormonal treatment (with diethylstilbestrol, estrogens, or progestogens) and adverse effects, including cancers in the mother or infant. A retrospective cohort of 2052 hormone-drug exposed mothers, 2038 control mothers, and their 4130 infants was collected from maternity centers in Helsinki covering the period from 1954 to 1963 (201). Cancer cases were sought in national registers through record linkage. Exposures were examined by the type of the drug (estrogen + progestogen or progestogen only) and by timing (early in pregnancy or only late in pregnancy). There were no statistically significant differences between the groups with regard to maternal cancers, whether total or specified hormone-dependent cancers. However, the total number of malformations recorded, as well as genital malformations in male infants, was higher among exposed children. The number of cancers among the offspring was small, and none of the differences between groups was statistically significant. The authors suggested that their study supported the conclusion that estrogen or progestogen therapy during pregnancy causes malformations among children who were exposed in utero, but not the hypothesis that it causes cancer later in life in the mother; the power to study cancers in offspring was too low to draw firm conclusions. Non-existence of the risk, negative confounding, weak exposure, or a low study power may have explained the negative findings.

Susceptibility Factors

Age

Occasionally, children are exposed unknowingly to estrogens. Precocious puberty has been observed in young girls after contact with hair lotions and other products containing estrogenic compounds (SED-12, 1032) (202,203).

The short-term complications of estrogens are unpleasant rather than dangerous. A questionnaire survey among American pediatric endocrinologists has showed that these effects commonly included weight gain, nausea or vomiting, areolar or nipple pigmentation, headache, and irregular menses (204). However, there seems to have been no methodical follow-up to determine the long-term consequences.

The longer-term consequences have in recent years given rise to rather greater concern. The use of estrogens to arrest excessive growth in height in girls was first reported in 1956 (205). While the estrogen is given continuously, the addition of a progestogen given cyclically around the time of the menarche is customary in order to induce (or permit) menstrual periods and to prevent metropathia hemorrhagica. The estrogen produces a mean reduction in predicted height, provided the treatment is begun at a bone age of 12 years and before the menarche (206). The duration of treatment is from 8 months to 3 years.

There has been an anecdotal report of thrombosis in a girl taking estrogens in addition to older evidence that they can reduce antithrombin activity, which could indeed raise the risk of thrombotic complications (207).

It was long thought that there was no impairment of subsequent fertility or of the pituitary–ovarian axis in tall healthy girls treated with estrogens, but this is now uncertain. In a retrospective cohort study in Tasmania, using medical record reviews and interviews, women who had been treated with estrogen to suppress growth were significantly more likely to be infertile and were more than twice as likely to have ever taken fertility drugs than women who were not treated in this way (208).

Estrogen treatment of girls in whom growth in height tends to be excessive is progressively losing favor. In 2002, after reviewing the possible risks, which in its view could include miscarriage, endometriosis, and ovarian cysts as well as infertility, the USA Physicians' Committee for Responsible Medicine petitioned the FDA to issue appropriate warnings (204).

Sex

Following castration for cancer of the prostate, a high proportion of men have hot flushes, and estrogens can provide relief. In a study in 12 such men, estrogen in a low dose (0.05 mg) or high dose (0.10 mg) given as patches twice-weekly for 4 weeks provided considerable improvement (209). In this dosage, mild painless breast swelling or nipple tenderness was noted in two and five of the 12 men treated with the low- and high-dose patches respectively. Estradiol concentrations increased from 12 pg/ml to 16 and 27 pg/ml with the low-dose and high-dose patches respectively. There were no significant changes in serum testosterone or luteinizing hormone concentrations. This was a small study, and data on the tolerability of this topical treatment in a larger series would be welcome.

There is evidence for a role of estrogen in male bone metabolism, notably from studies in a man with a genetic defect in estrogen receptors and in men with aromatase deficiencies. Estrogen is likely to affect bone turnover in men throughout life, and it has been suggested that older men could have reduced bone resorption in response to estrogen therapy. In a study of this possibility, in 14 men with osteopenia of the femoral neck using micronized estradiol 1 mg/day for 9 weeks, that is a dose that is effective in postmenopausal women, estradiol and estrone concentrations increased significantly by more than 6-fold and 15-fold respectively (210). Concentrations of serum hormone binding globulin increased significantly by 17%, but concentrations of total and unbound testosterone fell significantly, by 27% and 34% respectively. Markers of bone resorption showed wide variations both at baseline and during treatment; they were too inconsistent to justify conclusions as to the potential usefulness of the treatment. However, the adverse effects of treatment were minimal, including (as might be expected) breast tenderness and reduced libido, which reversed after treatment.

Hepatic disease

Women with even mild liver disease can have an increased risk of the adverse effects of some estrogens on the liver (211,212). Furthermore, estrogens can potentiate and aggravate the organic complications of

liver disease in other systems, for example increased cholesterol or lithogenesis (213,214).

Other features of the patient

Estrogens should be avoided in individuals with current thrombophlebitis or thromboembolism, estrogen-dependent tumors, abnormal genital bleeding without a diagnosis, and pregnancy. They are also contraindicated in apparently healthy women if they have an earlier history of jaundice in pregnancy, hepatic disease, thromboembolism, or porphyria.

Swedish workers have sought to develop a test system to define men who have a higher risk of cardiovascular complications when they take estrogens for cancer of the prostate (215). An investigational battery using exercise stress testing, evaluation of the peripheral circulation, blood volume estimation, chest X-ray, blood tests including hormonal status, lipoproteins, and antithrombin III, and history and physical examination taken by a cardiologist is claimed to make it possible to classify 84% of estrogen-treated patients as individuals with or without a particular risk of a cardiovascular complication and to identify an extremely high-risk subgroup.

Drug Administration

Drug formulations

Alternative means of administering estrogens continue to be investigated, particularly in the hope of reducing unwanted effects. If it is necessary to give estrogens shortly after delivery, one concern will be whether this will suppress lactation, the other whether undesirable amounts of estrogen may enter the milk and thus pass to the infant. A Finnish group has reported that by using transdermal estrogen a sufficient effect can be obtained to compensate for a hypoestrogenic state without significant passage into the milk (216). In 21 healthy breastfeeding women who had delivered 20 weeks earlier, all of whom had received transdermal estradiol (E2) 50, 75, or 100 micrograms/day or placebo for 2 weeks, none of the breast milk samples contained any measurable concentrations of estradiol. Serum estradiol concentrations were increased dose-dependently. Both serum FSH and LH concentrations were reduced in all treatment groups, with more pronounced suppression in those who took 75 and 100 micrograms/day. Serum inhibin B concentrations were not significantly suppressed.

In some instances, transdermal estrogens appear less likely to cause problems than other forms of administration. One group studied the treatment of polycystic ovary syndrome in 24 women, using transdermal or peroral administration of a combination of estradiol and cyproterone acetate in doses comparable to those used in oral contraceptives (217). The peroral treatment led to a significant impairment in insulin secretion and action whereas the transdermal application of estrogens did not significantly influence insulin sensitivity.

Another group has tested the hypothesis that continuous transdermal hormone replacement therapy with estrogen/progestogen combinations could have beneficial effects on risk markers for coronary heart disease without eliciting serious adverse effects. In a randomized study, 60 postmenopausal women received either transdermal oestradiol-17-beta 0.05 mg/day with norethisterone acetate 0.125 mg/day or an identical placebo (218). After 6 months, HRT resulted in highly significant reductions in E-selectin, angiotensin-converting enzyme, cholesterol, low-density lipoproteins, high-density lipoprotein 3, apolipoproteins AII, and fasting insulin. Factor VII coagulation activity fell, while plasminogen activator inhibitor-1 and fibrin D-dimer increased in the HRT group, while prothrombin fragments 1 + 2 fell, more so in the placebo group. There were no changes in matrix metalloproteinase (MMP)-2, or in LDL particle size. Transdermal HRT was therefore considered to have beneficial effects on vascular function and CHD risk markers. It is unfortunate that in this work there was no direct therapeutic comparison between effective doses of the transdermal and the oral forms.

Drug administration route

Well-designed studies of local, topical, and intradermal forms of estrogen as a means of attaining a general systemic effect have tended to show that when doses are therapeutically equivalent to those used orally the adverse effects are similar (219). However, this is a complex issue, which is discussed more extensively in connection with hormone replacement therapy.

Intranasal administration

Intranasal estradiol gives results comparable to transdermal estradiol, but substantially higher doses are needed. In 300 postmenopausal women, 17-β-estradiol 300 micrograms/day was as effective as two patches per week delivering 50 micrograms/day (220). Adverse events rates were similar but moderate, and severe mastalgia was significantly less frequent with intranasal estradiol (7.2%) than with the patch (15.5%); 66% of the patients chose to continue the intranasal therapy and 34% the transdermal therapy.

Subcutaneous implants

Implantable formulations of estrogens have been reviewed (221). Subcutaneous implants have as a rule durations of action of 4–12 months, depending on the dosage and formulation used; variations can be due to technical problems, such as disintegration or migration of an implant.

Transdermal patches

Typical patches of estradiol contain 50 micrograms, but there are important differences between the wanted and unwanted effects of the available products, because of the ways in which they are formulated. The wash-out period of estradiol after transdermal administration is about 6 weeks. Transdermal estrogens can also be supplemented periodically by an oral progestogen (222). New topical formulations of estrogens continue to be studied and

marketed, although most studies have shown little difference between the various formulations available (223).

The reported incidence of adverse skin reactions to transdermal estradiol varies from 2% to over 25%, depending on the transdermal system, climatic conditions, and individual sensitivity. Of 78 women 29 reported one or more adverse events and eight discontinued prematurely (224). The main reasons for premature withdrawal included problems of adhesion, skin reactions, or undesirable systemic effects, such as headache, breast tenderness, weight gain, leg cramps, and unacceptable withdrawal bleeding.

Poor adhesion and skin irritation, with erythema and itching, are the principal drawbacks of transdermal therapy (225). Skin irritation can be overcome in some cases by changing the application site every day. In a direct comparison of transdermal patches, the duration, severity, and number of skin reactions depended on the individual formulation and excipients.

Allergic contact dermatitis from transdermal estrogen has been described in Korea, where the reaction was found to be due to 17-β-estradiol itself and not to an excipient (226). In some cases, allergic reactions and systemic contact dermatitis are clearly attributable to the patch material or to excipients. Even natural estradiol given in this way can occasionally cause hypersensitivity reactions, as determined by patch tests (227).

All the systemic effects of estrogens can occur with transdermal administration, subject to some modification as a result of the liver being bypassed (228).

Transdermal absorption of estrogen can lead to pseudoprecocious puberty in young girls, and to symptoms in young boys and adult men such as gynecomastia, loss of libido, impotence, and galactorrhea (229–231).

In a randomized, placebo-controlled, crossover study for 12 weeks, the estrogen matrix patch Estraderm MX, which unlike some other patches contains no alcohol, significantly relieved climacteric symptoms in both lower and higher strengths (50 and 100 micrograms of estradiol) (232). Local tolerability was good, but there was a slight increase in estrogen-related adverse effects (breast tenderness, leukorrhea) with the higher dose; there was a 4.8% overall incidence of endometrial hyperplasia in patients with an intact uterus. In women who have local reactions to alcohol, a patch of this type may be helpful.

Other work has confirmed the similar value of two patch formulations, Menorest and Climara; the latter has been reported to cause a much higher incidence of local reactions, but they are mild (233). The Fem 7 patch, which delivers estradiol 50 micrograms/day, was also well tolerated (234). Another effective and well-accepted variant on the patch theme is Demestril, which releases estradiol 25 or 37.5 micrograms/day depending on the formulation used (235). Differences in effect and tolerability between all these various estradiol patches are primarily a question of dosage and release rate, but it also seems that acceptance may be better when the drug is incorporated into the adhesive rather than being stored in a separate reservoir. The former type of patch shows better adhesion and is cosmetically more acceptable (236).

When low-dose patch therapy results in breakthrough bleeding it is supposedly more likely to occur in women with large, thin-walled, superficial endometrial vessels (89). If this finding is correct it might also apply to breakthrough bleeding with other forms of hormonal therapy.

Transdermal estrogen for androgen-dependent prostatic cancer is increasingly preferred over the oral route because it avoids first-pass hepatic exposure. The effects of this form of treatment have been studied in an open phase II study in 24 men with prostatic carcinoma who were progressing after primary hormonal therapy and who received transdermal estradiol 0.6 mg (administered as six 24-hour patches of 0.1 mg each) replaced every 7 days (237). Three of the 24 had a confirmed reduction in prostate-specific antigen by more than half. Adverse effects were modest and there were no thromboembolic complications. The mean serum estradiol concentration rose from 17 (range 15–20) pg/ml to 461 (range 335–587) pg/ml. The total testosterone concentration remained stable in the anorchid range during treatment, but the free testosterone concentration fell as a result of increased sex hormone binding globulin. There were no changes in factor VIII activity, F 1.2, or resistance to activated protein C, but there was a modest reduction in the concentration of protein S.

Vaginal administration

Because weak estrogens, such as estriol and estrone (the main component of conjugated estrogens), are claimed to act primarily on the lower part of the genital tract, they have long been used topically for atrophic conditions of the vagina and vulva, and are reputed to have useful effects in doses that do not cause marked endometrial or systemic changes. However, everything may in fact be a question of dosage; it could well be that even a low dose of a potent estrogen would have a similarly selective effect. In 159 menopausal women with atrophic vaginitis who used either a conjugated equine estrogen vaginal cream (2 g/day containing conjugated estrogens 1.25 mg) or 17-β-estradiol pessaries 25 µg (one daily for 2 weeks), the two treatments provided equivalent relief of the symptoms of atrophic vaginitis, but at weeks 2, 12, and 24 there were increases in serum estradiol concentrations and suppression of follicle-stimulating hormone in significantly more patients who used the conjugated estrogen cream than in those who used the estradiol pessaries; the patients themselves rated the estradiol treatment more highly (238).

Another effective alternative to the use of weak estrogens is the administration of estradiol from an estradiol-releasing vaginal ring, which offers efficacy, safety, and tolerability with improved comfort and acceptability. The most frequent adverse events were vaginitis, breast tenderness, abdominal pain, pruritus, and vaginal discomfort (239). However, the incidence of these adverse events was similar to those of other estrogen vaginal delivery systems. In women with lower urinary tract symptoms after the menopause an estradiol-releasing vaginal ring was well tolerated and enjoyed better patient acceptance than local estriol (240).

With vaginal creams, used primarily in order to secure a marked local effect in arresting atrophy of the vulva and vagina, the degree of systemic effect can be variable, because of variations from day to day in vaginal vascularization and secretions (228).

In a study of micronized estradiol vaginal tablets 25 micrograms or placebo in 1612 women, with assessment at 4 and 12 months; the estrogen did not increase serum estrogen concentrations or stimulate endometrial growth (241). In a placebo-controlled study in the "urge syndrome" in 40 menopausal women an implant of 17-beta-estradiol 25 mg had no therapeutic effect, but nine women had vaginal bleeding (242).

References

1. Studd J, Pornel B, Marton I, Bringer J, Varin C, Tsouderos Y, Christiansen CAerodiol Study Group. Efficacy and acceptability of intranasal 17 beta-oestradiol for menopausal symptoms: randomised dose–response study. Lancet 1999;353(9164):1574–8.
2. Schmidt-Elmendorff H, Kammerling R. Vergleichende klinische Untersuchungen von Clomiphen. Cyclofenil und Epimestrol. [Comparative clinical studies on clomiphen, cyclofenil and epimestrol.] Geburtshilfe Frauenheilkd 1977;37(6):531–41.
3. Iida H, Miyamoto I, Noda Y, Sawaki M, Nagai Y. Adrenocortical insufficiency associated with long-term high-dose fosfestrol therapy for prostatic carcinoma. Intern Med 1999;38(10):804–7.
4. Liao E-Y, Luo X-H, Deng X-G, Wu X-P, Liao H-J, Wang P-F, Mao J-P, Zhu X-P, Huang G, Wei Q-Y. The effect of low dose nylestriol-levonorgestrel replacement therapy on bone mineral density in women with post-menopausal osteoporosois. Endocr Res 2003;29:217–26.
5. Ockene JK, Barad DH, Cochrane BB, Larson JC, Gass M, Wassertheil-Smoller S, Manson JE, Barnabei VM, Lane DS, Brzyski RG, Rosal MC, Wylie-Rosett J, Hays J. Symptom experience after discounting use of estrogen plus progestin. JAMA 2005;294(2):183–93.
6. Saunders-Pullman R. Estrogens and Parkinson disease: neuroprotective, symptomatic, neither, or both? Endocrine 2003;21:81–7.
7. Berlanga C, Mendieta D, Alva G, Del Carmen Lara M. Failure of tibolone to potentiate the pharmacological effect of fluoxetine in postmenopausal major depression. J Women's Health 2003;12:33–9.
8. Liu YK, Kosfeld RE, Marcum SG. Treatment of uraemic bleeding with conjugated oestrogen. Lancet 1984;2(8408):887–90.
9. Livio M, Mannucci PM, Vigano G, Mingardi G, Lombardi R, Mecca G, Remuzzi G. Conjugated oestrogens for the management of bleeding associated with renal failure. N Engl J Med 1986;315(12):731–5.
10. Koch HJ Jr, Escher GC, Lewis JS. Hormonal management of hereditary hemorrhagic talangiectasia. JAMA 1952;149(15):1376–80.
11. Vase P. Estrogen treatment of hereditary hemorrhagic telangiectasia. A double-blind controlled clinical trial. Acta Med Scand 1981;209(5):393–6.
12. Iversen P. Orchidectomy and oestrogen therapy revisited. Eur Urol 1998;34(Suppl 3):7–11.

13. Sonnenschein C, Soto AM. An updated review of environmental estrogen and androgen mimics and antagonists. J Steroid Biochem Mol Biol 1998;65(1–6):143–50.

14. Perez Gutthann S, Garcia Rodriguez LA, Castellsague J, Duque Oliart A. Hormone replacement therapy and risk of venous thromboembolism: population based case-control study. BMJ 1997;314(7083):796–800.

15. The Coronary Drug Project Research Group. The Coronary Drug Project. Findings leading to discontinuation of the 2.5-mg day estrogen group JAMA 1973;226(6):652–7.

16. Christodoulakos G, Lambrinoudaki I, Panoulis C, Papadias C, Economou E, Creatsas G. Effect of hormone therapy and raloxifene on serum VE-cadherin in postmenopausal women. Fertil Steril 2004;82:634–8.

17. Aitken DA, Daw EG. Allergic reaction to quinestrol. BMJ 1970;2(702):177.

18. Lake SR, Vernon SA. Emergency contraception and retinal vein thrombosis. Br J Ophthalmol 1999;83(5):630–1.

19. Murray DC, Christopoulou D, Hero M. Combined central retinal vein occlusion and cilioretinal artery occlusion in a patient on hormone replacement therapy. Br J Ophthalmol 2000;84(5):549–50.

20. Cahill M, O'Toole L, Acheson RW. Hormone replacement therapy and retinal vein occlusion. Eye 1999;13(Pt 6):798–800.

21. Kirwan JF, Tsaloumas MD, Vinall H, Prior P, Kritzinger EE, Dodson PM. Sex hormone preparations and retinal vein occlusion. Eye 1997;11(Pt 1):53–6.

22. Vastag O, Tornoczky J. Oralis anticoncipiens szedese soran kialakult szemfeneki arterias occlusio. [Arterial occlusion in the ocular fundus induced by oral contraceptives.] Orv Hetil 1984;125(51):3121–5.

23. Zeydler-Grzedzielewska L, Baszczynska-Zielinska B. Powiklania oczne po doustnym stosowaniu srodkow antykoncepcyjnych. [Ophthalmological complications after oral contraceptives.] Klin Oczna 1978;48(5):239–42.

24. Huismans H. Monolaterale rezidivierende Neuritis N. optici unter Langzeittherapie mit dem hormonalen Kontrazeptivum Anacyclin 28. [Recurring inflammation of optic nerve after long-time therapy with hormonal contraceptive anacyclin 28.] Klin Monatsbl Augenheilkd 1982;180(2):173–5.

25. Gierkowa A, Szaflik J, Samochowiec E, Halatek R. Estrogeny a cisnienie Wewntrz-gallkowc. [Oestrogens and intraocular pressure.] Klin Oczna 1977;47(3):113–5.

26. Kimura D. Estrogen replacement therapy may protect against intellectual decline in postmenopausal women. Horm Behav 1995;29(3):312–21.

27. Saletu B, Brandstatter N, Metka M, Stamenkovic M, Anderer P, Semlitsch HV, Heytmanek G, Huber J, Grunberger J, Linzmayer L, Kurz CH, Decker K, Binder G, Knogler W, Koll B. Double-blind, placebo-controlled, hormonal, syndromal and EEG mapping studies with transdermal oestradiol therapy in menopausal depression. Psychopharmacology (Berl) 1995;122(4):321–9.

28. Kay PAJ, Yurkow J, Forman LJ, Chopra A, Cavalieri T. Transdermal estradiol in the management of aggressive behavior in male patients with dementia. Clin Gerontol 1995;15:54–8.

29. Abdalla HI, Hart DM, Beastall GH. Reduced serum free thyroxine concentration in postmenopausal women receiving oestrogen treatment. BMJ (Clin Res Ed) 1984;288(6419):754–5.

30. Sturdee DW, Gustafson RC, Moore B. Glucose tolerance and hormone replacement therapy. A preliminary study. Postgrad Med J 1976;52(Suppl 6):52–4.

31. Weimann E, Brack C. Severe thrombosis during treatment with ethinylestradiol for tall stature. Horm Res 1996;45(6):261–3.

32. Malina L, Chlumsky J. Oestrogen-induced familial porphyria cutanea tarda. Br J Dermatol 1975;92(6):707–9.

33. Heinemann G. [Plasma iron, serum copper, and serum zinc during therapy with ovulation inhibitors.]Med Klin 1974;69(20):892–6.

34. Henriksson P, Blomback M, Bratt G, Edhag O, Eriksson A, Vesterqvist O. Effects of oestrogen therapy and orchidectomy on coagulation and prostanoid synthesis in patients with prostatic cancer. Med Oncol Tumor Pharmacother 1989;6(3):219–25.

35. Rosendaal FR, Helmerhorst FM, Vandenbroucke JP. Oral contraceptives, hormone replacement therapy and thrombosis. Thromb Haemost 2001;86(1):112–23.

36. Scarabin PY, Oger E, Plu-Bureau GEStrogen and THromboEmbolism Risk Study Group. Differential association of oral and transdermal oestrogen-replacement therapy with venous thromboembolism risk. Lancet 2003;362(9382):428–32.

37. Douketis JD, Julian JA, Kearon C, Anderson DR, Crowther MA, Bates SM, Barone M, Piovella F, Turpie AG, Middeldorp S, van Nguyen P, Prandoni P, Wells PS, Kovacs MJ, Macgillavry MR, Costantini L, Ginsberg JS. Does the type of hormone replacement therapy influence the risk of deep vein thrombosis? A prospective case-control study. J Thromb Haemost 2005;3(5):943–8.

38. Astedt B. Low fibrinolytic activity of veins during treatment with ethinyloestradiol. Acta Obstet Gynecol Scand 1971;50(3):279–83.

39. Beller FK, Nachtigall L, Rosenberg M. Coagulation studies of menopausal women taking estrogen replacement. Obstet Gynecol 1972;39(5):775–8.

40. Kroon UB, Silfverstolpe G, Tengborn L. The effects of transdermal estradiol and oral conjugated estrogens on haemostasis variables. Thromb Haemost 1994;71(4):420–3.

41. Casson PR, Carson SA. Androgen replacement therapy in women: myths and realities. Int J Fertil Menopausal Stud 1996;41(4):412–22.

42. Barlow DH. HRT and the risk of deep vein thrombosis. Int J Gynaecol Obstet 1997;59(Suppl 1):S29–33.

43. Barrett-Connor E, Timmons C, Young R, Wiita B. Estra Test Working Group. Interim safety analysis of a two year study comparing oral estrogen–androgen and conjugated estrogens in surgically menopausal women. J Women's Health 1996;5:593–602.

44. Sahdev P, Wolff M, Widmann WD. Mesenteric venous thrombosis associated with estrogen therapy for treatment of prostatic carcinoma. J Urol 1985;134(3):563–4.

45. McClennan BL. Ischemic colitis secondary to Premarin: report of a case. Dis Colon Rectum 1976;19(7):618–20.

46. Parker WA, Morris ME, Shearer CA. Oral contraceptive-induced ischemic bowel disease. Am J Hosp Pharm 1979;36(8):1103–7.

47. Grimaud JC, Bourliere M. Contraception et hépato-gastro-entérologie. [Contraception and hepatogastroenterology.] Fertil Contracept Sex 1989;17(5):407–13.

48. Eisalo A, Heino A, Rasanen V. Oestrogen, proestogen and liver function tests. Acta Obstet Gynecol Scand 1968;47(1):58–65.

49. Ottosson UB, Carlstrom K, Johansson BG, von Schoultz B. Estrogen induction of liver proteins and high-density lipoprotein cholesterol: comparison between estradiol valerate and ethinyl estradiol. Gynecol Obstet Invest 1986;22(4):198–205.

50. Underwood TW, Frye CB. Drug-induced pancreatitis. Clin Pharm 1993;12(6):440–8.

51. Orlander JD, Jick SS, Dean AD, Jick H. Urinary tract infections and estrogen use in older women. J Am Geriatr Soc 1992;40(8):817–20.

52. Kok AL, Burger CW, van de Weijer PH, Voetberg GA, Peters-Muller ER, Kenemans P. Micturition complaints in postmenopausal women treated with continuously combined hormone replacement therapy: a prospective study. Maturitas 1999;31(2):143–9.

53. Cooper SM, George S. Photosensitivity reaction associated with use of the combined oral contraceptive. Br J Dermatol 2001;144(3):641–2.

54. Horkay I, Tamasi P, Prekopa A, Dalmy L. Photodermatoses induced by oral contraceptives. Arch Dermatol Res 1975;253(1):53–61.

55. Corazza M, Mantovani L, Montanari A, Virgili A. Allergic contact dermatitis from transdermal estradiol and systemic contact dermatitis from oral estradiol. A case report. J Reprod Med 2002;47(6):507–9.

56. Smith AG, Shuster S, Thody AJ, Peberdy M. Chloasma, oral contraceptives, and plasma immunoreactive beta-melanocyte-stimulating hormone. J Invest Dermatol 1977;68(4):169–70.

57. Morgan MB, Raley BA, Vannarath RL, Lightfoot SL, Everett MA. Papillomatous melanocytic nevi: an estrogen related phenomenon. J Cutan Pathol 1995;22(5):446–9.

58. Ellis DL, Wheeland RG, Solomon H. Estrogen and progesterone receptors in melanocytic lesions. Occurrence in patients with dysplastic nevus syndrome. Arch Dermatol 1985;121(10):1282–5.

59. Baker VL. Alternatives to oral estrogen replacement. Transdermal patches, percutaneous gels, vaginal creams and rings, implants, other methods of delivery. Obstet Gynecol Clin North Am 1994;21(2):271–97.

60. Yang SG, Han KH, Cho KH, Lee AY. Development of erythema nodosum in the course of oestrogen replacement therapy. Br J Dermatol 1997;137(2):319–20.

61. Schmidt JB, Binder M, Demschik G, Bieglmayer C, Reiner A. Treatment of skin aging with topical estrogens. Int J Dermatol 1996;35(9):669–74.

62. Dei M, Verni A, Bigozzi L, Bruni V. Sex steroids and libido. Eur J Contracept Reprod Health Care 1997;2(4):253–8.

63. Graziottin A. Libido: the biologic scenario. Maturitas 2000;34(Suppl 1):S9–S16.

64. Lethaby A, Suckling J, Barlow D, Farquhar CM, Jepson RG, Roberts H. Hormone replacement therapy in postmenopausal women: endometrial hyperplasia and irregular bleeding. Cochrane Database Syst Rev 2004;(3):CD000402.

65. Bazex A, Salvador R, Dupré A, et al. Gynécomastie et hyperpigmentation aréolaire après locale anti-séborrhéique. Bull Soc Fr Dermatol Syphiligr 1967;74:466.

66. Venn A, Bruinsma F, Werther PG, Pyett P, Baird D, Jones P, Rayner J, Lumley PJ. Oestrogen treatment to reduce the adult height of tall girls: long-term effects on fertility. Lancet 2004;364:1513–8.

67. Styrt B, Sugarman B. Estrogens and infection. Rev Infect Dis 1991;13(6):1139–50.

68. Klinger G, Graser T, Mellinger U, Moore C, Vogelsang H, Groh A, Latterman C, Klinger G. A comparative study of the effects of two oral contraceptives containing dienogest or desogestrel on the human immune system. Gynecol Endocrinol 2000;14(1):15–24.

69. Andre F, Veysseyre-Balter CE, Rousset H, Descos L, Andre C. Exogenous oestrogen as an alternative to food allergy in the aetiology of angioneurotic oedema. Toxicology 2003;185:155–60.

70. Searcy CJ, Kushner M, Nell P, Beckmann CR. Anaphylactic reaction to intravenous conjugated estrogens. Clin Pharm 1987;6(1):74–6.

71. Ford LG, Brawley OW, Perlman JA, Nayfield SG, Johnson KA, Kramer BS. The potential for hormonal prevention trials. Cancer 1994;74(Suppl 9):2726–33.

72. Coker AL, Harlap S, Fortney JA. Oral contraceptives and reproductive cancers: weighing the risks and benefits. Fam Plann Perspect 1993;25(1):17–2136.

73. Oda K, Oguma N, Kawano M, Kimura A, Kuramoto A, Tokumo K. Hepatocellular carcinoma associated with long-term anabolic steroid therapy in two patients with aplastic anemia. Nippon Ketsueki Gakkai Zasshi 1987;50(1):29–36.

74. Greer T. Hepatic adenoma and oral contraceptive use. J Fam Pract 1989;28(3):322–6.

75. Brooks JJ. Hepatoma associated with diethylstilbestrol therapy for prostatic carcinoma. J Urol 1982;128(5):1044–5.

76. Heresbach D, Deugnier Y, Brissot P, Bourel M. Dilatations sinusoidales et prise de contraceptifs oraux. A propos d'un casavec revue de la litterature. [Sinusoid dilatation and the use of oral contraceptives. Apropos of a case with a review of the literature.] Ann Gastroenterol Hepatol (Paris) 1988;24(4):189–91.

77. Christopherson WM. Liver tumours and the pill. BMJ 1975;4(5999):756.

78. Buhler H, Pirovino M, Akobiantz A, Altorfer J, Weitzel M, Maranta E, Schmid M. Regression of liver cell adenoma. A follow-up study of three consecutive patients after discontinuation of oral contraceptive use. Gastroenterology 1982;82(4):775–82.

79. Marks WH, Thompson N, Appleman H. Failure of hepatic adenomas (HCA) to regress after discontinuance of oral contraceptives. An association with focal nodular hyperplasia (FNH) and uterine leiomyoma. Ann Surg 1988;208(2):190–5.

80. Glinkova V, Shevah O, Boaz M, Levine A, Shirin H. Hepatic haemangiomas: possible association with female sex hormones. Gut 2004;53:1352–5.

81. Ross RK, Bernstein L, Garabrant D, Henderson BE. Avoidable nondietary risk factors for cancer. Am Fam Physician 1988;38(2):153–60.

82. La Vecchia C, Negri E, Parazzini F. Oral contraceptives and primary liver cancer. Br J Cancer 1989;59(3):460–1.

83. Neuberger J, Forman D, Doll R, Williams R. Oral contraceptives and hepatocellular carcinoma. BMJ (Clin Res Ed) 1986;292(6532):1355–7.

84. World Health Organization. Combined oral contraceptives and liver cancer. The WHO Collaborative Study of Neoplasia and Steroid Contraceptives. Int J Cancer 1989;43(2):254–9.

85. Hsing AW, Hoover RN, McLaughlin JK, Co-Chien HT, Wacholder S, Blot WJ, Fraumeni JF Jr. Oral contraceptives and primary liver cancer among young women. Cancer Causes Control 1992;3(1):43–8.

86. Prentice RL, Thomas DB. On the epidemiology of oral contraceptives and disease. Adv Cancer Res 1987;49:285–401.

87. Stanford JL, Thomas DB. Reproductive factors in the etiology of hepatocellular carcinoma. The WHO Collaborative Study of Neoplasia and Steroid Contraceptives. Cancer Causes Control 1992;3(1):37–42.

88. Parazzini F, Negri E, La Vecchia C, Bruzzi P, Decarli A. Population attributable risk for endometrial cancer in northern Italy. Eur J Cancer Clin Oncol 1989;25(10):1451–6.

89. McGavigan CJ, Metaxa-Mariatou V, Dockery P, Rodger MW, Cameron IT, Campbell S. Large, thin walled, superficial endometrial vessels: the cause of breakthrough bleeding in women with Mirena? Br J Fam Plann 2000;26:235–6.

90. Horwitz RI, Feinstein AR. Estrogens and endometrial cancer. Responses to arguments and current status of an epidemiologic controversy. Am J Med 1986;81(3):503–7.

91. Rubin GL, Peterson HB, Lee NC, Maes EF, Wingo PA, Becker S. Estrogen replacement therapy and the risk of endometrial cancer: remaining controversies. Am J Obstet Gynecol 1990;162(1):148–54.

92. Horwitz RI, Feinstein AR. Alternative analytic methods for case-control studies of estrogens and endometrial cancer. N Engl J Med 1978;299(20):1089–94.

93. Antunes CM, Strolley PD, Rosenshein NB, Davies JL, Tonascia JA, Brown C, Burnett L, Rutledge A, Pokempner M, Garcia R. Endometrial cancer and estrogen use. Report of a large case-control study. N Engl J Med 1979;300(1):9–13.

94. Buring JE, Bain CJ, Ehrmann RL. Conjugated estrogen use and risk of endometrial cancer. Am J Epidemiol 1986;124(3):434–41.

95. Jick H, Watkins RN, Hunter JR, Dinan BJ, Madsen S, Rothman KJ, Walker AM. Replacement estrogens and endometrial cancer. N Engl J Med 1979;300(5):218–22.

96. Ziel HK, Finkle WD. Association of estrone with the development of endometrial carcinoma. Am J Obstet Gynecol 1976;124(7):735–40.

97. Spengler RF, Clarke EA, Woolever CA, Newman AM, Osborn RW. Exogenous estrogens and endometrial cancer: a case-control study and assessment of potential biases. Am J Epidemiol 1981;114(4):497–506.

98. Persson I. Climacteric Treatment with Estrogens and Estrogen–Progestogen Combinations: the Risk of Endometrial Neoplasia. Results of a Cohort Study. Thesis, University of UppsalaStockholm: Almqvist and Wiksell;. 1983.

99. Levi F, La Vecchia C, Gulie C, Franceschi S, Negri E. Oestrogen replacement treatment and the risk of endometrial cancer: an assessment of the role of covariates. Eur J Cancer 1993;29A(10):1445–9.

100. Jacobs HS, Loeffler FE. Postmenopausal hormone replacement therapy. BMJ 1992;305(6866):1403–8.

101. Woodruff JD, Pickar JHThe Menopause Study Group. Incidence of endometrial hyperplasia in postmenopausal women taking conjugated estrogens (Premarin) with medroxyprogesterone acetate or conjugated estrogens alone. Am J Obstet Gynecol 1994;170(5 Pt 1):1213–23.

102. Sulak PJ. Endometrial cancer and hormone replacement therapy. Appropriate use of progestins to oppose endogenous and exogenous estrogen. Endocrinol Metab Clin North Am 1997;26(2):399–412.

103. Battistini M. Estrogen and the prevention and treatment of osteoporosis. J Clin Rheumatol 1997;3:S28–33.

104. Beresford SA, Weiss NS, Voigt LF, McKnight B. Risk of endometrial cancer in relation to use of oestrogen combined with cyclic progestagen therapy in postmenopausal women. Lancet 1997;349(9050):458–61.

105. Suriano KA, McHale M, McLaren CE, Li KT, Re A, DiSaia PJ. Estrogen replacement therapy in endometrial cancer patients: a matched control study. Obstet Gynecol 2001;97(4):555–60.

106. Debus G, Schuhmacher I. Endometrial adenocarcinoma arising during estrogenic treatment 17 years after total abdominal hysterectomy and bilateral salpingo-oophorectomy: a case report. Acta Obstet Gynecol Scand 2001;80(6):589–90.

107. Kurman RJ, Felix JC, Archer DF, Nanavati N, Arce J, Moyer DL. Norethindrone acetate and estradiol-induced endometrial hyperplasia. Obstet Gynecol 2000;96(3):373–9.

108. Turner RT, Riggs BL, Spelsberg TC. Skeletal effects of estrogen. Endocr Rev 1994;15(3):275–300.

109. Kafonek SD. Postmenopausal hormone replacement therapy and cardiovascular risk reduction. A review. Drugs 1994;47(Suppl 2):16–24.

110. Garuti G, Grossi F, Cellani F, Centinaio G, Colonnelli M, Luerti M. Hysteroscopic assessment of menopausal breast-cancer patients taking tamoxifen; there is a bias from the mode of endometrial sampling in estimating endometrial morbidity? Breast Cancer Res Treat 2002;72(3):245–53.

111. Sturdee DW, van de Weijer P, von Holst T. Endometrial safety of a transdermal sequential estradiol–levonorgestrel combination. Climacteric 2002;5(2):170–7.

112. The Centers for Disease Control Cancer and Steroid Hormone Study. Oral contraceptive use and the risk of endometrial cancer. JAMA 1983;249(12):1600–4.

113. The WHO Collaborative Study of Neoplasia and Steroid Contraceptives. Epithelial ovarian cancer and combined oral contraceptives. The WHO Collaborative Study of Neoplasia and Steroid Contraceptives. Int J Epidemiol 1989;18(3):538–45.

114. Schlesselman JJ. Oral contraceptives and neoplasia of the uterine corpus. Contraception 1991;43(6):557–79.

115. The Cancer and Steroid Hormone Study of the Centers for Disease Control and the National Institute of Child Health and Human Development. The reduction in risk of ovarian cancer associated with oral-contraceptive use. N Engl J Med 1987;316(11):650–5.

116. Beral V, Hannaford P, Kay C. Oral contraceptive use and malignancies of the genital tract. Results from the Royal College of General Practitioners' Oral Contraception Study. Lancet 1988;2(8624):1331–5.

117. Brinton LA, Huggins GR, Lehman HF, Mallin K, Savitz DA, Trapido E, Rosenthal J, Hoover R. Long-term use of oral contraceptives and risk of invasive cervical cancer. Int J Cancer 1986;38(3):339–44.

118. Slattery ML, Overall JC Jr, Abbott TM, French TK, Robison LM, Gardner J. Sexual activity, contraception, genital infections, and cervical cancer: support for a sexually transmitted disease hypothesis. Am J Epidemiol 1989;130(2):248–58.

119. Gram IT, Macaluso M, Stalsberg H. Oral contraceptive use and the incidence of cervical intraepithelial neoplasia. Am J Obstet Gynecol 1992;167(1):40–4.

120. Bosch FX, Munoz N, de Sanjose S, Izarzugaza I, Gili M, Viladiu P, Tormo MJ, Moreo P, Ascunce N, Gonzalez LC, et al. Risk factors for cervical cancer in Colombia and Spain. Int J Cancer 1992;52(5):750–8.

121. Macnab JC, Walkinshaw SA, Cordiner JW, Clements JB. Human papillomavirus in clinically and histologically normal tissue of patients with genital cancer. N Engl J Med 1986;315(17):1052–8.

122. World Health Organization. Oral contraceptives and neoplasia: report of a WHO Scientific Group. WHO Tech Rep Ser 1992;817.

123. Anonymous. Oral contraceptives. Risk of cervical cancer with long-term use in woman with high risk type of HPV. WHO Pharmaceuticals Newslett 2002;2:3–4.

124. Kjaeldgaard A, Larsson B. Long-term treatment with combined oral contraceptives and cigarette smoking associated

with impaired activity of tissue plasminogen activator. Acta Obstet Gynecol Scand 1986;65(3):219–22.

125. Myles JL, Hart WR. Apoplectic leiomyomas of the uterus. A clinicopathologic study of five distinctive hemorrhagic leiomyomas associated with oral contraceptive usage. Am J Surg Pathol 1985;9(11):798–805.

126. Riman T, Dickman PW, Nilsson S, Correia N, Nordlinder H, Magnusson CM, Weiderpass E, Persson IR. Hormone replacement therapy and the risk of invasive epithelial ovarian cancer in Swedish women. J Natl Cancer Inst 2002;94(7):497–504.

127. Royal College of General Practitioners. Oral Contraceptives and HealthLondon: RCGP;. 1974.

128. Vessey M, Doll R, Peto R, Johnson B, Wiggins P. A long-term follow-up study of women using different methods of contraception—an interim report. J Biosoc Sci 1976;8(4):373–427.

129. Weiss NS, Lyon JL, Liff JM, Vollmer WM, Daling JR. Incidence of ovarian cancer in relation to the use of oral contraceptives. Int J Cancer 1981;28(6):669–71.

130. Hankinson SE, Colditz GA, Hunter DJ, Spencer TL, Rosner B, Stampfer MJ. A quantitative assessment of oral contraceptive use and risk of ovarian cancer. Obstet Gynecol 1992;80(4):708–14.

131. Mack TM. Hormone replacement therapy and cancer. Baillières Clin Endocrinol Metab 1993;7(1):113–49.

132. Nisker JA, Siiteri PK. Estrogens and breast cancer. Clin Obstet Gynecol 1981;24(1):301–22.

133. WHO Scientific Group. Steroid contraception and the risk of neoplasia. World Health Organ Tech Rep Ser 1978;619:1–54.

134. Royal College of General Practitioners. Oral Contraceptive StudyLondon: RCGP;. 1981.

135. Pike MC, Henderson BE, Casagrande JT, Rosario I, Gray GE. Oral contraceptive use and early abortion as risk factors for breast cancer in young women. Br J Cancer 1981;43(1):72–6.

136. Vessey MP, McPherson K, Doll R. Breast cancer and oral contraceptives: findings in Oxford–Family Planning Association contraceptive study. BMJ (Clin Res Ed) 1981;282(6282):2093–4.

137. Hulka BS, Chambless LE, Deubner DC, Wilkinson WE. Breast cancer and estrogen replacement therapy. Am J Obstet Gynecol 1982;143(6):638–44.

138. Ory GW, Layde OM, et al. Long term oral contraceptive use and the risk of breast cancer. Paper presented at 31st Annual Epidemic Service ConferenceAtlanta, Georgia;. 1982.

139. Brinton LA, Hoover R, Szklo M, Fraumeni JF Jr. Oral contraceptives and breast cancer. Int J Epidemiol 1982;11(4):316–22.

140. Drife J. Which pill? BMJ (Clin Res Ed) 1983;287(6403):1397–9.

141. Janerich DT, Polednak AP, Glebatis DM, Lawrence CE. Breast cancer and oral contraceptive use: a case-control study. J Chronic Dis 1983;36(9):639–46.

142. Rosenberg L, Miller DR, Kaufman DW, Helmrich SP, Stolley PD, Schottenfeld D, Shapiro S. Breast cancer and oral contraceptive use. Am J Epidemiol 1984;119(2):167–76.

143. Stadel BV, Rubin GL, Webster LA, Schlesselman JJ, Wingo PA. Oral contraceptives and breast cancer in young women. Lancet 1985;2(8462):970–3.

144. The Cancer and Steroid Hormone Study of the Centers for Disease Control and the National Institute of Child Health and Human Development. Oral-contraceptive use and the risk of breast cancer. N Engl J Med 1986;315(7):405–11.

145. Ellery C, MacLennan R, Berry G, Shearman RP. A case-control study of breast cancer in relation to the use of steroid contraceptive agents. Med J Aust 1986;144(4):173–6.

146. Meirik O, Lund E, Adami HO, Bergstrom R, Christoffersen T, Bergsjo P. Oral contraceptive use and breast cancer in young women. A joint national case-control study in Sweden and Norway. Lancet 1986;2(8508):650–4.

147. Shapiro S. Oral contraceptives—time to take stock. N Engl J Med 1986;315(7):450–1.

148. Stadel BV, Lai SH, Schlesselman JJ, Murray P. Oral contraceptives and premenopausal breast cancer in nulliparous women. Contraception 1988;38(3):287–99.

149. Lee NC, Rosero-Bixby L, Oberle MW, Grimaldo C, Whatley AS, Rovira EZ. A case-control study of breast cancer and hormonal contraception in Costa Rica. J Natl Cancer Inst 1987;79(6):1247–54.

150. Hulman G, Trowbridge P, Taylor CN, Chilvers CE, Sloane JP. Oral contraceptive use and histopathology of cancerous breasts in young women. Members of the U.K. National Case-Control Study Group J Pathol 1992;167(4):407–11.

151. Barrett-Connor E, Grady D. Hormone replacement therapy, heart disease, and other considerations. Annu Rev Public Health 1998;19:55–72.

152. Colditz GA, Hankinson SE, Hunter DJ, Willett WC, Manson JE, Stampfer MJ, Hennekens C, Rosner B, Speizer FE. The use of estrogens and progestins and the risk of breast cancer in postmenopausal women. N Engl J Med 1995;332(24):1589–93.

153. Althuis MD, Brogan DR, Coates RJ, Daling JR, Gammon MD, Malone KE, Schoenberg JB, Brinton LA. Hormonal content and potency of oral contraceptives and breast cancer risk among young women. Br J Cancer 2003;88:50–7.

154. Brinton LA, Daling JR, Liff JM, Schoenberg JB, Malone KE, Stanford JL, Coates RJ, Gammon MD, Hanson L, Hoover RN. Oral contraceptives and breast cancer risk among younger women. J Natl Cancer Inst 1995;87:827–35.

155. Claus EB, Stowe M, Carter D. Oral contraceptives and the risk of ductal breast carcinoma in situ. Breast Cancer Res Treat 2003;81:129–36.

156. Brinton LA. Hormone replacement therapy and risk for breast cancer. Endocrinol Metab Clin North Am 1997;26(2):361–78.

157. Willis DB, Calle EE, Miracle-McMahill HL, Heath CW Jr. Estrogen replacement therapy and risk of fatal breast cancer in a prospective cohort of postmenopausal women in the United States. Cancer Causes Control 1996;7(4):449–57.

158. Grodstein F, Stampfer MJ, Colditz GA, Willett WC, Manson JE, Joffe M, Rosner B, Fuchs C, Hankinson SE, Hunter DJ, Hennekens CH, Speizer FE. Postmenopausal hormone therapy and mortality. N Engl J Med 1997;336(25):1769–75.

159. Holli K, Isola J, Cuzick J. Hormone replacement therapy and biological aggressiveness of breast cancer. Lancet 1997;350(9092):1704–5.

160. Colditz GA, Stampfer MJ, Willett WC, Hunter DJ, Manson JE, Hennekens CK, Rosner BA, Speizer FE. Type of postmenopausal hormone use and risk of breast cancer. 12-year follow-up from the Nurses' Health Study. Cancer Causes Control 1992;3:433–9.

161. Bergkvist L, Adami HO, Persson I, Hoover R, Schairer C. The risk of breast cancer after estrogen and estrogen-progestin replacement. N Engl J Med 1989;321(5):293–7.

162. MacLennan AH. Hormone replacement therapy and the menopause. Australian Menopause Society. Med J Aust 1991;155(1):43–4.

163. Gambrell RD. Estrogen replacement therapy and breast cancer risk. A new look at the data. Female Patient 1993;18:55.

164. Colditz GA, Egan KM, Stampfer MJ. Hormone replacement therapy and risk of breast cancer: results from epidemiologic studies. Am J Obstet Gynecol 1993;168(5):1473–80.

165. Stewart GR. Hormone replacement therapy and breast cancer. Med J Aust 1993;158:146.

166. Stanford JL, Weiss NS, Voigt LF, Daling JR, Habel LA, Rossing MA. Combined estrogen and progestin hormone replacement therapy in relation to risk of breast cancer in middle-aged women. JAMA 1995;274(2):137–42.

167. Newcomb PA, Longnecker MP, Storer BE, Mittendorf R, Baron J, Clapp RW, Bogdan G, Willett WC. Long-term hormone replacement therapy and risk of breast cancer in postmenopausal women. Am J Epidemiol 1995;142(8):788–95.

168. Persson I, Thurfjell E, Bergstrom R, Holmberg L. Hormone replacement therapy and the risk of breast cancer. Nested case-control study in a cohort of Swedish women attending mammography screening. Int J Cancer 1997;72(5):758–61.

169. Gapstur SM, Morrow M, Sellers TA. Hormone replacement therapy and risk of breast cancer with a favorable histology: results of the Iowa Women's Health Study. JAMA 1999;281(22):2091–7.

170. Beral V. Million Women Study Collaborators. Breast cancer and hormone-replacement therapy in the Million Women Study. Lancet 2003;362(9382):419–27.

171. Diamanti-Kandarakis E. Hormone replacement therapy and risk of malignancy. Curr Opin Obstet Gynecol 2004;16:73–8.

172. Practice Committee of the American Society for Reproductive Medicine. Estrogen and progestogen therapy in postmenopausal women. Fertil Steril 2004;82 Suppl 1:S70–80.

173. Newcomer LM, Newcomb PA, Potter JD, Yasui Y, Trentham-Dietz A, Storer BE, Longnecker MP, Baron JA, Daling JR. Postmenopausal hormone therapy and risk of breast cancer by histologic type (United States). Cancer Causes Control 2003;14:225–33.

174. Jernstrom H, Bendahl P-O, Lidfeldt J, Nerbrand C, Agardh C-D, Samsioe G. A prospective study of different types of hormone replacement therapy use and the risk of subsequent breast cancer: the women's health in the Lund area (WHILA) study (Sweden). Cancer Causes Control 2003;14:673–80.

175. Bulbul NH, Ozden S, Dayicioglu V. Effects of hormone replacement therapy on mammographic findings. Arch Gynecol Obstet 2003;268:5–8.

176. Fleming RM. Do women taking hormone replacement therapy (HRT) have a higher incidence of breast cancer than women who do not? Integr Cancer Ther 2003;2:235–7.

177. Gertig DM, Erbas B, Fletcher A, Amos A, Kavanagh AM. Duration of hormone replacement therapy, breast tumour size and grade in a screening programme. Breast Cancer Res Treatment 2003;80:267–73.

178. Pritchard KI. Hormone replacement in women with a history of breast cancer. Oncologist 2001;6(4):353–62.

179. Marttunen MB, Hietanen P, Pyrhonen S, Tiitinen A, Ylikorkala O. A prospective study on women with a history of breast cancer and with or without estrogen replacement therapy. Maturitas 2001;39(3):217–25.

180. Zera RT, Danielson D, Van Camp JM, Schmidt-Steinbrunn B, Hong J, McCoy M, Anderson WR, Linzie BM, Rodriguez JL. Atypical hyperplasia, proliferative fibrocystic change, and exogenous hormone use. Surgery 2001;130(4):732–7.

181. Miyagawa A, Yuba Y, Haga H, Nishimura S, Kobashi Y. Fibrous tumor of the breast in a postmenopausal woman receiving estrogen. Pathol Int 2001;51(2):123–6.

182. Garton M. Breast cancer and hormone-replacement therapy: the Million Women Study. Lancet 2003;362(9392):1328.

183. Sacchini V, Zurrida S, Andreoni G, Luini A, Galimberti V, Veronesi P, Intra M, Viale G, Veronesi U. Pathologic and biological prognostic factors of breast cancers in short- and long-term hormone replacement therapy users. Ann Surg Oncol 2002;9(3):266–71.

184. Stahlberg C, Pedersen AT, Andersen ZJ, Keiding N, Hundrup YA, Obel EB, Moller S, Rank F, Ottesen B, Lynge E. Breast cancer with different prognostic characteristics developing in Danish women using hormone replacement therapy. Br J Cancer 2004;91:644–50.

185. Lillie EO, Bernstein L, Ingles SA, Gauderman WJ, Rivas GE, Gagalang V, Krontiris T, Ursin G. Polymorphism in the androgen receptor and mammographic density in women taking and not taking estrogen and progestin therapy. Cancer Res 2004;64:1237–41.

186. Lundstrom E, Christow A, Kersemaekers W, Svane G, Azavedo E, Soderqvist G, Mol-Arts M, Barkfeldt J, von Schoultz B. Effects of tibolone and continuous combined hormone replacement therapy on mammographic breast density. Am J Obstet Gynecol 2002;186(4):717–22.

187. Fournier A, Berrino F, Riboli E, Avenel V, Clavel-Chapelon F. Breast cancer risk in relation to different types of hormone replacement therapy in the E3N-EPIC cohort. Int J Cancer 2005;114:448–54.

188. Coombs NJ, Taylor R, Wilcken N, Boyages J. HRT and breast cancer: impact on population risk and incidence. Eur J Cancer 2005;41:1775–8.

189. Reed SD, Voigt LF, Beresford SAA, Hill DA, Doherty JA, Weiss NS. Dose of progestin in postmenopausal-combined hormone therapy and risk of endometrial cancer. Am J Obstet Gynecol 2004;191:1146–51.

190. Horn L-C, Dietel M, Einenkel J. Hormone replacement therapy (HRT) and endometrial morphology under consideration of the different molecular pathways in endometrial carcinogenesis. Eur J Obstr Gynec Reprod Biol 2005;122:4–12.

191. Carruthers R. Chloasma and oral contraceptives. Med J Aust 1966;2(1):17–20.

192. Beral V, Ramcharan S, Faris R. Malignant melanoma and oral contraceptive use among women in California. Br J Cancer 1977;36(6):804–9.

193. Beral V, Evans S, Shaw H, Milton G. Oral contraceptive use and malignant melanoma in Australia. Br J Cancer 1984;50(5):681–5.

194. Gallagher RP, Elwood JM, Hill GB, Coldman AJ, Threlfall WJ, Spinelli JJ. Reproductive factors, oral contraceptives and risk of malignant melanoma: Western Canada Melanoma Study. Br J Cancer 1985;52(6):901–7.

195. Hartge P, Tucker MA, Shields JA, Augsburger J, Hoover RN, Fraumeni JF Jr. Case-control study of female hormones and eye melanoma. Cancer Res 1989;49(16):4622–5.

196. Beiderbeck AB, Holly EA, Sturkenboom MCJM, Coebergh JW, Stricker BHCh, Leufkens HGM. No increased risk of non-Hodgkin's lymphoma with steroids, estrogens and psychotropics (Netherlands). Cancer Causes Control 2003;14:639–44.

197. Fernandez E, Gallus S, Bosetti C, Franceschi S, Negri E, La Vecchia C. Hormone replacement therapy and cancer risk: a systematic analysis from a network of case-control studies. Int J Cancer 2003;105:408–12.

198. Levgur M. Hormone therapy for women after breast cancer: a review. J Reprod Med Obst Gynaecol 2004;49:510–26.

199. Sharpe RM, Skakkebaek NE. Are oestrogens involved in falling sperm counts and disorders of the male reproductive tract? Lancet 1993;341(8857):1392–5.

200. World Health Organization Scientific Group. The effect of female sex hormones on fetal development and infant health. World Health Organ Tech Rep Ser 1981;657:1–76.

201. Hemminki E, Gissler M, Toukomaa H. Exposure to female hormone drugs during pregnancy: effect on malformations and cancer. Br J Cancer 1999;80(7):1092–7.

202. Ramos AS, Bower BF. Pseudoisosexual precocity due to cosmetic ingestion. JAMA 1969;207(2):368–9.

203. Landolt R, Murset G. Vorzeitige Pubertatsmerkmale als Folge unbeabsichitiger Ostrogenverabreichung. [Premature puberty signs as result of unintensional estrogen administration.] Schweiz Med Wochenschr 1968;98(17):638–41.

204. Barnard ND, Scialli AR, Bobela S. The current use of estrogens for growth-suppressant therapy in adolescent girls. J Pediatr Adolesc Gynecol 2002;15(1):23–6.

205. Denke MA. Hormone replacement therapy: benefit and safety issues. Curr Opin Lipidol 1996;7(6):369–73.

206. Sotos JF. Overgrowth disorders. Clin Pediatr (Phila) 1996;35(10):517–29.

207. Blomback M, Hall K, Ritzen EM. Estrogen treatment of tall girls: risk of thrombosis? Pediatrics 1983;72(3):416–9.

208. Venn A, Bruinsma F, Werther G, Pyett P, Baird D, Jones P, Rayner J, Lumley J. Oestrogen treatment to reduce the adult height of tall girls: long-term effects on fertility. Lancet 2004;364(9444):1513–8.

209. Gerber GS, Zagaja GP, Ray PS, Rukstalis DB. Transdermal estrogen in the treatment of hot flushes in men with prostate cancer. Urology 2000;55(1):97–101.

210. Taxel P, Kennedy D, Fall P, Willard A, Shoukri K, Clive J, Raisz LG. The effect of short-term treatment with micronized estradiol on bone turnover and gonadotrophins in older men. Endocr Res 2000;26(3):381–98.

211. O'Donohue J, Williams R. Hormone replacement therapy in women with liver disease. Br J Obstet Gynaecol 1997;104(1):1–3.

212. Hannaford PC, Kay CR, Vessey MP, Painter R, Mant J. Combined oral contraceptives and liver disease. Contraception 1997;55(3):145–51.

213. Lindberg MC. Hepatobiliary complications of oral contraceptives. J Gen Intern Med 1992;7(2):199–209.

214. Knopp RH. Cardiovascular effects of endogenous and exogenous sex hormones over a woman's lifetime. Am J Obstet Gynecol 1988;158(6 Pt 2):1630–43.

215. Henriksson P, Johansson SE. Prediction of cardiovascular complications in patients with prostatic cancer treated with estrogen. Am J Epidemiol 1987;125(6):970–8.

216. Perheentupa A, Ruokonen A, Tapanainen JS. Transdermal estradiol treatment suppresses serum gonadotropins during lactation without transfer into breast milk. Fertil Steril 2004;82:903–7.

217. Vrbikova J, Stanicka S, Dvorakova K, Hill M, Vondra K, Bendlova B, Starka L. Metabolic and endocrine effects of treatment with peroral or transdermal oestrogens in conjunction with peroral cyproterone acetate in women with polycystic ovary syndrome. Eur J Endocrinol 2004;150:215–23.

218. Stevenson JC, Oladipo A, Manassiev N, Whitehead MI, Guilford S, Proudler AJ. Randomized trial of effect of transdermal continuous combined hormone replacement therapy on cardiovascular risk markers. Br J Haematol 2004;124:802–8.

219. Al-Azzawi F, Buckler HM. Comparison of a novel vaginal ring delivering estradiol acetate versus oral estradiol for relief of vasomotor menopausal symptoms. Climacteric 2003;6:118–27.

220. Lopes P, Merkus HM, Nauman J, Bruschi F, Foidart JM, Calaf J. Randomized comparison of intranasal and transdermal estradiol. Obstet Gynecol 2000;96(6):906–12.

221. French RS, Cowan FM, Mansour DJ, Morris S, Procter T, Hughes D, Robinson A, Guillebaud J. Implantable contraceptives (subdermal implants and hormonally impregnated intrauterine systems) versus other forms of reversible contraceptives: two systematic reviews to assess relative effectiveness, acceptability, tolerability and cost-effectiveness. Health Technol Assess 2000;4(7):1–107.

222. Cerin A, Heldaas K, Moeller BThe Scandinavian LongCycle Study Group. Adverse endometrial effects of long-cycle estrogen and progestogen replacement therapy. N Engl J Med 1996;334(10):668–9.

223. Rovati LC, Setnikar I, Genazzani AR. Dose–response efficacy of a new estradiol transdermal matrix patch for 7-day application: a randomized, double-blind, placebo-controlled study. Italian Menopause Research Group. Gynecol Endocrinol 2000;14(4):282–91.

224. Young P, Purdie D, Jackman L, Molloy D, Green A. A study of infertility treatment and melanoma. Melanoma Res 2001;11(5):535–41.

225. Selby PL, Peacock M. The effect of transdermal oestrogen on bone, calcium-regulating hormones and liver in postmenopausal women. Clin Endocrinol (Oxf) 1986;25(5):543–7.

226. Shin Taek Oh, Dong Won Lee, Jun Young Lee, Baik Kee Cho. A case of allergic contact dermatitis to transdermal estradiol system. Korean J Dermatol 2001;39:111–3.

227. Goncalo M, Oliveira HS, Monteiro C, Clerins I, Figueiredo A. Allergic and systemic contact dermatitis from estradiol. Contact Dermatitis 1999;40(1):58–9.

228. Jewelewicz R. New developments in topical estrogen therapy. Fertil Steril 1997;67(1):1–12.

229. Schmidt KU, Wagner G, Mensing H. Ostrogen-induzierte Gynakomastie nach Anwendung ostrogenhaltiger Lokaltherapeutika. [Estrogen-induced gynecomastia following use of estrogen-containing local agents.] Dtsch Med Wochenschr 1987;112(23):926–8.

230. Gottswinto JM, Korth-Schutz S, Tummers B, Ziegler R. Gynäkomastie durch östrogen-haltiges Haarwasser. Med Klin 1984;79:181–3.

231. Langer J. Gynäkomastie durch Pharmaka. [Gynecomastia caused by drugs.] Derm Beruf Umwelt 1989;37(4):121–47.

232. de Vrijer B, Snijders MP, Troostwijk AL, The S, Iding RJ, Friese S, Smit DA, Schierbeek JM, Brandts H, van Kempen PJ, van Buuren I, Monza G. Efficacy and

tolerability of a new estradiol delivering matrix patch (Estraderm MX) in postmenopausal women. Maturitas 2000;34(1):47–55.

233. Andersson TL, Stehle B, Davidsson B, Hoglund P. Bioavailability of estradiol from two matrix transdermal delivery systems: Menorest and Climara. Maturitas 2000;34(1):57–64.

234. von Holst T, Salbach B. Efficacy and tolerability of a new 7-day transdermal estradiol patch versus placebo in hysterectomized women with postmenopausal complaints. Maturitas 2000;34(2):143–53.

235. De Aloysio D, Rovati LC, Giacovelli G, Setnikar I, Bottiglioni F. Efficacy on climacteric symptoms and safety of low dose estradiol transdermal matrix patches. A randomized, double-blind placebo-controlled study. Arzneimittelforschung 2000;50(3):293–300.

236. Lake Y, Pinnock S. Improved patient acceptability with a transdermal drug-in-adhesive oestradiol patch. Aust NZ J Obstet Gynaecol 2000;40(3):313–6.

237. Bland LB, Garzotto M, DeLoughery TG, Ryan CW, Schuff KG, Wersinger EM, Lemmon D, Beer TM. Phase II study of transdermal estradiol in androgen-independent prostate carcinoma. Cancer 2995;103:717–23.

238. Rioux JE, Devlin C, Gelfand MM, Steinberg WM, Hepburn DS. 17 beta-estradiol vaginal tablet versus conjugated equine estrogen vaginal cream to relieve menopausal atrophic vaginitis. Menopause 2000;7(3):156–61.

239. Bachmann G. Estradiol-releasing vaginal ring delivery system for urogenital atrophy. Experience over the past decade. J Reprod Med 1998;43(11):991–8.

240. Lose G, Englev E. Oestradiol-releasing vaginal ring versus oestriol vaginal pessaries in the treatment of bothersome lower urinary tract symptoms. BJOG 2000;107(8):1029–34.

241. Simunic V, Banovic I, Ciglar S, Jeren L, Pavicic Baldani D, Sprem M. Local estrogen treatment in patients with urogenital symptoms. Int J Gynaecol Obstet 2003;82:187–97.

242. Rufford J, Hextall A, Cardozo L, Khullar V. A double-blind placebo-controlled trial on the effects of 25 mg estradiol implants on the urge syndrome in postmenopausal women. Int Urogynecol J Pelvic Floor Dysfunct 2003;14:78–83.

Gonadotropins

General Information

Human chorionic gonadotropin (HCG, hCG), extracted from the urine of pregnant women, has mainly luteinizing hormone (LH) activity. Human menopausal gonadotropin (HMG, hMG) contains both follicle-stimulating hormone (FSH) and luteinizing hormone in about equal amounts. Where materials of natural origin are used, the relative amounts of follicle-stimulating hormone and luteinizing hormone in pituitary gonadotropin extracts vary with the extraction procedure used. However, in recent years, both pure recombinant versions of human FSH and human LH (rhFSH, rhLH) have become available and have increasingly replaced the natural products.

Luteinizing hormone-releasing hormone (LHRH) is used in the treatment of infertility (1). It induces pulsatile release of gonadotropin, and excessive stimulation can

result. However, if used over a period of time, the receptors cease to respond and there can be a fall in the concentrations of luteinizing hormone and follicle-stimulating hormone and a fall in sex steroid concentrations to the castrato range.

Treatment schedules for induction of ovulation have been described in a number of papers, but individual sensitivity of the ovaries varies greatly. Complications are generally considered more likely when the dose is excessive compared with individual needs; their incidence varies greatly from clinic to clinic, apparently because of differences in formulations and the dosage schedule used. Problems include superovulation, multiple pregnancy, and the hyperstimulation syndrome, which consists of rapid ovarian enlargement with intraperitoneal effusion (2). Ascites and hydrothorax are occasionally seen, probably due to an increase in vascular permeability at high estrogen concentrations (3). Vascular accidents have been reported, namely thrombophlebitis (4) and obstruction of the basilar artery (SED-12, 1033) (5). Gonadotropins have also been stated, although with much less certainty, to cause cardiomyopathy and behavioral and intellectual disturbances (SED-12, 1033; 6,7).

Observational studies

The European Metrodin HP Study Group has assessed the efficacy and safety of a highly purified urinary FSH in combination with human chorionic gonadotropin in inducing spermatogenesis in 28 men with primary complete isolated hypogonadotrophic hypogonadism, of whom 25 achieved spermatogenesis (8). Mean testicular volume increased by about 7 ml during treatment. Adverse events considered to be related to human chorionic gonadotropin were acne (n = 3), weight gain (n = 2), and gynecomastia (n = 1). Acne can be attributed to increased testosterone. Gynecomastia is an adverse effect of human chorionic gonadotropin treatment (9), and it may be caused by raised serum estradiol concentrations.

In 71 women undergoing in vitro fertilization and embryo transfer using recombinant human follicle-stimulating hormone in doses sufficient to attain a pregnancy rate of 24% (10), the main adverse effect was mild pain at the site of injection (less than 20% of patients) but there were two cases of ovarian hyperstimulation syndrome. In less than 10% of patients, redness, swelling, or bruising was seen and one patient developed headache.

The efficacy of recombinant human luteinizing hormone (rhLH) for supporting follicular development induced by recombinant human follicle-stimulating hormone (rhFSH) has been investigated in hypogonadotropic hypogonadal women (11). A total of 42 adverse events were reported in 14 of the 53 cycles in this study. Of these, 32 adverse events occurred in 11 of the 42 cycles treated with rhLH, and 10 occurred in three of the 11 cycles not treated with rhLH. The most frequent adverse events were pelvic and abdominal pain, headache, breast pain, nausea, ovarian enlargement, and somnolence. These adverse events are similar to those reported during therapy with follicle-stimulating hormone alone (11).

Comparative studies

When recombinant and urinary versions of follicle-stimulating hormone were compared under double-blind conditions in an in vitro fertilization program in a randomized, multicenter study (12), the former was more potent. There were no clinically relevant differences in safety between the two products and no cases of ovarian hyperstimulation syndrome.

The efficacy and safety of recombinant human follicle-stimulating hormone (r-hFSH) has been compared with that of highly purified urinary follicle-stimulating hormone (u-hFSH HP) in women undergoing ovarian stimulation for in vitro fertilization, including intracytoplasmic sperm injection, in a prospective, randomized study in 278 patients, who were treated with gonadotropin-releasing hormone and then received one of the two formulations in doses of 150 IU/day subcutaneously for the first 6 days; on day 7 the dose was adjusted, if necessary, according to the ovarian response (13). Human chorionic gonadotropin (10 000 IU subcutaneously) was administered once there was more than one follicle 18 mm in diameter and two others of 16 mm or larger. Rr-hFSH was more effective than u-hFSH HP in inducing multiple follicular development. There were seven cases (5.0%) of ovarian hyperstimulation syndrome in those given r-hFSH and three (2.2%) in those given u-hFSH HP; this difference was not significant.

General adverse effects

The short- and long-term effects of ovulation induction have been reported (8). In the short term, clomiphene and gonadotropins cause ovarian hyperstimulation syndrome (ovarian enlargement, bloating, and nausea) and multiple pregnancies; gonadotropins also cause ectopic pregnancy. In the long term, clomiphene may cause an increased risk of ovarian cancer.

Recombinant human chorionic gonadotropin

Recombinant human luteinizing hormone has now very largely replaced the product prepared from the urine of pregnant women (uhCG). In an open, randomized trial in 297 ovulatory infertile women in 20 US infertility centers, recombinant hCG 250 micrograms and 500 micrograms was compared with urinary hCG 10 000 U USP in assisted reproduction (14). The women were treated for a single cycle with one or the other. The mean numbers of oocytes retrieved per treatment group were equivalent (13–14). Although the numbers of fertilized oocytes on day 1 after oocyte retrieval and of cleaved embryos on the day of embryo transfer were significantly higher with 500 micrograms of recombinant hCG than with 250 micrograms, the incidence of the anticipated adverse events also tended to be higher.

More exact data on the adverse effects and relative safety of the recombinant and urinary formulations have been provided in a similar investigation in 259 women (15). In terms of safety, rhCG was well tolerated at a dose of up to 30 000 IU. Moderate ovarian hyperstimulation syndrome was reported in 12% of patients who received uhCG and 12% of those who received two injections of rhCG. There were no moderate or severe complications in patients who received a single dose of rhCG up to 30 000 IU. The results seem to show that a single dose of rhCG is effective in inducing final follicular maturation and early luteinization in in vitro fertilization and embryo transfer patients and is comparable with uhCG 5000 IU. The dose of rhCG that gave the highest efficacy to safety ratio was 15 000–30 000 IU.

The recombinant and urinary forms of human chorionic gonadotropin have also been compared in an international multicenter study, with similar findings (16), but it was notable that significantly more patients who were given uhCG reported local reactions (particularly inflammation and pain), presumably because of the presence of biological impurities.

Organs and Systems

Metabolism

What may be the first case in which an attack of acute porphyria was triggered by gonadotrophic stimulation of the ovary has been reported (17).

- A 36-year-old woman who had undergone a standard course of gonadotrophin treatment for infertility developed severe pelvic pain and hyponatremia. She had a family history of porphyria and it was thought that the treatment had fired an acute attack of the condition.

This case once more underlines the need to take a complete personal history before using this or any other form of intensive hormonal therapy. It also recalls the instances in which porphyria or pseudoporphyric incidents have been triggered by oral contraceptives.

Hematologic

Resistance of activated protein C and deep calf vein thrombosis has been reported during controlled ovarian stimulation for in vitro fertilization (18). The thrombosis occurred on the eighth day of human menopausal gonadotropin use and before human chorionic gonadotropin was given.

Reproductive system

There is a risk of ovarian hyperstimulation when an ovulation-inducing drug is followed by rapid ovarian enlargement with peritoneal effusion. The incidence of these complications varies with the product and dosage schedule used; in experienced hands, the frequency of complications may be no more than about 4%.

- In an unusual case reported in detail from Saudi Arabia, a 28-year-old woman receiving gonadotropins developed acute respiratory distress, abdominal pain, and severe hyponatremia associated with the syndrome of inappropriate antidiuretic hormone secretion (SIADH) (19). A multiple pregnancy nevertheless resulted and three fetuses went to term successfully.

While it is possible that the gonadotropins themselves induced SIADH, it seems more likely that it was a secondary complication of ovarian hyperstimulation.

The dangers of ovarian hyperstimulation with gonadotropins should not be underestimated. Quite apart from the risks of abdominal complications and even myocardial infarction, it can cause marked changes in liver function tests (20). It has been suggested that ultrasonographic monitoring is a means of detecting impending ovarian hyperstimulation, so that treatment can be suspended in good time (21).

- A 33-year-old woman developed severe symptomatic ovarian hyperstimulation after being given 10 000 IU of urinary human chorionic gonadotropin for empty follicle syndrome (22).

Although it has generally been thought that ovarian hyperstimulation would not occur when treating cases of empty follicle syndrome, this suggests that even when dealing with such patients, particularly if there is any reason to think that they are at risk of ovarian hyperstimulation, it is wise to take the usual precautions, using a much lower dose of human chorionic gonadotropin and adding progesterone for luteal support.

Just how dangerous and even life-threatening such hyperstimulation can be is illustrated by a recent case (23).

- A 28-year-old woman who had undergone attempted hormonal induction of ovulation presented some days later with ascites, oliguria, and vomiting. Over 2 weeks she developed severe hypoalbuminemia, due to a combination of intractable vomiting, intravenous rehydration, paracentesis, hypercatabolism, and proteinuria, with gross edema and progressively worsening liver function. Her serum albumin dropped to 9 g/l with liver function abnormalities: aspartate transaminase 462 IU/l, alkaline phosphatase 706 IU/l, bilirubin 26 µmol/l, prothrombin time 19 seconds. Paracentesis and total parenteral nutrition coincided with rapid clinical improvement.

Other presenting signs of ovarian hyperstimulation include ascites, hydrothorax, thrombophlebitis, and, as in one recently reported case, acute dyspnea (24).

A technique known as "prolonged coasting" has been developed over the last 20 years to reduce the incidence of severe ovarian hyperstimulation (SEDA-20, 389). It involves withdrawing exogenous gonadotrophins and postponing hCG administration if the patient's serum estradiol concentration becomes "dangerous"; treatment is resumed once the concentration is again acceptable (25). A full description of the various techniques used would go beyond the scope of this review, but it is important to realize that in principle they do considerably reduce the risk of hyperstimulation (26). However, experience to date shows that it is not foolproof and that spontaneous abortions can result where pregnancies have already started.

The effects of this technique have been examined objectively in women at risk of hyperstimulation by measurement of both follicular size and vascular endothelial growth factor (VEGF) in 22 women who had been coasted and 26 women who had not (27). Average follicular size was significantly less and VEGF concentrations

significantly lower. It is possible that coasting alters the capacity of granulosa cells to produce VEGF and/or their response to hCG and in this way acts to reduce the severity and incidence of severe hyperstimulation.

Various other low-dose approaches have been tested in an attempt to reduce the risk of complications. Recombinant FSH (rhFSH, onal-F) has been compared with urinary human FSH (uhFSH, Metrodin) in a randomized study in a low-dose step-up protocol for ovulation induction in 20 infertile clomiphene-resistant patients with polycystic ovaries (28). The starting dose was 75 IU of rhFSH or uhFSH. Human chorionic gonadotropin (hCG) 10 000 IU was administered if 1–3 follicles achieved a diameter of 16 mm or more, and both sonographic and hormonal monitoring were carried out. All the six pregnancies induced were in the rhFSH group, but two of them ended in miscarriage. There were no differences between the two groups concerning the intensity or duration of treatment or the hormonal response. Three patients had grade II and one patient grade III hyperstimulation. These results support earlier evidence that rhFSH is superior to uhFSH regarding pregnancy rates when using this low-dose protocol.

There is ever more evidence that the results obtained with low doses can equal those earlier obtained with larger doses, while in principle reducing the risk of overstimulation. Where human chorionic gonadotropin is concerned, a dose of 3300 IU now appears to be sufficient, at least in high responders, to provide adequate oocyte maturation and fertilization (29), whereas doses of 5000 or 10 000 U have often been used.

Attempts to identify hyper-responders continue. There is a significant predictive association between serum estradiol (E2) concentrations measured on stimulation days 3 and 5 and both ovarian hyper-responses and "extreme responses" in in vitro fertilization. However, the practical clinical value of stimulated serum estradiol (E2) concentrations for the prediction of hyper-responses is low, because of modest sensitivity and a high false-positive rate. For prediction of "extreme responses" the clinical value of stimulated E2 concentrations is moderate (30).

A German group has described two patients in whom severe ovarian hyperstimulation occurred, with severe and persistent ascites. In both cases it became necessary to terminate the early pregnancy, but because the grossly enlarged ovaries made laparoscopic termination impossible, mifepristone had to be used. In one case it was unsuccessful and had to be followed by curettage. In both cases ascites persisted for many months. This is not a familiar complication of ovarian hyperstimulation, and it is possible that the use of mifepristone at least aggravated and prolonged the ascites (31).

In a study of the relevance of the serum concentration of human chorionic gonadotrophin in 849 IVF cycles there were no significant relations between hCG concentrations and the proportion of follicles yielding oocytes, the fertilization rate, blastulation rate, or the probabilities of embryo transfer, implantation, or clinical pregnancy (32). This result again stresses the desirability of using moderate doses of hCG, which seems to reduce the risk of ovarian hyperstimulation while maintaining efficacy.

In vitro maturation of immature oocytes represents a potential alternative for fertility treatment in patients who are likely to suffer hyperstimulation. In two patients considered to be at risk of hyperstimulation, because of polycystic ovaries, priming with hCG 10 000 IU (specified only as the IVF-C brand) was followed by removal of the oocytes 36 hours later (33). Oocytes considered to be mature at the time of collection were inseminated using in vitro fertilization or intracytoplasmic sperm injection (ICSI), and the resulting embryos were cultured to the blastocyst stage. Transfer of these blastocysts resulted in pregnancy in both patients. Immature oocytes were matured in a culture medium containing 30% human follicular fluid, recombinant follicle-stimulating hormone 1 IU/ml, hCG 10 IU/ml, and recombinant epidermal growth factor (rhEGF) 10 ng/ml. ICSI was then carried out. Two and five expanded blastocysts were obtained after 5 days of culture and were cryopreserved. The findings suggested that one can avoid the risk of ovarian hyperstimulation when using hCG in women with polycystic ovaries and that (at least when using mature oocytes) pregnancy can be established.

Urine-derived urofollitropin and recombinant FSH appear to be equally effective and well tolerated for induction of ovulation (34). However, it is unclear whether human menopausal gonadotropins have a higher risk of overstimulation and ovarian hyperstimulation syndrome than urofollitropin in women with polycystic ovary syndrome.

As recombinant luteinizing hormone (rLH) becomes more widely available it will be important to determine whether, as has been suggested, it is less likely to lead to ovarian hyperstimulation than are the chorionic gonadotropins used up to now, in view of its shorter half-life (35). However, a recent examination of the clinical data submitted for registration of rLH in France showed no evidence to date that it is any safer in this respect that human chorionic gonadotrophin; the usual precautions to avoid ovarian hyperstimulation still need to be adopted (36). Various means have been developed to predict ovarian hyperstimulation by gonadotrophins; one of them involves rheometry (37). In 25 volunteers using a damped oscillation rheometer for blood measurements before and during administration of a regimen of human menopausal gonadotropin + human chorionic gonadotropin (hGM + hCG) there were detectable changes in blood rheometry well before the onset of frank changes in blood coagulation (38).

A mesothelial cyst in the round ligament has been attributed to ovarian stimulation (39).

- A 31 year old woman developed left lower quadrant pain after gonadotropin stimulation for IUI and a tender left inguinal mass after increasing ovarian stimulation for IVF/intracytoplasmic sperm injection. The mass was successfully removed.

Immunologic

Gonadotropins of natural origin contain various allergens, which can give rise to hypersensitivity reactions.

This was a serious problem with the "PMS" gonadotropin formulations formerly made from the serum of pregnant mares but now apparently obsolete; it was also described in the past with an FSH formulation of porcine origin. However hypersensitivity reactions can also occur to extracts of human material.

- A generalized allergic reaction to human menopausal gonadotropin (Pergonal) has been described during controlled ovarian hyperstimulation (40). In this case a desensitization protocol allowed the patient to complete her treatment cycle without further problems. Subsequently recombinant follicle stimulating hormone was used successfully and uneventfully.

On occasion, there have even been such reactions to highly purified human products, notably FSH; they can be managed by changing the treatment to intramuscular recombinant follicle stimulating hormone (41).

Long-Term Effects

Tumorigenicity

In a prospective study of 1200 infertile women in Israel, including a subgroup of women who developed breast cancer, there was no statistical association with the use of fertility-inducing drugs (42).

A subfertile man treated with human menopausal gonadotropin + human chorionic gonadotropin (hMG + hCG) developed a malignant teratoma of the testis; however, in view of his history a cause-and-effect relation was dubious (43).

Malignant melanoma

Concern that the drug treatment of female infertility might predispose the user to malignant melanoma was first engendered by a US study published in 1995 (44). Among women who had used clomiphene citrate for infertility the incidence of melanoma was higher (RR = 1.8; 95% CI = 0.8, 3.5) than among American women in general. However, in a case-cohort study of nearly 4000 infertile women there was a similar increase in the incidence of melanoma among those who had been treated with human chorionic gonadotropin compared with the rest; there was no association with the use of clomiphene.

Quite apart from the inherent discrepancy in these findings, several pieces of evidence have confused the debate. In the first place, the cohort of melanoma cases was small—barely a handful. In the second place, some earlier papers had suggested that infertility in women might of itself have an association with melanoma. The same impression came from various studies, in which the incidences of cancers in infertile women were examined (45–47). If that were true, it could affect the initial findings in either direction: a high spontaneous incidence might mask a real drug effect, or it might provide a predisposition to melanoma, which the drugs might then more readily trigger.

In the meantime, data from Australia have shown no greater incidence of melanoma among women who had used fertility drugs and undergone in vitro fertilization than in the country's general female population (48). Since then there has been one more significant paper, again from Australia, using data from a specialized fertility clinic in Queensland, relating to all women who attended the center over a decade (49). Whenever possible, the women were traced and their subsequent history noted. Originally intended as a retrospective case-cohort study using a subcohort, the approach had to be amended because no cases of melanoma were found in the subcohort. The work therefore proceeded as a matched case-control study; all the data were taken and set against publicly available figures on melanoma in Queensland. After some necessary exclusions, 3186 women were included; care was taken to minimize recall bias. Fourteen women developed melanoma after fertility treatment, eight cases being invasive. The expected incidence in the general population would have been 15.8 cases in the same period. The incidence actually observed was therefore only 0.89 of that anticipated (95% CI = 0.54, 1.48). The numbers of women who had used clomiphene or human menopausal gonadotropin were too small to make more differentiated calculations, but the incidence of melanoma seemed to correspond to that in the general population.

On current evidence, there seems no reason to discourage fertility-promoting drug treatments because of any risk of melanoma; they may even reduce it to some extent. However, this does not alter the fact that the data are deficient in various ways. Quite apart from the small numbers of melanoma cases that have been recorded, all the work to date has been performed in relatively sunny parts of the world; it is not known what would happen in other climates. Within countries, there are sharp differences in melanoma figures; in the USA, where about 32 000 new cases of skin melanoma were projected for 1994 (50), the highest melanoma rates occur among light-skinned populations in areas of intense sunlight, for example Arizona; the same applies to Queensland, Australia. In the USA as a whole there is a melanoma incidence among whites of 12.4 per 100 000 (51), while mortality rates vary inversely with latitude (52). Furthermore, in whites there has been a recent increase in the incidence of melanoma, during the precise period that this type of treatment has become popular, but probably for entirely different reasons, which may be associated with lifestyles and holiday habits; the reported incidence in whites rose by no less than 102% from 1973 to 1991 (52). Finally, as the Australian authors themselves stressed, the fact that the Queensland clinic was a private institution specializing in IVF/GIFT therapy means that women with endocrine- or ovulation-associated infertility may not so readily have been referred to it.

All this makes it very difficult to find a baseline incidence for melanoma with which cases treated for infertility can be compared. It is to be hoped that data of this type will continue to arrive from other centers, so that a definitive judgement will become possible.

Ovarian cancer

The hypothesis that the use of fertility drugs, including human gonadotropins and clomiphene, which increase the endogenous secretion of gonadotropins, might increase the risk of ovarian cancer appears to have come first clearly into the open in 1996 (53). However one can distil similar suggestions from other work from 1992 onwards (54–56), and anecdotal reports of an association have accumulated. The hypothesis has emerged that the increased number of ovulations (or the high concentrations of estrogen and gonadotropin) induced by drugs given to treat infertility could promote the development of ovarian cancers.

Ovarian cancer is much less common in married women, and during the last 30 years a direct inverse association has been found between the number of pregnancies and the duration of use of oral contraception on the one hand and the occurrence of ovarian cancer on the other. In 1971 a Lancet reviewer suggested that incessant ovulation might be a causal factor for the development of cancer of the ovary, in that the repeated rupture of follicles involved a cycle of damage to the surface epithelium, alternating with repair involving mitogenic activity and thereby in turn a risk of mutations (57). On the other hand, as has been pointed out, no correlation has been found between the risk of ovarian cancer and the age at menarche and menopause, that is the length of the fertile period, which might be anticipated if the so-called "ovulation hypothesis" is correct.

An alternative suggestion has been that gonadotropins, by enhancing the transformation of ovarian epithelial cells, also increase the risk of malignant transformation in this tissue. This idea is compatible with the inverse relations between ovarian cancer and pregnancy or oral contraception, since the latter processes suppress the secretion of gonadotropins.

Both the hypothesis of ovarian injury and that of gonadotropic influence seem to provide tempting explanations for any relation that there may be between infertility treatment and ovarian cancer, since such treatment both induces further ovarian "injury" by ovulation (sometimes multiple) and increases circulating gonadotropin concentrations. However, the existence of a possible mechanism does not prove that there actually is an association.

The stumbling block in either proving or disproving a link between the drugs and the cancers is the fact that infertility itself proves to be a risk factor for ovarian cancer. Women who fail to become pregnant have a higher risk of ovarian malignancy than other women, irrespective of whether they are taking drugs or not. A study from Denmark in 1997 showed that among infertile women the overall risk of ovarian cancer was not influenced by the use (or otherwise) of treatment with antifertility drugs (58). There is also American work that shows that among infertile women with a high risk of ovarian cancer circulating gonadotropin concentrations are low, which is what one would expect in such a group, but which does not tally well with the theory of gonadotropic causation (59).

Given current evidence, and with anecdotal reports that add nothing to the discussion of a possible cause-and-effect relation, one can discern considerable polarization in the discussion. It is not irrelevant, nor is it uncharitable, to point out that whereas fully independent academic workers have been most vocal in expressing concern, the papers that seek to dismiss an association between the drugs and the cancers have tended to emerge from groups that acknowledge support from pharmaceutical companies that produce the drugs used in this field. That is natural, and it results in the sort of argument and counter-argument that may do something to promote the emergence of the truth. However, it is currently unhelpful to the physician who is treating women for infertility and who is anxious to know what to tell the concerned patient, as well as finding some way of reducing whatever risks treatment may carry. However, bearing in mind the fact that the use of high doses of fertility drugs certainly brings with it other risks (for example that of sometimes dangerous overstimulation), this could be a reason for applying some of the more restrained available dosage schemes, and for avoiding persisting with this inherently abrasive treatment when it has failed to produce results on two or more occasions.

Breast cancer

The possibility that gonadotrophins used for the treatment of infertility might in later life lead to an increased risk of breast cancer has been examined in the USA using findings from the National Institute of Child Health and Human Development Women's Contraceptive and Reproductive Experiences Study (60). The investigators identified a population of 4575 patients with primary invasive breast cancer and 4682 healthy control subjects from the same environment, and examined their medical histories. A history of infertility drug use was not associated with a risk of breast cancer. However, compared with women who had never used any fertility medication, women who had used human menopausal gonadotropin for 6 months or more, or for at least six cycles, had a relative risk of breast cancer of 2.7-3.8. The authors therefore considered that long-term use of certain infertility drugs could increase the risk of breast cancer, but they pointed out that additional confirmatory studies are needed.

Data from the French E3N prospective cohort study have been analysed in the hope of throwing further light on this question (61). Of 92 555 women in the study population, 6602 were treated for infertility. During the 10-year follow-up period, 2571 cases of primary invasive breast cancer were diagnosed (183 in treated women). Analysis showed no significant overall association between the risk of breast cancer and treatment of any type for infertility (RR = 0.95, 95%CI = 0.82, 1.11). However, in the subgroup of women with a family history of breast cancer, infertility treatment was associated with a very slight further increase, of borderline significance, in the risk of breast cancer.

There is, however, a possibility that an increased risk of breast cancer might be associated with the state of infertility itself and not with the agents administered to treat it. In a retrospective study of data on 12 193 women evaluated for infertility between 1965 and 1988 at five clinical sites, 292were identified and followed up to the end of 1999. The standardized incidence ratios for in situ and invasive breast cancers in these women were compared with the breast cancer risks in a cohort from the general population (62). Infertile patients as a group had a significantly higher risk of breast cancer (RR = 1.29, 95%CI

= 1.1, 1.4). Analyses for types of treatment within the cohort showed adjusted relative risks of 1.02 for clomiphene citrate and 1.07 for gonadotropins, and no substantial relations to dosage or cycles of use. There were slight and non-significant increases in risk for both drugs after 20 years or more of follow-up (RR = 1.39 for clomiphene and 1.54 for gonadotropins). However, the risk associated with clomiphene for invasive breast cancers was statistically significant (RR = 1.60, 95%CI = 1.0, 2.5).

Second-Generation Effects

Pregnancy

A US group, working prospectively, has sought to develop a prediction model to assess the risk of inducing high-order multiple pregnancies (triplets or more) by gonadotrophic stimulation of the ovaries in 849 consecutive infertile women who underwent a total of 1542 cycles of treatment with gonadotrophins without the use of in vitro fertilization (63). Using a series of criteria considered to point to an increased risk of multiple pregnancy, treatment was cancelled in those cycles in which there appeared to be a substantially increased risk of multiple pregnancy. The use of this predictive routine was estimated to have reduced the number of overall treatment successes by some 8% (95% CI = 6.8, 9.2), but it very markedly reduced the number of high-order multiple pregnancies, by 285% (95% CI = 279, 291).

Drug Administration

Drug formulations

The composition of different formulations of hCG is not entirely consistent, and could account for some discrepancies in clinical studies, as well as introducing risks. For example, previously, formulations of hCG have been shown to be toxic to Kaposi's sarcoma (KS) cells. However, clinical studies using commercial hCG formulations in the human sarcoma are highly contradictory (64). The apparent discrepancies between different studies may be because both pro- and anti-KS components are present in varying proportions in different hCG formulations. As certain hCG formulations may not only lack the ability to control Kaposi's sarcoma, but also contain contaminant KS growth factor(s), the authors suggested caution when using crude hCG for the treatment of Kaposi's sarcoma.

These findings point to the need to reconsider the international standards applicable to the standardization, formulation, and marketing of hCG products, whether of natural or recombinant origin.

Drug dosage regimens

The incidence of ovarian hyperstimulation is highly dependent on the therapeutic regimen. In one study (65) the following methods were compared:

- a conventional human menopausal gonadotropin + human chorionic gonadotropin (hMG + hCG) program;

- the hMG step-down method, in which the daily dose of hMG was reduced from 150 IU to 75 IU when the follicle diameter reached 11–13 mm;
- the sequential hMG + gonadotropin-releasing hormone (GnRH) method, in which hMG injection was switched to pulsatile GnRH administration (20 micrograms/120 minutes subcutaneously) when the follicle diameter reached 11–13 mm;
- a new, modified hMG + GnRH method, in which pulsatile GnRH was injected together with hMG; daily hMG was stopped and the GnRH dosage was changed from 10 to 20 micrograms when the follicle diameter reached 11–13 mm.

Initially, the established methods were used randomly to treat 34 cycles in 20 women; subsequently, five patients who failed to conceive after treatment with sequential hMG + GnRH were then treated by the new method. More than eight growing follicles and multiple pregnancies were observed during treatment by the conventional method. The incidence of ovarian hyperstimulation syndrome was 26% with the conventional method, 20% with the step-down method, and 0% with the sequential hMG + GnRH method; however, the rate of ovulation was only 50% with the sequential hMG + GnRH method. By contrast, with the new method fewer than three growing follicles occurred in 82% of patients, there was a 100% rate of ovulation, and there were no multiple pregnancies or ovarian hyperstimulation syndrome. Moreover, the new method induced pregnancy in three out of five patients. The authors considered their modified method suitable for the treatment of severe hypogonadotrophic amenorrhea. In view of the risks attached to ovarian hyperstimulation, this type of program certainly merits further evaluation.

References

1. Reissmann T, Felberbaum R, Diedrich K, Engel J, Comaru-Schally AM, Schally AV. Development and applications of luteinizing hormone-releasing hormone antagonists in the treatment of infertility: an overview. Hum Reprod 1995;10(8):1974–81.
2. Engel T, Jewelewicz R, Dyrenfurth I, Speroff L, Vande Wiele RL. Ovarian hyperstimulation syndrome. Report of a case with notes on pathogenesis and treatment. Am J Obstet Gynecol 1972;112(8):1052–60.
3. Mroueh A, Kase N. Acute ascites and hydrothorax after gonadotropin therapy. Report of a case. Obstet Gynecol 1967;30(3):346–9.
4. Nwosu UC, Corson SL, Bolognese RJ. Hyperstimulation and multiple side-effects of menotropin therapy: a case report. J Reprod Med 1974;12(3):117–20.
5. Humbert G, Delaunay P, Leroy J, Robert M, Schuhl JF, Poussin A, Augustin P. Accident vasculaire cérébral au cours d'un traitement par les gonadotrophines. [Cerebrovascular accident during treatment with gonadotropins.] Nouv Presse Méd 1973;2(1):28–30.
6. Lovel TW, Porter GD. Cardiomyopathy after gonadotrophin treatment. BMJ 1977;1(6059):511.
7. Servais JF, Mormont C, Bostem F, Legros JJ. Perturbations neuropsychiques graves chez un jeune adolescent soumis à une thérapeutique endocrinienne. [Severe neuropsychic disturbances in a young adolescent treated with an endocrine therapy.] Acta Psychiatr Belg 1976;76(1):97–106.
8. Vollenhoven BJ, Healy DL. Short- and long-term effects of ovulation induction. Endocrinol Metab Clin North Am 1998;27(4):903–14.
9. European Metrodin HP Study Group. Efficacy and safety of highly purified urinary follicle-stimulating hormone with human chorionic gonadotropin for treating men with isolated hypogonadotropic hypogonadism. Fertil Steril 1998;70(2):256–62.
10. Strowitzki T, Kentenich H, Kiesel L, Neulen J, Bilger W. Ovarian stimulation in women undergoing in-vitro fertilization and embryo transfer using recombinant human follicle stimulating hormone (Gonal-F) in non-down-regulated cycles. Hum Reprod 1995;10(12):3097–101.
11. Loumaye E, Piazzi A, Warne D, Kalubi M, Cox P, Lancaster S, Rotere S, Sauvage M, Ursicino G, Baird D, et alThe European Recombinant Human LH Study Group. Recombinant human luteinizing hormone (LH) to support recombinant human follicle-stimulating hormone (FSH)-induced follicular development in LH- and FSH-deficient anovulatory women: a dose-finding study. J Clin Endocrinol Metab 1998;83(5):1507–14.
12. Out HJ, Mannaerts BM, Driessen SG, Coeling H, Bennink HJ. A prospective, randomized, assessor-blind, multicentre study comparing recombinant and urinary follicle stimulating hormone (Puregon versus Metrodin) in in-vitro fertilization. Hum Reprod 1995;10(10):2534–40.
13. Frydman R, Howles CM, Truong F. A double-blind, randomized study to compare recombinant human follicle stimulating hormone (FSH; Gonal-F) with highly purified urinary FSH (Metrodin) HP) in women undergoing assisted reproductive techniques including intracytoplasmic sperm injection. The French Multicentre Trialists. Hum Reprod 2000;15(3):520–5.
14. Chang P, Kenley S, Burns T, Denton G, Currie K, DeVane G, O'Dea L. Recombinant human chorionic gonadotropin (rhCG) in assisted reproductive technology: results of a clinical trial comparing two doses of rhCG (Ovidrel) to urinary hCG (Profasi) for induction of final follicular maturation in in vitro fertilization–embryo transfer. Fertil Steril 2001;76(1):67–74.
15. Loumaye EEuropean Recombinant LH Study Group. Human recombinant luteinizing hormone is as effective as, but safer than, urinary human chorionic gonadotropin in inducing final follicular maturation and ovulation in in vitro fertilization procedures: results of a multicenter double-blind study. J Clin Endocrinol Metab 2001;86(6):2607–18.
16. Hugues JNInternational Recombinant Human Chorionic Gonadotropin Study Group. Induction of ovulation in World Health Organization group II anovulatory women undergoing follicular stimulation with recombinant human follicle-stimulating hormone: a comparison of recombinant human chorionic gonadotropin (rhCG) and urinary hCG. Fertil Steril 2001;75(6):1111–8.
17. Seiden WB, Kelly LP, Ali R. Acute intermittent porphyria associated with ovarian stimulation: a case report. J Reprod Med 2003;48:201–3.
18. Ludwig M, Felberbaum RE, Diedrich K. Deep vein thrombosis during administration of HMG for ovarian stimulation. Arch Gynecol Obstet 2000;263(3):139–41.
19. Samman Y, Ghoneim H, Hashim IA. Syndrome of inappropriate ADH as a manifestation of severe ovarian hyperstimulation syndrome. J Obstet Gynaecol 2001;21:201–3.
20. Borgaonkar MR, Marshall JK. Marked elevation of serum transaminases may be associated with ovarian hyperstimulation syndrome. Am J Gastroenterol 1999;94(11):3373.

21. Grio R, Patriarca A, Ramondini L, Ferrara L, Curti A, Piacentino R. Il monitoraggio ecografico come metodo di prevenzione dei rischi da iperstimolazione ovarica in corso di trattamento farmacologico. [Ultrasonic monitoring as a method of preventing risks of ovarian hyperstimulation during drug therapy.] Minerva Ginecol 1999;51(1–2):15–7.

22. Evbuomwan IO, Fenwick JD, Shiels R, Herbert M, Murdoch AP. Severe ovarian hyperstimulation syndrome following salvage of empty follicle syndrome. Hum Reprod 1999;14(7):1707–9.

23. Davis AJ, Pandher GK, Masson GM, Sheron N. A severe case of ovarian hyperstimulation syndrome with liver dysfunction and malnutrition. Eur J Gastroenterol Hepatol 2002;14(7):779–82.

24. Garrett CW, Gaeta TJ. Ovarian hyperstimulation syndrome: acute onset dyspnea in a young woman. Am J Emerg Med 2002;20(1):63–4.

25. Levinsohn-Tavor O, Friedler S, Schachter M, Raziel A, Strassburger D, Ron-El R. Coasting—what is the best formula? Hum Reprod 2003;18:937–40.

26. Al-Shawaf T, Grudzinskas JG. Prevention and treatment of ovarian hyperstimulation syndrome. Best Pract Res Clin Obstet Gynaecol 2003;17:249–61.

27. Tozer AJ, Iles RK, Iammarrone E, Gillott CMY, Al-Shawaf T, Grudzinskas JG. The effects of "coasting" on follicular fluid concentrations of vascular endothelial growth factor in women at risk of developing ovarian hyperstimulation syndrome. Hum Reprod 2004;19:522–8.

28. Szilagyi A, Bartfai G, Manfai A, Koloszar S, Pal A, Szabo I. Low-dose ovulation induction with urinary gonadotropins or recombinant follicle stimulating hormone in patients with polycystic ovary syndrome. Gynecol Endocrinol 2004;18:17–22.

29. Schmidt DW, Maier DB, Nulsen JC, Benadiva CA. Reducing the dose of human chorionic gonadotropin in high responders does not affect the outcomes of in vitro fertilization. Fertil Steril 2004;82:841–6.

30. Hendriks DJ, Klinkert ER, Bancsi LFJMM, Looman CWN, Habbema JDF, Te Velde ER, Broekmans FJ. Use of stimulated serum estradiol measurements for the prediction of hyperresponse to ovarian stimulation in in vitro fertilization (IVF). J Assist Reprod Genet 2004;21:65–72.

31. Gnoth C, Halbe E, Freundl G. Persistent ascites after ovarian hyperstimulation syndrome and administration of mifepristone (RU 486) for the termination of pregnancy. Arch Gynecol Obstet 2003;268:65–8.

32. Shapiro BS, Daneshmand ST, Garner FC, Aguirre M, Ross R, Morris S. Effects of the ovulatory serum concentration of human chorionic gonadotropin on the incidence of ovarian hyperstimulation syndrome and success rates for in vitro fertilization. Fert Steril 2005;84:93–8.

33. Son WY, Yoon SH, Lee SW, Ko Y, Yoon HG, Lim JH. Blastocyst development and pregnancies after IVF of mature oocytes retrieved from unstimulated patients with PCOS after in-vivo HCG priming. Hum Reprod 2002;17(1):134–6.

34. Van Wely M, Andersen CY, Bayram N, Van Der Veen F. Urofollitropin and ovulation induction. Treatm Endocrin 2005;4:155–65.

35. Ludwig M, Westergaard L.G, Diedrich K, Andersen CY. Developments in drugs for ovarian stimulation. Best Pract Res Clin Obstet Gynecol 2003;17:231–47.

36. Anonymous. Lutropin alfa: combined with follitropin for follicular development: no better than menotropin. Prescrire Int 2003;12:91–2.

37. Braude P, Rowell P, Taylor A. ABC of subfertility. Assisted conception. III—Problems with assisted conception. Ovarian hyperstimulation syndrome. BMJ 2003;327:920.

38. Watanabe T. Early prediction of ovarian hyperstimulation syndrome during gonadotropin therapy by means of a damped oscillation rheometer. Biorheology 2002;39:767–86.

39. Ryley DA, Moorman DW, Hecht JL, Alper MM. A mesothelial cyst of the round ligament presenting as an inguinal hernia after gonadotropin stimulation for in vitro fertilization. Fertil Steril 2004;82:944–6.

40. Harrison S, Wolf T, Abuzeid MI. Administration of recombinant follicle stimulating hormone in a woman with allergic reaction to menotropin: a case report. Gynecol Endocrinol 2000;14(3):149–52.

41. Battaglia C, Salvatori M, Regnani G, Primavera MR, Genazzani AR, Artini PG, Volpe A. Allergic reaction to a highly purified urinary follicle stimulating hormone preparation in controlled ovarian hyperstimulation for in vitro fertilization. Gynecol Endocrinol 2000;14(3):158–61.

42. Potashnik G, Lerner-Geva L, Genkin L, Chetrit A, Lunenfeld E, Porath A. Fertility drugs and the risk of breast and ovarian cancers: results of a long-term follow-up study. Fertil Steril 1999;71(5):853–9.

43. Rubin SO. Malignant teratoma of testis in a subfertile man treated with HCG and HMG. A case report. Scand J Urol Nephrol 1973;7(1):81–4.

44. Rossing MA, Daling JR, Weiss NS, Moore DE, Self SG. Risk of cutaneous melanoma in a cohort of infertile women. Melanoma Res 1995;5(2):123–7.

45. Ron E, Lunenfeld B, Menczer J, Blumstein T, Katz L, Oelsner G, Serr D. Cancer incidence in a cohort of infertile women. Am J Epidemiol 1987;125(5):780–90.

46. Brinton LA, Melton LJ 3rd, Malkasian GD Jr, Bond A, Hoover R. Cancer risk after evaluation for infertility. Am J Epidemiol 1989;129(4):712–22.

47. Modan B, Ron E, Lerner-Geva L, Blumstein T, Menczer J, Rabinovici J, Oelsner G, Freedman L, Mashiach S, Lunenfeld B. Cancer incidence in a cohort of infertile women. Am J Epidemiol 1998;147(11):1038–42.

48. Venn A, Watson L, Lumley J, Giles G, King C, Healy D. Breast and ovarian cancer incidence after infertility and in vitro fertilisation. Lancet 1995;346(8981):995–1000.

49. Young P, Purdie D, Jackman L, Molloy D, Green A. A study of infertility treatment and melanoma. Melanoma Res 2001;11(5):535–41.

50. Boring CC, Squires TS, Tong T, Montgomery S. Cancer statistics, 1994. CA Cancer J Clin 1994;44(1):7–26.

51. In: Rees LAG, Eisner MP, Kosary CL, Hankey BF, Miller BA, Clegg L, Edwards BK, editors. SEER Cancer Statistics Review, 1973-1999. Bethesda MD: National Cancer Institute, 2002:23–124 http://seer.cancer.gov/csr/1973-1999/37.

52. Glass AG, Hoover RN. The emerging epidemic of melanoma and squamous cell skin cancer. JAMA 1989;262(15):2097–100.

53. Shushan A, Paltiel O, Iscovich J, Elchalal U, Peretz T, Schenker JG. Human menopausal gonadotropin and the risk of epithelial ovarian cancer. Fertil Steril 1996;65(1):13–8.

54. Whittemore AS, Harris R, Itnyre J. Characteristics relating to ovarian cancer risk: collaborative analysis of 12 US case-control studies. II. Invasive epithelial ovarian cancers in white women. Collaborative Ovarian Cancer Group. Am J Epidemiol 1992;136(10):1184–203.

55. Banks E, Beral V, Reeves G. The epidemiology of epithelial ovarian cancer: a review. Int J Gynecol Cancer 1997;7:425–38.

56. Rossing MA, Daling JR, Weiss NS, Moore DE, Self SG. Ovarian tumors in a cohort of infertile women. N Engl J Med 1994;331(12):771–6.

57. Fathalla MF. Incessant ovulation—a factor in ovarian neoplasia. Lancet 1971;2(7716):163.

58. Mosgaard BJ, Lidegaard O, Kjaer SK, Schou G, Andersen AN. Infertility, fertility drugs, and invasive ovarian cancer: a case-control study. Fertil Steril 1997;67(6):1005–12.

59. Helzlsouer KJ, Alberg AJ, Gordon GB, Longcope C, Bush TL, Hoffman SC, Comstock GW. Serum gonadotropins and steroid hormones and the development of ovarian cancer. JAMA 1995;274(24):1926–30.

60. Burkman R, Tang M-TC, Malone KE, Marchbanks PA, McDonald JA, Folger SG, Norman SA, Strom BL, Bernstein L, Ursin G, Weiss LK, Daling JR, Simon MS, Spirtas R. Infertility drugs and the risk of breast cancer: findings from the National Institute of Child Health and Human Development Women's Contraceptive and Reproductive Experiences Study. Fertil Steril 2003;79:844–851.

61. Gauthier E, Paoletti X, Clavel-Chapelon F, Fangon M, Follain Y. Hoang L, Niravong M, Evans G. Breast cancer risk associated with being treated for infertility: results from the French E3N cohort study. Hum Reprod 2004;19:2216–21.

62. Brinton LA, Scoccia B, Moghissi KS, Westhoff CL, Althuis MD, Mabie JE, Lamb EJ. Breast cancer risk associated with ovulation-stimulating drugs. Hum Reprod 2004;19:2005–13.

63. Tur R, Barri PN, Coroleu B, Buxaderas R, Parera N, Balasch J. Use of a prediction model for high-order multiple implantation after ovarian stimulation with gonadotropins. Fert Steril 2005;83:116–21.

64. Simonart T, Van Vooren JP, Meuris S. Treatment of Kaposi's sarcoma with human chorionic gonadotropin. Dermatology 2002;204(4):330–3.

65. Yokoi N, Uemura T, Murase M, Kondoh Y, Ishikawa M, Hirahara F. A modified hMG-GnRH method for the induction of ovulation in infertile women with severe hypogonadotropic amenorrhea. Endocr J 2002;49(2):159–64.

Hormonal contraceptives— emergency contraception

General Information

For a complete account of the adverse effects of estrogens, readers should consult the following monographs as well as this one:

- Diethylstilbestrol
- Estrogens
- Hormonal contraceptives—oral
- Hormone replacement therapy—estrogens
- Hormone replacement therapy—estrogens + androgens
- Hormone replacement therapy—estrogens + progestogens

A review of the English language literature has shown that in the USA, the source of most of the evidence, the two most commonly used forms of emergency contraception are the Yuzpe regimen (high-dose ethinylestradiol + high-dose levonorgestrel) and "Plan B" (high-dose levonorgestrel alone) (1). Although both methods sometimes stop

ovulation, they may also act by reducing the probability of implantation, through an effect on the endometrium (the "post-fertilization effect"). The available evidence for the latter mechanism is moderately strong. If this is the manner in which development of a zygote is prevented one would anticipate a certain proportion of failures, with the possibility of second-generation injury. This finding also has potential implications in such areas as informed consent, emergency department protocols, and conscience clauses, since it is more in the character of abortion than true contraception, making the term "emergency contraception" or "post-coital contraception" a slight misnomer.

Estrogens

Various estrogens and estrogen + progestogen combinations have been used in post-coital contraception. Courses of high-dose oral diethylstilbestrol, ethinylestradiol, conjugated estrogens, or combinations of estrogen and progestogen for 4–6 days are all effective. Estrogens are postovulatory rather than post-coital contraceptives, and so it is necessary to know the exact time of unprotected intercourse in relation to a woman's menstrual cycle (2). Depending on the frequency and timing of intercourse, a 5-day course of post-coital estrogen, introduced within 72 hours, gives a pregnancy rate of 0.03–0.3%.

Diethylstilbestrol has been widely used as a post-coital contraceptive. However, it is no longer in use in many countries for this purpose, because of the possible adverse effect on the development of a surviving fetus (see separate monograph).

Ethinylestradiol has been used in the past as a post-coital contraceptive, with a daily dose of 5 mg/day for 5 days. This method has a high incidence of adverse reactions, nausea, vomiting, and breast tenderness being the most frequent (3); the first menstrual cycle after treatment is likely to be abnormal.

Progestogens

Clinical trials of desogestrel implants showed that they were effective, but with bleeding irregularities and ovarian cysts as the primary adverse effects (4).

The "morning after" method of suppressing pregnancy is usually less well tolerated than normal hormonal contraception, and variants on the dosage schedule continue to be studied in an attempt to improve tolerability without undermining the reliability of the method.

Two regimens for emergency contraception started within 72 hours of unprotected coitus have been studied: (a) the progestogen levonorgestrel in two separate doses each of 0.75 mg; (b) the Yuzpe regimen of combined oral contraceptives—ethinylestradiol 100 micrograms + levonorgestrel 0.5 mg repeated 12 hours later (5). The relative risk of pregnancy for levonorgestrel compared with the Yuzpe regimen was 0.36 (95% Cl = 0.18, 0.70). Nausea and vomiting were significantly less frequent with the levonorgestrel regimen. Adverse effects of both regimens were nausea, vomiting, dizziness, fatigue, headache, breast tenderness, and low abdominal pain. However, all of these adverse effects were less frequent with levonorgestrel.

Estrogen + progestogen combinations

In recent years it has become common to use a combination of estrogen and progestogen for post-coital contraception. For example, a tablet containing ethinylestradiol 100 micrograms and levonorgestrel 0.5 mg (or norgestrel 1 mg) taken twice with an interval of 12 hours has been used (6). This treatment must begin within 72 hours of unprotected intercourse. The approach seems to be as effective as ethinylestradiol alone, while producing somewhat less nausea and vomiting (7). Apart from this the adverse effects most commonly experienced are as with estrogen alone. Overall failure rates are about 2–3%, with perhaps twice this failure rate when taken at mid-cycle. However, bearing in mind the rate of pregnancy after unprotected intercourse, the protective effect is not impressive; the chance of pregnancy is probably only halved.

It is probably impossible to define an ideal dose for this purpose. Essentially the aim is to provide a sufficient hormonal jolt to derange nidation and the development of the zygote, and this might be attained in various ways; the most acceptable dosage schemes will be those that are best tolerated. Because oral contraceptives are generally more readily available than specially formulated products, they have sometimes been used for this purpose in deliberate overdose. Even low-dose oral contraceptives, if taken in sufficient quantities, will prove effective post-coital contraception (8); progestogen-only tablets are also effective in a single dose, for example levonorgestrel 0.6 mg taken within 12 hours, but irregular bleeding, nausea, and dizziness are common adverse effects (SEDA-16, 466).

The FDA has approved a marketing application for the Prevent Emergency Contraceptive Kit (Gynetics), which contains tablets for post-coital emergency contraception, packaged with a urinary pregnancy test. The application is based on a regimen that consists of two tablets containing ethinylestradiol and levonorgestrel to be taken within 72 hours of unprotected intercourse and two tablets to be taken 12 hours later. This regimen is about 75% effective in preventing pregnancy. The most common adverse effects are nausea, vomiting, menstrual irregularities, breast tenderness, headache, abdominal pain and cramps, and dizziness (9).

Androgens

The synthetic androgen danazol has also been evaluated for post-coital use, but with inconsistent results (8); doses of twice 400 mg or twice 600 mg seem to be reliable while a single dose of 600 mg seems to be insufficient. A 10% incidence of vomiting, headache, and breast tenderness has been reported and a lower incidence (1–2%) of vomiting (10).

Antiprogesterones

The antiprogesterone mifepristone, almost exclusively used as an abortifacient, has also been tried as a post-coital contraceptive (11). In one randomized comparative trial, a single dose of mifepristone 600 mg was at least as effective as the usual hormonal method (12). Women who took mifepristone had lower rates of adverse effects, particularly nausea and vomiting, but their next menstrual period was more likely to be delayed. In another randomized trial, both methods were equally effective (SEDA-16, 466). The use of an estrogen + a progestogen had a higher total incidence of adverse effects, but mifepristone was associated with the greatest cycle disruption. If mifepristone was given in the follicular phase, 52% of women had a delay of 4 days or more in the onset of their next menstrual period (indicating that ovulation had been inhibited); when it was given in the luteal phase, 84% of women menstruated on time.

Physical methods

A non-hormonal approach to emergency contraception is insertion of an intrauterine contraceptive device up to 7 days after ovulation in a cycle during which unprotected intercourse has occurred (13).

Comparison of methods

The combined estradiol + levonorgestrel (Yuzpe regimen), the levonorgestrel-only regimen, and post-coital copper intrauterine devices have been compared by the Clinical Practice Gynaecology and Social and Sexual Issues Committees of the Society of Obstetricians and Gynaecologists of Canada. Sponsor: The Society of Obstetricians and Gynaecologists of Canada (13) and the following recommendations made:

1. Women who have had unprotected intercourse and want to prevent pregnancy should be offered hormonal emergency contraception up to 5 days after intercourse.
2. A copper IUCD can be used up to 7 days after intercourse in women who have no contraindications.
3. Women should be advised that the levonorgestrel regimen is more effective and causes fewer adverse effects than the Yuzpe regimen.
4. Either one double dose of the levonorgestrel regimen (1.5 mg) or the regular two-dose levonorgestrel regimen (0.75 mg each dose) can be used, as they have similar efficacy with no difference in adverse effects.
5. Hormonal emergency contraception should be started as soon as possible after unprotected sexual intercourse.
6. Women of reproductive age should be provided with a prescription for hormonal emergency contraception in advance of need.
7. The woman should be evaluated for pregnancy if menses have not begun within 21 days after emergency contraception.
8. A pelvic examination is not indicated for the provision of hormonal emergency contraception.

Organs and Systems

Cardiovascular

With the estrogen + progestogen type of emergency post-coital product (commonly norgestrel 500 micrograms + ethinylestradiol 50 micrograms) estrogenic complications can occasionally arise. Stroke has been reported after this type of oral contraception (14,15) and there were earlier isolated cases of retinal vein thrombosis (16) and occlusion of the right common carotid artery.

Gastrointestinal

Nausea and vomiting, which are common after use of the "morning after" pill, appear to be influenced by the timing of food and medication. With the standard Yuzpe regimen or modifications of it (substituting norethindrone as the progestogen or eliminating the second dose), taking the first dose within 1 hour of a meal or snack was associated with increased nausea and vomiting; while taking the second dose within 1 hour of a meal or snack was associated with decreased nausea and vomiting (17). At present many of these women use antiemetics; it is possible that the need for these drugs could be reduced by better timing of medication and food intake, but this is at present no more than a hypothesis.

Second-Generation Effects

Pregnancy

The "progestogen only" form of emergency post-coital contraception appears to share some of the problems of the progestogen-only pre-coital products: some 35 years after its initial introduction, the "progestogen-only pill" remains a contraceptive of limited merit, because it is less reliable than progestogen + estrogen combinations and because of the rather higher risk that any pregnancy that occurs will be ectopic (18). Essentially the same applies when a progestogen-only product is taken after coitus as a form of emergency contraception (the "morning after pill"). The most widely used product of this type comprises two tablets of levonorgestrel 0.75 mg, which was approved for sale in various countries in 1999. The main study available at that time related to 976 women; there were 11 failures, but all the resulting pregnancies were intrauterine. However, ectopic pregnancy has been previously reported after failure of post-coital progestogen treatment and there have been other unpublished cases among the "spontaneous reports" reaching the regulatory authorities (19). There were 12 such reports from the UK and others from the USA, New Zealand, and Sweden. There have since been three more cases of ectopic pregnancy after use of levonorgestrel for emergency contraception (20).

It is impossible to estimate the degree of risk, but it is probably higher in women who have had ectopic pregnancies in the past. Regulatory authorities are now ensuring that users of emergency post-coital contraceptives are warned, through package inserts, of the possibility of ectopic pregnancy, and they should consult a physician if they have a history of ectopic pregnancy or if they start to have abdominal or pelvic pain (21).

Susceptibility Factors

Post-coital contraception should not be used when there are absolute contraindications to estrogen; these include pregnancy, unstable angina, transient ischemic attacks, liver disease, undiagnosed genital bleeding, or a history of thromboembolism. Some absolute contraindications to long-term use, such as breast cancer and arterial disease, are not contraindications to short-term use (22).

References

1. Kahlenborn C, Stanford JB, Larimore WL. Postfertilization effect of hormonal emergency contraception. Ann Pharmacother 2002;36(3):465–70.
2. Notelovitz M. Estrogens and postcoital contraception. Female Patient 1981;6(7):36–8.
3. Haspels AA, Van Santen MR. Post coital contraception. J Gynaecol Endocrinol 1986;2(1–2):17–24.
4. Diaz S, Pavez M, Moo-Young AJ, Bardin CW, Croxatto HB. Clinical trial with 3-keto-desogestrel subdermal implants. Contraception 1991;44(4):393–408.
5. Grimes D, Von Hertzen H, Piaggio G, Van Look PFA. Randomised controlled trial of levonorgestrel versus the Yuzpe regimen of combined oral contraceptives for emergency contraception. Task Force on Postovulatory Methods of Fertility Regulation. Lancet 1998;352(9126):428–33.
6. Anonymous. Norsk Legemiddelhaåndbok 1998, 1999 for HelsepersonellOslo: Norsk Legemiddelhaåndbok;. 1998.
7. Haspels AA, Van Santen MR. Postcoital contraception. Pediatr Adolesc Gynecol 1984;2:63.
8. Trussell J, Stewart F, Guest F, Hatcher RA. Emergency contraceptive pills: a simple proposal to reduce unintended pregnancies. Fam Plann Perspect 1992;24(6):269–73.
9. Anonymous. Oral contraceptives—approved for emergency use. WHO Newslett 1998;9/10:12.
10. Anzen B, Zetterstrom J. Post-coital Contraception. In: Workshop on Contraceptive Methods. Uppsala: Swedish Medical Products Agency, 1994:2.
11. Glasier A, Thong KJ, Dewar M, Mackie M, Baird DT. Postcoital contraception with mifepristone. Lancet 1991;337(8754):1414–5.
12. Glasier A, Thong KJ, Dewar M, Mackie M, Baird DT. Mifepristone (RU 486) compared with high-dose estrogen and progestogen for emergency postcoital contraception. N Engl J Med 1992;327(15):1041–4.
13. Dunn S, Guilbert E, Lefebvre G, Allaire C, Arneja J, Birch C, Fortier M, Jeffrey J, Vilos G, Wagner MS, Grant L, Beaudoin F, Cherniak D, Pellizzari R, Sadownik L, Saraf-Dhar R, Turnbull V. Clinical Practice Gynaecology and Social Sexual Issues Committees, Society of Obstetricians and Gynaecologists of Canada (SOGC). Emergency contraception. J Obstet Gynaecol Can 2003;25(8):673–87.
14. Sanchez-Guerra M, Valle N, Blanco LA, Combarros O, Pascual J. Brain infarction after postcoital contraception in a migraine patient. J Neurol 2002;249:774.
15. Hamandi K, Scolding NJ. Emergency contraception and stroke. J Neurol 2003;250:615–6.
16. Lake SR, Vernon S. Emergency contraception and retinal vein thrombosis. Br J Ophthalmol 1999;83:630–1.
17. Shochet T, Blanchard K, King H, Henchcliffe B, Hunt J, McCaig C, Weaver K, Stirling A, Glasier A, Webb A, Ellertson C. Side effects of the Yuzpe regimen of

emergency contraception and two modifications. Contraception 2004;69:301–7.

18. Anonymous. Oral contraceptives. Ectopic pregnancy following emergency oral contraceptive failure. WHO Pharmaceuticals Newslett 2002;4:10.

19. Vinson DR. Emergency contraception and risk of ectopic pregnancy: is there need for extra vigilance? Ann Emerg Med 2003;42:306–7.

20. Sheffer-Mimouni G, Pauzner D, Maslovitch S, Lessing J.B, Gamzu R. Ectopic pregnancies following emergency levonorgestrel contraception. Contraception 2003;67:267–9.

21. Harrison-Woolrych M, Woolley J 2003 Progestogen-only emergency contraception and ectopic pregnancy. J Fam Plann Reprod Health Care;29:5–6.

22. Reader FC. Emergency contraception. BMJ 1991;302(6780):801.

Hormonal contraceptives— intracervical and intravaginal

General Information

The intracervical and intravaginal methods of contraception have not come into regular use, and experience with them has therefore been limited.

For a complete account of the adverse effects of progestogens, readers should consult the following monographs as well as this one:

- Hormonal contraceptives—progestogen implants
- Hormonal contraceptives—progestogen injections
- Hormonal contraceptives—oral
- Hormone replacement therapy—estrogens + progestogens
- Medroxyprogesterone
- Progestogens.

Intracervical contraceptives

When an intracervical device releasing levonorgestrel 20 mg/day was studied in 198 women over 2 years of use, a total of seven pregnancies occurred (1). All began during the first year and six occurred after the unnoticed expulsion of the device. One pregnancy occurred in an epileptic woman taking carbamazepine, while the intracervical device remained in place. In three cases the device was removed because of infection, in all three instances during the first year of use; in one case *Neisseria gonorrhoeae* was found and in another *Chlamydia trachomatis*. During the study, mean body weight increased, but remarkably there was a statistically significant reduction in the mean diastolic and systolic blood pressures after 1 and 2 years of use compared with the pre-insertion values.

Intravaginal contraceptives

As early as 1978, the vaginal administration of steroids for contraceptive purposes was attempted, at that time using vaginal rings containing medroxyprogesterone acetate or both norgestrel and estradiol. It was later found that complete inhibition of ovulation could as a rule be attained by the daily intravaginal application of a product containing norethisterone 1 mg and mestranol 50 micrograms (2).

Progestogen-only vaginal rings

Vaginal administration of steroid-containing polymer rings has been studied for at least 25 years as a means of contraception, without gaining wide acceptance. In a large multicenter WHO trial with a levonorgestrel ring, releasing 20 micrograms/day, the 1-year pregnancy rate was 4.5% (3). The main reason for discontinuation was menstrual disturbances (17%), followed by frequent expulsion of the ring and vaginal symptoms.

The finding of erythematous lesions in the vagina in some women has led to the development of a more flexible device. The Population Council has also developed a vaginal ring containing Nestorone progestin (16-methylene-17α-acetoxy-19-norpregn-4-ene-3,20-dione) for 6 months of continuous use (4). Ovulation inhibition was achieved in over 97% of the segments studied, with rings releasing 50, 75, or 100 micrograms/day. No pregnancies occurred in women who used the low-dose ring, while one pregnancy each occurred with the intermediate-dose and high-dose rings, for 6-month cumulative pregnancy rates of 0.0, 1.9, and 2.1% respectively; it is not clear why the reported pregnancy rates were higher with the higher doses. However, bleeding irregularities were common, and this form of contraception still demands further development work.

A low-dose levonorgestrel vaginal ring has also been studied. Women using vaginal rings releasing levonorgestrel 20 mg/day had more bleeding or spotting days than women using other hormonal contraceptives, with menstrual patterns similar to those of progestogen-only tablet users (5). Irregular and infrequent bleeding was also recorded by some women. Analysis of menstrual calendar data from WHO phase III clinical trials showed that the percentage of women who experience bleeding patterns defined as "acceptable" increases steadily from 39% in the first 3 months to 56% during months 10–12 (6). Frequent and irregular bleeding were the most common problems. In another study in 108 women there were four pregnancies during 1 year of investigation, with a discontinuation rate of 71%. Menstrual disturbances were the main adverse effects and also the most common reason for discontinuation, occurring in 45% of cycles during the first month (7).

References

1. Ratsula K. Clinical performance of a levonorgestrel-releasing intracervical contraceptive device during the first two years of use. Contraception 1989;39(2):187–93.

2. Coutinho EM, Silva AR, Carreira C, Barbosa I. Ovulation inhibition following vaginal administration of pills containing norethindrone and mestranol. Contraception 1984;29(2):197–202.

3. Brache V, Alvarez-Sanchez F, Faundes A, Jackanicz T, Mishell DR Jr, Lahteenmaki P. Progestin-only contraceptive rings. Steroids 2000;65(10–11):687–91.

4. British National Formulary. 2001;September:624.

5. Belsey EM. Vaginal bleeding patterns among women using one natural and eight hormonal methods of contraception. Contraception 1988;38(2):181–206.
6. Fraser IS. Vaginal bleeding patterns in women using once-a-month injectable contraceptives. Contraception 1994;49(4):399–420.
7. Gao J, Sun HZ, Song GY, Ma LY. Clinical investigation of a low-dose levonorgestrel-releasing vaginal ring. Fertil Steril 1986;46(4):626–30.

Hormonal contraceptives—male

General Information

The notion that an oral contraceptive closely similar to that used in women might be developed for men has been discussed for about 45 years, but the concept has not yet found wide acceptance. Delays in putting the concept into practice have related variously to difficulties in finding an effective combination, complaints of reduced libido or potency, and the long delay between the start of treatment and the attainment of azoospermia.

Of the many possible formulations tested all have proved to have unacceptable facets, generally including a very slow onset of action, uncertain reliability, and undesirable effects on biochemistry, body weight, or sexual function. However, some progress has been made with the combination of oral desogestrel and intramuscular testosterone.

In a study of the effects of various combinations of desogestrel and testosterone, including a sequential pattern, the optimal dosage to induce azoospermia seemed to be desogestrel 300 micrograms/day by mouth and testosterone enanate 50 mg weekly by intramuscular injection (1). Among 24 subjects, there were no withdrawals clearly related to the treatment. During weeks 1–3, adverse effects were reduced sex drive ($n = 4$), tiredness ($n = 1$), and a sensation of depression ($n = 1$); during weeks 4–24 they included mild acne ($n = 10$), increased sexual interest ($n = 3$), emotional lability ($n = 2$), tiredness ($n = 2$), night sweats ($n = 1$), and headache ($n = 1$). However, laboratory studies showed that desogestrel had clear effects on lipid metabolism in dosages of 150 micrograms/day or more, with reductions in HDL cholesterol, apolipoprotein, A1 lipoprotein, sex hormone binding globulin, and to some extent total cholesterol and LDL cholesterol. If this approach can be developed to provide a more convenient dosage scheme, these biochemical changes will be among those that need to be followed carefully

A combination of oral desogestrel 150 or 300 micrograms + intramuscular testosterone 50 or 100 mg has been tested in 24 young men and compared with historical data from studies on a combination of oral levonorgestrel + intramuscular testosterone (2). All the doses tested achieved azoospermia. All the groups tended to gain weight compared with their baseline, but the weight gain was greatest (and statistically significant) in men who received the higher dose of testosterone. Adverse effects

were acceptably low; acne occurred in occasional cases, but no one developed gynecomastia.

In a similar study limited to 8 weeks, the various formulations rapidly suppressed LH and FSH to a similar extent, irrespective of dosage, while testosterone concentrations fell slightly during treatment, with evidence of a linear dose-response relation (3). There were minor changes in plasma concentrations of inhibin B, but in seminal fluid it was suppressed, becoming undetectable in all the men who took desogestrel 300 micrograms/day. There were no significant changes in lipoproteins, fibrinogen, or sexual behavior during treatment, and only minor falls in hematocrit and hemoglobin concentration.

Organs and Systems

Endocrine

Attempts to develop a hormonal contraceptive for men have been in progress for at least 40 years, with only limited success. The most common problems have related to unreliability, slow onset of the effect, and loss of libido. It has been postulated that the addition of dutasteride, a combined inhibitor of 5-alpha-reductase type I and type II, or a long-acting gonadorelin receptor antagonist (acyline) to combination testosterone + levonorgestrel treatment may be advantageous in suppressing spermatogenesis (4). In a phase I study, 22 men received intramuscular testosterone enanthate 100 mg weekly for 8 weeks combined with one of the following: (1) oral levonorgestrel 125 micrograms/day; (2) oral levonorgestrel 125 micrograms/day + dutasteride 0.5 mg/day; (3) subcutaneous acyline 300 micrograms/kg every 2 weeks (as a comparator for any additional progestogenic effects); or (4) oral levonorgestrel 125 micrograms/day plus subcutaneous acyline 300 micrograms/kg every 2 weeks. Serum gonadotropin concentrations were suppressed to a similar degree by all four treatments, falling to nadirs of 1.2–3.4% for FSH and 0.5–0.8% for LH. Serum dihydrotestosterone concentrations were significantly reduced by dutasteride to a nadir of 31% at week 7. There were no significant differences in sperm concentrations across the groups.

Sexual function

In the study mentioned above under Endocrine, there was severe oligospermia (0.1–3 million/ml) or azoospermia in none of five and four of five men taking testosterone + levonorgestrel; two of six and four of six of those taking testosterone + levonorgestrel + dutasteride; two of six and four of six of those taking testosterone + acyline; and one of five and three of five of those taking testosterone + levonorgestrel + acyline. There was one non-responder each with testosterone + levonorgestrel and testosterone + levonorgestrel + acyline.

References

1. Wu FC, Balasubramanian R, Mulders TM, Coelingh-Bennink HJ. Oral progestogen combined with testosterone as a potential male contraceptive: additive effects between

desogestrel and testosterone enanthate in suppression of spermatogenesis, pituitary-testicular axis, and lipid metabolism. J Clin Endocrinol Metab 1999;84(1):112–22.

2. Anawalt BD, Herbst KL, Matsumoto AM, Mulders TM, Coelingh-Bennink HJ, Bremner WJ. Desogestrel plus testosterone effectively suppresses spermatogenesis but also causes modest weight gain and high-density lipoprotein suppression. Fertil Steril 2000;74(4):707–14.
3. Martin CW, Riley SC, Everington D, Groome NP, Riemersma RA, Baird DT, Anderson RA. Dose-finding study of oral desogestrel with testosterone pellets for suppression of the pituitary-testicular axis in normal men. Hum Reprod 2000;15(7):1515–24.
4. Matthiesson KL, Amory JK, Berger R, Ugoni A, McLachlan RI, Bremner WJ. Novel male hormonal contraceptive combinations: the hormonal and spermatogenic effects of testosterone and levonorgestrel combined with a 5alpha-reductase inhibitor or gonadotropin-releasing hormone antagonist. J Clin Endocrinol Metab 2005;90:91–7.

Hormonal contraceptives—oral

General Information

For a complete account of the adverse effects of estrogens, readers should consult the following monographs as well as this one:

- Diethylstilbestrol
- Estrogens
- Hormonal contraceptives—emergency contraception
- Hormone replacement therapy—estrogens
- Hormone replacement therapy—estrogens + androgens
- Hormone replacement therapy—estrogens + progestogens.

For a complete account of the adverse effects of progestogens, readers should consult the following monographs as well as this one:

- Hormonal contraceptives—implants
- Hormonal contraceptives—progestogen injections
- Hormonal contraceptives—intracervical and intravaginal
- Hormone replacement therapy—estrogens + progestogens
- Medroxyprogesterone
- Progestogens.

Hormonal contraception relies on the actions of estrogens and progestogens, of which oral contraceptives contain a mixture. The adverse effects of the separate components are discussed in other monographs.

The commonly available combinations of oral contraceptives include (estrogen first):

- ethinylestradiol + desogestrel
- ethinylestradiol + levonorgestrel
- ethinylestradiol + norethisterone
- ethinylestradiol + norgestimate
- mestranol + norethisterone.

Other forms of administration include:

- implantation
- intracervical administration
- intramuscular injection
- intravaginal administration
- transdermal administration.

These forms of contraception are covered in other monographs.

Efficacy

Hormonal contraceptives based on combinations of estrogen + progestogen, administered cyclically each month, are among the most effective forms of contraception. During typical use, only some 3% of women using combined oral contraceptives become pregnant in the first year of use, despite the failures of compliance that inevitably occur (1). The pregnancy rate for progestogen-only oral contraceptives is somewhat higher, about 5% (2). Compared with the original high-dose combination products, the lower dosages now in current use offer a smaller margin for error if tablets are missed; the efficacy of progestogen-only contraceptives is even more dependent on correct use. The accidental pregnancy rates for injectable and implanted hormonal contraceptives are lower than for the oral products, primarily because they do not depend on the daily taking of a tablet. The 1-year pregnancy rate for depot medroxyprogesterone acetate (injectable) is 0.3% and for levonorgestrel implants 0.09%.

Mechanisms of action

Estrogen and progestogen together inhibit gonadotropin secretion and thus prevent ovulation. Estrogen also stabilizes the endometrium and potentiates the action of the progestogen. In addition, the progestogen has contraceptive effects on the cervical mucus (thickening the mucus to make it hostile to sperm penetration), the endometrium (interfering with implantation), and the fallopian tubes (altering ovum transport). The original fixed-dose combinations have given way to formulations that contain lower doses, as well as to variants on the principle. The estrogen dosage, originally 150 micrograms or more, today normally lies in the range of 30–35 micrograms ethinylestradiol; even lower doses have been investigated, but these result in an unsatisfactory bleeding pattern and have little effect on ovulation. Doses of progestogens have fallen from the 5 mg (or even 10 mg) originally in use in 1960 to 1 mg or less today. To calculate the dose of progestogen that offers the highest benefit-to-harm balance is not easy, particularly since the relative potency of any progestogen can be expressed in various ways (for example in terms of its effect on the human endometrium, its androgenic or corticosteroid potency, or its ability to inhibit ovulation); these do not run parallel to one another and it is not at all clear which of these activities are relevant to the various long-term safety issues.

Progestogen-only products do not have inhibition of ovulation as their main effect; up to half of all cycles are ovulatory, and the contraceptive potential relates largely to changes in the consistency of the cervical mucus and the creation of a hostile environment for the sperm, as well as changes in tubal motility and ovum transport; after a period of treatment, endometrial atrophy occurs, rendering nidation unlikely.

Unusual combinations

Ethinylestradiol + chlormadinone acetate
In 19 650 women who had received six cycles of treatment with chlormadinone acetate 2 mg and ethinylestradiol 30 micrograms, cycle control was good, with beneficial reductions in intracyclic bleeding, severe withdrawal bleeding, dysmenorrhea, and amenorrhea (3). At baseline, 70% of the women had androgen-related skin disorders. After six cycles of chlormadinone acetate 2 mg + ethinylestradiol 30 micrograms, these disorders were improved in 87% of patients, including 29% who had complete resolution. The incidence of greasy or very greasy hair fell from 47 to 17%. There were two cases of venous thromboembolism. Breast pain (3.6%) and migraine or headache (2.6%) were the most frequently reported adverse events, but these symptoms disappeared in most women (85 and 80%) who had had them before treatment.

Ethinylestradiol + drospirenone
The effects of a monophasic oral contraceptive containing drospirenone 3 mg and ethinylestradiol 30 micrograms on pre-existing premenstrual symptoms has been studied in 326 women during 13 menstrual cycles (4). There were beneficial effects on water retention and appetite. Concentration was not significantly affected, and assessments of undesired hair changes and feelings of well-being did not change appreciably. There were no adverse effects of note.

Cyproterone acetate + a progestogen
There has been a single report of autoimmune hepatitis with the combination of cyproterone acetate and a progestogen (5). Similar events have been described very occasionally with other oral contraceptives and with diethylstilbestrol; they are not unique to cyproterone.

General adverse effects

The incidence of common adverse reactions to oral contraceptives varies with population and product. Many users have some mild reactions during the initial months of treatment, which disappear entirely as use continues; a small proportion of users withdraw at an early phase, because of individual intolerance, and turn to other methods of contraception. Relatively common adverse effects of combined oral contraceptives include intermenstrual bleeding, nausea or vomiting, breast tenderness, and headaches, although reactions are highly individual and problems can often be overcome by changing to a formulation with a greater or lesser content of active substances. Some women develop mild fever. Occasionally, oral contraceptive users report depression (or more usually a vague sensation of malaise), reduced libido, acne, or weight gain. Women taking combined oral contraceptives are also at greater risk of *Chlamydia* infection and of modest impairments of glucose and lipid metabolism. The

most serious complications attributable to oral contraceptives are cardiovascular diseases, but these are extremely rare and are even less common now, with lower-dose formulations, than in earlier decades; these much discussed risks are reviewed separately above. Hypersensitivity reactions have been observed, but only very rarely.

Tumor-inducing effects are discussed in the monograph on estrogens. The risks of epithelial ovarian and endometrial cancer are reduced by combined oral contraceptives. Effects on other cancers are slight.

Overall benefit-to-harm balance of combined oral contraceptives

A comprehensive analysis by The Alan Guttmacher Institute in the USA in 1991 evaluated the health risks of various contraceptive methods, as well as the health risks of a normal female reproductive life without contraceptives (6). Because combined oral contraceptives are highly effective, they prevent pregnancy-related deaths, particularly those associated with ectopic pregnancy. This factor more than offsets the small increased risk of cardiovascular disease related to current use, resulting in averted deaths at all ages (ranging from 3.9 per 100 000 current users at ages 15–19 up to 19 per 100 000 at ages 40–44 in the USA). They also prevent future deaths from ovarian and endometrial cancers (from 23 per 100 000 at ages 15–19 to 10 per 100 000 at ages 40–44). Current oral contraceptive use also prevents 1614 hospitalizations per 100 000 users annually. Most of these avoided hospital admissions are because of prevention of the complications of pregnancy, but they also include a reduced rate of hospitalization due to ovarian cysts, benign breast disease, upper genital tract infection, urinary tract infection, and invasive cancers of the ovary and endometrium. The conditions for which hospitalization rates may be slightly increased among combined oral contraceptive users include: myocardial infarction; stroke; venous thrombosis and embolism; invasive cancers of the breast, cervix, and liver; cervical intraepithelial neoplasia; and gallbladder disease.

Data from the classic Nurses' Health Study, followed up in 1994, reflected no difference in all-cause mortality between women who had ever used oral contraceptives and those who had never used them (7). There was also no increase in mortality associated with duration of use and no relation with time since first use or time since last use. Similarly, in the OFPA (Oxford) study, the overall 20-year mortality risk for oral contraceptive users compared with women using diaphragms or IUCDs was 0.9, suggesting no effect (8). Although the number of deaths from each cause was small, the pattern is consistent with the risks found in other studies. Oral contraceptive users had somewhat higher death rates from ischemic heart disease and cervical cancer, but lower rates of ovarian cancer mortality. Breast cancer mortality was similar for oral contraceptive users and non-users.

In developing countries, wherever there is a high maternal mortality rate, the risk of oral contraception is low in comparison (9). For all women in developing countries below the age of 40, oral contraceptive use is substantially safer than no method at all or traditional methods, about as safe as IUCDs, but not as safe as sterilization or as traditional methods backed by legal abortion performed by trained physicians.

Some of the risks have only become evaluable with much longer experience, for example those relating to the development of malignancies (covered in the monograph on estrogens). Data on these matters, too, seem reassuring; any cancer-promoting effect in one direction is at least counterbalanced by the reduction of risk in another.

Any consideration of major issues relating to the balance of benefit and harm, such as cancer or mortality rates, should be supplemented by a consideration of less prominent ones, for example, a reduction in disorders of the menstrual cycle (such as dysmenorrhea, menorrhagia, and the premenstrual syndrome) and the reduced risks of iron deficiency anemia, functional ovarian cysts, uterine fibroids, benign breast disease, pelvic inflammatory disease, and ectopic pregnancy (10,11).

Finally, since much of the work relates to high-dose products, it is important to stress that more recent work and reviews have confirmed the even greater relative safety of lower-dose products, although one must now express concern that the third-generation products may have increased certain risks once more. All the same, the broad picture of the safety of oral contraception is reassuring. Even at an earlier stage, such authoritative workers as Vessey and Doll (12) emphasized that the medical and social benefits of using oral contraceptives considerably outweighed the risks, while emphasizing the need to contain such risks as there are, that is by careful patient selection and supervision and by the use of oral contraceptives with the lowest possible dosages.

Progestogen-only oral contraceptives

Progestogen-only oral contraceptives are taken continuously and not cyclically. They not only lack the estrogen component of combined oral contraceptives but also have a lower dose of progestogen than even the current low-dose combined oral contraceptives. Progestogen-only contraceptives are therefore indicated for women who desire oral contraception but who have contraindications to or poor experience with the estrogen in combined oral contraceptives, who are breastfeeding, who are older (especially smokers), or who simply wish to keep their exogenous hormone doses to a minimum (11). The drawbacks of progestogen-only contraceptives are that menstrual irregularity is common and that careful compliance is necessary in order to achieve high efficacy.

The pharmacokinetics of progestogens in progestogen-only contraceptives are somewhat different from those in combined oral contraceptives, because of the interaction of estrogen and progestogen in the combination products. One of the major differences is that, as noted above, the plasma concentrations of progestogen rise over time in users of combined oral contraceptives; this does not happen in women taking progestogen-only contraceptives. The change is due in part to estrogen stimulation of serum hormone-binding globulin (SHBG) production, increased binding of progestogen to SHBG, and reduced progestogen clearance with combined oral contraceptives.

In contrast, progestogen-only contraceptives cause reduced SHBG concentrations and modest falls in progestogen concentrations over time.

Organs and Systems

Cardiovascular

The cardiovascular complications of oral contraceptives include venous thrombosis and thromboembolism, arterial damage, and hypertension.

Venous thromboembolism

A central issue almost from the beginning of the oral contraceptive era has been the undoubted ability of these products to increase the risk of thromboembolic and allied complications. It was the dominant reason for the progressive reduction in hormonal content of these products during their first 20 years; it led at one point to a precipitate and poorly motivated replacement of mestranol by ethinylestradiol as the estrogenic component; and rightly or wrongly it has played a central role in the recent debate concerning modified products based on newer progestogens.

History
The fact that some women could develop thromboembolic complications as a result of taking oral contraceptives first emerged in 1961, although at that time the evidence was anecdotal and poorly quantified. The first reasonably quantified investigation conducted on a sufficient scale to merit conclusions was published in 1967 by the UK Medical Research Council (13). This and other large studies conducted during the early years (and considered in older volumes in this series) concluded that women using oral contraceptives ran a greater risk than non-users of developing deep venous thrombosis, pulmonary embolism, cerebral thrombosis, myocardial infarction, and retinal thrombosis. Later papers and case reports described deep venous thrombosis, portal venous thrombosis, and pulmonary embolism (14–16). The Boston Collaborative Drug Surveillance Program follow-up study of more than 65 000 healthy women in 1980–82 found a positive association between current oral contraceptive use and venous thromboembolism (rate ratio 2.8); there was also a positive association between current oral contraceptive use and stroke or myocardial infarction (17). A UK study using data from 1978, by which time lower-dose products were increasing in use, pointed to an approximate doubling of the risk of thromboembolism compared with controls (SEDA-7, 387). The early 1980s were nevertheless marked by a series of critical papers that sought to question the entire concept of there being a link.

Much of the work on both sides of the argument was less than watertight. Some studies failed to consider the confounding effects of other risk factors (notably smoking) or the likelihood of detection bias (particularly for venous thromboembolism, which is much more common in young women than myocardial infarction or stroke). The results of some studies were also confounded by uncertainties in the history of drug exposure. A landmark paper to resolve the issue concluded that the link with venous thromboembolism in subjects without predisposition had been consistently observed in case-control and cohort studies (18). However, the evidence regarding myocardial infarction, various types of stroke, and cardiovascular mortality was less consistent. By 1990, an international Consensus Development Meeting reached agreement on the following statement regarding the relation between oral contraceptive use and cardiovascular disease (19):

> The majority of epidemiological studies strongly suggest an association between current oral contraceptive use and certain cardiovascular deaths. Although the relative risk is increased, the absolute risk is small. Because the risk of myocardial infarction is apparent in current users, disappears on cessation of use, and is not associated with duration of use, there is no epidemiologic support for the hypothesis that risk of cardiovascular diseases is of atherogenic origin · · ·. Whether particular formulations or progestogens have qualitative advantages or disadvantages merits further study. Estrogens and progestogens interact at many levels, and in epidemiologic studies of users of combined oral contraceptives it is difficult to assign a risk to either component separately. Moreover, it is physiologically unsound to do so · · ·. Alterations in plasma lipid, carbohydrate, and hemostasis variables are of major importance for the development of cardiovascular diseases, and their concentrations can be influenced by sex steroids, including artificial steroids contained in oral contraceptives. The pharmacodynamic responses · · · are dependent on not only the type and dosage of sex steroids, but also on intra- and interindividual variability in pharmacokinetics.

Frequency

It has been confirmed that the incidence and mortality rates of thrombotic diseases among young women are low (20). However, the risk is increased by oral contraceptives and there is variation in the degree of risk, depending on the accompanying progestogen. The spontaneous incidence of venous thromboembolism in healthy non-pregnant women (not taking any oral contraceptive) is about five cases per 100 000 women per year of use. The incidence in users of third-generation formulations is about 15 per 100 000 women per year. The incidence in users of third-generation formulations is about 25 per 100 000 women per year: this excess incidence has not been satisfactorily explained by bias or confounding. The risks of venous thromboembolism increase with age and is likely to be increased in women with other known factors for venous thromboembolism, such as obesity. The risk in pregnancy has been estimated at 60 cases per 100 000 pregnancies.

The Medicines Commission of the UK has reviewed all currently available relevant data and has confirmed that the incidence of venous thromboembolism is about 25 per 100 000 women per year of use (21). The incidence of venous thrombembolism in users of second-generation combined oral contraceptives is about 15 per 100 000 women per year of use. This indicates a small excess risk

of about 100 000 women-years for women using third-generation combined oral contraceptives containing desogestrel or gestodene, which has not been satisfactorily explained by bias or confounding. However, the absolute risk of venous thromboembolism in women taking combined oral contraceptives containing desogestrel or gestodene is very small and is much less than the risk of venous thromboembolism in pregnancy.

The incidence of venous thromboembolic disease in about 540 000 women born between 1941 and 1981 and taking oral contraceptives was 4.1–4.2 cases per 10 000 woman-years (22).

In another study, the figures ranged from 1895 events per 100 000 women-years when norgestimate was used to 3969 per 100 000 women-years when desogestrel was used (23). Although the authors did not find the difference statistically significant, it runs parallel to findings from other work regarding a higher risk when third-generation progestogens are used.

In women aged 15–29 years who used oral contraceptives containing third-generation progestogens, venous thromboembolism was twice as common as arterial complications. In women aged 30–44 years of age the number of arterial complications exceeded the number of venous complications by about 50%. However, in women under 30 years, deaths from arterial complications were 3.5 times more common than deaths from venous complications and in women aged 30–44 years 8.5 times more common. Women over 30 years of age who take oral contraceptives containing third-generation progestogens may have a lower risk of thrombotic morbidity, disability, and mortality than users of second-generation progestogens. However, a weighted analysis such as this does not result in any consistent recommendation of a particular progestogen type.

Nevertheless, some groups continue to produce data from their own systems that fail to confirm this. Some of these studies, including unpublished data circulated to experts for purposes of special pleading, have used selected material, and one can only consider them flawed. On the other hand, Jick et al. may be entirely right in their finding that, insofar as the special risk of idiopathic cerebral hemorrhage is concerned, no material difference in risk has been demonstrated between products of the second generation and those of the third generation (24).

And in another study it was found that users of oral contraceptives with second-generation progestogens have 30% greater increased risk of thrombotic diseases, a 260% greater increased risk of thrombotic deaths, and a 220% greater increased risk of post-thrombotic disability than users of oral contraceptives with third-generation progestogens (20).

Cyproterone acetate in combination with ethinylestradiol is indicated for the treatment of women with severe acne and moderately severe hirsutism. This product has been associated with a greater risk of venous thromboembolism than oral contraceptives. However, in a rigorous case-control study the risk of venous thromboembolism with cyproterone acetate + ethinylestradiol was not significantly greater than the risk in women who took conventional oral contraceptives (25).

Effects of dosage and formulation

As noted above, the early recognition of thromboembolic complications had repercussions for the formulation of the oral contraceptives; the progestogen and estrogen contents were both progressively reduced, and in 1969/70 mestranol was replaced by ethinylestradiol, on the grounds that the dose could thereby be halved (although it is not at all certain that this reduced the estrogenic contribution to thromboembolic events). By the late 1980s, when a major cohort study based in Oxford examined the problem (8), products containing estrogen 50 micrograms accounted for about 70% of the woman-years of tablet use, most of the remainder being accounted for by lower doses.

By the mid-1990s it was reasonably well proven that progressive dose reduction had reduced the risk of thrombotic complications (26). Epidemiological studies showed that users of low-dose combined products had small, and often statistically non-significant, rises in the risks of myocardial infarction (SEDA-16, 465) (27,28), thrombotic stroke (29–31), venous thromboembolism (32), and subarachnoid hemorrhage (29,31,33). Several of these studies compared the risks presented by different doses and found somewhat higher rates for products containing more than 50 micrograms of estrogen but somewhat lower rates among women currently using the lower-dose formulations (27,29,30,34).

A group in The Netherlands has stressed the fact that even though the risk of venous thrombosis is small in absolute terms, oral contraceptives form the major cause of thrombotic disease in young women. The risk is higher during the first year of use (up to one per 1000 per year), among women with a prothrombotic predisposition, and with third-generation progestogens (35).

Presentation

The commonest presentation is deep venous thrombosis in the leg, which can lead to pulmonary embolism. Fatal pulmonary embolism has even been reported after intravenous injections of conjugated estrogens (36). Despite the improvement noted with reduced doses, incidental case reports of severe cardiovascular events during the use of low-dose products have continued to appear. They include incidents of cerebral venous thrombosis and subarachnoid hemorrhage, fatal central angiitis, sinus thrombosis, and cerebral ischemia. In one series of 22 cases of cerebral infarction involving either arteries or veins, all the oral contraceptives that had been used contained a low dose of ethinylestradiol (37). Thromboembolism in other veins, such as the hepatic vein, that is Budd–Chiari syndrome, has occasionally been reported (38); the first 10 such cases were reported as long ago as 1972 and the increasing number since then has at times raised some concern (SEDA-6, 344) (SEDA-7, 386). A case of renal vein thrombosis has also occurred (39). Incidental reports continue to appear of thrombotic incidents in relatively unusual forms, including a further case of mesenteric thrombosis leading to intestinal necrosis (40) and a report of fatal pulmonary embolism following intravenous injections of conjugated estrogens (36).

The incidence of hepatic veno-occlusive disease in 249 consecutive women treated with norethisterone who underwent allogenic hemopoietic stem cell transplantation was 27% compared with 3% in women without this treatment (41). One-year survival rates were 17% and 73% in patients with ($n = 24$) or without veno-occlusive disease ($n = 225$) respectively. Because of this adverse effect, norethisterone should not be used in patients undergoing bone-marrow transplantation. Heparin prophylaxis does not affect the risk of death from veno-occlusive disease.

Susceptibility factors

By 1980 it was considered clear that the risk of thromboembolic events was further increased under particular conditions. It was higher in smokers, in older women, and in the obese, and appropriate warnings were issued. The fact that these warnings to a large extent eliminated the high-risk individuals who had formed part of the early population of oral contraceptive users means that data from the early period cannot be used to provide a valid historical comparison with later findings (42,43).

Thrombotic diathesis

Early epidemiological data on the recurrence of thrombosis (44) indicated something of an inherited predisposition, and others found a low content of fibrinolytic activators in the vessel wall of women who 6–12 months earlier had experienced a thrombotic complication while using oral contraceptives (45); high doses of estrogen affected the concentrations of such activators (46). However, such lesions are apparently not exclusive to users of oral contraceptives (SEDA-8, 360) and examination of the vessel wall is not of predictive value in determining risk.

The risk of venous thrombosis among carriers of the factor V Leiden mutation is increased eight-fold overall and 30-fold among carriers who take an oral contraceptive (47,48). This mutation results in resistance to activated protein C and thereby potentiates the prothrombotic effect of oral contraceptives. Early work suggested a greater risk after major surgery (49,50). However, epidemiological studies of postoperative venous thromboembolism are limited and disputed (51). There is no documented excess risk of postoperative thrombosis associated with low-dose combined oral contraceptives among women without other risk factors (52). If it is correct that some effects on coagulation persist for several weeks, it is wise to withdraw these products a month before surgery (51). From a practical point of view, any decision regarding possible discontinuation of combined oral contraceptives before surgery should take into consideration the need for alternative and adequate contraception during the interim. If the woman chooses to stop taking combined oral contraceptives, progestogen-only formulations (as well as barrier methods) are deemed suitable (51). A recommended alternative to discontinuation of a combined oral contraceptive is heparin in low doses (52).

Ethnicity

Much of the evidence on the occurrence of thromboembolic complications with oral contraceptives or hormone replacement therapy has been gathered from European or American populations, and it can be helpful to identify data from other parts of the world, where factors such as body weight, climate, or diet could affect the incidence. When a Japanese group sought to obtain national data by mailing questionnaires to a large number of institutes monitoring these forms of treatment, 771 (71%) of 1083 institutes responded (53). Follow-up questionnaires were sent to 39 institutions that reported having experienced in all 53 cases of thromboembolism during hormone therapy; 29 cases related to oral contraceptives and 13 to hormone replacement therapy, while 11 had taken other forms of hormone treatment. Of the 29 patients taking contraceptives, eight had developed arterial thromboembolism (including two with myocardial infarctions).

Age

The increase in risk with age is clear (6), although the underlying risk of cardiovascular disease also rises as age progresses. The US Food and Drug Administration has concluded that the benefits may outweigh the risks in healthy non-smoking women over age 40, and it has in most countries been common for over two decades to advise reticence in the use of oral contraceptives after the age of 35.

Obesity

Obesity has repeatedly been shown to play a role, and its relevance to particular types of complication has been demonstrated. The Oxford Family Planning Association's 1987 data showed that the risk of myocardial infarction or angina increased significantly with weight (54).

Smoking

Smoking has been very clearly incriminated as a susceptibility factor for thromboembolism and arterial thrombosis in women taking the oral contraceptive, and its apparently synergistic role has been well defined and quantified (55,56). The 1989 case-control analysis of the RCGP cohort study estimated the relative risk of myocardial infarct during current oral contraceptive use at only 0.9 for non-smokers, but at 3.5 for women smoking under 15 cigarettes per day, and as much as 21 for users of more than 15 cigarettes per day (57). Smoking increases not only the risk of myocardial infarction among oral contraceptive uses (28), but also the risk of angina pectoris (54), thrombotic stroke (29,30), and subarachnoid hemorrhage, and it can double or treble mortality (58–60). There has also been further confirmation that the effect is dose-related, light smokers having twice the risk of coronary heart disease and heavier smokers having up to four times the risk, compared with non-smokers; cessation of smoking is accompanied by a reduction in risk of coronary heart disease to the level prevalent among non-smokers within 3–5 years (56).

Smoking contributes to effects on the procoagulation process in young women (61). The effects of oral contraceptives on the coagulation system are much greater in smokers than non-smokers (45). Oral contraceptive users who were smokers generally have significantly lower fibrinolytic activity than non-smokers (62), but not consistently (63).

Others

Women of blood group O have less of a risk of thromboembolism (15). The risk of thromboembolic complications may be greater where there is a history of diabetes, hypertension, and pre-eclamptic toxemia. In some studies there has been an association with type II hyperlipoproteinemia, hypercholesterolemia, and atheroma (64–68). Hypertension may be an additional risk factor when considered in relation to oral contraceptive use.

Mechanisms

Study of the mechanisms that might underlie the link between oral contraceptives and thromboembolic events is of importance in developing safer formulations, but also in identifying, if possible, individuals at particular risk who should be advised to change to alternative contraceptive methods.

The 1990 international consensus statement cited above noted that: "Oral contraceptives induce alterations in hemostasis variables. There are changes in the concentrations of a large number of specific plasma components of the coagulation and fibrinolytic systems, although usually within the normal range ···. It is conceivable that these effects are estrogen-mediated because they have not been demonstrated in progestogen-only preparations. There is a dose-dependent relationship in the case of estrogen, although in combination tablets, the progestogens might exert a modifying effect ···. Further attention should be given to changes in factor VIIc and fibrinogen induced by oral contraceptives and also to the association between carbohydrate metabolism and fibrinolysis."

Quantification of coagulation factors is notoriously difficult, because of the interrelations among the various components of the coagulation cascade, the broad range of normal values, and considerable inter-laboratory variability (52). This variability is illustrated by a WHO study of users of combined oral contraceptives, conducted on several continents, which showed statistically significant differences among clinical centers in prothrombin time, fibrin plate lysis, plasminogen, and activated partial thromboplastin time (SEDA-16, 464). Effects also vary between different populations, users of different doses, users of different products, and tests performed at different periods of the medication cycle (63,69).

The term "hypercoagulability" has been used to describe a supposed pre-thrombotic state, identifiable by certain changes in the hemostatic system, but to date there is no broad-spectrum laboratory test for assessing the risk of thrombosis in a given individual, although coagulation changes in vitro have sometimes been regarded as proof of a thrombotic state. Deviations in laboratory data from patients with thromboses have often been interpreted as demonstrating the cause of the thrombosis, whereas they may simply be a consequence.

Despite the variations that are found, the overall conclusion is that oral contraceptives cause an increase in coagulation factors I (fibrinogen), II, VII, IX, X, and XII, and a reduction in antithrombin III concentrations, which would be expected to predispose to venous thromboembolism, especially if not counterbalanced by an increase either in fibrinolytic activity or of other inhibitory proteins of the coagulation, such as protein C (70).

There is also fairly strong evidence that immunological mechanisms play a role in thrombotic episodes associated with oral contraceptives, especially when they occur in the absence of risk factors for vascular disease (71), although this has been contested (72). In one series of reports on cerebral infarction, circulating immune complexes and/or specific antihormone antibodies were found in 15 of 20 patients (37). In a large series of women with venous or arterial thrombosis, anti-ethinylestradiol antibodies were absent in non-users but present in 72% of users; they were also present in 33% of healthy oral contraceptive users without thrombosis (SEDA-16, 465). In half of the cases there were both anti-ethinylestradiol antibodies and a history of smoking were found jointly in half of the cases.

There is a significant rise in fibrinogen concentrations during the early months of oral contraceptive use, and concentrations return to baseline after withdrawal (73). Prolonged use of oral contraception also seems to lower concentrations of antiaggregatory prostacyclin (74).

Some work that was considered to show severe acquired plasma resistance to activated protein C among users of third-generation (as opposed to second-generation) products has been re-examined by a French group (75). In their view the technical measures used to demonstrate the effect of activated protein C introduced a bias of interpretation and hence false results; they have further argued that such a test cannot demonstrate the presence of a raised thromboembolic risk in asymptomatic women taking these contraceptives, since it is non-specific and subject to changes in the plasma concentrations of many coagulation factors that are themselves increased or decreased by estrogens and progestogens. They point, for example, to protein S (76), changes in which account for the differential effect of oral contraceptives on Rosing's assay (77), but which are in their view irrelevant to issues of thromboembolic risk with oral contraceptives; the androgenic potential of the progestogen may further counteract the effect of estrogens in the test. More generally, in such a complex situation in which there is a "modification of the modification," there is no hemostasis-related test that provides a risk indicator for thrombosis. This argument is sound, but it naturally remains theoretical; the question of thromboembolism with the third-generation products must, as pointed out above, be resolved on the basis of epidemiological data, and certainly those data now strongly point to an increased risk.

Relative roles of estrogens and progestogens

The risk of thrombosis is closely associated with the estrogen component (78) for both arterial and venous events and with the progestogen for arterial events; however, if a particular progestogen is metabolized to estrogen or raises estrogen concentrations, it will make a contribution to venous complications. Estrogen alone has after all been incriminated as a cause of thromboembolism when given to men (79); the risk of puerperal thromboembolism after estrogen inhibition of lactation has been shown in several studies (80); non-contraceptive estrogens clearly increase the risk of acute myocardial infarction in women under 46 years of age (81). Changes in coagulation factors appear to be related to the estrogen dose (45,46,82,83).

Progestogen-only formulations do not have any significant effect on the coagulation system.

Prognosis

Despite the vast literature on thromboembolic complications of oral contraceptives, little attention has been paid to factors that may determine the ultimate prognosis and risk of death. Data from the Swedish Adverse Reactions Monitoring Bureau and other sources have now been used to study this question in regard to pulmonary embolism, as well as estimating the incidence (84). Over 36 years (during which the spectrum and usage of oral contraceptives naturally changed) 248 cases of suspected pulmonary embolism were reported. The presence of thromboembolism was confirmed in all fatal cases and 83% of non-fatal cases. The medical records showed that the presence of nausea or abdominal pain, age above 35 years, concomitant treatment with other drugs that increase the risk of thromboembolism, vein or lymph vessel malformations, and a deep vein thrombosis above the knee were positively associated with a fatal outcome. Chest pain and previous use of a combined oral contraceptive were negatively associated with a fatal outcome. Using pharmacy records to estimate sales, the incidence of verified pulmonary embolism was calculated as 1.72 per 100 000 treatment years; the figure for fatal cases was 0.25 per 100 000 treatment years.

Third-generation oral contraceptives and thromboembolism

There are now reasons to doubt whether the third-generation oral contraceptives are indeed safer than their predecessors in respect to thromboembolism and substantial grounds for believing that they present greater risks.

The first reason is theoretical. The demonstrated effects of the new substances and combinations on lipids and carbohydrates do not have any major relevance to the thromboembolic process. The latter is linked primarily to changes in the hemostatic system and blood coagulation, involving platelet aggregation, coagulation factors, fibrinogen concentrations, and blood viscosity.

The second reason is kinetic. It is true that the dose of estrogen (probably the main instrument in inducing thromboembolism) has been kept to a minimum, but the new progestogen gestodene tends to accumulate in the system with continued use, and the concentrations of ethinylestradiol increase simultaneously; this increase is due to the ability of gestodene to inhibit cytochrome P450 and therefore to inhibit the breakdown of estrogen, as well as its own metabolism (85). Similar findings emerged with desogestrel, although they were somewhat less marked (86).

The third reason is hematological. The third-generation contraceptives have greater adverse effects on the clotting system than those of the second generation. In particular, women using the third-generation products have a greater resistance to activated protein C (87), a shift that is associated with a higher risk of thrombosis.

The fourth reason is epidemiological. During the period 1987–88, when the third-generation products were relatively new, anecdotal reports of thromboembolic events appeared, including at least one death, and partly for this reason a series of large controlled studies were set up. The findings of three such studies (British, European, and global) became available to the drug control authorities late in 1995 and were subsequently published. The UK Committee on Safety of Medicines, considering all three, concluded that the risk of venous thromboembolic events in these third-generation oral contraceptives was about double that in users of the previous generation of products using the older progestogens (30 as opposed to 15 per 100 000 woman-years, the risk in healthy women being only five per 100 000). Despite the different populations studied, the individual studies produced broadly consistent results. The global study on four continents found a relative risk of 2.6 when comparing the desogestrel/gestodene products with the older variety, while the European study found a relative risk of 1.5–1.6. Various later papers pointed in the same direction. In Denmark, there was an increase in hospital admissions for primary venous thromboembolism in young women coinciding with the introduction of the third-generation products (88). Papers from The Netherlands have confirmed the main trend (89,90).

Authoritative reviews and editorials have further confirmed the correctness of the above findings. There has been some criticism of the individual studies on various points of detail, but it is difficult to see that this in any way undermines what is now very consistent evidence that the third-generation oral contraceptives increase the risk of thromboembolic events to a substantially greater degree than previous products. Some work that has been advanced as pointing to the safety of third-generation products (91) proves to relate primarily to the second-generation combinations, with only a few late entrants using the more recent oral contraceptives, and other work was performed on a very small scale.

As a rule, the study of adverse reactions must relate to current and emergent issues. However, now and again it can be instructive to look back into recent history. When a drug problem has been fairly clearly defined, and particularly when it has for a time been the subject of debate and even frank controversy, one can learn something from the processes involved. How did the facts become known? Why did the controversy emerge? And could the risk have been detected and eliminated earlier?

Since their appearance in the late 1950s, oral contraceptives have gone through several stages of development. What are now in retrospect referred to as first-generation oral contraceptives were high-dose combinations of progestogens (more particularly norethynodrel, norethisterone, and lynestrenol in doses of 2.5 mg or more) and the estrogen mestranol 75 micrograms. A decade later a second generation emerged, with substantially lower doses, commonly half of those used earlier and some new progestogens, notably the more potent levonorgestrel. Finally, in the early 1980s some manufacturers introduced so-called third-generation products, a particular characteristic of which was the use of entirely new, very potent progestogens, among them desogestrel and gestodene. Clinical studies of contraceptives that contained gestodene and desogestrel suggested that they are very similar to one

another, although differences in dosage and potency could account for reports that products that contain gestodene provide better cycle control (92).

Almost from the earlier years, the risk of thromboembolic complications among users of "the pill" was recognized, and by the mid-1960s it was well documented (93,94). Progressive reductions in dosage, in particular that of the estrogenic component, during the period that first- and second-generation products held sway were widely regarded as having reduced this risk to manageable proportions, although it was not eliminated. The relative risk with first-generation products was highly variable (2–11), but the best work in the UK and the USA fairly consistently reached an estimate of 4–6 (95–97). With the second-generation products the relative risk of thromboembolic complications was again variously estimated, but a large cohort study published in 1991 set it at 1.5 with products containing the lowest doses of estrogen, and 1.7 with products containing intermediate doses of estrogen (34).

The fact that both prescribers and users of medicines are likely to anticipate that new drugs will be in some way better than those that have gone before means that both groups are in principle receptive to potentially spurious claims and suggestions. By the time the third-generation oral contraceptives were marketed, this type of contraception had been around for a quarter of a century; the risk of thromboembolism, the most widely publicized problem in the field, seemed by that time to have receded with progressive reductions in dosage. There was every reason to hope that it would recede further with the newest generation of products. That expectation was further nurtured by the even lower doses latterly attainable. It also seems to have been fostered by some of the suggestive promotion that appeared, although that in fact related as a rule merely to an improved lipid spectrum, which in turn raised the theoretical possibility, also discussed but not documented by some clinical investigators (98), that arterial and cardiac risks might be less.

What in fact happened was that by 1989 alarm bells began to ring in Germany, where the regulatory authorities were alerted to the submission of an unusually high number of spontaneous reports of thromboembolic complications thought to be associated with the new products. Cases continued to accumulate, long-term studies already begun were completed, and in 1995 Britain's Committee on Safety of Medicines made a public statement to the effect that the risk of thromboembolic complications among hitherto healthy users of third-generation products was approximately twice than that seen with second-generation products (SEDA-19, xix). The studies in question, including work by the World Health Organization and others (SED-14, 1410), were subsequently published and confirmed that conclusion, as did later work (99). It was further reinforced by others (100), who worked on a smaller scale but provided well-documented evidence that while a factor V Leiden mutation or a biased family history could increase the risk in individual cases, they did not explain the higher thrombosis risk seen with a product based on desogestrel than with contraceptives that incorporated levonorgestrel, norethisterone, or lynestrenol.

Currently one must ask why the particular risk of the third-generation contraceptives was identified so late. These third-generation products had been in development since the late 1970s and the first had been marketed in 1981–82, some 14 years before the Committee on Safety of Medicines issued its statement. Could society not have done better and thereby reduced the risks to which women were exposed? There are two principal answers, both of them at least partly in the affirmative.

The first is that products of this type could well have been entered at an earlier date into large studies of oral contraception and their effects. A series of university centers around the world, as well as bodies such as Britain's Royal College of Physicians and Royal College of General Practitioners, have throughout the oral contraceptive era either sponsored or participated in prolonged cohort and case-control studies of these products. Experience with data on thromboembolism suggests that significant data are likely to be obtainable in a cohort study of manageable size within some 5–7 years. The use of third-generation products may have been small in the early years, but they were aggressively promoted in major oral contraceptive markets to ensure rapid growth, in all probability sufficient to provide adequate recruitment. One would hesitate to argue that such studies should be a universal condition of the marketing of drugs, but when the products concerned have immense social significance and considerable potential for good and harm, as the oral contraceptives do, and when the compounds involved are entirely new, there is at least a sound medical reason for such work in every case. That work was performed with successive forms of the earlier oral contraceptive products, in which dosages were progressively reduced, and there was particular reason to set it in motion on the introduction of products that contained new chemical components with some significant structural and pharmacological differences from the older progestogens. A straightforward statistical calculation shows that an early cohort study involving some 30 000–50 000 women taking a third-generation product could within 2 years have shown the degree of increase in the thrombotic risk, which was actually not elicited until much later.

The second answer with respect to the earlier acquisition of risk data must come from the laboratory. Not from animal studies, which in this field are of very restricted value, but from biochemical and particularly hematological work. When during the 1990s various groups began to examine in detail the effects of the third-generation contraceptives on processes related to the clotting system, they identified a series of properties that could very well explain an increased incidence of thrombosis.

The first of these was an increase in circulating concentrations of factor VII produced by the desogestrel plus estrogen combination, which was some 20–30% higher than that seen with a second-generation product based on levonorgestrel (101). The methods used to carry out this work were available before 1988 (102), and it is not at all clear from the published material whether there was a failure to compare the two generations in this respect at an early date, or whether such work was performed and either overlooked or misinterpreted.

A second finding related to the effects of activated protein C on thrombin generation in low-platelet plasma via the intrinsic or extrinsic clotting pathways. Using a method developed on the basis of work first published in 1997 (103), a Dutch group in Maastricht found that all types of combined oral contraceptives induced acquired resistance to activated protein C. With the third-generation contraceptives, however, the effect was significantly more marked than with those of the second generation: in other words, these drugs significantly reduced the ability of activated protein C to down-regulate the formation of thrombin (87). However, this work only became feasible in the late 1990s.

A third underlying mechanism seems to involve a reduction in concentrations of free protein S, again more pronounced with third-generation products. When protein S falls, the antifibrinolytic effect of the so-called thrombin-activated fibrinolysis inhibitor is increased; in other words, fibrinolysis is impeded, with an increased risk of clotting problems (104). Again, however, these are recent methods, which were not available when the third-generation products were launched.

The laboratory findings therefore suggest that a greater thrombosis-inducing effect of the third-generation oral contraceptives can be explained and even anticipated on the basis of known mechanisms. Not all the relevant methods were available in the early years, but that relating to factor VII most certainly was. It is unfortunate, to say the least, that such work was either not performed or not properly interpreted.

All in all, had a combination of hematological methods and field studies been initiated sufficiently soon, the increased risk of thromboembolism with the third-generation oral contraceptives could have been detected some years earlier, sufficient for society to take decisions on the benefit-to-harm balance of these drugs before so much needless injury was incurred.

The third-generation oral contraceptives: a judicial assessment

It was extraordinary to find a major epidemiological dispute regarding drug safety being handled by the High Court in England in late July 2002, when the Court handed down its decision regarding thromboembolic events induced by the third-generation oral contraceptives (105). Essentially, a group of women who claimed to have been injured as a consequence of having using this latest version of "the pill," based on two new progestogens, had sought to reclaim extensive damages from the manufacturers, since in their view the product did not possess the degree of safety which, in the words of European law, the user was legitimately entitled to expect. Since the safety achieved with the widely used products of the second generation was so widely regarded as acceptable, the Court had to decide whether the newer products had significantly failed to meet that standard. Faced with a long procession of expert epidemiological witnesses from both sides, and with some flat contradictions, the judge was obliged to rule on their arguments.

However, that it was an English court in which the issue came to be debated was not surprising, for it was in

England that the Committee on Safety of Medicines had written to prescribers in 1995 stating that three unpublished studies on the safety of combined oral contraceptives in relation to venous thromboembolism had indicated about "a two-fold increase in the risk of such conditions" compared with the preceding generation of products. This issue of a "two-fold increase" became crucial to the case. "For reasons of causation," as the Judge put it, the claimants had accepted the burden of proving that the increase in risk was not less than two-fold.

In fact, the English authorities, having rejected a vigorous defence of these products by the manufacturers, were by 1999 speaking more precisely of an increase in risk, as compared with the earlier products "of about 1.7–1.8 after adjustment," which was "not fully explained by bias or confounding"; appropriate label warnings were therefore imposed. These new warnings, summarized, said that an increased risk associated with combined oral contraceptives generally was well established, but was smaller than that associated with pregnancy (60 cases per 100 000 pregnancies). In healthy non-pregnant women who were not taking any combined contraceptive it was about five cases per 100 000 woman-years; in those taking the second-generation products it was about 15; and for third-generation products it was about 25. By September 2001, the European Union's Committee on Proprietary Pharmaceutical Products had formed its own view, and here too it was concluded that the "best estimate of the magnitude of the increased risk is in the range of 1.5–2.0."

In Court to support the claimants, Professor Alexander Walker assessed the relative risk of the third-generation products at 2.2, Dame Margaret Thorogood at 2.1, and Professor Klim McPherson at about 1.9. The experts for the defendants took the view that the relative risk was well below two, and could well be zero. As Mr Justice Mackay noted, having listened to these experts: " ⋯ the debate between them has been unyielding, at times almost rancorous in tone, and with a few honourable exceptions ⋯ devoid of willingness to countenance that there may be two sides to the question. So, science has failed to give women clear advice spoken with one voice."

There was also fundamental disagreement on confidence intervals when calculating relative risks in such matters: "The Defendants say that to establish causation in the individual, and therefore a relative risk which is greater than two, there must be seen not just a point estimate but also a lower confidence interval which is greater than two in order for the result to be significantly different from two."

The Court was faced with "a series of studies with different point estimates and largely overlapping confidence intervals. Time after time experts have had their attention drawn to point estimates from studies that appear, to the layman's eye, to be very different. Almost invariably they have dismissed those apparent differences by reference to the overlapping confidence intervals, saying that the figures are statistically compatible and there is no significant difference." Confronted with such material, the Court chose to set aside as inexact and theoretical much of the statistical rhetoric. Having done that, the Judge felt himself in a position to emerge "from that forest into broader more open country where the simpler

concept of the balance of probabilities rules." Constructing his judgement in that way, Mr Justice Mackay advanced in the course of 100 pages to the conclusion that the claimants had failed to demonstrate a doubling of the risk. In his view, "the most likely figure to represent the relative risk is around 1.7."

This extraordinary and wise judgement merits most careful reading by anyone anxious to understand the safety issues surrounding oral contraceptives. First, because of the insight that it demonstrates into the manner—not always edifying—in which evidence in this vital matter has been adduced, interpreted, and argued over in the course of more than a decade. Secondly, because it arrives, through a process of tight reasoning, at what is for the moment the most reliable conclusion we have. It seems beyond all possible doubt that the third generation of oral contraceptives is primarily characterized by an increased risk of thromboembolic complications. Whether that risk is great enough to warrant financial compensation is a matter for lawyers to decide. But given the lack of any tangible benefit to the user, the risk is clearly significant in human terms, and it is hard to see that there is any valid reason at all for continuing to use these products.

Arterial complications

Arterial disease and acute arterial disorders and their links to oral contraception have long been a matter of concern, partly because of actual reported instances of apparent complications, but largely because of the metabolic changes caused by the oral contraceptives. In particular, it has been thought that the effects of these products in raising blood pressure, affecting clotting, or changing the circulating concentrations of blood lipids and carbohydrates could result in cardiac and arterial risks, including an earlier onset of atherosclerosis and the occurrence of myocardial infarction and stroke. Basilar artery occlusion secondary to thrombosis (106), cerebral infarction (107,108), retinal vascular complications (109), and encephalopathy with renovascular hypertension (110) and acute myocardial infarction (111,112) have all been reported. There have been over 40 reports of intestinal ischemia and infarction in oral contraceptive users, with a high mortality rate (40,113).

The initial question must be whether the clinical data point to the emergence of complications of this type. The 1990 International Consensus Meeting found an increase in acute cardiovascular accidents during use of oral contraceptives, but not persisting after they had been discontinued. There is also a great deal of anecdotal evidence, although in view of the massive scale on which oral contraceptives have been used over 40 years, coincidence alone would lead to the accumulation of many reports of adverse events. Other evidence suggesting an increase in arterial thrombotic events has been noted incidentally in the discussion of venous events above. There is also evidence that the chance of unexpected cardiovascular death is lower in oral contraceptive users who have been taking a product based on one of the new progestogens in particular. In over 300 000 women there was a cardiovascular death rate of 4.3 per 100 000 women-years among users of combined oral contraceptives containing levonorgestrel, 1.5 per 100 000 among users of those based on desogestrel, and 4.8 per 100 000 among users of oral contraceptives containing gestodene (114). The relative risk estimates compared with levonorgestrel were 0.4 (95% CI = 0.1, 2.1) and 1.4 (0.5, 4.5) for desogestrel and gestodene respectively. However, it should be added that this is precisely one of the studies that concluded that the new progestogens substantially increased the incidence of venous thromboembolism.

However, a fatal flaw of most such studies was their failure to provide an adequate analysis of co-existent risk factors other than oral contraception. In fact, there is not a great deal of evidence of appreciable risks of this type among oral contraceptive users, unless other risk factors are present. The 1989 case-control analysis of the Royal College of General Practitioners cohort study showed that current oral contraception increased the risk of acute myocardial infarction, but only among smokers. The large cohort study from the Oxford Family Planning Association (OFPA) similarly found no significantly increased risk of myocardial infarction or angina pectoris among either current or former use of oral contraceptives, but a strong dose-related effect of current smoking. In an analogous manner, many studies have shown that the risk of coronary heart disease in oral contraceptive users or other women increases directly with body weight (54,56) and with age (6), but not clearly with oral contraceptive use alone. Nor does one find any published evidence that the risk of late arterial disease, notably atherosclerosis, is higher among users of oral contraceptives, despite the fact that with some 40 years of experience one would expect any such trend to have become evident by the end of the 20th century.

Alongside this clinical material one is faced with the biochemical evidence of changes in the oral contraceptive user. However, various findings make it impossible to draw clear pathogenetic conclusions from these biochemical data. As far as lipids are concerned, there is no doubt that oral contraceptives as a group increase low-density lipoprotein and reduce high-density lipoprotein and cholesterol; this shift is usually regarded as inducing a propensity to atherosclerosis, but here its significance is not so simple to assess. HDL cholesterol, for example, can be divided into subfractions, of which HDL2 seems to be more responsive to estrogens and progestogens; the concentration of HDL2 has been thought to correlate better with a reduced risk of cardiovascular disease than does total HDL cholesterol (115). The picture is further complicated by the fact that when estrogens are used in postmenopausal women they can raise HDL, a change that might be considered to have a favorable effect (116–118). What is more, the effects of these products on lipids change with time, rendering short-term studies useless as a basis for risk assessment. It could be that the older oral contraceptives raise the risk in the short term, as suggested above, but actually lower it in the long term.

It is by no means impossible that the overall effect of oral contraceptives on the arterial system is exercised through a complex of different mechanisms. In this respect it is worth recalling the "insulin resistance syndrome" or "metabolic syndrome," which comprises a set of metabolic risk factors for cardiovascular disease (specifically coronary heart disease and arterial disease) (119). These interrelated risk factors include hyperinsulinemia and impaired glucose tolerance, hypertriglyceridemia, reduced high-density lipoprotein (HDL) concentrations, and hypertension, with insulin resistance as a potential underlying factor. Hormonal contraceptives can variously affect these metabolic conditions, and the effect depends in part on steroid type and dose. Lower doses and newer formulations do not change HDL concentrations or increase blood pressure, but insulin resistance and hypertriglyceridemia still occur. These latter changes are caused primarily by the estrogen component of combined oral contraceptives, but the progestogen component can also modify these effects. The formulations with the least unfavorable metabolic effects are those that contain norethindrone or that are based on the newer progestogens, such as desogestrel, gestodene, or norgestimate. However, as noted elsewhere, it has yet to be determined whether the metabolic changes confer any clinical benefit.

Finally, it is fair to set the possible adverse effects of these hormonal products, and particularly of estrogen, against the fact that estrogen also has certain favorable effects on the arterial wall. It has been suggested that estrogen has a calcium channel blocking effect that relaxes the vessel walls, thus increasing blood flow (120). Others have documented in monkeys the fact that estrogens dilate the coronary arteries, an effect unrelated to plasma lipid concentrations, blood pressure, or heart rate (SED-13, 1217) (121). They have also found evidence in their animal studies that estrogen + progestogen administration to hypercholesterolemic animals reduces both their HDL cholesterol concentrations and their arterial lesions.

Frequency

West German data over the period 1955–80 showed no community-wide increase in the incidence of ischemic heart disease, cerebral vascular embolism, or pulmonary embolism, despite the rapid growth in oral contraceptive use (and the prevalence of high-dose products) during much of that period (122). The Oxford Family Planning Association's 1989 paper on its cohort study, which had followed up more than 17 000 women for an average of nearly 16 years, found no significant overall effect of oral contraceptive use on mortality, with a relative risk of 0.9 (8). Mortality from diseases of the circulatory system had slightly increased; the relative risk of death from ischemic heart disease in current or past oral contraceptive users was 3.3 (95% CI = 0.9–17.9), while data on fatal cerebrovascular disease were too few to be interpreted.

Similarly, a massive Finnish mortality study, covering 1 585 000 women-years of oral contraceptive use and two million women-years of copper-bearing intrauterine device use, showed no increase in relative risk among oral contraceptive users for myocardial infarction or cerebral hemorrhage deaths; however, there might have been an increased risk of death from pulmonary embolism among users of oral contraceptives (43).

An analysis of the cardiovascular mortality risk associated with low-dose oral contraceptives (under 50 micrograms of ethinylestradiol) in the USA showed that among non-smokers and light smokers the mortality among current oral contraceptive users was likely to be lower than the mortality due to pregnancy (26). Only among heavier smokers over 30 years old did the risk of oral contraceptive use exceed the risk of pregnancy. The researchers noted that in countries with higher maternal mortality rates than the USA, even older women who are both heavy smokers and oral contraceptive users would have a lower mortality risk than that associated with pregnancy.

A 5-year case-control study involving all Danish hospitals has once more quantified the thromboembolic risks associated with oral contraceptives as a whole; the risk with third-generation products was some 30% higher than with second-generation products (RR = 1.3; CI = 1.0, 1.8) (123). However, data on cerebral thrombosis from the same study showed that with third-generation products the mean risk was some 40% lower than with second-generation products (RR = 0.6; CI = 0.4, 0.9) (124).

Susceptibility factors

The effect of smoking has been investigated on a large scale in Denmark, where the incidence of smoking among women is much higher than in many other countries (125). Evidence has emerged that the combination of smoking with oral contraceptive use may have a synergistic effect on the risks of acute myocardial infarction and cerebral thromboembolism (but not of venous thromboembolism), particularly among users of high doses (50 micrograms). The authors therefore suggested that the very low-dose products, which in Denmark contain 20 micrograms of ethinylestradiol, should be preferred in smokers. While this conclusion is clear and defensible, the situation is somewhat complicated by the fact that in Denmark the only products that contain this low dose of estrogen are those in which it is combined with either desogestrel or gestodene, that is third-generation progestogens. It could well be that the safest combined oral contraceptives for smokers will prove to be those in which the 20 micrograms dose of estrogen is combined with a more traditional progestogen.

For current or potential users of oral contraceptives the question arises whether it is not wise to examine the individual's possible predisposition to thromboembolism (thrombophilia) before deciding for or against this form of birth control. It has been suggested that in teenage users who might prove to be carriers of the Factor V Leiden mutation, routine screening would not be economically justified (126). It was instead the author's view that clinicians can use thoughtful screening questions to identify potentially high-risk patients for thrombophilia and consider testing for inherited risk factors case by case.

Estrogens versus progestogens

As far as the estrogens are concerned, the original estrogen, mestranol, was abruptly replaced by ethinylestradiol in most or all products after a wide-scale panic relating to the thrombosis issue in 1969. The motive lay entirely in the fact that the ethinylestradiol was about twice as potent, so that the dose could be halved. Whether this in fact led to any reduction in cardiovascular thromboembolic risk was never specifically examined. The choice of estrogen might still be relevant to the extent that (physiological) 17-β-estradiol in microcrystalline form later became available for oral use and in theory might prove safer in some respects than semisynthetic estrogens, since it seems to have less effect on the fibrinolytic system.

The question of the progestogens has come acutely to the fore as a result of the debate regarding the third-generation progestogens gestodene and desogestrel. At the time of marketing, no specific claim appears to have been made that they would present a lesser degree of risk of thromboembolism. However, emphasis was placed on experimental findings that might indicate a better cardiovascular prognosis. The older oral contraceptives produce an increase in low density lipoprotein and a reduction in high density lipoprotein and cholesterol; those changes may have some relevance to the occurrence of arterial disease. By avoiding them, and having the lowest possible estrogen content, the new combinations were expected to be safer, although this had in no sense been proven. However, the manner in which this information was presented could have introduced a degree of confusion in the minds of prescribers and users, and the belief appears to have arisen that these third-generation oral contraceptives might prove less likely than their predecessors to cause thromboembolic disorders. That this is not so in relation to venous thromboembolism is discussed above. The theoretical argument that the risk of atherosclerosis and its associated complications might in the long run be less is so far entirely unproven, and with the fall in use of these products following these unfavorable findings (127), it seems uncertain whether the data necessary to examine that hypothesis will ever be accumulated.

Persistence of risk after discontinuation

Most, but not all, studies have concluded that the effect of oral contraception on the risk of cardiovascular disorders disappears after withdrawal (6,42,56,128–130). The Nurses' Health Study found no differences in either incidence of or mortality from various cardiovascular diseases between never-users and past-users, regardless of the duration of use, or the time since last use (7). The nested case-control analysis of the RCGP study showed that, although stroke risk was higher among current oral contraceptive users regardless of smoking status, former users had an increased risk only if they were current smokers. Such conclusions are supported most strongly by a 1990 meta-analysis of published studies on the relation between past use of oral contraceptives and myocardial infarction, which produced an adjusted relative risk estimate of 1.01, suggesting no association (131). Thus, there does not appear to be a long-term mechanism at work, such as atherosclerosis, but rather an effect confined to current use, such as thrombosis (42,56). However, there have been only a few studies of stroke in relation to previous oral contraceptive use, and those studies have produced inconsistent results; thus, meta-analysis of stroke data is precluded.

With some of the newer drugs, the effects may (as seems to be the case with the older drugs) persist for a number of weeks and justify the withdrawal of these products some time before surgery or other risks. A study of changes in hemostasis after withdrawal of the newer combined oral contraceptives (ethinylestradiol 30 micrograms plus either desogestrel or gestodene) (42) showed that several weeks elapsed before plasma concentrations of fibrinogen, factor X, and antithrombin III returned to baseline.

It should be noted that a few studies have produced deviant conclusions, for reasons that are not clear. Some found that the risk of fatal myocardial infarction was similar for current and past users (27), whereas others actually reported a lower risk of cerebral thromboembolic attack in former users compared with never users (30).

In summary, the final chapter in the story of oral contraceptives and arterial lesions has not yet been written. However, in the light of long experience there is currently reason for optimism. There is no reasonable evidence that oral contraceptives, whatever their biochemical effects, actually do increase the risk of atherosclerosis; as to the occurrence of acute arterial events, these are explained largely or entirely by the presence of risk factors other than oral contraception.

Hypertension

The association between combined oral contraceptives and hypertension, noted and confirmed as early as 1961, has been explored in a multicenter clinical trial carried out by the WHO (132,133) and on a lesser scale in many other reports, yet the facts remain surprisingly puzzling. It has become clear that the use of oral contraceptives in any dose can cause a mean increase in blood pressure, the effect being much more marked in some individuals than others. With the current range of oral contraceptives a substantial proportion of users show some increase in blood pressure compared with their pre-treatment condition (134), but the rise is rarely of clinical significance. Clinical hypertension seems unlikely to occur in more than 1–5% of women (135). The incidence may have been higher with the older high-dose products, but that is not entirely clear. The figures have to be set against the incidence of hypertension in a population of otherwise healthy women of fertile age, which is about 2%. The rise in blood pressure can appear at any time during treatment and persists for at least as long as the drug is taken, sometimes for several months longer, but even then it generally returns to normal. In order to detect women who react poorly, blood pressure measurements should be an integral part of the follow-up care of all women taking oral contraceptives. Considerable research has shown no overall increase in blood pressure or in the prevalence of hypertension associated with use of progestogen-only contraceptives; nor does the available information point to any increase in other cardiovascular disorders.

It is not clear why many women remain normotensive while others have a rise in blood pressure. No confirmation has been obtained of early beliefs that hypertension during oral contraception was more likely to occur in black American women, or in women with a history of hypertension during pregnancy (58,136). However, there is clinical evidence that this can occur and that the women involved

may have a defect in dopaminergic transmission affecting blood pressure and prolactin secretion (137); pre-existent abnormalities of platelet function and fibrinolysis have also been linked with this complication (SEDA-6, 348).

Published studies, in which various doses have been used, show that there is no clear relation between blood pressure and estrogen intake. The progestogens seem to be involved, but here too most specific studies fail to detect a dose–response relation (134). However, some do: in a 1977 analysis of data from the large prospective study by the Royal College of General Practitioners (RCGP), with oral contraceptives containing ethinylestradiol 50 micrograms and norethisterone acetate 1, 3, or 4 mg, the risk of hypertension increased with increasing progestogen dose (138).

The rise in blood pressure might reflect water retention caused by the mineralocorticoid effect of progestogens, but that is probably not the complete explanation. These drugs have an effect on the renin-angiotensin system, but there actually seems to be some fall in responsiveness to plasma renin activity. Other possible pathophysiological mechanisms discussed so far include insufficient adaptation to increased production of angiotensin and aldosterone, an increase in cardiac output, and changes in the metabolism of catecholamines. The estrogenic component of oral contraceptives has been stated to be the more important factor in producing abnormalities in the renin system, but the progestogen may also play a role. Some workers have found higher estrogen concentrations in oral contraceptive users who develop hypertension (139).

As might be expected, the few women with severe hypertension during oral contraceptive use, whether or not they were hypertensive before that time, run a somewhat greater risk of acute secondary complications due to hypertension, such as subarachnoid hemorrhage. If the hypertension is severe and persistent one might anticipate long-term effects on the cardiovascular system and kidneys. Nested case-control studies using data from the RCGP study showed that hypertension was an independent risk factor for both stroke (29) and myocardial infarction (57); after controlling for other variables, including oral contraceptive use, the odds ratios (or estimated relative risks) associated with hypertension were 2.8 for stroke and 2.4 for myocardial infarction. In that study, oral contraceptive use did not further increase the risk associated with either hypertension or a history of toxemia of pregnancy. Nevertheless, hypertensive women who take oral contraceptives should be monitored carefully.

Respiratory

Oral contraception is not considered to be relevant to the induction or aggravation of respiratory disorders, although the fact that a very few women have allergic reactions to these formulations could in theory be relevant to the occurrence of asthma.

Nervous system

Headache has long been reported as a reaction to oral contraceptives, just as it occurs unpredictably with many other forms of drug treatment; it is probable that women who are susceptible to headaches at certain phases of the menstrual cycle are more likely to react to oral contraceptives in this way. However, it does not seem to be in any sense consistent; in a placebo-controlled trial conducted as long ago as 1971, when doses of estrogens were high, headache was not found to be associated with use of combined oral contraceptives containing mestranol either 50 or 100 mg (140). In many other studies of the adverse effects of oral contraceptives, it is not possible to ascertain whether the prevalence of specific complaints, such as headache, is actually increased, because there is no appropriate comparison group.

Because migraine headaches are of vascular origin and are sometimes linked to the menstrual cycle, it is pertinent to consider whether hormonal contraception is appropriate in women suffering from this condition (141). No association of migraine headache with stroke has been demonstrated. However, some women with migraine have an increase in the severity and frequency of headache when they take combined oral contraceptives, just as some other migraine sufferers describe a relation to the menstrual cycle. As a precaution, women who have migraine headaches with focal neurological symptoms should not take combined oral contraceptives.

A systematic review of published data on the occurrence of headache with the more modest combination products now used has shown little indication that they have a clinically important effect on headache in most women (142). Headache that occurs during early cycles of oral contraceptive use tends to improve or disappear with continued use. No clear evidence supports the common clinical practice of switching from one oral contraceptive to another in the hope of attaining a lower incidence of headache. However, manipulating the extent or duration of estrogen withdrawal during the cycle may provide benefit.

Despite initial concern (SEDA-6, 349), combined oral contraceptives do not appear to worsen seizure control in most women with epilepsy, although seizure frequency should be carefully monitored. The primary consideration in selecting a contraceptive method for an epileptic woman is the need for dependability, but antiepileptic drugs that are enzyme inducers reduce the effectiveness of hormonal contraceptives. Women who wish to take combined oral contraceptives, but for whom enzyme-inducing drugs provide the best seizure control, should be given combined oral contraceptives with a relatively high dose of estrogen (for example ethinylestradiol 50 micrograms). Fewer seizures occur during the luteal phase (low estrogen) of the menstrual cycle, suggesting that estrogens (or oral contraceptives) may be epileptogenic.

Reversible electroencephalographic changes, probably due to progestogenic effects (143), have been observed in 25–60% of oral contraceptive users.

There are various reports of chorea (144,145), hemichorea (146), and paraballism (147). In one case, chorea was the first sign of lupus erythematosus (148). Although it has been suggested that in such cases the contraceptive simply triggered the reactivation of latent Sydenham's chorea, there has been a report of a case with no evidence of pre-existing chorea or recent streptococcal infection (149). However, the patient had positive antibasal ganglia antibodies, which supports an immunological basis for the pathophysiology of this complication.

Acute abdominal symptoms in users of hormonal contraceptives suggest embolism or infarction at some site, but there can be unusual explanations.

- Right-sided lower abdominal pain occurred in a 15-year-old girl, and had been present throughout the 3 months that she had used the product but it had now become so severe as to demand emergency care. The problem was traced to cutaneous nerve entrapment in the abdominal wall (150).

It is not clear how this could have resulted from the treatment, but it might have entailed fluid redistribution in or around an old appendicectomy scar. It may be noted that nerve entrapment is recognized as a possible adverse effect of oral contraceptives in the carpal tunnel syndrome.

Results from the Oxford Family Planning Association Study showed no relation between oral contraceptive use and the incidence of multiple sclerosis (151). Conversely, multiple sclerosis is no longer considered to be a contraindication to hormonal contraceptive use.

Sensory systems

Eyes

It is still difficult to judge whether there is a correlation between ocular pathology and the use of oral contraceptives, with the exception of thromboembolic incidents that affect the retinal circulation. Oral contraceptives have several times been reported to reduce the tolerability to contact lenses, but in any case this abates in some people as the years pass. However, pregnancy itself may result in loss of contact lens tolerance both for scleral and corneal lenses, lenses often having to be refitted after pregnancy; a similar effect of oral contraceptives is thus not entirely unlikely (152), even though other workers have failed to detect any such change (153). Similar doubts relate to the induction of macular hole with retinal detachment, but in one study 20 of 24 women with this complication were using oral contraceptives (SEDA-6, 348). Finally, there is one case report of retinal migraine linked to the end of oral contraceptive treatment cycles (154).

Ears

Aggravation of existing otosclerosis has been observed several times; in one series of five cases, withdrawal of the medication stabilized four cases while the fifth improved (155). There is no reason to expect a reduction in hearing except in cases of otosclerosis; indeed, in a study of several thousand American women, hearing was generally found to be better among current oral contraceptive users than in never-users, and was intermediate in past users (156). A long-term study of chronic oral contraceptive users, which included otological, audiological, and vestibular examinations, found no impairment of the function of the healthy internal ear (157).

Psychological, psychiatric

Psychiatric symptoms have been described in women taking oral contraceptives in isolated case reports (158,159), probably reflecting non-specific effects in susceptible individuals. As to psychological effects, many physicians have found that certain women react to oral contraceptives by becoming morose or unhappy (160), but this does not necessarily mean that they meet the clinical criteria of true depression, the incidence of which has not been found to be increased (161). Several possible biological mechanisms for mood changes have been suggested; however, when nervousness and depression among combined oral contraceptive users are carefully evaluated over time, the pattern is so inconsistent that it is difficult to study. If one looks for anything like consistent depression one is unlikely to find it (140).

Many women who change to an oral contraceptive after unsatisfactory experience with other forms of contraception find greater sexual satisfaction (161) because of relief from worry about pregnancy.

Endocrine

Both long-term and short-term progestational therapy can suppress pituitary ACTH production to some extent, as studied with the metyrapone test. Medroxyprogesterone and chlormadinone suppress the reaction to metyrapone almost completely. Recovery was rapid after withdrawal of therapy. However, no conclusion was drawn as to the relative effect of the ethinylestradiol that was also given. The cortisol secretion rate is depressed in women taking norethindrone and mestranol, and the suggestion has been made that the gluconeogenic effect of glucocorticoids is markedly potentiated in subjects taking estrogens or estrogen-like substances. Adrenal cortical insufficiency has been related to the use of ethinylestradiol and dimethisterone taken during 1 year. The ascorbic acid content of the anterior pituitary is reduced in the presence of estrogen-induced adenohypophyseal hypertrophy.

Fasting growth hormone concentrations are higher in women using a contraceptive agent than in controls (162).

Oral contraceptives can cause an increase in total thyroxine (163) and a fall in the percentage of free thyroxine (164). The uptake of radioactive iodine in the thyroid is usually normal; total uptake of radioactive iodine may be reduced (164). The effect of progestogens on thyroxine-binding globulin may possibly counteract the estrogenic action. The net result will be a rise in protein-bound iodine and a fall in resin triiodothyronine uptake (165). It has been suggested that oral contraceptives may actually have some protective effect against thyroid disease.

Metabolism

Lipid metabolism

The 1990 report of the International Consensus Development Meeting stated the following regarding the effects of oral contraceptives on carbohydrate and lipid metabolism (19): "All currently used oral contraceptives can cause deterioration in glucose tolerance accompanied by hyperinsulinemia. There is no evidence that the use of combined oral contraceptives is accompanied by overt symptoms of diabetes ⋯. The progestogen component is mainly responsible for the effects of oral contraceptives on carbohydrate metabolism, but the estrogen component may modulate the influence. The magnitude of the impact on glucose metabolism depends on the type of progestogen and also on the doses of a given steroid."

As has become clear since that time, these effects do not run parallel for all oral contraceptives; the third-generation products, which contain either desogestrel or gestodene, have rather different effects, the significance of which is unclear.

Lipid changes seen with the most widely used combined oral contraceptives comprise an increase in low density lipoprotein and reductions in high density lipoprotein and cholesterol. The third-generation products have these effects to a much smaller extent, leading to claims that they would be less likely to have long-term adverse cardiovascular effects related to atherosclerosis. However, such a claim reflects an all too readily adopted belief that the lipid changes produced by the more traditional combined oral contraceptives are in this respect capable of causing this type of (primarily arterial) cardiovascular disease. This is of itself far from certain.

Changes in lipid metabolism among users of progestogen-only contraceptives are minimal. Some studies have shown very small falls in HDL and HDL2 cholesterol, but no effect on other parameters of lipid metabolism. The androgenicity of progestogens parallels their effect on lipoprotein metabolism, but dosage must also be taken into account. For example, although levonorgestrel is more androgenic than norethindrone, its progestational potency is also greater, and levonorgestrel is therefore given in a lower dose for contraceptive purposes; the net result is that there is no clinical difference in lipid effects, as has been shown conclusively (166).

Adolescents with polycystic ovary syndrome are regarded as candidates for long-term combined hormonal treatment using a product of the oral contraceptive type, and there has been some concern about possible unfavorable late metabolic effects, notably on lipids. The risks with two combined products, one based on cyproterone acetate 2 mg and the other on desogestrel 0.15 mg, both with an estrogen, have been estimated in 24 women (98). After 12 months the hirsutism score was improved, but while triglycerides and HDL cholesterol were significantly increased by cyproterone, the only relevant effect of the desogestrel combination was a raised concentration of apolipoprotein A1. The authors concluded that the desogestrel combination was therefore to be preferred in such patients.

Carbohydrate metabolism

Carbohydrate metabolism was known at an early date to be affected by combined oral contraceptives. A mild to moderate degree of insulin resistance was found in some investigations (167,168). However, the considerably impaired glucose tolerance described in some users in the 1960s was directly dose-dependent. Although findings since then have not been entirely consistent (169), it is clear that the low-dose products introduced after the first decade of use had much less marked effects (170), as did the third-generation products based on newer progestogens. The clinical significance of these effects is limited. Even for the second-generation products, no difference was found across the board between ever users and never users in the incidence of diabetes mellitus. Prospective studies in England in 1979 and 1989 (171,172) showed no increased risk of diabetes in oral contraceptive users compared with controls or ex-users. These are, however, population-wide findings, and in some high-risk individuals, the effects on carbohydrate metabolism can be undesirable, with a significant deterioration in glucose tolerance (173); patients with serious or brittle diabetes should therefore not use these forms of contraception (174). It may also be wise to advise other contraceptive methods in women with a history of gestational diabetes, who might possibly be sensitive to these effects of the oral products (175). However, because of the increased risk of pregnancy complications in diabetic women, a highly effective contraceptive method such as the combined oral contraceptive is usually desirable, and it has been reasonably well demonstrated that there is no reason to avoid this type of formulation completely in a woman with stable and well-controlled diabetes. A clinical study of young women with insulin-dependent diabetes mellitus showed no significant differences between women using various combined oral contraceptives (containing up to 50 micrograms of ethinylestradiol) and non-users in hemoglobin A_{1c} concentrations, albumin excretion rates, and diabetic retinopathy (176). Possible very long-term consequences of changes in carbohydrate (and lipid) metabolism are considered further in this record and in connection with the cardiovascular system.

Most studies of carbohydrate metabolism have shown little effect of progestogen-only contraceptives, but there is a suggestion of slight deterioration in glucose tolerance and raised plasma insulin concentrations. Women with diabetes mellitus can generally take progestogen-only contraceptives without a change in insulin requirements.

Weight

Body weight tends to increase in some women without a clear explanation, although it could be attributable in some individuals to improved appetite, water retention, or conceivably the anabolic effect of an androgenic progestogen. The increase is usually less than 2 kg and occurs during the first 6 months of use. Studies that record weight change over time have generally found similar fluctuations in oral contraceptive users and non-users (140). Cyclic weight gain purely due to fluid retention can also occur.

Nutrition

Alterations in plasma vitamin concentrations have been observed in oral contraceptive users, and attributed to reduced absorption and changes in plasma protein-binding capacity (177).

Vitamin A

While most vitamin concentrations in the blood fall (173), vitamin A concentrations increase, although carotene concentrations fall. Curiously, an isolated report of hypercarotenemia has been published (178).

Vitamin B_6

Alterations in vitamin B_6 metabolism have been discussed, particularly in connection with the suspicion that an oral contraceptive might cause depression. An additional daily intake of pyridoxine has long been suggested as a means of correcting the complex changes observed during use of oral contraceptives (179,180); there are no firm data proving that such medication has any useful effect in most women, but the approach may be tried empirically when mood changes are a problem (181).

Vitamin B_{12}

Vitamin B_{12} deficiency has been seen in healthy oral contraceptive users in whom serum vitamin B_{12} binding proteins were not altered.

Folate

Both sequential and non-sequential types of oral contraceptives impair the absorption of polyglutamic folate but not that of monoglutamic folate; the change can result in megaloblastic anemia in predisposed subjects, for example those with celiac disease or having a deficient diet (182).

Vitamin C

Some studies have suggested that ascorbic acid concentrations are lower in the leukocytes and platelets of oral contraceptive users (183); however, this has not been confirmed (184).

Vitamin D

Studies of the effects of oral contraceptives on serum concentrations of vitamin D derivatives have given variable results.

Wintertime concentrations of 25-hydroxycolecalciferol were measured in 66 young women aged 20–40 years who did and did not use oral contraceptives (185). The initial mean 25-hydroxycolecalciferol concentration in the 26 users was 41% higher than in the 40 non-users before adjustment for age and vitamin D intake (83 versus 59 nmol/l), and 39% higher after adjustment. In five women who stopped taking oral contraceptives during the year after the initial measurement the 25-hydroxycolecalciferol concentrations fell by an average of 26 nmol/l, whereas the concentrations in women whose use or non-use of oral contraceptives was constant did not change. The effect on 25-hydroxycolecalciferol concentrations was not related to the dosage of ethinylestradiol, the type of oral contraceptive, or the duration of use.

However, in another study there was no difference in the concentrations of 25-hydroxycolecalciferol between controls and women who took oral contraceptives containing ethinylestradiol 30–50 micrograms for more than 1 year (186).

The time of year and the point during the menstrual cycle during which vitamin D derivatives are measured may be important. In seven women there was a two-fold rise in the serum concentration of 1,25-dihydroxycolecalciferol on day 15 of the menstrual cycle compared with days 1 and 8, without a detectable change in the serum calcium concentration (187). This increase did not occur in five women taking oral contraceptives, and there was a small but significant fall in the serum calcium concentration.

Mineral balance

Users of oral contraceptives excrete significantly less calcium than non-users (188) and estrogen treatment prevents bone loss in postmenopausal women (189); it is thus likely that the diminished urinary calcium excretion observed in women using oral contraceptives results from suppression of bone resorption by exogenous estrogens. Long-term use of oral contraceptives may therefore affect skeletal bone stores and prevent the development of osteoporosis. In line with these findings is an investigation showing an increase in radio-opacities in the mandibles of women using oral contraceptives (190).

Metal metabolism

Sex hormones can cause changes in metal metabolism, including both increased and reduced plasma zinc concentrations and raised serum copper; however, serum magnesium is not affected (191). The clinical importance of these effects is not known.

Hematologic

Iron status is improved in most oral contraceptive users because of reduced menstrual blood loss; an important benefit of oral contraceptive use is therefore a reduction in the prevalence of iron deficiency anemia (192). Much of the relevant research has been with higher dosages than are currently used. However, a study of a low-dose combined oral contraceptive (ethinylestradiol 30 micrograms plus desogestrel 0.15 mg) documented significantly lower menstrual blood loss than at baseline (193). Most women had normal values of hemoglobin, hematocrit, erythrocyte index, and serum ferritin both before and during oral contraceptive administration, with no significant changes. However, two women who had menorrhagia (defined as menstrual blood loss greater than 80 ml) and low serum ferritin before oral contraceptive use experienced improvement in both of these parameters while taking oral contraceptives. The cyclic variation in serum iron during the menstrual cycle has also been found to be less pronounced during the use of anovulatory agents (194).

The binding capacity of serum proteins is altered by oral contraceptives (195) and leads to alterations in the serum concentrations of various substances, including thyroxine, cortisol, and serum iron (196), and in serum iron binding capacity, which are all increased.

Erythrocyte enzymopathies have rarely been observed during pregnancy and oral contraceptive treatment (197) and in these cases a cause and effect relation seems likely.

Hemostatic variables have been reviewed in women taking oral contraceptives containing desogestrel and gestodene in comparison with oral contraceptives containing levonorgestrel (198). The database of 17 comparative studies was homogeneous. There were no differential effects for coagulation and fibrinolysis parameters, except for factor VII, which was consistently increased by 20% among users of third-generation oral contraceptives than among users of second-generation oral contraceptives. Factor VII is not a risk marker for venous thrombotic disease.

Data from the Leiden Thrombophilia Study have been used to construct a case-control study, based on contraceptive users who had experienced a first episode of objectively proven deep vein thrombosis (100). Patients and controls were considered thrombophilic when they had protein C deficiency, protein S deficiency, antithrombin deficiency, factor V Leiden mutation, or a prothrombin 20210 A mutation. Among healthy women, the risk of developing deep vein thrombosis was trebled in the first 6 months and doubled in the first year of contraceptive use. Among women with thrombophilia, the risk of deep vein thrombosis was increased 19-fold during the first 6 months and 11-fold (95% CI = 2.1, 57) in the first year of use. Venous thrombosis during the first period of oral contraceptive use might actually point to the presence of an inherited clotting defect.

Coagulation factors in users of progestogen-only contraceptives have not been studied extensively using current laboratory methods, but there appears to be little effect. Perhaps the most informative study is a randomized clinical trial of two progestogen-only contraceptives (norethindrone 0.35 mg and levonorgestrel 0.03 mg) (166), which showed a reduction in several coagulation factors among women who switched from a combined oral contraceptive, but no change among women who had not previously been using a hormonal contraceptive. Thus progestogen-only contraceptives appear to be particularly suitable for women who desire oral contraception but who are at increased risk of thrombosis, including older women who are smokers.

The judicial conclusion cited above that with third-generation oral contraceptives the risk of thromboembolic complications is substantially raised compared with that of second-generation products, continues to be corroborated in authoritative literature (199). Yet despite all the evidence, there is a surprising degree of optimism in some quarters, especially when results rely only on one or two measurements. Hypercoagulability has been assessed using thromboelastography in 43 women taking low-dose oral contraceptives (ethinylestradiol 35 micrograms or less, combined with various progestogens) for 3 months (200). The 3-month R time (a thromboelastographic parameter) was significantly reduced compared with pre-treatment values, although the authors argued that the magnitude of this change was not characteristic of hypercoagulability. The outcome was not affected by the type of progestogen used. The small size and limited duration of the study, and the limited range of measures used, inevitably throw some doubt on the significance of the findings.

Mouth

Gingivitis, of varying degrees of severity, is sometimes associated with oral contraceptive use, apparently because the steroids alter the microbial flora in the mouth (201). A case of gingival hyperplasia is described under "Reproductive system".

Even a low-dose oral contraceptive combination has an effect on the composition of saliva (202); although large individual variations were noted, protein, sialic acid, hexosamine, fucose, hydrogen ion concentration, and total electrolyte concentration fell, while the secretion rates increased. The sodium and hydrogen ion concentrations increased in parotid gland secretion and sodium in submandibular gland secretion. To what extent these changes might affect the dental status of the patient is unknown.

Oral pyogenic granulomata have been reported both in pregnant patients and in patients using oral contraceptives (203).

Progestogens, alone or together with estrogen, cause an increase in the width and tortuosity of peripheral blood vessels in the oral mucosa, which become more susceptible to local irritants and show increased permeability (204).

Gastrointestinal

Mild gastrointestinal complaints, such as nausea, vomiting and vague abdominal pain, were seen in 10–30% of patients in earlier studies when high-dose products were in use. A placebo-controlled clinical trial in 1971 documented a higher prevalence of nausea and vomiting among combined oral contraceptive users than among women taking either a placebo or a progestogen-only oral contraceptive; the prevalence was also higher for the combined oral contraceptive containing mestranol 100 micrograms than for the combination product containing mestranol 50 micrograms (140). Such effects are much less common with the low doses used today. Nausea, if it occurs, is associated with the estrogen component of combined oral contraceptives; its frequency and severity generally decline over time.

The relation between oral contraceptive use and inflammatory bowel disease was analysed in two case-control studies published in the 1990s (205,206). Both found a significantly increased risk among current users compared with never users for Crohn's disease, but only the former study detected an increased risk of ulcerative colitis; a dose–response effect was suggested for Crohn's disease. When the data were stratified by smoking status in the latter study, the increased risk was found only among current smokers.

Reversible ischemic colitis, an unusual condition in young people, has been described in 17 young women, with evidence for an association with oral contraceptives (207). Ischemic colitis occurs uncommonly in younger people. The median duration of illness was 2.1 days (range 1–4 days). All recovered with supportive care. Ten women (59%) were using low-dose estrogenic oral contraceptive agents, compared with the 1988 US average of 19% oral contraceptive users among women aged 15–44 years. The odds ratio showed a greater than 6-fold relative risk for the occurrence of ischemic colitis among oral contraceptive users.

Diarrhea, probably coincidental, is bound to occur on occasion in the very large population of oral contraceptive users; when it does so, the efficacy of the product is likely to be diminished and additional contraceptive methods may need to be used.

Liver

During the early years of oral contraception, with high-dose products in use, jaundice and other hepatic complications were a source of concern; with current products this is no longer the case. Most women experience no adverse effects on liver function, but occasional hepatic changes can occur, including intrahepatic cholestasis, cholelithiasis, vascular complications, and even tumors, which are discussed in the record on estrogens. It has been argued (38) that women with a history of liver disease whose liver function tests have returned to normal can take oral contraceptives with careful monitoring. However, it is widely considered that oral contraception should be avoided in women with a history of cholestatic jaundice of pregnancy; past or current benign or malignant hepatic tumors; active hepatitis; or familial defects of biliary excretion.

The most common change is a short-term rise in serum transaminases (208), which often abates if treatment is continued. An increase in serum alkaline phosphatase is usual, while serum transaminases can be normal to markedly increased (209). Long-term use leads to changes in hepatic ultrastructure, with involvement of the mitochondria, which develop crystalline inclusions. Furthermore, hypertrophy of the smooth endoplasmic reticulum and changes in the biliary canaliculi have been shown (210,211). These changes are not usually accompanied by any clinical symptoms. The Budd–Chiari syndrome can occur in connection with thromboembolism.

Benign liver tumors (hepatocellular adenoma and focal nodular hyperplasia) are extremely rare conditions that appear to be related to oral contraceptive use (212).

Jaundice as a result of oral contraceptive treatment has been repeatedly described. Whereas in the Swedish population figures between 1:100 and 1:4000 were published when the early high-dose formulations were still in use (213), the overall incidence was estimated in 1979 at about 1:10 000 (9), and the current incidence is certainly further reduced. When such hepatic symptoms occur, they usually do so within the first month of medication (214), and jaundice may be accompanied by anorexia, malaise, and pruritus. Very few cases arise after the third month of medication and those reported are regarded by some as unlikely to be due to oral contraceptives. Microscopic examination of the liver shows intrahepatic cholestasis. When medication is stopped, symptoms usually disappear rapidly and the reaction does not seem to leave any sequelae (215). Genetic components seem to be important for the development of the reaction; women who have experienced jaundice or severe pruritus in late pregnancy seem to be especially susceptible to jaundice or gallbladder disease when using oral contraceptives (216). Discussion of mechanisms has related mostly to estrogens (217), but cases have been described in individuals taking progestogens only (213); the explanation might be the conversion of the latter to estrogens in vivo (218). The cause of cholestasis is unknown, but animal data suggest that there is inhibition of bile flow and of the biliary excretion of bilirubin and bile salts.

Peliosis hepatis has been described in association with contraceptive-induced hepatic tumors and has sometimes developed in isolation, perhaps as a herald of more serious changes to follow, for example cirrhosis and portal hypertension; one such case ultimately required an orthotopic liver transplant (219).

Sinusoidal dilatation in the liver has been reported rarely.

- A 23-year-old woman developed an acute painful syndrome with cytolysis after 7 years of oral contraceptive use; she recovered promptly after oral contraceptive withdrawal (220).

Hepatic adenomatosis, which seems to have been reported only some 38 times, is a condition with a female preponderance; in earlier work it was noted that in 46% of the female patients oral contraception had been used. This means, however, that in the other 54% it had not, and it should be borne in mind that the condition can also occur in men.

- A 35-year-old woman, who had been fitted with Norplant 2 years before and had used oral contraceptives for some 20 years before that, developed epigastric and right upper quadrant abdominal pain (221). A liver mass was found and at surgery proved to consist of multiple adenomata; part of the liver had to be resected.

What is of potential concern is that in this case, as in a very few previously described, there was also evidence of hepatocellular dysplasia, which could be a pre-malignant condition. However, with widespread use of Norplant, some reported adverse events, such as this, may be purely coincidental.

Results in 1977 from the Boston Collaborative Drug Surveillance Program suggested that oral contraceptive users are more often diagnosed as having acute hepatitis than are non-users (222). There was no similar finding in the similarly early study by the UK Royal College of General Practitioners (138).

Biliary tract

The Boston Collaborative Drug Surveillance Program found in 1973 that of a large series of 212 patients with gallbladder disease 31% were using oral contraceptives, compared with only 20% of controls (223). In another study, the risk of gallbladder surgery was twice as high in oral contraceptive users as in non-users (224). A decade later, after dosages had fallen, a 1982 study from the UK Royal College of General Practitioners showed that there was no overall increased risk of gallbladder disease in the long term and that the previously demonstrated short-term increase in risk is due to acceleration of the onset of gallbladder disease in women already susceptible

to it (138). The risk may also be age-related, the relative risk of gallstone disease being higher in young women using oral contraceptives than in older users (225–227).

- A 21-year-old woman developed increasing jaundice, with severe pruritus and weight loss, after a bout of dyspepsia (228). She had been taking contraceptives for 4 years (cyproterone acetate 2 mg, ethinylestradiol 0.035 mg). Laboratory tests at first suggested cholestatic hepatitis, but ultrasonography showed biliary sludge in the gallbladder and dilatation of the common bile duct and the smaller biliary passages. There was a occupying lesion near the papilla: it was not fixed and had no vascular supply. At endoscopic retrograde cholangiopancreatography the lesion was removed. It consisted of jelly-like viscous streaky bile without calculi. Within a few days the jaundice disappeared, the pruritus ceased, and liver function returned to normal.

A meta-analysis in 1993 of the relation between combined oral contraceptives and gallbladder disease yielded a small increased risk for women who had ever used oral contraceptives (pooled estimated RR = 1.38) (229). There was a dose-related effect in the therapeutic range of doses, suggesting that, although the risk is less with lower-dose combined oral contraceptives, there may still be a weak relation. The increased risk appears to be concentrated in the early years of oral contraceptive use, suggesting that oral contraceptives accelerate the development of the disease. On the other hand, the 1994 findings in the Nurses' Health Study II showed no substantial increase in risk associated with ever use of oral contraceptives, but relative risks of 1.6 for longterm use and for current use, after adjusting for body mass index and several other confounding variables (225). A 1994 report from the Oxford FPA study similarly suggested no relation with ever use of oral contraceptives (230).

The finding that oral contraceptive use causes an increase in the cholesterol concentration in bile and a shift in the chenodeoxycholic/cholic acid ratio suggests a biochemical basis for the increase in gallbladder disease among oral contraceptive users (231,232). Effects on gallstone formation may well be due to the estrogen content, for example since exogenous estrogens seem to increase the risk of gallbladder disease in men (233), while in women they can increase the cholesterol saturation of bile and hence the lithogenic index (234).

Pancreas

Acute pancreatitis has been reported as a very unusual complication of oral contraceptive treatment (235), as have increases in serum amylase (236).

Urinary tract

Over the years a few reports have suggested a higher incidence of urinary infections in users of oral contraceptives. There has always been some uncertainty as to whether these sporadic reports reflect an adverse effect or simply a different pattern of sexual behavior among major users of these products. Some have found an increased incidence of urinary infections, others have not. The effect of local estrogens has been explored in a pilot study in 30 young women taking oral contraceptives, mean age 23 years, with a long-standing history of recurrent urinary tract infections (237). Vaginal estrogen therapy consisted of estriol 1 mg/day for 2 weeks and then twice a week for 2 weeks. The patients had a mean history of infection over 2.3 years, while the mean period of oral contraceptive use was 3.2 years. In the follow-up period of 11 months after treatment, 24 of the 30 reported no symptoms of cystitis and used no additional medications. There was normal bladder epithelium at control cystoscopy after estriol in all patients in whom trigonal metaplasia although vulnerable highly vascularized urothelium had been found at the initial investigation. These findings led the authors to conclude that in most young women taking oral contraceptives with a long-standing history of recurrent urinary infections a considerable infection-free period can be achieved after vaginal application of estrogen, perhaps because of improved bladder perfusion. However, they did not provide any new evidence as to whether urinary infections are a significant problem in young users of oral contraceptives.

Hemolytic–uremic syndrome seen in one very long-term user may have been due to antisteroid hormone antibodies (238).

Skin

Various types of skin reactions can occur during oral contraceptive treatment, but bearing in mind the vast number of women who take oral contraceptives, major skin reactions due to oral contraceptive treatment seem to be rare. The incidence, even including all minor complications, has been estimated at 5% (239), but field experience suggests that that is a generous figure. The figure includes chloasma, seborrhea, hirsutism, pruritus, herpes gestationis, porphyria cutanea tarda, and allergic reactions such as urticaria.

Low-dose combined oral contraceptive use generally results in improvement of acne, although occasionally a user has worsening of acne owing to the androgenic potency of the progestin used. Use of a less androgenic progestogen, for example norgestimate (240) or desogestrel or the antiandrogen cyproterone acetate (241,242), can have a favorable effect in patients with pre-existing acne, reducing the severity of the condition; an oral contraceptive in which cyproterone acetate replaces the progestogen has proved helpful in women with pre-existing acne.

The efficacy and adverse effects of oral cyproterone acetate 2 mg in combination with ethinylestradiol 35 micrograms in facial acne tarda have been studied in 890 women aged 15–50 years, of whom 96 withdrew prematurely from the study (243). Of these 96 women, only 30 withdrew because of adverse events: menstrual problems ($n = 11$), headache ($n = 10$), increased body weight ($n = 3$), and thrombophlebitis ($n = 1$). Five women withdrew because of poor efficacy. In all, 260 patients had adverse events during treatment. The incidence fell as the study progressed. Of those events that first occurred during treatment, the most frequently cited were breast tension (12%), headache (8.9%), nausea (5.8%), nervousness (4.0%), and dizziness (2.6%). There were no serious adverse events. There were no clinical significant changes in body weight or blood pressure.

There is a possible association of oral contraceptives with erythema nodosum, which has been linked to the use of either estrogens or progestogens or a combination of the two; however, probably neither hormone directly causes the condition but merely creates a fertile background for its generation by other antigens.

Pre-existing condyloma acuminata have been stated to increase during oral contraception, with regression after withdrawal (244).

Increased pigmentation of areas exposed to sunlight, as well as photosensitivity, has been incidentally observed in some users, and is probably analogous to the pigment changes that can occur in pregnancy.

In one case, pityriasis lichenoides disappeared after withdrawal of oral contraceptives (245).

Sweet's syndrome (acute febrile neutrophilic dermatosis) has been attributed to an oral contraceptive (246). However, bearing in mind that the syndrome has a variable presentation and is thought to represent a form of hypersensitivity reaction, it is not at all clear that there was a true cause-and-effect relation.

Pseudoporphyria has been described in a woman taking an oral contraceptive (247).

- A 40-year-old white woman with skin type II who for 4 months had been taking a low-dose combined oral contraceptive based on levonorgestrel and ethinylestradiol developed skin fragility on her sun-exposed forearms, with blisters, erosions, and scars. Histology led to a diagnosis of pseudoporphyria, since porphyrin concentrations were not raised. After the oral contraceptive was withdrawn the lesions healed slowly, despite continuing sun exposure.

Although there have been no previous reports attributing pseudoporphyria to oral contraceptives, in earlier reports of this condition (for example in users of sun-ray beds) a fair proportion of the women were in fact taking estrogens or oral contraceptives. One is also reminded of cases in which true porphyria was precipitated by hormonal treatment.

Hair

Contraceptives induce a condition of pseudopregnancy, and alopecia during treatment and after withdrawal has been seen. Of five women who developed diffuse alopecia while taking oral contraceptives, three had male pattern baldness while they were taking the treatment; two began to lose their hair after having stopped taking treatment, and these resembled postpartum baldness (248). One woman did not regain her hair 20 months after having stopped taking the oral contraceptive. However, the incidence of alopecia among users of oral contraceptives is very low, and the association may be coincidental, since there are also case reports of improvement in the quality of the hair (249).

Musculoskeletal

Although some studies have shown that combined oral contraceptives increase bone mineral density, the available evidence suggests that any beneficial effect is rather small (250), and is presumably related to the dosage of estrogen. The effects may depend in part on the age of women being studied, as normally bone mass density continues to increase until it peaks in women in their 20s and 30s, and then remains constant until the pre-menopausal period, when it begins to fall. For example, a study of young women (aged 19–22 years) showed that those taking very low-dose combined oral contraceptives (with as little as 20 micrograms of ethinylestradiol) had no change in bone density over 5 years, whereas non-users had a significant increase (251).

In one study of combinations of levonorgestrel 100 micrograms with ethinylestradiol 20 or 30 micrograms there was no change in bone mineral density over 3 years (252), and it is possible that formulations with even lower estrogen contents would be satisfactory in this respect, although not necessarily in others (such as cycle control).

There were some early reports of localized mandibular osteitis in women using oral contraceptives subsequent to surgery of the mandibular molar teeth (SEDA-2, 316). It has been suggested that changes in the hemostasis could be the cause.

It appears that oral contraceptive use reduces the prevalence of severe disabling rheumatoid arthritis. Although studies of this have produced discrepant results, a meta-analysis of studies that met specific methodological criteria produced an overall adjusted pooled odds ratio of 0.73 (253). The authors suggested that oral contraceptives do not actually prevent rheumatoid arthritis, but modify the disease process to prevent progression to severe disease. Pregnancy has similar effects. It is unclear whether it is the estrogen or the progestogen component of oral contraceptives that is responsible.

Sexual function

Occasionally, women report reduced libido, which may have a hormonal basis. One study showed that users of oral contraceptives had no rise in female-initiated sexual activity at the time when ovulation should have occurred, whereas non-users did show such an increase in sexual activity (254).

Reproductive system

Tumor-inducing effects of hormonal contraceptives are dealt with in the record on estrogens.

Breasts

Breast tenderness or pain can occur in some women (255,256), especially with estrogen-dominant formulations, although it is notable that other women with a history of breast discomfort experience improvement when they begin to take oral contraceptives.

- A woman with Wilson's disease treated with penicillamine developed severe hirsutism (257). After treatment with oral contraceptives, her breasts enlarged rapidly, and she had cyclic mastodynia. Around the same time she also developed gingival hyperplasia.

Benign breast disease (including fibroadenoma and cystic change) is less common among users of combined oral contraceptive than in the general population (212).

Ovaries

Women currently taking oral contraceptives are less likely than non-users to have functional ovarian cysts. This protective effect appears to be more modest with lower dose monophasic formulations than with those containing 35 micrograms or more of estrogen (258,259). Functional ovarian cysts (or persistent ovarian follicles) occur more often in users of progestogen-only contraceptives than in combined oral contraceptive users or in women using no hormonal contraceptive method. Follicular development is delayed and the follicle continues to grow for a period of time, but these enlarged follicles usually regress spontaneously and are not of clinical significance.

When a woman with polycystic ovary syndrome requires treatment with flutamide and metformin, the question arises whether the effects of this treatment could be deranged by simultaneous use of an oral contraceptive. In 36 women with polycystic ovary syndrome, of whom 12 were also taking a low-dose oral contraceptive the beneficial effects of flutamide 125 mg/day and metformin 1275 mg/day on hyperandrogenemia, hyperinsulinemia, and dyslipidemia were maintained when an oral contraceptive (ethinylestradiol 20 micrograms + gestodene 75 micrograms) was used, and in the latter there was an additional increase in sex hormone-binding globulin, and thus a further fall in the free androgen index (260). These workers concluded that in such patients combined treatment is in fact ideal.

Uterus

Effects on menstrual function depend on the dose used and the sensitivity of the individual user; they may be welcome or unwelcome (193,261). Menses generally become more regular and predictable, and dysmenorrhea is less common and less severe. The number of days of blood loss in each menstrual period is often reduced, as is the amount of menstrual flow; thus women who previously had iron deficiency anemia associated with menorrhagia have increased iron stores. A comparison of women who kept menstrual diary records as part of WHO trials has confirmed that users of combined oral contraceptives in adequate dosages have more regular menstrual cycles than do users of other hormonal methods (262). None of the combined oral contraceptive users in these studies had amenorrhea (defined as the absence of bleeding throughout a 90-day reference period), although shorter periods of amenorrhea have occasionally been reported in other studies, particularly with very low-dosage formulations and with longer-term use.

Intermenstrual bleeding (breakthrough bleeding or spotting) often occurs, especially during the first few cycles of treatment, and is often the reason that women choose to stop taking an oral contraceptive. When using products based on newer progestogens it seems that better control may be offered by formulations that contain gestodene compared with desogestrel and by levonorgestrel compared with norethindrone (263), but the absence of standardized methods makes such conclusions tentative. Research on triphasic formulations is too sparse to allow firm conclusions on this point. One study confirmed the long-standing experience that intermenstrual bleeding rates vary inversely with both estrogen and progestogen dose (264). However, one finds no evidence that breakthrough bleeding is an indication of reduced contraceptive efficacy, despite speculation regarding a possible relation.

Dysmenorrhea is less common and less severe among women who use oral contraceptives of any type, provided that ovulation is inhibited; this emerges both from experience and from prospective studies; the effect seems to be maintained as long as the oral contraceptive is continued. There seem to be no significant differences in this respect between monophasic products with low or high progestogen doses, those with high progestogen doses, or triphasic products (261).

Since post-treatment amenorrhea of more than 6 months duration was first suggested as an adverse reaction in around 1965, much work has been devoted to delineating the risk and prognosis of menstrual changes after the withdrawal of hormonal contraception. It is now recognized that post-treatment amenorrhea occurs in 0.7–0.8% of women, but this is no different from the background rate of spontaneous secondary amenorrhea. No cause and effect relation between oral contraceptive use and subsequent amenorrhea has been documented.

Menstrual irregularities are common among women taking progestogen-only contraceptives and are often the reason a user chooses to discontinue the method (265,266). Users of progestogen-only contraceptives are more likely than users of other hormonal contraceptive methods to have frequent bleeding (262). Infrequent bleeding, amenorrhea, and irregular bleeding among progestogen-only contraceptive users are more likely than among combined oral contraceptive users, but less prominent than among women using levonorgestrel-releasing vaginal rings or DMPA.

There has been concern at various times that prolonged oral contraception might cause permanent changes in the genital system. When high-dose products were in use, various studies showed condensation of the superficial cortical layers of the ovary (SEDA-8, 863). Severe atrophy of the endometrium after a period of oral contraception has been described (267), but the report usually quoted is one that dates from a period when high doses were in use, and the incidence is not known, since the endometrium is not usually examined. Certainly, the endometrium will go into a resting phase in women who have amenorrhea, but there is no reason to believe that it will become permanently unresponsive.

Epidemiological studies of the relation between oral contraceptive use and pelvic endometriosis have variously shown an increased risk, a reduced risk, and no effect (268). For example, an Italian study showed an increased risk among ever users of oral contraceptives, but this increase occurred only among former users, not current users (269). Furthermore, the authors noted that a similar pattern had been shown in several large cohort studies (OFPA, RCGP, and Walnut Creek). There was no association in the Italian study with recency, latency, or

duration of use, suggesting that any relation to oral contraceptive use is not a true biological relation but instead the result of selection and other biases.

Pelvic inflammatory disease, often resulting in infertility, ectopic pregnancy, or chronic pelvic pain, is a well-known pathological state that actually occurs at a somewhat lower incidence in oral contraceptive users and also tends to be less severe in these women compared with non-users (270–272). The biological mechanism for this protective effect may be the changes in cervical mucus or reduced menstrual bleeding (and thus reduced retrograde menstrual blood in the uterus). On the other hand, the relevant reviews have concluded that combined oral contraceptives provide no protection against lower reproductive tract infection (particularly cervical infections with *Chlamydia* or gonococcus) and may even have an adverse effect. This possible increased risk appears to be the result of an increase in the area of cervical ectropion associated with the estrogen in combined oral contraceptives. Candidiasis of the vagina in oral contraceptive users without evidence of diabetes mellitus has often been reported.

Immunologic

There is a sex difference in immune responsiveness, but little attention has been paid to the possible role played by sex hormones in its regulation. This lack of insight has led to the question of whether the use of oral contraceptives might affect the immune response, for better or for worse. An authoritative review of the immunological effects of estrogens and progestogens has concluded that, although understanding of any effect is incomplete, it is not likely that the low doses used in oral contraceptives would have negative effects on the immune system (273).

If that is the case, there must be another explanation for periodic reports that suggest an increased risk of systemic infections in oral contraceptive users. In a 1974 study by the British Royal College of General Practitioners oral contraceptive users had a higher than average incidence of certain infectious diseases (138).

Support for the concept that oral contraceptives might increase the risk of infection has been presented in other studies, and workers in the tropics have remarked that pregnant women appear to be unduly sensitive to malarial infestation (WHO, unpublished data).

The antibody response to tetanus toxoid in women is considerably lower in oral contraceptive users than in controls (274).

A depressed lymphocyte response to phytohemagglutinin has been observed in a series of women taking oral contraceptives (275); the reduction in phytohemagglutinin response reflects impaired T cell function, and this finding is of interest in view of the fact that a deficiency of T cell function is important in certain autoimmune diseases. Another consequence of prolonged impairment of T cell function would be an increased susceptibility to infectious diseases.

There have been several studies of the effect of sex hormones on serum immunoglobulin titers. In a study of the effect of four different oral contraceptives on the serum concentration of IgA, IgG, and IgM, the concentrations of all three immunoglobulins fell during the first course of treatment and returned to normal during subsequent cycles (276). There was some evidence that the steroid-induced reduction in immunoglobulins was predominantly caused by the estrogenic component. Subsequently, a study was conducted in which plasma from women currently taking combined oral contraceptives, past users of such products, women who had never used them, and non-users with a history of venous thrombosis was examined for the presence of immunoglobulin G (IgG) that showed specific binding of ethinylestradiol (277). There was no increase in "specific" IgG and no evidence of ethinylestradiol binding in oral contraceptive users compared with non-users. This study therefore provided no support for the hypothesis that a significant percentage of oral contraceptive users develop a specific IgG with high binding affinity for ethinylestradiol, which might be causally linked to the development of thrombotic phenomena in oral contraceptive users.

Numerous case reports have suggested that combined oral contraceptives can cause systemic lupus erythematosus (148,278). However, systematic examination of this issue in a 1994 case-control study showed no association (279).

Aggravation of bronchial asthma, eczema, rashes, angioedema, and vasomotor rhinitis have been incidentally observed, and cold urticaria has been reported in women taking oral contraceptives (280). It is not known whether in any particular individual the hypersensitivity reaction is due to the hormones themselves or to other ingredients in the tablet. Nasal provocation tests with suspensions of contraceptive steroids in patients with allergic rhinitis or pollinosis who had been taking these products showed a positive response in one-third of cases; the same patients also reacted to topical estrogens (281). Life-threatening anaphylaxis with a positive rechallenge test occurred in a young woman using oral contraceptives, but this must be extraordinarily rare (282).

According to anecdotal reports published over the years, recurrent angioedema has sometimes been associated with the use of oral contraceptives and hormone replacement therapy. In a recent study the supposed link was investigated (283). Of 516 women with recurrent angioedema, 228 (44%) had used oral contraceptives or hormone replacement therapy, and of this group 103 (45%) had urticaria-related angioedema, while 50 (22%) had idiopathic angioedema, 39 (17%) had hereditary angioedema type III, and 32 (14%) had hereditary angioedema type I. Oral contraceptives or hormone replacement therapy led to attacks of angioedema in 46 women (20%), including 20 (63%) of the women with hereditary angioedema type I, 24 (62%) of those with hereditary angioedema type III, and 2 (4%) of those with idiopathic angioedema. These 46 women included 26 in whom symptoms occurred for the first time after the use of these medications and 20 in whom pre-existing recurrent angioedema worsened considerably. However, it should be remembered that these conditions are not contraindications; many women with these diseases

tolerate these medications without any effects on their angioedema.

The immunological effects of two contraceptive combinations, namely Valette (ethinylestradiol 0.03 mg + dienogest 2.0 mg) and Lovelle (ethinylestradiol 0.02 mg + desogestrel 0.15 mg), have been examined during one treatment cycle (284). The latter significantly increased the numbers of lymphocytes, monocytes, and granulocytes. Valette reduced the CD4 lymphocyte count after 10 days and Lovelle did the opposite. Lovelle increased CD19 and CD23 cell counts after 21 days. Phagocytic activity was unaffected by either treatment. After 10 days, both contraceptives reduced the serum concentrations of IgA, IgG, and IgM, which remained low at day 21 with Lovelle but returned to baseline with Valette. Secretory IgA was unaffected by either contraceptive. Neither treatment affected concentrations of interleukins, except for a significant difference between the treatment groups in interleukin-6 after 10 days, which resolved after 21 days. Concentrations of non-immunoglobulin serum components fluctuated; macroglobulin was increased by Valette. However, total protein and albumin concentrations were reduced more by Lovelle than Valette. Complement factors also fluctuated. There was no evidence of sustained immunosuppression with either Valette or Lovelle.

Infection risk

Data on the risk of infection with HIV (human immunodeficiency virus) with combined oral contraceptives are sparse; some studies suggest an adverse effect and others show no association (270,285).

Body temperature

Body temperature tends to rise slightly in some users of oral contraceptives (286,287) Progesterone has a mild thermogenic effect, reflected in changes in body temperature during the normal menstrual cycle. Mild pyrexia in users of oral contraceptives may reflect this, but the patient should always be examined to exclude infection.

Long-Term Effects

Drug abuse

Children under 6 years who have accidentally ingested oral contraceptives have experienced nausea and vomiting for 10–15 hours after ingestion (SEDA-1, 306). Occasionally, apathy, drowsiness, and slight increases in transaminase activities have been reported.

Drug withdrawal

Although it was originally believed that women who stopped taking oral contraceptives, particularly after a long period of use, were more likely to have amenorrhea, careful analysis has shown that that is not the case. The likelihood of conception is reduced during the first 1–2 months after discontinuation, but cumulative conception rates after several months are not affected.

Tumorigenicity

The carcinogenic effects of oral contraceptives are covered in the monograph on estrogens.

Second-Generation Effects

Fertility

The return of fertility after a period of oral contraception has been differently assessed at different times. Although there can be a delay of 1–2 months in the return of fertility after withdrawal of a combined oral contraceptive, within a few months conception rates are similar to those of women who stop using non-hormonal contraception (42,288,289). In 48 patients classified as having amenorrhea after oral contraceptive use the subsequent conception rate was no lower than in a control group not with amenorrhea (290). There appears to be a shorter delay with low-dose than high-dose products (291). Delay in the return of ovulation has on occasion led to the erroneous conclusion that the first pregnancy after oral contraceptive use might be unduly prolonged (SEDA-6, 351).

There does not appear to be any clinically significant delay in return of fertility after discontinuation of progestogen-only contraceptives. Although there have been no large studies, data from several small studies suggest no effect. Furthermore, because progestogen-only contraceptives prevent ovulation in only about half of cycles, and because the pregnancy prevention effects fall rapidly if a tablet is taken late, the normal reproductive physiology presumably returns quickly after tablet discontinuation.

Pregnancy

The likelihood of ectopic pregnancy in women taking oral contraceptives has to be set against the normal incidence in the population, taking care to use the same denominator; one can express it as the proportion of women who experience such an event, or as the proportion of pregnancies that occur and prove to be ectopic (292). The proportion of pregnancies that implant at an extrauterine site is 0.005 for both combined oral contraceptive users and women using no contraception, but, because oral contraceptive users are much less likely to conceive, their rate of ectopic pregnancy is much lower (0.005 per 1000 woman years, compared with 2.6 per 1000 woman years for women using no contraception). The incidence of ectopic pregnancies is also somewhat lower for combined oral contraceptives than for other contraceptive methods. In the past there was some concern about a possible increased risk of ectopic gestation after withdrawal of oral contraceptives (293), but this is no longer considered to be an issue.

Up to 10% of pregnancies among users of progestogen-only contraceptives implant outside the uterus; this is not greatly different to the ectopic pregnancy rate in unprotected women, but it is much higher than among users of adequate combined oral contraception (292). The reasons may relate to changes in tubal motility and delay in ovum transport.

Teratogenicity

Oral contraceptives are neither teratogenic nor mutagenic, and there is little concern about the risk of congenital anomalies if an oral contraceptive is accidentally taken during an early unrecognized pregnancy. The American College of Obstetrics and Gynecology concluded in 1993 that there was no causal link (294). Reviews have come to the same conclusion (295,296), as has a meta-analysis completed in 1995 (297). In theory the androgenicity of a progestogen could result in virilization, but it is most unlikely to be taken sufficiently late or in sufficiently high doses to have this effect.

Gene toxicity

The fear that oral contraceptives might prove to induce chromosomal abnormalities was expressed when they were relatively new, but has largely been laid to rest. When aborted fetuses from women who used oral contraceptives were compared with those from non-users, there was no difference in the frequency of abnormal karyotypes or in sex ratio between the two groups. Certainly, data have been presented showing a slightly raised frequency of minor chromosomal changes in children whose mothers had been exposed to oral contraceptives before pregnancy, but from a genetic point of view, these scattered findings are not alarming.

Sex of the offspring

There was early minor evidence that the use of oral contraceptives might result in a predominance of female births (298). However, later evidence has been indecisive (299,300). If there is any effect at all it must be extremely small.

Congenital anomalies

A number of early American studies appeared to show that children exposed in utero to oral contraceptives ran a slightly increased risk of being born with certain types of birth defects; in particular a syndrome was described comprising multiple malformations involving the vertebrae, anus, cardiac structures, trachea, esophagus, renal structures and limbs (abbreviated to VACTERL) (301). The entire VACTERL syndrome was in fact seldom or never encountered; clusters of defects falling within this group were seen, but the associations were very variable. Furthermore, virilization of the female fetus and some of the other elements in the VACTERL group have been described after exposure to certain progestogens, hormonal pregnancy tests, or (rarely) to oral contraceptives taken in error in early pregnancy.

In a 1983 retrospective study of 155 children with congenital limb reductions 18 mothers (12%) were found to have taken oral contraceptives inadvertently during early pregnancy compared with only one mother in a control group, a relative risk of 24; adjustment for smoking hardly altered the figure (301). However, other work has suggested that smoking carries a higher risk of malformations than the use of oral contraceptives (SED-12, 1022) (302).

The results of such studies have led some reviewers to conclude that oral contraceptives are slightly teratogenic, but caution is needed. The conclusion of the 1980 WHO report cited above that such an effect is slight or absent probably remains valid for all widely used oral contraceptives; naturally, newer products might have other effects.

Congenital malformations may occur after the use of hormonal (estrogen + progestogen) pregnancy tests, now obsolete, since these high doses of a hormonal combination represented aggressive interference with any early pregnancy. A 1967 report suggested some association with meningomyelocele or hydrocephalus, and later retrospective studies provided some evidence of cardiac defects or limb reduction anomalies. Such studies always raise methodological doubts, but it is not unthinkable that these tests were harmful, since they sometimes induced bleeding even in early pregnancy; they could thus impair embryonic nutrition.

Lactation

The effects of combined oral contraceptives on lactation have been examined carefully (303,304), since estrogens are well-known inhibitors of ovulation in large doses. Even products containing 30 micrograms of ethinylestradiol reduce the volume of milk (305); the composition of the milk is also slightly altered, but again one has the impression that the effect is not important, except in a very poorly nourished population. Both progestogens and estrogens are excreted in the milk, their proportions correlating with those in plasma, but the absolute concentrations are lower. The plasma/milk ratio varies from compound to compound, probably owing to variations in the degree of protein binding and (for progestogens) also to the variable amount of fat in the milk. The amount of steroid transferred in 600 ml of milk is estimated at 0.1% or less of the daily dose taken. Although newborn infants might be relatively sensitive to these hormonal substances, because of the immaturity of their detoxification systems, no adverse effects have been found when they were looked for systematically; nevertheless, isolated cases of gynecomastia have been noted in babies when their mothers were taking oral contraceptives during lactation.

In an 8-year follow-up of Swedish children whose mothers used combined oral contraceptives while breast-feeding, there were no negative effects on health, growth, or development (306). It should be realized that the hormonal content of natural human milk and cows' milk is not negligible. If hormonal contraception is to be used during lactation, it would be sensible to prefer low-dose progestogens rather than combinations with estrogens; they are not the most effective contraceptives, but probably sufficient to supplement the contraceptive effect of lactation itself and they are unlikely to inhibit lactation.

There is much evidence that progestogen-only contraceptives (including tablets, injectables, and implants) have no adverse effects on milk production (307); they reach the milk in negligible amounts and have no adverse effects on the breast-fed infant (308).

Susceptibility Factors

There are no hard and fast rules about prescribing oral contraceptives in women at risk of complications; the degree of risk resulting from a particular factor has to be considered from case to case.

Absolute contraindications

Combined oral contraceptives should not be used by women with the following absolute contraindications:

1. thrombophlebitis or venous thromboembolic disorders (current or past)
2. cerebrovascular disease (current or past)
3. coronary artery or ischemic heart disease (current or past)
4. breast cancer (current or past)
5. endometrial cancer or other estrogen-dependent neoplasia (current or past)
6. hepatic adenoma or carcinoma (current or past)
7. impaired liver function (current)
8. less than 2 weeks postpartum
9. breastfeeding and less than 6 weeks postpartum
10. known or suspected pregnancy
11. use of enzyme-inducing drugs, specifically the antimicrobial drugs rifampicin and griseofulvin and many anticonvulsants.

Relative contraindications

Combined oral contraceptives should be used only with caution and careful monitoring by women with the following relative contraindications:

1. aged over 35 years and/or obese and/or currently smoking 15 or more cigarettes per day; when all three factors are present this can be regarded as an absolute contraindication
2. migraine, particularly with focal neurological symptoms
3. hypertension (current, controlled)
4. diabetes, particularly with retinopathy, neuropathy, or vascular disease
5. familial hyperlipidemia or current treatment for hyperlipidemia
6. gallbladder disease (current)
7. cholestatic jaundice of pregnancy or with prior oral contraceptive use
8. unexplained abnormal vaginal bleeding
9. breastfeeding, particularly if less than 6 months postpartum
10. major surgery, with prolonged immobility.

Although sickle cell disease is sometimes listed as a contraindication to oral contraceptive use, it has been suggested that this may not be justified (309). Women with sickle cell disease need highly effective contraception, because pregnancy is associated with increased morbidity and mortality to both mother and fetus, as well as the increased likelihood that the infant will have sickle cell disease. Theoretically, combined oral contraceptives should be given with caution, because of the increased risk of thrombosis associated with both sickle cell disease and combined oral contraceptives, but the limited available evidence indicates no change in hematological parameters among women using hormonal contraceptives. Progestogen-only formulations may be preferred, not only to avoid the potential risk of thrombosis but also because studies suggest that sickle cell crises may be inhibited.

The Oxford Family Planning Association's continuing study has shown convincingly that death from all causes is more than doubled in oral contraceptive users who smoke 15 or more cigarettes daily (310).

Drug Administration

Drug formulations

Low-dose oral contraceptives based on the older progestogens are relatively well tolerated in the short term, better so than the products that preceded them and those that came later. Two placebo-controlled studies with the combination of levonorgestrel 100 micrograms and ethinylestradiol in 704 patients over six cycles showed no differences in unwanted effects compared with placebo; in particular there was no evidence of weight gain (311).

After nearly 50 years, new variants on the theme of two-component oral contraceptives continue to appear in an attempt to improve tolerance. Especially when these involve the use of lower doses than hitherto, one may be skirting the limits of efficacy in the cause of safety. When assessing studies of these newer combinations it can therefore be relevant to consider the average body weight of participants. For example, in Thailand there were therapeutically excellent contraceptive results with a daily combination of drospirenone 3 mg and ethinylestradiol 30 micrograms compared with a combination of levonorgestrel 150 micrograms and ethinylestradiol 30 micrograms (312). The rates of spotting and breakthrough bleeding were low and not different between the two regimens. There were no pregnancies and no menorrhea in either group. The most common adverse events in both groups were nausea, headache, and breast tenderness. Drospirenone + ethinylestradiol had a more favorable effect on body weight and blood pressure: mean body weight and mean blood pressure remained lower than baseline mean. However, all of these findings have to be read in the light of the fact that the body weight of Thai women is substantially less than that of women in Europe or the USA, and that both the efficacy and adverse reaction pattern could differ between such populations.

Drug dosage regimens

Different schemes of administration have been studied and compared with one another without identifying any pattern of use that is ideal for all women. Various sequential programs of use, intended to mimic more closely the physiological changes in hormone secretion during the normal cycle rather than using a fixed combination throughout, have given better cycle control in some women, but others react better to the traditional pattern, in which the same combination is used throughout the 20-day period of use. The normophasic formulations use a popular sequential scheme; in these products the seven first tablets contain only estrogen and the next 14 tablets both estrogen and progestogen, giving an endometrium of a more normal secretory phase type; this in turn leads to more pronounced withdrawal bleeding. A further development of this principle, the triphasic type of product, involves administering a three-step regimen, in which the change from estrogenic to progestogenic dominance is more gradual; it appears to be helpful in avoiding excessive intermenstrual bleeding when this has been a problem, and it is apparently less likely than monophasic products to cause an unwanted reduction in HDL cholesterol (313). However, there is evidence that triphasic formulations based on norgestrel could carry the same increased risk of thromboembolic disorders as that seen with the third-generation oral contraceptives, because of a higher resistance to activated protein C than with the corresponding monophasic products (314).

In the "estrophasic" form of administration, ethinylestradiol 20 micrograms is given on days 1–5 of the cycle, 30 micrograms on days 6–12, and 35 micrograms on days 13–21. Norethisterone acetate 1 mg is also given throughout this period. The literature to date has not shown that this regimen, although claimed to be more "physiological" in its composition, is in fact better tolerated than a comparable combination in which ethinylestradiol is given in a dose of 30 micrograms throughout (315). However, the reduction in what may at some phases of the cycle be an unnecessarily high estrogen dose, that is more than is needed to maintain cycle control, is a healthy step, and it may be useful to have a further alternative product for women who do not find any existing formulation fully satisfactory.

There is continued interest in natural 17-β-estradiol in a form suitable for oral use, in view of the likelihood that it will produce fewer adverse effects than the synthetic estrogens used in most oral contraceptives. The particular problem has been to secure adequate cycle control with 17-β-estradiol, which is rapidly metabolized to estrone in the intestinal wall and liver; the degradation process is actually accelerated by progestogens. One approach under development in Germany involves combining this estrogen with dienogest, a progestogen that is reported to have no antiestrogenic activity (316). Preliminary work suggests that this can be successful, but one must be cautious in assuming that the end-product will be safer in all respects. There is evidence of a lesser effect of the natural estrogen on fibrinolysis, liver function, and lipid metabolism, but one must bear in mind that the true incidence of thromboembolic and other complications of the existing oral contraceptives is only now emerging after many years of worldwide use.

It has long been believed that a woman who intends to use oral contraception should wait for her next menstrual period before beginning the treatment, since by attuning the treatment to the existing cyclical rhythm the bleeding pattern will be more physiological. An alternative approach is to begin treatment immediately it is prescribed, whatever the menstrual phase. From recent randomized controlled work it now seems clear that either approach is acceptable; immediately starting treatment does not produce a less acceptable pattern of vaginal bleeding (317).

Drug–Drug Interactions

General

Two categories of drug interactions have been reported with oral contraceptives (318).

Interactions in which other drugs influence the effects of contraceptive steroids

The best known interactions are those in which another drug impairs the effect of the contraceptive steroids, leading to breakthrough bleeding and even pregnancy; such interactions are due primarily (but not exclusively) to enzyme induction, resulting in accelerated breakdown of the contraceptive steroids (319). This is a greater problem today than it was when higher-dose contraceptives with a larger reserve of contraceptive potency were in use. Many reported interactions of this type are single cases, and in some such instances it is likely that contraceptive failure was in fact due to poor adherence to therapy, diarrhea, or vomiting, rather than a direct interaction (320). However, with at least the enzyme-inducing anticonvulsants and rifampicin there are well-established major interactions.

In a few cases the activity of oral contraceptives is enhanced by other drugs; this is less likely to cause problems, but if the effect is very marked or prolonged one might suffer the consequences of hyperestrogenicity (320).

Interactions in which oral contraceptives interfere with the metabolism of other drugs

Studies in animals and in vitro studies in human liver microsomes have shown that oral contraceptives can inhibit the metabolism of other drugs that undergo various forms of oxidative metabolism. In contrast, oral contraceptives seem to induce glucuronidation. For example, oral contraceptives reduce the clearance of aminophenazone (aminopyrine) (321), phenazone (antipyrine) (322,323), and pethidine (324). It has been suggested that the estrogenic component of oral contraceptives is necessary for inhibition of drug oxidation, since women taking progestogens alone had a normal clearance of phenazone, whereas those taking a combination tablet had impaired elimination of phenazone (325). However, such interactions are rarely of clinical significance.

Alcohol

Women taking oral contraceptives have a significant fall in the absolute elimination rate of ethanol (105 mg/kg/hour) compared with controls (121 mg/kg/hour). The percentage elimination rate of ethanol is also significantly reduced in women taking oral contraceptives (0.015% per hour) compared with control subjects (0.019% per hour). These results are consistent during the three phases of the menstrual cycle and when body leanness is taken into consideration (326).

Antacids

Antacids apparently do not affect the systemic availability of oral contraceptives, but since magnesium-containing antacids can cause diarrhea, they might reduce absorption of contraceptive steroids.

Anticoagulants

Oral contraceptives have been reported to reduce the effect of anticoagulants, probably because oral contraceptives have an antagonistic effect on certain clotting factors, although they potentiate the action of acenocoumarol (SEDA-5, 371).

One study showed a significant increase in the clearance of phenprocoumon, owing to accelerated glucuronidation. As phenprocoumon is metabolized by hydroxylation as well as by direct glucuronidation, the increased clearance may mean that induction of the latter process over-rides inhibition of the former (327).

Antiepileptic drugs

Enzyme inducers

Failure of contraceptive therapy and breakthrough bleeding have been noted repeatedly in patients concurrently taking various enzyme-inducing anticonvulsant drugs (319,328). These include phenytoin, primidone, ethosuximide, phenobarbital, and carbamazepine. The specific isozyme responsible for metabolic 2-hydroxylation of ethinylestradiol is CYP3A4, which is induced by anticonvulsants (318). However, in addition to enzyme induction, the anticonvulsants can increase the binding of sex hormone- binding globulin. Since sex steroids bind with high affinity to sex hormone-binding globulin and since phenobarbital increases sex hormone-binding globulin capacity, unbound active steroid concentrations will tend to fall during treatment with phenobarbital (329). In addition, in animals, phenobarbital increases steroid metabolism in both the gut wall and liver (330).

The newer anticonvulsants have not been studied as intensively as the older drugs, but felbamate, oxcarbazepine, and topiramate have enzyme-inducing activity and reduce plasma steroid concentrations (331).

Non-enzyme inducers

Valproic acid, which is not an enzyme inducer, has no detectable effect on the pharmacokinetics of progestogens and estrogens (332).

The newer anticonvulsants have not been studied as intensively as the older drugs as regards the possibility of interference with the effects of oral contraceptives. The available data suggest that women taking oral contraceptives can also take gabapentin, lamotrigine, tiagabine, and vigabatrin without significant pharmacokinetic interactions; the effect of zonisamide is uncertain (327).

Management

The use of an alternative contraceptive method has long been advised in women taking antiepileptic drugs, unless they can be treated with the traditional high-dose oral products, for example containing 80–100 micrograms of estradiol (328); for effective protection they may also need a shortened tablet-free interval. A fair test is to see whether a woman taking oral contraceptives and anticonvulsants has adequate cycle control; if not, for example if there is mid-cycle spotting, this is a sign of interference and an alternative method will certainly be advisable.

Ascorbic acid

Ascorbic acid (vitamin C) is extensively sulfated in the gastrointestinal mucosa and competes with ethinylestradiol, which is also extensively sulfated. Plasma ethinylestradiol concentrations are increased by ascorbic acid in women, both after a single dose of ethinylestradiol and during long-term oral contraceptive use, but the results are not consistent. On one occasion it was claimed that this effectively transformed a low-dose oral contraceptive into a high-dose formulation (333). It seems very dubious whether ascorbic acid in fact interferes significantly with the effects of oral contraceptives.

Benzodiazepines

Oral contraceptives alter the metabolism of some benzodiazepines that undergo oxidation (chlordiazepoxide, alprazolam, diazepam) or nitroreduction (nitrazepam) (334). Oral contraceptives inhibit enzyme activity and reduce the clearances of these drugs. There is nevertheless no evidence that these interactions are of clinical importance. For other benzodiazepines that undergo oxidative metabolism, such as bromazepam and clotiazepam, no change has ever been found in oral contraceptive users.

Some other benzodiazepines are metabolized by glucuronic acid conjugation. Of these, the clearance of temazepam was increased when oral contraceptives were administered concomitantly, but the clearance of lorazepam and oxazepam was not (335). Again, it is unlikely that these are interactions of clinical importance.

Beta-blockers

Oral contraceptives increase the AUC and plasma concentrations of metoprolol, oxprenolol, and propranolol, but statistical significance is reached only with metoprolol. The changes are consistent with inhibition of hydroxylating enzymes, but are unlikely to be of clinical relevance (336).

Broad-spectrum antibiotics

There are sporadic, but well documented, reports of women using oral contraceptive steroids who became pregnant while taking a variety of antibiotics (337). However, there is much interindividual variation, which

may explain the fact that some studies have shown no interference between oral contraceptives and antibiotics. Current suspicion focuses primarily on the broad-spectrum antibiotics (338), including ampicillin and the tetracyclines. The purported mechanism is apparently not enzyme induction but interference with the enterohepatic circulation of ethinylestradiol. Ethinylestradiol can be conjugated with both sulfate and glucuronic acid; sulfation occurs primarily in the small intestinal mucosa, while glucuronidation occurs mainly in the liver. These conjugates are excreted in the bile and then reach the colon, where they may be hydrolysed by gut bacteria to liberate unchanged ethinylestradiol, which can be reabsorbed (318). Broad-spectrum antibiotics may suppress this bacterial effect, resulting in reduced plasma hormone concentrations. The antibiotics doxycycline (339) and tetracycline (256) have been shown to have no effect on serum concentrations of exogenous   estrogens and progestogens in women taking combined oral contraceptives containing ethinylestradiol 35 micrograms; however, in one of these studies endogenous progesterone was also assessed and there was no mid-cycle rise suggestive of ovulation.

Ciclosporin

Several case reports have suggested that the elimination of ciclosporin can be impaired by oral contraceptives, resulting in increased plasma ciclosporin concentrations. Ciclosporin undergoes hydroxylation and N-demethylation, in which cytochrome P450 is involved, so competitive enzyme inhibition probably explains the interaction. Dosages of ciclosporin should be reviewed carefully (340).

Clofibric acid

Oral contraceptives increase the plasma clearance of clofibric acid, which is mainly metabolized by glucuronidation (341,342).

Fluconazole

The effect of fluconazole 150 mg on circulating ethinylestradiol concentrations has been studied on day 6 of one of two cycles in women taking oral contraceptives (343). The serum concentrations of ethinylestradiol (C_{max} and AUC) were significantly increased by fluconazole, but t_{max} was not affected. These findings suggest that there is a potential for a clinically significant interaction between fluconazole and ethinylestradiol, by inhibition of estrogen metabolism.

Since oral contraceptive users sometimes need to be treated for vaginal candidiasis, the question arises which of the available treatments can be used without risk of impairing contraception. In a crossover placebo-controlled study, fluconazole 300 mg weekly for two cycles has been studied in 21 healthy women using Ortho-Novum 7/7/7 as a contraceptive (344). Fluconazole in this dose, which is twice that ordinarily recommended, produced small but statistically significant increases in the AUC_{0-24} for both ethinylestradiol (mean 24% increase) and norethindrone (mean 13%). The C_{max} of ethinylestradiol was slightly, but just significantly, higher with fluconazole than placebo. The C_{max} for norethindrone was not different between the two groups. There were no adverse events related to fluconazole. These changes are such that one should not anticipate any increased risk of contraceptive failure when fluconazole is given simultaneously.

Glucocorticoids

In standard reference works, oral contraceptives are commonly listed as increasing the circulating concentrations of glucocorticoids (82), but variable effects have been reported with different glucocorticoids.

In oral contraceptive users there is a 30–50% reduction in the clearance of prednisolone and a prolonged half-life (345). These alterations result from changes in both protein binding, which is increased, presumably owing to increased concentrations of glucocorticoid-binding globulin, and unbound drug clearance, which is reduced, presumably owing to inhibition of metabolism. It has therefore been suggested that lower doses of prednisolone should be used in oral contraceptive users.

In 40 healthy women oral contraceptives had a greater effect on prednisolone than on budesonide (45). In oral contraceptive users, the average plasma concentration of simultaneously administered prednisolone was 131% higher than in a control group, whereas the average plasma concentration of budesonide was only 22% higher. Mean plasma cortisol concentrations were suppressed by 90% and 82% with prednisolone and by 22% and 28% with budesonide in oral contraceptive users and controls, respectively. Ethinylestradiol plasma concentrations were not affected by either glucocorticoid. The authors concluded that the oral contraceptive made no difference to the plasma concentrations of budesonide or cortisol suppression after the administration of budesonide capsules. These findings suggest that oral budesonide can be used in the usual doses without problems in women using oral contraceptives.

Griseofulvin

Griseofulvin modifies hepatic enzyme activity in mice, and although there is no good evidence of a major enzyme-inducing effect in humans, several case reports of pregnancies in women taking both oral contraceptives and griseofulvin suggest an interaction; the authorities in several countries have warned that the contraceptive effect may be diminished (346).

Isotretinoin

Isotretinoin is a potent teratogen, and when it is prescribed it is vital to use one or more reliable contraceptive methods. It is therefore important to determine whether isotretinoin itself might interfere with the efficacy of hormonal contraception. In 26 women who were to be treated with isotretinoin and expected to use oral contraceptives, serum concentrations of the two components of Ortho Novum (ethinylestradiol and norethindrone) were used as markers for any direct kinetic effect of isotretinoin, while concentrations of serum progesterone, luteinizing hormone, and follicle-stimulating hormone were taken as indicators of hormonal effectiveness) (347). Adding isotretinoin to the oral contraceptive regimen resulted in small and inconsistent, but statistically significant, reductions in the concentrations of both ethinylestradiol (9% reduction in AUC) from time 0 to 24 hours after the dose on day 6) and norethindrone (11% reduction in C_{max} on day 20). Isotretinoin did not cause any statistically significant increases in pharmacodynamic markers. One woman in each study phase (one before and one during isotretinoin treatment) had a rise in progesterone consistent with possible ovulation. There were no serious or unexpected adverse events. These findings do not indicate any substantial ability of isotretinoin in therapeutic doses to render oral contraception less reliable, but the variability of the figures recorded underlines once more the need to use two contraceptive methods during isotretinoin treatment.

Methylxanthines

The clearances of both theophylline and caffeine are reduced in oral contraceptive users and half-lives are increased, probably because of inhibition of hepatic metabolism by cytochrome P450 (348). Caution in dosage is advisable.

Neuroleptic drugs

A single case of neuroleptic malignant syndrome has been described in a woman taking haloperidol and thioridazine, 12 hours after she started to take an oral contraceptive. The authors suggested that this could have been a pharmacodynamic interaction involving dopaminergic neurotransmission (349).

A kinetic study in which ziprasidone (40 mg/day) or placebo were co-administered with a second-generation oral contraceptive has provided evidence that ziprasidone is unlikely to interfere with oral contraception (350).

Omeprazole

Since hormonal contraceptives are potent inhibitors of some CYP isozymes, they can interfere with the metabolic breakdown of various drugs and thus potentiate their effects. The possibility that a contraceptive containing ethinylestradiol 40 micrograms + levonorgestrel 75 micrograms or levonorgestrel 60 micrograms only, given for 10 days, might interfere with the metabolism of omeprazole has been investigated (351). The progestogen alone did not cause any interaction but the combined product led to a 38% increase in the AUC of omeprazole, which is metabolized by CYP2C19, in all 10 subjects studied. There was no interference with the following stage of elimination, which is mediated by CYP3A4. The authors did not comment on the possible clinical consequences, but one would expect the degree of interaction to be sufficient to reduce the dose of omeprazole needed for an optimal effect.

Opioid analgesics

Increased glucuronidation may explain the fact that oral contraceptives enhance morphine clearance (352).

Paracetamol

Paracetamol might have a similar effect to ascorbic acid, that is competition with ethinylestradiol for sulfation capacity in the gut. Paracetamol significantly reduced the AUC of ethinylestradiol sulfate but had no effect on plasma levonorgestrel concentrations

In six healthy women, a single dose of paracetamol 1 g significantly increased the AUC of ethinylestradiol by 22% and reduced the AUC of ethinylestradiol sulfate (353). Plasma concentrations of levonorgestrel were unaltered. This interaction could be of clinical significance in women taking oral contraceptives who take paracetamol regularly or suddenly stop taking it, but it is doubtful whether it has any practical repercussions.

The clearance of paracetamol was 22% greater in men than women, entirely because of increased glucuronidation, there being no sex-related differences in the sulfation or oxidative metabolism of paracetamol (354). Paracetamol clearance in women using oral contraceptive steroids was 49% greater than in the control women. Glucuronidation and oxidative metabolism were both induced in contraceptive users (by 78% and 36% respectively) but sulfation was not altered. Although sex-related differences in paracetamol metabolism are unlikely to be of clinical importance, induction of paracetamol metabolism by oral contraceptive steroids may have clinical and toxicological consequences.

Rifamycins

Increased intermenstrual or breakthrough bleeding and pregnancy have been reported in women taking rifampicin in conjunction with contraceptive steroids (355). There is evidence that rifampicin increases the rate of metabolism of both the estrogenic and progestogenic components of oral contraceptives through hepatic microsomal enzyme induction (356) involving the same CYP isozyme as that induced by anticonvulsants, CYP3A. A four-fold increase in the rate of steroid metabolism has been shown; it is therefore unwise for women taking rifampicin to rely on steroid contraception and an alternative method should be used.

Roxithromycin

Roxithromycin does not interfere with the pharmacokinetics of oral contraceptives (357).

Salicylates

In a small study, the degree of erythrocyte aggregation during oral contraception was, at least in the short term, partly reversed by treatment with acetylsalicylic acid 100 mg/day (358).

Salicylic acid clearance is higher in users of oral contraceptives, owing to increases in the glycine and glucuronic acid conjugation pathways. In eight men, eight women, and eight women taking oral contraceptive steroids, the clearance of salicylic acid after an oral dose of aspirin 900 mg was 61% higher in the men than in the control women, largely because of increased activity of the glycine conjugation pathway (salicyluric acid formation) (359). Salicylic acid clearance was 41% higher in contraceptive users than in the control women, because of increases in both the glycine and glucuronic acid conjugation pathways. These data confirm the importance of hormonal factors in the regulation of drug conjugation reactions and suggest that sex-related differences in the disposition of salicylic acid and aspirin may be of clinical importance.

Tricyclic antidepressants

Oral contraceptives reduce the clearance of imipramine, probably by reducing hepatic oxidation, and thus increase its half-life. Hydroxylation of amitriptyline is inhibited by contraceptive steroids. The clinical significance is uncertain, but there is at least anecdotal evidence of an increase in antidepressant adverse effects (360). Caution should be exercised when tricyclic antidepressants are used long term in women taking oral contraceptives.

Troleandomycin

There have been several reports of hepatic cholestasis in women taking both troleandomycin and oral contraceptives (361). Oxidation of troleandomycin by CYP3A4 produces a derivative (probably a nitrosylated derivative) that binds tightly to the enzyme and thereby causes inactivation. This inhibition is highly selective for CYP3A4, and hepatic accumulation of ethinylestradiol is possible.

Smoking

The polycyclic hydrocarbons in cigarette smoke are potent inducers of certain cytochrome P450 isozymes. There is a marked increase in the 2-hydroxylation of natural estradiol in smokers, but not of ethinylestradiol, suggesting that the two estrogens are metabolized by different P450 enzymes. There is thus probably no pharmacokinetic interaction between smoking and oral contraceptives, but women taking oral contraception should be encouraged to avoid heavy smoking because of the risks to the cardiovascular system.

References

1. Hatcher RA, Trussell J, Stewart F, Stewart OK, Kowal D, Guest F, Cates W Jr, Policar MS. Contraceptive Technology. 16th rev ed.. New York: Irvington Publishers;. 1994.
2. McCann MF, Potter LS. Progestin-only oral contraception: a comprehensive review. Contraception 1994;50(6 Suppl 1):S1–S195.
3. Schramm G, Steffens D. Contraceptive efficacy and tolerability of chlormadinone acetate 2 mg/ethinylestradiol 0.03 mg (Belara): results of a post-marketing surveillance study Clin Drug Invest 2002;22:221–31.

4. Brown C, Ling F, Wan J. A new monophasic oral contraceptive containing drospirenone. Effect on premenstrual symptoms. J Reprod Med 2002;47(1):14–22.

5. Kacar S, Akdogan M, Kosar Y, Parlak E, Sasmaz N, Oguz P, Aydog G. Estrogen and cyproterone acetate combination-induced autoimmune hepatitis. J Clin Gastroenterol 2002;35(1):98–100.

6. Harlap S, Kost K, Forrest JD. Preventing Pregnancy, Protecting Health: a New Look at Birth Control Choices in the United StatesNew York: The Alan Guttmacher Institute;. 1991.

7. Colditz GA. Oral contraceptive use and mortality during 12 years of follow-up: the Nurses' Health Study. Ann Intern Med 1994;120(10):821–6.

8. Vessey MP, Villard-Mackintosh L, McPherson K, Yeates D. Mortality among oral contraceptive users: 20 year follow up of women in a cohort study. BMJ 1989;299(6714):1487–91.

9. Population Information Program. Update on Usage, Safety and Side EffectsBaltimore, MD: John Hopkins University;. 1979 Population Reports, Oral Contraceptives, Ser. A, No. 5.

10. DaVanzo J, Parnell AM, Foege WH. Health consequences of contraceptive use and reproductive patterns. Summary of a report from the US National Research Council. JAMA 1991;265(20):2692–6.

11. Szarewski A, Guillebaud J. Contraception. BMJ 1991;302(6787):1224–6.

12. Vessey MP, Doll R. Evaluation of existing techniques: is "the pill" safe enough to continue using? Proc R Soc Lond B Biol Sci 1976;195(1118):69–80.

13. A preliminary communication to the Medical Research Council by a Subcommittee. Risk of thromboembolic disease in women taking oral contraceptives. BMJ 1967;2(548):355–9.

14. Miwa LJ, Edmunds AL, Shaefer MS, Raynor SC. Idiopathic thromboembolism associated with triphasic oral contraceptives. DICP 1989;23(10):773–5.

15. Lamy AL, Roy PH, Morissette JJ, Cantin R. Intimal hyperplasia and thrombosis of the visceral arteries in a young woman: possible relation with oral contraceptives and smoking. Surgery 1988;103(6):706–10.

16. Scolding NJ, Gibby OM. Fatal pulmonary embolus in a patient treated with Marvelon. J R Coll Gen Pract 1988;38(317):568.

17. Porter JB, Hunter JR, Jick H, Stergachis A. Oral contraceptives and nonfatal vascular disease. Obstet Gynecol 1985;66(1):1–4.

18. Realini JP, Goldzieher JW. Oral contraceptives and cardiovascular disease: a critique of the epidemiologic studies. Am J Obstet Gynecol 1985;152(6 Pt 2):729–98.

19. Skouby SOCommittee Chairman. Consensus Development Meeting: Metabolic aspects of oral contraceptives of relevance for cardiovascular diseases. Am J Obstet Gynecol 1990;162:1335.

20. Lidegaard O. Thrombotic diseases in young women and the influence of oral contraceptives. Am J Obstet Gynecol 1998;179(3 Pt 2):S62–7.

21. Anonymous. Oral contraceptives containing gestodene or desogestrel-up-date: revised product information. WHO Pharm Newslett 1999;7/8:3.

22. Farmer RD, Lawrenson RA. Oral contraceptives and venous thromboembolic disease: the findings from database studies in the United Kingdom and Germany. Am J Obstet Gynecol 1998;179(3 Pt 2):S78–86.

23. Burnhill MS. The use of a large-scale surveillance system in Planned Parenthood Federation of America clinics to monitor cardiovascular events in users of combination oral contraceptives. Int J Fertil Womens Med 1999;44(1):19–30.

24. Jick SS, Myers MW, Jick H. Risk of idiopathic cerebral haemorrhage in women on oral contraceptives with differing progestagen components. Lancet 1999;354(9175): 302–303.

25. Seaman H, de Vries C, Farmer R. Venous thromboembolism associated with cyproterone acetate in combination with ethinyloestradiol (Dianette): observational studies using the UK General Practice Research Database. Pharmacoepidemiol Drug Saf 2004;13:427–36.

26. Schwingl PJ, Ory HW, King TDN. Modeled estimates of cardiovascular mortality risks in the US associated with low dose oral contraceptives. 1995 Unpublished draft.

27. Thorogood M, Mann J, Murphy M, Vessey M. Is oral contraceptive use still associated with an increased risk of fatal myocardial infarction? Report of a case-control study. Br J Obstet Gynaecol 1991;98(12):1245–53.

28. Rosenberg L, Palmer JR, Shapiro S. Use of lower dose oral contraceptives and risk of myocardial infarction. Circulation 1991;83:723.

29. Hannaford PC, Croft PR, Kay CR. Oral contraception and stroke. Evidence from the Royal College of General Practitioners' Oral Contraception Study. Stroke 1994;25(5):935–42.

30. Lidegaard O. Oral contraception and risk of a cerebral thromboembolic attack: results of a case-control study. BMJ 1993;306(6883):956–63.

31. Thorogood M, Mann J, Murphy M, Vessey M. Fatal stroke and use of oral contraceptives: findings from a case-control study. Am J Epidemiol 1992;136(1):35–45.

32. Thorogood M, Mann J, Murphy M, Vessey M. Risk factors for fatal venous thromboembolism in young women: a case-control study. Int J Epidemiol 1992;21(1):48–52.

33. Longstreth WT, Nelson LM, Koepsell TD, van Belle G. Subarachnoid hemorrhage and hormonal factors in women. A population-based case-control study. Ann Intern Med 1994;121(3):168–73.

34. Gerstman BB, Piper JM, Tomita DK, Ferguson WJ, Stadel BV, Lundin FE. Oral contraceptive estrogen dose and the risk of deep venous thromboembolic disease. Am J Epidemiol 1991;133(1):32–7.

35. Rosendaal FR, Helmerhorst FM, Vandenbroucke JP. Oral contraceptives, hormone replacement therapy and thrombosis. Thromb Haemost 2001;86(1):112–23.

36. Zreik TG, Odunsi K, Cass I, Olive DL, Sarrel P. A case of fatal pulmonary thromboembolism associated with the use of intravenous estrogen therapy. Fertil Steril 1999;71(2):373–5.

37. Chopard JL, Moulin T, Bourrin JC, et al. Contraception orale et accident vasculaire cérébral ischémique. Semin Hop (Paris) 1988;64:2075.

38. Lindberg MC. Hepatobiliary complications of oral contraceptives. J Gen Intern Med 1992;7(2):199–209.

39. Bohler J, Hauenstein KH, Hasler K, Schollmeyer P. Renal vein thrombosis in a dehydrated patient on an oral contraceptive agent. Nephrol Dial Transplant 1989;4(11):993–5.

40. Hassan HA. Oral contraceptive-induced mesenteric venous thrombosis with resultant intestinal ischemia. J Clin Gastroenterol 1999;29(1):90–5.

41. Hagglund H, Remberger M, Klaesson S, Lonnqvist B, Ljungman P, Ringden O. Norethisterone treatment, a major risk-factor for veno-occlusive disease in the liver after allogeneic bone marrow transplantation. Blood 1998;92(12):4568–72.

42. Grimes DA. The safety of oral contraceptives: epidemiologic insights from the first 30 years. Am J Obstet Gynecol 1992;166(6 Pt 2):1950–4.

43. Hirvonen E, Idanpaan-Heikkila J. Cardiovascular death among women under 40 years of age using low-estrogen oral contraceptives and intrauterine devices in Finland from 1975 to 1984. Am J Obstet Gynecol 1990;163(1 Pt 2):281–4.

44. Cirkel U, Schweppe KW. Fettstoffwechsel und orale Kontrazeptiva. Arztl Kosmetol 1985;15:253.

45. Fruzzetti F, Ricci C, Fioretti P. Haemostasis profile in smoking and nonsmoking women taking low-dose oral contraceptives. Contraception 1994;49(6):579–92.

46. Thorogood M, Villard-Mackintosh L. Combined oral contraceptives: risks and benefits. Br Med Bull 1993;49(1):124–39.

47. Machin SJ, Mackie IJ, Guillebaud J. Factor V Leiden mutation, venous thromboembolism and combined oral contraceptive usage. Br J Fam Planning 1995;21:13–4.

48. Rosenberg L, Palmer JR, Sands MI, Grimes D, Bergman U, Daling J, Mills A. Modern oral contraceptives and cardiovascular disease. Am J Obstet Gynecol 1997;177(3):707–15.

49. Vessey MP, Doll R, Fairbairn AS, Glober G. Postoperative thromboembolism and the use of oral contraceptives. BMJ 1970;3(715):123–6.

50. Greene GR, Sartwell PE. Oral contraceptive use in patients with thromboembolism following surgery, trauma, or infection. Am J Public Health 1972;62(5):680–5.

51. Whitehead EM, Whitehead MI. The pill, HRT and postoperative thromboembolism: cause for concern? Anaesthesia 1991;46(7):521–2.

52. Beller FK. Cardiovascular system: coagulation, thrombosis, and contraceptive steroids is there a link? In: Goldzieher JW, Fotherby K, editors. Pharmacology of the Contraceptive Steroids. New York: Raven Press, 1994:309.

53. Adachi T, Sakamoto S. Thromboembolism during hormone therapy in Japanese women. Sem Thromb Hemostas 2005;31:272–80.

54. Mant D, Villard-Mackintosh L, Vessey MP, Yeates D. Myocardial infarction and angina pectoris in young women. J Epidemiol Community Health 1987;41(3):215–9.

55. Frederiksen H, Ravenholt RT. Thromboembolism, oral contraceptives, and cigarettes. Public Health Rep 1970;85(3):197–205.

56. Rich-Edwards JW, Manson JE, Hennekens CH, Buring JE. The primary prevention of coronary heart disease in women. N Engl J Med 1995;332(26):1758–66.

57. Croft P, Hannaford PC. Risk factors for acute myocardial infarction in women: evidence from the Royal College of General Practitioners' oral contraception study. BMJ 1989;298(6667):165–8.

58. Jain AK. Cigarette smoking, use of oral contraceptives, and myocardial infarction. Am J Obstet Gynecol 1976;126(3):301–7.

59. Beral V. Mortality among oral-contraceptive users. Royal College of General Practitioners' Oral Contraception Study. Lancet 1977;2(8041):727–31.

60. Petitti DB, Wingerd J. Use of oral contraceptives, cigarette smoking, and risk of subarachnoid haemorrhage. Lancet 1978;2(8083):234–5.

61. Bruni V, Rosati D, Bucciantini S, Verni A, Abbate R, Pinto S, Costanzo G, Costanzo M. Platelet and coagulation functions during triphasic oestrogen–progestogen treatment. Contraception 1986;33(1):39–46.

62. Kjaeldgaard A, Larsson B. Long-term treatment with combined oral contraceptives and cigarette smoking associated with impaired activity of tissue plasminogen activator. Acta Obstet Gynecol Scand 1986;65(3):219–22.

63. Von Hugo R, Briel RC, Schindler AE. Wirkung oraler Kontrazeptiva auf die Blutgerinnung bei rauchenden und nichtrauchenden Probandinnen. Aktuel Endokrinol Stoffwechsel 1989;10:6.

64. Inman WH, Vessey MP. Investigation of deaths from pulmonary, coronary, and cerebral thrombosis and embolism in women of child-bearing age. BMJ 1968;2(599):193–9.

65. Arthes FG, Masi AT. Myocardial infarction in younger women. Associated clinical features and relationship to use of oral contraceptive drugs. Chest 1976;70(5):574–83.

66. Koenig W, Gehring J, Mathes P. Orale Kontrazeptiva und Myokardinfarkt bei jungen Frauen. Herz Kreisl 1984;16:508.

67. Zatti M. Contraccettivi orali: alterazioni delle variabili fisiologiche. C Ital Chim Clin 1983;8:249.

68. Leone A, Lopez M. Rôle du tabac et de la contraception orale dans l'infarctus du myocarde de la femme: description d'un cas. [Role of tobacco and oral contraception in myocardial infarction in the female. Description of a case.] Pathologica 1984;76(1044):493–8.

69. Gevers Leuven JA, Kluft C, Bertina RM, Hessel LW. Effects of two low-dose oral contraceptives on circulating components of the coagulation and fibrinolytic systems. J Lab Clin Med 1987;109(6):631–6.

70. Poller L. Oral contraceptives, blood clotting and thrombosis. Br Med Bull 1978;34(2):151–6.

71. Plowright C, Adam SA, Thorogood M, Beaumont V, Beaumont JL, Mann JI. Immunogenicity and the vascular risk of oral contraceptives. Br Heart J 1985;53(5):556–61.

72. Syner FN, Moghissi KS, Agronow SJ. Study on the presence of abnormal proteins in the serum of oral contraceptive users. Fertil Steril 1983;40(2):202–9.

73. Ernst E. Oral contraceptives, fibrinogen and cardiovascular risk. Atherosclerosis 1992;93(1–2):1–5.

74. Ylikorkala O, Puolakka J, Viinikka L. Oestrogen containing oral contraceptives decrease prostacyclin production. Lancet 1981;1(8210):42.

75. Gris JC, Jamin C, Benifla JL, Quere I, Madelenat P, Mares P. APC resistance and third-generation oral contraceptives: acquired resistance to activated protein C, oral contraceptives and the risk of thromboembolic disease. Hum Reprod 2001;16(1):3–8.

76. Marque V, Alhenc-Gelas M, Plu-Bureau G, Oger E, Scarabin PY. The effects of transdermal and oral estrogen/progesterone regimens on free and total protein S in postmenopausal women. Thromb Haemost 2001;86(2):713–4.

77. Rosing J, Middeldorp S, Curvers J, Christella M, Thomassen LG, Nicolaes GA, Meijers JC, Bouma BN, Buller HR, Prins MH, Tans G. Low-dose oral contraceptives and acquired resistance to activated protein C: a randomised cross-over study. Lancet 1999;354(9195):2036–40.

78. Porter JB, Hunter JR, Danielson DA, Jick H, Stergachis A. Oral contraceptives and nonfatal vascular disease—recent experience. Obstet Gynecol 1982;59(3):299–302.

79. Bailar JC 3rd, Byar DP. Estrogen treatment for cancer of the prostate. Early results with 3 doses of diethylstilbestrol and placebo. Cancer 1970;26(2):257–61.

80. Badaracco MA, Vessey MP. Recurrence of venous thromboembolic disease and use of oral contraceptives. BMJ 1974;1(901):215–7.

81. Jick H, Dinan B, Herman R, Rothman KJ. Myocardial infarction and other vascular diseases in young women. Role of estrogens and other factors. JAMA 1978;240(23):2548–52.

82. Stadel BV. Oral contraceptives and cardiovascular disease (first of two parts). N Engl J Med 1981;305(11):612–8.

83. Bottiger LE, Boman G, Eklund G, Westerholm B. Oral contraceptives and thromboembolic disease: effects of lowering oestrogen content. Lancet 1980;1(8178):1097–101.

84. Hedenmalm K, Samuelsson E, Spigset O. Pulmonary embolism associated with combined oral contraceptives: reporting incidences and potential risk factors for a fatal outcome. Acta Obstet Gynecol Scand 2004;83:576–85.

85. Jung-Hoffmann C, Kuhl H. Interaction with the pharmacokinetics of ethinylestradiol and progestogens contained in oral contraceptives. Contraception 1989;40(3):299–312.

86. Guengerich FP. Mechanism-based inactivation of human liver microsomal cytochrome P-450 IIIA4 by gestodene. Chem Res Toxicol 1990;3(4):363–71.

87. Rosing J, Tans G, Nicolaes GA, Thomassen MC, van Oerle R, van der Ploeg PM, Heijnen P, Hamulyak K, Hemker HC. Oral contraceptives and venous thrombosis: different sensitivities to activated protein C in women using second- and third-generation oral contraceptives. Br J Haematol 1997;97(1):233–8.

88. Mellemkjaer L, Sorensen HT, Dreyer L, Olsen J, Olsen JH. Admission for and mortality from primary venous thromboembolism in women of fertile age in Denmark, 1977–95. BMJ 1999;319(7213):820–1.

89. Vandenbroucke JP, Bloemenkamp KW, Helmerhorst FM, Rosendaal FR. Mortality from venous thromboembolism and myocardial infarction in young women in the Netherlands. Lancet 1996;348(9024):401–2.

90. Herings RM, Urquhart J, Leufkens HG. Venous thromboembolism among new users of different oral contraceptives. Lancet 1999;354(9173):127–8.

91. Hannaford PC, Kay CR. The risk of serious illness among oral contraceptive users: evidence from the RCGP's oral contraceptive study. Br J Gen Pract 1998;48(435):1657–62.

92. Bruni V, Croxatto H, De La Cruz J, Dhont M, Durlot F, Fernandes MT, Andrade RP, Weisberg E, Rhoa MGestodene Study Group. A comparison of cycle control and effect on well-being of monophasic gestodene-, triphasic gestodene- and monophasic desogestrel-containing oral contraceptives. Gynecol Endocrinol 2000;14(2):90–8.

93. Marks LV. Sexual chemistry. In: A history of the contraceptive pill. New Haven: Yale University Press, 2001:138–57.

94. Sartwell PE, et al. Oral contraceptives and relative risk of death from venous and pulmonary thromboembolism in the United States; an epidemiologic case-control study. Am J Epidemiol 1969;90:365.

95. Royal College of General Practitioners. Oral contraception and thrombo-embolic disease. J R Coll Gen Pract 1967;13(3):267–79.

96. Vessey MP, Doll R. Investigation of relation between use of oral contraceptives and thromboembolic disease. BMJ 1968;2(599):199–205.

97. Vessey MP, Doll R. Investigation of relation between use of oral contraceptives and thromboembolic disease. A further report. BMJ 1969;2(658):651–7.

98. Creatsas G, Koliopoulos C, Mastorakos G. Combined oral contraceptive treatment of adolescent girls with polycystic ovary syndrome. Lipid profile. Ann NY Acad Sci 2000;900:245–52.

99. Jick H, Kaye JA, Vasilakis-Scaramozza C, Jick SS. Risk of venous thromboembolism among users of third generation oral contraceptives compared with users of oral contraceptives with levonorgestrel before and after 1995: cohort and case-control analysis. BMJ 2000;321(7270):1190–5.

100. Bloemenkamp KW, Rosendaal FR, Helmerhorst FM, Buller HR, Vandenbroucke JP. Enhancement by factor V Leiden mutation of risk of deep-vein thrombosis associated with oral contraceptives containing a third-generation progestagen. Lancet 1995;346(8990):1593–6.

101. Kemmeren JM, Algra A, Grobbee DE. Third generation oral contraceptives and risk of venous thrombosis: meta-analysis. BMJ 2001;323(7305):131–4.

102. Bonnar J, Daly L, Carroll E. Blood coagulation with a combination pill containing gestodene and ethinyl estradiol. Int J Fertil 1987;32(Suppl):21–8.

103. Nicolaes GA, Thomassen MC, Tans G, Rosing J, Hemker HC. Effect of activated protein C on thrombin generation and on the thrombin potential in plasma of normal and APC-resistant individuals. Blood Coagul Fibrinolysis 1997;8(1):28–38.

104. Meijers JC, Middeldorp S, Tekelenburg W, van den Ende AE, Tans G, Prins MH, Rosing J, Buller HR, Bouma BN. Increased fibrinolytic activity during use of oral contraceptives is counteracted by an enhanced factor XI-independent down regulation of fibrinolysis: a randomized cross-over study of two low-dose oral contraceptives. Thromb Haemost 2000;84(1):9–14.

105. High Court. XYZ and others (Claimants) versus (1) Schering Health Care Limited, (2) Organon Laboratories Limited and (3) John Wyeth & Brother Limited. Judgement by the Hon. Mr Justice Mackay. London, 29 July 2002. Case No: 0002638. Neutral Citation No: (2002) EWHC 1420 (QB).

106. Biller J, Haberland C, Toffol GJ, O'Reilly D, Tentler RL. Basilar artery occlusion in an adolescent girl: a risk of oral contraceptives? J Child Neurol 1986;1(4):347–50.

107. Iuliano G, Di Domenico G, Masullo C, et al. Terapia contracettiva trifasica et ictus cerebri. Riv Neurobiol 1985;85:231.

108. Sanchez-Guerra M, Valle N, Blanco LA, Combarros O, Pascual J. Brain infarction after postcoital contraception in a migraine patient. J Neurol 2002;249(6):774.

109. Lalive d'Epinai SP, Trub P. Retinale vaskuläre Komplikationen bei oralen Kontrazeptiva. Klin Mbl Augenheilkd 1986;188:394.

110. Bradley JR, Reynolds J, Williams PF, Appleton DS. Encephalopathy in renovascular hypertension associated with the use of oral contraceptives. Postgrad Med J 1986;62(733):1031–3.

111. Landau E, Lessing JB, Weintraub M, Michowitz M. Acute myocardial infarction in a young woman taking oral contraceptives. A case report. J Reprod Med 1986;31(10):1008–10.

112. Janion M, Wojtacha P, Wozakowska-Kaplon B, Kurzawski J, Klank-Szafran M, Ciuraszkiewicz K. Myocardial infarction in a female patient using oral contraceptives—a case report. Kardiol Pol 2002;56:75–8.

113. Schneiderman DJ, Cello JP. Intestinal ischemia and infarction associated with oral contraceptives. West J Med 1986;145(3):350–5.

114. Jick H, Jick SS, Gurewich V, Myers MW, Vasilakis C. Risk of idiopathic cardiovascular death and nonfatal venous

thromboembolism in women using oral contraceptives with differing progestagen components. Lancet 1995;346(8990):1589–93.

115. Fotherby K. Oral contraceptives and lipids. BMJ 1989;298(6680):1049–50.

116. Burch JC, Byrd BF Jr, Vaughn WK. The effects of long-term estrogen on hysterectomized women. Am J Obstet Gynecol 1974;118(6):778–82.

117. Gordon T, Kannel WB, Hjortland MC, McNamara PM. Menopause and coronary heart disease. The Framingham Study. Ann Intern Med 1978;89(2):157–61.

118. Hammond CB, Jelovsek FR, Lee KL, Creasman WT, Parker RT. Effects of long-term estrogen replacement therapy. I. Metabolic effects. Am J Obstet Gynecol 1979;133(5):525–36.

119. Godsland IF, Crook D. Update on the metabolic effects of steroidal contraceptives and their relationship to cardiovascular disease risk. Am J Obstet Gynecol 1994;170(5 Pt 2):1528–36.

120. Collins P, Rosano GM, Jiang C, Lindsay D, Sarrel PM, Poole-Wilson PA. Cardiovascular protection by oestrogen—a calcium antagonist effect? Lancet 1993;341(8855):1264–5.

121. Williams JK, Adams MR, Herrington DM, Clarkson TB. Short-term administration of estrogen and vascular responses of atherosclerotic coronary arteries. J Am Coll Cardiol 1992;20(2):452–7.

122. Detering K, Kallischnig G. The cardiovascular risk of oral contraception with special reference to German mortality statistics. New Trends Gynecol Obstet 1985;1:360.

123. Lidegaard O, Edstrom B, Kreiner S. Oral contraceptives and venous thromboembolism: a five-year national case-control study. Contraception 2002;65(3):187–96.

124. Lidegaard O, Kreiner S. Contraceptives and cerebral thrombosis: a five-year national case-control study. Contraception 2002;65(3):197–205.

125. Lidegaard O. Smoking and use of oral contraceptives: impact on thrombotic diseases. Am J Obstet Gynecol 1999;180(6 Pt 2):S357–63.

126. Sass AE, Neufeld EJ. Risk factors for thromboembolism in teens: when should I test? Curr Opin Pediatr 2002;14(4):370–8.

127. Skjeldestad FE. Pillesal, fødslar og svangerskapsavbrøt før og etter "Marvelon saken". [Sale of oral contraceptives, births and abortions prior to and after the "Marvelon issue".] Tidsskr Nor Laegeforen 2000;120(3):339–44.

128. Collaborative Group for the Study of Stroke in Young Women. Oral contraception and increased risk of cerebral ischemia or thrombosis. N Engl J Med 1973;288(17):871–8.

129. Inman WH. Oral contraceptives and fatal subarachnoid haemorrhage. BMJ 1979;2(6203):1468–70.

130. Helmrich SP, Rosenberg L, Kaufman DW, Strom B, Shapiro S. Venous thromboembolism in relation to oral contraceptive use. Obstet Gynecol 1987;69(1):91–5.

131. Stampfer MJ, Willett WC, Colditz GA, Speizer FE, Hennekens CH. Past use of oral contraceptives and cardiovascular disease: a meta-analysis in the context of the Nurses' Health Study. Am J Obstet Gynecol 1990;163(1 Pt 2):285–91.

132. WHO Special Programme of Research, Development and Research Training in Human Reproduction. The WHO multicentre trial of the vasopressor effects of combined oral contraceptives: 1. Comparisons with IUD. Task Force on Oral Contraceptives. Contraception 1989;40(2):129–45.

133. WHO Special Programme of Research, Development and Research Training in Human Reproduction. The WHO multicentre trial of the vasopressor effects of combined oral contraceptives: 2. Lack of effect of estrogen. Task Force on Oral Contraceptives. Contraception 1989;40(2):147–56.

134. Woods JW. Oral contraceptives and hypertension. Hypertension 1988;11(3 Pt 2):11–5.

135. Connell EB. Oral contraceptives. The current risk-benefit ratio. J Reprod Med 1984;29(Suppl 7):513–23.

136. Pritchard JA, Pritchard SA. Blood pressure response to estrogen–progestin oral contraceptive after pregnancy-induced hypertension. Am J Obstet Gynecol 1977;129(7):733–9.

137. Lehtovirta P, Ranta T, Seppala M. Elevated prolactin levels in oral contraceptive pill-related hypertension. Fertil Steril 1981;35(4):403–5.

138. Royal College of General Practitioners' Oral Contraception Study. Effect on hypertension and benign breast disease of progestagen component in combined oral contraceptives. Lancet 1977;1(8012):624.

139. Kaul L, Curry CL, Ahluwalia BS. Blood levels of ethynylestradiol, caffeine, aldosterone and desoxycorticosterone in hypertensive oral contraceptive users. Contraception 1981;23(6):643–51.

140. Goldzieher JW, Moses LE, Averkin E, Scheel C, Taber BZ. A placebo-controlled double-blind crossover investigation of the side effects attributed to oral contraceptives. Fertil Steril 1971;22(9):609–23.

141. Mattson RH, Rebar RW. Contraceptive methods for women with neurologic disorders. Am J Obstet Gynecol 1993;168(6 Pt 2):2027–32.

142. Loder EW, Buse DC, Golub JR. Headache as a side effect of combination estrogen-progestin oral contraceptives: a systematic review. Am J Obstet Gynecol 2005;193:636–49.

143. Lobo RA, Gibbons WE. The role of progestin therapy in breast disease and central nervous system function. J Reprod Med 1982;27(Suppl 8):515–21.

144. Asherson RA, Harris NE, Gharavi AE, Hughes GR. Systemic lupus erythematosus, antiphospholipid antibodies, chorea, and oral contraceptives. Arthritis Rheum 1986;29(12):1535–6.

145. Leys D, Destee A, Petit H, Warot P. Chorea associated with oral contraception. J Neurol 1987;235(1):46–8.

146. Buge A, Vincent D, Rancurel G, Cheron F. Hémichorée et contraceptifs oraux. [Hemichorea and oral contraceptives.] Rev Neurol (Paris) 1985;141(10):663–5.

147. Driesen JJ, Wolters EC. Oral contraceptive induced paraballism. Clin Neurol Neurosurg 1987;89(1):49–51.

148. Mathur AK, Gatter RA. Chorea as the initial presentation of oral contraceptive induced systemic lupus erythematosus. J Rheumatol 1988;15(6):1042–3.

149. Miranda M, Cardoso F, Giovannoni G, Church A. Oral contraceptive induced chorea: another condition associated with anti-basal ganglia antibodies. J Neurol Neurosurg Psychiatry 2004;75:327–8.

150. Peleg R. Abdominal wall pain caused by cutaneous nerve entrapment in an adolescent girl taking oral contraceptive pills. J Adolesc Health 1999;24(1):45–7.

151. Villard-Mackintosh L, Vessey MP. Oral contraceptives and reproductive factors in multiple sclerosis incidence. Contraception 1993;47(2):161–8.

152. Soni PS. Effects of oral contraceptive steroids on the thickness of human cornea. Am J Optom Physiol Opt 1980;57(11):825–34.

153. De Vries Reilingh A, Reiners H, Van Bijsterveld OP. Contact lens tolerance and oral contraceptives. Ann Ophthalmol 1978;10(7):947–52.

154. Byrne E. Retinal migraine and the pill. Med J Aust 1979;2(12):659–60.

155. Jorge A, Schwartzman Y. Efectos de los anticonceptivos sobre la otosclerosis. Rev Bras Oto-Rino-Laringol 1975;41:46.

156. Loveland DB. Auditory levels according to use of oral contraceptives in 5449 women. J Am Aud Soc 1975;1:28.

157. Zanker K, Kessler L. Innenohrstörung durch orale hormonale Kontrazeptive? Z Klin Med 1985;40:1897.

158. Calanchini C. Die Auslösung eines Zwangssyndroms durch Ovulationshemmer. [Development of a compulsive syndrome by ovulation inhibitors.] Schweiz Arch Neurol Psychiatr 1986;137(4):25–31.

159. Van Winter JT, Miller KA. Breakthrough bleeding in a bulimic adolescent receiving oral contraceptives. Pediat Adolesc Gynecol 1986;4:39.

160. Chang AM, Chick P, Milburn S. Mood changes as reported by women taking the oral contraceptive pill. Aust NZ J Obstet Gynaecol 1982;22(2):78–83.

161. Fleming O, Seager CP. Incidence of depressive symptoms in users of the oral contraceptive. Br J Psychiatry 1978;132:431–40.

162. Jacobs AJ, Odom MJ, Word RA, Carr BR. Effect of oral contraceptives on adrenocorticotropin and growth hormone secretion following CRH and GHRH administration. Contraception 1989;40(6):691–9.

163. Walden CE, Knopp RH, Johnson JL, Heiss G, Wahl PW, Hoover JJ. Effect of estrogen/progestin potency on clinical chemistry measures. The Lipid Research Clinics Program Prevalence Study. Am J Epidemiol 1986;123(3):517–31.

164. Barsivala V, Virkar K. Thyroid functions of women taking oral contraceptives. Contraception 1974;9(3):305–14.

165. WHO Task Force on Oral Contraceptives. Oral and injectable hormonal contraceptive and signs and symptoms of vitamin deficiency and goitre: prevalence studies in five centres in the developing and developed world. WHO Bull. 1983.

166. Ball MJ, Ashwell E, Gillmer MD. Progestagen-only oral contraceptives: comparison of the metabolic effects of levonorgestrel and norethisterone. Contraception 1991;44(3):223–33.

167. Ramamoorthy R, Saraswathi TP, Kanaka TS. Carbohydrate metabolic studies during twelve months of treatment with a low-dose combination oral contraceptive. Contraception 1989;40(5):563–9.

168. Simon D, Senan C, Garnier P, Saint-Paul M, Garat E, Thibult N, Papoz L. Effects of oral contraceptives on carbohydrate and lipid metabolisms in a healthy population: the Telecom study. Am J Obstet Gynecol 1990;163(1 Pt 2):382–7.

169. Spellacy WN. Carbohydrate metabolism during treatment with estrogen, progestogen, and low-dose oral contraceptives. Am J Obstet Gynecol 1982;142(6 Pt 2):732–4.

170. Elkind-Hirsch K, Goldzieher JW. Metabolism: carbohydrate metabolism. In: Goldzieher JW, Fotherby K, editors. Pharmacology of the Contraceptive Steroids. New York: Raven Press, 1994:345.

171. Wingrave SJ, Kay CR, Vessey MP. Oral contraceptives and diabetes mellitus. BMJ 1979;1(6155):23.

172. Hannaford PC, Kay CR. Oral contraceptives and diabetes mellitus. BMJ 1989;299(6711):1315–6.

173. World Health Organization. Oral Contraceptives: Technical and Safety Aspects. WHO Offset Publications, 64Geneva: World Health Organization;. 1982.

174. Gaspard U. Contraception orale, métabolisme glucidique et critères de surveillance. [Oral contraception, glucid metabolism and monitoring criteria.] Contracept Fertil Sex (Paris) 1988;16(2):113–8.

175. Speroff L, Darney PD. A Clinical Guide for ContraceptionBaltimore, Maryland: Williams & Wilkins;. 1992.

176. Garg SK, Chase HP, Marshall G, Hoops SL, Holmes DL, Jackson WE. Oral contraceptives and renal and retinal complications in young women with insulin-dependent diabetes mellitus. JAMA 1994;271(14):1099–102.

177. Amatayakul K. Metabolism: vitamins and trace elements. In: Goldzieher JW, Fotherby K, editors. Pharmacology of the Contraceptive Steroids. New York: Raven Press, 1994:363.

178. Malnick SD, Halperin M, Geltner D. Hypercarotenemia associated with an oral contraceptive. DICP 1989;23(10):811.

179. Rose DP. The influence of oestrogens on tryptophan metabolism in man. Clin Sci 1966;31(2):265–72.

180. Price SA, Toseland PA. Oral contraceptives and depression. Lancet 1969;2(7612):158–9.

181. Anonymous. Depression and oral contraceptives: the role of pyridoxine. Drug Ther Bull 1978;16(22):86–7.

182. Kornberg A, Segal R, Theitler J, Yona R, Kaufman S. Folic acid deficiency, megaloblastic anemia and peripheral polyneuropathy due to oral contraceptives. Isr J Med Sci 1989;25(3):142–5.

183. Rivers JM. Oral contraceptives and ascorbic acid. Am J Clin Nutr 1975;28(5):550–4.

184. Weininger J, King JC. Effect of oral contraceptives on ascorbic acid status of young women consuming a constant diet. Nutr Rep Int 1977;15(3):255–64.

185. Harris SS, Dawson-Hughes B. The association of oral contraceptive use with plasma 25-hydroxyvitamin D levels. J Am Coll Nutr 1998;17(3):282–4.

186. Schreurs WH, van Rijn HJ, van den Berg H. Serum 25-hydroxycholecalciferol levels in women using oral contraceptives. Contraception 1981;23(4):399–406.

187. Gray TK, McAdoo T, Hatley L, Lester GE, Thierry M. Fluctuation of serum concentration of 1,25-dihydroxyvitamin D3 during the menstrual cycle. Am J Obstet Gynecol 1982;144(8):880–4.

188. Goulding A, McChesney R. Diminished urinary calcium excretion by women using oral contraceptives. Aust NZ J Med 1976;6:251.

189. Recker RR, Saville PD, Heaney RP. Effect of estrogens and calcium carbonate on bone loss in postmenopausal women. Ann Intern Med 1977;87(6):649–55.

190. Darzenta NC, Giunta JL. Radiographic changes of the mandible related to oral contraceptives. Oral Surg Oral Med Oral Pathol 1977;43(3):478–81.

191. Prasad AS, Oberleas D, Moghissi KS, Lei KY, Stryker JC. Effect of oral contraceptive agents on nutrients: I. Minerals. Am J Clin Nutr 1975;28(4):377–84.

192. Amatayakul K. Metabolism: vitamins and trace elements. In: Goldzieher JW, Fotherby K, editors. Pharmacology of the Contraceptive Steroids. New York: Raven Press, 1994:23–124.

193. Larsson G, Milsom I, Lindstedt G, Rybo G. The influence of a low-dose combined oral contraceptive on menstrual blood loss and iron status. Contraception 1992;46(4):327–334.

194. Mardell M, Zilva JF. Effect of oral contraceptives on the variations in serum-iron during the menstrual cycle. Lancet 1967;2(7530):1323–5.

195. Lucis OJ, Lucis R. Oral contraceptives and endocrine changes. Bull World Health Organ 1972;46(4):443–50.
196. Rahman HA, et al. A report on the effect of oral contraceptives on blood picture, serum iron and TIBC in twenty cases of healthy Egyptian women. Bull Alexandr Fac Med 1982;.
197. Kendall AG, Charlow GF. Red cell pyruvate kinase deficiency: adverse effect of oral contraceptives. Acta Haematol 1977;57(2):116–20.
198. Winkler UH. Effects on hemostatic variables of desogestrel- and gestodene-containing oral contraceptives in comparison with levonorgestrel-containing oral contraceptives: a review. Am J Obstet Gynecol 1998;179(3 Pt 2):S51–61.
199. Bloemenkamp KWM, Helmerhorst FM, Rosendaal FR, Vandenbroucke JP. Thrombophilias and gynaecology. Best Pract Res Clin Obstet Gynaecol 2003;17:509–28.
200. Zahn CM, Gonzalez DI Jr, Suto C, Kennedy S, Hines JF. Low-dose oral contraceptive effects on thromboelastogram criteria and relationship to hypercoagulability. Am J Obstet Gynecol 2003;189:43–7.
201. Zachariasen RD. Ovarian hormones and gingivitis. J Dent Hyg 1991;65(3):146–50.
202. Magnusson I, Ericson T, Hugoson A. The effect of oral contraceptives on the concentration of some salivary substances in women. Arch Oral Biol 1975;20(2):119–26.
203. Mussalli NG, Hopps RM, Johnson NW. Oral pyogenic granuloma as a complication of pregnancy and the use of hormonal contraceptives. Int J Gynaecol Obstet 1976;14(2):187–91.
204. Delaunay P, Commissionat Y. Contraception orale et muqueuse buccale. [Oral contraception and oral mucosa.] Actual Odontostomatol (Paris) 1980;34(129):149–56.
205. Boyko EJ, Theis MK, Vaughan TL, Nicol-Blades B. Increased risk of inflammatory bowel disease associated with oral contraceptive use. Am J Epidemiol 1994;140(3):268–78.
206. Sandler RS, Wurzelmann JI, Lyles CM. Oral contraceptive use and the risk of inflammatory bowel disease. Epidemiology 1992;3(4):374–8.
207. Deana DG, Dean PJ. Reversible ischemic colitis in young women. Association with oral contraceptive use. Am J Surg Pathol 1995;19(4):454–62.
208. Hargreaves T. Oral contraceptives and liver function. J Clin Pathol 1970;23(Suppl):3.
209. Stoll BA, Andrews JT, Mofferam R. Liver damage from oral contraceptives. BMJ 1966;1:960.
210. Larsson-Cohn U, Stenram U. Liver ultrastructure and function in icteric and non-icteric women using oral contraceptive agents. Acta Med Scand 1967;181(3):257–64.
211. Perez V, Gorodisch S, De Martire J, Nicholson R, Di Paola G. Oral contraceptives: long-term use produces fine structural changes in liver mitochondria. Science 1969;165:1805.
212. WHO Scientific Group. Oral contraceptives and neoplasia. World Health Organ Tech Rep Ser 1992;817:1–46.
213. Westerholm B. Oral contraceptives and jaundice: Swedish experience. In: Baker SB de C, Tripot J, editors. Proceedings, European Society for the Study of Drug Toxicity, Oxford, 1968. Amsterdam: Excerpta Medica, 1968:158–63.
214. Ockner RK, Davidson CS. Hepatic effects of oral contraceptives. N Engl J Med 1967;276(6):331–4.
215. Briggs MH, Briggs M. Metabolic effects of hormonal contraceptives. In: Chang CF, Griffin D, Woolman A, editors. Recent Advances in Fertility Regulation 81 1980:83–111 Beijing.

216. Dalen E, Westerholm B. Occurrence of hepatic impairment in women jaundiced by oral contraceptives and in their mothers and sisters. Acta Med Scand 1974;195(6):459–63.
217. Adlercreutz H, Tenhunen R. Some aspects of the interaction between natural and synthetic female sex hormones and the liver. Am J Med 1970;49:630–48.
218. Brown JB, Blair HAF. Urinary oestrogen metabolites of 17-norethisterone and esters. Proc R Soc Med 1960;53:433.
219. van Erpecum KJ, Janssens AR, Kreuning J, Ruiter DJ, Kroon HM, Grond AJ. Generalized peliosis hepatis and cirrhosis after long-term use of oral contraceptives. Am J Gastroenterol 1988;83(5):572–5.
220. Heresbach D, Deugnier Y, Brissot P, Bourel M. Dilatations sinusoi_dales et prise de contraceptifs oraux. A propos d'un cas avec revue de la litterature. [Sinusoid dilatation and the use of oral contraceptives. Apropos of a case with a review of the literature.] Ann Gastroenterol Hepatol (Paris) 1988;24(4):189–91.
221. Suarez AA, Brunt EM, Di Bisceglie AM. A 35-year-old woman with progesterone implant contraception and multiple liver masses. Semin Liver Dis 2001;21(3):453–9.
222. Morrison AS, Jick H, Ory HW. Oral contraceptives and hepatitis. A report from the Boston Collaborative Drug Surveillance Program, Boston University Medical Center. Lancet 1977;1(8022):1142–3.
223. Anonymous. Oral contraceptives and venous thromboembolic disease, surgically confirmed gallbladder disease, and breast tumours. Report from the Boston Collaborative Drug Surveillance Programme. Lancet 1973;1(7817):1399–404.
224. Stolley PD, Tonascia JA, Tockman MS, Sartwell PE, Rutledge AH, Jacobs MP. Thrombosis with low-estrogen oral contraceptives. Am J Epidemiol 1975;102(3):197–208.
225. Grodstein F, Colditz GA, Hunter DJ, Manson JE, Willett WC, Stampfer MJ. A prospective study of symptomatic gallstones in women: relation with oral contraceptives and other risk factors. Obstet Gynecol 1994;84(2):207–14.
226. Scragg RK, McMichael AJ, Seamark RF. Oral contraceptives, pregnancy, and endogenous oestrogen in gall stone disease—a case-control study. BMJ (Clin Res Ed) 1984;288(6433):1795–9.
227. Strom BL, Tamragouri RN, Morse ML, Lazar EL, West SL, Stolley PD, Jones JK. Oral contraceptives and other risk factors for gallbladder disease. Clin Pharmacol Ther 1986;39(3):335–41.
228. Riederer J. Verschlussikterus durch sludge im Ductus choledochus. [Obstructive jaundice due to sludge in the common bile duct.] Dtsch Med Wochenschr 2000;125(1–2):11–4.
229. Thijs C, Knipschild P. Oral contraceptives and the risk of gallbladder disease: a meta-analysis. Am J Public Health 1993;83(8):1113–20.
230. Vessey M, Painter R. Oral contraceptive use and benign gallbladder disease; revisited. Contraception 1994;50(2):167–73.
231. Bennion LJ, Ginsberg RL, Gernick MB, Bennett PH. Effects of oral contraceptives on the gallbladder bile of normal women. N Engl J Med 1976;294(4):189–92.
232. Tritapepe R, Di Padova C, Zuin M, Bellomi M, Podda M. Lithogenic bile after conjugated estrogen. N Engl J Med 1976;295(17):961–2.
233. Coronary Drug Project. Gallbladder disease as a side effect of drugs influencing lipid metabolism. N Engl J Med 1977;296(21):1185–90.

234. Kern F Jr, Everson GT, DeMark B, McKinley C, Showalter R, Braverman DZ, Szczepanik-Van Leeuwen P, Klein PD. Biliary lipids, bile acids, and gallbladder function in the human female: effects of contraceptive steroids. J Lab Clin Med 1982;99(6):798–805.

235. Mungall IP, Hague RV. Pancreatitis and the pill. Postgrad Med J 1975;51(602):855–7.

236. Burke M. Pregnancy, pancreatitis and the pill. BMJ 1972;4(839):551.

237. Pinggera G-M, Feuchtner G, Frauscher F, Rehder P, Strasser H, Bartsch G, Herwig R. Effects of local estrogen therapy on recurrent urinary tract infections in young females under oral contraceptives. Eur Urol 2005;47:243–9.

238. Schillinger F, Montagnac R, Birembaut P, Hopfner C. Syndrome hémolytique et urémique au décours d'une contraception orale. [Hemolytic–uremic syndrome during oral contraception.] Rev Fr Gynecol Obstet 1986;81(12):721–5.

239. Barrière H, Roubeix Y. Dermatoses et oestroprogestatifs. Gaz Med Fr 1977;84:1485.

240. Lucky AW, Henderson TA, Olson WH, Robisch DM, Lebwohl M, Swinyer LJ. Effectiveness of norgestimate and ethinyl estradiol in treating moderate acne vulgaris. J Am Acad Dermatol 1997;37(5 Pt 1):746–54.

241. Charoenvisal C, Thaipisuttikul Y, Pinjaroen S, Krisanapan O, Benjawang W, Koster A, Doesburg W. Effects on acne of two oral contraceptives containing desogestrel and cyproterone acetate. Int J Fertil Menopausal Stud 1996;41(4):423–9.

242. Wendler J, Siegert C, Schelhorn P, Klinger G, Gurr S, Kaufmann J, Aydinlik S, Braunschweig T. The influence of Microgynon and Diane-35, two sub-fifty ovulation inhibitors, on voice function in women. Contraception 1995;52(6):343–8.

243. Gollnick H, Albring M, Brill K. The efficacy of oral cyproterone acetate in combination with ethinylestradiol in acne tarda of the facial type. J Dermatol Treat 1998;9:71–9.

244. Mariotti F, Ruocco V. Oral contraceptives and sharpened condylomas. Riforma Med 1971;85:429.

245. Hollander A, Grots IA. Mucha–Habermann disease following estrogen–progesterone therapy. Arch Dermatol 1973;107(3):465.

246. Saez M, Garcia-Bustinduy M, Noda A, Guimera F, Dorta S, Escoda M, Fagundo E, Sanchez R, Martin-Herrera A, Garcia Montelongo R. Sweet's syndrome induced by oral contraceptive. Dermatology 2002;204(1):84.

247. Silver EA, Silver AH, Silver DS, McCalmont TH. Pseudoporphyria induced by oral contraceptive pills. Arch Dermatol 2003;139:227–8.

248. Greenwald AE. Anovulatorios y alopecia. [Oral contraceptives and alopecia.] Dermatol Iber Lat Am 1970;12:29–36.

249. Schoberberger R, Husslein P, Kunze M. Akzeptanz und Befindlichkeit unter einer norgestimathaltigen Kombinationspille. [Acceptance and subjective well-being with a norgestimate combination pill.] Gynakol Rundsch 1991;31(2):65–76.

250. Fortney JA, Feldblum PJ, Talmage RV, Zhang J, Godwin SE. Bone mineral density and history of oral contraceptive use. J Reprod Med 1994;39(2):105–9.

251. Polatti F, Perotti F, Filippa N, Gallina D, Nappi RE. Bone mass and long-term monophasic oral contraceptive treatment in young women. Contraception 1995;51(4):221–4.

252. Endrikat J, Mih E, Dusterberg B, Land K, Gerlinger C, Schmidt W, Felsenberg D. A 3-year double-blind, randomized, controlled study on the influence of two oral contraceptives containing either in combination with levonorgestrel on bone mineral density. Contraception 2004;69:179–87.

253. Spector TD, Hochberg MC. The protective effect of the oral contraceptive pill on rheumatoid arthritis: an overview of the analytic epidemiological studies using meta-analysis. J Clin Epidemiol 1990;43(11):1221–30.

254. Adams DB, Gold AR, Burt AD. Rise in female-initiated sexual activity at ovulation and its suppression by oral contraceptives. N Engl J Med 1978;299(21):1145–50.

255. Rozenbaum H. Petits problèmes de la contraception Mastodynies et contraceptifs oraux. [Little problems of contraception. Mastodynia and oral contraceptives.] Concours Med 1979;101(20):3341–2.

256. Mutti P, Cesarini R. Considerazioni sulle principali complicanze e controindicazioni dell'uso dei contraccettivi orali. [Principle complications and contraindications of the use of oral contraceptives.] Minerva Ginecol 1979;31(5):363–75.

257. Rose BI, LeMaire WJ, Jeffers LJ. Macromastia in a woman treated with penicillamine and oral contraceptives. A case report. J Reprod Med 1990;35(1):43–5.

258. Holt VL, Daling JR, McKnight B, Moore D, Stergachis A, Weiss NS. Functional ovarian cysts in relation to the use of monophasic and triphasic oral contraceptives. Obstet Gynecol 1992;79(4):529–33.

259. Lanes SF, Birmann B, Walker AM, Singer S. Oral contraceptive type and functional ovarian cysts. Am J Obstet Gynecol 1992;166(3):956–61.

260. Ibanez L, De Zegher F. Low-dose combination of flutamide, metformin and an oral contraceptive for non-obese, young women with polycystic ovary syndrome. J Hum Reprod (Oxf) 2003;18:57–60.

261. Milsom I, Sundell G, Andersch B. The influence of different combined oral contraceptives on the prevalence and severity of dysmenorrhea. Contraception 1990;42(5):497–506.

262. Belsey EM. Vaginal bleeding patterns among women using one natural and eight hormonal methods of contraception. Contraception 1988;38(2):181–206.

263. Rosenberg MJ, Long SC. Oral contraceptives and cycle control: a critical review of the literature. Adv Contracept 1992;8(Suppl 1):35–45.

264. Saleh WA, Burkman RT, Zacur HA, Kimball AW, Kwiterovich P, Bell WK. A randomized trial of three oral contraceptives: comparison of bleeding patterns by contraceptive types and steroid levels. Am J Obstet Gynecol 1993;168(6 Pt 1):1740–5.

265. Mall-Haefeli M. Was bringt die Micropille?. [What does the micropill bring?.] Ther Umsch 1986;43(5):365–71.

266. Fraser IS. Menstrual changes associated with progestogen-only contraception. Acta Obstet Gynecol Scand Suppl 1986;134:21–7.

267. Toth F, Kerenyin T. Changes of endometrium during contraceptive treatment. Acta Morphol Acad Sci Hung 1973;14:114.

268. Vercellini P, Ragni G, Trespidi L, Oldani S, Crosignani PG. Does contraception modify the risk of endometriosis? Hum Reprod 1993;8(4):547–51.

269. Parazzini F, Ferraroni M, Bocciolone L, Tozzi L, Rubessa S, La Vecchia C. Contraceptive methods and risk of pelvic endometriosis. Contraception 1994;49(1):47–55.

270. Cates W Jr, Stone KM. Family planning, sexually transmitted diseases and contraceptive choice: a literature update—Part II. Fam Plann Perspect 1992;24(3):122–8.

271. Expert Committee on Pelvic Inflammatory Disease. Pelvic inflammatory disease. Research directions in the 1990s. Sex Transm Dis 1991;18(1):46–64.

272. McGregor JA, Hammill HA. Contraception and sexually transmitted diseases: interactions and opportunities. Am J Obstet Gynecol 1993;168(6 Pt 2):2033–41.

273. Schuurs AHWM, Geurts TBP, Goorissen EM. Immunologic effects of estrogens, progestins, and estrogen–progestin combinations. In: Goldzieher JW, Fotherby K, editors. Pharmacology of the Contraceptive Steroids. New York: Raven Press, 1994:379–99.

274. Joshi UM, Rao SS, Kora SJ, Dikshit SS, Virkar KD. Effect of steroidal contraceptives on antibody formation in the human female. Contraception 1971;3:327.

275. Hagen C, Froland A. Depressed lymphocyte response to P.H.A. in women taking oral contraceptives Lancet 1972;1(7761):1185.

276. Klinger G, Schubert H, Stelzner A, Krause G, Carol W. Zum Verhalten der Serumimmunoglobulin Titer von IgA, IgG und IgM bei Kurz- und Langzeitapplikation verschiedener hormonaler Kontrazeptiva. [Serum immunoglobulin titer of IgA, IgG and IgM during short- and long-term administration of contraceptive hormones.] Dtsch Gesundheitsw 1978;33(23):1057–62.

277. Huang NH, Li C, Goldzieher JW. Absence of antibodies to ethinyl estradiol in users of oral contraceptive steroids. Fertil Steril 1984;41(4):587–92.

278. Kulisevsky Bojarski J, Rodriguez de la Serna A, Rovira Gols A, Roig Arnall C. Migraña acompañada como manifestación del lupus eritematoso sistemicon: presentación de 2 casos. [Complicated migraine as a manifestation of systemic lupus erythematosus. Presentation of 2 cases.] Med Clin (Barc) 1986;87(3):112–4.

279. Strom BL, Reidenberg MM, West S, Snyder ES, Freundlich B, Stolley PD. Shingles, allergies, family medical history, oral contraceptives, and other potential risk factors for systemic lupus erythematosus. Am J Epidemiol 1994;140(7):632–42.

280. Burns MR, Schoch DR, Grayzel AI. Cold urticaria and an oral contraceptive. Ann Intern Med 1983;98(6):1025–6.

281. Pelikan Z. Possible immediate hypersensitivity reaction of the nasal mucosa to oral contraceptives. Ann Allergy 1978;40(3):211–9.

282. Scinto J, Enrione M, Bernstein D, Bernstein IL. In vitro leukocyte histamine release to progesterone and pregnanediol in a patient with recurrent anaphylaxis associated with exogenous administration of progesterone. J Allergy Clin Immunol 1990;85:228.

283. Bork K, Fischer B, Dewald G. Recurrent episodes of skin angioedema and severe attacks of abdominal pain induced by oral contraceptives or hormone replacement therapy. Am J Med 2003;114:294–8.

284. Klinger G, Graser T, Mellinger U, Moore C, Vogelsang H, Groh A, Latterman C, Klinger G. A comparative study of the effects of two oral contraceptives containing dienogest or desogestrel on the human immune system. Gynecol Endocrinol 2000;14(1):15–24.

285. Howe JE, Minkoff HL, Duerr AC. Contraceptives and HIV. AIDS 1994;8(7):861–71

286. Anonymous. Verhoging lichaamstemperatuur bij orale anticonceptiva. Geneesmiddelenbulletin 1998;32:85–6.

287. Rogers SM, Baker MA. Thermoregulation during exercise in women who are taking oral contraceptives. Eur J Appl Physiol Occup Physiol 1997;75(1):34–8.

288. Vessey MP, Wright NH, McPherson K, Wiggins P. Fertility after stopping different methods of contraception. BMJ 1978;1(6108):265–7.

289. Harlap S, Davies AM. The Pill and Births: The Jerusalem Study, Final Report. In: US Department of Health, Education and Welfare, National Institute of Child Health and Development. Bethesda, MD: Center for Population Research, 1978:219.

290. Hull MG, Bromham DR, Savage PE, Jackson JA, Jacobs HS. Normal fertility in women with post-pill amenorrhoea. Lancet 1981;1(8234):1329–32.

291. Bracken MB, Hellenbrand KG, Holford TR. Conception delay after oral contraceptive use: the effect of estrogen dose. Fertil Steril 1990;53(1):21–7.

292. Franks AL, Beral V, Cates W Jr, Hogue CJ. Contraception and ectopic pregnancy risk. Am J Obstet Gynecol 1990;163(4 Pt 1):1120–3.

293. Weiss DB, Aboulafia Y, Milewidsky A. Ectopic pregnancy and the pill. Lancet 1976;2(7978):196–7.

294. American College of Obstetricians and Gynecologists (ACOG). Contraceptives and congenital anomalies. ACOG Committee Opinion: Committee on Gynecologic Practice. Number 124-July 1993. Int J Gynaecol Obstet 1993;42(3):316–7.

295. Bracken MB. Oral contraception and congenital malformations in offspring: a review and meta-analysis of the prospective studies. Obstet Gynecol 1990;76(3 Pt 2):552–7.

296. Simpson JL, Phillips OP. Spermicides, hormonal contraception and congenital malformations. Adv Contracept 1990;6(3):141–67.

297. Raman-Wilms L, Tseng AL, Wighardt S, Einarson TR, Koren G. Fetal genital effects of first-trimester sex hormone exposure: a meta-analysis. Obstet Gynecol 1995;85(1):141–9.

298. Keseru TL, Maraz A, Szabo J. Oral contraception and sex ratio at birth. Lancet 1974;1(7853):369.

299. Rothman KJ, Liess J. Gender of offspring after oral-contraceptive use. N Engl J Med 1976;295(16):859–61.

300. Janerich DT, Piper JM. Sex of offspring after use of oral contraceptives. N Engl J Med 1977;296(23):1360–1.

301. McCredie J, Kricker A, Elliott J, Forrest J. Congenital limb defects and the pill. Lancet 1983;2(8350):623.

302. Nikschick S, Goretzlehner G, Boldt O, Leineweber B, Radzuweit H, Hagen A, Born B, Melzer H, Nowak M, Fischer R, et al. Fehlbildungshaufigkeit nach Anwendung hormonaler Kontrazeptiva. [Incidence of abnormalities following the use of hormonal contraceptives.] Zentralbl Gynakol 1989;111(17):1152–9.

303. Nilsson S, Nygren KG. Transfer of contraceptive steroids to human milk. Res Reprod 1979;11(1):1–2.

304. McCann MF, Liskin LS, Piotrow PT, Rinehard W, Fox G, editors. Breast-feeding, fertility, and family planning. Population Reports, Series J, No. 24. Baltimore, Maryland, Population Information Program, 1984.

305. World Health Organization (WHO) Task Force on Oral Contraceptives. Effects of hormonal contraceptives on breast milk composition and infant growth. Stud Fam Plann 1988;19(6 Pt 1):361–9.

306. Nilsson S, Mellbin T, Hofvander Y, Sundelin C, Valentin J, Nygren KG. Long-term follow-up of children breast-fed by mothers using oral contraceptives. Contraception 1986;34(5):443–57.

307. World Health Organization Task force for Epidemiological Research on Reproductive HealthSpecial Programme of Research, Development and Research Training in Human Reproduction. Progestogen-only contraceptives during lactation: I. Infant growth. Contraception 1994;50(1):35–53.

308. World Health Organization, Task Force for Epidemiological Research on Reproductive

HealthSpecial Programme of Research, Development, and Research Training in Human Reproduction. Progestogen-only contraceptives during lactation: II. Infant development. Contraception 1994;50(1):55–68.

309. Howard RJ, Tuck SM. Haematological disorders and reproductive health. Br J Fam Plann 1993;19:147.

310. Vessey M, Painter R, Yeates D. Mortality in relation to oral contraceptive use and cigarette smoking. Lancet 2003;362(9379):185–91.

311. Coney P, Washenik K, Langley RG, DiGiovanna JJ, Harrison DD. Weight change and adverse event incidence with a low-dose oral contraceptive: two randomized, placebo-controlled trials. Contraception 2001;63(6):297–302.

312. Suthipongse W, Taneepanichskul S. An open-label randomized comparative study of oral contraceptives between medications containing 3 mg drospirenone (DRSP)/30 mug ethinylestradiol and 150 mug levonogestrel (LNG)/30 mug EE in Thai women. Contraception 2004;69:23–6.

313. Fotherby K, Caldwell AD. New progestogens in oral contraception. Contraception 1994;49(1):1–32.

314. Kluft C, de Maat MP, Heinemann LA, Spannagl M, Schramm W. Importance of levonorgestrel dose in oral contraceptives for effects on coagulation. Lancet 1999;354(9181):832–3.

315. Rowan JP. "Estrophasic" dosing: A new concept in oral contraceptive therapy. Am J Obstet Gynecol 1999;180(2 Pt 2):302–6.

316. Hoffmann H, Moore C, Kovacs L, Teichmann AT, Klinger G, Graser T, Oettel M. Alternatives for the replacement of ethinylestradiol by natural 17 beta-estradiol in dienogest-containing oral contraceptives. Drugs Today 1999;35(Suppl C):105–13.

317. Westhoff C, Morroni C, Kerns J, Murphy P.A. Bleeding patterns after immediate vs. conventional oral contraceptive initiation: a randomized, controlled trial. Fertil Steril 2003;79:322–9.

318. Back DJ, Orme ML. Pharmacokinetic drug interactions with oral contraceptives. Clin Pharmacokinet 1990;18(6):472–84.

319. Back DJ, Orme MLE. Drug interactions. In: Goldzieher JW, Fotherby K, editors. Pharmacology of the Contraceptive Steroids. New York: Raven Press, 1994:407.

320. Shenfield GM, Griffin JM. Clinical pharmacokinetics of contraceptive steroids. An update. Clin Pharmacokinet 1991;20(1):15–37.

321. Sonnenberg A, Koelz HR, Herz R, Benes I, Blum AL. Limited usefulness of the breath test in evaluation of drug metabolism: a study in human oral contraceptive users treated with dimethylaminoantipyrine and diazepam. Hepatogastroenterology 1980;27(2):104–8.

322. Homeida M, Halliwell M, Branch RA. Effects of an oral contraceptive on hepatic size and antipyrine metabolism in premenopausal women. Clin Pharmacol Ther 1978;24(2):228–32.

323. Teunissen MW, Srivastava AK, Breimer DD. Influence of sex and oral contraceptive steroids on antipyrine metabolite formation. Clin Pharmacol Ther 1982;32(2):240–6.

324. Crawford JS, Rudofsky S. Some alterations in the pattern of drug metabolism aociated with pegnancy, oral contraceptives, and the newly-born. Br J Anaesth 1966;38(6):446–54.

325. Chambers DM, Jefferson GC, Chambers M, Loudon NB. Antipyrine elimination in saliva after low-dose combined or progestogen-only oral contraceptive steroids. Br J Clin Pharmacol 1982;13(2):229–32.

326. Jones MK, Jones BM. Ethanol metabolism in women taking oral contraceptives. Alcohol Clin Exp Res 1984;8(1):24–8.

327. Monig H, Baese C, Heidemann HT, Ohnhaus EE, Schulte HM. Effect of oral contraceptive steroids on the pharmacokinetics of phenprocoumon. Br J Clin Pharmacol 1990;30(1):115–8.

328. Crawford P, Chadwick DJ, Martin C, Tjia J, Back DJ, Orme M. The interaction of phenytoin and carbamazepine with combined oral contraceptive steroids. Br J Clin Pharmacol 1990;30(6):892–6.

329. Nilsson S, Victor A, Nygren KG. Plasma levels of d-norgestrel and sex hormone binding globulin during oral d-norgestrel medication immediately after delivery and legal abortion. Contraception 1977;15(1):87–92.

330. Back DJ, Breckenridge AM, Crawford FE, Orme ML, Rowe PH. Phenobarbitone interaction with oral contraceptive steroids in the rabbit and rat. Br J Pharmacol 1980;69(3):441–52.

331. Wilbur K, Ensom MH. Pharmacokinetic drug interactions between oral contraceptives and second-generation anticonvulsants. Clin Pharmacokinet 2000;38(4):355–65.

332. Crawford P, Chadwick D, Cleland P, Tjia J, Cowie A, Back DJ, Orme ML. The lack of effect of sodium valproate on the pharmacokinetics of oral contraceptive steroids. Contraception 1986;33(1):23–9.

333. Briggs MH. Megadose vitamin C and metabolic effects of the pill. BMJ (Clin Res Ed) 1981;283(6305):1547.

334. Jochemsen R, van der Graaff M, Boeijinga JK, Breimer DD. Influence of sex, menstrual cycle and oral contraception on the disposition of nitrazepam. Br J Clin Pharmacol 1982;13(3):319–24.

335. Patwardhan RV, Mitchell MC, Johnson RF, Schenker S. Differential effects of oral contraceptive steroids on the metabolism of benzodiazepines. Hepatology 1983;3(2):248–53.

336. Kendall MJ, Quarterman CP, Jack DB, Beeley L. Metoprolol pharmacokinetics and the oral contraceptive pill. Br J Clin Pharmacol 1982;14(1):120–2.

337. Hughes BR, Cunliffe WJ. Interactions between the oral contraceptive pill and antibiotics. Br J Dermatol 1990;122(5):717–8.

338. Friedman CI, Huneke AL, Kim MH, Powell J. The effect of ampicillin on oral contraceptive effectiveness. Obstet Gynecol 1980;55(1):33–7.

339. Neely JL, Abate M, Swinker M, D'Angio R. The effect of doxycycline on serum levels of ethinyl estradiol, norethindrone, and endogenous progesterone. Obstet Gynecol 1991;77(3):416–20.

340. Deray G, le Hoang P, Cacoub P, Assogba U, Grippon P, Baumelou A. Oral contraceptive interaction with cyclosporin. Lancet 1987;1(8525):158–9.

341. Liu HF, Magdalou J, Nicolas A, Lafaurie C, Siest G. Oral contraceptives stimulate the excretion of clofibric acid glucuronide in women and female rats. Gen Pharmacol 1991;22(2):393–7.

342. Miners JO, Robson RA, Birkett DJ. Gender and oral contraceptive steroids as determinants of drug glucuronidation: effects on clofibric acid elimination. Br J Clin Pharmacol 1984;18(2):240–3.

343. Sinofsky FE, Pasquale SA. The effect of fluconazole on circulating ethinyl estradiol levels in women taking oral contraceptives. Am J Obstet Gynecol 1998;178(2):300–4.

344. Hilbert J, Messig M, Kuye O, Friedman H. Evaluation of interaction between fluconazole and an oral contraceptive in healthy women. Obstet Gynecol 2001;98(2):218–23.

345. Legler UF, Benet LZ. Marked alterations in dose-dependent prednisolone kinetics in women taking oral contraceptives. Clin Pharmacol Ther 1986;39(4):425–9.

346. van Dijke CP, Weber JC. Interaction between oral contraceptives and griseofulvin. BMJ (Clin Res Ed) 1984;288(6424):1125–6.

347. Hendrix CW, Jackson KA, Whitmore E, Guidos A, Kretzer R, Liss CM, Shah LP, Khoo K-C, McLane J, Trapnell CB. The effect of isotretinoin on the pharmacokinetics and pharmacodynamics of ethinyl estradiol and norethindrone. Clin Pharmacol Ther 2004;75:464–75.

348. Patwardhan RV, Desmond PV, Johnson RF, Schenker S. Impaired elimination of caffeine by oral contraceptive steroids. J Lab Clin Med 1980;95(4):603–8.

349. Rivera JM, Iriarte LM, Lozano F, Garcia-Bragado F, Salgado V, Grilo A. Possible estrogen-induced NMS. DICP 1989;23(10):811.

350. Muirhead GJ, Harness J, Holt PR, Oliver S, Anziano RJ. Ziprasidone and the pharmacokinetics of a combined oral contraceptive. Br J Clin Pharmacol 2000;49(Suppl 1):S49–56.

351. Palovaara S, Tybring G, Laine K. The effect of ethinyloestradiol and levonorgestrel on the CYP2C19-mediated metabolism of omeprazole in healthy female subjects. Br J Clin Pharmacol 2003;56:232–7.

352. Watson KJR, Ghabrial H, Mashford ML, Harman PJ, Breen KJ, Desmond PV. The oral contraceptive pill increases morphine clearance but does not increase hepatic blood flow. Gastroenterology 1986;90:1779.

353. Rogers SM, Back DJ, Stevenson PJ, Grimmer SF, Orme ML. Paracetamol interaction with oral contraceptive steroids: increased plasma concentrations of ethinyloestradiol. Br J Clin Pharmacol 1987;23(6):721–5.

354. Miners JO, Attwood J, Birkett DJ. Influence of sex and oral contraceptive steroids on paracetamol metabolism. Br J Clin Pharmacol 1983;16(5):503–9.

355. Skolnick JL, Stoler BS, Katz DB, Anderson WH. Rifampin, oral contraceptives, and pregnancy. JAMA 1976;236(12):1382.

356. Bolt HM, Kappus H, Bolt M. Effect of rifampicin treatment on the metabolism of oestradiol and 17 alpha-ethinyloestradiol by human liver microsomes. Eur J Clin Pharmacol 1975;8(5):301–7.

357. Archer JS, Archer DF. Oral contraceptive efficacy and antibiotic interaction: a myth debunked. J Am Acad Dermatol 2002;46(6):917–23.

358. El Bouhmadi A, Laffargue F, Raspal N, Brun JF. 100 mg acetylsalicylic acid acutely decreases red cell aggregation in women taking oral contraceptives Clin Hemorheol Microcirc 2000;22(2):99–106.

359. Miners JO, Grgurinovich N, Whitehead AG, Robson RA, Birkett DJ. Influence of gender and oral contraceptive steroids on the metabolism of salicylic acid and acetylsalicylic acid. Br J Clin Pharmacol 1986;22(2):135–142.

360. Krishnan KR, France RD, Ellinwood EH Jr. Tricyclic-induced akathisia in patients taking conjugated estrogens. Am J Psychiatry 1984;141(5):696–7.

361. Miguet JP, Vuitton D, Pessayre D, Allemand H, Metreau JM, Poupon R, Capron JP, Blanc F. Jaundice from troleandomycin and oral contraceptives. Ann Intern Med 1980;92(3):434.

Hormonal contraceptives—progestogen injections

General Information

For a complete account of the adverse effects of progestogens, readers should consult the following monographs as well as this one:

- Hormonal contraceptives—intracervical and intravaginal
- Hormonal contraceptives—oral
- Hormonal contraceptives—progesterone implants
- Hormone replacement therapy—estrogens + progestogens
- Medroxyprogesterone
- Progestogens.

Injectable hormonal contraceptives, which are normally composed of long-acting esters of progestogens, have obvious practical advantages over oral products when user compliance is poor, for example in illiterate or mentally subnormal women or in some populations in developing countries. However, the fact that they are used in this type of patient has led to some social protest against their use, as if they were intended to undermine free will or provide cheap but unpleasant contraception for the underprivileged. This may in turn explain some unbalanced criticism of these products in terms of efficacy and safety. Their sometimes incomplete cycle control is indeed a practical disadvantage, but not a risk, and the fact that they contain no estrogen actually means that they are safer in those respects when risks of hormonal contraception are due mainly to estrogenic effects, particularly thromboembolic complications. All in all, the injectable hormonal contraceptives provide effective, reversible, and relatively safe contraception, which can well be used not only in the populations named above but also, for example, in some women who smoke or when an estrogen is contraindicated (1,2).

General adverse effects

The degree to which women tolerate the adverse effects of long-acting injectable contraceptives seems to vary from one population to another, and it can be important to examine the frequency and severity of complaints in different environments. Particularly in developed countries, these products are often stated to cause mood changes, weight gain, and demineralization, but in developing countries they are very widely used. A worldwide review has surveyed the incidence of these conditions in users and has compared some of the figures with those found with an implantable product (Norplant; see the monograph on Hormonal contraceptives–progestogen injections) (3). Perhaps surprisingly, a consensus seems to be emerging that depot medroxyprogesterone acetate implants do not in fact result in an increase in the incidence of depression or in the severity of pre-existing depression, even after 1 or 2 years, nor do they cause significant weight gain. Similarly, Norplant did not cause depression.

Subgroups of users of depot medroxyprogesterone acetate may have reduced spinal bone density, but this seems to be reversible after withdrawal, even after several years of drug exposure (4). Bone mineral density in one cross-sectional study was lower among users of depot medroxyprogesterone acetate, but withdrawal was followed by complete recovery of normal bone density (4). A current study in the USA is expected to provide further data on this matter in women who have used medroxyprogesterone acetate for as long as 10 years.

Norethisterone enantate

The adverse effects of norethisterone enantate when used as a 2-monthly injectable contraceptive have been compared in various populations with those of depot medroxyprogesterone acetate and were found to be closely similar (5,6).

The largest single trial conducted with norethisterone enantate, covering some 9000 women-months of use, provided a fair picture of its adverse effects. Menstrual irregularity (prolonged bleeding, spotting, or amenorrhea) was the main complaint. Other adverse effects were periodic abdominal bloating and tender breasts, both of which were thought to be due to water retention and were relieved by diuretics. There was no associated weight gain. More than 50 of the women had pre-existing hypertension, and in these users the injections did not significantly affect blood pressure, which generally remained below 140/90 mmHg. Blood clotting was also not affected. High density lipoprotein cholesterol concentrations in the women treated were significantly lower than in the controls. The results of glucose tolerance tests did not differ significantly (7).

Three studies carried out in Bangladesh (8), Pakistan (9), and China (10) showed similar adverse reactions patterns. In the Bangladeshi study, nine of 254 women had a rise in both systolic and diastolic blood pressures, but five had a reduction of the same magnitude. In the Chinese women there were no significant changes in blood pressure. However, five Chinese women developed abnormal liver function tests and three of these women had liver enlargement after treatment for more than 2 years.

Other compounds and combinations

Other progestogen-only injectables have been tested, but those examined so far appear to have similar properties to the formulations that are already available.

Combined estrogen + progestogen injectables have been the subject of much experimentation. Administered monthly, they were developed in order to provide more dependable patterns of vaginal bleeding. Many formulations have been evaluated, and two of these have undergone phase III clinical trials by the WHO: one contains medroxyprogesterone acetate 25 mg with estradiol cipionate 5 mg and the other norethisterone enantate 50 mg plus estradiol valerate 5 mg. Analysis of daily menstrual diary record cards for women using these methods, compared with several other contraceptive methods and no method, showed that bleeding patterns for women receiving monthly injections were more regular, but not entirely normal (11). Although the median experience was similar to that of women not using contraception, the range of menstrual patterns was much wider. The outcome in this respect was found to be acceptable in only 70% of cycles during the first year of use, but later this figure rose to 85–90%. Under 10% of women discontinued use during the first year because of bleeding irregularities or amenorrhea, a rate that is presumably related in part to thorough counselling.

References

1. DaVanzo J, Parnell AM, Foege WH. Health consequences of contraceptive use and reproductive patterns. Summary of a report from the US National Research Council. JAMA 1991;265(20):2692–6.
2. Szarewski A, Guillebaud J. Contraception. BMJ 1991;302(6787):1224–6.
3. Kaunitz AM. Long-acting hormonal contraception: assessing impact on bone density, weight, and mood. Int J Fertil Womens Med 1999;44(2):110–7.
4. Cundy T, Cornish J, Evans MC, Roberts H, Reid IR. Recovery of bone density in women who stop using medroxyprogesterone acetate. BMJ 1994;308(6923):247–8.
5. Salem HT, Salah M, Aly MY, Thabet AI, Shaaban MM, Fathalla MF. Acceptability of injectable contraceptives in Assiut, Egypt. Contraception 1988;38(6):697–710.
6. Kazi AI. Comparative evaluation of two once-a-month contraceptive injections. J Pak Med Assoc 1989;39(4):98–102.
7. Howard G, Blair M, Fotherby K, Elder MG, Bye P. Seven years clinical experience of the injectable contraceptive, norethisterone enanthate. Br J Fam Plann 1985;11:9.
8. Chowdhury TA. A clinical study on injectable contraceptive Noristerat. Bangladesh Med J 1985;14(2–3):28–35.
9. Kazi A, Holck SE, Diethelm P. Phase IV study of the injection Norigest in Pakistan. Contraception 1985;32(4):395–403.
10. Frederiksen H, Ravenholt RT. Thromboembolism, oral contraceptives, and cigarettes. Public Health Rep 1970;85(3):197–205.
11. Fraser IS. Menstrual changes associated with progestogen-only contraception. Acta Obstet Gynecol Scand Suppl 1986;134:21–7.

Hormonal contraceptives— progestogen implants

General Information

Hormonal formulations for implantation contain progestogens, including the following:

- levonorgestrel
- etonogestrel
- desogestrel
- megestrol
- norethisterone.

For a complete account of the adverse effects of progestogens, readers are urged to consult the following monographs as well as this one:

- Hormonal contraceptives—progestogen injections
- Hormonal contraceptives—intracervical and intravaginal

- Hormonal contraceptives—oral
- Hormone replacement therapy—estrogens + progestogens
- Medroxyprogesterone
- Progestogens.

The two principal implants that release levonorgestrel, i.e. the six-capsule Norplant and the two-rod Jadelle are considered by authoritative reviewers to have essentially equal rates of drug release, pregnancy, and adverse events over 5 years of use (1).

Levonorgestrel

Subdermal implanted silastic rods containing levonorgestrel (Norplant) have been widely studied and used with the support of the Population Council, but have fallen out of favor in a number of industrialized countries, because of complications. Six rods are inserted subdermally into the arm using a special device; each contains 35 mg of levonorgestrel, which is released into the circulation over 5 years. The total amount of levonorgestrel released daily during the first 500 days averages about 60 micrograms, falling to a plateau of 30 micrograms/day for the remainder of the 5-year period during which the product remains effective. It then has to be removed and replaced. The contraceptive effect of the implant does not seem to be caused primarily by ovulation inhibition, since after about the first year of use the hormone concentrations are too low to have this effect (2,3).

A product similar in approach to Norplant is the biodegradable subdermal capsular implant Capronor, which releases levonorgestrel over 12–18 months. Doses of 12 and 21.6 mg in capsules of differing size have been compared (4). Ovulation occurred in all cycles at the lower dose and in a quarter of cycles at the higher dose, so it is likely that the contraceptive effect results essentially from other progestogen-induced changes. Several users had local swelling or itching of the skin at the capsule insertion site, relieved by topical glucocorticoids.

The effectiveness, adverse events, and acceptability of the FDA-approved variant of levonorgestrel capsule implants in the USA over 5 years and the determinants of these outcomes have been studied (5). There were three pregnancies, yielding a 5-year cumulative rate of 1.3 per 100 users, an average annual rate of three per 1000 women. Ectopic pregnancy occurred at a rate of 0.6 per 1000 woman-years. There were no pregnancies in women who weighed less than 79 kg. Medical conditions that most often led to removal of the implant were prolonged or irregular menstrual bleeding, followed by headache, weight gain, and mood changes. Weight gain averaged 1 kg/year.

Etonogestrel

Implanon, which became available in 1999, is a subdermal implant that contains 68 mg of etonogestrel, the active metabolite of desogestrel. The product and field experience is therefore still limited. During the first 2 years after implantation, there is no ovulation; ovulation occurs occasionally in the third year, and it is recommended that the implant be removed after this time. As with Norplant, the principal problem is the occurrence of irregular bleeding (6), which leads some 25–30% of users to ask that the implant be removed. After some time, amenorrhea occurs in some 20% of users. There was a clinically significant increase in bodyweight in 20% of women carrying the implant (7). There may also be some local irritation from the implant, and minor scarring at the implantation site (8,9). In clinical trials the implant had no effect on coagulation measures, hemostasis, fat metabolism, or hepatic function, but according to the approved product information sheet the possibility of a slight increase in insulin resistance cannot be excluded.

Desogestrel

In clinical trials, implants containing desogestrel were effective, but with bleeding irregularities and ovarian cysts as the primary adverse effects (10).

Megestrol

Implants filled with megestrol acetate gave an unexpectedly high incidence of tubal pregnancies, while the absolute number of ectopic pregnancies was clearly greater than that expected for the general population (11). This finding reflects the same type of effect as has been described from time to time with oral progestogen-only products.

Norethisterone

A biodegradable delivery system using subcutaneous implants of fused pellets made from norethisterone and pure cholesterol has been tested (12).

General adverse effects

Generally speaking, the systemic effects of progestogen implants are very similar to those of low-dose oral progestogen-only contraception, except for variations due to the progressive change in the amount of hormone released. Many studies using various metabolic measures have shown no significant pattern of deviation from normal values (13,14), either during use of the implant or after removal (15).

Adverse effects of levonorgestrel implants are similar to those observed with progestogen only and combined oral contraceptives. The risks of ectopic pregnancy, other pregnancy complications, and pelvic inflammatory disease are reduced in comparison with those in women who use copper or non-medicated intrauterine devices. The risks of gallbladder disease and frank or borderline hypertension, although small, are respectively about 1.5 and 1.8 times greater in women using levonorgestrel implants than in women not using hormonal contraception. Other serious diseases do not occur significantly more often in users of levonorgestrel implants than in women not using hormonal contraception. The great majority of levonorgestrel implant users have menstrual problems, but serious bleeding problems are not more frequent than in controls. In 16 000 women other health problems reported more frequently by users of levonorgestrel implants than by women not using hormonal contraception included skin conditions, headache, upper limb neuropathies, dizziness, nervousness, malaise, minor visual disturbances, respiratory conditions, arthropathies, weight change, anxiety, and non-clinical depression. Clinical depression is stated to be no more frequent in women using implants compared with those not using hormonal contraception (i.e. intrauterine devices or sterilization), but one must doubt this; certain women with a tendency to depression do experience triggering or aggravation of their condition with hormonal contraceptives, and it is not clear how this could differ between the various products. Problems with removing the device appear to be less frequent with Jadelle than with Norplant.

While the Norplant device has lost favor in some countries because of local intolerance and difficulties with removal, it continues to be widely used elsewhere. The difference in usage of Norplant between countries seems to reflect in part the degree of sophistication of users. Where, as in many western countries, low-dose oral contraceptives are very widely used and have become the standard by which users judge the acceptability of other means of contraception, the Norplant method has remained popular where expectations are somewhat lower.

Acceptability

As in the case of injectable depot contraceptives (SED-14, 1433) subdermal contraceptive implants are more likely to be used in developing countries, in order to overcome social and compliance problems, and that this can in principle involve risks to which underprivileged populations may be especially subject. All the same, acceptance is strikingly good (16). In a survey of data from eight developing countries, information was available on 7977 women starting Norplant, of whom 6625 used intrauterine devices and 1419 had been sterilized; most of the participants were followed for 5 years. All of the methods produced satisfactory degrees of contraception and, with a few exceptions, no characteristic morbidity was detected among Norplant users compared with the other groups. The two principal exceptions concerned gallbladder disease, which was 50% more common in women who used Norplant, and hypertension and borderline hypertension, the incidence of which was markedly raised in current implant users (RR = 1.81; 95% CI = 1.12, 2.92). Other unexpected findings were increased rates of respiratory disease and reduced risks of inflammatory disease of the genital tract in users of Norplant compared with sterilized women and those who used an intrauterine device (17).

In Burkina Faso, experience in 1660 women over 4 years has been critically reviewed (18). There were 247 withdrawals before the fourth year, for various reasons, including cycle disorders (60 withdrawals), unspecified medical reasons (n = 53), personal objections (n = 47), weight gain (n = 14), and contraceptive failure (n = 2). Menstrual disorders, including amenorrhea, spotting, and hypermenorrhea, occurred in 51% of the cases. The

investigators stressed the need for a good information and sensitization campaign to reduce the number of implant withdrawals before the fourth year of use, since the product often seems to be withdrawn for insufficient reasons.

A study in Senegal produced similar findings over 5 years; the method was safe and effective, but dissatisfaction with cycle control was again a prominent reason for requesting removal of the implant (19).

A Thai study in 88 asymptomatic, young, HIV-1-positive women immediately after delivery has similarly confirmed the good acceptability of Norplant in a developing country, despite the high incidence of irregular bleeding and some instances of headache and hair loss (20).

In 10 718 women in China, Norplant was reliable and no serious or fatal effects were reported (21). When pregnancies did occur, only 3.1 per 100 were ectopic, which is higher than for the general population in Beijing but much lower than in US studies of Norplant (presumably because of lower rates of pelvic inflammatory disease in China). The 5-year continuation rate was 72 per 100 acceptors. Hemoglobin concentrations increased during the first year of use and remained high, presumably because of a reduction in menstrual blood loss. Although early findings suggested a reduction in platelet counts, follow-up work showed that in this population these were already low on admission to the study. Insertion-related complications necessitated removal in only 21 users.

In a study in Greece the method was well accepted by adolescents, although the study was small (13 subjects) (22). No significant problems arose during the 24-month follow-up period.

On the other hand, Norplant has been criticized in some Western countries, primarily because of adverse effects at the implantation site. An overview of adverse events reported to the FDA over 3 years, during which more than 700 000 implants were estimated to be in place, cited reports of 24 women hospitalized for infections at the insertion site and 14 who were either hospitalized or disabled because of difficulties associated with capsule removal (23). Fourteen women (two per 100 000) were reportedly hospitalized because of strokes. Three women developed thrombotic thrombocytopenic purpura and six developed thrombocytopenia. Finally, 39 Norplant users developed pseudotumor cerebri (benign intracranial hypertension), an incidence of 5.5 per 100 000; this condition is associated with obesity or recent weight gain, conditions that were present in most of the women for whom data were given. Although the rates of stroke and pseudotumor cerebri were slightly less than the expected rates in the general population of women of reproductive age, one has to take into account the well-known under-reporting of adverse events to agencies such as the FDA; the figures could therefore mean that Norplant users are actually at increased risk.

Reviewing the overall scene in Britain, Hannaford has pointed to the considerable difference in acceptance rates for Norplant in the industrialized world and developing countries and has stressed the fact that the adverse reaction incidence is, according to the best evidence, low (24).

Rapid rejection of implantable progestogen-based contraceptives by some users, because of discomfort and local complications (for example because of breakage or migration of the device, or less than expert placement and removal), has attracted much attention in past reviews.

Organs and Systems

Cardiovascular

Norplant does not alter the blood pressure (25).

Nervous system

Headache is fairly common in women using progestogen implants (26).

Psychological, psychiatric

Two cases of major depression and panic disorder, developing soon after insertion of Norplant and resolving after removal, have been reported, but a causal association was not proven (27).

Five women using the Norplant system developed major depression, two of whom also developed obsessive-compulsive disorder and one of whom also developed agoraphobia (28). They had no prior psychiatric history but developed major depression within 1–3 months after insertion of Norplant. The depression worsened over time and in all cases resolved within 1–2 months after removal of Norplant. There was no recurrence of depression after 7–8 months in four cases available for follow-up. In addition to major depression, obsessive-compulsive disorder developed in two women and symptoms of agoraphobia developed in one woman during Norplant treatment, which resolved after removal.

Metabolism

Norplant does not alter body weight (29).

Hematologic

Research on blood coagulation has produced inconsistent results, usually showing little effect, as one would expect from a progestogen-based method without an estrogen component (30).

During 1 year of observation of 23 healthy fertile African women, beginning at the time that a Norplant device was inserted, the mean packed cell volume rose slightly but significantly from 40.5 to 42.2, but the mean total leukocyte, neutrophil, and lymphocyte counts all fell significantly, as did the mean platelet count (31). In four patients, the platelet counts were only $50–80 \times 10^9/l$. The rise in packed cell volume might, according to the authors, help to counter anemia in people in developing countries. However, the fall in the platelet count is hard to explain.

Skin

Some women who use progestogen implants develop acne, because of the androgenic activity of levonorgestrel. Three women developed severe acne vulgaris within

several weeks to a few months after either insertion of a levonorgestrel IUCD (two women, 27 and 33 years of age) or subcutaneous implantation of etonogestrel (a 26-year-old woman) (32).

Reproductive system

The most frequent adverse effect of progestogen implants is irregular menstrual bleeding (33), which in some countries has reduced the acceptability of the treatment (34). It is common during the first year of use but tends to become much less marked thereafter (13,29,35). In one study, the incidence of menstrual irregularity in Norplant users was 73% compared with only 5% in a comparable population using oral contraceptives (36). There is also a fairly high incidence of breakthrough bleeding or amenorrhea (37). The cause of the irregular bleeding is not fully understood, but there is evidence that an increase in endometrial vascular fragility might precipitate vessel breakdown and hence breakthrough bleeding (38).

Of 756 Norplant users (mean duration of use 3.08 years) most had previously used coitus interruptus as a contraceptive method and chose Norplant because of its effectiveness, despite the fact that adverse effects were detected in 80% (39). There were bleeding problems in 70%. Pregnancy occurred in only one case. Discontinuation because of bleeding problems occurred in 38%.

It has been reported that the irregular bleeding or spotting that may be experienced with this device is to some extent alleviated by intermittent administration of mifepristone, based on a double-blind, randomized, placebo-controlled trial in 120 Norplant users (40). From the second to the seventh month one group of users received intermittent mifepristone (100 mg/day on 2 consecutive days in every month). Women who used mifepristone recorded the same frequency of bleeding/spotting episodes as controls, but the bleeding episodes were significantly less prolonged, the total number of bleeding days being reduced by 35%. After the end of mifepristone use, bleeding patterns were similar in both groups. One pregnancy occurred in the mifepristone-treated group, in month 6 of treatment; the outcome was a healthy male baby. The authors concluded that intermittent administration of mifepristone can offer a clinically significant improvement in the vaginal bleeding pattern in Norplant users. Clearly, more experience is needed if mifepristone is to be used over long periods for this purpose.

It is not clear why some women are more susceptible to this complication than others. In a Thai study in a large number of Norplant users irregular bleeding was characterized by low estradiol concentrations, absence of luteal activity, and a thin hyperechoic pattern in the endometrium (41). The possible role of cellular apoptosis in the endometrial response to Norplant has been investigated using immunohistochemistry, but with negative results (42). However, among Norplant users the superficial endometrial blood vessels are more fragile than in controls and even more fragile than in untreated women with dysfunctional uterine bleeding (43).

An unusual approach to dealing with this irregular bleeding has been to give an antiprogestogen simultaneously. In 50 Chinese women with implants, mifepristone 50 mg once every 4 weeks has been compared with placebo (44). In all the women, regardless of treatment, the frequency of bleeding fell significantly over 1 year of observation, as it commonly does. However, women who took mifepristone had significantly shorter episodes of bleeding during treatment than during the 90 days before treatment started; the duration of bleeding episodes fell more gradually in the controls. Women who used mifepristone were more likely to find the treatment acceptable than the women who used placebo. Despite concerns that antiprogestogenic effects may jeopardize contraception, there were no pregnancies. In the view of the investigators, this approach may offer a useful strategy to relieve unwanted adverse effects of implants until bleeding patterns improve spontaneously with time.

A second unusual approach to the bleeding problem has been to give vitamin E. There is evidence that there is a poor angiogenic response in the endometrium of users of Norplant, and it has been hypothesized that this might be caused by an imbalance of pro-oxidant and antioxidant processes. A placebo-controlled study has suggested that vitamin E (200 mg/day for 10 days monthly) significantly reduces the number of monthly bleeding days (45). However, there was also some reduction in bleeding days with placebo, and this approach would need further study before the results could be accepted as clinically useful.

Amenorrhea is uncommon in women with progestogen implants, but the monthly blood loss is usually reduced rather than increased (46). Menstrual irregularity does not appear to be correlated with body mass index.

The appearance of enlarged ovarian follicles is a recognized complication of Norplant, but the reported incidence varies, probably because different methods are used to recognize them. Serial ultrasonography produces much higher figures than clinical methods and has led to exaggerated concern; the enlarged follicles are transient and do not require intervention (47).

Breast discharge has been reported in some women with progestogen implants (48).

Infection risk

Insertion-related complications include infection, hematoma formation, local irritation, scar formation, early implant expulsions, and allergic reactions to the dressing. A pooled analysis of insertion site complications in multi-country studies showed that 0.8% of women develop infection after insertion of Norplant, generally within the first week, but sometimes several months later (49). Implant expulsion occurred at some stage in 0.4% of users, often because of infection but sometimes because of poor placement. Two-thirds of expulsions were reported more than 2 months after insertion. The rates of such complications vary widely between practices and between countries.

Second-Generation Effects

Fertility

As with other progestogen-based contraceptive methods, the return of fertility after withdrawal is rapid: serum levonorgestrel concentrations are undetectable within a week after implant removal, and normal cycles usually resume during the first month.

Teratogenicity

Because the pregnancy rate among users of Norplant is quite low, the rate of ectopic pregnancy is also very low. There is no evidence that infants conceived during Norplant use are at higher risk of birth defects.

Lactation

One particular advantage of progestogen-only contraception is its suitability for use during breastfeeding, since there are no estrogens to impede lactation. The infant's intake of steroids is low and appears to be acceptable; its daily intake of steroids (estimated from concentrations in maternal milk during the first month of use) has been estimated to be 90–100 nanograms of levonorgestrel (Norplant), 75–120 nanograms of etonogestrel (Implanon), and 50 and 110 nanograms of nestorone (Nestorone and Elcometrine implants respectively) (50). However, it is still considered advisable to defer the implantation of these devices until 6 weeks after delivery, in view of the theoretical possibility of an adverse influence on the neonate.

Drug Administration

Drug formulations

The practical problems associated with Norplant have related to its physical form rather than its pharmacological profile. Practitioners specially trained in the insertion and removal of the device usually handle it without major problems, but without this special instruction it can be difficult to ensure that the rods are properly placed and that they are removed without scarring or other complications. Even given appropriate handling, the rods can cause problems as a result of migration or breakage in situ.

An implant can usually be removed in under a quarter of an hour under local anesthesia, but removal can be more difficult if the clinician is inexperienced, if the rods were not positioned properly at insertion, or if fibrous tissue has grown around them. If removal is not expertly handled in problematic cases, considerable scarring can result, and some users have proceeded to litigation as a consequence of such complications. Complications in the removal of Norplant capsules have been evaluated in 3416 cases from 11 countries (51). Complications were reported in 4.5% of removals, usually attributable to implants being broken during removal (1.7%) or being embedded below the subdermal plane (1.2%). Logistic regression analysis showed that the most important risk factors for complicated removals were complications at insertion and an infection at the implant site (before or at the time or removal). For women without complications, the mean removal time was 12 minutes, but for those with complications the mean increased to 30 minutes. These results illustrate the necessity of proper insertion technique, under aseptic conditions. Capsules become surrounded by a fibrous sheath within 3 months after implantation; beyond a few months, there is no difference in complication rate by duration of use.

Modified Norplant

A modified system, Norplant-2, requires only two instead of six rods. In 140 women using the Norplant-2 contraceptive subdermal implant system there were no accidental pregnancies over 3 years (52). Adverse effects that caused withdrawal from the study were acne, headache, and pain at the implant site. The termination rate for these medical reasons in year 3 of the study was 4.6%. The other main reason for termination was prolonged menstrual flow; the 3-year cumulative termination rate for menstrual irregularities was 3.8%.

References

1. Sivin I. Risks and benefits, advantages and disadvantages of levonorgestrel-releasing contraceptive implants. Drug Saf 2003;26:303–35.
2. Alvarez F, Brache V, Tejada AS, Faundes A. Abnormal endocrine profile among women with confirmed or presumed ovulation during long-term Norplant use. Contraception 1986;33(2):111–9.
3. Sivin I, Diaz S, Holma P, Alvarez-Sanchez F, Robertson DN. A four-year clinical study of NORPLANT implants. Stud Fam Plann 1983;14(6–7):184–91.
4. Darney PD, Monroe SE, Klaisle CM, Alvarado A. Clinical evaluation of the Capronor contraceptive implant: preliminary report. Am J Obstet Gynecol 1989;160(5 Pt 2):1292–5.
5. Sivin I, Mishell DR Jr, Darney P, Wan L, Christ M. Levonorgestrel capsule implants in the United States: a 5-year study. Obstet Gynecol 1998;92(3):337–44.
6. Affandi B. An integrated analysis of vaginal bleeding patterns in clinical trials of Implanon. Contraception 1998;58(Suppl 6):S99–S107.
7. Croxatto HB, Urbancsek J, Massai R, Coelingh Bennink H, van Beek AImplanon Study Group. A multicentre efficacy and safety study of the single contraceptive implant Implanon. Hum Reprod 1999;14(4):976–81.
8. Anonymous. Etonorgestrel. Geneesmiddelenbulletin 1999;33:123–4.
9. Admiraal PJJ, Luers JFJ. Etonogestrel implantaat. Pharma Selecta 1999;15:152–5.
10. Diaz S, Pavez M, Moo-Young AJ, Bardin CW, Croxatto HB. Clinical trial with 3-keto-desogestrel subdermal implants. Contraception 1991;44(4):393–408.
11. Croxatto HD, Diaz S, Rosati S, Croxatto HB. Adnexal complications in women under treatment with progestogen implants. Contraception 1975;12(6):629–37.
12. Gupta G, Saxena BB, Landesman R, Ledger WJ. Preparation, properties, and release rate of norethindrone (NET) from subcutaneous implants. In: Zatuchni GI, Goldsmith A, Shelton JD, Seiarra JJ, editors. Long-Acting Contraceptive Delivery Systems. Philadelphia: Harper and Row, 1984:425.
13. Croxatto HB. NORPLANT: levonorgestrel-releasing contraceptive implant. Ann Med 1993;25(2):155–60.
14. Singh K, Viegas OA, Loke D, Ratnam SS. Effect of Norplant-2 rods on liver, lipid and carbohydrate metabolism. Contraception 1992;45(5):463–72.
15. Singh K, Viegas OA, Loke DF, Ratnam SS. Evaluation of liver function and lipid metabolism following Norplant-2 rods removal. Adv Contracept 1993;9(3):233–9.
16. Glasier A. Implantable contraceptives for women: effectiveness, discontinuation rates, return of fertility, and outcome of pregnancies. Contraception 2002;65(1):29–37.
17. Meirik O, Farley TM, Sivin I. Safety and efficacy of levonorgestrel implant, intrauterine device, and sterilization. Obstet Gynecol 2001;97(4):539–47.
18. Kone B, Lankoande J, Ouedraogo CM, Ouedraogo A, Bonane B, Dao B, Sanou J. La Contraception par les implants sous-cutanes de lévonorgestral (Norplant). Experience africaine du Burkina Faso. [Contraception with levonorgestrel (Norplant) subcutaneous implants. African experience in Burkina Faso.] Contracept Fertil Sex 1999;27(2):162–3.
19. Ba MG, Moreau JC, Sokal D, Dunson R, Dao B, Kouedou D, Diadhiou F. A 5-year clinical evaluation of Norplant implants in Senegal. Contraception 1999;59(6):377–81.
20. Taneepanichskul S, Tanprasertkul C. Use of Norplant implants in the immediate postpartum period among asymptomatic HIV-1-positive mothers. contraception 2001;64(1):39–41.
21. Gu SJ, Du MK, Zhang LD, Liu YL, Wang SH, Sivin I. A 5-year evaluation of NORPLANT contraceptive implants in China. Obstet Gynecol 1994;83(5 Pt 1):673–8.
22. Cardamakis E, Georgopoulos A, Fotopoulos A, Sykiotis GP, Pappas AP, Lazaris D, Tzingounis VA. Clinical experience with Norplant subdermal implant system as long-term contraception during adolescence. Eur J Contracept Reprod Health Care 2002;7(1):36–40.
23. Wysowski DK, Green L. Serious adverse events in Norplant users reported to the Food and Drug Administration's MedWatch Spontaneous Reporting System. Obstet Gynecol 1995;85(4):538–42.
24. Hannaford P. Postmarketing surveillance study of Norplant in developing countries. Lancet 2001;357(9271):1815–6.
25. Davies GC, Newton JR. Subdermal contraceptive implants—a review: with special reference to Norplant. Br J Fam Plann 1991;17:4.
26. Population Council, Center for Biomedical Research, New York, New York 10021, USA. sivin@popcbr.rockefeller.edu.
27. Wagner KD, Berenson AB. Norplant-associated major depression and panic disorder. J Clin Psychiatry 1994;55(11):478–80.
28. Wagner KD. Major depression and anxiety disorders associated with Norplant. J Clin Psychiatry 1996;57(4):152–7.
29. Pasquale SA, Knuppel RA, Owens AG, Bachmann GA. Irregular bleeding, body mass index and coital frequency in Norplant contraceptive users. Contraception 1994;50(2):109–16.
30. Shaaban MM, Elwan SI, el-Kabsh MY, Farghaly SA, Thabet N. Effect of levonorgestrel contraceptive implants, Norplant, on blood coagulation. Contraception 1984;30(5):421–30.
31. Aisien AO, Sagay AS, Imade GE, Ujah IA, Nnana OU. Changes in menstrual and haematological indices among Norplant acceptors. Contraception 2000;61(4):283–6.

32. Cohen EB, Rossen NN. Acne vulgaris bij gebruik van progestagenen in een hormoonspiraal of een subcutaan implantaat. [Acne vulgaris in connection with the use of progestagens in a hormonal IUD or a subcutaneous implant.] Ned Tijdschr Geneeskd 2003;147(43):2137–9.

33. Singh K, Viegas OA, Liew D, Singh P, Ratnam SS. Norplant-2 rods: one year experience in Singapore. Contraception 1988;38(4):429–40.

34. Rehan N, Inayatullah A, Chaudhary I. Norplant: reasons for discontinuation and side-effects. Eur J Contracept Reprod Health Care 2000;5(2):113–8.

35. Shoupe D, Mishell DR Jr, Bopp BL, Fielding M. The significance of bleeding patterns in Norplant implant users. Obstet Gynecol 1991;77(2):256–60.

36. Berenson AB, Wiemann CM, Rickerr VI, McCombs SL. Contraceptive outcomes among adolescents prescribed Norplant implants versus oral contraceptives after one year of use. Am J Obstet Gynecol 1997;176(3):586–92.

37. Brache V, Faundes A, Alvarez F, Cochon L. Nonmenstrual adverse events during use of implantable contraceptives for women: data from clinical trials. Contraception 2002;65(1):63–74.

38. Hickey M, d'Arcangues C. Vaginal bleeding disturbances and implantable contraceptives. Contraception 2002;65(1):75–84.

39. Tugrul S, Yavuzer B, Kayahan A, Yildirim G. Norplant insertions at the Zeynep Kamil Gynecologic and Pediatric Training Research Hospital in Istanbul. Contraception 2004;69:323–6.

40. Massai MR, Pavez M, Fuentealba B, Croxatto HB, D'Arcangues C. Effect of intermittent treatment with mifepristone on bleeding patterns. Contraception 2004;70:47–54.

41. Kaewrudee S, Taneepanichskul S. Norplant users with irregular bleeding. Ultrasonographic assessment and evaluation of serum concentrations of estradiol and progesterone. J Reprod Med 2000;45(12):983–6.

42. Rogers PA, Lederman F, Plunkett D, Affandi B. Bcl-2, Fas and caspase 3 expression in endometrium from levonorgestrel implant users with and without breakthrough bleeding. Hum Reprod 2000;15(Suppl 3):152–61.

43. Hickey M, Dwarte D, Fraser IS. Superficial endometrial vascular fragility in Norplant users and in women with ovulatory dysfunctional uterine bleeding. Hum Reprod 2000;15(7):1509–14.

44. Cheng L, Zhu H, Wang A, Ren F, Chen J, Glasier A. Once a month administration of mifepristone improves bleeding patterns in women using subdermal contraceptive implants releasing levonorgestrel. Hum Reprod 2000;15(9):1969–72.

45. Subakir SB, Setiadi E, Affandi B, Pringgoutomo S, Freisleben HJ. Benefits of vitamin E supplementation to Norplant users—in vitro and in vivo studies. Toxicology 2000;148(2–3):173–8.

46. Balogh SA, Klavon SL, Basnayake S, Puertollano N, Ramos RM, Grubb GS. Bleeding patterns and acceptability among Norplant users in two Asian countries. Contraception 1989;39(5):541–53.

47. Alvarez-Sanchez F, Brache V, de Oca VM, Cochon L, Faundes A. Prevalence of enlarged ovarian follicles among users of levonorgestrel subdermal contraceptive implants (Norplant). Am J Obstet Gynecol 2000;182(3):535–9.

48. Segal M. Norplant: Birth Control at Arm's Reach. FDA: Office of Women's Health Website. 2001 http://www.fda.gov/bbs/topics/CONSUMER/CON00009.html.

49. Klavon SL, Grubb GS. Insertion site complications during the first year of NORPLANT use. Contraception 1990;41(1):27–37.

50. Diaz S. Contraceptive implants and lactation. Contraception 2002;65(1):39–46.

51. Dunson TR, Amatya RN, Krueger SL. Complications and risk factors associated with the removal of Norplant implants. Obstet Gynecol 1995;85(4):543–8.

52. Chompootaweep S, Kochagarn E, Tang-Usaha J, Theppitaksak B, Dusitsin N. Experience of Thai women in Bangkok with Norplant-2 implants. Contraception 1998;58(4):221–5.

Hormonal contraceptives—transdermal

Just as with estrogens and hormone replacement therapy, it has sometimes been suggested that the metabolic effects of estrogen + progestogen contraceptives administered transdermally are qualitatively different in one way or another from those of the equivalent oral products. A study by the Johnson and Johnson company using its contraceptive patch (which delivers norelgestromin 150 micrograms and ethinylestradiol 20 micrograms to the circulation in the course of a week) was performed primarily to examine the effects on blood lipids (1). There was a double-blind comparison with a placebo patch. At cycles 3, 6, and 9, there were increases from baseline in high density lipoprotein cholesterol, HDL3 cholesterol, total cholesterol, and total triglycerides, and reductions in the concentrations of low density lipoprotein and HDL. These findings were very similar to those seen with oral contraceptives based on norgestimate + ethinylestradiol.

Reference

1. Creasy GW, Fisher AC, Hall N, Shangold GA. Transdermal contraceptive patch delivering norelgestromin and ethinyl estradiol: effects on the lipid profile. J Reprod Med 2003;48:179–86.

Hormone replacement therapy—estrogens

General Information

For a complete account of the adverse effects of estrogens, readers should consult the following monographs as well as this one:

- Diethylstilbestrol
- Estrogens
- Hormonal contraceptives—emergency contraception
- Hormonal contraceptives—oral
- Hormone replacement therapy—estrogens + androgens
- Hormone replacement therapy—estrogens + progestogens.

Estrogen replacement therapy was until recently widely recommended for the prevention of osteoporosis in middle-aged and older women (1). Long-term estrogen therapy also reduces the incidence of ischemic heart disease in such women (2). However, it has always been difficult to know in which women such prophylactic use is likely to be needed, and this dilemma is compounded by the prospect of adverse reactions, which can include any of the acute effects listed in the estrogen monograph, but also in some cases long-term effects such as tumors.

The multiplicity of hormone replacement therapy regimens in use (involving one or two drugs, continuous or intermittent treatment, and various forms of administration) has made it difficult to express any general conclusion about the benefit-to-harm balance (3), and there has been a thoughtful review of the obstacles to assessing these matters objectively and scientifically, including questions of both ethics and trial design (4). Even the ultimate effect of hormone replacement therapy on the incidence of ischemic heart disease remains subject to dispute (5), and incidental reports of cardiac complications, sometimes in women with entirely healthy coronary vessels, continue to cause concern (6). For such reasons, much work has been devoted to determining the lowest effective dose of estrogen needed to achieve particular results.

An extraordinarily thorough review of all significant controlled studies of estrogen replacement therapy has been published by the Cochrane Collaboration (7). The participants totalled 2511 and the trials lasted 0.25–3 years. The primary purpose was to confirm efficacy, but data on adverse effects were also collected. Withdrawal because of adverse events, commonly breast tenderness, edema, joint pains, and psychological symptoms, was not significantly higher with HRT than placebo (OR = 1.38; 95% CI = 0.87, 2.21). Breast tenderness and withdrawal bleeding were the only significant problems in terms of frequency. The studies did not justify the conclusion that there are serious adverse effects, such as thrombosis and malignancies.

The desirability of limiting treatment to the minority of women who really need it is now regularly echoed (8–12). As has been stressed in a brief review (13), the Women's Health Initiative study was stopped because of safety concerns regarding combined treatment with estrogens + progestogens, and it was an entirely fair conclusion that the risks of the treatment outweighed the benefits. The outcome of the Women's Health Initiative has had drastic consequences for the acceptance of hormone replacement therapy among women who have been informed of the findings (14). All the same, the risks were difficult to express in exact terms, and this has led to criticism of the work and its conclusions (15). There was undoubtedly an increase in breast cancer among users, but no greater than the increase reported in observational studies; there was an increase in vascular events, but many of the women in the study had risk factors for cardiovascular disease. Since no further long-term trials of combined hormone replacement therapy appear to be in progress, the ultimate truth regarding the benefit to harm balance may remain in doubt for very long time. "Hormone replacement therapy can still be prescribed for menopausal symptoms and for osteoporosis prevention,

but the need for continued use should be reviewed annually" (13), and "a consensus is growing that postmenopausal women may be treated with HRT only ⋯ for disturbing symptoms of the ovarian hormone insufficiency syndrome, rather than ⋯ for menopause per se" (16).

A number of groups continue to stress the possibility, raised in the Nurses Health Study and elsewhere, that by reducing the dosages used in hormonal replacement one might eliminate the risks while retaining efficacy (17), but so long as this has not been shown to be true it will not provide a way ahead.

The Million Women Study in the UK (18) has been criticized on various grounds by some proponents of hormone replacement therapy, notably because in their view the number of deaths from breast cancer was too small and the follow-up too short to justify the belief that HRT increases the risk of death from breast cancer; discrepancies between this and other studies have also been stressed (19). The interpretation of the study in the editorial that accompanied it has also been criticized as being unduly pessimistic. However, the fact remains that the study is not the only source of serious doubts about the benefit to harm balance of hormone replacement therapy.

With such disagreements and doubts it can be difficult to provide a woman with the properly balanced information which she needs if "informed consent" to hormonal replacement treatment is to be meaningful (20).

The evidence of adverse effects emerging from randomized trials in and around 2002 has resulted in a dramatic fall in the use of hormone replacement therapy, the use of some formulations falling by two-thirds (21). Continuing debate on the benefit to harm balance of hormonal therapy at the time of the menopause or subsequently has in the recent past hardly yielded new conclusions (22).

Assessment of the efficacy and safety of hormonal replacement therapy has always been bedevilled by the question of adherence to therapy, which is often poorly recorded. Particularly after the acute symptoms of the menopause have passed and been forgotten, some women lose their motivation to continue hormonal treatment. Added to this is the now incontrovertible evidence that HRT can in some cases be harmful, and presentation of the risks in the mass media has undoubtedly further reduced adherence. An Italian group examined this problem prospectively in 138 women who agreed to be enrolled in a longitudinal study intended to last for 24 months (23). Only 72 were still taking the treatment after 1 year and only 56 at the end of the study, although only three reported that they had experienced no benefit. Type of work, surgical menopause, and previous use of oral contraceptives were significantly associated with better adherence. The occurrence of real or supposed adverse effects and a fear of breast cancer were the commonest reasons cited for early discontinuation.

Observational studies

A Japanese study of the use of estriol 2 mg/day for 12 months in 68 postmenopausal women with climacteric symptoms showed a significant effect in relieving hot flushes, night sweats, and insomnia (24,25). There were significant falls in serum follicle stimulating hormone (FSH) and luteinizing hormone (LH) concentrations, but no effect on lipids, bone demineralization, or blood pressure. There was slight vaginal bleeding in 14% of women treated during a natural menopause, but histological and ultrasound evaluation showed no changes in the endometrium or breasts. It is evident, however, that higher doses might be needed when treating women of other races with a higher body weight. Other workers have found that when given with a progestogen over long periods, estriol 2.0 mg/day seems much less likely to cause undesirable lipid changes than are equine conjugated estrogens, which can cause increased HDL cholesterol and triglyceride concentrations (26).

Comparative studies

In a randomized, multicenter study in Denmark 376 perimenopausal women with climacteric symptoms were randomly allocated to oral sequential combined treatment with regimens based on estrogen plus either desogestrel or medroxyprogesterone acetate (27). Both treatments effectively alleviated menopausal complaints within 6 months and gave good cycle control. Bleeding pattern and mood disturbances were more favorably affected by desogestrel, but overall the differences in adverse effects (irregular bleeding and a slight tendency to hypotension) were not large. It should be noted, however, that with cyclic combined hormone replacement therapy treatment, the bleeding pattern alone does not seem to be a reliable means of distinguishing cases in which the endometrium is atrophic or inactive from those in which it is proliferative or hyperplastic (28).

Organs and Systems

Cardiovascular

The overall benefit to harm balance for medium-term hormone (estrogen + progestogen) replacement therapy (2 years) has been assessed in a novel although theoretical study using a Markov model. Data from the Women's Health Initiative were used to simulate the effect of short-term treatment on life expectancy and quality-adjusted life expectancy (QALE) in 50-year-old menopausal women with intact uteri (29). Quality-of-life (QOL) utility scores were derived from the literature. The investigators assumed that HRT affected quality of life only during the perimenopause, when it reduced symptoms by 80%. Among asymptomatic women, short-term therapy was associated with net reductions in life expectancy and QALE of 1–3 months, depending on the risk of cardiovascular disease. Women with mild or severe menopausal symptoms gained 3–4 months or 7–8 months of QALE respectively. Among women at low risk of cardiovascular complications, HRT extended QALE, even if menopausal symptoms lowered quality of life by as little as 4%. Among women at increased risk of cardiovascular disease, HRT extended QALE only if symptoms lowered quality of life by at least 12%. The authors'

conclusion was that hormone therapy is associated with reduced survival but gains in QALE for women with menopausal symptoms, and that women who are expected to benefit from short-term HRT can be identified by the severity of their menopausal symptoms and their risk of cardiovascular disease.

Coronary heart disease

The continuing debate about the relation, if any, between HRT and coronary heart disease has been reviewed (30,31). A paradoxical finding in the Women's Health Initiative (WHI) study was that while HRT resulted in an improvement in blood lipid concentrations there was no reduction in the incidence of coronary heart disease. A re-examination of the findings in 2005 generated the hypothesis that the key to the paradox could lie in effects on specific lipid subgroups rather than on lipids as a whole (32). This hypothesis was tested by an evaluation of differences in coronary calcification, lipids, and lipoprotein subclasses among menopausal HRT users and non-users in a longitudinal study. Lipoprotein subclasses and coronary artery calcification (the latter measured using electron beam computed tomography) were studied in HRT users (49%) and non-users in a total of 243 women from the Healthy Women Study, who were about 8 years postmenopausal. The distribution of calcification scores was not significantly different between users and non-users and neither were there differences between the groups as regards any LDL subclass. However, regardless of HRT use, women with detectable calcification of the coronary arteries had higher concentrations of VLDL and small LDL particles, higher LDL particle concentration, and smaller mean LDL size compared with women with no detectable calcification. The fact that HRT users had higher concentrations of VLDL particles (triglycerides) and did not have a better LDL subclass distribution could explain the fact that HRT was not associated with a difference in coronary calcification in this study or with a reduction in coronary heart disease risk in randomized clinical trials.

Thromboembolic disease

One of the most serious aspects of the thromboembolic complications now widely acknowledged as being associated with HRT is that their emergence coincides with the development of the conclusion that the role of HRT in reducing the risk of coronary heart disease is at best unproven. A form of treatment that was originally viewed as potentially beneficial to the cardiovascular system is at present on balance perhaps harmful (33).

A US group examined potential risk factors for venous thromboembolic events in women assigned to HRT in the Postmenopausal Estrogen/Progestin Interventions (PEPI) study, a 3-year double-blind study in 875 postmenopausal women designed to assess the effects of HRT on heart disease risk factors (HDL cholesterol, fibrinogen, blood pressure, and insulin) (34). Women with a history of estrogen-associated venous thromboembolic events were excluded. Ten women, all assigned to HRT, had a venous thromboembolic event during the study. Only baseline fibrinogen varied significantly between those who had a venous thromboembolic event while assigned to HRT event (mean 2.49 g/l) and those who did not have an event (mean 2.81 g/l). Adjusting for covariates did not affect this finding. As the authors remarked, the lower fibrinogen concentrations among women who subsequently reported venous thromboembolic events may be a marker for a specific, but as yet undefined, coagulopathy that is magnified in the presence of exogenous hormones. However, larger studies are needed to confirm this hypothesis.

Since much of the evidence of thromboembolic complications with HRT relates to the use of conjugated equine estrogens, the degree of risk when natural 17-beta-estradiol was used instead has been examined in Norway in a population-based case-control study involving consecutive women, aged 44–70 years, discharged from a University Hospital between 1990 and 1996 with a diagnosis of deep venous thrombosis or pulmonary embolism (35). Women with cancer-associated thrombosis were excluded. Random controls were used. The material comprised 176 cases and 352 controls, that is two controls for each case. All the women who received HRT had been given estradiol. The frequency of HRT use was 28% (50/176) in cases and 26% (93/352) in controls. The estimated matched crude odds ratio was 1.13 (CI = 0.71, 1.78), which shows no significant association of overall use of estradiol-based HRT and thromboembolism. However, when the duration of exposure to HRT was taken into account by stratification, there was an increased risk of thromboembolism during the first year of use, with a crude odds ratio of 3.54 (CI = 1.54, 5.2). This effect was reduced by extended use to a crude odds ratio of 0.66 (CI = 0.39, 1.10) after the first year of use. The authors concluded that the use of estradiol for HRT was associated with a three-fold increase in the risk of venous thromboembolism, but that this increased risk was restricted to the first year of use. One is bound to wonder whether this shift in risk was genuine or reflects only the limitations of the study.

Among the less common forms of thromboembolism that have been reported is occlusion of the retinal vein, familiar with the oral contraceptives but unusual with HRT (36).

QT interval prolongation
Hormone replacement therapy can cause prolongation of the QT interval on the electrocardiogram. In a prospective study set of the incidence and extent of this effect 3103 women were followed at intervals over 9 years and data were collected on their use of hormonal replacement and the QT interval, prolongation being defined as an increase of not less than 10% (37). The QT$_c$ interval was moderately but significantly longer in users of hormone replacement therapy, the risk of QT prolongation being nearly twice that in never-users. The consequences of these changes for the user's health could not be assessed.

The effects of HRT on cardiovascular function have been prospectively studied over 1 year in 46 healthy postmenopausal women, mean age 55 years, who took either estrogen replacement therapy alone (n = 23) or progestogen + estrogen replacement therapy (n = 23) (38). The doses used were 0.625 mg/day of conjugated equine estrogen with or without medroxyprogesterone acetate 2.5 mg/day. The controls were 25 health premenopausal women, mean age 35 years. Long-term estrogen-only replacement increased the QT interval, QT dispersal, and the index of parasympathetic activity; there was also a small non-significant increase in the incidence of dysrhythmias. Long term use of progestogen + estrogen did not affect the QT interval, QT dispersion, or the frequencies of ventricular dysrhythmias or parasympathetic activity, but it did increase the incidence of supraventricular tachycardias. These findings support the idea that estrogen may directly modulate ventricular repolarization and that progestogens do not.

Respiratory

Since female reproductive hormones appear to influence respiratory disease in some as yet poorly defined way, a prospective cohort study over 8 years sought to determine whether postmenopausal hormone use was associated with an increased rate of newly diagnosed asthma or chronic obstructive pulmonary disease (39). During 546 259 person-years of follow-up, current use of estrogen alone was associated with an increased rate of asthma (multivariate rate ratio = 2.29; 95%CI = 1.59, 3.29) compared with those who never used hormones. Current users of estrogen + progestogen had a similarly increased rate of newly diagnosed asthma. Rate ratios increased with certainty of diagnosis of asthma. In contrast, rates of newly diagnosed obstructive pulmonary disease were the same among hormone users and non-users.

Ear, nose, throat

Visual hallucinations have been associated with estrogen in a patient with Charles Bonnet syndrome (40).

- An 84-year-old woman with poor visual acuity secondary to bilateral, non-exudative, age-related macular degeneration had non-threatening visual hallucinations 2 weeks after starting oral estrogen for osteoporosis. The estrogen was withdrawn and the hallucinations subsided. She was given estrogen twice more and each time the hallucinations recurred.

In this patient estrogen may have promoted release phenomena and triggered the hallucinatory episodes.

Nervous system

Over the years there have been reports that headache or classical migraine is either alleviated or exacerbated by HRT. This has been studied in 50 menopausal women with headaches who were randomized to either transdermal estradiol 50 micrograms for 7 days a month or oral conjugated estrogens 0.625 mg/day for 28 days, both regimens being supplemented with medroxyprogesterone acetate 10 mg/day during the latter half of each month (41). In patients with episodic tension headache there was no significant change in headache pattern. However, in women with migraine without aura the frequency and duration of the attacks increased significantly during HRT in the subgroup using the oral formulation; the transdermal formulation had no effect on the migraine pattern.

Sensory systems

The possibility that estrogen replacement therapy might cause dryness of the eyes has been reviewed in the light of data from the large Women's Health Study in the USA (42), and this work has been further reviewed (43). Questionnaires were sent to 25 665 participants. For every 3-year increase in the duration of replacement therapy there was a 15% increase in the incidence of dry eye syndrome. The risk was greater in women who used estrogen alone than in those who used combined estrogen + progestogen regimens. The evidence was not statistically strong, but it suggests that there is some correlation and that users and prescribers should be aware of it.

Psychological

The mechanisms underlying the mood changes that are often associated with menstruation, the menopause, and hormonal therapy are not understood, but there is now some evidence that they have an association with the response to the neuroactive steroid pregnanolone and that progestogens and estrogens might alter this response. In a randomized, double-blind, crossover study 26 postmenopausal women with climacteric symptoms took oral estradiol 2 mg/day continuously for two cycles and either vaginal progesterone 800 mg or a placebo during the last 14 days of each cycle (44). Before treatment and again at the end of each treatment cycle pregnanolone was administered intravenously, and its effects on saccadic eye velocity, saccade acceleration, saccade latency, and self-rated sedation were examined. During treatment with either estradiol alone or with added progesterone the effect of pregnanolone on saccadic eye movements and self-rated sedation was increased. Saccadic eye velocity, saccade acceleration, and sedation responses to pregnanolone were also increased in women who usually experienced cyclicity of mood during HRT treatment, but not in those with no history of mood cyclicity.

Metabolism

Lipids

Changes in lipids have been observed with both HRT and oral contraceptives and have sometimes been promoted as potentially advantageous, but it is not clear how significant such changes are, at least in biochemical terms. A review and pooled analysis of 248 prospective studies available up to the year 2000 has provided data on this issue in postmenopausal women (45). All estrogen-only regimens raised HDL cholesterol and lowered LDL and total cholesterol. Oral estrogens raised triglycerides. Transdermal 17-beta-estradiol lowered triglycerides.

The unfavorable effects of estrogens on blood lipids are particularly serious in women with hypertriglyceridemia. The changes in women with previously raised lipids have been quantified (46). In 56 women, median age 52 years,

with serum triglyceride concentrations over 4.5 mmol/l (400 mg/dl) despite diet and drug treatment, or with a history of hypertriglyceridemic acute pancreatitis. Of the 56 women, 23 had taken some form of hormone replacement therapy and one had been treated with selective estrogen receptor modulators; in these women at entry the median fasting triglyceride concentration averaged 1270 mg/dl and in the previously untreated women 1087 mg/dl. After baseline testing, the hormonal treatment was withdrawn and they received a very low fat diet, gemfibrozil 1.2–1.5 mg/day, and omega-3-fatty acids 4–12 g/day. After 2-4 weeks of this treatment, the median triglyceride concentration in those who had taken hormones fell from 1270 to 284 mg/dl and in the non-hormone group from 1087 to 326 mg/dl. The authors stressed the seriousness of the lipid complications that can occur with estrogens when women already have a tendency, familial or otherwise, to hypertriglyceridemia. Triglycerides must be measured before beginning hormone therapy; hormone therapy is contraindicated in women with a triglyceride concentration of 500 mg/dl or more. Triglyceride-lowering diets and drugs are likely to fail as long as hormones are being given.

Glucose tolerance

The effects of therapeutic doses of estrogens on glucose tolerance are probably only slight, although the available data are inconsistent. In a study of the effects of transdermal and peroral oestrogen in conjunction with cyproterone acetate on metabolic and hormonal parameters in 24 women with polycystic ovary syndrome, peroral estrogens (at doses comparable to those currently used in combined oral contraceptives) significantly impaired insulin secretion and action (47). In contrast, transdermal estrogens did not significantly alter insulin sensitivity. It is doubtful whether these effects are of clinical importance.

Weight

Weight gain is widely believed to be a common consequence of HRT, and the desire to avoid obesity is a major reason why some women decline treatment. However, the potential effects of HRT need to be distinguished from effects that could be due to changing lifestyle or ageing. The effects of short-term hormone replacement and age on alterations in weight, body composition, and energy balance have therefore been studied in a prospective study in 18 healthy women aged 45–55 years and in 15 aged 70–80 years, with measurements at baseline, repeated after 1 month of transdermal estrogen (Estraderm 50 micrograms/day), and again after a further month of transdermal estrogen with vaginal progesterone (100 mg bd) added for the final 7 days (48). In neither age group did estrogen treatment correlate with anthropometric changes. Resting energy expenditure and activity were positively correlated with fat-free mass, while energy intake was not. Resting energy expenditure, energy intake, and activity were lower in older women when adjusted for fat-free mass. Changes in weight during treatment were not statistically significant. In addition, there was no difference between the groups in body mass index, fat mass, fat-free mass, total body water, or waist-to-hip ratio. This work has confirmed the reduction in energy expenditure that occurs with ageing, and it suggests that there is no effect of HRT on resting energy expenditure or body weight.

Hematologic

There has been a randomized, placebo-controlled study in 25 postmenopausal women to investigate the mechanisms that could underlie the induction of thrombosis by unopposed estrogens (49). Fasting and fat-load-stimulated plasma concentrations of clotting factor VII were measured after 8 weeks of oral 17-beta-estradiol (2 mg/day). Estradiol increased the mean fasting and postprandial plasma concentrations of total factor VII by 17 and 21% respectively, but did not affect the fasting and/or postprandial plasma concentrations of active factor VII. These findings argue against the idea that raised concentrations of total factor VII underlie the increased risk of arterial thromboembolism in these women.

It has been firmly concluded, in the light of prior evidence, that HRT increases the risk of venous thrombosis, this risk not being outweighed by any demonstrable benefit in terms of arterial cardiovascular disease (50). This conclusion is now being increasingly accepted, and the effects of postmenopausal HRT on blood coagulation have been intensively studied and documented over the years. However, the effects in older women, who have the highest risk of thromboembolism, are not well defined, and a US group has studied the association between HRT and concentrations of natural anticoagulant proteins in this subpopulation in a cross-sectional study in women of 65 years or older participating in the Cardiovascular Health Study (51). Protein C antigen and antithrombin were measured in HRT users (230 taking an unopposed estrogen and 60 taking an estrogen with a progestogen) and a comparison group of 196 non-users. Estrogen use was associated with significantly higher protein C concentrations (4.80 versus 4.30 micrograms/ml); the results were similar with estrogen/progestogen. In both user groups, antithrombin was significantly lower than in non-users (109% for each treatment group versus 115% in non-users). Adjustment for factors related to prescription of HRT and to anticoagulant protein concentrations had little impact on the results. For antithrombin, the association with HRT was larger for thinner Caucasian women and black women. The authors concluded that venous thrombosis from HRT may be partly mediated by alterations in antithrombin, but not by protein C concentrations.

Although the thrombogenic potential of oral estrogen in postmenopausal women is well documented, it has been argued that direct studies of the effect of estrogen replacement on hemostasis are largely lacking and not well known (52). A review of a series of randomized trials has shown that the treatment has no significant effect on concentrations of fibrinogen and factor VII. Plasma concentrations of antithrombin and protein S fell with oral estrogen but not with transdermal estrogen. No form of replacement affected protein C concentrations, but there

was activation of coagulation in the presence of oral estrogen, as reflected by a rise in the concentration of prothrombin fragment 1 + 2. As far as fibrinolysis is concerned, oral estrogen reduces plasma PAI-1 and tPA, leading to an increase in fibrinolytic potential. The absence of an effect of transdermal estrogen on coagulation and fibrinolysis suggests that the route of estrogen administration is important, but it has not to date been convincingly shown that transdermal estrogen in equieffective doses is less thrombogenic than the oral form.

The effect of continuously administered low-dose 17-beta-estradiol (E2) + norethisterone acetate (NETA) on coagulation and fibrinolytic factors has been studied in 120 menopausal women, using two dosage variations (1 mg of E2 with 0.25 mg or 0.5 mg of NETA) compared with placebo over a year (53). In either dose, the combination significantly lowered plasma concentrations of factor VII, fibrinogen, antithrombin, and plasminogen activator inhibitor-1 (PAI-1) compared with placebo. These changes appear favorable, since they may lead to increased fibrinolytic activity and could reduce the risk of coronary heart disease. However, antithrombin activity was also reduced, which may increase the risk of venous thromboembolism.

In 27 postmenopausal subjects who took estradiol for 8 weeks, either alone or in combination with the progestogen norethisterone, there was an increase in plasma thromboxane beta$_2$ concentration, possibly determined by platelet activation, which suggests an increased short-term risk of thrombosis; P-selectin expression was not affected (54).

It is not surprising to see further evidence emerging, this time from Japan, as to *why* the risk of venous thromboembolism during HRT is likely to be greater in hypertensive women than in others. In 38 hypertensive (but treated) women and 32 normotensive subjects, who took a course of conjugated equine estrogen 0.625 mg/day + medroxyprogesterone acetate 2.5 mg/day for 12 months, and 19 other hypertensive subjects and 15 normotensive women who took no hormone replacement at all, antithrombin concentrations in the hypertensive and normotensive women who took HRT fell significantly at 6 and 12 months, their D-dimer concentrations fell at 12 months, and their plasminogen concentrations fell at 6 and 12 months (55). There were no changes in hemostatic factors in either control group. This meticulous study must lead one to conclude that this form of HRT activates blood coagulation and fibrinolysis in both hypertensive and normotensive postmenopausal women. This may well be related to the risk of thromboembolic events.

Gastrointestinal

Since hormone status could be involved in the occurrence of irritable bowel syndrome, the risk has been examined in women using hormone replacement therapy (56).

A population of women aged 50-69 years old with at least one prescription for HRT were identified from Britain's General Practice Research Database, and a cohort of 50 000 women who had never used HRT was sampled from the same source population. The incidence of irritable bowel syndrome per 1000 person-years was 1.7 in the cohort of never-users and 3.8 among HRT users. Both current and past users of HRT had an increased risk of irritable bowel syndrome compared with non-users, after adjusting for co-morbidity and consultation patterns. The increased risk was unaffected by treatment duration, regimen, or route of administration. This result suggests that HRT is associated with an increased risk of irritable bowel syndrome similar to that observed among younger premenopausal women with endogenous estrogenic activity.

Biliary tract

Hormone replacement therapy is associated with an increased risk of gallstones. In 16 postmenopausal women with no history of gallstones, fasting and residual gall-bladder volumes increased and the ejection fraction fell significantly were examined after 3 months of treatment with HRT (conjugated estrogen 0.625 mg/day, + medroxyprogesterone acetate 2.5 mg/day) (57). There was no change in measures of lithogenicity, such as nucleation time.

Urinary tract

Since microalbuminuria can be regarded as being associated with renal and cardiovascular disease, evidence that the incidence of microalbuminuria is higher during treatment with oral contraceptives or hormone replacement therapy deserves to be taken seriously. A Dutch group has performed a case-control study of baseline and dispensing data relating to 4301 women participating in a study on the prevention of renal and vascular disease; the main outcome measure was microalbuminuria (30–300 mg/day) (58). After adjusting for age, hypertension, diabetes, obesity, hyperlipidemia, and smoking, the odds ratio for microalbuminuria was 1.90 (CI = 1.23, 2.93) for premenopausal oral contraceptive users and 2.05 (1.12, 3.77) for postmenopausal hormone replacement therapy users. The point estimate increased dose-dependently, albeit insignificantly, according to the estrogen content of the oral contraceptives (30–50 micrograms) and was greater in oral contraceptives with a second-generation progestogen (OR = 2.04) than those using a third-generation progestogen (OR = 1.39; CI = 0.63, 3.06). In the case of HRT, the odds ratio increased with the duration of HRT, that in women who had used the product for more than 5 years being double that in others.

At various times evidence has appeared that HRT reduces the risk of urinary infections, while other reports have suggested that the risk is increased. The same seems to apply to urinary incontinence; it has often been stated that incontinence is reduced by HRT, but a brief report has shown that in some cases existing urinary incontinence becomes more frequent and severe (59).

Skin

- A 54-year-old woman developed melasma, macular hyperpigmentation associated with increased estrogen

states, in atypical sites after starting to take HRT; on withdrawal it began to fade (60).

Musculoskeletal

Despite the evidence that estrogens can be of value in countering osteoporosis, some studies have suggested that women who use them are more likely to have back pain than those who do not; the possible causal link has remained unclear, and continues so despite recent confirmation of the phenomenon. Baseline information on estrogen replacement therapy, functional status, back pain and function, and other variables has been obtained in 7209 elderly white American women (mean age 71 years) enrolled in a study of osteoporotic fractures; X-rays were also taken at baseline and an average of 3.7 years later (61). A total of 1039 women were using estrogen replacement therapy at baseline, 2016 reported former use, and 4154 had never used estrogen replacement therapy. Compared with never-users, a significantly higher percentage of current estrogen users reported clinical back pain (53 versus 43%) and back impairment (12 versus 9.2%) at baseline and at the follow-up visit (pain 51 versus 41; impairment 16 versus 12%). This occurred despite a higher prevalence of vertebral fractures in never-users of estrogen at the baseline visit. The increased likelihood of back pain and impairment of function in current and former estrogen users remained in evidence, despite statistical adjustment for possibly interfering factors. The relative risks for impaired back function in former and current users at follow-up were 1.1 (0.9, 1.3) and 1.6 (1.3, 2.0) respectively (62).

Reproductive system

Breasts
Two doses of transdermal estrogen, 50 and 100 micrograms/day, have been compared with placebo in preventing bone loss in postmenopausal women over 24 months (63). Bone mineral density in the lumbar spine was only marginally better with the higher dose; the slightly better effect was largely offset by a higher incidence of breast pain, reported by 8% of women on placebo, by 6% of those who took 50 micrograms/day, and by 17% of women who took 100 micrograms/day.

Uterus
It has long been recognized that periodic or irregular uterine bleeding will occur in some women using HRT. While it is simple to dismiss this merely as a reactivation of endometrial proliferation and shedding, some workers have sought to examine the precise mechanism of this unwanted complication, particularly because it might prove to be the harbinger of more serious events involving the endometrium. From recent work in the UK it has been concluded that estrogen treatment appears to alter the endometrial expression of matrix metalloprotease 9 (MMP-9) and the tissue inhibitor of metalloproteases (TIMP-1) as well as the local balance between these molecules (64). This alteration may promote breakdown of the endometrial extracellular matrix and blood vessels and hence bleeding.

There could be fairly simple ways of screening for endometrial disorders in women using HRT. A study in 93 such women has confirmed the earlier finding that if a Papanicolaou smear is taken from the vagina the presence of endometrial cells in the smear gives some (non-specific) indication that there are endometrial changes, which may range from hyperplasia or polyps to endometrial carcinoma (65).

The incidence of endometrial hyperplasia in a large series of women using different forms of HRT over 12 months has been examined (66). Subgroups each received one of six blinded norethindrone acetate + ethinylestradiol combinations (0/5 mg, 0.25/5 mg, 1/5 mg, 0/10 mg, 0.5/10 mg, or 1/10 mg) or open conjugated equine estrogens 0.625 mg with medroxyprogesterone acetate 2.5 mg. Endometrial hyperplasia, assessed by biopsy, developed in 26 subjects, 23 of these being in the subgroup who took ethinylestradiol 10 micrograms without norethindrone acetate. Norethindrone acetate thus appears to have protected the endometrium from estrogen-induced hyperplasia and changes in proliferative status. Those who took norethindrone acetate + ethinylestradiol had significantly less endometrial proliferation than those who took conjugated equine estrogens + medroxyprogesterone acetate.

Several groups have successfully used transvaginal ultrasonography to examine the state of the endometrium, although experience is still limited (67). In one series of 702 women measurements of endometrial thickness, using transvaginal ultrasound, provided a helpful but not infallible indication of those women in whom hysterectomy may be advisable; increased endometrial thickness (in excess of 4.5 mm) during HRT tends to run parallel with other endometrial abnormalities, such as polyps or endocavitary fibroids (68). In interpreting these findings it is important to bear in mind that medical and female attitudes to hysterectomy differ markedly between countries; for example, the operation is performed and accepted much more readily in the USA than in Europe.

Immunologic

Two healthy young women took estrogen supplements for some 3 years and then developed classic Sjögren's syndrome (69). The syndrome was most severe in the woman who had taken the higher dose. These cases seem to have confirmed earlier reports that estrogens can play a role in the pathogenesis of Sjögren's syndrome in susceptible patients.

Allergy to steroids of any type is unusual, but it has been reported with both corticosteroids and sex hormones, and cross-allergy can occur.

- A woman with a persistent dermatitis of the hands and feet developed multiple contact allergies to topical steroids (70). She had a past history of allergic contact dermatitis to a hormone replacement patch containing both estrogen and progesterone. Patch testing showed positive reactions to hydroxyprogesterone, progesterone, estradiol, and multiple corticosteroids.

Long-Term Effects

Drug dependence

While the effects of estrogen treatment on mental function and mood are generally assessed as positive, work in Britain has raised the possibility of some form of psychological dependence. The starting point was the finding in various studies that a proportion of women in whom hormone replacement therapy was terminated had a return of psychological symptoms, such as low mood and tiredness, despite the fact that their circulating estrogen concentrations were high. A questionnaire-based study was therefore carried out in 600 women, mean age 46 years; in most of them, HRT with implants had been undertaken after hysterectomy, and the mean duration of use was 5 years. Among those with high circulating estradiol concentrations (more than 500 pmol/l) 40% reported a need to use top-up doses of HRT to cope with daily activities, 78% spoke of low mood and tiredness (apparently when estrogen concentrations were falling), 80% experienced a "buzz" (which was undefined) 1–2 weeks after receiving a new implant, and 75% claimed that life without an implant would be "terrible." These effects, interpreted as evidence of dependence, were almost absent in women with lower circulating estrogen concentrations. The authors were of the opinion that circulating concentrations of some 300 pmol/l, which are sufficient to maintain bone mass, should be the therapeutic aim, and that there will then be much less of a dependence problem than when higher concentrations are attained (71,72).

Drug withdrawal

Sudden withdrawal of estrogen replacement therapy can result in very rapid boe loss, and patients who abandon this treatment should be carefully monitored and provided with alternative care to avoid a serious risk of fractures (73).

Mutagenicity

A finding that needs further study is that when estrogens are used for the treatment of osteoporosis they may have some genotoxic potential, as evidenced by their ability to cause an increased frequency of sister chromatid exchange (74).

Tumorigenicity

The associations between hormone replacement therapy and breast, endometrial, and ovarian cancers are discussed in the monograph on estrogens.

Susceptibility Factors

The choice of an optimal and reasonably safe dose of a hormonal product varies with race and population, at least because of variations in body weight and possibly also differences in metabolic processes. Dosage studies, for example with very low-dose estrogen treatment, must therefore of necessity be conducted in different populations. In menopausal Chinese women, a daily dose of

1 mg of estradiol has been found to be as effective as 2 mg in reducing the risk of osteoporosis (75), but it would be unwise to accept these conclusions as being valid for typical European or American women.

Age

When a young woman undergoes a surgical menopause it is clear that estrogen replacement treatment, if given at all, is likely to be needed for many years, and in the present state of knowledge this is probably justifiable, provided that the effects are monitored. The dilemma that the physician faces in such cases has been discussed in the light of a patient in whom gross obesity compounded the possible risk of thrombosis; the patient was nevertheless treated with an implant and remained well for 4 years (76).

Renal disease

Estrogen replacement therapy may have untoward effects in patients with renal disease, including an increased risk of thrombosis of dialysis access and potentially worsening of coronary artery disease, probably because the excretion of estrogens is impaired (77).

Transplantation

There is evidence that in women who have been treated with allogeneic stem cell transplantation for hematological malignancies, hormone replacement therapy may introduce particular risks. Premature ovarian failure in 30 women who were followed up in a single center 12–120 months after stem cell transplantation was treated with HRT (estrogen + progestogen) (78). Three of the women who were affected by chronic graft versus host disease (cGVHD) developed hemocolpometra after hormonal treatment. Local application of estrogens consistently improved the gynecological complication, but the vaginal synechiae tended to relapse when local treatment was interrupted, despite the apparent absence of other evidence of active cGVHD. These workers urged that all women with cGVHD should undergo gynecological examination before the introduction of HRT, in order to avoid the risk of inducing hemocolpometra. Vaginal and cervical synechiae should be treated with prolonged local treatments, and temporary use of continuous HRT regimens may be advisable. Moreover, close monitoring by pelvic examination and ultrasonography is advisable during the initial cycles to detect any complication caused by possible intrauterine adhesions undetected during gynecological examination.

Drug Administration

Drug formulations

Throughout the 40-year history of HRT efforts have been made to improve the benefit to harm balance by modifications in the pattern of drug administration. In most cases it is not clear that improved tolerance to a particular drug, when this is claimed, is due to anything other than a reduction in total dosage or circulating concentrations, although there are exceptions.

Vaginal rings

Vaginal rings loaded with estrogen and/or progestogen, as they are currently produced, provide steady delivery of the steroid over a period of up to 3 months; they have been used primarily as a means of treating menopausal symptoms. Resting on the pelvic floor muscles in a nearly horizontal position, the rings are as a rule imperceptible and cause no local symptoms. Over 5700 healthy US women who evaluated an unmedicated ring as a drug delivery platform found it very acceptable independent of age or prior use of barrier contraceptives (79). The fact that the estrogen can in this way be delivered directly into the systemic circulation is thought to result from there being less interference with the processes of coagulation and fibrinolysis than when estrogens are given transdermally. When progesterone is administered in this form, there are fewer adverse effects than with other routes of use, possibly due to lower serum concentrations of metabolites such as alloprenanolone.

Drug dosage regimens

The amount of estrogen taken during estrogen replacement is usually about one quarter of that found in oral contraceptives, and is intended to be sufficient to restore physiological amounts of endogenous estrogens. During the physiological cycle, menstrual discomfort of all types is at its mildest (and usually absent) during the mid-follicular phase when plasma estradiol concentrations are 60–150 pg/ml (80). In replacement therapy some workers seek to titrate the dose of estrogen individually in order to maintain this level, hoping thereby not only to avoid adverse effects associated with hyper- or hypo-estrogenicity but also to optimize the therapeutic effect. Strictly speaking this individualized treatment is called for because of the variability of estrogen clearance, but in normal women plasma levels are rarely measured, an approximate adaptation of dosage being undertaken purely on the basis of subjective reactions.

The variety of hormonal replacement products is considerable, and many have closely similar records as regards both efficacy and safety. The principal merit of many of them is simply that they offer alternatives—a woman who does not react well to one may fare better with another, sometimes for no apparent reason. Some of the published comparisons serve little more than promotional purposes and the basic data produced merely underline the similarity of the various products.

One study illustrates the point and is typical of many—a comparison of three sequential regimens in what is described as a randomized double-blind study; however, the 1218 women involved during the first year and the 531 subjects who continued for a further year were spread over multiple centers in eight countries, which makes valid comparisons difficult (81). The first regimen was 17-beta-estradiol 1 mg on days 1–14 and then either 17-beta-estradiol 1 mg + trimegestone 0.125 mg or 17-beta-estradiol 1 mg + trimegestone 0.25 mg on days 15–28.

The second regimen was estradiol valerate 1 mg on days 1–16 and then estradiol valerate 1 mg + norethisterone 1 mg on days 17–28. The authors thought that the bleeding profile was more favorable with 17-beta-estradiol 1 mg + trimegestone 0.25 mg than with the lower dose of trimegestone. However, both of the trimegestone regimens had a good protective effect on endometrial proliferation, and the higher dose had a lower incidence of proliferative endometrium with an overall favorable bleeding profile. The mean percentage of women who reported withdrawal bleeding during the week after withdrawal of progestogen was higher with 17-beta-estradiol 1 mg + trimegestone 0.25 mg, which had a more efficient progestogen effect on the endometrium and good predictability of bleeding. Although the authors expressed a preference for one product, the data showed that the mean numbers and average lengths of bleeding episodes were similar in the three groups.

There is no benefit and sometimes a disadvantage to giving estrogen alone for only 25 days a month; in particular, estrogen withdrawal symptoms such as decreased well being, headaches, and hot flushes can occur each time the treatment is interrupted.

It is widely recommended that estrogen replacement therapy, if it is to be used at all, should be initiated at the time of menopause or within 3 years of it, since it is at this time that bone loss can be most severe. Many physicians go on to argue that once it has been started hormonal replacement therapy should continue for at least 20 years and perhaps indefinitely, in view of evidence that withdrawal may be followed by accelerated bone loss, at least comparable to that observed after the menopause. Later use of estrogen, once bone has already been lost, does not result in appreciable recovery of bone, although further loss can still be prevented. Large comparative studies have suggested that a series of alternative regimens for hormone replacement therapy should be available, so that for each individual woman the most appropriate form of treatment can be chosen; no one regimen is ideal for all, and finding the best approach for a given patient may be a matter of trial and error (82).

For the acute treatment of climacteric vasomotor symptoms it seems clear that micronized 17-beta-estradiol in a dose as low as 0.25 mg can be sufficient; however, a starting dose of 1 mg is advisable, with subsequent adjustments as necessary. At a dose of 2 mg the proportion of women who withdraw from treatment with the active product because of adverse effects was twice that seen with placebo (83). To provide longer-term protection against early postmenopausal bone loss, treatment with estradiol in a dose of 1 mg/day, balanced by a progestogen, is adequate (84). Most workers believe that the estrogen is best counterbalanced by a progestogen when used in the long term, but here there is still some disagreement about the doses needed.

Drug administration route

Transdermal administration

The oft-repeated hypothesis that transdermal hormone therapy might be safer than oral treatment in equivalent doses has been put to the test in several studies. It seems possible that certain effects of estrogens will vary with the route of administration because of first-pass metabolism in the liver. On the other hand, when comparing the effects of oral and transdermal treatment one has to be sure that the concentrations reaching the system by the two routes are truly therapeutically equivalent before one can draw any conclusion regarding such a dissociation of effect. The various forms of transdermal hormone formulations have been reviewed (85). The authors concluded that while the transdermal route offers various practical advantages, adverse effects are about the same as with oral products.

Oral post-menopausal estrogen replacement therapy increases circulating concentrations of C-reactive protein, but in 68 women who took a combination of transdermal 17-beta-estradiol and micronized progesterone there was no significant effect of transdermal estrogen on C-reactive protein concentrations compared with placebo (86).

Another study, in the Netherlands, looked primarily at effects of various types and routes of replacement therapy on the hemostatic variables associated with venous thrombosis (87). In a double-blind, randomized, placebo-controlled study, 152 healthy hysterectomized postmenopausal women received 13 monthly cycles of placebo, transdermal 17-beta estradiol (50 micrograms/day), oral estradiol 1 mg, or a combination of oral estradiol + gestodene 25 micrograms/day. In all the actively treated groups, there were increases in resistance to activated protein C, which were more marked in those who took oral treatment. The effect was not explained by changes in protein S, protein C, or prothrombin, but it could contribute to the increased incidence of venous thrombosis in users of hormone replacement therapy. This is not the first study in which increases in activated protein C have been observed with HRT; they seem to occur irrespective of the progestogen used. However, these new results contrast with some earlier work in which transdermal estradiol was actually claimed to reduce resistance to activated protein C, an effect that might be favourable as regards clotting.

There is other evidence that transdermal estrogen replacement therapy has relatively little effect on hemostasis. In a case control study, 155 consecutive patients with a first documented episode of idiopathic venous thromboembolism, 92 of whom had had a pulmonary embolism and 63 a deep venous thrombosis, were compared with 381 healthy matched controls (88). Overall, 32 (21%) of the cases and 27 (7%) of the controls were current users of oral estrogen replacement therapy, whereas 30 (19%) cases and 93 (24%) controls were current users of transdermal estrogen replacement therapy. After adjustment for potential confounding variables, the odds ratios for venous thromboembolism in current users of oral and transdermal estrogen replacement therapy compared with non-users were 3.5 (95% CI = 1.8, 6.8) and 0.9 (0.5, 1.6) respectively. Estimated risk for venous thromboembolism in current users of oral estrogen replacement therapy compared with transdermal users was 4.0 (1.9, 8.3).

Because C-reactive protein is synthesized in the liver, It has been hypothesized that the estrogen-induced rise in

C-reactive protein is related to first-pass hepatic metabolism (89). In a randomized, crossover, placebo-controlled study in 21 postmenopausal women, transdermal estradiol had no effect on C-reactive protein or on concentrations of the anti-inflammatory growth factor IGF-1, whereas oral conjugated estrogens for 8 weeks caused a more than two-fold increase in C-reactive protein and a significant reduction in IGF-1. The magnitude of increase in C-reactive protein was inversely correlated to the fall in IGF-1. Neither transdermal estradiol nor oral conjugated estrogens had any effects on the plasma concentrations of cytokines that promote the synthesis of C-reactive protein. The authors concluded that in postmenopausal women, oral but not transdermal estrogen increased C-reactive protein by a first-pass hepatic effect. Because C-reactive protein is a powerful predictor of an adverse prognosis in otherwise healthy postmenopausal women, they considered that the route of administration may be an important consideration in minimizing the adverse effects of estrogens on cardiovascular outcomes.

In 35 postmenopausal women who had been amenorrheic for at least 1 year, two consecutive 2-month courses of transdermal estrogen (estradiol patches 25 micrograms and 50 micrograms) were randomly followed by a 2-month course of treatment with either an estradiol patch 100 micrograms/day or an estradiol patch 50 micrograms/day combined with either progesterone 300 mg/day or medroxyprogesterone acetate 5 mg/day during the last 14 days (90). Neither transdermal estradiol alone nor transdermal estradiol plus progestogen altered the lipoprotein profile, LDL resistance to oxidation, or LDL particle size. However, all treatments similarly reduced myeloperoxidase protein concentrations.

In a case-control study 155 postmenopausal women who had had venous thromboembolism were compared with 381 matched controls (91). In all, 32 cases and 27 controls were current users of oral replacement therapy, whereas 30 cases and 93 controls were current users of transdermal products. After adjustment for potential confounding variables, the estimated risk ratio for venous thromboembolism in current users of the oral products compared with the transdermal users was 4.0 (1.9–8.3). This is strong evidence that the transdermal route was considerably safer. However, the conclusions of different studies continue to conflict with one another, no doubt in part because of variations in the formulations and patterns of use of the products.

There is some evidence that in women with osteoporosis an increase in bone density can be obtained by giving estrogens transdermally in such low doses that there is little risk of endometrial hyperplasia (92).

Pulsed intranasal therapy

"Pulsed" (i.e. intermittent) estrogen treatment, given by the intranasal route, has been examined as a means of reducing the risk or rate of postmenopausal bone loss and hence osteoporosis. In a 2-year randomized, placebo-controlled study, in 386 women, hysterectomized patients received 17-beta-estradiol, 150 or 300 micrograms/day for 2 years, and women with an intact uterus received micronized progesterone 200 mg/day over 14 days of each 28-day cycle (93). Bone marrow density, measured at two sites, increased significantly in women who used the active treatment in a dose-related manner, the differences compared with placebo were 5.2% and 6.7% at the spine and 3.2% and 4.7% at the hip with 150 and 300 micrograms/day respectively. On the other hand, there were reductions versus baseline of −3.2% and −3.3% at the spine and hip respectively in women who took placebo. In the patients with at least one risk factor for osteoporotic fractures, the difference between placebo and estradiol was even higher. Tolerance was good in all cases.

One would wish to see a side-by-side comparison of this and other routes and patterns of estrogen use before concluding whether there is indeed any dissociation of wanted and unwanted effects; in view of current concern regarding estrogen use after the menopause, comparisons with non-hormonal treatment for osteoporosis (e.g. alendronate) would also be desirable.

Intrauterine administration

The effects of the Fibroplant intrauterine device, which releases some 14 micrograms/day of levonorgestrel and is given alongside estrogen therapy, have been evaluated in an open study over 3 years in 150 perimenopausal and postmenopausal women, most of whom also took an estimated 1.5 mg of estradiol, released from a percutaneous administration form (94). In all, 132 women (88%) were satisfied with the treatment and wanted to have a further intrauterine device inserted at the end of the study. Histological examination of endometrial biopsies from 101 women showed a predominantly inactive endometrium characterized by a pseudodecidual reaction of the endometrial stroma with endometrial atrophy, which is in keeping with the effects seen with progestogens. No specimens showed signs of proliferation. While one can accept this as evidence that the Fibroplant device is an acceptable means of administering levonorgestrel for hormone replacement therapy, one is bound to question the authors' further conclusion that it is less likely than other forms of administration to produce such systemic adverse effects as those involving the breast and cardiovascular system; it is hard to see how this could be so.

Drug–Drug Interactions

Dexamfetamine

Preclinical studies (as well as anecdotal clinical reports in the course of the years) seem to show that estrogens, through their effects on the central nervous system, can affect behavioral responses to psychoactive drugs. In an unusual crossover study, the subjective and physiological effects of oral dexamfetamine 10 mg have been assessed after pretreatment with estradiol (95). One group of healthy young women used estradiol patches (Estraderm TTS, total dose 0.8 mg), which raised plasma estradiol concentrations to about 750 pg/ml, and a control group used placebo patches. Most of the subjective and physiological effects of dexamfetamine were not affected by acute estradiol treatment, but the estrogen did increase the magnitude of the effect of dexamfetamine on subjective ratings of "pleasant stimulation" and reduced ratings of "want more." Estradiol also produced some subjective effects when used alone, raising ratings of "feel drug," "energy and intellectual efficiency," and "pleasant stimulation."

Food-Drug Interactions

It has sometimes been suspected that food might interfere sufficiently with the availability of progestogen + estrogen combinations, especially low-dose formulations, to impair the effects of treatment. One crossover study in 18 women taking a low-dose combination (containing norethindrone acetate 1 mg and ethinylestradiol 10 micrograms) showed that a single high-fat meal, while changing the absorption pattern, did not affect it to a sufficient degree to interfere with the effects of the combination (96).

References

1. Turner RT, Riggs BL, Spelsberg TC. Skeletal effects of estrogen. Endocr Rev 1994;15(3):275–300.
2. Grey AB, Cundy TF, Reid IR. Continuous combined oestrogen/progestin therapy is well tolerated and increases bone density at the hip and spine in post-menopausal osteoporosis. Clin Endocrinol (Oxf) 1994;40(5):671–7.
3. Barrett-Connor E, Stuenkel CA. Hormone replacement therapy (HRT)—risks and benefits. Int J Epidemiol 2001;30(3):423–6.
4. Ylikorkala O. Balancing between observational studies and randomized trials in prevention of coronary heart disease by estrogen replacement: HERS study was no revolution. Acta Obstet Gynecol Scand 2000;79(12):1029–36.
5. Lloyd G. Hormone replacement therapy and ischaemic heart disease: continuing questions but still no answers. Int J Clin Pract 2000;54(7):416–7.
6. Steiner MK, Clarkson PB, Lip GY. Myocardial infarction complicating hormone replacement therapy in a young woman with normal coronary arteries. Int J Clin Pract 2000;54(7):475–7.
7. MacLennan A, Lester S, Moore V. Oral estrogen replacement therapy versus placebo for hot flushes: a systematic review. Climacteric 2001;4(1):58–74.
8. Kaweski S; Plastic Surgery Educational Foundation DATA Committee. Anti-aging medicine. Part I. Hormone replacement therapy in women. Plast Reconstr Surg 2003;111:935–8.
9. Gabriel-Cox K. Hormone replacement therapy and primary prevention: alas, again. Prev Cardiol 2003;6:61–2.
10. Michels KB, Manson JE. Postmenopausal hormone therapy: a reversal of fortune. Circulation 2003;107:1830–3.
11. Grady D Postmenopausal hormones—therapy for symptoms only. New Engl J Med 2003;348:1835–7.
12. Cranney A, Wells GA. Hormone replacement therapy for postmenopausal osteoporosis. Clin Geriatr Med 2003;19:361–70.
13. MacLennan AH, Sturdee D. Is hormone therapy still an option for the management of osteoporosis? Climacteric 2003;6:89–91.
14. Lawton B, Rose S, McLeod D, Dowell A. Changes in use of hormone replacement therapy after the report from the Women's Health Initiative: cross sectional survey of users. BMJ 2003;327:845–6.
15. La Vecchia C. Menopause, hormone therapy and breast cancer risk. Eur J Cancer Prev 2003;12:437–8.
16. Verhaeghe J. Turbulent times for hormone replacement therapy: is there a way out? Gynecol Obstet Invest 2003;56:43–50.
17. Sanada M, Higashi Y, Nakagawa K, Tsuda M, Kodama I, Kimura M, Chayama K, Ohama K. A comparison of low-dose and standard-dose oral estrogen on forearm endothelial function in early postmenopausal women. J Clin Endocrinol Metab 2003;88:1303–9.
18. Beral V. Breast cancer and hormone-replacement therapy in the Million Women Study. Lancet 2003;362:419–27.
19. Gambacciani M, Genzzani AR. The study with a million women (and hopefully fewer mistakes). Gynecol Endocrinol 2003;17:359–62.
20. Hendrix SL. Menopausal hormone therapy informed consent. Am J Obstet Gynecol 2003;189:S31-2; discussion S32–6.
21. Hersh AL, Stefanick ML, Stafford RS. National use of postmenopausal hormone therapy: annual trends and response to recent evidence. JAMA 2004;291:47–53.
22. Levgur M. Estrogen and combined hormone therapy for women after genital malignancies: a review. J Reprod Med 2004;49(10):837–48.
23. Corrado F, D'Anna R, Caputo F, Cannata ML, Zoccali MG, Cancellieri F. Compliance with hormone replacement therapy in postmenopausal Sicilian women. Eur J Obstet Gynecol Reprod Biol 2005;118:225–8.
24. Takahashi K, Manabe A, Okada M, Kurioka H, Kanasaki H, Miyazaki K. Efficacy and safety of oral estriol for managing postmenopausal symptoms. Maturitas 2000;34(2):169–77.
25. Takahashi K, Okada M, Ozaki T, Kurioka H, Manabe A, Kanasaki H, Miyazaki K. Safety and efficacy of oestriol for symptoms of natural or surgically induced menopause. Hum Reprod 2000;15(5):1028–36.
26. Itoi H, Minakami H, Iwasaki R, Sato I. Comparison of the long-term effects of oral estriol with the effects of conjugated estrogen on serum lipid profile in early menopausal women. Maturitas 2000;36(3):217–22.
27. Saure A, Planellas J, Poulsen HK, Jaszczak P. A double-blind, randomized, comparative study evaluating clinical effects of two sequential estradiol–progestogen combinations containing either desogestrel or medroxyprogesterone acetate in climacteric women. Maturitas 2000;34(2):133–42.
28. Burch D, Bieshuevel E, Smith S, Fox H. Can endometrial protection be inferred from the bleeding pattern on combined cyclical hormone replacement therapy. Maturitas 2000;34(2):155–60.
29. Col NF, Weber G, Stiggelbout A, Chuo J, D'Agostino R, Corso P. Short-term menopausal hormone therapy for symptom relief: an updated decision model. Arch Int Med 2004;164:1634–40.
30. Petitti D. Hormone replacement therapy and coronary heart disease: four lessons. Int J Epidemiol 2004;33:461–3.
31. Lawlor DA, Smith GD, Ebrahim S. The hormone replacement–coronary heart disease conundrum: is this the death of observational epidemiology? Int J Epdemiol 2004;33:464–7.
32. Mackey R.H, Kuller L.H, Sutton-Tyrrell K, Evans R.W, Holubkov R, Matthews K.A. Hormone therapy, lipoprotein subclasses, and coronary calcification: The Healthy Women Study. Arch Int Med 2005;165:510–5.
33. Rossouw JE. Hormone replacement therapy and cardiovascular disease. Curr Opin Lipidol 1999;10(5):429–34.

34. Whiteman MK, Cui Y, Flaws JA, Espeland M, Bush TL. Low fibrinogen level: A predisposing factor for venous thromboembolic events with hormone replacement therapy. Am J Hematol 1999;61(4):271–3.

35. Hoibraaten E, Abdelnoor M, Sandset PM. Hormone replacement therapy with estradiol and risk of venous thromboembolism—a population-based case-control study. Thromb Haemost 1999;82(4):1218–21.

36. Cahill M, O'Toole L, Acheson RW. Hormone replacement therapy and retinal vein occlusion. Eye 1999;13(Pt 6):798–800.

37. Carnethon MR, Anthony MS, Cascio WE, Folsom AR, Rautaharju PM, Liao D, Evans GW, Heiss G. A prospective evaluation of the risk of QT prolongation with hormone replacement therapy: the atherosclerosis risk in communities study. Ann Epidemiol 2003;13:530–6.

38. Gokce M, Karahan B, Yilmaz R, Orem C, Erdol C, Ozdemir S. Long term effects of hormone replacement therapy on heart rate variability, QT interval, QT dispersion and frequencies of arrhythmia. Int J Cardiol 2005;99:373–9.

39. Barr RG, Wentowski CC, Grodstein F, Somers SC, Stampfer MJ, Schwartz J, Speizer FE, Camargo CA Jr. Prospective study of postmenopausal hormone use and newly diagnosed asthma and chronic obstructive pulmonary disease. Arch Int Med 2004;164:379–86.

40. Fernandes LH, Scassellati-Sforzolini B, Spaide RF. Estrogen and visual hallucinations in a patient with Charles Bonnet syndrome. Am J Ophthalmol 2000;129(3):407.

41. Nappi RE, Cagnacci A, Granella F, Piccinini F, Polatti F, Facchinetti F. Course of primary headaches during hormone replacement therapy. Maturitas 2001;38(2):157–63.

42. Schaumberg DA, Buring JE, Sullivan DA, Dana MR. Hormone replacement therapy and dry eye syndrome. JAMA 2001;286(17):2114–9.

43. Barney NP. Can hormone replacement therapy cause dry eye? Arch Ophthalmol 2002;120(5):641–2.

44. Wihlback A-C, Nyberg S, Backstrom T, Bixo M, Sundstrom-Poromaa I. Estradiol and the addition of progesterone increase the sensitivity to a neurosteroid in postmenopausal women. Psychoneuroendocrinology 2005;30:38–50.

45. Godsland IF. Effects of postmenopausal hormone replacement therapy on lipid, lipoprotein, and apolipoprotein (a) concentrations: analysis of studies published from 1974–2000. Fertil Steril 2001;75(5):898–915.

46. Goldenberg NM, Wang P, Glueck CJ. An observational study of severe hypertriglyceridemia, hypertriglyceridemic acute pancreatitis, and failure of triglyceride-lowering therapy when estrogens are given to women with and without familial hypertriglyceridemia. Clin Chim Acta 2003;332:11–19.

47. Vrbikova J, Stanicka S, Dvorakova K, Hill M, Vondra K, Bendlova B, Starka L. Metabolic and endocrine effects of treatment with peroral or transdermal oestrogens in conjuction with peroral cyproterone acetate in women with polycystic ovary syndrome. Eur J Endocrinol 2004;150:215–23.

48. Anderson EJ, Lavoie HB, Strauss CC, Hubbard JL, Sharpless JL, Hall JE. Body composition and energy balance: lack of effect of short-term hormone replacement in postmenopausal women. Metabolism 2001;50(3):265–9.

49. de Valk-de Roo GW, Stehouwer CD, Emeis JJ, Nicolaas-Merkus A, Netelenbos C. Unopposed estrogen increases total plasma factor VII, but not active factor VII—a short-term placebo-controlled study in healthy postmenopausal women. Thromb Haemost 2000;84(6):968–72.

50. Rosendaal FR, Helmerhorst FM, Vandenbroucke JP. Oral contraceptives, hormone replacement therapy and thrombosis. Thromb Haemost 2001;86(1):112–23.

51. Cushman M, Psaty BM, Meilahn EN, Dobs AS, Kuller LH. Post-menopausal hormone therapy and concentrations of protein C and antithrombin in elderly women. Br J Haematol 2001;114(1):162–8.

52. Petit L, Alhenc-Gelas M, Aiach M, Scarabin PY. Hormone replacement therapy of the menopause and haemostasis. Sang Thromb Vaiss 2002;14:32–8.

53. Borgfeldt C, Li C, Samsioe G. Low-dose oral combination of 17beta-estradiol and norethisterone acetate in postmenopausal women decreases factor VII, fibrinogen, antithrombin and plasminogen activator inhibitor-1. Climacteric 2004;7:78–85.

54. Oliveira RLS, Aldrighi JM, Gebara OE, Rocha TRF, D'Amico E, Rosano GMC, Ramires JAF. Postmenopausal hormone replacement therapy increases plasmatic thromboxane beta2. Int J Cardiol. 2005;99:449–54.

55. Sumino H, Ichikawa S, Sawada Y, Sakamoto H, Kumakura H, Takayama Y, Sakamaki T, Kurabayashi M. Effects of hormone replacement therapy on blood coagulation and fibrinolysis in hypertensive and normotensive postmenopausal women. Thromb Res 2005;115:359–66.

56. Ruigomez A, Garcia Rodriguez LA, Johansson S, Wallander M-A. Is hormone replacement therapy associated with an increased risk of irritable bowel syndrome? Maturitas 2003;44:133–40.

57. Dhiman RK, Sarkar PK, Sharma A, Vasishta K, Kohli KK, Gupta S, Suri S, Chawla Y. Alterations in gallbladder emptying and bile retention in the absence of changes in bile lithogenicity in postmenopausal women on hormone replacement therapy. Dig Dis Sci 2004;49:1335–41.

58. Monster TB, Janssen WM, de Jong PE, de Jong-van den Berg LTPrevention of Renal Vascular End Stage Disease Study Group. Oral contraceptive use and hormone replacement therapy are associated with microalbuminuria. Arch Intern Med 2001;161(16):2000–5.

59. Hendrix SL, Cochrane BB, Nygaard IE, Handa VL, Barnabei VM, Iglesia C, Aragaki A, Naughton MJ, Wallace RB, McNeeley SG, Waetjen LE. Estrogen therapy increased the incidence and severity of urinary incontinence symptoms in postmenopausal women. Evid Based Obstet Gynec 2005;7:149–50.

60. Covic A, Goldsmith DJ, Segall L, Stoicescu C, Lungu S, Volovat C, Covic M. Rifampicin-induced acute renal failure: a series of 60 patients. Nephrol Dial Transplant 1998;13(4):924–9.

61. Musgrave DS, Vogt MT, Nevitt MC, Cauley JA. Back problems among postmenopausal women taking estrogen replacement therapy: the study of osteoporotic fractures. Spine 2001;26(14):1606–12.

62. Symmons DP, van Hemert AM, Vandenbroucke JP, Valkenburg HA. A longitudinal study of back pain and radiological changes in the lumbar spines of middle aged women. I. Clinical findings. Ann Rheum Dis 1991;50(3):158–61.

63. Arrenbrecht S, Boermans AJ. Effects of transdermal estradiol delivered by a matrix patch on bone density in hysterectomized, postmenopausal women: a 2-year placebo-controlled trial. Osteoporos Int 2002;13(2):176–83.

64. Hickey M, Higham J, Sullivan M, Miles L, Fraser IS. Endometrial bleeding in hormone replacement therapy users: preliminary findings regarding the role of matrix metalloproteinase 9 (MMP-9) and tissue inhibitors of MMPs. Fertil Steril 2001;75(2):288–96.

65. Montz FJ. Significance of "normal" endometrial cells in cervical cytology from asymptomatic postmenopausal women receiving hormone replacement therapy. Gynecol Oncol 2001;81(1):33–9.

66. Portman DJ, Symons JP, Wilborn W, Kempfert NJ. A randomized, double-blind, placebo-controlled, multicenter study that assessed the endometrial effects of norethindrone acetate plus ethinyl estradiol versus ethinyl estradiol alone. Am J Obstet Gynecol 2003;188:334–42.

67. Ferrazzi E, Leone FPG. Investigating abnormal bleeding on HRT or tamoxifen: the role of ultrasonography. Best Pract Res Clin Obst Gynaecol 2004;18:145–56.

68. Omodei U, Ferrazzi E, Ramazzotto F, Becorpi A, Grimaldi E, Scarselli G, Spagnolo D, Spagnolo L, Torri W. Endometrial evaluation with transvaginal ultrasound during hormone therapy: a prospective multicenter study. Fertil Steril 2004;81:1632–7.

69. Nagler RM, Pollack S. Sjögren's syndrome induced by estrogen therapy. Semin Arthritis Rheum 2000;30(3):209–14.

70. Lamb SR, Wilkinson SM. Contact allergy to progesterone and estradiol in a patient with multiple corticosteroid allergies. Dermatitis 2004;15:78–81.

71. O'Leary A, Bowen-Simpkins P, Tejura H, Rajesh U. Are high levels of oestradiol after implants associated with features of dependence? Br J Obstet Gynaecol 1999;106(9):960–3.

72. Bewley S, Granleese J. Repeat oestradiol implants: features of dependence? J Obstet Gynaecol 1999;19(2):190–1.

73. Miller E. Therapeutic options: an evidence-based approach to prevention and treatment of osteoporosis. Int J Fertil Women's Med 2003;48:122–6.

74. Sahin FI, Sahin I, Ergun MA, Saracoglu OF. Effects of estrogen and alendronate on sister chromatid exchange (SCE) frequencies in postmenopausal osteoporosis patients. Int J Gynaecol Obstet 2000;71(1):49–52.

75. Haines CJ, Yim SF, Chung TKH, Lam CWK, Lau EWC, Ng MHL, Chin R, Lee DTS. A prospective, randomized, placebo-controlled study of the dose effect of oral estradiol on bone mineral density in postmenopausal Chinese women. Maturitas 2003;45:169–73.

76. Ewies AAA, Olah KSJ. Endometrial adenocarcinoma treated by hysterectomy and bilateral salpingo-oophorectomy at age 22-the dilemma of long-term HRT. J Obstet Gynaecol 2000;20:639–40.

77. Mattix H, Singh AK. Estrogen replacement therapy: implications for postmenopausal women with end-stage renal disease. Curr Opin Nephrol Hypertens 2000;9(3):207–14.

78. Tauchmanova L, Selleri C, Di Carlo C, De Rosa G, Bifulco G, Sammartino A, Lombardi G, Colao A, Rotoli B, Nappi C. Estrogen–progestogen induced hematocolpometra following allogeneic stem cell transplant. Gynecol Oncol 2004;93:112–5.

79. Ballagh SA. Vaginal rings for menopausal symptom relief. Drugs Aging 2004;21:757–66.

80. de Lignieres B. Hormone replacement therapy: clinical benefits and side-effects. Maturitas 1996;23(Suppl):S31–6.

81. Koninckx PR, Spielmann D. A comparative 2-year study of the effects of sequential regimens of 1 mg 17-beta-estradiol and trimegestone with a regimen containing estradiol valerate and norethisterone on the bleeding profile and endometrial safety in postmenopausal women. Gynecol Endocrinol 2005;21:82–9.

82. Heikkinen JE, Vaheri RT, Ahomaki SM, Kainulainen PM, Viitanen AT, Timonen UM. Optimizing continuous-combined hormone replacement therapy for postmenopausal women: a comparison of six different treatment regimens. Am J Obstet Gynecol 2000;182(3):560–7.

83. Notelovitz M, Lenihan JP, McDermott M, Kerber IJ, Nanavati N, Arce J. Initial 17beta-estradiol dose for treating vasomotor symptoms. Obstet Gynecol 2000;95(5):726–31.

84. Bjarnason NH, Byrjalsen I, Hassager C, Haarbo J, Christiansen C. Low doses of estradiol in combination with gestodene to prevent early postmenopausal bone loss. Am J Obstet Gynecol 2000;183(3):550–60.

85. Henzl MR, Loomba PK. Transdermal delivery of sex steroids for hormone replacement therapy and contraception: a review of principles and practice. Reprod Med 2003;48:525–40.

86. Lacut K, Oger E, Le Gal G, Blouch M-T, Abgrall J-F, Kerlan V, Scarabin P-Y, Mottier D. Differential effects of oral and transdermal postmenopausal estrogen replacement therapies on C-reactive protein. Thromb Haemost 2003;90:124–31.

87. Post MS, Thomassen MCLGD, Van der Mooren M.J, Van Baal WM, Rosing J, Kenemans P, Stehouwer CDA. Effect of oral and transdermal estrogen replacement therapy on hemostatic variables associated with venous thrombosis: a randomized, placebo-controlled study in postmenopausal women. Arterioscl Thromb Vasc Biol 2003;23:1116–21.

88. Scarabin PY, Oger E, Plu-Bureau G. Differential association of oral and transdermal oestrogen-replacement therapy with venous thromboembolism risk. Lancet 2003;362:428–32.

89. Vongpatanasin W, Tuncel M, Wang Z, Arbique D, Mehrad B, Jialal I. Differential effects of oral versus transdermal estrogen replacement therapy on C-reactive protein in postmenopausal women. J Am Coll Cardiol 2003;41:1358–63.

90. Hermenegildo C, Garcia-Martinez MC, Valldecabres C, Tarin JJ, Cano A. Transdermal estradiol reduces plasma myeloperoxidase levels without affecting the LDL resistance to oxidation or the LDL particle size. Menopause 2002;9(2):102–9.

91. Scarabin PY, Oger E, Plu-Bureau GEStrogen and THromboEmbolism Risk Study Group. Differential association of oral and transdermal oestrogen-replacement therapy with venous thromboembolism risk. Lancet 2003;362(9382):428–32.

92. Ettinger B, Ensrud KE, Wallace R, Johnson KC, Cummings SR, Yankov V, Vittinghoff E, Grady D, Ravn P. Ultralow-dose transdermal estradiol increased bone mineral density, with a low rate of endometrial hyperplasia. Evid Based Obstet Gynecol 2005;7:162–3.

93. Nielsen TF, Ravn P, Bagger YZ, Warming L, Christiansen C. Pulsed estrogen therapy in prevention of postmenopausal osteoporosis: a 2-year randomized, double blind, placebo-controlled study. Osteoporos Int 2004;15:168–74.

94. Wildemeersch D, Janssens D, Schacht E, Pylyser K, De Wever N. Intrauterine levonorgestrel delivered by a frameless system, combined with systemic estrogen: acceptability and endometrial safety after 3 years of use in peri- and postmenopausal women. Gynecol Endocrinol 2005;20:336–42.

95. Justice AJ, de Wit H. Acute effects of estradiol pretreatment on the response to d-amphetamine in women. Neuroendocrinology 2000;71(1):51–9.

96. Boyd RA, Zegarac EA, Eldon MA. The effect of food on the bioavailability of norethindrone and ethinyl estradiol from norethindrone acetate/ethinyl estradiol tablets intended for continuous hormone replacement therapy. J Clin Pharmacol 2003;43:52–8.

Hormonal replacement therapy— estrogens + androgens

General Information

For a complete account of the adverse effects of estrogens, readers should consult the following monographs as well as this one:

- Diethylstilbestrol
- Estrogens
- Hormonal contraceptives—emergency contraception
- Hormonal contraceptives—oral
- Hormone replacement therapy—estrogens
- Hormone replacement therapy—estrogens + progestogens.

An estrogen + an androgen

This variant on the theme of estrogen replacement therapy has been propagated from various centers for different reasons (1,2).

The theoretical starting point is the observation that (particularly after oophorectomy) there are deficiencies of both testosterone and androstenedione (3) and from the observation that estrogens alone do not relieve all menopausal symptoms. While there may well be justification for androgen replacement after oophorectomy, it is not clear that most of the claims made for use of this approach following a natural menopause are sufficiently well founded to justify the risks involved.

Adding an androgen to estrogen replacement therapy in the menopause has been thought to provide supplementary benefit with respect to climacteric symptoms, fatigue, and impaired libido, as well as favorably affecting muscle mass, skin quality, and bone density. It is also stated that androgens improve relief of vasomotor symptoms and relieve depression and anxiety when they occur after the menopause in this group of patients. Some workers have concluded that in women who respond to conjugated estrogens with a rise in blood pressure (not a common response by any means), this effect could be avoided by the addition of an androgen. Yet others have asserted that when the hematocrit falls during estrogen therapy, the effect can be prevented by an androgen.

The main reason for caution with the use of androgens is the susceptibility of menopausal women to their virilizing effects, which can sometimes prove irreversible. Deepening of the voice, hirsutism, and acne can occur in many patients at an early stage of treatment and can prove distressing. There may be enlargement of the clitoris, although not consistently.

However, there are other reasons for caution. Statements with respect to the effect of estrogen + androgen combinations on blood lipids are, for example, contradictory, depending on the combinations used. If androgens are to be used, the effect on lipoproteins should at all events be monitored (1).

It is doubtful whether one can avoid unwanted androgenic effects by cautious dosing. For example, the published data seem to show that a desired effect on libido is only likely to occur at androgen doses sufficient to produce serum testosterone concentrations in the virilizing range (over 2 ng/ml), and that even after withdrawal of such doses virilizing concentrations of testosterone are maintained for many months.

Finally, androgens actually appear in some respects to counter the desired effects of estrogens in this patient group. Doppler flowmetry has been used to study the cardiovascular effects of adding an androgen to an estrogen in an open, randomized study in 40 patients over 8 months, all of whom were using transdermal estradiol (50 micrograms/day) and cyclic medroxyprogesterone acetate (10 mg/day) (4). Half of the subjects then received additional testosterone undecanoate (40 mg/day). The investigators concluded that while the androgen improved sexual desire and satisfaction and had no effect on endometrial thickness, it did in part counteract the beneficial effects of the estrogens on cerebral vascular activity and lipids. The most notable change was a significant increase in the pulsatility index of the middle cerebral artery. The androgen also resulted in a 10% reduction in HDL cholesterol concentration within 8 months. The authors therefore urged caution in using androgens, at least in the manner used in this study.

There are naturally some groups that have worked together with manufacturers to profile the supposed advantages of particular estrogen + androgen regimens, especially when these are available in the form of fixed combination formulations.

The adverse effects of estrogen + androgen therapy include mild hirsutism and acne (5). One group of workers, who examined the use of "Estratest" (an esterified combination of estrogen and methyltestosterone), concluded that in their experience under 5% of women developed acne or facial hirsutism, a frequency similar to that experienced when using conjugated estrogens 0.625 mg/day. Women had significantly less nausea with the estrogen + androgen treatment than with conjugated estrogen therapy. Cancers, cardiovascular disease, thromboembolism, and liver disease were stated to be rare among users of the combination. The only adverse events exceeding 4% of total reports were alopecia, acne, weight gain, and hirsutism (6). However, much higher rates of complications with such combinations have been reported from other centres (1).

The evident disadvantage of a fixed combination is that it renders it impossible to carry out any fine adjustment of dosages, such as might be called for in the light of the clinical response and adverse effects in a given individual.

All in all, it seems very doubtful whether any of the supposed benefits of androgen therapy justify the risks involved, except possibly as a transitional measure in those recently oophorectomized women who have acute symptoms of sudden androgen withdrawal.

An estrogen + an androgen + a progestogen

Another variant on hormone replacement therapy involves using all three types of sex steroid in parallel, starting from the argument that during the fertile period all three are synthesized by the ovary (7). A "natural" version of this therapy uses estradiol, testosterone (with or without dehydroepiandrosterone), and progesterone in an appropriate pharmaceutical form (for example micronized), so that absorption is attained without the need for 17-substitution. This approach naturally avoids some of the undesirable effects of the synthetic steroids, and has been stated to improve menopausal depression and anxiety. However, the adverse effects of all three types of component can be experienced.

References

1. Kaunitz AM. The role of androgens in menopausal hormonal replacement. Endocrinol Metab Clin North Am 1997;26(2):391–7.
2. Casson PR, Carson SA. Androgen replacement therapy in women: myths and realities. Int J Fertil Menopausal Stud 1996;41(4):412–22.
3. Davis S. Testosterone deficiency in women. J Reprod Med 2001;46(Suppl 3):291–6.
4. Penotti M, Sironi L, Cannata L, Vigano P, Casini A, Gabrielli L, Vignali M. Effects of androgen supplementation of hormone replacement therapy on the vascular reactivity of cerebral arteries. Fertil Steril 2001;76(2):235–40.
5. Cameron DR, Braunstein GD. Androgen replacement therapy in women. Fertil Steril 2004;82(2):273–89.
6. Barrett-Connor E. Efficacy and safety of estrogen/androgen therapy. Menopausal symptoms, bone, and cardiovascular parameters. J Reprod Med 1998;43(Suppl 8):746–52.
7. Hargrove JT, Osteen KG. An alternative method of hormone replacement therapy using the natural sex steroids. Infert Reprod Med Clin North Am 1995;6:653–74.

Hormone replacement therapy—estrogens + progestogens

General Information

For a complete account of the adverse effects of estrogens, readers should consult the following monographs as well as this one:

- Diethylstilbestrol
- Estrogens
- Hormonal contraceptives—emergency contraception
- Hormonal contraceptives—oral
- Hormone replacement therapy—estrogens
- Hormone replacement therapy—estrogens + androgens.

For a complete account of the adverse effects of progestogens, readers should consult the following monographs as well as this one:

- Hormonal contraceptives—intracervical and intravaginal
- Hormonal contraceptives—oral
- Hormonal contraceptives—progestogen implants
- Hormonal contraceptives—progestogen injections
- Medroxyprogesterone

- Progestogens.

Two alternatives to long-term estrogen therapy have been proposed, because of the fear of certain risks (particularly malignancy) that might result in postmenopausal women:

- combined estrogen + progestogen regimens with a monthly interruption to allow for withdrawal bleeding
- long-term therapy with estrogens alone periodically interrupted by a cycle of combined treatment.

In those few countries in which hysterectomy is still endemic it has been argued that in the residual minority of women with an intact uterus combination therapy should be the normal form of HRT. Therapeutic benefits have also been claimed from using the combination. Unfortunately, some of the publications that have made claims for the therapeutic advantages of adding progestogens to estrogens in HRT have not provided exact comparative data, and the beneficial effects which are described are not clearly different from those claimed for estrogen alone.

The dispute about the benefit to harm balance of the various competing forms of HRT for use in the climacteric or postmenopausally is becoming increasingly intense, with a sharp division of opinion between protagonists and critics of the individual patterns of treatment. The view was often defended by earlier workers that, at least for certain classes of users, some form of combined estrogen + progestogen treatment is likely to be more appropriate and perhaps more physiological than estrogen replacement alone. Many variants have been used and none is likely to be ideal for all subjects. Some have argued that in the climacteric there are sound reasons for using estrogen with intermittent progestogen and that it is much underused, despite the fact that uterine bleeding and other adverse progestogenic effects are, with some combined formulations (but not all), major reasons for patient non-compliance and early withdrawal (1).

Observational studies

In 104 women with established postmenopausal osteoporosis, continuous estrogen + progestogen therapy resulted in increases in bone mineral density of the femoral neck and a fall in systolic blood pressure; the most common adverse effects were mastalgia (44%) and vaginal bleeding (29%) (2).

The combined use of estradiol and dydrogesterone reduce both diastolic and systolic blood pressures in post menopausal women in whom the diastolic pressure had been raised (3). Evidence is also advanced from various quarters that adding a progestogen to adequate dosages of an estrogen promotes new bone formation, restores bone that has been lost and reduces the risk of carcinoma of the breast.

When 16 diabetic and hypertensive postmenopausal women aged 47–57 years were treated cyclically with estradiol plus norgestrel, existing proteinuria and even creatinine clearance often improved (4). The effects were unrelated to conventional risk factors for vascular complications, such as raised blood pressure, plasma glucose, or serum cholesterol.

General adverse effects

Of 206 postmenopausal women who took the oral combination of estradiol valerate plus norethisterone (5) eight withdrew because of bleeding during year 1; during years 2 and 3 there were no withdrawals because of bleeding. By the end of year 3, 133 patients had completed the study. There were serious adverse effects in 24, but there was no definite relation to therapy. The numbers of adverse events reported each year by the patients who completed the study are shown in Table 1. The authors concluded that this combination was effective in the majority of patients and was well tolerated.

Distinguishing adverse effects due to estrogens or progestogens

When patients have adverse effects during combined hormone replacement therapy it is necessary to determine whether the progestogen or the estrogen is causing the problem. If heavy bleeding or breast tenderness is the primary complaint, the estrogen component is probably the problem and therefore the dose should be reduced. If the patient complains of irritability, depression, water retention, or headaches, the problems are probably due to the progestogen component and the latter should in that case be changed or the dose adjusted; since several different progestogens are in use (particularly norethindrone, norethindrone acetate, medroxyprogesterone acetate, and micronized progesterone) there is a degree of choice.

Benefit to harm balance

With increasing concern over the long-term safety of hormone replacement therapy, the benefit to harm balance has to be continually reassessed, and conclusions as to its prophylactic or therapeutic value need to be adjusted as experience accumulates. Not all the promises held out for the benefits of this therapy have been confirmed. For example, while estrogens prevent peripheral bone loss they do not prevent vertebral fractures (6) and in a 2-year placebo-controlled, crossover study in 34 healthy postmenopausal women, treatment with transdermal estrogen alone (Menorest 50 micrograms/day) did not improve lipid profiles or any indices of arterial function (7).

It is remarkable that, despite decades of accumulated observational evidence, the balance of benefits and harms for hormone use in healthy postmenopausal women remains uncertain (8). Quite apart from the constantly changing spectrum of the available data, one explanation for the confusion is the relatively high proportion of poor-quality clinical work, particularly studies that are designed to promote particular commercialized forms of treatment from among the many alternatives available.

A study that cannot be faulted on that score is the Women's Health Initiative, a randomized, controlled, primary prevention trial (planned to last for 8.5 years), in which 16 608 postmenopausal women aged 50–79 years with an intact uterus at baseline were recruited at 40 US clinical centers over the period 1993–98 (9). In one part of this study, 8506 participants received conjugated equine estrogens 0.625 mg/day plus medroxyprogesterone acetate 2.5 mg/day; 8102 were given placebo. The primary desired outcome was reduction of coronary heart disease (non-fatal myocardial infarction and death), with invasive

Table 1   The numbers of adverse events in 3 successive years in patients taking estradiol valerate + norethisterone (5)

Adverse event	Year 1 (n = 164)	Year 2 (n = 144)	Year 3 (n = 133)
Cardiovascular			
Hypertension	5	3	—
Palpitation	4	4	3
Phlebitis	3	—	—
Respiratory			
Breathlessness	3	0	1
Metabolism			
Weight gain	10	5	2
Gastrointestinal			
Abdominal pain	2	2	—
Musculoskeletal			
Fractures	7	1	1
Joint/bone pain	6	3	6
Reproductive system			
Menopausal symptoms	4	1	5
Breast tenderness	63	4	3
Breast lumps	2	4	2
Bleeding/spotting	91	60	24
Abnormal smear	—	2	—
Ovarian cysts	1	1	4
Other adverse events	105	53	34
Total	306	143	85

breast cancer as the primary anticipated adverse outcome. After a mean of 5.2 years, the data and safety monitoring board recommended stopping the trial of estrogen plus progestogen versus placebo because the test statistic for invasive breast cancer exceeded the stopping boundary for this adverse effect and the global index statistic supported harms exceeding benefits. The estimated hazard ratios (and 95% confidence intervals) were:

- coronary disease 1.29 (1.02, 1.63; $n = 286$)
- breast cancer 1.26 (1.00, 1.59; $n = 290$)
- stroke 1.41 (1.07, 1.85; $n = 212$)
- pulmonary embolism 2.13 (1.39, 3.25; $n = 101$)
- colorectal cancer 0.63 (0.43, 0.92; $n = 112$)
- endometrial cancer 0.83 (0.47, 1.47; $n = 47$)
- hip fracture 0.66 (0.45, 0.98; $n = 106$)
- death due to other causes 0.92 (0.74, 1.14; $n = 331$).

What the above amounts to is that the absolute excess risks per 10 000 woman-years attributable to the use of an estrogen plus a progestogen were seven more coronary heart disease events, eight more strokes, eight more pulmonary embolisms, and eight more invasive breast cancers, while the risk reductions per 10 000 woman-years were six fewer colorectal cancers and five fewer hip fractures. The absolute excess risk of events included in the global index was 19 per 10 000 woman-years. The overall harms in this study thus clearly exceeded the benefits. All-cause mortality was not affected.

Other published studies, many of which are of limited scope, do not run closely parallel to the above findings from the Women's Health Initiative, and the data on cardiovascular effects remain particularly confusing. However, Beral and colleagues have pointed out optimistically that "substantial new data should soon be available from randomized trials of estrogen-alone hormonal replacement therapy versus placebo," although they added that "few additional trial data on combined hormone replacement therapy are expected for about a decade" (10). They also pointed out that existing randomized trials are too small to provide reliable evidence on some basic matters, including the relative risks of the various compounds in use.

Organs and Systems

Cardiovascular

Despite biologically plausible mechanisms whereby estrogens might be expected to confer cardioprotection in postmenopausal women, as well as observational data suggesting cardiovascular benefit, the literature continues to provide contradictory outcomes on this. Electrocardiographic work has suggested that not only the estrogen but also the progestogen component of HRT can have some impact on the electrophysiological properties of the heart (11), the clinical significance of which, if any, is not understood. The picture is further confused by evidence that a particular regimen may initially increase the risk, yet confer long-term benefit, as in the Heart and Estrogen/progestin Replacement Study

(HERS), while in other well-planned work, such as the recent Estrogen Replacement and Atherosclerosis trial (ERA), there was no benefit (12).

There has been a randomized trial in 270 postmenopausal women to evaluate the effects on cardiovascular risk markers of two continuous combined estrogen + progestogen replacement products (17-beta-estradiol 1 mg with or without norethindrone acetate 0.25 or 0.5 mg) compared with unopposed estrogen or placebo (13). LDL cholesterol was reduced to a similar extent in all those who took the active treatment (10–14% from baseline). Compared with unopposed 17-beta-estradiol, 17-beta-estradiol plus norethindrone acetate 0.5 mg enhanced the reductions in total cholesterol and apolipoprotein B concentrations. The combination of 17-beta-estradiol plus norethindrone blunted or reversed the increases in concentrations of high-density lipoprotein cholesterol, apolipoprotein A-I, and triglycerides produced by 17-beta-estradiol alone. The effects of 17-beta-estradiol plus norethindrone on hemostatic variables were similar to those of 17-beta-estradiol alone, except for factor VII activity, which was significantly reduced by 17-beta-estradiol plus norethindrone acetate 0.25 and 0.5 mg. The combination of 17-beta-estradiol plus norethindrone blunted reductions in C peptide and insulin concentrations produced by unopposed 17-beta-estradiol, but did not affect them compared with placebo. The authors concluded that 17-beta-estradiol plus norethindrone produced favorable changes in most cardiovascular risk markers and had a profile distinct from that of unopposed estrogen.

The findings of the randomized HERS suggested that in women with clinically recognized heart disease, HRT might be associated with early harm but late benefit in terms of coronary events. The findings of that study seem in the meantime to have been confirmed by some further US work. In one study the histories and subsequent course of 981 postmenopausal women who had survived a first myocardial infarct and had thereafter used estrogen or estrogen + progestogen were examined (14). Relative to the risk in a parallel group of women not currently using hormones there was a suggestion of increased risk during the first 60 days after starting hormone therapy (RR = 2.16; CI = 0.94, 4.95) but of reduced risk with current hormone use for longer than 1 year (RR = 0.76), although the confidence intervals were wide.

However, in a second study, data on 1857 women from the Coumadin Aspirin Reinfarction Study were used to assess the incidence of cardiac deaths or unstable angina as related to the use of HRT. Of the population studied, 524 (28%) had used HRT at some point and 111 of the latter (21%) had started HRT after suffering a myocardial infarct ("new users"). Women who began HRT after their first myocardial infarct had a significantly higher subsequent incidence of unstable angina than women who had never used hormones (39 versus 20%); however, these new hormone users suffered death or recurrence of myocardial infarct at a much lower rate than never-users (4 versus 15%). These differences are striking. Prior/current users had no excess risk of the composite end-point after adjustment. Users of estrogen plus progestogen had a lower incidence of death, infarct, or unstable angina during follow-up than users of estrogen only (RR = 0.56) (15). As Grady and Hulley have commented in an editorial, current data seem to make it clear that "postmenopausal hormone therapy should not be used for the purpose of preventing coronary disease unless future data from well-designed randomized trials document such benefit" (16).

The thrombotic complications of combined HRT in a potentially high-risk group have been assessed in a randomized, multicenter study in the USA in 2763 women, average age 67 years (17). All had some degree of pre-existing coronary heart disease but no previous venous thromboembolism, and none had undergone hysterectomy. They took either conjugated equine estrogens 0.625 mg + medroxyprogesterone acetate 2.5 mg or a placebo. During an average 4.1 years of follow-up, 34 women in the hormone therapy group and 13 in the placebo group had venous thromboembolism (relative risk = 2.7, excess risk = 3.9 per 1000 woman-years). The mean risk for venous thromboembolism was increased among women who had leg fractures (RR = 18) or cancer (RR = 4) and it was also raised several-fold for 3 months after inpatient surgery or non-surgical hospitalization. The risk was approximately halved by the use of aspirin or statins.

Metabolism

Hyperlipidemic postmenopausal women taking combined sequential estrogen + progestogen replacement therapy have large fluctuations in lipid and lipoprotein concentrations. These fluctuations depend on the hormonal phase, that is estrogen alone or combined with progestogen. Progestogens blunt or even overwhelm the estrogenic effects on lipoproteins (18).

Progestogen has also been claimed to produce more favorable concentrations of HDL cholesterol (19), but this is a questionable conclusion; most work seems to show that whereas estrogen alone increases HDL concentrations (for example by some 7%), combined treatment weakens this favorable effect and actually can reduce HDL concentrations by some 16%.

Changes in lipids have been observed with both HRT and oral contraceptives and have sometimes been promoted as potentially advantageous, but it is not clear how significant such changes are, at least in biochemical terms. A review and pooled analysis of 248 prospective studies available up to the year 2000 has provided data on this issue in postmenopausal women (20). All estrogen-only regimens raised HDL cholesterol and lowered LDL and total cholesterol. Oral estrogens raised triglycerides. Transdermal 17-beta-estradiol lowered triglycerides. Progestogens had little effect on estrogen-induced reductions in LDL and total cholesterol. Estrogen-induced increases in HDL and triglycerides were opposed according to the type of progestogen in the following order (from least to greatest effect): dydrogesterone and medrogestone, progesterone, cyproterone acetate, medroxyprogesterone acetate, transdermal norethindrone acetate,

norgestrel, and oral norethindrone acetate. Tibolone reduced HDL cholesterol and triglyceride concentrations. Raloxifene reduced LDL cholesterol concentrations. In 41 studies of 20 different formulations, HRT generally lowered lipoprotein (a). Thus, the route of estrogen administration and the type of progestogen used determine the effects of HRT on lipid and lipoprotein concentrations.

In another study an estrogen + progestogen combination produced no adverse effects on serum lipids or lipoproteins (21), but this again may depend very much on the exact combination and duration of treatment.

Whatever the truth, the question arises whether the modifications in lipid effects resulting from the addition of progestogen will not interfere with the favorable impact of estrogen on coronary artery disease; there has been some earlier evidence that the combined therapy is rather less effective than plain estrogen in preventing cardiac disorders (SEDA-16, 459).

Female sex hormones can also have effects on lipids when they are given transdermally, and this has been studied retrospectively in 159 women who used transdermal or oral replacement therapy (22). All used either transdermal estradiol 0.05 mg twice weekly or oral conjugated estrogen 0.625 mg/day, each combined with oral medroxyprogesterone acetate 2.5 mg/day. The mean increases in HDL cholesterol in the first year and second year averaged 10 and 31% with oral treatment, the corresponding figures for transdermal therapy being 14 and 34%. With oral therapy the mean reductions in total cholesterol in the first and second years were 2.9 and 15%, and with transdermal treatment 5.6 and 5.7%. With oral treatment, the mean falls in LDL cholesterol in the first and second years were 6.2 and 18% and with transdermal treatment 7.9 and 16% respectively. Transdermal treatment reduced triglyceride concentrations by 34%, whereas oral estrogen treatment increased them by 19% at the end of 2 years. Both treatments changed serum lipids favorably. Nevertheless, triglycerides were increased by oral estrogen but reduced by transdermal treatment at 2 years.

It has been hypothetically suggested that the use of HRT could slow the progression of atherosclerosis by an effect on lipids. In a 1-year study of 321 women with increased thickness of the carotid intima media who were using either various forms of HRT or none at all, there was no slowing in the progression of subclinical atherosclerosis and no unfavorable effect on the process (23). HRT significantly reduced LDL cholesterol, fibrinogen, and FSH.

Reproductive system

Adding a progestogen to estrogen therapy means that regular withdrawal bleeding occurs, probably in some 97% of users up to the age of 60 years. This could explain why such combinations, although increasingly advocated, have not been used on a wider scale; few women relish the prospect of regular "menstrual" bleeding persisting for many years after the menopause, and it might introduce new and unforeseen risks, particularly to the aging uterus.

However, on theoretical and practical grounds, such combinations have been developed and used for relatively short periods of treatment during the climacteric itself to regularize bleeding and to relieve menopausal symptoms. The pattern of short-term adverse effects of these products is very similar to that of the combined oral contraceptives.

Some cases have underlined the need to use an estrogen in combination with a progestogen, rather than unopposed estrogen, when treating women who have undergone radical surgery (removal of both the ovaries and uterus) for endometriosis. If unopposed estrogen replacement is given, any residual area of endometriosis will rapidly expand (24).

Continuous administration of an estrogen + progestogen combination is effective in achieving amenorrhea with prolonged use (75% at 6 months). An adverse effect of such a regimen is a high incidence of unpredictable break-through bleeding, particularly during the initial months of treatment (25).

Mammary tension and mastodynia are adverse effects related to the action of estrogens (26). In postmenopausal women estrogen + progestogen replacement therapy can be associated with an increase in mammographic density and with the onset or worsening of mastodynia. Tibolone, a steroid with estrogenic, progestogenic, and some androgenic activity, does not seem to affect breasts of normal structure and can be considered a first-rate replacement therapy in women whose breasts are rather dense or who have benign mastopathy (26).

Various companies and investigational groups continue to examine the relative efficacy and safety of different forms of combined postmenopausal treatment. In a randomized, placebo-controlled trial 579 women were treated for 26 cycles with sequential combinations of 17-beta-estradiol 1 mg plus dydrogesterone 5 or 10 mg or 17-beta-estradiol 2 mg with dydrogesterone 10 or 20 mg (27). The effects of these treatments in the 442 women who underwent biopsy were considered satisfactory in terms of cycle control and endometrial response, but the 1 mg dose of 17-beta-estradiol was associated with more intermittent uterine bleeding than the 2 mg dose. Higher doses of dydrogesterone were associated with a higher incidence of cyclical bleeds and a later time of onset.

Long-Term Effects

Tumorigenicity

Breast cancer

The complexity of the relation between hormonal replacement therapy and breast cancer has been stressed in previous volumes (SED-14, 1454) (SEDA-22, 465), and much depends on the type of replacement therapy given and the class of tumor studied. This latter point has been underscored by a US study that provided evidence that the use of combined hormonal replacement therapy increases the risk of lobular, but not ductal, breast carcinoma in middle-aged women (28).

An American cohort study designed to determine whether increases in risk associated with an estrogen + progestogen regimen are greater than those associated with estrogen alone has been carried out based on follow-up data for 1980–1995 from the National Breast Cancer Detection Demonstration Project (29). From 46 355 postmenopausal women, mean age at the start of follow-up was 58 years, 2082 cases of breast cancer were identified. Increases in risk with estrogen only and estrogen + progestogen were restricted to use within the previous 4 years, the relative risks being 1.2 and 1.4 respectively. The relative risk increased by 0.01 with each year of estrogen use and by 0.08 with each year of estrogen + progestogen use. Among women with a BMI of 24.4 kg/m^2 or less, the mean increases in relative risk were 0.03 and 0.12 with each year of estrogen use and estrogen + progestogen use respectively. These associations were evident for the majority of invasive tumors with ductal histology and regardless of the extent of invasive disease. The risk in heavier women did not increase with the use of estrogen only or estrogen + progestogen. These data suggest that estrogen + progestogen increases the risk of breast cancer beyond that associated with estrogen alone.

Endometrial cancer

Because sequential combined hormone replacement therapy with estrogen + progestogen for 10–24 days per month can increase the risk of endometrial cancer in the long run, attention has been devoted to the possibility of giving the two types of hormone continuously. In one retrospective case-control study in the USA it was concluded that the risk of endometrial cancer among users of continuous combined treatment, relative to women who had never used hormone replacement therapy, was 0.6 (95% CI = 0.3, 1.3); the risk relative to women who used intermittent combined therapy was 0.4 (CI = 0.2, 1.1) (30). The authors' conclusions were cautious, since most continuous combined hormonal therapy had been fairly short-term (under 72 months), but the figures suggested that women taking continuous combined hormone replacement therapy for several years were not at an increased risk of endometrial cancer compared with women who had never taken hormone replacement therapy and might in fact be at reduced risk of endometrial cancer.

In the meantime, others have concluded that the risk of endometrial cancer is present, but is less with combined therapy than with unopposed estrogen. However, the picture is not simple; the contradictions could be explained by the fact that risks appear to vary both by usage patterns and by patient characteristics, such as body weight and a history of diabetes (31).

Susceptibility Factors

Genetic factors

In a population-based, case-control study in 232 postmenopausal women who had had a non-fatal myocardial infarct during the previous 3 years, a stratified random sample of 723 postmenopausal women without a history of infarction acted as controls (32). Among hypertensive women, the presence of the prothrombin 20210 G→A variant was a significant risk factor for infarct (OR = 4.32; 95% CI = 1.52, 12) and in this group there was also a significant interaction between the use of HRT and the presence of the prothrombin variant in increasing the risk of infarction. Compared with non-users of HRT with the wild-type genotype, women who were current users and who had the prothrombin variant (n = 8) had a nearly 11-fold increase in the risk of a non-fatal myocardial infarct. The interaction was absent among non-hypertensive women. No interaction with HRT was found for factor V Leiden in either hypertensive or non-hypertensive women. These findings suggest that screening for the prothrombin variant may allow a better assessment of the risks and benefits associated with HRT in individual postmenopausal women.

Other features of the patient

While the extent of vaginal bleeding when using estrogens plus progestogens varies somewhat with the exact formulation and dose, another determining factor is the pretreatment state of the endometrium: a thick endometrium at the start of treatment results in significantly more bleeding days than a thin endometrium (33). This might be a helpful predictor of the extent to which a particular woman will find this type of HRT acceptable.

Drug Administration

Drug formulations

The impact of a new formulation of low-dose micronized medroxyprogesterone plus 17-beta-estradiol on lipid profiles in menopausal women has been studied for 12 months. Total cholesterol concentrations fell 8.4%, low-density lipoprotein cholesterol fell 18%, and high-density lipoprotein cholesterol increased 6.9%; total triglycerides increased 12%. The most frequently reported adverse events were menorrhagia, breast tenderness, cervical polyps or cysts, bloating, fatigue or lethargy, influenza or a flu-like syndrome, back pain, headaches, irritability, and depression (34).

Drug dosage regimens

In 438 postmenopausal women, randomly assigned to either constant 17-beta-estradiol (1 mg/day) plus inter mittent norgestimate 90 micrograms (3 days off, 3 days on) or a fixed combination of 17-beta-estradiol (2 mg/day) with norethisterone acetate (1 mg), the two regimens had similar bleeding profiles and provided comparable relief from vasomotor symptoms (1). However, breast discomfort and edema were experienced by twice as many subjects who used the fixed combination. The intermittent regimen was notably free of endometrial hyperplasia.

Drug administration route

In an open, non-comparative study, the efficacy of a low dose transdermal estrogen (Oesclim 25 transdermal

patches, releasing 17-beta-estradiol 25 micrograms/day) was tested in 60 women with postmenopausal symptoms over 8 weeks (35). The dosage could be doubled if required and sequential treatment with an oral progestogen was also given for 12 days or more each month in all non-hysterectomized women. Of the 60 patients, 53 reacted satisfactorily to the basic dose and all the various treatments were said to be well tolerated. One could cite a dozen similar papers from the recent past in which the findings were so amorphous that they have not made a serious contribution to the evolution of knowledge.

In two multicenter, double-blind, randomized, controlled trials of three once-a-week transdermal systems delivering continuous combined 17-beta-estradiol + levonorgestrel (estrogen 45 micrograms/day + progestogen 15, 30, or 40 micrograms/day) to treat vasomotor symptoms and prevent estrogen-induced endometrial hyperplasia in 1138 women, all were highly effective (36). Reactions at the site of application, vaginal hemorrhage, and breast pain were the most common adverse events, and the proportion of women with amenorrhea increased over time in all the treatment groups.

Drug–Drug Interactions

Statins

With growing interest in the use of statins in women, the question naturally arises whether hormonal replacement could have any effect on their efficacy or safety. Data from the HERS (conducted in women with cardiac disorders) seem to have shown that there is no interaction (37). Estrogen replacement itself resulted in a significant increase in the early risk of primary events in women who did not use statins but not in statin users. Adjustment for statin use after randomization showed no adverse effect of estrogen on the efficacy of statins, in terms of either cardiovascular events or mortality.

References

1. Rozenberg S, Caubel P, Lim PC. Constant estrogen, intermittent progestogen vs. continuous combined hormone replacement therapy: tolerability and effect on vasomotor symptoms. Int J Gynaecol Obstet 2001;72(3):235–43.
2. Grey AB, Cundy TF, Reid IR. Continuous combined oestrogen/progestin therapy is well tolerated and increases bone density at the hip and spine in post-menopausal osteoporosis. Clin Endocrinol (Oxf) 1994;40(5):671–7.
3. Foster RH, Balfour JA. Estradiol and dydrogesterone. A review of their combined use as hormone replacement therapy in postmenopausal women. Drugs Aging 1997;11(4):309–32.
4. Mattix H, Singh AK. Estrogen replacement therapy: implications for postmenopausal women with end-stage renal disease. Curr Opin Nephrol Hypertens 2000;9(3):207–14.
5. Perry W, Wiseman RA, Cullen NM. Combined oral estradiol valerate–norethisterone treatment over three years in postmenopausal women. 1. Clinical aspects and endometrial histology. Gynecol Endocrinol 1998;12(2):109–22.
6. Gutteridge DH, Stewart GO, Prince RL, Price RI, Retallack RW, Dhaliwal SS, Stuckey BG, Drury P,

Jones CE, Faulkner DL, Kent GN, Bhagat CI, Nicholson GC, Jamrozik K. A randomized trial of sodium fluoride (60 mg) +/− estrogen in postmenopausal osteoporotic vertebral fractures: increased vertebral fractures and peripheral bone loss with sodium fluoride; concurrent estrogen prevents peripheral loss, but not vertebral fractures Osteoporos Int 2002;13(2):158–70.

7. Teede HJ, Liang YL, Kotsopoulos D, Zoungas S, Craven R, McGrath BP. Placebo-controlled trial of transdermal estrogen therapy alone in postmenopausal women: effects on arterial compliance and endothelial function. Climacteric 2002;5(2):160–9.

8. Rossouw JE, Anderson GL, Prentice RL, LaCroix AZ, Kooperberg C, Stefanick ML, Jackson RD, Beresford SA, Howard BV, Johnson KC, Kotchen JM, Ockene J. Writing Group for the Women's Health Initiative Investigators. Risks and benefits of estrogen plus progestin in healthy postmenopausal women: principal results From the Women's Health Initiative randomized controlled trial. JAMA 2002;288(3):321–33.

9. Lanzone A. The puzzle of hormone replacement therapy (HRT) and cardiovascular disease (CVD). J Endocrinol Invest 2002;25(1):1–3.

10. Beral V, Banks E, Reeves G. Evidence from randomised trials on the long-term effects of hormone replacement therapy. Lancet 2002;360(9337):942–4.

11. Haseroth K, Seyffart K, Wehling M, Christ M. Effects of progestin–estrogen replacement therapy on QT-dispersion in postmenopausal women. Int J Cardiol 2000;75(2–3):161–5.

12. Wenger NK. Hormonal and nonhormonal therapies for the postmenopausal woman: what is the evidence for cardioprotection? Am J Geriatr Cardiol 2000;9(4):204–9.

13. Davidson MH, Maki KC, Marx P, Maki AC, Cyrowski MS, Nanavati N, Arce JC. Effects of continuous estrogen and estrogen-progestin replacement regimens on cardiovascular risk markers in postmenopausal women. Arch Intern Med 2000;160(21):3315–25.

14. Heckbert SR, Kaplan RC, Weiss NS, Psaty BM, Lin D, Furberg CD, Starr JR, Anderson GD, LaCroix AZ. Risk of recurrent coronary events in relation to use and recent initiation of postmenopausal hormone therapy. Arch Intern Med 2001;161(14):1709–13.

15. Alexander KP, Newby LK, Hellkamp AS, Harrington RA, Peterson ED, Kopecky S, Langer A, O'Gara P, O'Connor CM, Daly RN, Califf RM, Khan S, Fuster V. Initiation of hormone replacement therapy after acute myocardial infarction is associated with more cardiac events during follow-up. J Am Coll Cardiol 2001;38(1):1–7.

16. Grady D, Hulley SB. Postmenopausal hormones and heart disease. J Am Coll Cardiol 2001;38(1):8–10.

17. Grady D, Wenger NK, Herrington D, Khan S, Furberg C, Hunninghake D, Vittinghoff E, Hulley S. Postmenopausal hormone therapy increases risk for venous thromboembolic disease. The Heart and Estrogen/progestin Replacement Study. Ann Intern Med 2000;132(9):689–96.

18. Weintraub MS, Grosskopf I, Charach G, Eckstein N, Ringel Y, Maharshak N, Rotmensch HH, Rubinstein A. Fluctuations of lipid and lipoprotein levels in hyperlipidemic postmenopausal women receiving hormone replacement therapy. Arch Intern Med 1998;158(16):1803–6.

19. Gambrell RD Jr. Progestogens in estrogen-replacement therapy. Clin Obstet Gynecol 1995;38(4):890–901.

20. Godsland IF. Effects of postmenopausal hormone replacement therapy on lipid, lipoprotein, and apolipoprotein (a) concentrations: analysis of studies published from 1974–2000. Fertil Steril 2001;75(5):898–915.

21. Jensen J, Christiansen C. Dose-response effects on serum lipids and lipoproteins following combined oestrogen-progestogen therapy in post-menopausal women. Maturitas 1987;9(3):259–66.

22. Erenus M, Karakoc B, Gurler A. Comparison of effects of continuous combined transdermal with oral estrogen and oral progestogen replacement therapies on serum lipoproteins and compliance. Climacteric 2001;4(3):228–34.

23. Angerer P, Stork S, Kothny W, Schmitt P, von Schacky C. Effect of oral postmenopausal hormone replacement on progression of atherosclerosis: a randomized, controlled trial. Arterioscler Thromb Vasc Biol 2001;21(2):262–8.

24. Taylor M, Bowen-Simpkins P, Barrington J. Complications of unopposed oestrogen following radical surgery for endometriosis. J Obstet Gynaecol 1999;19(6):647–8.

25. Cameron ST, Critchley HOD. Continuous oestrogen and interrupted progestogen in HRT bleed-free regimens. Contemp Rev Obstet Gynaecol 1998;10:151–5.

26. Colacurci N, Mele D, De Franciscis P, Costa V, Fortunato N, De Seta L. Effects of tibolone on the breast. Eur J Obstet Gynecol Reprod Biol 1998;80(2):235–8.

27. Ferenczy A, Gelfand MM, van de Weijer PH, Rioux JE. Endometrial safety and bleeding patterns during a 2-year study of 1 or 2 mg 17 beta-estradiol combined with sequential 5–20 mg dydrogesterone Climacteric 2002;5(1):26–35.

28. Li CI, Weiss NS, Stanford JL, Daling JR. Hormone replacement therapy in relation to risk of lobular and ductal breast carcinoma in middle-aged women. Cancer 2000;88(11):2570–7.

29. Schairer C, Lubin J, Troisi R, Sturgeon S, Brinton L, Hoover R. Menopausal estrogen and estrogen-progestin replacement therapy and breast cancer risk. JAMA 2000;283(4):485–91.

30. Hill DA, Weiss NS, Beresford SA, Voigt LF, Daling JR, Stanford JL, Self S. Continuous combined hormone replacement therapy and risk of endometrial cancer. Am J Obstet Gynecol 2000;183(6):1456–61.

31. Jain MG, Rohan TE, Howe GR. Hormone replacement therapy and endometrial cancer in Ontario, Canada. J Clin Epidemiol 2000;53(4):385–91.

32. Psaty BM, Smith NL, Lemaitre RN, Vos HL, Heckbert SR, LaCroix AZ, Rosendaal FR. Hormone replacement therapy, prothrombotic mutations, and the risk of incident nonfatal myocardial infarction in postmenopausal women. JAMA 2001;285(7):906–13.

33. Odmark IS, Jonsson B, Backstrom T. Bleeding patterns in postmenopausal women using continuous combination hormone replacement therapy with conjugated estrogen and medroxyprogesterone acetate or with 17beta-estradiol and norethindrone acetate. Am J Obstet Gynecol 2001;184(6):1131–8.

34. Harrison RF, Magill P, Kilminster SG. Impact of a new formulation of low-dose micronised medroxyprogesterone and 17-beta estradiol, on lipid profiles in menopausal women. Clin Drug Invest 1998;16:93–9.

35. Gadomska H, Barcz E, Cyganek A, Leocmach Y, Chadha-Boreham H, Marianowski L. Efficacy and tolerability of low-dose transdermal estrogen (Oesclim) in the treatment of menopausal symptoms. Curr Med Res Opin 2002;18(2):97–102.

36. Shulman LP, Yankov V, Uhl K. Safety and efficacy of a continuous once-a-week 17beta-estradiol/levonorgestrel transdermal system and its effects on vasomotor symptoms and endometrial safety in postmenopausal women: the results of two multicenter, double-blind, randomized, controlled trials. Menopause 2002;9(3):195–207.

37. Herrington DM, Vittinghoff E, Lin F, Fong J, Harris F, Hunninghake D, Bittner V, Schrott HG, Blumenthal RS, Levy RHERS Study Group. Statin therapy, cardiovascular events, and total mortality in the Heart and Estrogen/Progestin Replacement Study (HERS). Circulation 2002;105(25):2962–7.

Medroxyprogesterone

General Information

Other information on medroxyprogesterone will be found in other monographs that deal with progestogens:

- Hormonal contraceptives—intracervical and intravaginal
- Hormonal contraceptives—oral
- Hormonal contraceptives—progestogen implants Hormonal contraceptives—progestogen injections
- Hormone replacement therapy—estrogens + progestogens
- Progestogens.

Medroxyprogesterone acetate is given in a relatively high dose for hormonal contraception and acts primarily by inhibiting ovulation. However, as with the other progestogen-only contraceptives, other mechanisms probably play a very significant role. It is extremely effective, with less than one pregnancy per 100 woman-years.

Depot medroxyprogesterone acetate is by far the most widely used formulation of this compound; the World Health Organization's assessment of it in 1983 (1) remains valid, as confirmed by later studies and reviews (2–4). By 1994 it was estimated that the drug had been used by 30 million women in more than 90 countries, and at the turn of the century it continues to be used on a large scale.

In addition to its use as a contraceptive, medroxyprogesterone acetate has also been used to treat benign prostatic hyperplasia, in which intermediate doses (for example 150 mg) are used (5), and to stimulate the appetite in patients receiving palliative care for cancer, although little published work can be found to support the latter indication.

General adverse effects

Reports on adverse reactions to lower doses of medroxyprogesterone acetate are not entirely consistent, probably because of differences in pharmaceutical formulation which markedly affect the drug's systemic availability. However, high doses of medroxyprogesterone acetate are extensively used for the treatment of hormone-dependent carcinomas (notably of the breast) and marked adverse effects occur consistently under these conditions (SEDA-12, 343). Such doses are likely to bring out the compound's glucocorticoid potency. At a dose of some 800 mg/day, effects are likely to include excessive weight gain (in 4090% of cases), Cushingoid facies (10–20%), worsening of diabetes mellitus (up to 8%), edema

(10–20%), and other effects suggestive of Cushing's syndrome. The changes are especially marked in women treated for more than 5 weeks; effects are less severe at lower doses. Smaller numbers of patients can develop rash, thromboembolism, dysuria, nervousness, headache, or nausea and vomiting.

In a condition such as benign prostatic hyperplasia, common complications are reduced libido, a reduced volume of ejaculate, and impotence; within 3 days of starting treatment, serum testosterone can reach castration concentrations.

The contraceptive efficacy of depot medroxyprogesterone acetate does not appear to be affected by interactions with other drugs; some interactions are known (6), but the doses used for contraceptive purposes are sufficient to remain effective even if metabolism is increased, for example by aminoglutethimide or phenytoin.

Organs and Systems

Cardiovascular

To date medroxyprogesterone does not seem to have been associated with thrombosis, but an authoritative review has pointed out that this remains a possible risk (7).

Medroxyprogesterone has been reported to have variable effects on blood pressure. In some studies it had no effect on blood pressure at all (8) or reduced diastolic pressure slightly (9). In 24 women (21 normotensive and three hypertensive) aged 16–35 years who received injections of medroxyprogesterone acetate 150 mg for contraception mean blood pressure fell from 124/79 to 120/75 mmHg; the change was attributable to effects in the women with hypertension (10).

Nervous system

For women with epilepsy, depot medroxyprogesterone acetate is a particularly useful contraceptive method, because it reduces seizure frequency (11). The dosage is so high that reduced efficacy due to enzyme-inducing anti-epileptic medication is not an issue. As with other hormonal contraceptives, some women tend to have headaches and mood changes.

Psychological, psychiatric

Mental or personality changes, a typical glucocorticoid effect, have been reported to be more severe and more frequent with combined aminoglutethimide plus medroxyprogesterone acetate treatment than with monotherapy in patients with bone metastases from breast cancer. The increased frequency of depressive syndromes on the two-drug therapy could not be attributed to the physical adverse effects of the combination, since the mental disorders appeared only during the first weeks of treatment, whereas the Cushingoid features did not become apparent until some 6–8 weeks of treatment had been given (12).

Endocrine

Medroxyprogesterone, while suppressing spermatogenesis, also depresses release of growth hormone induced by insulin or arginine (13).

Medroxyprogesterone reportedly increases basal growth hormone concentrations (14).

Metabolism

Treatment with low-dose medroxyprogesterone acetate (50 and 150 mg/day) for endometriosis reduces HDL cholesterol (15) confined to the HDL2 subfraction, which was lowered by as much as 58% after 24 weeks of treatment; the effect was clearly dose-related in the therapeutic dosage range.

A multicenter study of lipid metabolism conducted by the WHO showed considerable differences in serum lipids and apolipoproteins among the centers, with overall small falls in HDL cholesterol and increases in LDL concentrations (16).

In undernourished lactating women in one developing country, metabolic effects were more pronounced than among healthy users (17); serum cholesterol concentrations were somewhat higher with medroxyprogesterone during their first 6 months of lactation, but there were no alterations in glucose tolerance, serum triglycerides, or total protein concentrations during 1 year of treatment.

There is a disputed effect on carbohydrate metabolism, but it is at most mild and there is certainly no precipitation of diabetes in healthy women. Carbohydrate metabolism was unaffected by medroxyprogesterone in one study in which there was modest impairment of glucose tolerance among users of levonorgestrel-containing, low-dose combined oral contraceptives and progestogen-only tablets (18).

Depot medroxyprogesterone acetate contraception is widely used by women of the Navajo tribe of American Indians, and they constitute a high-risk population for diabetes mellitus. However, medroxyprogesterone can cause weight gain and independently reduce sensitivity to insulin, which would be particularly undesirable in such women. Contraceptive use has been studied in 284 Navajo women with diabetes and 570 non-diabetic controls. Users of depot medroxyprogesterone were more likely to develop diabetes than those who had used combination estrogen + progestogen oral contraception only (OR = 3.8; 95% CI = 1.8, 7.9). The excess risk persisted after adjustment for body mass index and it became more pronounced with longer use (19).

Metabolic effects seen when the drug is used in high doses for other purposes (notably the treatment of breast and endometrial cancer) are unlikely to be seen in contraceptive use. This applies to the glucocorticoid potency that medroxyprogesterone undoubtedly possesses to some degree; at the higher doses adrenal suppression can be observed (20) but not at contraceptive doses (21).

Fluid balance

Medroxyprogesterone acetate has a degree of mineralocorticoid potency (22). However, in 10 patients with advanced hormone-sensitive and non-hormone sensitive tumors high-dose medroxyprogesterone acetate (over 500 mg/day) had no effects on body weight, lean body mass, blood pressure, plasma sodium concentration, urinary sodium excretion, or the exchangeable sodium pool (8).

Hematologic

Medroxyprogesterone acetate, administered either orally or by injection, has little or no effect on blood coagulation (23).

The suitability of medroxyprogesterone for women with sickle cell disease has been evaluated in a controlled crossover trial, which showed that both hematological and clinical parameters were improved (24).

Liver

No consistent effects of medroxyprogesterone acetate on liver function have been found, and primary biliary cirrhosis and chronic active hepatitis have appeared to improve during treatment (25).

Musculoskeletal

Subgroups of users of depot medroxyprogesterone acetate may have reduced spinal bone density, but this seems to be reversible after withdrawal, even after several years of drug exposure (26). Bone mineral density in one cross-sectional study was lower among users of depot medroxyprogesterone acetate, but withdrawal was followed by complete recovery of normal bone density (26). A current study in the USA is expected to provide further data on this matter in women who have used medroxyprogesterone acetate for as long as 10 years.

Reproductive system

Poor cycle control is a problem with medroxyprogesterone acetate. Most women using the product have at first either irregular or excessive bleeding and spotting or amenorrhea linked to endometrial atrophy (27); however, only one woman in a thousand bleeds sufficiently to warrant aggressive therapy, such as curettage. As the duration of use increases, amenorrhea becomes more common. Depot medroxyprogesterone acetate is associated with greater variability in menstrual patterns than other hormonal contraceptives (28,29). Bleeding/spotting episodes are infrequent but are prolonged when they occur, and the prevalence of amenorrhea increases over time to more than half of users after the first year. Under 10% of users have bleeding patterns defined as fully satisfactory and acceptable, compared with 85–90% of women not using contraception and the majority of women taking appropriate doses of oral contraceptives. However, with appropriate patient selection and counselling, many users view amenorrhea positively and are content to continue with the medroxyprogesterone. Indeed, because they are often amenorrheic, they may experience improvements in such menstrual cycle conditions as menorrhagia and dysmenorrhea and in iron deficiency anemia. Other potential benefits include reduction in the risk of pelvic inflammatory disease, improvement in sickle cell disease parameters, and lessened seizure frequency in women with epilepsy.

Other effects are generally less prevalent with progestogen-only contraceptives than with combined oral contraceptives because of the absence of an estrogen and a lower dose of the progestogen. Headache, breast tenderness, and less commonly nausea and dizziness have been reported by users of progestogen-only contraceptives, but it is not clear whether progestogen-only contraceptives actually play a causal role. Androgenic adverse effects, such as acne, hirsutism, and weight gain, occur, but rarely.

The reduced penetrability of cervical mucus, which contributes to the contraceptive effect, may well provide some small degree of protection against pelvic inflammatory disease. However, this effect is likely to be less than that exerted by combined oral contraceptives, since the expanded cervical ectropion found among combined oral contraceptive users is not present in users of progestogen-only contraceptives.

Immunologic

Anaphylactic reactions to medroxyprogesterone are very rare.

- A 40-year-old woman developed anaphylactic shock after receiving depot medroxyprogesterone acetate 150 mg intramuscularly (30). She was not taking any other medications, and there was no history of allergy to food or cosmetics. She responded fully to immediate resuscitation. She had another episode when she received another dose 12 weeks later.

Long-Term Effects

Tumorigenicity

The effects of depot medroxyprogesterone acetate on reproductive cancers appear to be similar to those of combined oral contraceptives. Most notably, despite initial concerns about breast cancer in beagle dogs that were given large doses of medroxyprogesterone, a pooled analysis of epidemiological studies concluded that women using medroxyprogesterone are not at increased risk of breast cancer (31). Furthermore, the risk did not increase with increasing duration of use. However, women who had begun use within the past 5 years had significantly increased risk, perhaps because of accelerated growth of pre-existing tumors or increased surveillance.

Another review, dating from 1994, concluded that depot medroxyprogesterone acetate has a protective effect against endometrial cancer that is at least as strong as for combined oral contraceptives, but that, based on the limited available evidence, there is no association with ovarian cancer (32). Regarding cervical neoplasia, studies of depot medroxyprogesterone acetate do not show a strong adverse effect, but as with combined oral contraceptives it is uncertain whether there is no association or a slightly increased risk (33).

Second-Generation Effects

Fertility

Return of fertility may be delayed for several months after withdrawal of medroxyprogesterone acetate. The length of the delay is not related to the duration of use. There is no evidence of permanent impairment of fertility (2,34).

Teratogenicity

If a breakthrough pregnancy occurs during the use of depot medroxyprogesterone acetate, the developing embryo and fetus will continue to be exposed to it for months, and an adverse effect cannot be entirely excluded, but little concrete information has emerged. Clitoral hypertrophy has been described in three infants exposed to medroxyprogesterone in utero. In view of the hormonal spectrum of medroxyprogesterone, this is a conceivable adverse effect, but there is no confirmation, nor is it clear whether the drug harms the fetus in any other way (25).

Lactation

Many studies have shown that lactation is not adversely affected by depot medroxyprogesterone acetate and that breast-milk production may even be increased (35). Because of the low binding affinity of medroxyprogesterone to sex hormone binding globulin, the concentration of steroids in the milk is close to that in the maternal plasma, unlike the 19-nortestosterone derivatives.

Children whose mothers used depot medroxyprogesterone acetate while breastfeeding have been followed up in Thailand for 17 years and in Chile for 4.5 years, with no documented effect on growth or development (36). In undernourished lactating women the metabolic effects seem to be more pronounced than among healthy users (17).

Susceptibility Factors

Depot medroxyprogesterone acetate should not be used in women with breast cancer, genital cancer, undiagnosed uterine bleeding, or suspected pregnancy (37), but these are merely logical precautions.

The only study of depot medroxyprogesterone acetate and HIV infection, conducted among Thai prostitutes, showed an increased risk after adjustment for other variables (38).

Drug Administration

Drug administration route

An injection of medroxyprogesterone acetate 150 mg provides contraception for some 3 months. Peak concentrations in the blood are reached on around the 10th day after injection, but the drug is still detectable in the blood at the 90th day, although with wide interindividual variation.

References

1. World Health Organization. Injectable Hormonal Contraceptives. In: Technical and Safety Aspects. Geneva: WHO Publication, 1982:65.
2. Kaunitz AM. Long-acting injectable contraception with depot medroxyprogesterone acetate. Am J Obstet Gynecol 1994;170(5 Pt 2):1543–9.
3. Landgren BM. In: Gestagen Methods (Depo-Provera, Mini-pill and Norplant). Uppsala: Swedish Medical Products Agency, 1994:2.
4. American College of Obstetricians and Gynecologists (ACOG). In: Hormonal Contraception. Washington, DC: ACOG Technical Bulletin, 1994:198.
5. Onu PE. Depot medroxyprogesterone in the management of benign prostatic hyperplasia. Eur Urol 1995;28(3):229–35.
6. Tatro DS. Drug interaction facts. In: Facts and Comparisons. Missouri: St Louis, 1999:908–10.
7. Anonymous. Medroxyprogesterone and palliative care: new indication. No impact on quality of life. Prescrire Int 2001;10(51):3–4.
8. Lelli G, Angelelli B, Zanichelli L, Strocchi E, Mondini F, Monetti N, Piana E, Pannuti F. The effect of high dose medroxyprogesterone acetate on water and salt metabolism in advanced cancer patients. Chemioterapia 1984;3(5):327–9.
9. Harvey PJ, Molloy D, Upton J, Wing LM. Dose response effect of cyclical medroxyprogesterone on blood pressure in postmenopausal women. J Hum Hypertens 2001;15(5):313–21.
10. Black HR, Leppert P, DeCherney A. The effect of medroxyprogesterone acetate on blood pressure. Int J Gynaecol Obstet 1978;17(1):83–7.
11. Mattson RH, Rebar RW. Contraceptive methods for women with neurologic disorders. Am J Obstet Gynecol 1993;168(6 Pt 2):2027–32.
12. Wander HE, Nagel GA, Blossey HC, Kleeberg U. Aminoglutethimide and medroxyprogesterone acetate in the treatment of patients with advanced breast cancer. A phase II study of the Association of Medical Oncology of the German Cancer Society (AIO). Cancer 1986;58(9):1985–9.
13. Simon S, Schiffer M, Glick SM, Schwartz E. Effect of medroxyprogesterone acetate upon stimulated release of growth hormone in men. J Clin Endocrinol Metab 1967;27(11):1633–6.
14. Gershberg H, Zorrilla E, Hernandez A, Hulse M. Effects of medroxyprogesterone acetate on serum insulin and growth hormone levels in diabetics and potential diabetics. Obstet Gynecol 1969;33(3):383–9.
15. Teichmann AT, Cremer P, Wieland H, Kuhn W, Seidel D. Lipid metabolic changes during hormonal treatment of endometriosis. Maturitas 1988;10(1):27–33.
16. Kongsayreepong R, Chutivongse S, George P, Joyce S, McCone JM, Garza-Flores J, Valles de Bourges V, de La Cruz DL, Perez-Palacios G, Rosseneu M, et al. A multi-centre comparative study of serum lipids and apolipoproteins in long-term users of DMPA and a control group of IUD users. World Health Organization. Task Force on Long-Acting Systemic Agents for Fertility Regulation Special Programme of Research, Development and Research Training in Human Reproduction. Contraception 1993;47(2):177–91.
17. Joshi UM, Virkar KD, Amatayakul K, Singkamani R, Bamji MS, Prema K, Whitehead TP, Belsey MA, Hall P, Parker RA. Metabolic side-effects of injectable depot-medroxyprogesterone acetate, 150 mg three-monthly, in undernourished lactating women. WHO Task Force on Long-acting Agents for Fertility Regulation Bull World Health Organ 1986;64(4):587–94.
18. Kamau RK, Maina FW, Kigondu C, Mati JK. The effect of low-oestrogen combined pill, progestogen-only pill and medroxyprogesterone acetate on oral glucose tolerance test. East Afr Med J 1990;67(8):550–5.
19. Kim C, Seidel KW, Begier EA, Kwok YS. Diabetes and depot medroxyprogesterone contraception in Navajo women. Arch Intern Med 2001;161(14):1766–71.
20. Mahlke M, Grill HJ, Knapstein P, Wiegand U, Pollow K. Oral high-dose medroxyprogesterone acetate (MPA) treatment: cortisol/MPA serum profiles in relation to breast cancer regression. Oncology 1985;42(3):144–9.
21. World Health Organization. Oral contraceptives: technical and safety aspects. WHO Offset Publ 1982;(64):1–45.
22. Thomas CP, Liu KZ, Vats HS. Medroxyprogesterone acetate binds the glucocorticoid receptor to stimulate {alpha}ENaC and sgk1 expression in renal collecting duct epithelia. Am J Physiol Renal Physiol 2005;.
23. Beller FK. Cardiovascular system: coagulation, thrombosis, and contraceptive steroids is there a link? In: Goldzieher JW, Fotherby K, editors. Pharmacology of the Contraceptive Steroids. New York: Raven Press, 1994:309.
24. De Ceulaer K, Gruber C, Hayes R, Serjeant GR. Medroxyprogesterone acetate and homozygous sickle-cell disease. Lancet 1982;2(8292):229–31.
25. World Health Organization. Multinational comparative clinical trial of long-acting injectable contraceptives: norethisterone enanthate given in two dosage regimens and depot-medroxyprogesterone acetate. Final report. Contraception 1983;28(1):1–20.
26. Cundy T, Cornish J, Evans MC, Roberts H, Reid IR. Recovery of bone density in women who stop using medroxyprogesterone acetate. BMJ 1994;308(6923):247–8.
27. Hyjazi Y, Maes E, Hurlet A, Masure R, Vekemans M. Acétate de médroxyprogestérone-dépôt: effets cliniques et métaboliques (lipides, glucose, hémostase). [Depot medroxyprogesterone acetate: clinical and metabolic effects (lipids, glucose, hemostasis).] J Gynecol Obstet Biol Reprod (Paris) 1985;14(1):93–103.
28. Belsey EM. Vaginal bleeding patterns among women using one natural and eight hormonal methods of contraception. Contraception 1988;38(2):181–206.
29. Fraser IS. Vaginal bleeding patterns in women using once-a-month injectable contraceptives. Contraception 1994;49(4):399–420.
30. Selo-Ojeme DO, Tillisi A, Welch CC. Anaphylaxis from medroxyprogesterone acetate. Obstet Gynecol 2004;103(5 Pt 2):1045–6.
31. Skegg DC, Noonan EA, Paul C, Spears GF, Meirik O, Thomas DB. Depot medroxyprogesterone acetate and breast cancer. A pooled analysis of the World Health Organization and New Zealand studies. JAMA 1995;273(10):799–804.
32. Lumbiganon P. Depot-medroxyprogesterone acetate (DMPA) and cancer of the endometrium and ovary. Contraception 1994;49(3):203–9.
33. La Vecchia C. Depot-medroxyprogesterone acetate, other injectable contraceptives, and cervical neoplasia. Contraception 1994;49(3):223–30.
34. Fotherby K, Howard G. Return of fertility in women discontinuing injectable contraceptives. J Obstet Gynaecol 1986;6(Suppl 2):S110–5.
35. McCann MF, Liskin LS, Piotrow PT, Rinehart W, Fox G. Breast-feeding, fertility, and family planning. Popul Rep J 1981;(24):J525–J75.

36. McCann MF, Potter LS. Progestin-only oral contraception: a comprehensive review. Contraception 1994;50(6 Suppl 1):S1–S195.

37. Fraser I, Holck SE. Depot-medroxyprogesterone acetate. In: Mishell D, editor. Advances in Contraceptive Technology 1982:23–124.

38. Rehle T, Brinkmann UK, Siraprapasiri T, Coplan P, Aiemsukawat C, Ungchusak K. Risk factors of HIV-1 infection among female prostitutes in Khon Kaen, Northeast Thailand. Infection 1992;20(6):328–31.

Mifepristone

General Information

Mifepristone (RU-486) has become best known as an abortifacient. It is a potent antagonist at progesterone receptors and glucocorticoid receptors. The abortifacient effect is thought to be primarily due to blockade of endometrial progesterone receptors, but mifepristone also impedes the production of human chorionic gonadotropin and progesterone in the placenta. When given in a single dose of 10 mg/kg by mouth to induce menses, heavy bleeding was reported in some cases (1).

Whatever the adverse effects of mifepristone, the risks have to be looked at realistically and compared with those of the alternatives available to a particular woman in particular circumstances. Particularly in rural areas in developing countries, the risks of surgical and non-professional abortion are high, whereas, as has been shown in a study in rural India, a regimen of mifepristone plus misoprostol can be used as effectively and safely, through family planning clinics and country hospitals, as in a European environment (2).

The use of mifepristone and misoprostol for termination of pregnancy was approved relatively late in the USA, and only now is American experience with this mode of treatment accumulating. With data on some 80 000 courses to hand, experience is characterized as favourable (3). Thirteen patients required blood transfusions, 10 were treated with antibiotics for infections, and six had a generalized allergic reaction. In 50 patients the pregnancy continued despite treatment, and in 48 of these suction curettage was carried out; 39 other patients required suction curettage for heavy or prolonged vaginal bleeding.

Controversy surrounding the use of mifepristone as an abortifacient has continued, particularly in the USA. Many of the objections raised reflect ethical or religious views, but various papers have stressed the risks involved, such as the fact that in the USA at least two preventable deaths have occurred, as well as other life-threatening complications. It has also been argued that approval of mifepristone as an abortifacient breached the FDA's procedural rules. In 2002 a Citizen Petition to the Congress called for a revocation of the drug's approval (4).

Observational studies

The effective oral doses of mifepristone are 100–600 mg, and at any dose the bulk of recipients abort. Of 150 healthy women who received the higher dose, 131 attained a complete abortion. Three women reported bleeding for more than 2 weeks after abortion; 16 women had a reduced hemoglobin concentration of under 11 g/dl, justifying iron therapy. Other adverse effects were uterine contractions and pelvic pain ($n = 4$), transient asthenia ($n = 3$), and nausea ($n = 2$) (5). These findings seem to be typical, even though dosage schemes have varied; as little as 100 mg orally has been used successfully with similar adverse effects (SED-12, 1037; 6).

Various anti-progestogenic routines for the termination of pregnancy continue to be compared. Of 354 women who were given mifepristone 200 mg in the clinic and then sent home with two tablets of misoprostol 200 micrograms to take 48 hours later, 324 (91.5%) had a successful termination (7). The most common adverse effects were pain or cramps (93%) and nausea (67%), followed by weakness (55%), headache (46%), and dizziness (44%). Overall acceptability of the regimen was high: 63% of women reported that it was "very satisfactory" and another 23% found it "satisfactory". There were no serious complications and the simplified routine, with a much reduced duration of hospital care, was considered acceptable.

A Chinese group has sought to compare the efficacy and safety of different dosage schemes and dosage forms of mifepristone with misoprostol for early termination (8). In a randomized double-blind trial in 480 women, one group took two mifepristone 150 mg tablets in the morning and 150 mg 12 hours later for 2 days, while another group took three 75 mg capsules orally twice daily for 2 days. In both groups, misoprostol 600 micrograms was given 48 hours later. There were no significant differences between the two groups in the rates of complete abortion (95% or more) or incomplete abortion (3.3% or more), vaginal bleeding, or the incidence of adverse effects, such as vomiting, nausea, headache, diarrhea, and lower abdominal pain.

However, there are still groups who have concluded that higher doses are required, and alternative schemes of treatment with mifepristone are being compared to attain an optimal efficacy/safety balance in different circumstances. In a prospective study in 104 women, the best means of using mifepristone combined with oral misoprostol in the management of first trimester miscarriage (missed abortion and blighted ovum) was investigated (9). The women took either oral mifepristone 600 mg ($n = 44$) or 200 mg ($n = 60$), in both groups followed after 48 hours by oral misoprostol. Successful treatment (i.e. an empty uterus on scan and no bleeding after 10 days) was attained in some two-thirds of he women in both groups. In the high-dose group, the adverse effects were nausea in 25% and diarrhea in 16%; in the low-dose group, there was nausea in 7% and diarrhea in 7%. Since the therapeutic effects were similar the low-dose regimen seems preferable, and the method as a whole may provide a valid alternative to surgery in these cases.

The adverse effects of these medicinal approaches to abortion have been studied in 15 clinics in 11 countries in 2219 healthy women requesting medical abortion within 63 days of the onset of amenorrhea (10). Mifepristone 200 mg was given orally on day 1, followed by misoprostol 0.8 mg either orally or vaginally on day 3. Oral of misoprostol was associated with a higher frequency of nausea and vomiting than vaginal administration at 1 hour after administration. With oral misoprostol, diarrhea was more frequent at 1, 2, and 3 hours after administration than with vaginal administration. Misoprostol induced fever during at least 3 hours after administration in up to 6% of the women; the peak occurred slightly higher and later with the vaginal route. Lower abdominal pain peaked at 1 and 2 hours after oral misoprostol, and at 2 and 3 hours after vaginal misoprostol. In the two groups that continued misoprostol, 27% of the women had diarrhea between the misoprostol visit and the two-week follow up visit, compared with 9% in the placebo group. Among the women studied, 84% would have chosen medical abortion again, 9% would have chosen surgical abortion, and 7% did not know.

Comparative studies

No doubt in part because of ethical controversies it has sometimes been difficult to mount adequate controlled studies, especially in the USA. Many women and practitioners have retained a preference for dilatation and evacuation as a means of performing abortion rather than using a medicinal technique. In a pilot study at Chapel Hill, North Carolina oral mifepristone 200 mg followed 2 days later by vaginal and oral misoprostol was compared with the surgical method (11). Of 47 women eligible for the trial, 29 declined to participate, primarily because of a preference for dilatation and evacuation. Of the 18 participants enrolled, nine were randomized to treatment with mifepristone + misoprostol and 9 to dilatation and evacuation. Mifepristone + misoprostol caused more pain and adverse events, although none was serious.)

As so often happens in the hormonal field, drugs of this class have commonly been given in excessive doses, no doubt because of the over-riding need to ensure efficacy; as time goes by lower doses are proving effective and are better tolerated. For emergency contraception, for example, mifepristone 10 mg now appears to be as effective as the 25 mg that was recommended before (12).

Placebo-controlled studies

In a double-blind, randomized, controlled trial, 896 healthy women requesting a medical abortion (57–63 days gestation, mean age 25 years) were randomized to a single oral dose of mifepristone 200 mg or 600 mg, both followed in 48 hours by gemeprost 1 mg vaginally (13). The complete abortion rates were similar with the lower and higher doses of mifepristone (92 versus 92%). The incidences of adverse effects were similar, with the exception of nausea at 1 week, which was less frequent in the low-dose group (3.6 versus 7.6%).

Organs and Systems

Electrolyte balance

Severe hypokalemia has been attributed to long-term mifepristone (14).

- An extremely ill 51-year-old man with Cushing's syndrome, due to an ACTH-secreting pituitary macroadenoma, which had failed to respond to conventional surgical, medical, and radiotherapeutic approaches, responded dramatically in the short-term and long-term to high-dose mifepristone (up to 25 mg/kg/day) for 18 months. However, she developed severe hypokalemia, attributed to excessive cortisol activation of mineralocorticoid receptors; it responded to spironolactone.

This case shows the potential need for concomitant mineralocorticoid receptor blockade when mifepristone is used to treat Cushing's syndrome, since mineralocorticoid concentrations can rise markedly, reflecting corticotropin disinhibition.

Gastrointestinal

The safety and effectiveness of a combination of mifepristone + misoprostol in dealing with late uterine death have been studied using two different regimens, each in 20 women (15). In one, misoprostol was administered both vaginally and orally and in the other it was given only vaginally. There was no difference in the efficacy of the two regimens, but oral misoprostol was associated with a higher incidence of gastrointestinal adverse effects.

Reproductive system

Long-term mifepristone is primarily used as a means of treating uterine myomas, endometriosis (25–100 mg/day), and possibly inoperable meningiomas (200 mg/day) or inoperable Cushing's syndrome. While it is primarily regarded as an antiprogestogen, some of these uses reflect its antiglucocorticoid and antiproliferative effects. However, there are also data to suggest that, acting as an antiprogestogen, mifepristone can promote an unopposed estrogen milieu, and can thus have a proliferative effect on the endometrium.

- An adolescent girl with Cushingoid features and osteoporosis took mifepristone 400 mg/day for its antiglucocorticoid effect in an attempt to prevent further bone loss (16). Her striae, weight gain, and buffalo hump markedly improved, and further bone loss was halted. However, with each of the two 6-month courses of mifepristone (9 months apart) she developed massive simple endometrial hyperplasia and a markedly enlarged uterus. This reverted to normal after withdrawal of mifepristone.

The authors suggested that interval pelvic imaging may be advisable in women who take long-term mifepristone.

Since the contraceptive properties of low-dose mifepristone result from its antiprogestogenic properties, with no effect on follicular development, the user's endometrium remains exposed for long periods to unopposed estrogen. In 90 European and Asian (Chinese) women taking mifepristone 2 or 5 mg/day for 120 days the endometrial thickness increased significantly in the Europeans but decreased in the Asians (17). There were proliferative or cystic changes, with dense stroma and a significant reduction in markers of proliferation, i.e. mitotic index and Ki67 staining. It is not at all clear why the findings differed by race, although some earlier work pointed to a difference in the secretion or metabolism of estrogens between Caucasians and Chinese; the findings could also have reflected differences in body weight (and thus in relative dosage), but the absence of signs of hyperplasia or atypia led the authors to suggest that in this respect the product is safe.

From time to time mifepristone causes uterine rupture, sometimes even in unscarred uterus (18).

Infection risk

The frequency of infection after medical abortion is quite low. A major systematic review of the literature up to mid-2003 showed that in a total population of 46 421 cases, infection occurred only in 0.92%, with little variation between the various medical techniques used (19).

Long-Term Effects

Tumorigenicity

A rare case of a non-metastatic gestational trophoblastic tumor after induction of early abortion with mifepristone and misoprostol has been reported (20).

- Ultrasound before induction of an abortion suggested that the pregnancy was abnormal. The abortion was successfully induced and recovery appeared normal up to day 16, after which the patient declined further surveillance and was lost to follow-up. Sixty days after the initial treatment, she presented to a hospital with a history of intermittent bleeding and underwent curettage, revealing a complete hydatidiform mole. Chemotherapy was instituted when concentrations of human chorionic gonadotrophin plateaued. Complete gonadotrophin regression occurred after three weekly injections of methotrexate, and up to the time of writing surveillance was uneventful.

Second-Generation Effects

Pregnancy

When dealing with pre-term rupture of the membranes it is important to know the relative safety records of oxytocin alone or oral mifepristone preceding intravenous oxytocin, since these are the main therapeutic alternatives. In 65 pregnant women with spontaneous rupture of the membranes at or beyond the 36th week, who were randomly assigned to oxytocin alone or to oral mifepristone 200 mg followed by oxytocin infusion if there had been no induction within 18 hours, the average interval from start

of induction to delivery was 1194 minutes for mifepristone + oxytocin and 771 minutes for oxytocin given alone (21). Successful induction of labor with vaginal delivery was achieved within 24 hours in 78% of those who were given mifepristone compared with 52% of those given oxytocin alone. However, there was more fetal distress with mifepristone + oxytocin (9 versus 2; RR = 4.36; 95%; CI = 1.02, 19) and a trend toward more cesarean births (7 versus 3; RR = 2.26; 95% CI = 0.64, 7.99). Eleven infants of women who had been given mifepristone (33%) but only three infants of women who had been given oxytocin alone (9.4%) had to be admitted to the neonatal intensive care unit because of a generally poor condition (RR = 3.56; 95% CI = 1.09, 12). The authors concluded that oral mifepristone 18 hours before oxytocin infusion did not improve the stimulation of labor in women with premature rupture of membranes near term and was associated with more adverse fetal outcomes than oxytocin alone.

Drug Administration

Drug dosage regimens

There has sometimes been reluctance to use higher doses of mifepristone, because of a supposedly greater risk of severe adverse effects. However, in a randomized comparison of a single oral dose of mifepristone (either 200 mg or 600 mg) followed 48 hours later by oral misoprostol 400 µg the two regimens produced identical results as regards the induction of abortion and the incidence of adverse effects (22).

The optimal dose of mifepristone to secure an abortion without excessive adverse effects is not known. In a study in nearly 900 women there was no appreciable difference between oral doses of 200 or 600 mg, followed after 48 hours by gemeprost 1 mg vaginally (13). The similarity of adverse reactions with the lower and higher doses of mifepristone has been confirmed by others (23). However, in another study mifepristone 0.5 mg, which has sometimes been recommended on supposed safety grounds, was not sufficient to induce abortion (24). The frequencies of various adverse effects of mifepristone in effective doses have emerged from various studies. In one study nausea, vomiting, or diarrhea in women using a standard regimen occurred in 68%, 36%, and 20% respectively (25); these risks are not considered to be problematic. The combination of oral mifepristone and vaginal misoprostol is also effective and safe, has few serious adverse effects, and is well accepted by women (26).

References

1. Nieman LK, Choate TM, Chrousos GP, Healy DL, Morin M, Renquist D, Merriam GR, Spitz IM, Bardin CW, Baulieu EE, et al. The progesterone antagonist RU 486. A potential new contraceptive agent. N Engl J Med 1987;316(4):187–91.
2. Coyaji K, Elul B, Krishna U, Otiv S, Ambardekar S, Bopardikar A, Raote V, Ellertson C, Winikoff B. Mifepristone abortion outside the urban research hospital setting in India. Lancet 2001;357(9250):120–2.

3. Hausknecht R. Mifepristone and misoprostol for early medical abortion: 18 months experience in the United States. Contraception 2003;67:463–5.

4. Calhoun BC, Harrison DJ. Challenges to the FDA approval of mifepristone. Ann Pharmacother 2004;38:163–8.

5. Maria B, Stampf F, Goepp A, Ulmann A. Termination of early pregnancy by a single dose of mifepristone (RU 486), a progesterone antagonist. Eur J Obstet Gynecol Reprod Biol 1988;28(3):249–55.

6. Mishell DR Jr, Shoupe D, Brenner PF, Lacarra M, Horenstein J, Lahteenmaki P, Spitz IM. Termination of early gestation with the anti-progestin steroid RU 486: medium versus low dose. Contraception 1987;35(4):307–21.

7. Shannon CS, Winikoff B, Hausknecht R, Schaff E, Blumenthal PD, Oyer D, Sankey H, Wolff J, Goldberg R. Multicenter trial of a simplified mifepristone medical abortion regimen. Obstet Gynecol 2005;105:345–51.

8. Liao AH, Han XJ, Wu SY, Xiao DZ, Xiong CL, Wu XR. Randomized, double-blind, controlled trial of mifepristone in capsule versus tablet form followed by misoprostol for early medical abortion. Eur J Obstet Gynecol Reprod Biol 2004;116:211–6.

9. Coughlin LB, Roberts D, Haddad NG, Long A. Medical management of first trimester miscarriage (blighted ovum and missed abortion): is it effective? J Obstet Gynaecol 2004;24:69–71.

10. Honkanen H, Piaggio G, Von Hertzen H, Bartfai G, Erdenetungalag R, Gemzell-Danielsson K, Gopalan S, Horga M, Jerve F, Mittal S, Ngoc NTN, Peregoudov A, Prasad RNV, Pretnar-Darovec A, Shah RS, Song S, Tang OS, Wu SC. WHO multinational study of three misoprostol regimens after mifepristone for early medical abortion. II: Side effects and women's perceptions. Br J Obstet Gynaecol 2004;111:715–25.

11. Grimes DA, Smith MS, Witham AD. Mifepristone and misoprostol versus dilation and evacuation for midtrimester abortion: a pilot randomised controlled trial. Int J Obstet Gynaecol 2004;111:148–53.

12. Xiao BL, von Hertzen H, Zhao H, Piaggio G. 10 mg and 25 mg mifepristone for emergency contraception had similar efficacy and tolerability. Evidence-based Obstet Gynecol 2004;6:24.

13. Dhall GI, Calder A, Gomez-Alzugaray M, Ho PC, Pretnar Darovec A, Chen JK, Bygdeman M, Kovacs L, Albert SG, Kavkasidze G, Song LJ, Van Look PFA, Von Hertzen H, Noonan E, Ali M, Peregoudov A, Laperriere N, Grimes D. World Health Organization Task Force on Post-ovulatory Methods of Fertility Regulation. Medical abortion at 57 to 63 days' gestation with a lower dose of mifepristone and gemeprost. A randomized controlled trial. Acta Obstet Gynecol Scand 2001;80(5):447–51.

14. Chu JW, Matthias DF, Belanoff J, Schatzberg A, Hoffman AR, Feldman D. Successful long-term treatment of refractory Cushing's disease with high-dose mifepristone (RU 486). J Clin Endocrinol Metab 2001;86(8):3568–73.

15. Fairley TE, Mackenzie M, Owen P, Mackenzie F. Management of late intrauterine death using a combination of mifepristone and misoprostol—experience of two regimens. Eur J Obstet Gynecol 2005;118:28–31.

16. Newfield RS, Spitz IM, Isacson C, New MI. Long-term mifepristone (RU486) therapy resulting in massive benign endometrial hyperplasia. Clin Endocrinol (Oxf) 2001;54(3):399–404.

17. Baird DT, Brown A, Critchley HOD, Williams AR, Lin S, Cheng L. Effect of long-term treatment with low-dose mifepristone on the endometrium. Hum Reprod 2003;18:61–8.

18. Bagga R, Chaudhary N, Kalra J. Rupture in an unscarred uterus during second trimester pregnancy termination with mifepristone and misoprostol. Int J Gynecol Obstet 2004;87:42–3.

19. Shannon C, Brothers LP, Philip NM, Winikoff B. Infection after medical abortion: a review of the literature. Contraception 2004;70:183–90.

20. Lichtenberg ES. Gestational trophoblastic tumor after medical abortion. Obstet Gynec 2003;101:1137–9.

21. Wing DA, Guberman C, Fassett M. A randomized comparison of oral mifepristone to intravenous oxytocin for labor induction in women with prelabor rupture of membranes beyond 36 weeks' gestation. Am J Obst Gynecol 2005;192:445–51.

22. Wu YM, Gomez-Alzugaray M, Haukkamaa M, Ngoc NTN, Ho PC, Pretnar-Darovec A, Healy DL, Sotnikova E, Shah RS, Pavlova NG, Chen JK, Song S, Bygdeman M, Kovacs L, Khomasuridze A, Song LJ, Hamzaoui R, Alexaniants S, Von Hertzen H. Comparison of two doses of mifepristone in combination with misoprostol for early medical abortion: a randomised trial. World Health Organisation Task Force on Post-ovulatory Methods of Fertility Regulation. BJOG 2000;107(4):524–30.

23. Creinin MD, Pymar HC, Schwartz JL. Mifepristone 100 mg in abortion regimens Obstet Gynecol 2001;98(3):434–9.

24. Templeton A, Dhall GI, Calder A, Gomez-Alzugaray M, Ho PC, Pretnar-Darovec A, Sikazwe C, Jun-Kang C, Prasad RNV, Bygdeman M, Kovacs L, Kavkasidze G, Li-Juan S, Noonan E, Ali M, Peregoudov A, Laperriere N, Von Hertzen H, Grimes D, Ali MBR. Lowering the doses of mifepristone and gameprost for early abortion: a randomised controlled trial. World Health Organization Task Force on Post-ovulatory Methods for Fertility Regulation. BJOG 2001;108(7):738–42.

25. Creinin MD, Schwartz JL, Pymar HC, Fink W. Efficacy of mifepristone followed on the same day by misoprostol for early termination of pregnancy: report of a randomised trial. BJOG 2001;108(5):469–73.

26. Knudsen UB. First trimester abortion with mifepristone and vaginal misoprostol. Contraception 2001;63(5):247–50.

Progestogens

General Information

Most aspects of progestogens are dealt with in the monograph on hormonal contraception. For a complete account of the adverse effects of progestogens, readers should consult the following monographs as well as this one:

- Hormonal contraceptives—intracervical and intravaginal
- Hormonal contraceptives—oral
- Hormonal contraceptives—progestogen implants
- Hormonal contraceptives—progestogen injections
- Hormone replacement therapy—estrogens + progestogens
- Medroxyprogesterone.

While the progestogens have certain characteristic effects of their own, notably on the female menstrual cycle, the spectrum of adverse effects of any particular progestogen (particularly when given in high doses) is likely to depend heavily on the extent to which it also has glucocorticoid, mineralocorticoid, estrogenic, or androgenic properties.

The natural endogenous progestogen is progesterone (rINN), but most progestogens are semisynthetic. Progestogens belong to two main families:

- hydroxyprogesterone derivatives, which include hydroxyprogesterone caproate, dydrogesterone, medroxyprogesterone, chlormadinone, and cyproterone acetate (all rINNs), and which tend to be antiandrogenic
- ethisterone derivatives, which include norethisterone, norgestrel, levonorgestrel, desogestrel, and gestodene (all rINNs), which have some androgenic activity, and norgestimate (rINN), which has some estrogenic activity.

Water retention occasionally occurs and may reflect a degree of deoxycortone acetate (DOCA)-like activity; virilization of a female fetus is more likely to occur with a product that has some androgenic activity, and breast tenderness with a product that has estrogenic activity.

Some individuals taking progestogens for breast cancer will therefore experience, for example, not only painful swelling of the breast and prolonged amenorrhea (which are progestogenic), but also weight gain and hypercalcemia (which are likely to be glucocorticoid effects). Patients who take progestogens during pregnancy are said to be susceptible to prolonged postpartum bleeding, but this probably reflects the pregnancy disorder for which these drugs were at one time given, for example habitual or threatened abortion. Virilization of the female fetus has been described after administration of various progestogens in early pregnancy and is presumably an androgenic effect.

Progestogens given alone for contraceptive purposes can cause a number of adverse effects, some of which may reflect their other hormonal properties while others are non-specific. Headache, nausea and vomiting, breast tenderness, and pain in the back or abdomen can occur.

Animal studies cannot be regarded as providing a reliable indicator of the spectrum of activity of individual compounds; suggestions that derivatives of hydroxyprogesterone (such as megestrol acetate, medroxyprogesterone acetate) are more "natural" (because of their progesterone-like structure) than derivatives of 19-nortestosterone (such as norgestrel, lynestrenol, ethynodiol acetate, norethisterone, and allylestrenol) are not reflected in any biological findings. Experience, too, can be misleading; there is some suggestion that hydroxyprogesterone caproate can have adverse effects on the fetus when used in pregnancy, while similar reports about allylestrenol (used for the same purpose) are lacking, but one must bear in mind the anecdotal nature of such evidence and especially the fact that hydroxyprogesterone caproate appears to have been more widely used than allylestrenol and is hence more likely to have given rise to reports of adverse reactions.

Progestogens belonging to the ethisterone family (norethisterone, levonorgestrel, desogestrel) have some androgenic activity; those in the hydroxyprogesterone family (hydroxyprogesterone caproate, chlormadinone, cyproterone acetate) tend to be antiandrogenic, while norgestimate seems to be somewhat estrogenic. Water retention occasionally occurs and may reflect a degree of DOCA-like activity; virilization of a female fetus is more likely to occur with a product that has some androgenic activity, and breast tenderness with a product that has estrogenic activity.

In a multicenter, prospective, double-blind, randomized, parallel group study undertaken by general practitioners to compare progesterone pessaries with placebo in the relief of symptoms of premenstrual syndrome, spontaneous reports of adverse events were recorded (1). The 41 patients were randomized to treatment or placebo groups. Patients taking active therapy reported more frequent vaginal pruritus, headache, and irregularities of menstruation. However, when cyclical treatment with progestogen alone was given to postmenopausal women, there was no greater degree of endometrial hyperplasia than in untreated women (2).

Semisynthetic progestogens

Desogestrel (rINN)
Desogestrel, one of the so-called third-generation progestogenic steroids intended for use in oral contraceptives, is metabolized to estrogen. It was developed and introduced because of its relatively favorable effect on blood lipids in experimental work; this led to the hope that it might, in the long run, have a relatively favorable effect on the risk of atherogenesis. However, it is not clear that this does in fact happen, and the third-generation progestogens have been associated with an increased risk of thromboembolism.

Gestodene (rINN)
Gestodene is a third-generation progestogen that has been implicated in an increased risk of thromboembolism.

Gestonorone caproate (rINN)
Gestonorone (17-hydroxy-19-norprogesterone) has been used in doses of 200 mg intramuscularly weekly for benign prostatic hyperplasia (3). Mild adverse effects included loss of appetite and mild fever, but more remarkable were significant reductions in erythrocyte count, hemoglobin, and hematocrit, which normalized after drug withdrawal (4).

Hydroxyprogesterone caproate (rINN)
High doses of hydroxyprogesterone and the related norderivative have been used to treat benign prostatic hyperplasia. Very striking is the high incidence of impotence recorded in these studies, which can affect two-thirds of patients and seems to persist in some patients after withdrawal (5).

Levonorgestrel (rINN)
Extensive clinical trials and premarketing studies were conducted before the Norplant (levonorgestrel) implant was registered and approved, in order to elucidate its

mode of action, effectiveness, and adverse effects. However, none of these trials included either teenagers under 18 years of age or nulligravid women.

In an 18-month observational study of 136 adolescents (13–18 years) and 542 adults (19–46 years) who were given Norplant levonorgestrel contraceptive implants problems were reported by 110 patients, mostly irregular bleeding (53% of the adolescents and 38% of the adults) (6). Removal of the implant was requested by 11% of both adolescents and adults, most commonly for intolerable menstrual cycle changes, and in 6% of all the adults for irregular bleeding; the time from insertion to removal was 3–15 months for the adolescents and 1–17 months for the adults. Other problems that led to removal (in 5% of adolescents and 7.5% of adults), apart from a desire to become pregnant, included headache, weight gain, and acne.

Lynestrenol (rINN)

Lynestrenol is one of the older progestogens used in oral contraceptives and has been very widely and successfully employed for nearly 40 years; as monotherapy it has been used to treat irregularity of the menstrual cycle.

In a Finnish study analysis of the association between the prolonged use of lynestrenol (to suppress menstruation in mentally retarded women) and arterial disease detected at autopsy, the conclusion was that such treatment, here given for a mean of more than 6 years, increases the risk of arterial disease and that such treatment must be very carefully considered (7).

Medroxyprogesterone acetate (rINNM)

Medroxyprogesterone acetate is the subject of a separate monograph.

Megestrol (rINN)

Megestrol acetate, like medroxyprogesterone acetate, is used for metastatic breast cancer in postmenopausal women. Its commonest adverse effects are typical of the progestogens as a group, but glucocorticoid-like effects are less prominent than with medroxyprogesterone acetate. Typical effects and incidence figures for effective doses in cancer patients (SED-12, 1036) (8,9) have been cited as including weight gain in some 81–88% of cases, mild edema in up to 34%, and hypertension in up to 25%. There are lower but appreciable occurrences of constipation, dyspnea or chest tightness, heartburn, hyperglycemia, and increased urinary frequency; a few cases of phlebitis or thrombosis have been described. Vaginal bleeding, nervousness, sweating, vertigo, gastrointestinal symptoms, skin rash, pruritus, and thrombocytopenia have also been incidentally recorded.

Megestrol acetate has also proved of value in patients with metastatic prostatic cancer, epithelial ovarian cancer, or malignant melanoma and is therefore used in both sexes. The adverse effects are very similar in men to those seen with oncological doses in women; loss of libido and potency is likely to occur in male patients. In one clinical study of 43 men with recurrent and metastatic cancer of the prostate given megestrol acetate 160 mg/day orally, five developed a symptomatic rise in liver enzymes but it resolved during further treatment. In three patients, increasing bone pain occurred, no doubt relating to changes in bony metastases and requiring analgesia. Another patient developed hypercalcemia and one patient developed convulsive epilepsy (10). These latter problems are characteristic of the primary condition as it responds, and not typical for megestrol acetate. The glucocorticoid-induced gain in body weight when it occurs is often linked to improved appetite (11), which can be a positive advantage in cachectic patients with advanced cancers.

When megestrol acetate was used alongside diethylstilbestrol or ethinylestradiol in men with previously untreated metastatic carcinoma of the prostate, there was a high incidence of feminizing adverse effects (70–74%), no doubt attributable to the estrogens; a higher than expected rate of cardiovascular complications (18%) and an unexplained need for cortisone replacement (13%) were also observed (12).

Organs and Systems

Cardiovascular

Progestogens with a degree of mineralocorticoid activity will tend to cause water and salt retention and to increase blood pressure in susceptible subjects. However, effects on blood pressure can be variable; for example, medroxyprogesterone has been variously reported to cause a fall in blood pressure in some initially hypertensive patients while rapidly increasing diastolic pressure in some other women, or to have no effect on blood pressure at all.

Since thromboembolic complications can occur with progestogens, there may be a danger in using them in patients in whom there are other risk factors for thromboembolism. A Spanish group had to deal with patients with AIDS in whom megestrol acetate seems to be helpful in countering AIDS-related anorexia or cachexia. However, advanced HIV infection is itself a risk factor for thromboembolism, as is tuberculosis, which readily occurs in this population. Of 199 patients with AIDS followed for 2 years, 25 took megestrol 320 mg/day. Deep vein thrombosis occurred in seven patients in the entire series, four of them being in the megestrol group and three having tuberculosis. The duration of hormonal therapy up to the moment of thrombosis averaged 98 days. Tuberculosis was an independent risk factor. Statistical analysis led to the conclusion that in this high-risk population the use of megestrol had increased the risk of thrombosis by a factor of 7.6 (13).

Thromboembolism and third-generation progestogens

In October 1995 the UK Committee on Safety of Medicines (CSM) issued a warning that oral contraceptives containing the third-generation progestogens gestodene or desogestrel carry a higher risk of venous thromboembolism, and that women using these should consider changing to another brand (14).

The warning was based on three unpublished studies that had not at the time been formally peer reviewed. All three showed about double the risk of venous thromboembolism with gestodene and desogestrel products compared with oral contraceptives containing other progestogens. The first, a large WHO collaborative case-control study of cardiovascular disease and oral contraceptives was undertaken in 17 countries. It was completed in July 1995, and involved 829 cases of venous thromboembolism and 2641 controls from nine countries in which third-generation oral contraceptives had been used (15). The second, from the Boston Collaborative Drug Surveillance Program, was an analysis of the occurrence of venous thromboembolism in a UK general practice cohort of 238 130 women who had received a prescription for an oral contraceptive containing levonorgestrel, gestodene, or desogestrel (16). The third was a transnational case-control study conducted in five European countries, funded by Schering, the leading manufacturer of gestodene (17).

The WHO study was undertaken because the association between oral contraceptive use and venous thromboembolism had not been examined since the 1970s, when oral contraceptives contained higher doses of estrogen and progestogen than now, and because none of the earlier studies had been done in developing countries. The finding of a higher risk of venous thromboembolism with gestodene and desogestrel came as a surprise, and this, together with publicity in the media, prompted the CSM to commission the UK cohort study. The transnational study was set up at the request of the German regulatory authority to follow up German spontaneous reporting data that in 1990 had strongly suggested higher risks of thromboembolism with gestodene-containing oral contraceptives. This led to much controversy in the press and television. Schering had argued that highly publicized deaths had stimulated selective reporting, and that the claimed higher risk was an artefact.

The sudden announcement by the CSM in October 1995 caught prescribers and users of oral contraceptives completely unprepared. What some General Practitioners described as the "pill panic" in the media (18) drove thousands of women to consult their doctors (18–20), who had not been briefed. A heated debate ensued over whether the CSM's decision was justified, whether its announcement should have been delayed until the data were published, and over the dramatic and confusing way in which it was issued. Before long there was general agreement that the decision was necessary and correct, but that its communication had been handled badly, and the Health Minister said that the Government would review the incident to learn from it. Important suggestions for getting this kind of communication correct have subsequently been made (21–23). Official actions in other countries ranged from the imposition of stronger restrictions (in Germany) to decisions in the Netherlands and Canada to wait and consider the published studies, and in the USA not to advise switching to other products (24). The European Union's Committee on Proprietary Medicinal Products also decided to wait and see.

Although doubts about the relative safety of gestodene emerged in 1990, regulators did not publicly acknowledge them. Nor did they help independent scientists to examine all the relevant data (including prescribing figures, essential to provide denominators for the calculation of risk), perhaps because they were insufficient and might have been wrongly interpreted. In Germany, the regulatory authority privately asked Schering to undertake a case-control study; in the UK the Medicines Control Agency considered the available evidence inadequate and dismissed the doubts. Whether the CSM was consulted at that time or only later remains a minor official secret. The attitude changed early in July 1995, when the CSM saw the early results of the WHO Collaborative Study, and a highly critical UK television programme about gestodene-containing oral contraceptives was broadcast (Granada, "World in Action," 10 July). The CSM asked workers from the transnational case-control study to "expedite their results," and commissioned the cohort study using data routinely collected from General Practitioners. The analysis of venous thromboembolism in the transnational study was completed on 8 October, and was promptly discussed with members of the Medicines Control Agency and the CSM. The CSM quickly made its decision (17) and announced it on 18 October. The relevant data from the WHO study and the GP cohort study were published on 16 December; those from the transnational study were published on 13 January 1996 (25). A searching independent analysis of these three studies, and of a fourth (26) that the CSM had not considered, supported the decision (27).

In retrospect, what could the CSM and other authorities have done to alert the world to the potential problem during the 5 years of growing doubts about the relative safety of gestodene? To know about the doubts would have helped women and their doctors. They could then have begun to discuss among themselves whether to act on them or not, in order to weigh any real advantages of their gestodene oral contraceptive against the doubt and potential risk. A joint statement by regulators and manufacturers about their plans for further investigations would have made it clear that there was a problem to be resolved, instead of appearing to ignore or deny it. This would have allowed prescribers and independent experts to rethink their prescribing policies, for example deciding in what circumstances gestodene oral contraceptives should no longer be the first choice. That would not have pleased the manufacturers, since it would almost certainly have reduced the sales of their leading product in an uncontrollable way. The position of desogestrel creates additional complications, since its relative safety was not questioned until the data from the WHO study appeared in July 1995. If doubts had been officially expressed about the gestodene-containing products Femodene and Minulet, these oral contraceptives would meanwhile have lost some market share to Marvelon and Mercilon, the desogestrel-containing products. But greater openness from the start could have minimized the alarm and confusion.

Psychological

Progesterone, the physiological progestogen, has long been overshadowed in medical treatment by its synthetic analogues, because of their superior oral absorption.

However, it can be administered in other ways, particularly as a vaginal suppository, and the hypothesis has long existed that it might be more effective or better tolerated than the synthetic agents. In a double-blind, placebo-controlled, randomized study a Swedish group examined the mental effects of progesterone in 36 women with climacteric symptoms (28). All received estradiol 2 mg/day during three 28-day cycles. Vaginal progesterone suppositories (400 or 800 mg/day) or placebo were added sequentially for 14 days per cycle. Women without a history of premenstrual syndrome had cyclical variations in both negative mood and physical symptoms while taking progesterone 400 mg/day, but not the higher dose or the placebo. Women without a history of premenstrual syndrome had more physical symptoms on progesterone treatment compared with placebo. Women with prior premenstrual syndrome reported no progesterone-induced symptom cyclicity. The authors concluded that in women without prior premenstrual syndrome natural progesterone caused negative mood effects similar to those induced by synthetic progestogens, but the dose-effect relation was complex.

Liver

The progestogens as a group have little effect on the liver. However, some progestogens can increase non-conjugated bilirubin (29); norethisterone acetate has been implicated in this effect (30).

Skin

Progestogens have very occasionally been reported to cause hypersensitivity reactions or skin disorders. Pemphigus has been reported (31).

- A 34-year-old woman with a 3-month history of dysphagia, odynophagia, and conjunctivitis with bulbar injection, who had been taking an oral contraceptive containing a progestogen for 7 months, developed typical bullous lesions on her trunk and nose, typical of pemphigus. Ceftriaxone and ampicillin, which can aggravate pemphigus, exacerbated the lesions. There was reason to believe that the patient had a genetic predisposition to the disorder.

The circumstances pointed strongly to a drug association, but the identity of the oral contraceptive was not stated; it is likely to have contained a synthetic progestogen and not progesterone itself.

However progesterone-induced dermatitis certainly does occur.

- A 68-year-old woman who took a formulation containing hydroxyprogesterone acetate + conjugated estrogens had for many years an autoimmune dermatitis (32).

Autoimmune progesterone-induced dermatitis with purpura and petechiae has been reported (33).

Sweet's syndrome has been reported several times in women taking oral contraceptives, but a well-documented recent case concerned the use of the Mirena uterine system for the administration of menorrhagia, where the complication could only have been due to levonorgestrel (34).

- A 54-year-old woman fitted with a Mirena system soon developed fever and progressive skin lesions. A skin biopsy confirmed Sweet's syndrome. She was treatment with topical and oral glucocorticoids, but the condition relapsed on reduction of the dose. Her symptoms finally resolved on removal of the intrauterine system and she remained symptom free after 9 months.

A Japanese report has suggested that erythema multiforme may be induced by a product based on a progestogen alone (35).

Immunologic

Hypersensitivity to steroids used for contraceptive purposes has very occasionally been reported for many years.

- A 42-year-old woman who used the Mirena system to relieve heavy periods and spasmodic dysmenorrhea developed an itchy eruption on her shins on the day after insertion of the system, later spreading to her thighs, chest, and arms (36). A diagnosis of "autoimmune progesterone dermatitis" was made, although one is bound to wonder whether the reaction was to progesterone itself or to levonorgestrel. Treatment with glucocorticoids and antihistamines provided only temporary relief, and the Mirena system had to be removed.

Other complications (acne, alopecia, and pruritus) have been associated with Mirena, an intrauterine system containing levonorgestrel.

- Rosacea accompanied the use of Mirena in a 36-year-old woman for 2 years and disappeared within 6 months of removal (37).

However, one is bound to wonder whether this was a direct reaction to levonorgestrel or a stress reaction to the absence of menstrual periods. Like many other users of Mirena, this woman had amenorrhea associated with facial flushing and pustules; conditions such as urticaria, eczema, pompholyx, and erythema multiforme occur cyclically in some women in the second half of the menstrual cycle, irrespective of contraceptive use.

Long-Term Effects

Tumorigenicity

The effects of adding a progestogen on the carcinogenic effects of estrogens are discussed in the monograph on estrogens.

Second-Generation Effects

Teratogenicity

For a number of years from about 1950 onwards, progestogens were used in cases of threatened and habitual abortion. They were largely abandoned for this purpose because of the general conclusion that they were ineffective. There was no general conclusion as to any adverse effects that might have resulted, although some of the progestogens were suspected of having virilizing effects on the fetus. Subsequently, progestogens (usually natural progesterone) were used to provide "luteal support" for some 4 weeks after in vitro fertilization. In 283 women treated for this reason with injectable progesterone 300 mg/day, oral micronized progesterone 90 mg/day, or a sustained-release transvaginal gel, among the offspring there were incidental cases of facial teratoma associated with a cleft palate, a respiratory distress syndrome, and Pierre–Robin syndrome; there was no clear indication that in this respect one formulation was safer than another or that the effects observed were other than might have been anticipated in untreated controls with a similar history (38). Women who received the injectable progesterone tended to complain of drowsiness, reduced libido, dyspareunia, and vaginal irritability.

With regard to progestogens given alone to prevent threatened or habitual abortion, there is no good evidence that they are beneficial, and much evidence to the contrary; however, effects on the sexual development of the fetus cannot be excluded (39).

Tumors may possibly be induced in the second generation. Neuroblastoma in four infants has been attributed to pregnancy or to gonadotropins, clomiphene citrate, or progestational hormones (40), because these drugs result in increased exposure of the early pregnancy to estrogenic or progestogenic influences. Most of these neuroblastomas regress spontaneously, but when regression does not occur they may become malignant. Children born to women who have taken hormonal preparations in early pregnancy should therefore be screened for urinary vanillylmandelic acid concentrations at the age of 6 months.

Drug Administration

Drug formulations

As with estradiol, a case has been made for using natural progesterone, rather than synthetic analogues, largely because it is assumed that as a physiological substance it will be safer. Progesterone is unsuitable for oral use (unless given in a special micronized form), but it is used by other routes. These include systemic and intra-articular injection (41), an intranasal ointment (42), transdermal formulations (43), and intravaginal formulations (44). Apart from local irritation, the wanted and unwanted effects produced when using these modes of administration are the familiar manifestations of progestogen treatment and are proportional to the amount of the drug that actually enters the circulation.

Micronized oral formulations

The fact that progesterone when given by mouth has poor systemic availability can be largely overcome by micronization, and the first product based on this concept was marketed in France as long ago as 1980. Studies and reviews have appeared, particularly since 1997, suggesting that it is indeed less likely to cause adverse effects than

the synthetic progestogens are (45). The most frequently reported adverse reactions are stated to be dizziness or drowsiness, which could be related to the pregnenolone metabolites and do not seem to reflect vasoactive changes. It has been argued theoretically that there might be altered sodium metabolism, but no hypertensive effects have been seen. Unusually high doses of micronized progesterone given in pregnancy (in the hope of avoiding premature labor) have been suspected of causing intrahepatic cholestasis, at least in women with a genetic predisposition, but these doses are much higher that those in normal use. No changes in lipid profile appear to occur.

With these very positive conclusions it is not clear why micronized progesterone has not been more widely used. Commercial factors may well have played a role in maintaining the overwhelming dominance of the patented synthetic progestogens. On the other hand, despite the fact that there are estimated to be 500 000 current users of micronized progesterone in France alone, the worldwide scope of experience is still limited compared with that of the synthetic analogues, and one must be prepared for surprises if this product should ever be used more widely. It is a fact that in the 1970s, when studies in beagle dogs gave rise to much concern regarding progestogens and the induction of mammary tumors, the same effect was also observed with natural progesterone if sufficient doses were administered. Even a natural substance can have unpleasant effects when used in a manner not foreseen in nature.

Intrauterine release systems

Levonorgestrel is used in the form of intrauterine devices, both as a contraceptive and to treat menorrhagia. They are effective, but critical reviewers continue to point to the need to be alert to the possible development of pain and hypermenorrhea, and to warn patients of the possibility of expulsion or perforation (46).

Any intrauterine device can very occasionally perforate the uterine wall and enter the peritoneal cavity. When the device releases an active pharmacological agent it is relevant to know whether this is likely to cause adhesions. An investigation in Israel looked into this issue, examining the files of all patients with an intra-peritoneal intrauterine device over a twelve-year period (47). Eight such cases were identified, four of them involving a levonorgestrel-containing device and four a copper intrauterine device. Laparoscopy for removal of the intrauterine device disclosed mild local peritoneal adhesions between the omentum and the pelvic organs in all cases. There was no difference between the two devices as regards the appearance of the peritoneum. These few cases suggest that the potential of the levonorgestrel system to adhere to the peritoneum is low and similar to that of the copper-bearing device.

The fiber-based ("frameless") FibroPlant delivery system for levonorgestrel has been tested in an open study in 32 women as a means of relieving menorrhagia or for contraceptive purposes (48). The period of exposure was 1–23 months. This system, which releases levonorgestrel 14 micrograms/day, appeared to be effective for both purposes, and there were no cases of infection, expulsion, or perforation.

A 1-year study of the FibroPlant system in a mixed population of 141 peri- and post-menopausal women, including women with heavy or post-menopausal bleeding and women needing contraception, was too small and too heterogeneous to justify firm conclusions, and most of the women were in any case also using percutaneous 17-beta-estradiol 1.5 mg/day) (49). However, the results suggested that this regimen is well tolerated.

An alternative intrauterine delivery system (LNG-IUS) consists of an adapted Nova-T device with a silastic reservoir attached to the vertical arm; the reservoir is impregnated with levonorgestrel and is covered with a rate-limiting silastic membrane. The release rate of levonorgestrel is about 20 micrograms/day for at least 5 years. In a 5-year study in which 1821 women used the combined device and 937 others used the plain Nova-T device, the Pearl index (the number of unwanted pregnancies occurring in 100 couples using a given method for a period of one year) was 0.09/100 woman-years for the LNG-IUS and the ectopic pregnancy rate was 0.02/100 woman-years (50). There were fewer withdrawals because of bleeding problems and pelvic inflammatory disease with LNG-IUS compared with Nova-T, but there were more withdrawals because of hormonal adverse effects and absence of bleeding. One of the advantages claimed for LNG-IUS is that there will be less menstrual blood loss. However, all women who used LNG-IUS had some change in their bleeding pattern after the device had been inserted, and some had many days of spotting. Of another 30 women who used the LNG-IUS system to relieve menorrhagia and who were followed for a year, 13 reported one or more pelvic adverse event; there were six complaints of irregular bleeding, four of abdominal pain, three of breast tenderness, and occasional cases of headache, mood changes, or acne (51).

In a prospective non-comparative 6-month study of 34 women with mild to moderate endometriosis this approach gave marked relief of symptoms, and two-thirds of the women elected to continue treatment after the trial was completed (52). The staging of the disease was favorably affected. Administration of low doses in this manner seems to provide a means of avoiding significant systemic adverse effects while maintaining efficacy, but longer-term experience is required.

In another study of the LNG-IUS in 200 young nulliparous women, half of whom received the intrauterine system and the remainder an oral contraceptive for 1 year, 20% of those in the LNG-IUS group withdrew, one-third because of *pain*; the adverse effects in the oral group, in which 28% withdrew, were hormonal (53).

LNG-IUS has also been used for contraception immediately after termination of pregnancy in 20 nulliparous young women and was well accepted, although irregular vaginal bleeding was not uncommon (54).

When exposure to LNH-IUS continued for up to 4 years the system was well tolerated throughout, with a high continuation rate; in women with heavy menstrual bleeding some irregular bleeding and spotting can occur, but this is much more acceptable than the menorrhagia for which the treatment is used (55).

A systematic review of Mirena, an intrauterine progestogen release system (56), has attracted correspondence (57,58). Like other devices, Mirena releases levonorgestrel, in this case 20 micrograms/day. Since it had no greater efficacy than the Copper T device and was very much more costly, the debate has turned on safety. Amenorrhea is common with this device, as with others like it, and correspondents have pointed out that this is regarded by many women as an unwelcome complication.

In a study of the long-term acceptability of Mirena, 165 women were examined during and after 6 and 36 months of use. There were changes in menstrual bleeding pattern in 161 women (98%), with cessation or transient absence of menstruation in 75 (47%) and 14 (9%) women respectively. As in many other studies, amenorrhea was considered by most women (81%) as a welcome effect. The device had no disturbing effects on the women or their partners during sexual intercourse (59).

The fact that the Mirena system induces intermenstrual bleeding within the first few months after insertion is puzzling. It has been suggested that it is due to changes in vascular development, and a randomized study in 48 women using hysterectomy specimens has shown that the system has a localized effect on some vessels within the superficial endometrium. The cross-sectional diameters of the largest vascular lumina were significantly increased after treatment. However, there was no difference in the median values of vessel diameter or the vascular surface density (60). This may not necessarily be the only explanation for early intermenstrual bleeding during such treatment. Other authors have concluded that intrauterine levonorgestrel induces a decrease in expression of vascular endothelial growth factor but increased expression of adrenomedullin in the endometrial glands and stroma after 3 months of therapy (61).

Transdermal administration

An older 19-norprogesterone (ST 1435, Merck Darmstadt) was used experimentally in a transdermal form as a possible hormonal contraceptive. A dose of 0.8–1 mg/day was needed to inhibit ovulation in all subjects. There was some irregularity of bleeding, and some subjects had breast tenderness (62).

Vaginal gel and suppositories

To provide luteal support in ovarian stimulation protocols, especially when following the long procedure, progesterone can be administered by various routes. The oral route is relatively ineffective, since progesterone has a low oral systemic availability (below 10%), which may result in adverse effects such as somnolence. Intramuscular administration is painful and inconvenient. Some workers have therefore given progesterone in the form of an 8% vaginal gel, which is effective and better tolerated than alternative approaches. The gel adheres to the vaginal epithelium, and leakage is substantially less than when using capsules or suppositories; there are no local complications (63). No adverse reactions have been reported with the use of a modified-release vaginal gel containing polycarbophil-based progesterone (64).

Two different vaginal suppositories have been compared in 60 patients at risk of ovarian hyperstimulation (65). Cyclogest vaginal suppositories 400 mg bd and Crinone 8% vaginal gel od, both for 14 days were compared. Perineal irritation was reported by some 20% of patients in each group. Significantly more patients using the suppositories graded inconvenience of administration, leakage, and interference with coitus as moderate or severe.

Drug-drug interactions

Cocaine

It is unusual to find a study in which the use of a medicinal treatment is found to interact with "street drugs" or other agents used illicitly. The effects of progesterone on the drug experience of cocaine users have been studied (66). Ten adult cocaine users entered two experimental sessions. Before each session, they took either two oral doses of progesterone 200 mg or placebo. Two hours after the second dose, they received cocaine 0.3 mg/kg intravenously and started the self-administration period, in which five optional doses of cocaine were available. Progesterone attenuated the cocaine-induced increase in diastolic blood pressure without affecting the increases in systolic blood pressure and heart rate. Progesterone also attenuated the subjective ratings of the "high" and "feel" responses but did not affect cocaine self-administration behavior.

References

1. Magill PJProgesterone Study Group. Investigation of the efficacy of progesterone pessaries in the relief of symptoms of premenstrual syndrome. Br J Gen Pract 1995;45(400):589–93.
2. Rabe T, Mueck AO, Deuringer FU, Vladescu E, Runnebaum B. Spacing-out of progestin—efficacy, tolerability and compliance of two regimens for hormonal replacement in the late postmenopause. Gynecol Endocrinol 1997;11(6):383–92.
3. Iguchi H, Ikeuchi T, Kai Y, Yoshida H. [Influence of antiandrogen therapy for prostatic hypertrophy on lipid metabolism.]Hinyokika Kiyo 1994;40(3):215–9.
4. Okada K, Oishi L, Yoshida O. Effects on the pituitary–gonadal axis in the treatment of benign prostatic hypertrophy with gestoronone caproate. Curr Ther Res 1984;35:139.
5. Palanca E, Juco W. Conservative treatment of benign prostatic hyperplasia. Curr Med Res Opin 1977;4(7):513–20.
6. Cullins VE, Remsburg RE, Blumenthal PD, Huggins GR. Comparison of adolescent and adult experiences with Norplant levonorgestrel contraceptive implants. Obstet Gynecol 1994;83(6):1026–32.
7. Huovinen K, Autio S, Kaprio J. Peroral lynestrenol and arterial disease in mentally retarded women. A case-control study based on autopsy findings. Acta Obstet Gynecol Scand 1988;67(3):211–4.
8. Feliu J, Gonzalez-Baron M, Berrocal A, Artal A, Ordonez A, Garrido P, Zamora P, Garcia de Paredes ML, Montero JM. Usefulness of megestrol acetate in cancer cachexia and anorexia. A placebo-controlled study. Am J Clin Oncol 1992;15(5):436–40.
9. Tchekmedyian NS, Tait N, Aisner J. High-dose megestrol acetate in the treatment of postmenopausal women with advanced breast cancer. Semin Oncol 1986;13(4 Suppl 4):20–5.
10. Crombie C, Raghavan D, Page J, Woods R, Dalley D, Devine R, Rosen M. Phase II study of megestrol acetate for metastatic carcinoma of the prostate. Br J Urol 1987;59(5):443–6.
11. Loeffler TM, Weber FW, Hausamen TU. Einfluss von mittelhoch dosiertem Megestrolacetat auf Appetitstimulation und Gewichtszunahme bei gleichzeitiger zytostatische Therapie. Tumordiagn Ther 1992;13:72.
12. Johnson DE, Babaian RJ, Swanson DA, von Eschenbach AC, Wishnow KI, Tenney D. Medical castration using megestrol acetate and minidose estrogen. Urology 1988;31(5):371–4.
13. Force L, Barrufet P, Herreras Z, Bolibar I. Deep venous thrombosis and megestrol in patients with HIV infection. AIDS 1999;13(11):1425–6.
14. Carnall D. Controversy rages over new contraceptive data. BMJ 1995;311:1117–8.
15. World Health Organization Collaborative Study of Cardiovascular Disease and Steroid Hormone Contraception. Effect of different progestagens in low oestrogen oral contraceptives on venous thromboembolic disease. Lancet 1995;346(8990):1582–8.
16. Jick H, Jick SS, Gurewich V, Myers MW, Vasilakis C. Risk of idiopathic cardiovascular death and nonfatal venous thromboembolism in women using oral contraceptives with differing progestagen components. Lancet 1995;346(8990):1589–93.
17. Spitzer WO. Data from transnational study of oral contraceptives have been misused. BMJ 1995;311(7013):1162.
18. Armstrong JL, Reid M, Bigrigg A. Scare over oral contraceptives. Effect on behaviour of women attending a family planning clinic. BMJ 1995;311(7020):1637.
19. Seamark CJ. Scare over oral contraceptives. Effect on women in a general practice in Devon.··· BMJ 1995;311(7020):1637.
20. Davies AW, York JR, Jones SR. [Scare over oral contraceptives] ··· and south Wales.]BMJ 1995;311(7020):1637–8.
21. Ketting E. Third generation oral contraceptives. CSM's advice will harm women's health worldwide. BMJ 1996;312(7030):576.
22. Stewart-Brown S, Pyper C. Third generation oral contraceptives. CSM should rethink its approach for such announcements. BMJ 1996;312(7030):576.
23. Smith C. Third generation oral contraceptives. How one clinic's practice conforms with CSM's advice. BMJ 1996;312(7030):576–7.
24. Carnall D, Karcher H, Lie LG, Sheldon T, Spurgeon D, Josefson D, Zinn C. Third generation oral contraceptives—the controversy. BMJ 1995;311(7020):1589–90.
25. Spitzer WO, Lewis MA, Heinemann LA, Thorogood M, MacRae KD. Third generation oral contraceptives and risk of venous thromboembolic disorders: an international case-control study. Transnational Research Group on Oral Contraceptives and the Health of Young Women. BMJ 1996;312(7023):83–8.
26. Bloemenkamp KW, Rosendaal FR, Helmerhorst FM, Buller HR, Vandenbroucke JP. Enhancement by factor V Leiden mutation of risk of deep-vein thrombosis associated with oral contraceptives containing a third-generation progestagen. Lancet 1995;346(8990):1593–6.
27. McPherson K. Third generation oral contraception and venous thromboembolism. BMJ 19967;312(7023):68–9.

28. Andreen L, Bixo M, Nyberg S, Sundstrom-Poromaa I, Backstrom T. Progesterone effects during sequential hormone replacement therapy. Eur J Endocrinol 2003;148:571–7.

29. Boyer JL, Preisig R, Zbinden G, de Kretser DM, Wang C, Paulsen CA. Guidelines for assessment of potential hepatotoxic effects of synthetic androgens, anabolic agents and progestagens in their use in males as antifertility agents. Contraception 1976;13(4):461–8.

30. Werner T. Ikterus mit Worschluss-syndrom nach Behandlung mit Norethisteronazetat. Z Gastroenterol 1969;7:186.

31. Lo Schiavo A, D'Avino M. Progesterone, an unsuspected pemphigus inductor. G Ital Dermatol Venereol 1999;134:331–4.

32. Ingber A, Trattner A, David M. Hypersensitivity to an oestrogen–progesterone preparation and possible relationship to autoimmune progesterone dermatitis and corticosteroid hypersensitivity. J Dermatol Treat 1999;10:139–40.

33. Wintzen M, Goor-Van Egmond MBT, Noz KC. Autoimmune progesterone dermatitis presenting with purpura and petechiae. Clin Exp Dermatol 2004;29:316.

34. Hamill M, Bowling J, Vega-Lopez F. Sweet syndrome and a Mirena intrauterine system. J Fam Planning Reprod Health Care 2004;30:115–6.

35. Suzuki R, Matsumura Y, Kambe N, Fujii H, Tachibana T, Miyachi Y. Erythema multiforme due to progesterone in a low-dose oral contraceptive pill. Br J Dermatol 2005;152:370–1.

36. Pereira A, Coker A. Hypersensitivity to Mirena—a rare complication. J Obstet Gynaecol 2003;23:81.

37. Choudry K, Humphreys F, Menage J. Rosacea in association with the progesterone-releasing intrauterine contraceptive device. Clin Exp Dermatol 2001;26(1):102.

38. Pouly JL, Bassil S, Frydman R, Hedon B, Nicollet B, Prada Y, Antoine JM, Zambrano R, Donnez J. Luteal support after in-vitro fertilization: Crinone 8%, a sustained release vaginal progesterone gel, versus Utrogestan, an oral micronized progesterone. Hum Reprod 1996;11(10):2085–9.

39. World Health Organization. Treatment of threatened or habitual abortion. In: Drugs in Pregnancy and Delivery. 11th European Symposium on Clinical Pharmacological Evaluation in Drug Control. Copenhagen: WHO Regional Office for Europe, 1984:6.

40. Mandel M, Toren A, Rechavi G, Dor J, Ben-Bassat I, Neumann Y. Hormonal treatment in pregnancy: a possible risk factor for neuroblastoma. Med Pediatr Oncol 1994;23(2):133–5.

41. Cuchacovich M, Tchernitchin A, Gatica H, Wurgaft R, Valenzuela C, Cornejo E. Intraarticular progesterone: effects of a local treatment for rheumatoid arthritis. J Rheumatol 1988;15(4):561–5.

42. Dalton ME, Bromham DR, Ambrose CL, Osborne J, Dalton KD. Nasal absorption of progesterone in women. Br J Obstet Gynaecol 1987;94(1):84–8.

43. Persico N, Mancini F, Artini PG, Regnani G, Volpe A, de Aloysio D, Battaglia C. Transdermal hormone replacement therapy and Doppler findings in normal and overweight postmenopausal patients. Gynecol Endocrinol 2004;19(5):274–81.

44. Lightman A, Kol S, Itskovitz-Eldor J. A prospective randomized study comparing intramuscular with intravaginal natural progesterone in programmed thaw cycles. Hum Reprod 1999;14(10):2596–9.

45. de Lignieres B. Oral micronized progesterone. Clin Ther 1999;21(1):41–60.

46. Anonymous. Arzneimittelnebenwirkungen aktuell. Intern Praxis 2003;43:405.

47. Haimov-Kochman R, Doviner V, Amsalem H, Prus D, Adoni A, Lavy Y. Intraperitoneal levonorgestrel-releasing intrauterine device following uterine perforation: the role of progestins in adhesion formation. Hum Reprod 2003;18:990–993.

48. Wildemeersch D, Schacht E. Treatment of menorrhagia with a novel "frameless" intrauterine levonorgestrel-releasing drug delivery system: a pilot study. Eur J Contracept Reprod Health Care 2001;6(2):93–101.

49. Wildemeersch D, Schacht E, Wildemeersch P. Performance and acceptability of intrauterine release of levonorgestrel with a miniature delivery system for hormonal substitution therapy, contraception and treatment in peri- and postmenopausal women. Maturitas 2003;44:237–45.

50. Andersson K, Guillebaud J. The levonorgestrel intrauterine system: more than a contraceptive. Eur J Contracept Reprod Health Care 2001;6(Suppl 1):15–22.

51. Istre O, Trolle B. Treatment of menorrhagia with the levonorgestrel intrauterine system versus endometrial resection. Fertil Steril 2001;76(2):304–9.

52. Lockhat FB, Emembolu JO, Konje JC. The evaluation of the effectiveness of an intrauterine-administered progestogen (levonorgestrel) in the symptomatic treatment of endometriosis and in the staging of the disease. Hum Reprod 2004;19:179–84.

53. Suhonen S, Haukkamaa M, Jakobsson T, Rauramo I. Clinical performance of a levonorgestrel-releasing intrauterine system and oral contraceptives in young nulliparous women: a comparative study. Contraception 2004;69:407–12.

54. Li C-FI, Lee SSN, Pun TC. A pilot study on the acceptability of levonorgestrel-releasing intrauterine device by young, single, nulliparous Chinese females following surgical abortion. Contraception 2004;69:247–50.

55. Radesic B, Sharma A. Levonorgestrel-releasing intrauterine system for treating menstrual disorders: a patient satisfaction questionnaire. Aust NZ J Obstet Gynaecol 2004;44:247–51.

56. French RS, Cowan FM, Mansour D, Higgins JP, Robinson A, Procter T, Morris S, Guillebaud J. Levonorgestrel-releasing (20 microgram/day) intrauterine systems (Mirena) compared with other methods of reversible contraceptives. BJOG 2000;107(10):1218–25.

57. Gerber B, Reimer T, Krause A, Friese K, Muller H. Levonorgestrel-releasing intrauterine devices. Lancet 2001;357(9258):801.

58. Onyeka BA, French R, Mansour D, Robinson A, Guillebaud J. Levonorgestrel-releasing (20 mcg/day) intrauterine systems (Mirena) compared with other methods of reversible contraceptives BJOG 2001;108(7):770–1.

59. Baldaszti E, Wimmer-Puchinger B, Loschke K. Acceptability of the long-term contraceptive levonorgestrel-releasing intrauterine system Mirena: a 3-year follow-up. Contraception 2003;67:87–91.

60. McGavigan CJ, Dockery P, Metaxa-Mariatou V, Campbell D, Stewart CJR, Cameron IT, Campbell S. Hormonally mediated disturbance of angiogenesis in the human endometrium after exposure to intrauterine levonorgestrel. Hum Reprod 2003;18:77–84.

61. Laoag-Fernandez JB, Maruo T, Pakarinen P, Spitz IM, Johansson E. Effects of levonorgestrel-releasing intra-

uterine system on the expression of vascular endothelial growth factor and adrenomedullin in the endometrium in adenomyosis. Hum Reprod 2003;18:694–9.

62. Laurikka-Routti M, Haukkamaa M, Lahteenmaki P. Suppression of ovarian function with the transdermally given synthetic progestin ST 1435. Fertil Steril 1992;58(4):680–4.
63. Ludwig M, Diedrich K. Evaluation of an optimal luteal phase support protocol in IVF. Acta Obstet Gynecol Scand 2001;80(5):452–66.
64. Warren MP, Biller BM, Shangold MM. A new clinical option for hormone replacement therapy in women with secondary amenorrhea: effects of cyclic administration of progesterone from the sustained-release vaginal gel Crinone (4% and 8%) on endometrial morphologic features and withdrawal bleeding. Am J Obstet Gynecol 1999;180(1 Pt 1):42–8.
65. Ng EHY, Miao B, Cheung W, Ho P-C. A randomised comparison of side effects and patient inconvenience of two vaginal progesterone formulations used for luteal support in in vitro fertilisation cycles. Eur J Obstet Gynecol Reprod Biol 2003;111:50–4.
66. Sofuoglu M, Mitchell E, Kosten TR. Effects of progesterone treatment on cocaine responses in male and female cocaine users. Pharmacol Biochem Behav 2004;78:699–705.

Raloxifene

General Information

Raloxifene is a non-steroidal so-called "selective estrogen receptor modulator" (SERM), that is it binds to estrogen receptors, but this binding produces agonist effects at some sites and antagonist effects at others (1). It has estrogen agonist effects on bone and lipid metabolism but estrogen antagonist effects on the breast and endometrium; it is also claimed by its protagonists to have cardioprotective effects, perhaps through an effect on endothelial cells and a reduction in homocysteine concentrations (2).

Reports of adverse reactions to raloxifene should be considered alongside those reported for tamoxifen and other anti-estrogens. However, earlier reports have pointed to a considerable increase in thromboembolism, as has some recent large-scale work (3), and it would be premature to draw final conclusions about the conditions in which it can safely be used.

Raloxifene has been studied for its ability to reduce bone loss in postmenopausal women (4). Some specialized SERMs could reduce the risk of osteoporosis after the menopause without having other troublesome hormonal effects (5), but much more work is needed to determine whether they will fulfill this hope.

In a critical review of raloxifene, published in France, it was concluded that the compound has no advantages compared with a traditional estrogen, and that in view of certain findings in animal studies there is a possibility that it might increase the risk of ovarian cancer; there is also a need to determine whether it is sufficiently safe in women with a history of (or predisposition to) breast cancer (6).

One also finds a critical view expressed in the USA, where a survey of the literature up to the end of 1999 concluded that while raloxifene might carry a lesser risk of breast cancer than estrogen replacement therapy, it was also less effective in maintaining bone density, and that as regards cardiovascular risk the estrogenic treatment produced a more favorable outcome (7).

The uses and adverse effects of raloxifene have been reviewed (8–12). Current work seems to show an altogether positive effect of raloxifene (for example 60 mg/day) on bone metabolism and serum lipids in post-menopausal women on chronic hemodialysis, without significant adverse effects in the short term. However, even the authors of very promising work in this connection point to the difficulty in assessing the long-term safety of the treatment in such women (13). Longer-term work elsewhere has pointed particularly to the occurrence of thromboembolic disease, but also of hot flushes, influenza-like symptoms, peripheral edema, and leg cramps. With the exception of thromboembolism these are unpleasant rather than serious, but they still need to be recorded and studied in this very susceptible group of users.

Idoxifene is another of the newer selective estrogen receptor modulators (SERMs), and preclinical data show that it has greater antiestrogenic activity than tamoxifen but lower estrogenic activity. It is not yet clear whether this affects its degree of usefulness or safety when it is used, for example, in cases of metastatic breast cancer. In comparisons of the two drugs in such patients the desired effects were similar and the incidence of adverse effects was essentially the same (14).

In a randomized phase II trial in 47 such women in whom tamoxifen 20 mg/day had ceased to be effective, idoxifene showed only very slight evidence of activity; possible drug-related adverse effects were similar in frequency to those with tamoxifen (hot flushes/flashes 13% versus 15%, mild nausea 20% versus 15%) (15). Endocrine and lipid analysis in both groups showed similar changes.

Many centers continue to examine this and other SERMs, for example in countering menopausal bone loss (16), in the hope that they can take the place of tamoxifen and provide a means of avoiding the risks of such complications as endometrial cancer, cataract, and stroke (17–19).

Observational studies

An extensive literature review has provided a useful assessment of the benefit to harm balance of raloxifene (20). The findings were reassuring. One large fracture prevention trial provided the best evidence that raloxifene 60 mg/day for 3 years reduced the relative risk of vertebral fractures by 30–50% in women with prevalent fractures or osteoporosis. The extraskeletal effects of raloxifene include a reduction in total cholesterol and low density lipoprotein cholesterol concentrations. Raloxifene was not associated with endometrial hyperplasia, and there was a 72% reduction in the incidence of invasive breast cancer. Adverse events associated with raloxifene included an increase in the absolute risk of venous thromboembolism and increased risks of hot flushes (flashes) and leg cramps. Compared with other therapies for osteoporosis, raloxifene has a smaller impact on bone mineral density, a similar effect on the occurrence of vertebral fractures, and no effect on the frequency of non-vertebral fractures. In the present state of knowledge it seems clear that raloxifene can be recommended for prevention of vertebral fractures in women with osteopenia/osteoporosis who are not at high risk of non-vertebral fractures and who do not have a past history of venous thromboembolism.

Comparative studies

Since both raloxifene and the non-hormonal drug alendronate reduce the incidence of osteoporotic fractures in postmenopausal women it is relevant to determine which approach is better tolerated and thus most likely to promote long-term adherence to therapy. Adverse effects and compliance have been studied in a direct randomized comparison over 12 months in 902 women attending 154 treatment centres in Spain (21). They took either raloxifene 60 mg/day or alendronate 10 mg/day. Those who took raloxifene reported significantly better compliance than those who took alendronate; more patients discontinued alendronate prematurely than raloxifene (26% versus 16%. The main reason for premature discontinuation was adverse reactions, particularly gastrointestinal reactions (9.9% with alendronate, 3.4% with raloxifene).

Alendronate 70 mg once weekly and raloxifene 60 mg/day for 12 months have been compared in an international multicenter blinded trial in 487 women with low bone density (22). Bone mineral density increased much more with alendronate. Overall tolerability was similar, but the proportion of patients who reported vasomotor events was significantly higher with raloxifene (9.5%) than with alendronate (3.7%); the proportions of patients who reported gastrointestinal events were similar.

Organs and Systems

Cardiovascular

Evidence of the wanted or unwanted effects of antiestrogens on the cardiovascular system has been sought in an extensive literature study (23). In one published study there was a two- to three-fold rise in the incidence of thromboembolism, similar to that seen with estrogen treatment. There were also some cases of leg cramps and hot flushes (24).

There have been conflicting reports on the incidence and severity of symptoms such as hot flushes (also known as hot flashes) during long-term treatment with raloxifene for the prevention of osteoporosis. In fact the difference between raloxifene and placebo does not seem to be very great. In a review of three identical randomized trials in which raloxifene 60 mg was given for long periods to healthy postmenopausal women of various ages it was concluded that after 30 months the cumulative incidence of hot flushes was 21% for placebo and 28% for raloxifene, but the difference in frequency was confined to the first 6 months of therapy (25). There was no difference

between placebo and raloxifene in the maximum severity of symptoms or the rate of early discontinuation, while the period during which hot flushes continued was only a little shorter in the raloxifene group. In a US study in more than 1100 postmenopausal women who took raloxifene 30–150 mg/day the only significant adverse effect of therapy was hot flushes (25% with 60 mg/day and 18% in the placebo group) (26).

The effects of raloxifene on the vascular endothelium have been studied in 19 subjects who underwent endothelial function testing at baseline and after treatment with placebo or raloxifene (60 mg/day for 6 weeks) (27). The findings in this small short-term study were entirely positive. Brachial artery diameter change (flow-mediated dilatation) increased 5.0% with placebo and 8.6% with raloxifene in response to a hyperemic stimulus. The ratio of AUC response to AUC reference with the use of laser Doppler measures was 1.18 for placebo and 1.28 for raloxifene. Flow-mediated dilatation and AUC ratio correlated significantly. The authors concluded that raloxifene enhanced endothelial-mediated dilatation in brachial arteries and digital vessels in these women, and they discussed the drug's possible cardioprotective effect.

Endocrine

Some studies have suggested that raloxifene has a relatively favorable safety profile among the antiestrogens, notably as regards cardiovascular risk factors (SEDA-27, 431), but when used therapeutically it is generally considered likely to produce an increase in hot flushes/flashes, very much like tamoxifen. This has now been disputed on the basis of a double-blind study in 487 postmenopausal women who took raloxifene drug for 8 months to counter the development of osteoporosis (28). Treated patients took either raloxifene 60 mg/day throughout or raloxifene by slow-dose escalation for the first 2 months, followed by the standard dose for the rest of the study; another group took placebo. The baseline incidence of hot flushes/flashes (3–5 per week) was low. During treatment it increased by an average of less than one episode per week in both active treatment groups and reduced by less than one per week with placebo. The high proportion (about 60%) of asymptomatic patients at baseline had increased further by the end of treatment in all groups. The proportion of women whose pre-existing episodes abated during treatment was significantly greater with slow dose escalation and placebo but not with standard doses of raloxifene, when compared with the proportion with treatment-related episodes. There were no statistically significant between-group differences in the distribution of the number of episodes after 2 months. However one analyses these figures, it would seem that the effect of raloxifene in increasing hot flushes/flashes is not dramatic, although it exists; if it does prove problematical, slow dose escalation may reduce it.

Metabolism

LDL cholesterol and total cholesterol concentrations fell significantly in women taking raloxifene compared with placebo, but there was no change in HDL cholesterol or triglyceride concentrations, nor was endometrial thickness affected; the incidence of vaginal bleeding was not increased (29).

Reproductive system

Several sources have suggested that raloxifene can on occasion either cause uterine endometrial polyps or cause pre-existent polyps to enlarge considerably (30).

In one of the largest international multicenter studies of raloxifene it was found that, compared with combined hormone replacement therapy (with 17-beta-oestradiol 2 mg + norethisterone acetate 1 mg) 12 months of raloxifene treatment at 60 mg/day was not associated with increased endometrial thickness or uterine volume (31).

Susceptibility factors

Genetic

Most clinical work with raloxifene 60 mg/day for the treatment of osteoporosis and lipid disorders in the menopause has been performed in Western populations. A multinational multicenter study in 483 Asian women (and a similar placebo control group) treated for 1 year has now confirmed that the efficacy and the adverse effects of the treatment are very similar to those in western populations (32).

Age

There is a very proper reluctance today to interfere with hormonal processes during puberty and adolescence for fear of producing adverse long-term changes. Just as the use of estrogens in rapidly growing girls has largely fallen out of favor in most countries, so the safety of attempts to treat pubertal gynecomastia in boys is being questioned. However, this can be a distressing condition at a sensitive age, and some workers have cautiously used tamoxifen and raloxifene for this purpose. The results of different approaches have been compared in 38 patients with persistent pubertal gynecomastia at an average age of 14 years (33). They received reassurance alone or a 3- to 9-month course of an estrogen receptor modifier (tamoxifen 60 mg/day or raloxifene 10–20 mg bd). There were significant reductions in breast nodule size with both drugs, although the effect was more marked with raloxifene. In these doses, there were no adverse effects. If further work is to be performed it will be important to provide long-term follow-up to detect any unwanted later effects.

Drug–Drug Interactions

Estrogens

Because raloxifene acts as an estrogen receptor antagonist on some genitourinary tissues, one might expect it to block the vaginal effects of local estrogen therapy. A multicenter placebo-controlled US study in 91 post-menopausal women set out to determine whether oral raloxifene (60 mg/day), such as is used to counter post-

menopausal osteoporosis, might interfere with the efficacy of a low-dose estradiol-releasing vaginal ring used to relieve vaginal atrophy in women of a similar age. During the 6 months of treatment the signs of vaginal atrophy were assessed both objectively (vaginal histology and pH) and subjectively. There was no evidence of interference with local estrogen treatment (34).

A very similar conclusion was reached In another study of a possible interaction between raloxifene 60 mg/day and a conjugated estrogen cream used locally to treat vaginal atrophy (35).

Levothyroxine

An interaction of raloxifene with levothyroxine has been described (36).

- In a 79-year-old woman raloxifene 60 mg/day significantly interfered with the absorption of levothyroxine. The problem was observed clinically when it became necessary to raise her dose of levothyroxine progressively from 150 micrograms/day to 300 micrograms/day to maintain euthyroidism.

The interaction was later confirmed by specific testing but the mechanism is unclear.

Warfarin

To assess the potential for an interaction between raloxifene and warfarin, 15 healthy postmenopausal women each received single doses of warfarin 20 mg before and during 2 weeks of dosing with raloxifene 120 mg/day (37). Raloxifene reduced the oral clearance of R- and S-warfarin respectively by 7.1 and 14% and the oral volume of distribution by 7.4 and 9.8%. Raloxifene reduced the maximum prothrombin time by 10% and the area under the prothrombin versus time curve from 0–120 hours by an average of 8%. The authors concluded that raloxifene may produce a small increase in systemic warfarin exposure but a reduced pharmacodynamic effect. Since the effects are slight this interaction is unlikely to have clinical consequences.

References

1. Young RL. An introductiosn to SERMs and their gynecologic effects. Am J Managed Care 1999;5(Suppl):S146–55.
2. Saitta A, Morabito N, Frisina N, Cucinotte D, Corrado F, D'Anna R, Altavilla D, Squadrito G, Minutoli L, Arcoraci V, Cancellieri F, Squadrito F. Cardiovascular effects of raloxifene hydrochloride. Cardiovasc Drug Rev 2001;19(1):57–74.
3. Cauley JA, Norton L, Lippman ME, Eckert S, Krueger KA, Purdie DW, Farrerons J, Karasik A, Mellstrom D, Ng KW, Stepan JJ, Powles TJ, Morrow M, Costa A, Silfen SL, Walls EL, Schmitt H, Muchmore DB, Jordan VC, Ste-Marie LG. Continued breast cancer risk reduction in postmenopausal women treated with raloxifene: 4-year results from the MORE trial. Multiple outcomes of raloxifene evaluation. Breast Cancer Res Treat 2001;65(2):125–34.
4. Vignot E, Meunier PJ. Effets du raloxifène sur la perte osseuse et le risque fracturaire chez la femme menopausée. [Effects of raloxifene on bone loss and fracture risk in the

menopausal woman.] Contracept Fertil Sex 1999;27(12):858–60.

5. Albertazzi P, Purdie DW. Oestrogen and selective oestrogen receptor modulators (SERMs): current roles in the prevention and treatment of osteoporosis. Best Pract Res Clin Rheumatol 2001;15(3):451–68.

6. Anonymous. Raloxifene: new preparation. Not better than oestrogen. Prescrire Int 1999;8(44):165–7.

7. Umland EM, Rinaldi C, Parks SM, Boyce EG. The impact of estrogen replacement therapy and raloxifene on osteoporosis, cardiovascular disease, and gynecologic cancers. Ann Pharmacother 1999;33(12):1315–28.

8. Snyder KR, Sparano N, Malinowski JM. Raloxifene hydrochloride. Am J Health Syst Pharm 2000;57(18):1669–78.

9. Sismondi P, Biglia N, Roagna R, Ponzone R, Ambroggio S, Sgro L, Cozzarella M. How to manage the menopause following therapy for breast cancer is raloxifene a safe alternative? Eur J Cancer 2000;36(Suppl 4):S74–6.

10. Body JJ, Sternon J. Raloxifène (Celvista, Evista). Rev Med Brux 2000;21(1):35–41.

11. Heringa M. Review on raloxifene: profile of a selective estrogen receptor modulator. Int J Clin Pharmacol Ther 2003;41:331–45.

12. Cosman F. Selective estrogen-receptor modulators Clin Geriatr Med 2003;19:371–9.

13. Hernandez E, Valera R, Alonzo E, Bajares-Lilue M, Carlini R, Capriles F, Martinis R, Bellorin-Font E, Weisinger JR. Effects of raloxifene on bone metabolism and serum lipids in postmenopausal women on chronic hemodialysis. Kidney Int 2003;63:2269–74.

14. Arpino G, Krishnan MN, Dinesh CD, Bardou VJ, Clark GM, Elledge RM. Idoxifene versus tamoxifen: a randomized comparison in postmenopausal patients with metastatic breast cancer. Ann Oncol 2003;14:233–41.

15. Johnston SRD, Gumbrell LA, Evans TRJ, Coleman RE, Smith IE, Twelves CJ, Soukop M. Rea DW, Earl HM, Howell A, Jones A, Canney P, Powles TJ, Haynes BP, Nutley B, Grimshaw R, Jarman M, Halber GW, Brampton M, Haviland J, Dowsett M, Coombes RC. A cancer research (UK) randomized phase II study of idoxifene in patients with locally advanced/metastatic breast cancer resistant to tamoxifen. Cancer Chemother Pharmacol 2004;53:341–8.

16. Brandi ML. Raloxifene reduces vertebral fracture risk in postmenopausal women with osteoporosis. Clin Exp Rheumatol 2000;18(3):309–10.

17. Rosenbaum Smith SM, Osborne MP. Breast cancer chemoprevention. Am J Surg 2000;180(4):249–51.

18. Dardes RC, Jordan VC. Future directions in endocrine therapy for the treatment and prevention of breast cancer. Sem Breast Dis 2000;3:119–30.

19. Goldstein SR, Siddhanti S, Ciaccia AV, Plouffe L Jr. A pharmacological review of selective oestrogen receptor modulators. Hum Reprod Update 2000;6(3):212–24.

20. Cranney A, Adachi J.D. Benefit-risk assessment of raloxifene in postmenopausal osteoporosis. Drug Saf 2005;28:721–30.

21. Turbi C, Herrero-Beaumont G, Acebes JC, Torrijos A, Grana J, Miguelez R, Sacristan JA, Marin F. Compliance and satisfaction with raloxifene versus alendronate for the treatment of postmenopausal osteoporosis in clinical practice: an open-label, prospective, nonrandomized, observational study. Clin Ther 2004;26:245–56.

22. Sambrook PN, Geusens P, Ribot C, Solimano JA, Ferrer-Barriendos J, Gaines K. Verbruggen N, Melton ME. Alendronate produces greater effects than raloxifene on bone density and bone turnover in postmenopausal women with low bone density: Results of EFFECT (EFficacy of FOSAMAX versus EVISTA Comparison Trial). J Int Med 2004;255:503–11.

23. Blumenthal RS, Baranowski B, Dowsett SA Cardiovascular effects of raloxifene: the arterial and venous systems. Am Heart J 2004;147:783–9.

24. Compston JE. Selective oestrogen receptor modulators: potential therapeutic applications. Clin Endocrinol (Oxf) 1998;48(4):389–91.

25. Cohen FJ, Lu Y. Characterization of hot flashes reported by healthy postmenopausal women receiving raloxifene or placebo during osteoporosis prevention trials. Maturitas 2000;34(1):65–73.

26. Johnston CC Jr, Bjarnason NH, Cohen FJ, Shah A, Lindsay R, Mitlak BH, Huster W, Draper MW, Harper KD, Heath H 3rd, Gennari C, Christiansen C, Arnaud CD, Delmas PD. Long-term effects of raloxifene on bone mineral density, bone turnover, and serum lipid levels in early postmenopausal women: three-year data from 2 double-blind, randomized, placebo-controlled trials. Arch Intern Med 2000;160(22):3444–50.

27. Sarrel PM, Nawaz H, Chan W, Fuchs M, Katz DL. Raloxifene and endothelial function in healthy postmenopausal women. Am J Obstet Gynecol 2003;188:304–9.

28. Palacios S, Lucia F, Farias M, Luebbert H, Gomez G, Yabur JA, Quail DC, Turbi C, Kayath MJ, Almeida MJ, Monnig E, Nickelsen T. Raloxifene is not associated with biologically relevant changes in hot flushes in postmenopausal women for whom therapy is appropriate. Am J Obstet Gynecol 2004;191:121–31.

29. Delmas PD, Bjarnason NH, Mitlak BH, Ravoux AC, Shah AS, Huster WJ, Draper M, Christiansen C. Effects of raloxifene on bone mineral density, serum cholesterol concentrations, and uterine endometrium in postmenopausal women. N Engl J Med 1997;337(23):1641–7.

30. Maia H Jr, Maltez A, Oliveira M, Almeida M, Coutinho EM. Growth of an endometrial polyp in a postmenopausal patient using raloxifene. Gynaecol Endosc 2000;9:117–21.

31. Neven P, Lunde T, Benedetti-Panici P, Tiitinen A, Marinescu B, De Villiers T, Hillard T, Cano A, Peer E, Quail D, et al (89 other authors). A multicentre randomised trial to compare uterine safety of raloxifene with a continuous combined hormone replacement therapy containing oestradiol and norethisterone acetate. Br J Obstet Gynaecol 2003;110:157–67.

32. Kung AWC, Chao H-T, Huang K-E, Need AG, Taechakraichana N, Loh F-H, Gonzaga F, Sriram U, Ismail NMN, Farooqi A, Rachman IA, Crans GG, Wong M, Thiebaud D. Efficacy and safety of raloxifene 60 milligrams/day in postmenopausal Asian women. J Clin Endocrinol Metab 2003;88:3130–6.

33. Lawrence SE, Faught KA, Vethamuthu J, Lawson ML. Beneficial effects of raloxifene and tamoxifen in the treatment of pubertal gynecomastia. J Pediatr 2004;145(1):71–6.

34. Pinkerton JV, Shifren JL, La Valleur J, Rosen A, Roesinger M, Siddhanti S. Influence of raloxifene on the efficacy of an estradiol-releasing ring for treating vaginal atrophy in postmenopausal women. Menopause 2003;10:45–52.

35. Parsons A, Merritt D, Rosen A, Heath III H, Siddhanti S, Plouffe L Jr. Effect of raloxifene on the response to conjugated estrogen vaginal cream or nonhormonal moisturizers in postmenopausal vaginal atrophy. Obstet Gynecol 2003;101:346–52.

36. Siraj ES, Gupta MK, Reddy SSK. Raloxifene causing malabsorption of levothyroxine. Arch Intern Med 2003;163:1367–70.
37. Miller JW, Skerjanec A, Knadler MP, Ghosh A, Allerheiligen SR. Divergent effects of raloxifene HCl on the pharmacokinetics and pharmacodynamics of warfarin. Pharm Res 2001;18(7):1024–8.

Tamoxifen

General Information

Tamoxifen is an estrogen receptor partial agonist with antiestrogenic properties in the breast and estrogenic effects in tissues such as bone and the cardiovascular system. In most cases there is endometrial thickening on ultrasonography, and additional tests, such as hydrosonography or hysteroscopy, are required to confirm the presence of an empty atrophic uterus, as seen in most asymptomatic women taking tamoxifen.

Tamoxifen is commonly used in the treatment of breast carcinoma (1); the overall rates published for adverse effects vary very greatly, between 1 and 60% (2,3). It has also been used as a form of HRT to reduce bone loss and the incidence of fractures in high-risk cases (4). A combination of tamoxifen with ovarian suppression is as effective as the use of cytostatic drugs, and has been claimed to be better tolerated (5–7).

The use of tamoxifen to prevent breast cancer has been reviewed (8). The merits of using tamoxifen to prevent mammary carcinoma in women who have never had the disease but are believed to be at high risk have been disputed (9), but it is clear that it would involve very long treatment and that one's view of the adverse effects might need to be revised for this class of users. The available data after 5, 10, and 15 years of follow up confirmed an increase in the incidence of endometrial cancer and of thromboembolic complications and suggested ocular toxicity, but these effects were not common and should be more than balanced by the reduced risk of coronary heart disease and osteoporosis (8).

Tamoxifen also has beneficial side effects: it protects the myocardium, reduces the incidence of ischemic heart disease, reduces the loss of bone mineral density, and has beneficial effects on lipids (10). With evidence accumulating from major studies in several countries, there is still considerable optimism regarding the use of tamoxifen or its analogues to prevent breast cancer in high-risk groups, although the results of various studies are not consistent and much detail needs to be filled in (11,12). Chemoprevention with tamoxifen and the newer selective estrogen receptor modulators has to be weighed adequately against possible risks (13). This form of chemoprophylaxis has not been widely adopted; in the population as a whole the proportion of women who stand to benefit is low, and the risks of unnecessary drug treatment in the remainder have to be taken into account. In a survey in North Carolina 10% or less of women in all age groups were potentially eligible for chemoprevention while the maximum proportion of breast cancers prevented in eligible women was estimated at 6.0–8.3% (14). Clearly, the most desirable key to future policy on prophylaxis would be a means of selecting the subgroup at the highest risk, so that drug treatment could be limited to them.

Observational studies

The effect of high-dose tamoxifen as an adjunct to postoperative brain irradiation has been studied for 40 weeks in 12 patients with glioblastoma multiforme, but without controls (15). Two weeks after surgery, the patients were given high-dose oral tamoxifen (120 mg/m^2 bd for 3 months) and 2 weeks later external beam radiotherapy (59.4 Gy, three daily fractions every 6.5 weeks). In one patient tamoxifen was associated with severe vomiting, necessitating dosage reduction and subsequent withdrawal; another patient had bilateral deep venous thrombosis after 51 weeks, but a causal relation was not firmly established. The authors concluded that adjuvant high-dose tamoxifen is relatively well tolerated, although in this series it did not appear to improve the prognosis.

In a small study in the Mayo Clinic the acceptability of using tamoxifen alongside intravenous cisplatin was examined in 15 patients with lung cancer (16). Daily doses in various patients were 160 mg/m^2, 200 mg/m^2, or 250 mg/m^2 for 7 days. Grade 3 anemia occurred in one patient only, at the 200 mg/m^2 dose, while another patient, with an unfavorable cardiovascular history, had an embolic stroke 20 days after completing the course. On the basis of this small trial, the Clinic proposed to continue using high doses of tamoxifen alongside cisplatin in such patients. On present evidence from this and other centers, tamoxifen potentiates the cytostatic effects of cisplatin without clearly increasing the toxicity of the regimen; various mechanisms to explain this apparently useful interaction are being debated.

A short report has been published on the Italian Randomized Trial of Tamoxifen in 2700 women, which is intended to assess the success of the drug set against placebo, used in 2708 women, in preventing breast cancer in a population of hysterectomized post-menopausal women (17). After a median 81 months of follow-up, breast cancers had developed in 34 women in the tamoxifen group and 45 in the placebo group. The effect was highly significant in a subgroup of women considered, in the light of their reproductive and hormonal characteristics, as being at high risk of breast cancer, but was dubious in low-risk women, in whom the risk of cancer may actually have been marginally increased. However, the authors stressed that whatever usefulness the drug proves to have for this purpose must be set against its adverse effects, such as endometrial cancer and thromboembolic complications. As currently published, the findings did not indicate the incidence of these complications in the study itself.

Comparative studies

One of the many controversies surrounding the use of tamoxifen in elderly women is whether after lumpectomy it should be accompanied by radiotherapy to potentiate the desired effect. It has been suggested that there is not a great deal of merit in adding radiotherapy to tamoxifen, since radiotherapy plus tamoxifen reduces local recurrence of breast cancer in elderly women compared with tamoxifen alone, but survival rates are not improved and benefits are offset by an increase in adverse effects (18).

Tamoxifen versus aromatase inhibitors

While tamoxifen is still widely regarded as the standard adjuvant endocrine treatment for postmenopausal women with localized breast cancer, provided it is hormone receptor positive, there are problems with recurrence and adverse effects. Reservations have recently been expressed about the future place of tamoxifen, and the case has been made that it is time to move from tamoxifen to the oral aromatase inhibitors (19).

There has been a brief report of some of the results of the ATAC trial (part of the CORE study) in 9366 women, which was designed to continue for 5 years, part of which involved directly comparing tamoxifen with the aromatase inhibitor anastrozole (20). The conclusion was that anastrozole should be the preferred treatment in such cases. After a median follow-up of 68 months, anastrozole significantly prolonged disease-free survival (575 events with anastrozole versus 651 with tamoxifen; hazard ratio = 0.87; 95% CI = 0.78, 0.97), prolonged time to recurrence, and significantly reduced distant metastases (324 versus 375) and contralateral breast cancers. There were fewer withdrawals with anastrozole than with tamoxifen, apparently reflecting the fact that anastrozole was also associated with fewer adverse effects (especially gynecological problems and vascular events), although arthralgia and fractures were increased.

The roles of tamoxifen and the aromatase inhibitors as adjuvant therapy for early breast cancer in postmenopausal women have been reviewed, distinguishing three approaches: replacement of tamoxifen as adjuvant therapy for 5 years (early adjuvant therapy); sequencing of tamoxifen before or after an aromatase inhibitor during the first 5 years (early sequential adjuvant therapy); or the use of an aromatase inhibitor after 5 years of tamoxifen (extended adjuvant therapy) (21). Briefly, the conclusions were that at the time of the survey there was little to choose between the three methods in terms of the balance of benefit and harm. However, like others, the authors stressed that agents of this type are proving to be superior to tamoxifen in preventing recurrence of the disease.

There may well be a role for combined therapy with both tamoxifen and an aromatase inhibitor if an optimal benefit to harm balance is to be attained, as suggested by a study of a combination of tamoxifen and exemestane for 8 weeks in 33 postmenopausal women with breast cancer (22). There was a striking absence of endocrine adverse effects.

Others have suggested that patients be treated for a period with tamoxifen and then switched to anastrozole

for follow up. A report on the ABCSG 8 trial and the ARNO 95 trial (both of which were prospective open studies) has provided information on this approach (23). Women with hormone-sensitive early breast cancer who had taken adjuvant oral tamoxifen 20 or 30 mg/day for 2 years were randomized to oral anastrozole 1 mg/day (n = 1618) or tamoxifen 20 or 30 mg/day (n = 1606) for the remainder of their adjuvant therapy. At a median follow-up of 28 months, there was a highly significant 40% reduction in the risk of an event with anastrozole compared with tamoxifen (67 versus 110 events; hazard ratio = 0.60; 95% CI = 0.44, 0.81). There were significantly more fractures but significantly fewer case of thrombosis in those who took anastrozole than in those who took tamoxifen. These data lend support to a switch from tamoxifen to anastrozole in patients who have taken adjuvant tamoxifen for 2 years.

The unwanted effects of tamoxifen on the endometrium (including induction of fibroids, polyps, and endometrial cancer) have long been of concern, and attempts are now being made to find ways of preventing or reversing these complications, or finding an alternative treatment that does not involve these risks. Again, promising experience with the aromatase inhibitors features prominently in current recommendations.

In a prospective study in 77 consecutive women with postmenopausal breast cancer scheduled to start endocrine treatment for breast cancer, using either tamoxifen or an aromatase inhibitor tamoxifen treatment significantly increased endometrial thickness and uterine volume after 3 months (24). In additional, tamoxifen induced endometrial cysts and polyps and increased the size of pre-existing fibroids. In contrast, aromatase inhibitors did not stimulate endometrial growth and were not associated with endometrial pathology. Furthermore, they reduced endometrial thickness and uterine volume in patients who had previously taken tamoxifen.

This study has again confirmed that endometrial problems can be induced by tamoxifen early in the course of treatment; and that these problems do not arise with aromatase inhibitors, which may actually reduce the endometrial changes induced by tamoxifen. The idea that the new oral aromatase inhibitors might well replace tamoxifen in breast cancer was tentatively advanced in SEDA-26 (p. 445) and has now been supported by some of the material cited above, as well as by a panel consensus (25). Citing efficacy and safety data on anastrozole, exemestane, and letrozole, the authors concluded that third-generation aromatase inhibitors may be considered first-line therapy of hormone-receptor-positive advanced breast cancer in postmenopausal women and may also be used for preoperative therapy of breast cancer.

Placebo-controlled studies

In the Breast Cancer Prevention Trial (P-1), initiated by the National Surgical Adjuvant Breast and Bowel Project (NSABP) in 1992, more than 13 000 eligible women were randomized to tamoxifen 20 mg/day or placebo for 5 years (26). During 69 months of follow-up tamoxifen reduced the risk of both invasive and non-invasive cancer and reduced fractures of the hip, radius, and spine; however, the rate of endometrial cancer increased (RR = 2.53; 95% CI = 1.35, 4.97), as did the frequency of vascular events.

General adverse effects

The adverse effects of tamoxifen are largely those that one would expect to be associated with a reduction in estrogenic activity, that is hot flushes (which can be severe), dry skin, mental or nervous system effects (such as mild depression, headache, fatigue, nervousness, and tremor), oligomenorrhea and amenorrhea, loss of libido, vaginal discharge, and rare events, such as pruritus, migraine, and edema (SED-12, 1034) (27). Nausea and vomiting are not uncommon. There are also reports of hirsutism, weight gain, rashes, thrombocytopenia, and leukopenia (SED-12, 1034); the hirsutism could reflect a relative dominance of endogenous androgen activity as the degree of estrogenic activity declines. The most specific and dangerous complication of tamoxifen is hypercalcemia, a direct consequence of the successful treatment of mammary carcinoma with bony metastases; the incidence varies greatly. Liver dysfunction and peliosis hepatis have been incidentally reported.

When tamoxifen is used in men (28), common adverse effects have included weight gain (25%), mood alterations (21%), hot flushes (21%), reduced libido (29%), and deep vein thrombosis (4%). The hot flushes respond well to oral clonidine 0.1 mg/day (29).

One expert in the USA (30) has publicly defended the safety of tamoxifen on the grounds that some of its supposed adverse effects may in fact have other causes. It is a difficult argument to follow, since she postulates that several of the unwanted effects referred to are in fact menopausal. However, these are largely likely to be inevitable consequences of the very changes that treatment with tamoxifen is intended to induce, that is suppression of estrogenic effects. Virtually the opposite belief can be derived from a Canadian study, which showed that 25 women taking tamoxifen were diffident about attributing adverse events to the drug, and therefore tended to under-report adverse effects (31). Menopause-like problems with these drugs are clearly likely to persist unless or until more selective SERMs become available, for example substances that act exclusively on the breast tumor.

Organs and Systems

Cardiovascular

Both deep vein thrombosis and pulmonary embolism have been described with tamoxifen.

- Cerebral sinus thrombosis, progressing to hemorrhagic cerebral infarction, occurred in a 52-year-old woman (32).

Although the authors pointed to the absence of risk factors other than the drug, it must be remembered that cerebral venous thrombosis is a recognized complication of various malignancies. In this case the breast tumor had been treated with various cytostatic drugs and stem cell transplantation, and tamoxifen had been given as an adjuvant, and it was believed that the tumor had been eliminated. Nevertheless, in this complex case one should perhaps be hesitant in attributing the complication solely to the drug.

In the light of three further cases of thrombosis, it has been suggested that there may be a particular predisposition to this complication in patients with high circulating concentrations of homocysteine, and that these should be checked for in advance of treatment (33).

Some cases of thrombosis and pulmonary embolism may have been attributable to the primary condition being treated, and the risk must not be over-estimated (34).

An extensive literature survey covering a 7-year period sought to resolve doubts about whether the risk of venous thromboembolism is greater with tamoxifen than with other treatments used to prevent and treat breast cancer, taking careful account of other susceptibility factors that might distort the picture (35). Accurate determination of the rate of thromboembolism was impaired by the lack in most studies of routine assessments to detect asymptomatic cases. However, based on symptomatic cases the risk of thromboembolism was increased two- to three-fold during use of either tamoxifen or raloxifene to prevent breast carcinoma. It is not known whether the risk is increased further in women with inherited hypercoagulable states. In the case of early-stage breast carcinoma, the risk of thromboembolism is increased with both tamoxifen and anastrozole, although the problem appeared to be somewhat less when using anastrozole.

The effect of tamoxifen 20 mg/day on the incidence of venous thromboembolism has been assessed in a placebo-controlled breast cancer prevention trial for 5 years in 5408 hysterectomized women (36). There were 28 incidents of thromboembolism on placebo and 44 on tamoxifen (hazard ratio = 1.63; 95% CI = 1.02, 2.63), 80% of which involved only superficial phlebitis, which accounted for all of the excess due to tamoxifen within 18 months from randomization. Compared with placebo, the risk of venous thromboembolism with tamoxifen was higher in women aged 55 years or older, those with a body mass index of 25 kg/m^2 or more, those with a raised blood pressure or a total cholesterol of 6.50 mmol/l (250 mg/dl) or greater, current smokers, and those with a family history of coronary heart disease, all familiar risk factors for venous complications. Of the 685 women with a coronary heart disease risk score of 5 or greater, one in the placebo arm and 13 in the tamoxifen arm developed venous thromboembolism. In a multivariate regression analysis, age in excess of 60 years, height of 165 cm or more, and a diastolic blood pressure of 90 mmHg or higher all had independent detrimental effects on the risk of venous thromboembolism during tamoxifen therapy, whereas transdermal estrogen therapy concomitant with tamoxifen was not associated with any excess risk (HR = 0.64; 95% CI = 0.23, 1.82). The authors concluded that the increased risk of venous thromboembolism during the use of tamoxifen was largely associated with the

Table 1 Incidences of venous thromboembolism with and without breast cancer taking various treatments (37)

Population	Incidence of venous thromboembolism (per year unless otherwise stated)
General population without cancer	0.12%
Women without cancer	0.08% per year (DVT)
	0.03% per year (PE)
Women without cancer taking tamoxifen	0.12% (DVT)
	0.07% per year (PE)
Women without cancer taking HRT	0.23%
General population	0.6% over 3 years
General population with breast cancer	1.0%
Early-stage breast cancer, no adjuvant treatment	0.8% within 6 weeks after surgery
Early-stage breast cancer, no adjuvant treatment	0.4% over 5 years
Early-stage breast cancer taking tamoxifen	1.7% over 5 years
Early-stage breast cancer, taking adjuvant tamoxifen	1.4% over 5 years
Early-stage breast cancer receiving chemotherapy	2.1% within 6 weeks
Early-stage breast cancer, receiving chemotherapy and taking tamoxifen	11% over 5 years

well-known risk factors for this condition, and that this information should be part of pre-treatment counselling.

The risks of venous thromboembolism in women with and without breast cancer have been analysed and are summarized in Table 1 (37). In one case tamoxifen was associated with myocardial infarction (38).

Respiratory

An important synergistic reaction between radiation-related pulmonary fibrosis and tamoxifen has been described in 196 women followed for a minimum of 5 years, with a relative risk of 2.0 (39). However, others have shown that tamoxifen did not increase the pulmonary toxicity of agents such as carmustine and dacarbazine (40).

Nervous system

A short supplementary report on the US NSABP, originally published in 1999, later corrected the original data on adverse effects: among women who had used tamoxifen for an average of 29 months to complement irradiation after lumpectomy for intraductal carcinoma; there were five cases of stroke, compared with only one among the women who had not used tamoxifen (41). In a parallel study of breast cancer prevention there was also a slight but non-significant increase in the incidence of stroke in those taking tamoxifen. It may be wise to regard a history of stroke, transient ischemic attacks, uncontrolled hypertension, diabetes mellitus, or atrial fibrillation as relative contraindications to tamoxifen. On the other hand, other work showed that tamoxifen had precisely the same effect on myoinositol concentrations in the basal ganglia as estrogen replacement therapy did (SEDA-17, 432), which could suggest that there is no risk to brain function.

The effects of estrogen and tamoxifen on positron emission tomography (PET) measures of brain glucose metabolism and magnetic resonance imaging (MRI) have been evaluated as measures of hippocampal atrophy in three groups of postmenopausal women, women taking estrogen, women with breast cancer taking tamoxifen, and women not taking estrogen or tamoxifen (42). In those taking tamoxifen there were widespread areas of hypometabolism in the inferior and dorsal lateral frontal lobes relative to the other two groups. The untreated women had lower metabolism in the inferior frontal cortex and temporal cortex compared with those taking estrogen. Those taking tamoxifen also had significantly lower semantic memory scores than the other two groups. Finally, those taking tamoxifen had smaller right hippocampal volumes than those taking estrogen, an effect that was of borderline significance. Both right and left hippocampal volumes were significantly smaller than in those taking estrogen when a single outlier was removed. Those taking estrogen had hippocampal volumes that were intermediate to the other two groups. The authors concluded that these findings provide physiological and anatomical evidence for neuroprotective effects of estrogen. Biochemical changes are difficult to interpret in clinical terms, and there is now an evident need for longer-term controlled work correlating tamoxifen use and cognitive performance.

Sensory systems

There have been repeated reports of ophthalmic complications from tamoxifen, including irreversible retinopathy with seriously reduced visual acuity, refractile opacities, cystoid macular edema, retinal yellow-white dots, and keratopathy (SEDA-6, 356; SEDA-7, 391; SEDA-16, 466).

- Bilateral optic neuritis developed in a woman with breast cancer who was treated for 6 months with tamoxifen (43).

In a prospective study even in low doses (for example 10 mg/day or lower) tamoxifen caused ocular toxicity if given for a sufficiently long period; most of the changes were reversible but they justify very close monitoring (44). A related compound, MER-29 (triparanol), causes cataract and has various other adverse reactions in common with tamoxifen.

Estrogen receptors are present in the retina, and tamoxifen has been stated to affect color vision. In a further study of this phenomenon in 24 middle-aged women who were taking tamoxifen 20 mg/day as adjuvant therapy for early stage breast cancer, visual fields were measured using both short wavelength automated perimetry and frequency doubling perimetry (45). The visual fields were affected, the changes being detectable within 2 years. The effects of tamoxifen were more readily detected with short wavelength automated perimetry, suggesting that it affects some types of visual pathways preferentially, presumably the cone pathways, which are measured with this technique.

Some older work pointed to an increased risk of other ophthalmic complications, including cataract in patients with cancer who took tamoxifen for a longer period. The issue was later examined in Britain using a case-control study design and data collected in the General Practice Research Database relating to women taking tamoxifen for breast cancer, the comparators being women with other cancers who were not taking tamoxifen (46). Current tamoxifen users were not at increased risk of cataract and there was no evidence of an increased risk with increasing cumulative dose (AOR = 1.0, 95%CI = 0.7, 1.4).

Metabolism

Steatosis and adipose tissue distribution has been evaluated using CT scanning in a cross-sectional study of 32 women taking tamoxifen for breast cancer and a similar control group (47). Tamoxifen users generally had more visceral adipose tissue and more liver fat than controls, and had a higher risk of diabetes. It is still unclear whether tamoxifen causes long-term metabolic abnormalities in obese patients, or whether patients with the metabolic syndrome X of obesity are at increased risk of the complications of tamoxifen. In view of this finding, and earlier results pointing in the same direction, it would be wise in future studies of tamoxifen to monitor metabolic changes in obese women with or without breast cancer.

Tamoxifen has favorable effects on lipid and lipoprotein profiles, reducing concentrations of total and low-density lipoprotein cholesterol. However there is also evidence that it can cause increased serum triglyceride concentrations, which in some cases have risen dangerously. A Taiwan group has sought to determine whether this adverse effect might be avoided by using lower but still effective doses of the drug in women with early breast cancer (48). They found that in 115 patients with breast cancer taking tamoxifen 20 mg bd the serum triglyceride concentration rose significantly after 15 months of therapy, although the increase was only clinically dangerous (400 mg/dl or more) in 14 cases. In these patients the dose was halved to 10 mg/day, and in 10 of the 14 women the triglycerides fell markedly; in the other four they did not, and antilipemic therapy was needed. The authors did not evaluate the efficacy of lower doses, but there is some earlier literature that seems to show that efficacy is attainable at this level.

Hematologic

Thrombosis and pulmonary embolism have been described with tamoxifen (49,50); the number of cases is small, but the association would not be unexpected in view of what is known about the effects of other sex hormones. The primary condition might be responsible, at least in part, for the occurrence of such complications. Tamoxifen does reduce antithrombin III but not to a degree at which a major risk would be expected, and other measurable effects on the coagulation process seem to be slight.

When tamoxifen 20 mg/day was compared with equieffective doses of anastrozole in 668 patients with advanced breast tumors that were hormone receptor-positive or of unknown receptor status, tamoxifen produced too high a rate of thromboembolism and vaginal bleeding to be considered the treatment of choice (51,52).

There is some evidence that one might be able to maintain the therapeutic benefits of tamoxifen in breast cancer at much lower doses (for example 1 mg/day and 5 mg/day) than those generally used (20 mg/day), thus perhaps avoiding the risks associated with thrombogenesis (53). In a non-randomized study, all three doses were studied in 120 women with estrogen receptor-positive breast cancer, comparing the outcome over a 4-week period with that in controls. Expression of the tumor expression marker Ki-67 fell to a similar degree in all three tamoxifen dosage groups, with no difference in the magnitude of reduction among the different dosages. Effects on various blood markers (including insulin-like growth factor-I, sex hormone-binding globulin, low-density lipoprotein cholesterol, ultrasensitive C-reactive protein, fibrinogen, and antithrombin III concentrations) were too variable to draw clear conclusions about whether the lower doses were indeed safer, but they provide a reasonable basis for further examination of the matter (54).

Liver

Liver dysfunction and peliosis hepatis are occasional complications of tamoxifen. There have also been reports of cirrhosis with fatty liver in women taking tamoxifen after surgery for breast cancer (55). The condition is reversible, and liver tests are advisable so that the tamoxifen can be promptly withdrawn if necessary.

- An elderly woman with a history of breast cancer developed multifocal steatohepatitis, but after tamoxifen was withdrawn the CT features improved dramatically, and the hepatic transaminases normalized (56).

The frequency and course of hepatic steatosis due to tamoxifen has been studied using CT scans in 76 patients with breast cancer who took tamoxifen for 5 years (57). In all 29 women developed hepatic steatosis during the first 2 years, four to a severe degree. The liver:spleen ratio returned to normal within a mean of 1.2 years after the end of treatment in 23 of these women. The authors stressed that hepatic dysfunction can occur with tamoxifen, and that it is vital to differentiate the condition from hepatic metastases.

Pancreas

Severe acute pancreatitis has been attributed to tamoxifen (58).

- A woman with hypertriglyceridemia and breast cancer was given tamoxifen and various lipid-regulating agents after mastectomy. She stopped the latter of her own accord after 2 years and had a recurrence of hypertriglyceridemia and pancreatitis.

In this instance there were other possible precipitating factors, particularly hypertriglyceridemia, and it is hard to see why tamoxifen should have been held responsible.

Skin

Tamoxifen has several adverse effects on the skin, including edema, flushing, rashes, hyperhidrosis, urticaria, alopecia, and hypertrichosis. Radiation recall dermatitis, a severe painful inflammatory skin reaction in sites that have previously been exposed to ionized radiation, can occur in patients taking tamoxifen (59). In one case the tamoxifen was withdrawn and the skin healed spontaneously in 7 weeks (60). Toremifene, a tamoxifen analogue, was well tolerated: during 18 months of continuous treatment no signs of radiation recall developed.

Hair

Effects of hormonal or antihormonal products on the hair are reported sporadically.

- A woman taking tamoxifen for metastatic cancer (presumably from the breast) developed alopecia; she began to lose her hair within 3 months and was entirely bald after 13 months of treatment (61).

The authors did not make it clear whether cytostatic drugs, which can cause alopecia, were also used, but it is striking that there have been several earlier reports of baldness with tamoxifen.

Musculoskeletal

In principle an anti-estrogen might precipitate osteoporosis, but tamoxifen has not been shown to do so; indeed, there is reason to believe that it protects the skeleton against steroid-induced bone loss (62), and in some studies of the state of the bones during treatment with tamoxifen there was actually a higher bone density than in controls.

Sexual function

Tamoxifen can cause loss of libido (63). In 57 patients sexual desire, arousal, and the ability to achieve orgasm were unaffected by tamoxifen (64). There was a 54% incidence of dyspareunia, but this seemed to be a consequence of co-administration of chemotherapy, which can cause vaginal dryness and loss of libido, rather than an effect of tamoxifen.

Reproductive system

Breasts

Tamoxifen can cause a sudden rapid increase in the growth rate of uterine leiomyomas (65).

- A leiomyoma of the breast occurred in a 50-year-old woman taking tamoxifen. It appeared as a discrete mass and had a microscopic pattern akin to leiomyomas at other sites (66).

Ovaries

In premenopausal women, tamoxifen has complex effects on ovarian function, compatible with accelerated development of multiple follicles, with ovarian enlargement and cyst formation (67,68); this might be expected in view of its similarity to clomiphene. Ovarian cysts have also been seen in postmenopausal patients with breast cancer during long-term adjuvant therapy with tamoxifen. Some premenopausal women with breast cancer had very marked increase in estrogen concentrations as a result of increased ovarian estrogen synthesis caused by tamoxifen. All premenopausal women with breast cancer taking tamoxifen should be under close gynecological and ultrasonographic surveillance to detect such effects as soon as they occur.

Dutch workers concluded that patients who were still having a menstrual cycle had a high chance (81%) of developing ovarian cysts during tamoxifen treatment, but that postmenopausal women taking tamoxifen only developed ovarian cysts if their ovaries were able to respond to FSH stimulation, as shown by serum estradiol production (69). Differences in patient populations might explain why some workers (70) still find no association in their patients between tamoxifen and ovarian pathology.

Macroscopically visible cystic endosalpingiosis in the paraovarian region has been described in a woman who had been taking tamoxifen for breast cancer (71).

- A 2.5 cm multicystic lesion was seen on the external surface of the right ovary, and histological examination showed a mass of dilated glands lined by ciliated tubal-type epithelium and set in a fibrovascular stroma. Cystic endosalpingiosis resulting in a tumor-like mass is rarely described and is probably not well recognized by histopathologists.

Although unlikely to be mistaken for malignancy, this kind of lesion can result in diagnostic confusion. The role of tamoxifen in the development of the lesion in this case is not clear, but the estrogenic effects of tamoxifen may have contributed.

In one case, a complex cyst, thought to be due to ovarian hyperstimulation, resolved after monthly administration of a depot gonadorelin (GnRH) receptor agonist without abandoning tamoxifen (72). One might expect some patients to react to tamoxifen with ovarian hyperstimulation, since another non-steroidal antiestrogen (that is clomiphene) is used for ovarian stimulation and also on occasion produces cysts.

In one case reported from Japan, there was torsion of an ovarian cyst (73).

In a study of the mechanism and frequency of this complication, hormone concentrations in 20 premenopausal women taking tamoxifen (20 mg/day) were compared with those in untreated controls (74). Ovarian cysts were found in 80% of the treated patients but only in 8% of controls, and 17-beta-estradiol concentrations were significantly raised.

Uterus

Intermenstrual bleeding is a practical problem during tamoxifen therapy, particularly since it obliges the physician to undertake repeated endometrial investigations to exclude malignancy. Monitoring the uterine cavity in women taking tamoxifen is mandatory, especially when there is postmenopausal bleeding.

Some preliminary but well-designed work has suggested that by inserting a levonorgestrel-releasing intrauterine system it may be possible to limit considerably the problems posed by unscheduled uterine bleeding (75).

Benign thickening of the endometrium is common during tamoxifen treatment, but appears to be fully reversible within a few months of withdrawal (76,77).

The pathology of tamoxifen-associated cases of myometrial adenomyosis has been compared with that in five cases of postmenopausal adenomyosis not associated with tamoxifen. The tumors were not identical: morphological features more often present in the tamoxifen-associated cases were cystic dilatation of glands (which sometimes resulted in grossly visible intramural cystic lesions), fibrosis of the stroma, and various forms of epithelial metaplasia. The proliferative activity in the adenomyosis, as determined by MIB1 staining, was higher in the tamoxifen group (78), and this could be another mechanism of postmenopausal bleeding among tamoxifen users.

Whether one should routinely screen patients for endometrial changes is disputed; there seems to be no correlation between endometrial thickness and endometrial pathology, and complications could be easily overlooked (79).

The gynecological consequences of antiestrogens (tamoxifen and toremifene) have been evaluated in 167 postmenopausal breast cancer patients in a 3-year prospective study. There was a proliferative endometrium more often in the tamoxifen group than in the toremifene group, but this did not translate into an increase in the rate of endometrial cancer. The authors did not recommend routine surveillance of the endometrium.

Uterine polyps are not uncommon during postmenopausal treatment with tamoxifen (80), and up to 3% can show malignant changes. There has been an attempt to identify risk factors for the development of these polyps, by analysing the histories of 54 women in whom they occurred, as well as the histories of a larger control group without polyps (81). The women who developed polyps had a later menopause, had breast cancer for a longer period, and weighed more.

Endometrial polyps ("basilomas") can become malignant (82,83), perhaps because they lack progesterone receptors and are exposed to unopposed estrogen (84).

The susceptibility factors that predispose to polyps have been sought In 64 patients with polyps (85). The combination of shorter tamoxifen exposure before the diagnosis of primary polyps, lower parity, lower menopausal age at the time of diagnosis of primary polyps, and greater duration of tamoxifen treatment significantly increased the risk of recurrent endometrial polyps. One additional year of tamoxifen treatment increased the risk of recurrent polyps five-fold.

A Japanese study of DNA extracted from endometrial polyps in women treated with tamoxifen showed a three-fold increase in K-ras mutations compared with the incidence in cases of spontaneous endometrial hyperplasia. These findings could support the hypothesis that the endometrial polyps will prove an early indicator for the development of endometrial carcinoma in such patients (86).

Not only can endometrial polyps that arise during tamoxifen treatment undergo malignant degeneration, but in some cases they may be the site of metastases from the original breast cancer. Such polyps must always undergo thorough histological sampling to distinguish the two possibilities. Two cases with metastases from lobular breast carcinoma to a polyp have been described (87).

Tumorigenicity

A variety of uterine tumors have been associated with tamoxifen, Levine et al have now presented what is probably the first report of Tamoxifen-associated uterine liposarcoma has now been observed in a 62-year-old woman (88). The tumor cells were immunoreactive to vimentin, estrogen receptors, and S-100. Surgery was performed, but the tumor recurred 9 months later.

Immunologic

An acute inflammatory polyarthritis resembling rheumatoid arthritis has been reported in three women temporally related to the use of tamoxifen (89).

Long-Term Effects

Tumorigenicity

Several authors (90,91) have described a variety of cases, seven in all, of malignancies secondary to therapeutic dosages of tamoxifen given for 6 months to 10 years.

Uterine fibroids and endometrial polyps (sometimes with bleeding) have been reported in menopausal women who had taken tamoxifen for periods of months or years (SEDA-16, 466) (92,93). In view of this, the question of whether tamoxifen increases the risk of endometrial cancer has been widely discussed. The authors of a 1993 review of the outcome of six major trials tended strongly to the conclusion that tamoxifen can cause both endometrial hyperplasia and endometrial cancer proportional to the total dose (94); the figures pointed to an overall incidence of endometrial cancer of 0.5% in tamoxifen users and 0.1% in controls. Another major review up to 1992 concluded that in the world literature there were 70 cases of uterine malignancies with tamoxifen, including 61 cases of adenocarcinoma of the endometrium and four cases of uterine sarcoma (95).

Six cases of endometrial carcinoma were subsequently reported from France (96), and 36 cases in all had been reported up to that time (97). Although the effect can be caused by tamoxifen alone in women aged over 55, in younger women it is more likely to be an additive one, attributable to use of both tamoxifen and pelvic irradiation in the same subject.

Two distinct patterns of uterine cancer have been shown using magnetic resonance imaging of the tamoxifen-exposed uterus in 35 women (98). Patients with pattern 1 had homogeneous high signal intensity of the endometrium on T2-weighted images and enhancement of the endometrial–myometrial interface and a signal void in the lumen on gadolinium-enhanced images (18 patients). Patients with pattern 2 had heterogeneous endometrial signal intensity on T2-weighted images with enhancement of the endometrial–myometrial interface and lattice-like enhancement traversing the endometrial canal on gadolinium-enhanced images (17 patients).

Although the endometrial cancers associated with tamoxifen are usually pure adenocarcinomas, other types of rare tumors have also been reported. A pure uterine rhabdomyosarcoma has been reported (99), and a mesodermal mixed tumor of the endometrium occurred 5 years after 5 years of tamoxifen therapy (100). The tumor responded only to combined treatment with doxorubicin, cyclophosphamide, 5-fluorouracil, and carboplatin. It is possible that this type of tumor arises later than adenocarcinomas and should be looked for during long-term use of tamoxifen.

- Two well-documented cases of uterine carcinosarcoma have been reported in elderly women after 6 and 7 years of tamoxifen treatment (101). At laparotomy, a heterologous malignant mixed Mullerian tumor with peritoneal spread was found in each case and rapidly proved fatal; large uterine polyps with special histological features may represent an intermediate step in the formation of such tumors (102).

Ten similar cases have been described before.

When assessing the risk of endometrial malignancy in women with breast cancer taking tamoxifen, it is worth taking into account evidence that patients with breast cancer may at the outset have some endometrial pathology. In women with breast cancer scheduled for tamoxifen there were endometrial polyps in 9.3%, endometrial cysts in 16%, and synechiae in 12% at the outset. Tamoxifen significantly increased the incidence of these benign endometrial lesions, usually after less than 1 year of treatment. There were no cases of endometrial carcinoma in 34 patients who had taken tamoxifen for 12–24 months, and only one in 78 patients who had taken it for 5–72 months (103).

The risk that tamoxifen may cause endometrial cancer has been the subject of lively correspondence in the Lancet (104), fired by the paper published in 2000 by Bergman and her colleagues, who had concluded that the endometrial cancers seen with tamoxifen are unusually aggressive (105). Concern was expressed that such a conclusion could lead to even wider hesitation to use tamoxifen in breast cancer, despite the fact that it is already used very selectively, for example in women with positive estrogen

receptors. A contradiction between Bergman's results and those of the NSABP P-1 were also highlighted, and doubts expressed whether Bergman's findings justify restricting the use of tamoxifen as a preventive agent. However, a Canadian group adduced its own work to support Bergman's findings, while French workers suggested that her unfavorable results, which were not seen in their own patients, could have been due to selection bias. It was also argued that a progestogen-releasing intrauterine contraceptive device might be used to counter the undesirable effects of tamoxifen on the endometrium. Clearly the issue raised by Bergman is still subject to debate, but it is obvious that physicians who use tamoxifen in advanced breast cancer or as a preventive agent should continue to do so selectively and that ways of protecting the endometrium during tamoxifen therapy need to be found.

The effects of norethisterone on endometrial abnormalities have been studied in 463 postmenopausal women taking tamoxifen or placebo (106). As in other studies, the results showed that any increased risk of endometrial cancer caused by tamoxifen is low and that transvaginal ultrasound screening is probably not justified for asymptomatic women taking tamoxifen. The authors found that 26% of women taking tamoxifen have endometrial thickening of 8 mm or more. It is possible to identify cysts in 7% of these women, polyps in 3%, and both cysts and polyps in 8%. These changes are characteristic of tamoxifen and unlike those seen with estrogen replacement therapy.

Although it has been suggested that tamoxifen-associated endometrial carcinoma has a distinct gene expression profile, this has not been confirmed. There are two types of this cancer, with extremely different molecular profiles, but the distinction is not related to tamoxifen exposure (107). Much other work is being done to determine the characteristics of tamoxifen-associated endometrial tumors, in particular as regards their content of estrogen receptors (ER) and progesterone receptors. The pathological features and expression of ERα, ERβ, and progesterone receptors in these tumors have been compared with matched cases of non-tamoxifen-associated endometrial cancers (108). Compared with spontaneous tumors the drug-associated tumors were characterized by a lower expression of ERα, higher expression of progesterone receptors , and more frequent expression of ERβ. Differential expression of ERα and ERβ may alter the expression of key target genes (such as those induced by AP-1-dependent gene transcription) and contribute to the pathogenesis and clinical behavior of these tumors. Survival was significantly poorer in women with drug-associated tumors than in those with non-drug associated tumors.

The usefulness of transvaginal ultrasound in detecting serious uterine changes in tamoxifen users has been disputed. According to one group it is a dependable diagnostic method (109), whereas others found it disappointing, with a high proportion of false positive results, even when the assessment criteria were chosen so as to exclude mild endometrial thickening (110). Setting these two papers beside one another it seems that one can detect marked endometrial changes but that ultrasound is not a dependable means of determining whether there is malignancy.

Second-Generation Effects

Teratogenicity

Since animal studies suggested the possibility of fetal and neonatal malformations it has for a long time been customary to exclude pregnancy before giving tamoxifen. However, there is currently reason to believe that the risk presented by tamoxifen to the human fetus is very slight or non-existent.

Susceptibility Factors

Genetic factors

Certain women have a genetic predisposition to develop an endometrial malignancy during tamoxifen treatment. There were significant amounts of tamoxifen-DNA adducts in the endometrium in eight of 16 women who took the drug but none at all in others, suggesting that a genotoxic mechanism may be responsible for tamoxifen-induced endometrial cancer (111). However, there is biochemical and histological evidence that tamoxifen-associated endometrial carcinoma is likely to be similar to type I and will therefore have a relatively favorable prognosis (112).

Since tamoxifen is metabolized by CYP450 enzymes, including CYP3A5, and bearing in mind two genetic polymorphisms in CYP3A5 (CYP3A5*3 and CYP3A5*6), it has been suggested that the presence of such polymorphisms in some patients might have an effect on the incidence of adverse effects of tamoxifen. However, a recent study seems to have shown that this is not the case—the metabolism and adverse effects of tamoxifen were the same in subjects with these polymorphisms as in other women (113).

Whether the adverse effects of tamoxifen when used to treat breast cancer recurrence correlate with the quantities of circulating tamoxifen and its metabolites (N-desmethyltamoxifen and 4-hydroxytamoxifen has been studied in 99 women with breast cancer, who had been taking tamoxifen for at least 30 days (114). Women who had at least one tamoxifen-related adverse effect had significantly higher concentrations of tamoxifen than women not did not. Women who reported visual problems had significantly higher concentrations of both tamoxifen and N-desmethyltamoxifen compared with others. However, concentrations of 4-hydroxytamoxifen were negatively associated with vaginal discharge. The authors suggested that that patterns of tamoxifen metabolism and its adverse effects are in some respects related and that studies of the metabolism of tamoxifen could be of value in choosing better tolerated schemes of treatment for individual patients.

Age

There is a very proper reluctance today to interfere with hormonal processes during puberty and adolescence for fear of producing adverse long-term changes. Just as the use of estrogens in rapidly growing girls has largely fallen out of favor in most countries, so the safety of attempts to treat pubertal gynecomastia in boys is being questioned.

However, this can be a distressing condition at a sensitive age, and some workers have cautiously used tamoxifen and raloxifene for this purpose. The results of different approaches have been compared in 38 patients with persistent pubertal gynecomastia at an average age of 14 years (115). They received reassurance alone or a 3- to 9-month course of an estrogen receptor modifier (tamoxifen 60 mg/day or raloxifene 10–20 mg bd). There were significant reductions in breast nodule size with both drugs, although the effect was more marked with raloxifene. In these doses, there were no adverse effects. If further work is to be performed it will be important to provide long-term follow-up to detect any unwanted later effects.

Drug–Drug Interactions

Antidepressants

There is an impression, in the light of clinical experience, that antidepressants might reduce the clinical efficacy of tamoxifen (116), but more evidence is needed to confirm or reject this view.

Atracurium dibesilate

Tamoxifen has been associated with prolonged atracurium block in a patient with breast cancer (SEDA-12, 117) (117).

Cytotoxic drugs

An unusual case of rapidly fatal renal failure reported in 1993 could reflect an interaction between tamoxifen and one or more cytostatic agents, with mitomycin C a prime suspect; in a series of breast cancer patients some 10% of those treated both with tamoxifen and a cytostatic agent developed abnormal renal function, progressing towards various stages of hemolytic-uremic syndrome (118).

Diuretics

Many patients who take tamoxifen for breast cancer take other drugs for co-existing illnesses, and the possibility of interactions with these drugs has so far been incompletely studied. In a study of 98 treated women I was shown that co-medication can influence plasma concentrations of tamoxifen and its metabolites (N-desmethyltamoxifen and 4-hydroxytamoxifen) (119). Those taking diuretics had significantly higher plasma concentrations of tamoxifen and N-desmethyltamoxifen than others. Analgesics and anti-inflammatory drugs were negatively associated with plasma tamoxifen concentrations. Chemotherapeutic agents, allergy drugs, antidepressants, and medications for diabetes did not significantly alter plasma concentrations of tamoxifen or its metabolites.

Drug–Procedure Interactions

The use of tamoxifen in combination with radiotherapy appears to increase the risk of breast fibrosis, which is a known effect of irradiation. In a retrospective study of the records of 147 women with breast cancer who had taken part in a major prospective study of tamoxifen 20 mg/day and who had also received adjuvant radiotherapy, 90 were hormone receptor-positive (120). There was a statistically significant difference in terms of mean complication-relapse-free survival rates at 3 years (48% versus 66%) and at 2 years (51% versus 80%) in the tamoxifen and control groups respectively. In each group the mean complication-relapse-free survival rates were significantly lower in patients with low levels of CD8 radiation-induced apoptosis (20%, 66%, and 79% for CD8 < = 16%, 16–24%, and > 24% respectively). There were similar results for the complication-free survival rates. These findings pointed suggest that concomitant use of tamoxifen with irradiation is significantly associated with an increased incidence of grade 2 or higher subcutaneous fibrosis.

Management of adverse drug reactions

Hot flushes/flashes remain a problem when tamoxifen is used to treat breast cancer. In a 4-week study in 22 women with this problem considerable relief was obtained by simultaneous use of oral gabapentin 300 mg tds (121). Occasional side effects were nausea, rash and excessive sleepiness.

References

1. Jaiyesimi IA, Buzdar AU, Decker DA, Hortobagyi GN. Use of tamoxifen for breast cancer: twenty-eight years later. J Clin Oncol 1995;13(2):513–29.
2. Insler V, Lunenfeld B. Anovulation. Contrib Gynecol Obstet 1978;4:6–77.
3. De Muylder X, Neven P. Tamoxifen and potential adverse effects. Cancer J 1993;6:111.
4. Rosenfeld JA. Can the prophylactic use of raloxifene, a selective estrogen-receptor modulator, prevent bone mineral loss and fractures in women with diagnosed osteoporosis or vertebral fractures? West J Med 2000;173(3):186–8.
5. Boccardo F, Rubagotti A, Amoroso D, Mesiti M, Romeo D, Sismondi P, Giai M, Genta F, Pacini P, Distante V, Bolognesi A, Aldrighetti D, Farris A. Cyclophosphamide, methotrexate, and fluorouracil versus tamoxifen plus ovarian suppression as adjuvant treatment of estrogen receptor-positive pre-/perimenopausal breast cancer patients: results of the Italian Breast Cancer Adjuvant Study Group 02 randomized trial. J Clin Oncol 2000;18(14):2718–27.
6. Goldstein SR. Drugs for the gynecologist to prescribe in the prevention of breast cancer: current status and future trends. Am J Obstet Gynecol 2000;182(5):1121–6.
7. Reddy P, Chow MS. Safety and efficacy of antiestrogens for prevention of breast cancer. Am J Health Syst Pharm 2000;57(14):1315–25.
8. Bruzzi P. Tamoxifen for the prevention of breast cancer. Important questions remain unanswered, and existing trials should continue. BMJ 1998;316(7139):1181–2.
9. Kaufman CS, Bear HD. Another view of the tamoxifen trial. J Surg Oncol 1999;72(1):1–8.
10. Baum M. Tamoxifen—the treatment of choice. Why look for alternatives? Br J Cancer 1998;78(Suppl 4):1–4.
11. Cuzick J, Powles T, Veronesi U, Forbes J, Edwards R, Ashley S, Boyle P. Overview of the main outcomes in breast-cancer prevention trials. Lancet 2003;361:296–300.
12. Rastogi P, Vogel VG. Update on breast cancer prevention. Oncology (Huntingdon) 2003;17:799–805.
13. Biglia N, Defabiani E, Ponzone R, Mariani L, Marenco D, Sismondi P. Management of risk of breast carcinoma in postmenopausal women. Endocr Relat Cancer 2004;11:69–83.
14. Lewis CL, Kinsinger LS, Harris RP, Schwartz RJ. Breast cancer in primary care: implications for chemoprevention. Arch Intern Med 2004;164:1897–903.
15. Muanza T, Shenouda G, Souhami L, Leblanc R, Mohr G, Corns R, Langleben A. High dose tamoxifen and radiotherapy in patients with glioblastoma multiforme: a phase IB study. Can J Neurol Sci 2000;27(4):302–6.
16. Perez EA, Gandara DR, Edelman MJ, O'Donnell R, Lauder IJ, DeGregorio M. Phase I trial of high- dose tamoxifen in combination with cisplatin in patients with lung cancer and other advanced malignancies. Cancer Invest 2003;21:1–6.
17. Veronesi U, Maisonneuve P, Rotmensz N, Costa A, Sacchini V, Raviglini R, D'Aiuto G, Lovison F, Gucciardo G, Muraca MG. Pizzichetta MA, Conforti S, Decensi A, Robertson C, Boyle P, and the Italian Tamoxifen Study Group. Italian randomized trial among women with hysterectomy: tamoxifen and hormone-dependent breast cancer in high-risk women. J Natl Cancer Inst 2003;95:160–5.
18. Anonymous. After lumpectomy, overall survival is similar with tamoxifen alone compared with tamoxifen plus radiotherapy in elderly women with early stage breast cancer, Evid Based Health Care 2005;9:79–80.
19. Fricker J. Letrozole better than tamoxifen in postmenopausal women. Lancet Oncol 2005;6:247.
20. Bradbury J. Results of the ATAC (Arimidex, Tamoxifen, Alone or in Combination) trial after completion of 5 years' adjuvant treatment for breast cancer. Lancet 2005;365:60–2.
21. Mouridsen HT, Robert NJ. The role of aromatase inhibitors as adjuvant therapy for early breast cancer in postmenopausal women. Eur J Cancer 2005;41:1678–89.
22. Love RR, Hutson PR, Havighurst TC, Cleary JF. Endocrine effects of tamoxifen plus exemestane in postmenopausal women with breast cancer. Clin Cancer Res 2005;11:1500–3.
23. Jakesz R, Jonat W, Gnant M, Mittlboeck M, Greil R, Tausch C, Hilfrich J, Kwasny W, Menzel C, Samonigg H, Seifert M, Gademann G, Kaufmann M. Switching of postmenopausal women with endocrine-responsive early breast cancer to anastrozole after 2 years' adjuvant tamoxifen. Combined results of ABCSG trial 8 and the ARNO 95 trial. Lancet 2005;366:455–62.
24. Morales L, Timmerman D, Neven P, Konstantinovic ML, Carbonez A, Van Huffel S, Ameye I, Weltens C, Christiaens MR, Vergote I, Paridaens R. Third generation aromatase inhibitors may prevent endometrial growth and reverse tamoxifen-induced uterine changes in postmenopausal breast cancer patients. Ann Oncol 2005;16:70–4.
25. Joensuu H, Ejlertsen B, Lonning PE, Rutqvist L-E. Aromatase inhibitors in the treatment of early and advanced breast cancer. Acta Oncol 2005;44:23–31.
26. Dunn BK, Ford LG. Prevention of breast cancer. Sem Breast Dis 2000;3:90–9.
27. Sawka CA, Pritchard KI, Paterson AH, Sutherland DJ, Thomson DB, Shelley WE, Myers RE, Mobbs BG,

Malkin A, Meakin JW. Role and mechanism of action of tamoxifen in premenopausal women with metastatic breast carcinoma. Cancer Res 1986;46(6):3152–6.

28. Anelli TF, Anelli A, Tran KN, Lebwohl DE, Borgen PI. Tamoxifen administration is associated with a high rate of treatment-limiting symptoms in male breast cancer patients. Cancer 1994;74(1):74–7.

29. Pandya KJ, Raubertas RF, Flynn PJ, Hynes HE, Rosenbluth RJ, Kirshner JJ, Pierce HI, Dragalin V, Morrow GR. Oral clonidine in postmenopausal patients with breast cancer experiencing tamoxifen-induced hot flashes: a University of Rochester Cancer Center Community Clinical Oncology Program study. Ann Intern Med 2000;132(10):788–93.

30. Jones J. Tamoxifen side effects may be attributable to other causes. J Natl Cancer Inst 2001;93(1):11–2.

31. Arnold BJ, Cumming CE, Lees AW, Handman MD, Cumming DC, Urion C. Tamoxifen in breast cancer: symptom reporting. Breast J 2001;7(2):97–100.

32. Finelli PF, Schauer PK. Cerebral sinus thrombosis with tamoxifen. Neurology 2001;56(8):1113–4.

33. Tisman G. Thromboses after estrogen hormone replacement, progesterone or tamoxifen therapy in patients with elevated blood levels of homocysteine. Am J Hematol 2001;68(2):135.

34. Goldhaber SZ. Tamoxifen: preventing breast cancer and placing the risk of deep vein thrombosis in perspective. Circulation 2005;111:539–41.

35. Deitcher SR, Gomes MPV. The risk of venous thromboembolic disease associated with adjuvant hormone therapy for breast carcinoma: a systematic review. Cancer 2004;101:439–49.

36. Decensi A, Maisonneuve P, Rotmensz N, Bettega D, Costa A, Sacchini V, Salvioni A, Travaglini R, Oliviero P, D'Aiuto G, Gulisano M, Gucciardo G, Del Turco MR, Pizzichetta MA, Conforti S, Bonanni B, Boyle P, Veronesi U. Effect of tamoxifen on venous thromboembolic events in a breast cancer prevention trial. Circulation 2005;111:650–6.

37. Decensi A, Maisonneuve P, Rotmensz N, Bettega D, Costa A, Sacchini V, Salvioni A, Travaglini R, Oliviero P, D'Aiuto G, Gulisano M, Gucciardo G, Del Turco MR, Pizzichetta MA, Conforti S, Bonanni B, Boyle P, Veronesi U. Effect of tamoxifen on venous thromboembolic events in a breast cancer prevention trial. Circulation 2005;111:650–6.

38. Ludwig M, Tolg R, Richardt G, Katus HA, Diedrich K. Myocardial infarction associated with ovarian hyperstimulation syndrome. JAMA 1999;282(7):632–3.

39. Bentzen SM, Skoczylas JZ, Overgaard M, Overgaard J. Radiotherapy-related lung fibrosis enhanced by tamoxifen. J Natl Cancer Inst 1996;88(13):918–22.

40. Rusthoven JJ, Quirt IC, Iscoe NA, McCulloch PB, James KW, Lohmann RC, Jensen J, Burdette-Radoux S, Bodurtha AJ, Silver HK, Verma S, Armitage GR, Zee B, Bennett K. Randomized, double-blind, placebo-controlled trial comparing the response rates of carmustine, dacarbazine, and cisplatin with and without tamoxifen in patients with metastatic melanoma. National Cancer Institute of Canada Clinical Trials Group. J Clin Oncol 1996;14(7):2083–90.

41. Dignam JJ, Fisher B. Occurrence of stroke with tamoxifen in NSABP B-24. Lancet 2000;355(9206):848–9.

42. Eberling JL, Wu C, Tong-Turnbeaugh R, Jagust WJ. Estrogen- and tamoxifen-associated effects on brain structure and function. NeuroImage 2004;21:364–71.

43. Pugesgaard T, Von Eyben FE. Bilateral optic neuritis evolved during tamoxifen treatment. Cancer 1986;58(2):383–6.

44. Pavlidis NA, Petris C, Briassoulis E, Klouvas G, Psilas C, Rempapis J, Petroutsos G. Clear evidence that long-term, low-dose tamoxifen treatment can induce ocular toxicity. A prospective study of 63 patients. Cancer 1992;69(12):2961–4.

45. Eisner A, Austin DF, Samples JR. Short wavelength automated perimetry and tamoxifen use. Br J Ophthalmol 2004;88:125–30.

46. Bradbury BD, Lash TL, Kaye JA, Jick SS. Tamoxifen and cataracts: a null association. Breast Cancer Res Treat 2004;87:189–96.

47. Nguyen MC, Stewart RB, Banerji MA, Gordon DH, Kral JG. Relationships between tamoxifen use, liver fat and body fat distribution in women with breast cancer. Int J Obes Relat Metab Disord 2001;25(2):296–8.

48. Liu C-L, Yang T-L. Sequential changes in serum triglyceride levels during adjuvant tamoxifen therapy in breast cancer patients and the effect of dose reduction. Breast Cancer Res Treat 2003;79:11–16.

49. Ferrazzi E, Cartei G, De Besi P, Fornasiero A, Palu G, Paccagnella A, Sperandio P, Fosser V, Grigoletto E, Fiorentino M. Tamoxifen in disseminated breast cancer. Tumori 1977;63(5):463–8.

50. Millward MJ, Cantwell BM, Lien EA, Carmichael J, Harris AL. Intermittent high-dose tamoxifen as a potential modifier of multidrug resistance. Eur J Cancer 1992;28A(4–5):805–10.

51. Bonneterre J, Thurlimann B, Robertson JF, Krzakowski M, Mauriac L, Koralewski P, Vergote I, Webster A, Steinberg M, von Euler M. Anastrozole versus tamoxifen as first-line therapy for advanced breast cancer in 668 postmenopausal women: results of the Tamoxifen or Arimidex Randomized Group Efficacy and Tolerability study. J Clin Oncol 2000;18(22):3748–57.

52. Nabholtz JM, Buzdar A, Pollak M, Harwin W, Burton G, Mangalik A, Steinberg M, Webster A, von Euler MArimidex Study Group. Anastrozole is superior to tamoxifen as first-line therapy for advanced breast cancer in postmenopausal women: results of a North American multicenter randomized trial. J Clin Oncol 2000;18(22):3758–67.

53. Wu K, Brown P. Is low-dose tamoxifen useful for the treatment and prevention of breast cancer? J Natl Cancer Inst 2003;95:766–7.

54. Robertson C, Viale G, Pigatto F, Johansson H, Kisanga ER, Veronesi P, Torrisi R, Cazzaniga M, Mora S, Sandri MT, Pelosi G, Luini A, Goldhirsch A, Lien EA, Veronesi U. A randomized trial of low-dose tamoxifen on breast cancer proliferation and blood estrogenic biomarkers. J Natl Cancer Inst 2003;95:779–90.

55. Oien KA, Moffat D, Curry GW, Dickson J, Habeshaw T, Mills PR, MacSween RN. Cirrhosis with steatohepatitis after adjuvant tamoxifen. Lancet 1999;353(9146):36–7.

56. Cai Q, Bensen M, Greene R, Kirchner J. Tamoxifen-induced transient multifocal hepatic fatty infiltration. Am J Gastroenterol 2000;95(1):277–9.

57. Nishino M, Hayakawa K, Nakamura Y, Morimoto T, Mukaihara S. Effects of tamoxifen on hepatic fat content and the development of hepatic steatosis in patients with breast cancer: high frequency of involvement and rapid reversal after completion of tamoxifen therapy. Am J Radiol 2003;180:129–34.

58. Lin H-H, Hsu CH, Chao YC. Tamoxifen-induced severe acute pancreatitis. Dig Dis Sci 2004;49:997–9.
59. Parry BR. Radiation recall induced by tamoxifen. Lancet 1992;340(8810):49.
60. Bostrom A, Sjolin-Forsberg G, Wilking N, Bergh J. Radiation recall—another call with tamoxifen. Acta Oncol 1999;38(7):955–9.
61. Puglisi F, Aprile G, Sobrero A. Tamoxifen-induced total alopecia. Ann Intern Med 2001;134(12):1154–5.
62. Fentiman IS, Fogelman I. Breast cancer and osteoporosis—a bridge at last. Eur J Cancer 1993;29A(4):485–6.
63. Malinovszky KM, Cameron D, Douglas S, Love C, Leonard T, Dixon JM, Hopwood P, Leonard RC. Breast cancer patients' experiences on endocrine therapy: monitoring with a checklist for patients on endocrine therapy (C-PET). Breast 2004;13(5):363–8.
64. Mortimer JE, Boucher L, Baty J, Knapp DL, Ryan E, Rowland JH. Effect of tamoxifen on sexual functioning in patients with breast cancer. J Clin Oncol 1999;17(5):1488–92.
65. Leo L, Lanza A, Re A, Tessarolo M, Bellino R, Lauricella A, Wierdis T. Leiomyomas in patients receiving tamoxifen. Clin Exp Obstet Gynecol 1994;21(2):94–8.
66. Son EJ, Oh KK, Kim EK, Son HJ, Jung WH, Lee HD. Leiomyoma of the breast in a 50-year-old woman receiving tamoxifen. Am J Roentgenol 1998;171(6):1684–6.
67. Sherman BM, Chapler FK, Crickard K, Wycoff D. Endocrine consequences of continuous antiestrogen therapy with tamoxifen in premenopausal women. J Clin Invest 1979;64(2):398–404.
68. Powles TJ, Jones AL, Ashley SE, O'Brien ME, Tidy VA, Treleavan J, Cosgrove D, Nash AG, Sacks N, Baum M, McKinna JA, Davey JB. The Royal Marsden Hospital pilot tamoxifen chemoprevention trial. Breast Cancer Res Treat 1994;31(1):73–82.
69. Mourits MJ, de Vries EG, Willemse PH, ten Hoor KA, Hollema H, Sluiter WJ, de Bruijn HW, van der Zee AG. Ovarian cysts in women receiving tamoxifen for breast cancer. Br J Cancer 1999;79(11–12):1761–4.
70. McGonigle KF, Vasilev SA, Odom-Maryon T, Simpson JF. Ovarian histopathology in breast cancer patients receiving tamoxifen. Gynecol Oncol 1999;73(3):402–6.
71. McCluggage WG, Weir PE. Paraovarian cystic endosalpingiosis in association with tamoxifen therapy. J Clin Pathol 2000;53(2):161–2.
72. Turan C, Unal O, Dansuk R, Guzelmeric K, Cengizoglu B, Esim E. Successful management of an ovarian enlargement resembling ovarian hyperstimulation in a premenopausal breast cancer patient receiving tamoxifen with cotreatment of GnRH-agonist. Eur J Obstet Gynecol Reprod Biol 2001;97(1):105–7.
73. Nasu K, Miyazaki T, Kiyonaga Y, Kawasaki F, Miyakawa I. Torsion of a functional ovarian cyst in a premenopausal patient receiving tamoxifen. Gynecol Obstet Invest 1999;48(3):200–2.
74. Cohen I, Figer A, Tepper R, Shapira J, Altaras MM, Yigael D, Beyth Y. Ovarian overstimulation and cystic formation in premenopausal tamoxifen exposure: comparison between tamoxifen-treated and nontreated breast cancer patients. Gynecol Oncol 1999;72(2):202–7.
75. Gardner FJ, Konje JC, Abrams KR, Brown LJ, Khanna S, Al-Azzawi F, Bell SC, Taylor DJ. Endometrial protection from tamoxifen-stimulated changes by a levonorgestrel-releasing intrauterine system: a randomised controlled trial. Lancet 2000;356(9243):1711–7.
76. Love CD, Dixon JM. Thickened endometrium caused by tamoxifen returns to normal following tamoxifen cessation. Breast 2000;9(3):156–7.
77. Cohen I, Beyth Y, Azaria R, Flex D, Figer A, Tepper R. Ultrasonographic measurement of endometrial changes following discontinuation of tamoxifen treatment in postmenopausal breast cancer patients. BJOG 2000;107(9):1083–7.
78. McCluggage WG, Desai V, Manek S. Tamoxifen-associated postmenopausal adenomyosis exhibits stromal fibrosis, glandular dilatation and epithelial metaplasias. Histopathology 2000;37(4):340–6.
79. Seoud M, Shamseddine A, Khalil A, Salem Z, Saghir N, Bikhazi K, Bitar N, Azar G, Kaspar H. Tamoxifen and endometrial pathologies: a prospective study. Gynecol Oncol 1999;75(1):15–9.
80. Bakour SH, Khan KS, Newton JR. Evaluation of the endometrium in abnormal uterine bleeding associated with long-term tamoxifen use. Gynaecol Endosc 2000;9:19–22.
81. Cohen I, Azaria R, Bernheim J, Shapira J, Beyth Y. Risk factors of endometrial polyps resected from postmenopausal patients with breast cancer treated with tamoxifen. Cancer 2001;92(5):1151–5.
82. Schlesinger C, Silverberg SG. Tamoxifen-associated polyps (basalomas) arising in multiple endometriotic foci: A case report and review of the literature. Gynecol Oncol 1999;73(2):305–11.
83. Cohen I, Bernheim J, Azaria R, Tepper R, Sharony R, Beyth Y. Malignant endometrial polyps in postmenopausal breast cancer tamoxifen-treated patients. Gynecol Oncol 1999;75(1):136–41.
84. Maia H Jr, Maltez A, Calmon LC, Moreira K, Coutinho EM. Endometrial carcinoma in postmenopausal patients using hormone replacement therapy: a report on four cases. Gynaecol Endosc 1999;8:235–41.
85. Biron-Shental T, Tepper R, Fishman A, Shapira J, Cohen I. Recurrent endometrial polyps in postmenopausal breast cancer patients on tamoxifen. Gynecol Oncol 2003;90:382–6.
86. Hachisuga T, Miyakawa T, Tsujioka H, Horiuchi S, Emoto M, Kawarabayashi T. K-ras mutation in tamoxifen-related endometrial polyps. Cancer 2003;98:1890–7.
87. Houghton JP, Ioffe OB, Silverberg SG, McGrady B, McCluggage WG. Metastatic breast lobular carcinoma involving tamoxifen-associated endometrial polyps: report of two cases and review of tamoxifen-associated polypoid uterine lesions. Mod Pathol 2003;16:395–8.
88. Levine PH, Wei X-J, Gagner J-P, Flax H, Mittal K, Blank SV. Pleomorphic liposarcoma of the uterus. Case report and literature review. Int J Gynecol Pathol 2003;22:407–11.
89. Creamer P, Lim K, George E, Dieppe P. Acute inflammatory polyarthritis in association with tamoxifen. Br J Rheumatol 1994;33(6):583–5.
90. Clement PB, Oliva E, Young RH. Mullerian adenosarcoma of the uterine corpus associated with tamoxifen therapy: a report of six cases and a review of tamoxifen-associated endometrial lesions. Int J Gynecol Pathol 1996;15(3):222–9.
91. Orbo A, Lindal S, Mortensen E. Tamoxifen og endometriecancer. En kasuistikk. [Tamoxifen and endometrial cancer. A case report.] Tidsskr Nor Laegeforen 1996;116(16):1877–8.
92. Boudouris O, Ferrand S, Guillet JL, Madelenat P. Efféts paradoxaux du tamoxifène sur l'utérus de la femme. [Paradoxical effects of tamoxifen on the woman's uterus.

Apropos of 7 cases of myoma that appeared while under anti-estrogen treatment.] J Gynecol Obstet Biol Reprod (Paris) 1989;18(3):372–8.

93. Nuovo MA, Nuovo GJ, McCaffrey RM, Levine RU, Barron B, Winkler B. Endometrial polyps in postmenopausal patients receiving tamoxifen. Int J Gynecol Pathol 1989;8(2):125–31.

94. Rutqvist LE, Mattsson AThe Stockholm Breast Cancer Study Group. Cardiac and thromboembolic morbidity among postmenopausal women with early-stage breast cancer in a randomized trial of adjuvant tamoxifen. J Natl Cancer Inst 1993;85(17):1398–406.

95. Seoud MA, Johnson J, Weed JC Jr. Gynecologic tumors in tamoxifen-treated women with breast cancer. Obstet Gynecol 1993;82(2):165–9.

96. Treilleux T, Mignotte H, Clement-Chassagne C, Guastalla P, Bailly C. Tamoxifen and malignant epithelial-nonepithelial tumours of the endometrium: report of six cases and review of the literature. Eur J Surg Oncol 1999;25(5):477–82.

97. Ramondetta LM, Sherwood JB, Dunton CJ, Palazzo JP. Endometrial cancer in polyps associated with tamoxifen use. Am J Obstet Gynecol 1999;180(2 Pt 1):340–1.

98. Ascher SM, Johnson JC, Barnes WA, Bae CJ, Patt RH, Zeman RK. MR imaging appearance of the uterus in postmenopausal women receiving tamoxifen therapy for breast cancer: histopathologic correlation. Radiology 1996;200(1):105–10.

99. Okada DH, Rowland JB, Petrovic LM. Uterine pleomorphic rhabdomyosarcoma in a patient receiving tamoxifen therapy. Gynecol Oncol 1999;75(3):509–13.

100. Dumortier J, Freyer G, Sasco AJ, Frappart L, Zenone T, Romestaing P, Trillet-Lenoir V. Endometrial mesodermal mixed tumor occurring after tamoxifen treatment: report on a new case and review of the literature. Ann Oncol 2000;11(3):355–8.

101. Jessop FA, Roberts PF. Mullerian adenosarcoma of the uterus in association with tamoxifen therapy. Histopathology 2000;36(1):91–2.

102. Fotiou S, Hatjieleftheriou G, Kyrousis G, Kokka F, Apostolikas N. Long-term tamoxifen treatment: a possible aetiological factor in the development of uterine carcinosarcoma: two case-reports and review of the literature. Anticancer Res 2000;20(3B):2015–20.

103. Andia D, Lafuente P, Matorras R, Usandizaga JM. Uterine side effects of treatment with tamoxifen. Eur J Obstet Gynecol Reprod Biol 2000;92(2):235–40.

104. Tempfer C, Kubista E, Atkins CD, Narod SA, Pal T, Graham T, Mitchell M, Fyles A, Lasset C, Bonadona V, Mignotte H, Bremond A, Van Leeuwen FE, Bergman L, Beelen MLR, Gallee MPW, Hollema H, Dickson MJ, Pandiarajan T, Kairies P, Marsh F, Mayfield M. Tamoxifen and risk of endometrial cancer. Lancet 2001;357(9249):65–8.

105. Bergman L, Beelen ML, Gallee MP, Hollema H, Benraadt J, van Leeuwen FE. Risk and prognosis of endometrial cancer after tamoxifen for breast cancer. Comprehensive Cancer Centres' ALERT Group. Assessment of Liver and Endometrial cancer Risk following Tamoxifen. Lancet 2000;356(9233):881–7.

106. Powles TJ, Bourne T, Athanasiou S, Chang J, Grubock K, Ashley S, Oakes L, Tidy A, Davey J, Viggers J, Humphries S, Collins W. The effects of norethisterone on endometrial abnormalities identified by transvaginal ultrasound screening of healthy post-menopausal women on tamoxifen or placebo. Br J Cancer 1998;78(2):272–5.

107. Ferguson SE, Olshen AB, Viale A, Awtrey CS, Barakat RR, Boyd J. Gene expression profiling of tamoxifen-associated uterine cancers: evidence for two molecular classes of endometrial carcinoma. Gynecol Oncol 2004;92:719–25.

108. Wilder JL, Shajahan S, Khattar NH, Wilder DM, Yin J, Rushing RS, Beaven R, Kaetzel C, Ueland FR, Van Nagell JR, Kryscio RJ, Lele SM. Tamoxifen-associated malignant endometrial tumors: pathologic features and expression of hormone receptors estrogen-alpha, estrogen-beta and progesterone. A case controlled study. Gynecol Oncol 2004;92:553–8.

109. Strauss HG, Wolters M, Methfessel G, Buchmann J, Koelbl H. Significance of endovaginal ultrasonography in assessing tamoxifen-associated changes of the endometrium. A prospective study. Acta Obstet Gynecol Scand 2000;79(8):697–701.

110. Gerber B, Krause A, Muller H, Reimer T, Kulz T, Makovitzky J, Kundt G, Friese K. Effects of adjuvant tamoxifen on the endometrium in postmenopausal women with breast cancer: a prospective long-term study using transvaginal ultrasound. J Clin Oncol 2000;18(20):3464–70.

111. Shibutani S, Ravindernath A, Suzuki N, Terashima I, Sugarman SM, Grollman AP, Pearl ML. Identification of tamoxifen-DNA adducts in the endometrium of women treated with tamoxifen. Carcinogenesis 2000;21(8):1461–7.

112. Roy RN, Gerulath AH, Cecutti A, Bhavnani BR. Effect of tamoxifen treatment on the endometrial expression of human insulin-like growth factors and their receptor mRNAs. Mol Cell Endocrinol 2000;165(1–2):173–8.

113. Tucker AN, Tkaczuk KA, Lewis LM, Tomic D, Lim CK, Flaws JA. Management of late intrauterine death using a combination of mifepristone and misoprostol—experience of two regimens. Cancer Lett 2005;217:61–72.

114. Gallicchio L, Lord G, Tkaczuk K, Danton M, Lewis LM, Lim CK, Flaws JA. Association of tamoxifen (TAM) and TAM metabolite concentrations with self-reported side effects of TAM in women with breast cancer. Breast Cancer Res Treat 2004;85:89–97.

115. Lawrence SE, Faught KA, Vethamuthu J, Lawson ML. Beneficial effects of raloxifene and tamoxifen in the treatment of pubertal gynecomastia. J Pediatr 2004;145(1):71–6.

116. Ahmad K. Antidepressants may decrease tamoxifen efficacy. Lancet Oncol 2004;5:6.

117. Naguib M, Gyasi HK. Antiestrogenic drugs and atracurium—a possible interaction? Can Anaesth Soc J 1986;33(5):682–3.

118. Montes A, Powles TJ, O'Brien ME, Ashley SE, Luckit J, Treleaven J. A toxic interaction between mitomycin C and tamoxifen causing the haemolytic uraemic syndrome. Eur J Cancer 1993;29A(13):1854–7.

119. Gallicchio L, Tkaczuk K, Lord G, Danton M, Lewis LM, Lim CK, Flaws JA. Medication use, tamoxifen (TAM), and TAM metabolite concentrations in women with breast cancer. Cancer Lett 2004;211;57–67.

120. Azria D, Gourgou S, Sozzi WJ, Zouhair A, Mirimanoff RO, Kramar A, Lemanski C, Dubois JB, Romieu G, Pelegrin A, Ozsahin M. Concomitant use of tamoxifen with radiotherapy enhances subcutaneous breast fibrosis in hypersensitive patients. Br J Cancer 2004;91:1251–60.

121. Pandya KJ, Thummala AR, Griggs JJ, Rosenblatt JD, Sahasrabudhe DM, Guttuso TJ, Morrow GR, Roscoe JA. Pilot study using gabapentin for tamoxifen-induced hot flashes in women with breast cancer. Breast Cancer Res Treat 2004;83:87–9.

Tibolone

General Information

Tibolone is an agonist at estrogen and progestogen receptors, with weak androgenic activity. It is given as an alternative to hormone replacement therapy, without added progestogen, and has been in use for some 30 years to treat bone loss in post-menopausal women. Some long-term studies (for example over 10 years) appear to have confirmed its safety and relative freedom from adverse effects (1). In particular there is little or no increase in thrombotic events and the incidence of breast tenderness is low.

Studies and reviews sponsored by the manufacturer of tibolone have over many decades argued that, as one reviewer puts it, tibolone "may provide a safer alternative to traditional hormone replacement therapy", but even this review adds that "the impact of tibolone on the risk of breast cancer or cardiovascular and thromboembolic events is not well defined" (2). Bearing in mind that these are precisely the questions that have cast a shadow over other forms of hormone replacement therapy, this is a serious defect in the evidence about the drug's safety; it is possible that the extent of use of tibolone has been insufficient to provide well-documented answers.

Placebo-controlled studies

Despite the still uncertain adverse effects profile of tibolone, it continues to be used in relieving the hot flushes caused by anti-estrogen therapy, and does so in doses that cause no additional problems. In a further double-blind, placebo-controlled study of oral tibolone 2.5 mg/day in 70 postmenopausal women taking tamoxifen after breast cancer surgery tibolone reduced the severity of hot flushes and perhaps also their incidence (3).

Organ and Systems

Metabolism

The effects of 5 years of therapy with tibolone 2.5 mg/day on the lipid profile in 82 postmenopausal women with mild hypercholesterolemia have been examined (4). Total, low-density, and high-density lipoprotein cholesterol and lipoprotein(a) were very significantly reduced by tibolone group (n = 53) compared with controls (n = 29), by 18%, 32%, 16% and 12% respectively; triglycerides did not change. At this dose, which was sufficient to relieve menopausal symptoms, there were some adverse effects on hormone-dependent tissues (vaginal spotting in 11% and febrile hemorrhagic cystic mastopathy in 3.8%), but long-term therapy with tibolone was well tolerated and its effect on the concentrations of serum lipids appeared to be beneficial.

Musculoskeletal

A 2-year randomized controlled study in 90 women compared the effects of oral tibolone doses of 1.25 mg/day and 2.5 mg/day on bone loss in the early postmenopausal period; all took calcium 1000 mg/day. Vertebral and femoral bone density rose in both treated groups but fell in the control group, and bone turnover markers (urinary excretion of hydroxyproline/creatinine and plasma osteocalcin concentrations) were similarly affected favorably in the treated groups, as was the incidence of hot flushes/flashes (5). Studies such as this still leave open the question of the advisability of continuing tibolone treatment over a longer period. While tibolone has indeed been shown to benefit mineral bone density, few data are available to show whether it lowers fracture incidence; nor is it clear whether there is a link between tibolone and breast cancer (6).

Drug-drug interactions

Coumarin anticoagulants

Two patients taking oral anticoagulants developed excessive anticoagulant activity shortly after they had begun to take a course of tibolone (7). This seems to be a specific interaction, apparently similar to that seen with more potent estrogens, and the dose of anticoagulant may need to be reduced when tibolone is taken; the problem did not seem to arise consistently with other hormone replacement formulations.

References

1. Rymer J, Robinson J, Fogelman I. Tiz even keresztul naponta 2.5 mg dozisban adagolt tibolon hatasa a csontvesztesre postmenopauzas nokben. Magyar Nöorvosok Lapja 2003;66:101–8.
2. Swegle JM, Kelly MW. Tibolone: a unique version of hormone replacement therapy. Ann Pharmacother 2004;38:874–81.
3. Kroiss R, Fentiman IS, Helmond FA, Rymer J, Foidart JM, Bundred N, Mol-Arts M, Kubista E. The effect of tibolone in postmenopausal women receiving tamoxifen after surgery for breast cancer: a randomised, double-blind, placebo-controlled trial. BJOG 2005;112:228–33.
4. Kalogeropoulos S, Petrogiannopoulos C, Gagos S, Kampas N, Kalogeropoulos G. The influence of 5-year therapy with tibolone on the lipid profile in postmenopausal women with mild hypercholesterolemia. Gynecol Endocrinol 2004;18:227–32.
5. Gambacciani M, Ciaponi M, Cappagli B, Monteleone P, Benussi C, Bevilacqua G, Genazzani AR. A longitudinal evaluation of the effect of two doses of tibolone on bone density and metabolism in early postmenopausal women. Gynecol Endocrinol 2004;18:9–16.
6. Devogelaer J-P. A review of the effects of tibolone on the skeleton. Exp Opin Pharmacother 2004;5:941–9.
7. McLintock LA, Dykes A, Tait RC, Walker ID. Interaction between hormone replacement therapy preparations and oral anticoagulant therapy. Br J Obstet Gynaecol 2003;110:777–9.

IODINE AND DRUGS THAT AFFECT THYROID FUNCTION

Iodine-containing medicaments

General Information

Iodine is a non-metallic halogen element (symbol I; atomic no 53) which exists as a near-black solid but readily sublimates, giving a purple-colored vapor. It is found in nature both free (for example in large amounts in seaweeds such as kelp and in low concentrations in seawater) and in minerals such as iodyrite (silver iodide) and Chile saltpetre (sodium iodide).

Iodine-containing medicaments

Iodine must be present in the normal diet to prevent iodine-deficiency goiter or cretinism, and iodine deficiency-related disorders are still a worldwide (although preventable) group of diseases that affect about 150 million people in at least 40 countries. The WHO sponsored a program to control these disorders by the year 2000 (1,2), and since 1990 there has been a remarkable progress in prevention of iodine deficiency disorders. However, by the year 2000 one-third of the population affected by iodine deficiency disorders still did not have access to iodized salt (3).

Scepticism about the introduction of population-wide programs to prevent iodine-deficiency disorders is occasionally encountered in regions of mild iodine deficiency, especially in Europe (4). The main arguments against introduction of iodized salt are a temporary rise in the incidence of hyperthyroidism (5), a possible increase in the incidence of Graves' disease, and the fact that the remission rates with antithyroid drug therapy will fall (6). The value of preventing mild iodine deficiency has been supported by a longitudinal study from Switzerland, in which 109 000 people in a defined catchment area were studied before and for 9 years after correction of mild iodine deficiency (7). The incidence of toxic nodular goiter increased in the first year by 27%, but thereafter there was a steady fall in the incidence of both toxic nodular goiter (−73%) and Graves' disease (−33%). The range of optimal iodine intake is fairly narrow. Mild and moderate iodine excess are probably associated with higher frequency of hypothyroidism (8).

Some drugs contain iodine in amounts that considerably exceed the optimum daily intake of inorganic iodine. Such drugs include:

- most radiographic contrast media
- amiodarone and benziodarone
- iodoquinoline
- iodine-containing antiseptics (for example povidone-iodine).

Health Canada has advised consumers against using some products containing iodine (SEAVITE Premium Atlantic Kelp tablets), since these products, when consumed according to the label instructions, can provide 25 times the recommended daily allowance (RDA) of iodine for adults; this could lead to serious adverse health consequences (9). The RDA for iodine ranges from 90 micrograms/day for children aged 1–8 years to 150 micrograms/day for adults. Excessive iodine intake could lead to thyroid disorders and in turn to heart problems. Three reports of serious adverse events have been associated with the use of these products; one patient required hospitalization. The excessive iodine can cause hypothyroidism or hyperthyroidism. Individuals who are especially sensitive to the toxic effect of excess iodine include fetuses, children of all ages, pregnant women, breast fed babies, and people who are or have been those under supervision for thyroid disease. Anyone taking amiodarone may also be at increased risk.

Radioactive iodine

Different forms of radioiodine have been used at different times, including ^{123}I, ^{125}I, and ^{131}I. Radioactive iodine is used to scan the thyroid gland and in the treatment of thyrotoxicosis. See in the monograph on Radioactive iodine.

Potassium iodide and potassium iodate

Potassium iodide is the inorganic iodide most commonly used in high dosage for acute thyrotoxicosis. Indeed, large amounts of iodine cause reduced organification of iodine and a temporary block of thyroid hormone secretion (Wolff–Chaikoff effect) and therefore result in a more rapid thyrostatic effect than synthesis inhibitors. Potassium iodide is also used for preoperative treatment of goiter, especially to reduce preoperative bleeding. It can be used in combination with thyrostatic drugs but should never be prescribed in combination with potassium perchlorate, since each abolishes the other's effects. The thyrostatic effects of iodide are evident even at a dose of 6 mg/day, but doses between 50 and 100 mg/day are usually recommended. In some cases of intolerance to higher doses, perchlorate can be used, for example for preoperative treatment.

Potassium iodide has been widely used in asthma and chronic bronchitis as an expectorant. There is considerable controversy about its efficacy. It should not be used in adolescent patients because of its potential to aggravate and induce acne and its effect on the thyroid gland. In view of its doubtful efficacy and definite toxicity, it would be preferable if physicians stopped prescribing it as an expectorant.

Potassium iodide and potassium iodate are commonly added to table salt to prevent iodine deficiency and associated thyroid disease.

Iodine in protecting the thyroid against radioiodine

Accidents with nuclear reactors or nuclear bombs can expose large numbers of people to several decay products of uranium, and iodine isotopes are among the most abundant compounds released in such reactions. It is therefore logical to use salts of stable isotopes of iodine to prevent the accumulation of radioiodine in a person or population at risk of such exposure. The accidents in Windscale (UK), Three Mile Island (USA), and particularly Chernobyl (Ukraine) drew attention to such problems. The major question is therefore whether the potential adverse effects of stable iodine when given indiscriminately to large groups of people would outweigh the risk of radioiodine exposure. Stable iodine needs to be rapidly available when disasters occur, since, in order to be effective, it has to be given in sufficient amounts (100 mg) within a short time before or after (-12 to $+3$ hours) radioiodine exposure. Potassium iodate (KIO_3) is more stable than potassium iodide (KI), since the latter readily evaporates during prolonged storage. However, the dose recommended for radioprotection of 100 mg of iodine daily over several days (138 mg iodate per day) are close to retinotoxic doses of iodate reported in cases of accidental intoxication. In these doses iodate cannot be recommended. As an additive to salt for correcting iodine deficiency, much smaller doses of iodate are used (up to 1.7 mg/day), and in these doses iodate is probably safe (10).

The main adverse effects of stable iodine are shown in Table 1.

Iodine should be given to the general population if the risk of radioiodine exposure is sufficient (over 15–100 rem), but people with increased susceptibility to the adverse effects of iodine (previous thyroid disease or known serious allergies) should be excluded (11–16). In elderly people the benefit of stable iodine probably does not outweigh its potential adverse effects, while in pregnant women and infants the benefit to harm balance is not established; rapid evacuation of such people from fallout zones should be given the highest priority (SEDA-11, 358).

Tincture of iodine

Tincture of iodine (aqueous iodine oral solution, Lugol's solution) is a solution of iodine 5% plus potassium iodide 10% in water, which is used to reduce the vascularity of the thyroid gland in thyrotoxicosis before surgery.

Iodinated glycerol

Iodinated glycerol is used as a mucolytic agent in respiratory disorders, but its efficacy is controversial. Organically bound iodine is changed to unbound iodine after absorption.

Iodoform

Iodoform is a lemon-yellow-colored crystalline organic salt of iodine (CHI_3), analogous to chloroform, with a saffron-like odor, used as an antiseptic.

Iodophors

Iodophors are labile complexes of elemental iodine with macromolecular carriers that both increase the solubility and provide sustained release of iodine. Povidone-iodine is a water-soluble iodophor that is used as an antiseptic and is said to be free of the undesirable effects of iodine tincture. However, iodine can be absorbed from it through burned areas (17), vaginal mucosa (18), oral mucosa (19), and in children even with normal skin (20). Povidone-iodine is discussed in a separate monograph under the title Polyvidone.

Iodinated radiocontrast media (SED-15, 1848–96)

Many radiocontrast media contain iodine. These include iodixonal, iohexol, iomeprole, iopamidole, iopanoic acid, iopitridole, iopromide, iothalamate, iotrolan, ioversol, and ioxaglate.

General adverse effects

It has been estimated that in 1994 some 1.5 billion people in 118 countries were at risk of iodine deficiency, this being regarded as the world's most significant cause of preventable brain damage and mental retardation. Fortification of all salt for animal and human consumption has been chosen as the preferred method for the prevention of iodine deficiency disorders, and this approach is proving effective in reducing the incidence of such disorders. However, iodine supplementation is not without risks, which have been discussed (21) and which include allergic reactions and iodine-induced hyperthyroidism. It has been clearly shown that the benefits of iodine deficiency outweigh the risks on a population basis, but it is nevertheless evident that introduction of iodine supplementation is associated with clinical problems in individual subjects.

Because of its adverse effects, it is logical to omit iodine from all pharmaceutical formulations whenever possible, and at least clearly label its presence when it is necessary. The adverse effects of iodine include goiter and hypothyroidism (20,22), hyperthyroidism (SEDA-18, 176), neutropenia (23), metabolic acidosis (24), and generalized iododerma (17).

The term "iodism" covers a group of adverse effects that include irritation of the skin, the mucous membranes, and the conjunctiva. Allergic reactions are rare and

Table 1 Adverse effects of iodine given for protection against radioiodine

Adverse effect	Susceptible individuals
Iodine-induced goiter	
Iodine-induced hypothyroidism	Fetus and neonate
Iodine-induced hyperthyroidism	People living in iodine-deficient areas; people with a history of hyperthyroidism
Sialadenitis and taste disturbances	
Nausea and abdominal pain	
Skin rashes	
Edema (including face and glottis)	
Allergic-like reactions (iodine fever, eosinophilia, serum sickness-like symptoms, vasculitis)	People with hypocomplementemic vasculitis

mainly cause rashes, pruritus, fever, eosinophilia, and allergic vasculitis (25–28). Leukocytosis, swelling of the salivary glands, iodine coryza, and gastric upsets have also been reported. Headache can accompany the other reactions. In rare cases, jaundice, bleeding from the mucous membranes, and bronchospasm can occur. Inflammatory states may be aggravated by these adverse reactions.

Effects of iodine on thyroid function

Iodine excess can induce hyperthyroidism or hypothyroidism (SEDA-12, 355; SEDA-13, 378). Pharmacological amounts of iodine induce only a temporary inhibition of thyroid hormone secretion, since even during continuous administration of iodine normal thyroid function reappears ("escape from inhibition"), at least in most healthy subjects. For some unknown reasons, thyroid function can remain suppressed, resulting in hypothyroidism, secondary hypersecretion of TSH, and development of goiter (29). Patients with autoimmune thyroiditis or partial thyroid resection and very young infants (or fetuses) are especially susceptible to iodine-induced hypothyroidism. That therapeutic doses of iodine could induce hyperthyroidism was already known in the nineteenth century shortly after its introduction for the prevention and treatment of iodine deficiency (5,30). Thereafter, similar observations were made in several other parts of the world when iodine supplementation was introduced in iodine-deficient areas. Such iodine-induced hyperthyroidism (the "Jod-Basedow" phenomenon) can also occur in patients with other thyroid diseases (especially multinodular goiter), even when the diet was sufficient in iodine before the excess intake of iodine. This can even be found in patients with apparently normal thyroid glands. The Jod-Basedow phenomenon is usually associated with a slight goiter, high concentrations of both free levothyroxine (T4) and triiodothyronine (T3) and a very low uptake of radioactive iodine. The disease disappears spontaneously weeks or months after interruption of the excess iodine (31–33). Such a disorder should be differentiated from the temporary increase in T4 and reciprocal fall in T3 that can occur 1–2 weeks after the administration of iodine or iodine-containing drugs and that is not associated with symptoms of thyroid dysfunction (34).

Organs and Systems

Cardiovascular

Cardiac dysrhythmias have been seen after accidental ingestion of a large amount of potassium iodide solution (35). In one case administration of iodide was associated with pulmonary edema and iododerma (SEDA-7, 190).

Endocrine

It has been estimated that in 1990 iodine deficiency affected almost one-third of the world's population and represented the greatest single cause of preventable brain damage and mental retardation. Fortification of all salt for animal and human consumption has been chosen as the preferred method for the prevention of iodine

deficiency disorders, and this approach is effective in reducing the incidence of such disorders. However, iodine supplementation is not without risk, particularly iodine-induced hyperthyroidism and thyroiditis. The issue of benefit versus harm has been reviewed and the view, previously expressed, that the benefits of correcting iodine deficiency far outweigh risk of iodine supplementation has been reiterated (36). Complications of iodine administration are not confined to those taking dietary supplements to correct deficiency, but can also occur in those given iodine-containing contrast media and with the use of iodine-containing antiseptic solutions.

Shortly after the administration of iodine-containing drugs, there is a self-limited increase in serum thyroxine (T4), which sometimes exceeds the reference range, and a reciprocal fall in serum triiodothyronine (T3). This usually resolves spontaneously, but can persist during further treatment (so-called isolated hyperthyroxinemia). In some patients, true hyperthyroidism (increases in both T4 and T3 with clinical symptoms) occurs, for example in about 5% of patients taking long-term amiodarone, whereas evolution to iodine-induced hypothyroidism is less frequent (37–39). On the other hand, the frequency of iodine-induced hyperthyroidism can comprise about half of all cases of hyperthyroidism, at least in elderly patients taking several drugs (SEDA-7, 399).

The use of iodine has been held responsible for the increasing frequency of relapse of Graves' disease in the USA. Treatment of more severe cases of iodine-induced hyperthyroidism can be difficult, as thyroid synthesis inhibitors are not immediately active and ^{131}I cannot be used because of low thyroid uptake. The carefully supervised combination of perchlorate and methimazole is effective (40), but surgery has also occasionally been advocated.

A summary of the occurrence and epidemiology of iodine-induced hyperthyroidism has been published (41), based on the authors' experience in Tasmania, Zaire, Zimbabwe, and Brazil. Another review has more specifically examined the cardiac features of iodine-induced hyperthyroidism and has emphasized the importance of awareness, monitoring, and treatment of such hyperthyroidism in areas in which iodine supplementation has been recently introduced (42).

The complexity of the interaction between iodine intake and autoimmune thyroid disease has been highlighted by reports of evidence that iodide (compared with thyroxine) induces thyroid autoimmunity in patients with endemic (iodine deficient) goiter (43), while in those with pre-existing thyroid autoimmunity, evidenced by the presence of antithyroid (thyroid peroxidase) antibodies, administration of iodine in an area of mild iodine deficiency led to subclinical or overt hypothyroidism (44).

More importantly, in a study from Italy the use of iodine-containing disinfectants was responsible for transient neonatal hypothyroidism in more than 50% of cases identified (another common cause being transfer of maternal antibodies) (45). These findings led the authors to conclude that pregnant women should be advised of the adverse effects of using iodine-containing products and that their use should be generally discouraged.

Because of reports of severe hyperthyroidism after the introduction of iodized salt in two severely iodine-deficient African counties (Zimbabwe and the Democratic Republic of the Congo), a multicenter study has been conducted in seven countries in the region to evaluate whether the occurrence of iodine-induced hyperthyroidism after the introduction of iodized salt was a generalized phenomenon or corresponded to specific local circumstances in the two affected countries (46). Iodine deficiency had been successfully eliminated in all of the areas investigated and the prevalence of goiter had fallen markedly. However, it was clear that some areas were now exposed to iodine excess as a result of poor monitoring of the quality of iodized salt and of the iodine intake of the population. In these areas, iodine-induced hyperthyroidism occurred only when iodized salt had been recently introduced.

This complication of iodine administration is not confined to those receiving dietary supplements. Two of 788 unselected patients from a relatively iodine-deficient area of Germany who underwent coronary artery angiography with an iodine-containing radiographic contrast agent developed hyperthyroidism within 12 weeks (despite the absence of the typical risk factors of advanced age, preceding nodular goiter, or a low serum TSH) (47). While this represents a relatively low incidence, this series highlights the importance of recognizing the role of iodine-containing drugs in inducing hyperthyroidism, even in developed countries.

Iodinated glycerol

After the administration of iodinated glycerol organically bound iodine is changed to unbound iodide, causing thyrotoxicosis, hypothyroidism, or goiter in some patients (48). Reversible hypothyroidism has been reported in nursing-home residents, without a history of thyroid disease, who had been taking iodinated glycerol as an expectorant (49). Hypothyroidism has been reported after long-term treatment with iodinated glycerol (50).

Iodophors

Extensive iodine absorption from povidone-iodine can cause transient hypothyroidism or in patients with latent hypothyroidism the risk of destabilization and thyrotoxic crisis (SEDA-20, 226; SEDA-22, 263). Especially at risk are patients with an autonomous adenoma, localized diffuse autonomy of the thyroid gland, nodular goiter, latent hyperthyroidism of autoimmune origin, or endemic iodine deficiency (51).

Hyperthyroidism from povidone-iodine is rarer than hypothyroidism (SEDA-20, 226), but a history of long-term use of iodine-containing medications should be considered when investigating the cause of hyperthyroidism.

- A 48-year-old woman developed palpitation and insomnia (52). The clinical history, physical examination, and laboratory tests supported hyperthyroidism. Since July 1994 she had been combating constipation by improper use of an iodine-containing antiseptic cream for external use only. She had inserted povidone-iodine into her rectum by means of a cannula.

The iodine-containing cream was withdrawn and she was given a beta-blocker. The palpitation resolved within 2 weeks and her plasma thyroid hormone concentrations normalized within 1 month.

Hyperthyroidism in this patient was probably triggered by improper long-term use of an over-the-counter iodine-containing cream.

Potassium iodide

Iodine-induced hypothyroidism has been described as the result of prolonged intake of potassium iodide and iodinated glycerol as mucolytics (53).

Patients with an underlying disorder of the thyroid gland may be more predisposed to this complication.

The case of a severe iodine-induced thyrotoxicosis in a patient who had been using iodine-containing eye-drops for more than 10 years has been reported (54).

Mouth

Occasionally, after a high dose of iodine, sudden swelling of the parotid and submandibular glands develops (55).

- Acute sialadenitis ("iodide mumps") has been described in a 70-year-old man who underwent femoral artery angiography with an iodine-containing contrast agent; he gave a history of a similar episode 24 hours after a previous angiogram (56).

This effect is thought to be a hypersensitivity reaction due to formation of a complex between iodide and plasma proteins.

Gastrointestinal

Lugol's iodine spray is being increasingly used during diagnostic endoscopy to detect early mucosal changes of esophageal carcinoma. Transient acute gastric mucosal damage induced by iodine spray has been reported (57).

Urinary tract

Iodinated radiographic contrast media can cause acute renal insufficiency, perhaps as a result of reduced renal blood flow, an intrarenal osmotic effect, or direct tubular toxicity (58). Diuretics, calcium channel blockers, adenosine receptor antagonists, acetylcysteine, low-dose dopamine, the dopamine D_1 receptor agonist fenoldopam, endothelin receptor antagonists, and captopril have all been used to prevent contrast nephropathy.

Skin

A complication of the use of alcoholic iodine solution has been described in three women undergoing cesarean section, who developed painful, superficial, inflammatory reactions on their buttocks after skin preparation for surgery with 10% iodine in alcohol (59). These lesions were believed to have been caused by pooling of the solution underneath the patients, topical skin damage being exacerbated by heat and occlusive drapes.

Induction and aggravation of acne is a typical reaction to iodide (60).

Iododerma, which is thought to be an allergic reaction, starts with an acneiform lesion, localized in the area of the sebaceous glands, which spreads to form verrucous granulomatous lesions (61,62). After discontinuation of iodide, the skin clears over a few weeks. In addition to this typical picture of iodide sensitivity, iodide can cause urticaria and erythema and even hemorrhagic rashes. In order to verify the etiology of the skin conditions in certain cases, sensitivity testing may be required, but is not without risk.

Immunologic

Allergy to iodides can occur (63,64).

Of 126 participants in a study of the metabolism of radiolabelled proteins, four repeatedly developed urticaria and other symptoms after potassium iodide administration (65). Two of them were challenged with oral potassium iodide and developed urticaria, angioedema, polymyalgia, conjunctivitis, and coryza. Ten control patients were also challenged without adverse effects.

- Delayed hypersensitivity to potassium iodide occurred in a 66-year-old man who was given a cough syrup, Elixifilin, which contained potassium iodide (130 mg/15 ml), as well as theophylline and alcohol. Dyspnea, angioedema, itching, and erythema of the face and neck developed a few hours after the second dose. His symptoms disappeared 24 hours after treatment with parenteral glucocorticoids. Five hours after Elixifilin or iodide challenge, he developed edema of the face and neck, itching of the pharynx and eyes, and a sensation of heat (66).

Second-Generation Effects

Pregnancy

Iodine readily crosses the placenta, and the fetal concentration usually exceeds the maternal concentration. The placenta does not seem to have a regulating transfer mechanism, implying that excess maternal intake of iodine will also expose the fetus to iodine intoxication. This usually results in hypothyroidism and development of goiter. Such goiters may become very large and even create obstetrical problems during delivery or mechanical compression during early postnatal life (SEDA-4, 295) (SEDA-5, 328). In neonates iodine excess is a well-known cause of transient hypothyroidism. Iodine-containing antiseptics should therefore be avoided in both the delivery room and the neonatal ward. A similar warning against the use of iodine or iodine-containing drugs applies during lactation since iodine is actively secreted in milk.

Fetotoxicity

Large quantities of iodine reduce the organic binding of iodine (the Wolff–Chaikoff effect). Thus, the regular use of iodide during pregnancy can cause development of a goiter in the fetus. The size of the goiter in the child can be large enough to cause difficulty during delivery. Treatment of vaginitis with iodine-containing solutions in pregnant women can lead to goiter and hypothyroidism in the infant (18).

Neonatal goiter caused by the use of potassium iodine as an expectorant during pregnancy has been reported (67). The neonate, a girl, had acute hypothyroidism, with myxedema and respiratory distress. She was given levothyroxine for 6 months, with complete normalization of thyroid function.

Severe transient postnatal hypothyroidism has been reported in infants whose mothers have received high doses of iodine during pregnancy or multiple local applications of povidone-iodine during pregnancy and for delivery (SED-14, 472). Transient neonatal hypothyroidism during breastfeeding after postnatal maternal topical iodine treatment has also been reported (68).

- A baby girl was born prematurely at 29 weeks. Her weight, length, and head circumference were appropriate to her gestational age. Parenteral feeding was stopped at 20 days, and breastfeeding was gradually increased. TSH screening for congenital hypothyroidism on day 5 was negative (below 1 µU/ml; reference range 0.45–10.0), but a second screening on day 23 was high at 23 µU/ml. There were no signs of hypothyroidism and no palpable goiter. A confirmatory laboratory test on day 29 showed a high serum TSH concentration (288 µU/ml) and reduced concentrations of free thyroxine (2.8 ng/l; reference range 19–23) and free tri-iodothyronine (1.52 pg/ml; reference range 2.2–5.4). The mother had developed an abscess of the abdominal wall 1 week after cesarean section and had been treated with intravenous antibiotics and iodine tampons, 60 cm^2 daily to the abscess wound, containing about 10.5 mg of iodine. Maternal thyroid function was normal (TSH 1.59 µU/ml and free thyroxine 12 ng/l).
- Thyroid antibodies to thyroglobulin, TSH receptors, and thyroperoxidase were negative. Iodine concentrations in the maternal milk and infant urine were extremely high: 4410 (reference range 29–490) micrograms/l and 3932 (reference range below 185) micrograms/l respectively. Treatment with levothyroxine (25 micrograms/day) was started on day 32, breastfeeding was discontinued, and disinfection with iodine was stopped. Thyroid function normalized after 6 days, levothyroxine was withdrawn, and breastfeeding was restarted. Thyroid function remained normal over a follow-up period of 4 months.

Skin disinfection with iodine also caused goiter and hypothyroidism in five of 30 newborns under intensive care (69). Antiseptics containing iodine should be avoided not only during pregnancy and delivery but also after the delivery during breastfeeding.

Drug Administration

Drug administration route

Complications of iodine applied to the skin are well recognized and reflect absorption through the skin, especially in neonates. Two case reports have highlighted the fact that, even in adults, topical administration of povidone iodine can be associated with serious toxicity.

- A 45-year-old man with mediastinitis and renal and hepatic dysfunction was treated with mediastinal irrigation with povidone iodine (70). He developed toxic plasma iodine concentrations and clinical deterioration; hemodialysis and hemofiltration were effective in reducing plasma iodine concentrations.
- A 68-year-old man was treated for a subcutaneous infection of the thigh by subcutaneous irrigation with povidone iodine (71). Toxic plasma and urinary iodine concentrations were associated with abnormalities of cardiac conduction, lactic acidosis, acute renal insufficiency, hypocalcemia, and thyroid dysfunction.

These cases suggest that topical povidone iodine should be used with caution in patients in whom significant absorption can occur, especially in the presence of renal impairment.

Drug overdose

- A patient who deliberately took potassium iodide solution 50 ml and a small dose of mefenamic acid (six capsules) as part of a suicide attempt developed acute renal insufficiency necessitating hemodialysis (72). Normal renal function returned after 10 days of hemodialysis.

The authors postulated that iodide toxicity had resulted in hemolysis and hemoglobinuria, which, together with acute interstitial nephritis secondary to inhibition of prostaglandin synthesis from mefenamic acid ingestion, had resulted in acute renal insufficiency. The mechanism of hemolysis resulting from toxic doses of iodine is not clear, although it may reflect inhibition of various red cell enzymes.

Interference with Diagnostic Tests

Thyroid function tests

Estimation of protein-bound iodine and tracer studies for the estimation of thyroid function are interfered with by the use of iodine-containing compounds (73).

References

1. Anonymous. Prevention and control of iodine deficiency disorders. Lancet 1986;2(8504):433–4.
2. Hetzel BS. The Prevention and Control of Iodine Deficiency Disorders. Nutrition Policy Discussion Paper no. 3Rome: United Nations ACC/SCN;. 1988.
3. Delange F, Burgi H, Chen ZP, Dunn JT. World status of monitoring iodine deficiency disorders control programs. Thyroid 2002;12(10):915–24.
4. Laurberg P. Iodine intake—what are we aiming at? J Clin Endocrinol Metab 1994;79(1):17–9.
5. Kohn LA. A look at iodine-induced hyperthyroidism: Recognition. Bull NY Acad Med 1975;51(8):959–66.
6. Solomon BL, Evaul JE, Burman KD, Wartofsky L. Remission rates with antithyroid drug therapy: continuing influence of iodine intake? Ann Intern Med 1987;107(4):510–2.
7. Delange F. Correction of iodine deficiency: benefits and possible side effects. Eur J Endocrinol 1995;132(5):542–3.
8. Laurberg P, Bulow Pedersen I, Knudsen N, Ovesen L, Andersen S. Environmental iodine intake affects the type of nonmalignant thyroid disease. Thyroid 2001;11(5):457–69.
9. Anonymous. Iodine. Some products contain more than the RDA. WHO Pharm Newslett 2003;3:2.
10. Burgi H, Schaffner TH, Seiler JP. The toxicology of iodate: a review of the literature. Thyroid 2001;11(5):449–56.
11. Yalow RS. Risks in mass distribution of potassium iodide. Bull NY Acad Med 1983;59(10):1020–7.
12. Robbins J. Indications for using potassium iodide to protect the thyroid from low level internal irradiation. Bull NY Acad Med 1983;59(10):1028–38.
13. Shleien B, Halperin JA, Bilstad JM, Botstein P, Dutra EV Jr. Recommendations on the use of potassium iodide as a thyroid-blocking agent in radiation accidents: an FDA update. Bull NY Acad Med 1983;59(10):1009–19.
14. Crocker DG. Nuclear reactor accidents—the use of KI as a blocking agent against radioiodine uptake in the thyroid—a review. Health Phys 1984;46(6):1265–79.
15. Helsing E, Dukes MNG. The Safety of Stable Iodine When Used to Provide Protection against Nuclear Fallout. Internal Advisory ReportCopenhagen: WHO Regional Office for Europe;. 1986.
16. Wolff J. Risks for stable and radioactive iodine in radiation protection of the thyroid. In: Hall R, Kobberling J, editors. Thyroid Disorders Associated with Iodine Deficiency and Excess 22. New York: Raven Press, 1985:111 Serono Symposia Publications.
17. Bishop ME, Garcia RL. Iododerma from wound irrigation with povidone-iodine. JAMA 1978;240(3):249–50.
18. Vorherr H, Vorherr UF, Mehta P, Ulrich JA, Messer RH. Vaginal absorption of povidone-iodine. JAMA 1980;244(23):2628–9.
19. Ferguson MM, Geddes DA, Wray D. The effect of a povidone-iodine mouthwash upon thyroid function and plaque accumulation. Br Dent J 1978;144(1):14–6.
20. Block SH. Thyroid function abnormalities from the use of topical betadine solution on intact skin of children. Cutis 1980;26(1):88–9.
21. Delange F. Risks and benefits of iodine supplementation. Lancet 1998;351(9107):923–4.
22. Safran M, Braverman LE. Effect of chronic douching with polyvinylpyrrolidone-iodine on iodine absorption and thyroid function. Obstet Gynecol 1982;60(1):35–40.
23. Alvarez E. Neutropenia in a burned patient being treated topically with povidone-iodine foam. Plast Reconstr Surg 1979;63(6):839–40.
24. Pietsch J, Meakins JL. Complications of povidone-iodine absorption in topically treated burn patients. Lancet 1976;1(7954):280–2.
25. Friend DG. Iodide therapy and the importance of quantitating the dose. N Engl J Med 1960;263:1358–60.
26. Utiger RD. The diverse effects of iodide on thyroid function. N Engl J Med 1972;287(11):562–3.
27. Horn B, Kabins SA. Iodide fever. Am J Med Sci 1972;264(6):467–71.
28. Eeckhout E, Willemsen M, Deconinck A, Somers G. Granulomatous vasculitis as a complication of potassium iodide treatment for Sweet's syndrome. Acta Dermatol Venereol 1987;67(4):362–4.
29. Vagenakis AG, Braverman LE. Drug induced hypothyroidism. Pharmacol Ther (C) 1976;1:149.
30. Coindet JF. Découverte d'une remàde contre le goitre. Bibl Univ Sci BL Arts 1820;14:90.

31. Ingbar SH. Autoregulation of the thyroid: the effects of thyroid iodine enrichment and depletion. In: Hall R, Kobberling J, editors. Thyroid Disorders Associated with Iodine Deficiency and Excess 22. New York: Raven Press, 1985:153 Serono Symposia Publications.

32. Savoie JC, Massin P, Thomopoulos P, et al. Hyperthyroïde induite par l'iode: une variété mal connue de pathologie iatrogène. Concours Med 1977;99–20:3227.

33. Evered D, Yeo PP. Drug-induced endocrine disorders. Drugs 1977;13(5):353–65.

34. Burger A, Dinichert D, Nicod P, Jenny M, Lemarchand-Beraud T, Vallotton MB. Effect of amiodarone on serum triiodothyronine, reverse triiodothyronine, thyroxin, and thyrotropin. A drug influencing peripheral metabolism of thyroid hormones. J Clin Invest 1976;58(2):255–9.

35. Tresch DD, Sweet DL, Keelan MH Jr, Lange RL. Acute iodide intoxication with cardiac irritability. Arch Intern Med 1974;134(4):760–2.

36. Delange F, Lecomte P. Iodine supplementation: benefits outweigh risks. Drug Saf 2000;22(2):89–95.

37. Jonckheer MH. Amiodarone and the thyroid gland. A review. Acta Cardiol 1981;36(3):199–205.

38. Andersen ED. Long-term antiarrhythmic therapy with amiodarone: high prevalence of thyrotoxicosis (11%). Eur Heart J 1981;2:199.

39. Karpman BA, Rapoport B, Filetti S, Fisher DA. Treatment of neonatal hyperthyroidism due to Graves' disease with sodium ipodate. J Clin Endocrinol Metab 1987;64(1):119–23.

40. Martino E, Aghini-Lombardi F, Mariotti S, Bartalena L, Braverman L, Pinchera A. Amiodarone: a common source of iodine-induced thyrotoxicosis. Horm Res 1987;26(1–4):158–71.

41. Stanbury JB, Ermans AE, Bourdoux P, Todd C, Oken E, Tonglet R, Vidor G, Braverman LE, Medeiros-Neto G. Iodine-induced hyperthyroidism: occurrence and epidemiology. Thyroid 1998;8(1):83–100.

42. Dunn JT, Semigran MJ, Delange F. The prevention and management of iodine-induced hyperthyroidism and its cardiac features. Thyroid 1998;8(1):101–6.

43. Kahaly GJ, Dienes HP, Beyer J, Hommel G. Iodine induces thyroid autoimmunity in patients with endemic goitre: a randomised, double-blind, placebo-controlled trial. Eur J Endocrinol 1998;139(3):290–7.

44. Reinhardt W, Luster M, Rudorff KH, Heckmann C, Petrasch S, Lederbogen S, Haase R, Saller B, Reiners C, Reinwein D, Mann K. Effect of small doses of iodine on thyroid function in patients with Hashimoto's thyroiditis residing in an area of mild iodine deficiency. Eur J Endocrinol 1998;139(1):23–8.

45. Weber G, Vigone MC, Rapa A, Bona G, Chiumello G. Neonatal transient hypothyroidism: aetiological study. Italian Collaborative Study on Transient Hypothyroidism. Arch Dis Child Fetal Neonatal Ed 1998;79(1):F70–2.

46. Delange F, de Benoist B, Alnwick D. Risks of iodine-induced hyperthyroidism after correction of iodine deficiency by iodized salt. Thyroid 1999;9(6):545–56.

47. Delange F, de Benoist B, Alnwick D. Risks of iodine-induced hyperthyroidism after correction of iodine deficiency by iodized salt. Thyroid 1999;9(6):545–56.

48. Kalant H, Roschlan W. Organically bound iodine. In: Principles of Medical Pharmacology. 5th ed.. Washington DC: Decker, 1989:484–5.

49. Drinka PJ, Nolten WE. Effects of iodinated glycerol on thyroid function studies in elderly nursing home residents. J Am Geriatr Soc 1988;36(10):911–3.

50. Mather JL, Baycliff CD, Paterson NAM. Hypothyroidism secondary to iodinated glycerol. Can J Hosp Pharm 1993;46:177–8.

51. Gortz G, Haring R. Wirkung und Nebenwirkung von Polyvinylpyrrolidon-Jod (PVP-Jod). Therapiewoche 1981;31:4364.

52. Pagliaricci S, Lupattelli G, Mannarino E. Ipertiroidismo da uso impxoprio di iodio-povidone. [Hyperthyroidism due to the improper use of povidone-iodine.] Ann Ital Med Int 1999;14(2):124–6.

53. Gomolin IH. Iodinated glycerol-induced hypothyroidism. Drug Intell Clin Pharm 1987;21(9):726–7.

54. Andre F, Bielefeld P, Besancenot JF, Belleville I, Sgro C, Martin F. Fausse inocuite des collyres: à propos d'une observation de thyrotoxicose induite par l'iode. [False innocuousness of eye drops. Apropos of 1 case of thyrotoxicosis induced by iodine.] Therapie 1988;43(5):431–2.

55. Bernecker C. Potassium iodide in bronchial asthma. BMJ 1969;4(677):236.

56. Chuen J, Roberts N, Lovelock M, King B, Beiles B, Frydman G. "Iodide mumps" after angioplasty. Eur J Vasc Endovasc Surg 2000;19(2):217–8.

57. Sreedharan A, Rembacken BJ, Rotimi O. Acute toxic gastric mucosal damage induced by Lugol's iodine spray during chromoendoscopy. Gut 2005;54(6):886–7.

58. Ide JM, Lancelot E, Pines E, Corot C. Prophylaxis of iodinated contrast media-induced nephropathy: a pharmacological point of view. Invest Radiol 2004;39(3):155–70.

59. Chilvers RJ, Weisz MT. Side-effects of alcoholic iodine solution (10%). Br J Anaesth 2000;85(1):178.

60. Papa CM. Acne and hidden iodides. Arch Dermatol 1976;112(4):555–6.

61. Baumgartner TG. Potassium iodide and iododerma. Am J Hosp Pharm 1976;33(6):601–3.

62. Wilkin JK, Strobel D. Iododerma occurring during thyroid protection treatment. Cutis 1985;36(4):335–7.

63. Toman Z. Alergicka reakcepo sukcinylcholinjodidu Spofa behem celkove anestezie. [Allergic reaction after succinylcholine iodide Spofa during general anesthesia.] Rozhl chir 1976;55(12):836–8.

64. Sicherer SH. Risk of severe allergic reactions from the use of potassium iodide for radiation emergencies. J Allergy Clin Immunol 2004;114(6):1395–7.

65. Curd JG, Milgrom H, Stevenson DD, Mathison DA, Vaughan JH. Potassium iodide sensitivity in four patients with hypocomplementemic vasculitis. Ann Intern Med 1979;91(6):853–7.

66. Munoz FJ, Bellido J, Moyano JC, Alvarez MJ, Juan JL. Adverse reaction to potassium iodide from a cough syrup. Allergy 1997;52(1):111–2.

67. Bostanci I, Sarioglu A, Ergin H, Aksit A, Cinbis M, Akalin N. Neonatal goiter caused by expectorant usage. J Pediatr Endocrinol Metab 2001;14(8):1161–2.

68. Casteels K, Punt S, Bramswig J. Transient neonatal hypothyroidism during breastfeeding after post-natal maternal topical iodine treatment. Eur J Pediatr 2000;159(9):716–717.

69. Chabrolle JP, Rossier A. Goitre and hypothyroidism in the newborn after cutaneous absorption of iodine. Arch Dis Child 1978;53(6):495–8.

70. Kanakiriya S, De Chazal I, Nath KA, Haugen EN, Albright RC, Juncos LA. Iodine toxicity treated with hemodialysis and continuous venovenous hemodiafiltration. Am J Kidney Dis 2003;41:702–8.

71. Labbe G, Mahul P, Morel J, Jospe R, Dumont A, Auboyer
     C. Intoxication a l'iode apres irrigations sous-cutanées de
     povidone iodée. Ann Fr Anesth Reanim 2003;22:58–60.
72. Sinniah R, Lye WC. Acute renal failure from hemoglobinu-
     ric and interstitial nephritis secondary to iodine and mefe-
     namic acid. Clin Nephrol 2001;55(3):254–8.
73. Davies PH, Franklyn JA. The effects of drugs on tests of
     thyroid function. Eur J Clin Pharmacol 1991;40(5):439–51.

Iodine radioactive

General Information

Three radioactive isotopes of ^{127}I are currently used in clinical medicine:

1. ^{131}I (radioactive half-life of 8 days and a high-energy emitter), used mainly in the therapy of hyperthyroidism and thyroid cancer.
2. ^{123}I (radioactive half-life 13 hours) has replaced ^{131}I for diagnostic purposes; however, for in vivo imaging meta-stable technetium-99 (^{99m}Tc) is often preferred, because of its lower radiation dose, availability, and cost.
3. ^{125}I (radioactive half-life of 60 days and a low energy emitter), previously used in the treatment of hyperthyroidism, but now replaced by ^{131}I because of disappointing therapeutic results [1,2].

Radioactive isotopes of iodine are handled by the thyroid in the same way as stable iodine and are therefore actively concentrated, incorporated into thyroglobulin, stored, metabolized, and secreted as thyroid hormones. Small amounts of radioactive iodine are therefore ideal probes to analyse the uptake of iodine, the distribution of iodine in the gland, and possibly even its turnover and incorporation into thyroid hormones. Larger amounts of radioactive iodine selectively radiate the thyroid gland and therefore selectively impair the function of the follicular thyroid cells and eventually destroy them.

Doses

Three dosage ranges for radioactive forms of iodine are used:

1. For diagnostic purposes usually much less than 1 mCi (37 MBq) is given with thyroid radiation doses of a few rads of ^{123}I up to 50–200 rads (0.5–2.0 Gray) (^{131}I).
2. In the treatment of hyperthyroidism the dose of ^{131}I is usually a few millicuries and is either roughly estimated or calculated according to the size of the thyroid gland, the uptake of a tracer dose of iodine, and the type of thyroid disorder (diffuse or nodular), with doses ranging from 80 to 150 microCi (3.0–5.5 MBq) per gram of thyroid tissue [3,4].
3. In thyroid cancer, ^{131}I can be used to eliminate tumor tissue that cannot be removed surgically but still captures iodine; in such circumstances, amounts of 100 mCi (4000 MBq) of ^{131}I or more are not unusual;

with such high amounts, other tissues besides the thyroid gland can also receive substantial amounts of radiation.

The administration of ^{131}I requires safety measurements to reduce to a minimum the irradiation of medical personnel and to avoid contamination of rooms and relatives of patients. Capsules containing ^{131}I are therefore to be preferred to liquid iodine. At doses above 25 mCi (555 MBq), usually intended only for treatment of patients with thyroid cancer, isolation in a specially constructed room of a service for nuclear medicine is necessary. Waste disposal should also be carefully managed so as to avoid overall contamination [5,6].

General adverse effects

Radiation thyroiditis is an infrequent complication resulting in swelling and localized pain over the thyroid gland which subsides spontaneously or with anti-inflammatory or corticosteroid therapy (SEDA-1, 314).

Acute exacerbation of hyperthyroidism, resulting particularly in cardiac complications (arrhythmias or decompensation) or even "thyroid storm," has been reported several times (SEDA-1, 314) and should be avoided by treating very severely hyperthyroid patients with antithyroid drugs prior to the administration of ^{131}I. A temporary increase in serum triiodothyronine and l-thyroxine without clinical symptoms of exacerbation of hyperthyroidism, however, occurs much more frequently (SEDA-1, 314). In 71 patients given ^{131}I for differentiated thyroid carcinoma, short-term adverse effects included gastrointestinal complaints, salivary gland swelling with pain, change in taste and headache [7].

Organs and Systems

Cardiovascular

In a series of thyrocardiac patients, of those dying primarily from thyrotoxicosis more than 21% did so within 3 weeks of ^{131}I treatment [8], presumably reflecting too sudden a change in metabolic activity for patients with existing cardiac complications.

Respiratory

Acute respiratory embarrassment due to thyroid swelling or subsequently due to cicatrization occurs only rarely.

Nervous system

Although aseptic meningitis has been associated with the use of radioactive iodine, the products used were albumin complexes (^{131}I-RISA); this complication is almost certainly attributable to the protein content or to pyrogens rather than to the radioactive iodine itself [8].

Sensory systems

Several papers have reported that radioiodine therapy can lead to worsening of ophthalmopathy, possibly because of the release of thyroid antigens during the inflammatory reaction after ^{131}I therapy. The worsening can be prevented by glucocorticoid therapy (9).

Endocrine

The calcitonin-producing cells of the thyroid are usually destroyed by ^{131}I (SEDA-14, 369).

Both hyperfunction (10) and hypofunction of the parathyroid glands have been described after the use of ^{131}I (11).

Hypothyroidism

There is an increased incidence of late hypothyroidism in patients with autoimmune hyperthyroidism, but the risk increases markedly after extensive thyroid surgery and especially after ^{131}I treatment. Analysis of the cumulative incidence of hypothyroidism shows two phases: an early phase of radiation death of thyroid cells, depending on the ^{131}I dosage and occurring during the first 1–2 years after treatment; a second period of a lower (0.5–3.5% per year) but life-long risk of developing hypothyroidism for a variety of reasons (natural history of the disease, autoimmune processes) (see Table 1) (12–14).

The total incidence of hypothyroidism can therefore be reduced by lowering the therapeutic dose, but at the expense of a higher incidence of more prolonged or recurrent hyperthyroidism. Calculation of the therapeutic dose according to thyroid gland size, iodine uptake, or biological half-life and type of thyroid disorder can help to reduce the total incidence of hypothyroidism, although this is less well documented than many believe (15,16). Moreover, the occurrence of hypothyroidism after the use of ^{131}I should not be dramatized, since treatment is much simpler than abandoning the patient first to the prolonged risk of recurrent hyperthyroidism and thereafter to life-long follow-up for hypothyroidism. Hypothyroidism after ^{131}I can also be transient, and replacement therapy should not be started too early (17).

Hematologic

Leukemia does not occur more often in patients treated with ^{131}I for hyperthyroidism than in similar patients treated by surgery. After use of the high doses used in the treatment of thyroid cancer there was a definite increase in the incidence of leukemia (18).

Salivary glands

In 71 patients given ^{131}I for differentiated thyroid carcinoma, salivary gland swelling with pain occurred in 50% (7); women had a significantly higher incidence than men.

Gastrointestinal

Of 71 patients given ^{131}I for differentiated thyroid carcinoma, 65% had gastrointestinal complaints: appetite loss, nausea, and vomiting occurred in 61, 40, and 7.6% respectively and increased significantly in the patients who received doses above 55.5 MBq/kg and with rises in TSH (7).

Reproductive system

Large amounts of ^{131}I, as used in thyroid cancer therapy, can cause testicular damage as documented from hormonal and sperm analysis (19), but long-term results are nevertheless reassuringly normal (20).

Long-Term Effects

Mutagenicity

Mutagenic effects on the sexual organs are difficult to determine in practice. However, while the radiation dose to the ovary and testes is rather small after ^{131}I treatment for hyperthyroidism (maximum 5 roentgens) it can be substantial after the higher amounts of ^{131}I that are used for thyroid cancer. In any case, children born to mothers previously treated with ^{131}I did not have an increased incidence of congenital malformations. The number of such observations is too small, however, to allow definite conclusions about its safety (21). In patients treated for thyroid carcinoma there was no differences in fertility rate, birth weight, prematurity, or congenital malformations compared with healthy subjects, providing reassurance about the use of radioiodine to treat hyperthyroidism in women of child-bearing age (SEDA-20, 394).

Tumorigenicity

The total number of case reports of thyroid cancer after ^{131}I is very small (under 30 cases) (22) in relation to the estimated number of patients treated with ^{131}I since 1941 (over 1 000 000 patients). Moreover, systematic follow-up or retrospective studies did not show an increased risk of

Table 1 The risk of hypothyroidism after ^{131}I

N	^{131}I dose (mCi)	Total follow-up period (years)	Incidence of hypothyroidism (%)				Total annual cumulative incidence (% per year)	Reference
			One-year follow-up		End of follow-up			
			Diffuse goiter	Nodular goiter	Diffuse goiter	Nodular goiter		
4473	8–20	26	8	3	77	64	3	(12)
1369	9	17	6	3	26	14	3.5	(13)
248	6–10	10	38	11	70	18	0.5	(14)

Table 2 ^{131}I treatment and thyroid cancer: a comparison with thyroidectomy and antithyroid drugs

Incidence of thyroid cancer	Thyroidectomy (n = 11 732)	^{131}I (n = 21 714)	Antithyroid drugs (n = 1238)
Within 1 year of treatment	50	9	0
After 1 year of treatment	4	19	4
Total	54	28	4
Number of deaths from thyroid cancer	4	6	0

Table 3 ^{131}I treatment and thyroid cancer

Number of patients treated with ^{131}I	3000
Mean age	57 years
Mean dose of ^{131}I	13.3 mCi
Mean observation period	13 years
Thyroid cancer	
Observed incidence	4%
Expected incidence	3.2%
Thyroid cancer more than 5 years after ^{131}I	
Observed incidence	2.1%
Expected incidence	3%

thyroid carcinoma in patients treated with ^{131}I for hyperthyroidism. The results of two such studies are shown in more detail in Table 2 (23) and Table 3 (24).

In another follow-up study of 1005 women treated with ^{131}I there was no increase in total morbidity or in the incidence of thyroid cancer (20).

In 10 552 Swedish patients (mean age 57 years) who received ^{131}I for hyperthyroidism (mean follow-up 15 years) there were increases in overall cancer mortality and deaths due to carcinoma of the stomach, lung, and kidney. While the findings for stomach cancer may be of significance, for tumors at other sites, because of an association with time after ^{131}I treatment (58 cases at 10 years or more of follow-up against the expected 44 cases), the lack of a relation between cancer mortality and either the time from radioiodine treatment or the dose administered argues against a carcinogenic effect of radioiodine (SEDA-17, 475; 25).

The use of very high amounts of ^{131}I for thyroid cancer imposes special care and risks: the frequency of radiation thyroiditis is much higher (more than 20%) and similar symptoms of pain and swelling can also be observed in the salivary glands. Nausea and vomiting may also occur. The incidence of leukemia is increased: 15 cases being reported in 5000 patients treated with ^{131}I for thyroid cancer (18); it therefore seems wise to limit the total dose of ^{131}I in a single patient to 500 mCi unless the thyroid disease activity permits higher long-term risks. It is also important to keep such patients well hydrated to allow rapid elimination of ^{131}I not retained by thyroid tissue. The radiation dose to the

ovaries is not negligible, being approximately 200 roentgens after 500 mCi of ^{131}I, a dose sufficient to increase slightly the subsequent risk of miscarriage or congenital abnormalities. However, no apparent increase in the rate of abnormalities has been observed in the outcome of pregnancies among women previously treated for thyroid cancer.

The use of ^{131}I in children is different from its use in adults. Experience worldwide is much more limited as regards both the number of children treated and the total number of years of observation (SEDA-20, 394). The risk of eventual tumor-inducing effects in the thyroid or other tissues is real. The young thyroid is very sensitive to external radiation or to nuclear fall-out: 66% of young adults developed thyroid lesions 25 years after such exposure (26). One report on a high prevalence of hypothyroidism after ^{131}I showed no cases of thyroid or other malignancies after a mean follow-up period of almost 15 years (27). However, others found an increased frequency of thyroid nodules: among case reports on thyroid cancer after ^{131}I in the world literature the younger age group is largely over-represented, owing to the frequency of ^{131}I use in this age group (22). In view of the small number of long-term results in a young population with probably higher susceptibility for thyroid tumors it seems unwise to use ^{131}I as preferred treatment for adolescents or young adults with hyperthyroidism. Much longer follow-up periods will be necessary, preferably with central registration to allow a definite conclusion about treatment (21,18). However, many experts consider the current follow-up period sufficiently long to extend the use of ^{131}I to all patients with Graves' disease above the age of 25 (SEDA-14, 368; 28). There are, however, large discrepancies in treatment strategies globally.

Second-Generation Effects

Pregnancy

Radioactive iodine passes the placenta and accumulates in the fetal thyroid where the concentration probably exceeds that in the maternal thyroid. Detailed studies show that the fetal dose of iodine is virtually nil before the 90th day of gestation but sharply increases thereafter (29). This alone is sufficient reason to avoid the use of ^{131}I in pregnancy, but there is also some controversial evidence that various congenital deformities have been produced by the isotope (30).

Teratogenicity

Concern about possible second-generation effects of ^{131}I is difficult to allay but has not been substantiated, since there is an absence of obvious birth defects or genetic changes in the offspring of patients treated with ^{131}I (20,22,24,31,32). Moreover, the radiation dose to the ovaries in ^{131}I therapy for hyperthyroidism is usually below three roentgens and thus comparable to the radiation due to common radiographic abdominal examinations. If

[131]I is given during pregnancy, fetal hypothyroidism and chromosomal aberrations can occur (33).

Lactation

[131]I is transferred in the milk and should not be given during lactation. Even the diagnostic use of radioisotopes of iodine should be avoided (34).

Interference with Diagnostic Tests

Detection of pulmonary embolism

Injections of ^{131}I given to detect pulmonary embolism can result in false-negative results in the ^{125}I-labeled fibrinogen test for venous thrombosis.

References

1. Glanzmann C, Kaestner F, Horst W. Therapie der Hyperthyreose mit Radioisotopen des Jods: Erfahrungen bei über 2000 Patienten. [Radio-iodine treatment of hyperthyroidism. Experience in more than 2000 patients.] Klin Wochenschr 1975;53(14):669–78.
2. Glanzmann C, Horst W. Iodine-125 and iodine-131 in the treatment of hyperthyroidism. Clin Nucl Med 1980;5(7):325–33.
3. Holm LE, Lundell G, Dahlqvist I, Israelsson A. Cure rate after ^{131}I therapy for hyperthyroidism. Acta Radiol Oncol 1981;20(3):161–6.
4. Bliddal H, Hansen JM, Rogowski P, Johansen K, Friis T, Siersbaek-Nielsen K. [131]I treatment of diffuse and nodular toxic goitre with or without antithyroid agents. Acta Endocrinol (Copenh) 1982;99(4):517–21.
5. Thomas SR, Maxon HR, Fritz KM, Kereiakes JG, Connell WD. A comparison of methods for assessing patient body burden following ^{131}I therapy for thyroid cancer. Radiology 1980;137(3):839–42.
6. Radioprotection Committee. Radioprotection in radioactive iodine therapy. Belg Tijdschr Radiol 1980;63:39.
7. Kita T, Yokoyama K, Higuchi T, Kinuya S, Taki J, Nakajima K, Michigishi T, Tonami N. Multifactorial analysis on the short-term side effects occurring within 96 hours after radioiodine-131 therapy for differentiated thyroid carcinoma. Ann Nucl Med 2004;18(4):345–9.
8. Shani J, Atkins HL, Wolf W. Adverse reactions to radiopharmaceuticals. Semin Nucl Med 1976;6(3):305–28.
9. Bartalena L, Marcocci C, Bogazzi F, Panicucci M, Lepri A, Pinchera A. Use of corticosteroids to prevent progression of Graves' ophthalmopathy after radioiodine therapy for hyperthyroidism. N Engl J Med 1989;321(20):1349–52.
10. Triggs SM, Williams ED. Irradiation of the thyroid as a cause of parathyroid adenoma. Lancet 1977;1(8011):593–4.
11. Jialal I, Pillay NL, Asmal AC. Radio-iodine-induced hypoparathyroidism. A case report. S Afr Med J 1980;58(23):939–40.
12. Holm LE, Lundell G, Israelsson A, Dahlqvist I. Incidence of hypothyroidism occurring long after iodine-131 therapy for hyperthyroidism. J Nucl Med 1982;23(2):103–7.
13. Best JD, Chan V, Khoo R, Teng CS, Wang C, Yeung RT. Incidence of hypothyroidism after radioactive iodine therapy for thyrotoxicosis in Hong Kong Chinese. Clin Radiol 1981;32(1):57–61.
14. Kamphuis JJ. Behandeling van hyperthyreoïdie met [131]I: een retrospectief onderzoek. [Treatment of hyperthyroidism using [131]I: a retrospective study.] Ned Tijdschr Geneeskd 1980;124(26):1045–9.
15. Hayes MT. Hypothyroidism following iodine-131 therapy. J Nucl Med 1982;23(2):176–9.
16. Watson AB, Brownlie BE, Frampton CM, Turner JG, Rogers TG. Outcome following standardized 185 MBq dose ^{131}I therapy for Graves' disease Clin Endocrinol (Oxf) 1988;28(5):487–96.
17. MacFarlane IA, Shalet SM, Beardwell CG, Khara JS. Transient hypothyroidism after iodine-131 treatment for thyrotoxicosis. BMJ 1979;2(6187):421.
18. Blahd WH. Treatment of malignant thyroid disease. Semin Nucl Med 1979;9(2):95–9.
19. Handelsman DJ, Conway AJ, Donnelly PE, Turtle JR. Azoospermia after iodine-131 treatment for thyroid carcinoma. BMJ 1980;281(6254):1527.
20. Hoffman DA, McConahey WM, Diamond EL, Kurland LT. Mortality in women treated for hyperthyroidism. Am J Epidemiol 1982;115(2):243–54.
21. Maxon HR, Thomas SR, Chen IW. The role of nuclear medicine in the treatment of hyperthyroidism and well-differentiated thyroid adenocarcinoma. Clin Nucl Med 1981;6(10S):P87–98.
22. McDougall IR, Nelsen TS, Kempson RL. Papillary carcinoma of the thyroid seven years after I-131 therapy for Graves' disease. Clin Nucl Med 1981;6(8):368–71.
23. Wolff J. Risks for stable and radioactive iodine in radiation protection of the thyroid. In: Hall R, Kobberling J, editors. Thyroid Disorders Associated with Iodine Deficiency and Excess 22. New York: Raven Press, 1985:111 Serono Symposia Publications.
24. Holm LE, Dahlqvist I, Israelsson A, Lundell G. Malignant thyroid tumors after iodine-131 therapy: a retrospective cohort study. N Engl J Med 1980;303(4):188–91.
25. Holm LE, Hall P, Wiklund K, Lundell G, Berg G, Bjelkengren G, Cederquist E, Ericsson UB, Hallquist A, Larsson LG, et al. Cancer risk after iodine-131 therapy for hyperthyroidism. J Natl Cancer Inst 1991;83(15):1072–7.
26. Larsen PR, Conard RA, Knudsen K. Thyroid hypofunction appearing as a delayed manifestation of accidental exposure to radioactive fallout in a Marshallese population. In: Biological Effects of Ionizing Radiation 1. Vienna: International Atomic Energy Agency, 1978:101.
27. Freitas JE, Swanson DP, Gross MD, Sisson JC. Iodine-131: optimal therapy for hyperthyroidism in children and adolescents? J Nucl Med 1979;20(8):847–50.
28. Graham GD, Burman KD. Radioiodine treatment of Graves' disease. An assessment of its potential risks. Ann Intern Med 1986;105(6):900–5.
29. Johnson JR. Fetal thyroid dose from intakes of radioiodine by the mother. Health Phys 1982;43(4):573–82.
30. Nishimura H, Tanimura T. Clinical Aspects of Teratogenicity of Drugs Amsterdam: Excerpta Medica;. 1976.
31. Dobyns BM, Sheline GE, Workman JB, Tompkins EA, McConahey WM, Becker DV. Malignant and benign neoplasms of the thyroid in patients treated for hyperthyroidism: a report of the cooperative thyrotoxicosis therapy follow-up study. J Clin Endocrinol Metab 1974;38(6):976–98.
32. Sarkar SD, Beierwaltes WH, Gill SP, Cowley BJ. Subsequent fertility and birth histories of children and adolescents treated with ^{131}I for thyroid cancer. J Nucl Med 1976;17(6):460–4.

33. Goh KO. Radioiodine treatment during pregnancy: chromosomal aberrations and cretinism associated with maternal iodine-131 treatment. J Am Med Womens Assoc 1981;36(8):262–5.

34. Dydek GJ, Blue PW. Human breast milk excretion of iodine-131 following diagnostic and therapeutic administration to a lactating patient with Graves' disease. J Nucl Med 1988;29(3):407–10.

Polyvidone and povidone-iodine

General Information

Polyvidone (polyvinylpyrrolidone, povidone) is a variable-weight polymer of the monomer N-vinylpyrrolidinone. When it enters the body it causes histologically characteristic reactions in tissues with which it comes into contact (1,2).

Polyvidone co-polymers are used in cosmetics as antimicrobials, antistatics, binding compounds, stabilizers of emulsions, and film-forming, viscosity-controlling, hair-fixing, skin-conditioning, and skin-protective agents. It is used as a component of hair sprays and as a retardant for subcutaneous injections. It was formerly used as a plasma expander (3) and has been inappropriately used for intravenous injection as a "blood tonic", especially in Asian societies. Some products intended for parenteral administration contain polyvidone as an excipient. Polyvidone is widely used as a suspending and coating agent in tablets, for its film-forming properties in eye drops, and as a carrier molecule for iodine in disinfectants. About 20% of all tablets on the market contain polyvidone. It is also used in the cosmetics industry as a dispersing agent and as a lubricant in ointments.

Povidone-iodine

Povidone-iodine is a macromolecular complex (poly-I(I-vinyl-2-pyrrolidinone) that is used as an iodophor. It is formulated as a 10% applicator solution, a 2% cleansing solution, and in many topical formulations, for example aerosol sprays, aerosol foams, vaginal gels, ointments, and mouthwashes. Because it contains very little free iodine (less than 1 ppm in a 10% solution) its antibacterial effectiveness is only moderate compared with that of a pure solution of iodine.

Systemic absorption

The extent of systemic absorption of povidone-iodine depends on the localization and the conditions of its use (area, skin surface, mucous membranes, wounds, body cavities).

Healthy skin

Repeated surgical skin antisepsis and hand washing did not increase serum iodine concentrations, but produced a small increase in iodine content in the 24-hour urine (4).

Burns

The use of povidone-iodine for the treatment of burns, for peritoneal lavage in the treatment of purulent peritonitis, or as a rinsing solution for body cavities can increase serum iodine concentrations associated with increased urinary excretion of iodine. In people with burns the extent of iodine absorption depends on the extent of the burned body surface. It is not uncommon for serum iodine concentrations to rise to more than 1000 µg/ml. If renal function is intact, iodine elimination in the urine can be adequate. The serum iodine concentration returns to normal about 1 week after the last application.

The penetration of povidone-iodine has been studied in vivo in rabbits (5). The penetration from third-degree burns on the back was measured autoradiographically in tissues, blood, urine, and bandages. The results showed that about 20% of iodine is absorbed through fresh necrosis, whereas only 5% is absorbed through a clean wound or 24-hour old necrosis. The passage through burn necrosis was faster than through vital tissue. In repeated topical use on burns the extent of absorption seems to decrease with the treatment time.

Wounds

Povidone-iodine inhibits leukocyte migration and fibroblast aggregation in wounds. The effect on the wound healing process has been studied in 294 children undergoing surgery, 283 of whom had undergone appendectomy (6). In a first series using 5% povidone-iodine aerosol for preoperative disinfection the postoperative wound infection rate was 19% in the test group and only 8% in the controls. When a 1% povidone-iodine solution was used, only 2.6% of the patients were infected (control group 8.5%). Using a drain with a cellulose viscose sponge, 5% povidone-iodine by aerosol inhibited leukocyte migration, but no cell aggregates or fibroblasts were detected. A 5% solution allowed better cellular movement and attachment to the framework, polymorphonuclear leukocytes predominating. The excipients in the aerosol formula must be more toxic to the cell than those in the solution. If a 1% povidone-iodine solution was absorbed by the sponge, the aggregation phenomenon was only slightly averted and cell morphology was similar to that of the saline control.

Povidone-iodine reduced the number of wound infections only in patients with appendicitis in whom neither peritonitis nor a periappendicular abscess had yet developed (SED-11, 489).

Mucous membranes

The effect of a povidone-iodine mouthwash on thyroid function has been studied in 16 medically healthy volunteers (7). After they had used the mouthwash 4 times daily for a period of 14 days all thyroid tests were significantly changed, but there was no suppression of thyroid function. However, this was not to be expected, considering the short test period.

Body cavities

When povidone-iodine is used as a rinsing solution in body cavities, absorption of the whole macromolecular complex is possible. The complex has a molecular weight of about 60 000 and cannot be eliminated by the kidneys or metabolically. It is filtered by the reticuloendothelial system (4,8,9).

Although povidone-iodine is no longer used in dialysates, a povidone-iodine-containing cap is used to seal the Tenckhoff catheter during the day. Iodine-induced hypothyroidism occurred in a 3-year-old boy and an 18-month-old girl, in both cases due to the sealing cap (10). The povidone-iodine inside the cap diffused into the catheter and flushed into the peritoneal cavity at the next dialysis session.

Intravaginal administration

Systemic iodine absorption can occur after intravaginal administration of povidone-iodine (11). There were increases in serum iodine, protein-bound iodine, and inorganic iodine, but not serum thyroxine, after a 2-minute vaginal administration of povidone-iodine in non-pregnant women (12).

Guidelines for the safe use of povidone-iodine complexes

In 1985 a working group of the Federal German Medical Association issued a number of recommendations for the safe use of povidone-iodine complexes (13). They remain valid and can be summarized as follows:

1. The application of povidone-iodine formulations cannot be recommended for surgical hand disinfection, since active iodine-free formulations are available.
2. The activity of povidone-iodine in preoperative skin disinfection in adults is well proven.
3. Povidone-iodine is appropriate for skin disinfection before an incision, a puncture, with use of intravenous or arterial catheters, and for the prophylaxis of iatrogenic Clostridia infections.
4. In the case of superficial wounds, povidone-iodine can be applied occasionally or repeatedly in spite of increased iodine absorption through the broken skin surfaces.
5. Lavage of wound and body cavities with povidone-iodine or its instillation is not indicated because of increased iodine absorption.
6. Routine body washing of patients in intensive care units is not cost-beneficial.
7. Vaginal administration of povidone-iodine is not recommended.
8. Povidone-iodine is contraindicated in premature babies and neonates; this also applies to prophylactic disinfection of the umbilical stump.
9. The clinical usefulness of povidone-iodine in the treatment of burns is well proven.
10. Local mouth antiseptics serve no therapeutic purpose; this is also true for povidone-iodine.

Organs and Systems

Nervous system

- A 62-year-old man treated with continuous mediastinal irrigation with a 1:10 solution of povidone-iodine developed seizures on the fifth day of drainage (14). After the seizure, his serum iodine concentration was raised (120 µg/ml). Renal insufficiency developed at the same time. The electroencephalogram showed no evidence of epileptic activity or other abnormalities. The povidone-iodine irrigation was replaced by continuous irrigation with a solution of neomycin and polymyxin B. Renal function improved and the creatinine concentration returned to normal 3 days after the seizure.

Endocrine

Extensive iodine absorption can cause transient hypothyroidism or in patients with latent hypothyroidism the risk of destabilization and thyrotoxic crisis (SEDA-20, 226; SEDA-22, 263). Especially at risk are patients with an autonomous adenoma, localized diffuse autonomy of the thyroid gland, nodular goiter, latent hyperthyroidism of autoimmune origin, or endemic iodine deficiency (4).

Povidone-iodine-induced hyperthyroidism is rarer than hypothyroidism (SEDA-20, 226), but a history of long-term use of iodine-containing medications should be considered when investigating the cause of hyperthyroidism (15).

- A 48-year-old woman developed palpitation and insomnia. The clinical history, physical examination, and laboratory tests supported hyperthyroidism. Since July 1994 she had been combating constipation by improper use of an iodine-containing antiseptic cream for external use only. She had inserted povidone-iodine into her rectum by means of a cannula. The iodine-containing cream was withdrawn and she was given a beta-blocker. The palpitation resolved within 2 weeks and her plasma thyroid hormone concentrations normalized within 1 month.

Hyperthyroidism in this patient was probably triggered by improper long-term use of an over-the-counter iodine-containing cream.

Thyrotoxicosis related to iodine toxicity in a child with burns occurred after alternate-day povidone-iodine washes (16).

- A 22-month-old boy was admitted to a pediatric intensive care unit after partial and full thickness burns over 80% of his body surface area. After debridement he was given alternate day povidone-iodine (Betadine) washes. He became increasingly tachycardic, hypertensive, and hyperpyrexic, with sweating, agitation, and diarrhea and developed neutropenia. Daily sepsis screens were negative. Thyroid function tests showed evidence of iodine-induced thyrotoxicosis. He was given propranolol and carbimazole, and chlorhexidine was substituted for povidone-iodine. His tachycardia, hypertension, and diarrhea slowly improved and his neutropenia resolved. By day 42 his free thyroxine concentration was normal and he was given thyroxine. On day 63 the carbimazole, propranolol, and thyroxine were withheld. However thyroid function tests 1 week later showed hypothyroidism, and thyroxine was restarted. Repeat plasma and urine iodine concentrations on day 57 (a month after withdrawal of povidone-iodine) continued to show marked urinary excretion of iodine (urine concentration 65 μmol/l, reference range 0.39–1.97) with high but falling plasma iodine concentrations (5.9 μmol/l, reference range 0.32–0.63).

Hematologic

Severe neutropenia occurred in a patient in whom deep, second-degree burns, involving about 50% of the body surface, were being treated with Betadine Helafoam® twice a day (17).

Liver

There have been reports of liver damage from polyvidone (18).

Urinary tract

Povidone-iodine sclerosis has been suggested to be safe and effective in treating lymphoceles after renal transplantation, with only minor complications of the procedure, such as pericatheter cutaneous infections. However, a case of acute renal tubular necrosis has been reported (19).

- In a 23-year-old woman, a kidney allograft recipient with recurrent lymphoceles treated with povidone-iodine irrigations (50 ml of a 1% solution bd for 6 days), a metabolic acidosis occurred and renal function deteriorated. After a few days, despite suspension of irrigation, the patient developed oliguria, and dialysis was needed. A renal biopsy showed acute tubular necrosis.

Iodine-induced renal insufficiency has also been reported after the use of topical povidone-iodine on the skin and after intracavity irrigation.

- A 65-year-old man with second- and third-degree burns covering 26% of his body was given intravenous lactated Ringer solution and topical silver sulfadiazine in addition to debridement and skin grafting (20). However, he developed a wound infection with *Pseudomonas aeruginosa*, which was treated successfully with topical povidone-iodine gel. Persistent nodal bradycardia with hypotension, metabolic acidosis, and renal insufficiency occurred 16 days later. Iodine toxicosis was suspected and the serum iodine concentration was 206 μg/ml (reference range 20–90 μg/ml). The povidone-iodine gel was therefore withdrawn immediately. His family refused hemodialysis and he died 44 days after admission.
- A 57-year-old man developed renal insufficiency after triple coronary bypass grafting, 7 days after povidone-iodine mediastinal irrigation and required 3 days of renal replacement therapy (21). Complete resolution

occurred within 8 days and followed a short non-oliguric phase (4 days).

Although other common causes of acute renal insufficiency were present in the second case, the only significant change in management at the time of onset of renal insufficiency was the use of povidone-iodine.

Skin

Povidone-iodine causes concentration-dependent damage to cells and clusters. The effect is most pronounced for isolated cells, but it is also detectable in more complex tissues. Clinical experience with burn victims cannot rule out the possibility that the healing process may be slightly retarded. However, this deficiency may be balanced by an appropriate microbicidal effect on the healing edge (22).

Polyvidone storage disease

Polyvidone molecules that weigh less than 20 kD can be excreted by a normally functioning kidney, whereas larger polymers are phagocytosed and permanently stored in the mononuclear phagocytic system, causing so-called polyvidone storage disease. Polyvidone storage disease occurs in patients who have received polyvidone for prolonged periods of time. The large polymers deposit in the histiocytes and cause them to proliferate and infiltrate histiocytes in the reticuloendothelial system, including osteocytes. There is generally no significant damage to these organs except that prolonged administration can cause bone destruction, skin lesions, arthritis, and polyneuropathy. The first cutaneous case of polyvidone storage disease, reported in 1964 (23), was caused by local injection of polyvidone-containing posterior pituitary extracts for the treatment of diabetes insipidus. Similar cases, including those following local injection of porcine polyvidone to treat neuralgia, were documented, mostly in European reports (24,25). Localized cutaneous polyvidone storage disease was then known as Dupont–Lachapelle disease (26). Five cases of polyvidone storage disease with cutaneous involvement have been documented (27). Two patients presented with skin eruptions mimicking collagen vascular disease and chronic pigmented purpuric dermatosis. In one other polyvidone was found in a metastatic tumor and in the other in a pemphigus lesion. The fifth case was seen in a blind skin biopsy specimen taken to exclude Niemann–Pick disease after examination of a bone-marrow smear. The latter patient and the patient with a collagen vascular-like disease also had severe anemia and serious orthopedic and neurological complications due to massive infiltration of polyvidone-containing cells in the bone-marrow, with destruction of the bone. Polyvidone storage disease can easily be diagnosed by its histopathological features. Skin biopsy specimens show a variable number of characteristic blue-gray vacuolated cells around blood vessels and adnexal structures and stain positively with mucicarmine, colloidal iron, and alkaline Congo red, and negatively with periodic acid Schiff and Alcian blue.

Musculoskeletal

Pathological fractures of several bones, and destructive lesions seen radiologically in other bones, have been reported in patients who had received repeated intravenous injections of polyvidone for many years (28,29). Biopsies of the fracture sites showed both intracellular deposits of polyvidone and mucoid changes in the affected cells. If of sufficient severity, this may cause a virtual "melt down" of osseous tissue.

Immunologic

Polyvidone has been reported to cause anaphylaxis (30).

- A 32-year-old man took paracetamol (in Doregrippin) for flu-like symptoms and about 10 minutes later developed generalized urticaria, angioedema, hypotonia, and tachycardia, and became semiconscious. His symptoms were rapidly relieved by intravenous antihistamines and steroids. This was the first time he had taken Doregrippin,, but he had previously taken paracetamol-containing formulations, which had been well tolerated. He was not taking any regular medications. Subsequent testing of the various constituents of the analgesic tablets identified polyvidone as the cause of the anaphylactic reaction.

This report demonstrates a rare case of a type I allergic reaction towards a commonly used ingredient of tablets and widely used disinfectants.

In principle, all forms of the well-known iodine-induced allergic reactions, such as iododerma tuberosum, dermatitis, petechiae, and sialadenitis are possible with povidone-iodine, but the incidence seems to be very low (SEDA-11, 489; SEDA-12, 586; 4,31,32).

- A severe anaphylactoid reaction occurred immediately after the instillation of a 10% solution of povidone-iodine into a hydatid cyst cavity during surgery. Severe bronchospasm developed immediately and was followed by a coagulopathy and subsequent liver and renal insufficiency (33).

There have been only a few reports of contact allergy to povidone-iodine, despite its widespread use. In two cases there were positive patch test reactions on days 2, 3, and 7 to povidone-iodine (5% aqueous) and iodine (0.5% in petrolatum), but negative reactions to povidone itself (34).

Second-Generation Effects

Pregnancy

Routine vaginal douching with povidone-iodine during pregnancy causes maternal iodine overload and markedly increases the iodine content in amniotic fluid and of the fetal thyroid, as soon as the trapping mechanism of iodine by the thyroid has started to develop. Vaginal use of povidone-iodine is therefore not recommended during pregnancy (35,36) and labor (37).

The fetal thyroid starts to store iodine between the 10th and 13th weeks of gestation, and to secrete thyroid hormone between the 18th and 24th weeks. Especially after intravaginal administration during pregnancy, povidone-iodine can cause congenital goiter and hypothyroidism in newborn infants. However, hyperthyroidism can also occur.

In 99 of 9320 newborns TSH concentrations were above the reference range (20 mU/ml) on the fifth day of life, but between the 10th and 21st day all these infants had normal TSH concentrations and normal thyroid function (38). In 76 of the newborns with hyperthyrotropinemia, urinary iodine excretion was significantly raised (above 16 µg/ml). Most of them were born in obstetric departments where iodophores were routinely used for disinfection during labor.

In 66 mothers and their infants povidone-iodine was given during labor and delivery as a 1% or 2% solution pumped intravaginally through a plastic catheter until delivery (for 5–30 hours), urinary iodide concentrations on the first and the fifth day and serum iodine concentrations at birth were significantly raised in the mothers as well as in the neonates (39). At birth, the TSH concentrations in the mothers and infants were no different from those in the controls, but on the third and fifth days they were significantly higher. Thyroxine concentrations were significantly lower in the exposed mothers and infants (at birth and on the third and on the fifth days). One-fifth of the infants had high TSH concentrations (above 20 µU/ml) and low thyroxine values (below 7 µg/ml), which is suggestive of hypothyroidism. However, none of the infants developed clinical symptoms, and on the 14th day the values were normal again. In the iodine-exposed mothers and infants tri-iodothyronine (T3) concentrations were significantly reduced at birth, but not thereafter. The concentrations of reverse T3 did not differ from the controls at birth, but were significantly lower on succeeding days. This reduction in reverse T3 in the iodine-exposed infants was probably due to reduced thyroxine concentrations, causing a lack of substrates for monodeiodination to reverse T3.

Iodine concentrations in breast milk and in random urine in neonates and the serum concentrations of neonatal TSH and free thyroxine on day 5 after delivery were measured after the use of povidone-iodine for disinfection after delivery (36). Iodine concentrations in the breast milk and neonatal TSH were significantly raised. Perinatal iodine exposure causes transient hypothyroidism in a significant number of neonates, in whom careful monitoring and follow-up of thyroid gland function are needed. It is better to avoid the use of iodine-containing antiseptics in pregnancy and neonates, especially if follow-up cannot be guaranteed.

Susceptibility Factors

Age

Neonates

Hypothyroidism in neonates has been related to the use of small doses of iodine as an antiseptic. The high vulnerability of the neonatal thyroid is a reason for avoiding povidone-iodine for care of the umbilical stump or omphaloceles (SEDA-11, 488; SEDA-12, 585; 40).

Serum TSH and thyroxine concentrations have been measured 57 days after birth in 365 healthy newborns whose umbilical stump had been treated with 10% povidone-iodine (41). The prevalence of high TSH concentrations was significantly higher in this group than in the general population (3.1% versus 0.4%), as was the rate of transient hypothyroidism (2.7% versus 0.25%). All the children were normal when retested 1 week later. Transient hypothyroidism due to skin contamination with povidone-iodine occurred in a neonate with an omphalocele (42).

The postnatal iodine overload, measured as urinary iodine concentration, has been studied in ill neonates after the cutaneous application of povidone-iodine (0.96% I_2; Betadine) (SEDA-11, 488; 39). The mean iodine overload was 1297 µg/day in one povidone-iodine group and 1253 µg/day in a second group; in the control group 64% of the newborns had iodinuria of less than 100 µg/day, and of the 10 others three were born by cesarean section: in these cases the mothers received an iodine-containing curariform agent. There were 12 cases of hypothyroidism among the neonates exposed to iodine-containing antiseptics, but none in the control group. Very low-birth-weight infants admitted to a neonatal intensive care unit who had been given chlorhexidine-containing antiseptics ($n = 29$) were compared with infants in a comparable unit who had been given iodinated antiseptic agents ($n = 54$) (43). The latter had an up to 50-fold higher increase in urinary iodine excretion than the controls. The median serum TSH concentration was significantly higher in the iodine-exposed infants (4.6 mU/ml) than in the control infants (2.4 mU/ml). On day 14, TSH concentrations in nine of the 36 iodine-exposed infants were above 20 mU/ml, their mean thyroxine concentration was significantly lower (44 nmol/1) than the mean thyroxine concentrations (83 nmol/l) in both the exposed infants with normal TSH concentrations and the controls.

Renal disease

Since iodine is eliminated by the kidneys, renal insufficiency increases the risk of toxicity, and the risk may be further increased by metabolic acidosis (44,45).

Drug Administration

Drug contamination

Bacterial contamination of povidone-iodine formulations has been reported. *Pseudomonas cepacia* was discovered in the blood cultures of 52 patients in four hospitals in New York over 7 months, and of 16 patients in a Boston hospital over a 10-week period in 1980 (46). A contaminated povidone-iodine solution produced by one manufacturer was implicated as the source of the bacteria. It is not clear why this solution was contaminated, whereas other marketed povidone-iodine solutions

containing equivalent amounts of available or free iodine remained sterile.

Interference with Diagnostic tests

Povidone-iodine gives a positive reaction with an ortho-toluidine reagent used to detect blood in the urine, for example Hematest reagent tablets or dipsticks (SEDA-11, 488; 47).

Povidone-iodine used for skin disinfection before skin puncture blood was taken altered serum concentrations of potassium, phosphate, and uric acid.

References

1. Bergmann M, Flance IJ, Blumenthal HT. Thesaurosis following inhalation of hair spray: a clinical and experimental study. N Engl J Med 1958;258(10):471–6.
2. Bergmann M, Flance IJ, Cruz PT, Klam N, Aronson PR, Joshi RA, Blumenthal HT. Thesaurosis due to inhalation of hair spray. Report of twelve new cases, including three autopsies. N Engl J Med 1962;266:750–5.
3. Weese HG, Periston H. Ein never Blutluessigkeitsersatz. Münch Med Wochenschr 1943;90:11–15.
4. Gortz G, Haring R. Wirkung und Nebenwirkung von Polyvinylpyrrolidon-Jod (PVP-Jod). Therapiewoche 1981;31:4364.
5. Colcleuth RG. Distribution protein binding of betadine ointment in burn wounds. In: Altemeier WA, editor. II World Congress/Antisepsis Proceedings. New York: HP Publishing Co, 1980:122–3.
6. Viljanto J. Disinfection of surgical wounds without inhibition of normal wound healing. Arch Surg 1980;115(3):253–6.
7. Ferguson MM, Geddes DA, Wray D. The effect of a povidone-iodine mouthwash upon thyroid function and plaque accumulation. Br Dent J 1978;144(1):14–6.
8. Glick PL, Guglielmo BJ, Tranbaugh RF, Turley K. Iodine toxicity in a patient treated by continuous povidone-iodine mediastinal irrigation. Ann Thorac Surg 1985;39(5):478–80.
9. Campistol JM, Abad C, Nogué S, Bertrán A. Acute renal failure in a patient treated by continuous povidone-iodine mediastinal irrigation. J Cardiovasc Surg (Torino) 1988;29(4):410–2.
10. Vulsma T, Menzel D, Abbad FC, Gons MH, de Vijlder JJ. Iodine-induced hypothyroidism in infants treated with continuous cyclic peritoneal dialysis. Lancet 1990;336(8718):812.
11. Jacobson JM, Hankins GV, Murray JM, Young RL. Self-limited hyperthyroidism following intravaginal iodine administration. Am J Obstet Gynecol 1981;140(4):472–3.
12. Vorherr H, Vorherr UF, Mehta P, Ulrich JA, Messer RH Vaginal absorption of povidone-iodine. JAMA 1980;244(23):2628–9.
13. Wissenschaftlicher Beirat der Bundesärztekammer. Fur Anwendung von Polyvinylpyrrolidon-Jod Komplexen. Dtsch Ärztebl 1985;82:1434.
14. Zec N, Donovan JW, Aufiero TX, Kincaid RL, Demers LM. Seizures in a patient treated with continuous povidone-iodine mediastinal irrigation. N Engl J Med 1992;326(26):1784.
15. Grant JA, Bilodeau PA, Guernsey BG, Gardner FH. Unsuspected benzyl alcohol hypersensitivity. N Engl J Med 1982;306(2):108.

16. Robertson P, Fraser J, Shield J, Weir P. Thyrotoxicosis related to iodine toxicity in a paediatric burn patient. Intensive Care Med 2002;28:1369.

17. Alvarez E. Neutropenia in a burned patient being treated topically with povidone-iodine foam. Plast Reconstr Surg 1979;63(6):839–40.

18. Golightly LK, Smolinske SS, Bennett ML, Sutherland EW 3rd, Rumack BH. Pharmaceutical excipients. Adverse effects associated with 'inactive' ingredients in drug products (Part II). Med Toxicol Adverse Drug Exp 1988;3(3):209–40.

19. Manfro RC, Comerlato L, Berdichevski RH, Ribeiro AR, Denicol NT, Berger M, Saitovitch D, Kott WJ, Goncalves LF. Nephrotoxic acute renal failure in a renal transplant patient with recurrent lymphocoele treated with povidone–iodine irrigation. Am J Kidney Dis 2002;40: 655–7.

20. Aiba M, Ninomiya J, Furuya K, Arai H, Ishikawa H, Asaumi S, Takagi A, Ohwada S, Morishita Y. Induction of a critical elevation of povidone-iodine absorption in the treatment of a burn patient: report of a case. Surg Today 1999;29:157–9.

21. Ryan M, Al–Sammak Z, Phelan D. Povidone-iodine mediastinal irrigation: a case of acute renal failure. J Cardiothorac Vasc Anesth 1999 13:729–31.

22. Steen M. Review of the use of povidone-iodine (PVP-I) in the treatment of burns. Postgrad Med J 1993;69 Suppl 3:S84–92.

23. Dupont A, Lachapelle JM. Dermite due à un depot medicamenteux au cours du traitement d'un diabète insipide. [Dermatitis due to a medicamentous deposit during the treatment of diabetes insipidus.] Bull Soc Fr Dermatol Syphiligr 1964;71:508–9.

24. Lachapelle JM. Thesaurismose cutanée par polyvinylpyrrolidone. [Cutaneous thesaurismosis due to polyvinylpyrrolidone.] Dermatologica 1966;132(6):476–89.

25. Mensing H, Köster W, Schaeg G, Nasemann T. Zur klinischen Varianz der Polyvinylpyrrolidon-Dermatose. [Clinical variability of polyvinylpyrrolidone dermatosis.] Z Hautkr 1984;59(15):1027–37.

26. Bazex A, Geraud J, Guilhem A, Dupre A, Rascol A, Cantala P. Maladie de Dupont et Lachapelle (thesaurismose cutaneé par polyvinylpyrrolidone. [Dupont-Lachapelle disease (cutaneous thesaurismosis due to polyvinylpyrrolidone).] Arch Belg Dermatol Syphiligr 1966;22(4):227–33.

27. Kuo TT, Hu S, Huang CL, Chan HL, Chang MJ, Dunn P, Chen YJ. Cutaneous involvement in polyvinylpyrrolidone storage disease: a clinicopathologic study of five patients, including two patients with severe anemia. Am J Surg Pathol 1997;21(11):1361–7.

28. Kepes JJ, Chen WY, Jim YF. 'Mucoid dissolution' of bones and multiple pathologic fractures in a patient with past history of intravenous administration of polyvinylpyrrolidone (PVP). A case report. Bone Miner 1993;22(1):33–41.

29. Dunn P, Kuo T, Shih LY, Wang PN, Sun CF, Chang MJ. Bone marrow failure and myelofibrosis in a case of PVP storage disease. Am J Hematol 1998;57(1):68–71.

30. Ronnau AC, Wulferink M, Gleichmann E, Unver E, Ruzicka T, Krutmann J, Grewe M. Anaphylaxis to polyvinylpyrrolidone in an analgesic preparation. Br J Dermatol 2000;143:1055–8.

31. Zamora JL. Chemical and microbiologic characteristics and toxicity of povidone-iodine solutions. Am J Surg 1986;151(3):400–6.

32. Ancona A, Suárez de la Torre R, Macotela E. Allergic contact dermatitis from povidone-iodine. Contact Dermatitis 1985;13(2):66–8.

33. Okten F, Oral M, Canakici N, et al. An anaphylactoid induced with polyvinylpyrrolidone iodine. A case report. Turk Anesteziyol Reanim 1993;21:118–22.

34. Erdmann S, Hertl M, Merk HF. Allergic contact dermatitis from povidone-iodine. Contact Dermatitis 1999;40:331.

35. Melvin GR, Aceto T Jr, Barlow J, Munson D, Wierda D. Iatrogenic congenital goiter and hypothyroidism with respiratory distress in a newborn. S D J Med 1978;31(10):15–19.

36. Mahillon I, Peers W, Bourdoux P, Ermans AM, Delange F. Effect of vaginal douching with povidone-iodine during early pregnancy on the iodine supply to mother and fetus. Biol Neonate 1989;56(4):210–7.

37. Koga Y, Sano H, Kikukawa Y, Ishigouoka T, Kawamura M. Effect on neonatal thyroid function of povidone-iodine used on mothers during perinatal period. J Obstet Gynaecol 1995;21(6):581–5.

38. Grüters A, l'Allemand D, Heidemann PH, Schürnbrand P. Incidence of iodine contamination in neonatal transient hyperthyrotropinemia. Eur J Pediatr 1983;140(4):299–300.

39. l'Allemand D, Grüters A, Heidemann P, Schürnbrand P. Iodine-induced alterations of thyroid function in newborn infants after prenatal and perinatal exposure to povidone iodine. J Pediatr 1983;102(6):935–8.

40. Castaing H, Fournet JP, Léger FA, Kiesgen F, Piette C, Dupard MC, Savoie JC. Thyroïde du nouveau né et surcharge en iode après la naissance. [The thyroid gland of the newborn infant and postnatal iodine overload.] Arch Fr Pediatr 1979;36(4):356–68.

41. Arena J, Eguileor I, Emparanza J. Repercusion sobre la function tiroidea del RN a termino de la aplicacion de povidona iodada en el munon umbilical. [Repercussion of the application of povidone-iodine to the umbilical stump on thyroid function of the neonate at term.] An Esp Pediatr 1985;23(8):562–8.

42. Tummers RF, Krul EJ, Bakker HD. Passagere hypothyreoidie ten gevolge van huidinfectie met jodium bij een pasgeborene met een omfalokele. [Transient hypothyroidism due to skin contamination with iodine in a newborn infant with an omphalocele.] Ned Tijdschr Geneeskd 1985;129(20):958–9.

43. Smerdely P, Lim A, Boyages SC, Waite K, Wu D, Roberts V, Leslie G, Arnold J, John E, Eastman CJ. Topical iodine-containing antiseptics and neonatal hypothyroidism in very-low-birthweight infants. Lancet 1989;2(8664): 661–4.

44. Wilson JP, Solimando DA Jr, Edwards MS. Parenteral benzyl alcohol-induced hypersensitivity reaction. Drug Intell Clin Pharm 1986;20(9):689–91.

45. Shmunes E. Allergic dermatitis to benzyl alcohol in an injectable solution. Arch Dermatol 1984;120(9):1200–1.

46. Craven DE, Moody B, Connolly MG, Kollisch NR, Stottmeier KD, McCabe WR. Pseudobacteremia caused by povidone-iodine solution contaminated with *Pseudomonas cepacia*. N Engl J Med 1981;305(11):621–3.

47. Van Steirteghem AC, Young DS. Povidone-iodine ("Betadine") disinfectant as a source of error. Clin Chem 1977;23(8):1512.

Potassium perchlorate

General Information

Potassium perchlorate is a thyrostatic drug that is still used (in a dose of 1000 mg/day or more) as an alternative to the thionamides, especially in cases of allergy. It has also been used to treat the iodine-induced form of thyrotoxicosis, such as type 1 hyperthyroidism due to amiodarone (qv).

Compared with the thionamides, potassium perchlorate has two disadvantages:

1. treatment cannot be directly changed to radioiodine therapy, since perchlorate elimination lasts for some weeks;
2. brief high-dose iodine therapy cannot be used as a preoperative thyrostatic measure.

Potassium perchlorate produces goiter, as do the thionamides, but its effects on the hematological system are the main reason for using it sparingly.

Organs and Systems

Hematologic

Agranulocytosis and aplastic anemia have been described in patients taking potassium perchlorate (SED-8, 897) (1). Deaths have been recorded as a result (2,3).

Skin

Erythema nodosum associated with lupus erythematosus cells has been described as an adverse effect of potassium perchlorate (SED-8, 897) (1).

References

1. Rokke KE, Vogt JH. Combination of potassium perchlorate and propylthiouracil in the treatment of thyrotoxicosis. Acta Endocrinol (Copenh) 1968;57(4):565–77.
2. Johnson RS, Moore WG. Fatal aplastic anaemia after treatment of thyrotoxicosis with potassium perchlorate. BMJ 1961;5236:1369–71.
3. Krevans JR, Asper SP Jr, Rienhoff WF Jr. Fatal aplastic anemia following use of potassium perchlorate in thyrotoxicosis. JAMA 1962;181:162–4.

Protirelin

General Information

Protirelin is a synthetic tripeptide that stimulates the hypophyseal secretion of thyrotrophin (thyroid-stimulating hormone, TSH). It is used mainly for diagnostic purposes in dynamic tests of pituitary and hypothalamic function, but its use in the assessment of hyperthyroidism has been superseded by sensitive assays of thyrotrophin (SED-13, 1311) (1). Protirelin has neurotransmitter properties and has been used to treat a variety of neurological disorders, including intractable epilepsy (2). Some experiments have also been performed to evaluate its effects in mental disorders.

Protirelin is generally given intravenously (as a bolus of 200 micrograms), as absorption after oral and intranasal administration is unpredictable.

Comparative studies

Protirelin has been given antenatally in combination with a glucocorticoid, to accelerate fetal lung maturation in an attempt to reduce the incidence of infant respiratory distress syndrome. However, there was no improvement in outcome and the mothers experienced more adverse effects (particularly flushing, headache, nausea, and vomiting) in the protirelin group in two large prospective studies (3,4). The infants were reported to have mild developmental delay at 12 months of age (5): this finding was initially criticized because of methodological problems and there was no consensus that protirelin induces harmful effects in these infants (6).

Subsequently, the addition of protirelin to glucocorticoid therapy was the subject of a meta-analysis (7). In 1134 premature infants the serum TSH concentration was increased for the first 6 hours after the last maternal dose of protirelin, then suppressed for 36 hours before returning to control values (8). The largest controlled trial (in 1368 infants) reported a small delay in development at 12 months (5). However, developmental assessment was by questionnaire, with incomplete ascertainment, and these findings have been questioned (6). In the mothers, there was a three-fold increase in nausea, vomiting, or flushing and a two-fold increase in hypertension compared with glucocorticoid therapy alone.

General adverse effects

The adverse effects of protirelin are usually mild. These include facial flushing, urinary urgency, vaginal sensations, nausea, chest pain, and altered taste sensation (9).

Organs and Systems

Cardiovascular

A transient rise in blood pressure occurs immediately after the administration of protirelin (10). In very rare cases, transient amaurosis and bronchospasm have been reported, thought to be due to either vasopressor syncope or cardiac arrhythmias (11–13).

Nervous system

The most serious adverse effect of protirelin is pituitary apoplexy (pituitary hemorrhage or infarction, characterized by severe headache, visual loss, and often by pituitary failure, hypotension, and coma). This complication has been described in 15 cases after pituitary function testing with protirelin. Pituitary macroadenoma was present in all cases. Although insulin and gonadorelin were also used in these patients, protirelin was considered to be the most likely agent responsible, owing to its vasoactive properties (SED-13, 1311) (14).

- A woman developed severe bifrontal headache and visual blurring 5 minutes after the intravenous administration of protirelin 200 micrograms to investigate her pituitary macroadenoma (15). The symptoms resolved in less than 2 hours without sequelae.
- A patient developed a severe headache, nausea and vomiting, visual disturbance, and altered mental function 88 hours after a protirelin/gonadorelin stimulation test to investigate a pituitary macroadenoma (16). Bleeding into the tumor was seen on CT scan. The patient died 9 days later of pneumonia.

Loss of consciousness or convulsions occurred in a few patients who received high doses (400 micrograms) of protirelin intravenously.

References

1. Surks MI, Chopra IJ, Mariash CN, Nicoloff JT, Solomon DH. American Thyroid Association guidelines for use of laboratory tests in thyroid disorders. JAMA 1990;263(11):1529–32.
2. Takeuci Y. Thyrotropin-releasing hormone (protirelin). Role in the treatment of epilepsy. CNS Drugs 1996;6:341–350.
3. Australian Collaborative Trial of Antenatal Thyrotropin-releasing Hormone (ACTOBAT) for prevention of neonatal respiratory disease. Lancet 1995;345(8954):877–82.
4. Ballard RA, Ballard PL, Cnaan A, Pinto-Martin J, Davis DJ, Padbury JF, Phibbs RH, Parer JT, Hart MC, Mannino FL, Sawai SKNorth American Thyrotropin-Releasing Hormone Study Group. Antenatal thyrotropin-releasing hormone to prevent lung disease in preterm infants. N Engl J Med 1998;338(8):493–8.
5. Crowther CA, Hiller JE, Haslam RR, Robinson JSACTOBAT Study Group. Australian Collaborative Trial of Antenatal Thyrotropin-Releasing Hormone: adverse effects at 12-month follow-up. Pediatrics 1997;99(3):311–7.
6. McCormick MC. The credibility of the ACTOBAT follow-up study. Pediatrics 1997;99(3):476–8.
7. Gross I, Moya FR. Is there a role for antenatal TRH therapy for the prevention of neonatal lung disease? Semin Perinatol 2001;25(6):406–16.
8. Ballard PL, Ballard RA, Ning Y, Cnann A, Boardman C, Pinto-Martin J, Polk D, Phibbs RH, Davis DJ, Mannino FL, Hart M. Plasma thyroid hormones In premature infants effect of gestational age and antenatal thyrotropin-releasing hormone treatment. TRH Collaborative Trial Participants. Pediatr Res 1998;44(5):642–9.
9. Dolva LO, Riddervold F, Thorsen RK. Side effects of thyrotrophin releasing hormone. BMJ (Clin Res Ed) 1983;287(6391):532.
10. Devlieger R, Vanderlinden S, de Zegher F, Van Assche FA, Spitz B. Effect of antenatal thyrotropin-releasing hormone on uterine contractility, blood pressure, and maternal heart rate. Am J Obstet Gynecol 1997;177(2):431–3.
11. McFadden RG, McCourtie DR, Rodger NW. TRH and bronchospasm. Lancet 1981;2(8249):758–9.
12. Drury PL, Belchetz PE, McDonald WI, Thomas DG, Besser GM. Transient amaurosis and headache after thyrotropin releasing hormone. Lancet 1982;1(8265):218–9.
13. Cimino A, Corsini R, Radaeli E, Bollati A, Giustina G. Transient amaurosis in patient with pituitary macroadenoma after intravenous gonadotropin and thyrotropin releasing hormones. Lancet 1981;2(8237):95.
14. Masago A, Ueda Y, Kanai H, Nagai H, Umemura S. Pituitary apoplexy after pituitary function test: a report of two cases and review of the literature. Surg Neurol 1995;43(2):158–64.
15. Sachmechi I, Bitton RN, Patel D, Schneider BS. Transient headache and impaired vision after intravenous thyrotropin-releasing hormone in a patient with pituitary macroadenoma. Mt Sinai J Med 1999;66(5–6):330–3.
16. Dokmetas HS, Selcuklu A, Colak R, Unluhizarci K, Bayram F, Kelestimur F. Pituitary apoplexy probably due to TRH and GnRH stimulation tests in a patient with acromegaly. J Endocrinol Invest 1999;22(9):698–700.

Thionamides

General Information

Several natural or synthetic substances interfere with the synthesis and/or secretion of the thyroid hormones. Two types of thionamides are used in the treatment of hyperthyroidism:

1. derivatives of thiouracil, especially propylthiouracil (rINN); methylthiouracil and iodothiouracil have been used in the past, but are not currently used clinically;
2. derivatives of thioimidazole, especially thiamazole (rINN; methimazole) and its carbethoxy derivative carbimazole (rINN), which is converted in the body to thiamazole (1,2).

All of these drugs interfere with the thyroid peroxidase system and inhibit the synthesis of the thyroid hormones, reducing their overproduction in hyperthyroidism. However, if they are used in too high dosages, they can cause hypothyroidism and hypersecretion of thyrotrophin (TSH) which in turn will stimulate thyroid growth and the development of goiter. To avoid these problems, regular dosage adjustment or combination with synthetic thyroid hormones is necessary as soon as the euthyroid state is obtained.

Antithyroid drugs may also suppress lymphocytic infiltration into the thyroid and thereby directly modulate the basic disorder of autoimmune hyperthyroidism (SEDA-6, 364; SEDA-9, 344). Propylthiouracil, but not the thioimidazoles, also inhibits the conversion of thyroxine to its more active derivative triiodothyronine. This effect is significant during high-dose treatment, and propylthiouracil may therefore be preferred if a more rapid onset of action is desired, for example thyrotoxic crisis, although clear experimental proof of the advantageous effect is still lacking (3).

The antithyroid drugs are well absorbed from the intestinal tract, but the half-life of propylthiouracil is much shorter (2 hours) than that of the thioimidazoles (6 hours). However, the in vivo half-life may be longer due to accumulation and retention of the drug in the thyroid gland (4).

General adverse effects

Both the thiouracils and the thioimidazoles can produce hypothyroidism and goiter. Most of their other adverse effects are allergic rather than toxic. The overall frequency of untoward reactions is 2–14%, but severe reactions occur in less than 1% of patients. Some data suggest that the thioimidazoles have a lower incidence of adverse effects than the thiouracils (5). An association between the dosage of thionamide and the development of untoward reactions has been found in several studies (6). It has therefore been proposed that the initial dose of carbimazole should not exceed 30 mg/day and that of propylthiouracil 300 mg/day (SEDA-17, 474). Allergic reactions include drug fever, lymphadenopathy, arthralgia, agranulocytosis, thrombocytopenia, leukopenia, and skin reactions (1,7). In view of the in vivo conversion of carbimazole to thiamazole, cross-allergy between the two compounds can be expected and has been observed. Cross-allergy between thiouracil and thioimidazoles is rare, but a few cases have been reported. Tumor-inducing effects have not been reported.

Organs and Systems

Nervous system

Neuritis has been described in patients taking thiamazole (8,9).

Sensory systems

Eyes

In contrast to ^{131}I, antithyroid drugs do not seem to increase the risk of new or worse exophthalmos in patients with Graves' disease (10,11).

Retrobulbar neuritis has been reported in a patient taking thiamazole (12).

Ears

Ototoxicity has rarely been attributed to antithyroid drugs (13). In one case progressive bilateral sensorineural hearing loss attributed to propylthiouracil was associated with myeloperoxidase-antineutrophil cytoplasmic antibodies (MPO-ANCA) (14).

Taste

Taste disturbance has been described in patients taking antithyroid drugs and has been attributed to zinc deficiency (SEDA-7, 398; SEDA-11, 357).

Endocrine

Overtreatment with antithyroid drugs can cause hypothyroidism (15,16).

Metabolism

A specific form of hypoglycemia occurs in Hirata disease, a rare autoimmune syndrome in which large amounts of insulin can be released from autoantibodies. In a Japanese series of 197 cases, 43% of the patients had been taking medications before diagnosis: thiamazole for Graves' disease, alpha-mercaptopropionyl glycine for cataracts, liver disease, or rheumatoid arthritis, or glutathione for liver disease, all of which are sulfhydryl compounds. After these drugs were withdrawn, the hypoglycemic attacks subsided (17).

Hematologic

Neutropenia, agranulocytosis, aplastic anemia, and thrombocytopenia are the most important adverse effects of antithyroid drugs.

Neutropenia and agranulocytosis

There are two different types of neutropenia due to antithyroid drugs: a mild dose-related reduction in leukocyte count and a true allergic agranulocytosis (SEDA-10, 368; 18).

Allergic agranulocytosis

DoTS classification (BMJ 2003;327:1222–5)
Dose-relation: hypersusceptibility effect
Time-course: intermediate
Susceptibility factors: genetic (HLA DRB1*08032 allele); age (over 40); sex (women)

Severe agranulocytosis (or more rarely pancytopenia) is usually only observed during the first few months of therapy. Since agranulocytosis can develop very rapidly, periodic leukocyte counts are usually considered to be of little help, but it has been suggested that weekly leukocyte counts during the first month of treatment can detect presymptomatic cases and allow more rapid intervention (19). Patients should therefore be warned to seek immediate medical help if a fever or sore throat develops during antithyroid drug treatment. If the drug is withdrawn immediately recovery is the rule, but fatal cases have also been reported (20,21). In one case agranulocytosis unusually occurred after a second exposure to the drug, in this case propylthiouracil (22).

Frequency

The risk of agranulocytosis has been estimated during several surveys. A large European–Israeli study (23) showed a risk of about 3 per 10 000 users. However, the mortality in this survey was small (one in 45 cases) (SEDA-13, 376). In two hospital surveys of agranulocytosis (24,25) there was an increased risk in women aged over 40 years and when the dose of thiamazole (thiamazole) was more than 40 mg/day. In vitro lymphocyte testing can confirm the sensitization of the immune system to the antithyroid drugs and can occasionally indicate cross-sensitivity between thiamazole and propylthiouracil (SEDA-8, 372; SEDA-9, 344). In a Japanese study, using an adverse drug reactions database, 24 of 91 cases of presumed drug-induced leukopenia were associated with thiamazole (26). The estimated overall risk was 3 per 10 000, largely in the first 3 months (RR = 182, 95% CI = 74, 449).

A UK study used drug prescribing data recorded on the General Practice Research Database to identify the incidence of idiosyncratic neutropenia and agranulocytosis (27). The incidences of neutropenia and agranulocytosis in England and Wales were estimated to be 120 and 7 cases per million per year respectively. Current users of drugs classed as "thyroid inhibitors" had the highest adjusted odds ratios for neutropenia (adjusted OR = 35; 95% CI = 12, 100) and for agranulocytosis (OR = 21; 95% CI = 3.3, ∞) compared with other classes of drug associated with this complication. The increased risk of neutropenia was highest in those who had received two or three prior prescriptions (OR = 58; CI = 7.4, 454), compared with one prior prescription (OR = 14; CI = 1.6, 119) or those who had received four or more prior prescriptions (OR = 34; 7.7, 154). The increased risk of neutropenia associated specifically with carbimazole was higher in those taking 20 mg/day or more (OR = 33; CI = 8.0, 136), compared with those taking 5-15 mg/day (OR = 17; CI = 4.2, 72).

Another important UK study has examined data spontaneously reported to the Medicines and Healthcare products Regulatory Agency through the Yellow Card system (28). Between 1981 and 2003 there were 5.23 million prescriptions for thionamide drugs in England and Scotland, 94% of which were for carbimazole. Neutrophil dyscrasias (agranulocytosis and neutropenia) accounted for 49% of all deaths ascribed to these drugs. They were more frequently fatal in those over 65 years, and since 1981 reports of neutrophil dyscrasias were significantly more frequent per prescription of propylthiouracil than carbimazole. The latter finding may reflect a genuine difference in risk, relative unfamiliarity with the use of propylthiouracil, or higher use of this drug in certain patient groups.

The findings from these two UK studies support the view that agranulocytosis remains the most important complication of antithyroid drugs, remembering that neutropenia may in part reflect underlying hyperthyroidism rather than an adverse drug effect. A study of 109 cases of antithyroid drug-induced agranulocytosis has introduced the concept of "normal white cell count agranulocytosis" by describing a significant number of cases in whom total white cell counts were normal despite the presence of symptomatic agranulocytosis (29). This observation highlights the importance of measuring neutrophil counts in addition to total white cell count if there is clinical suspicion of bone marrow suppression.

Mechanism
Laboratory studies have provided insights into the immune mechanisms underlying the hematological complications of antithyroid drugs (30). Sera from five

patients taking thiamazole who presented with immune thrombocytopenia showed antibodies to the platelet cell adhesion molecule-1. Similar antibodies were present in the serum of a patient with carbimazole-associated neutropenia and mild thrombocytopenia, together with antibodies to the neutrophil-specific Fc gamma receptor IIIb (31). Antibodies against the rhesus component of erythrocyte proteins have also been described in patients with carbimazole-associated anemia, leading to the conclusion that carbimazole can induce cell lineage-specific drug-dependent antibodies that cause cytopenias.

In 24 patients with Graves' disease with thiamazole-induced agranulocytosis, 68 patients with Graves' disease without agranulocytosis, and 525 healthy controls, there was a strong positive association of the HLA DRB1*08032 allele with susceptibility to methimazole-induced agranulocytosis, suggesting that cellular autoimmunity may be involved in its development (32).

Time-course
In 18 cases of antithyroid drug-induced agranulocytosis in China, previous evidence that most cases occur early in treatment (2–12 weeks in 17 of 18 cases) and in those taking high doses was confirmed (33). This series also confirmed that agranulocytosis develops abruptly, arguing against routine monitoring of white cell count, and that fever and sore throat are the earliest symptoms.

Outcomes have been reported in a consecutive series of 91 patients hospitalized with non-chemotherapy drug-induced agranulocytosis from 1985–2000 (34). All but two survived. Antithyroid drugs were the cause of agranulocytosis in 20% of cases. Univariate and multivariate analyses failed to reveal a specific effect of antithyroid drugs on the time to neutrophil recovery. In contrast, hemopoietic growth factor treatment was associated with speedier hematological recovery.

Management
The treatment of this complication is controversial. There have been at least 15 reports of the use of granulocyte colony stimulating factor (G-CSF) in severe cases (granulocyte count under 100×10^6/l) of thionamide-induced agranulocytosis with the objective of shortening the period of neutropenia and hence the risk of infection (35). In another case the use of G-CSF in thionamide-induced agranulocytosis was associated with a number of iatrogenic complications (35). A review of treatment with G-CSF has shown that the average time to recovery from agranulocytosis is 8.2 days, not obviously different from the reported range of 7–14 days without the drug, leading the authors to argue against its routine use in afebrile patients, even in the face of a severe reduction in granulocyte count.

Administration of granulocyte colony-stimulating factor (G-CSF) is reported to shorten the recovery period (36), although others have reported it to be ineffective in severe agranulocytosis (37). In a further study the efficacy of G-CSF has been investigated in 109 patients with agranulocytosis caused by antithyroid drugs (38). G-CSF significantly reduced the recovery period from 9.2 to 2.3 days.

However, it was ineffective in symptomatic patients with granulocyte counts below $0.1 \times 10^9/l$.

In 24 patients with Graves' disease who developed agranulocytosis during antithyroid drug therapy, randomized to receive G-CSF ($n = 14$) or an antibiotic only, recovery time (defined as the number of days required for neutrophil counts to exceed $0.5 \times 10^9/l$) did not differ between the treatments in patients with moderate or severe agranulocytosis, arguing against its routine use (39). These conclusions have been supported by retrospective data from a further 12 patients, four of whom received G-CSF (40). Again, there was no significant difference in terms of the speed of hematological recovery, the number of days of antibiotic treatment, or the duration of hospitalization.

In a retrospective cohort study of 90 cases of drug-induced agranulocytosis in Strasbourg, antithyroid drugs were implicated in 23% of cases, second only to antibiotics in terms of frequency of prescription in the affected cohort (41). The clinical presentation was often severe and included isolated fever (41% of cases), septicemia or septic shock (31%), and pneumonia (10%). The outcome was favorable in 98% of cases. All the patients were treated with broad-spectrum antibiotics and 42 received hemopoietic growth factors; in those given growth factors the mean durations for hematological recovery, antibiotic therapy, and hospitalization were significantly reduced. While patient selection may have contributed to these findings, they do suggest a useful role for such growth factors in supporting patients with this potentially life-threatening complication of thionamide therapy.

Aplastic anemia

Aplastic anemia due to antithyroid drugs is very rare and has been said to occur as an adverse effect of thionamide therapy with about one-tenth of the frequency of agranulocytosis.

- Aplastic anemia developed in a 58-year-old woman taking thiamazole for the third time; she responded well to drug withdrawal and treatment with human granulocyte colony stimulating factor (42).
- A 16-year-old girl who had taken thiamazole for 1 month (30 mg/day) developed a sore throat and dysphagia and had pancytopenia (43). Instead of the expected picture of hypoplasia, bone marrow aspiration showed replacement with plasma cells, a finding suggestive of myeloma and representing a picture not previously described in this context. Thiamazole was withdrawn and she was given antibiotics, dexamethasone, and granulocyte colony stimulating factor. Her hematology and bone marrow findings normalized within days and she was well at follow-up at 24 months.
- A 53 year old took methimazole 30 mg/day for 3 weeks and developed aplastic anemia associated with an increased peripheral blood lymphocyte count and a hypocellular bone marrow with plasmacytosis (44).

There have been anecdotal reports of the use of G-CSF in cases of thionamide-induced agranulocytosis (45). In a retrospective review (46) the outcomes in 10 severe cases treated with G-CSF and in 10 treated without were reviewed. The time to hematological recovery, the duration of antibiotic use, and the duration of hospitalization were all shorter in those treated with G-CSF, although there were no deaths in either group. These findings are in accord with the results of other non-randomized studies of the use of G-CSF in drug-induced agranulocytosis, but conflict with the results of one randomized study that showed no benefit (39). The latest findings must therefore be interpreted with caution, although it is notable that this study was confined to those with severe suppression of leukocyte counts and clinical evidence of infection.

Liver

Both carbimazole and propylthiouracil can cause liver damage, sometimes as part of a hypersensitivity reaction associated with pruritus, rash, fever, and arthralgia. Severe liver injury is believed to be rare, with only 20 reported cases up to 1993 (47). In contrast, subclinical hepatic dysfunction, characterized by a rise in hepatic enzymes, may be common and does not necessitate drug withdrawal in the absence of symptoms (47).

Of 14 cases of suspected drug-induced liver disease presenting to a gastroenterology department over a 3-year period, one was thought to be related to thiamazole, with a hepatitic pattern of liver function tests in a 39-year-old woman 6 days after the start of therapy; recovery was swift and complete (48). Delayed cholestatic hepatitis without antineutrophil cytoplasmic antibodies has been reported (49), and there have been fatal cases of hepatic necrosis (SEDA-21, 438) (7).

In a retrospective review of 497 patients taking propylthiouracil for hyperthyroidism, clinically overt hepatitis developed in six patients at 12–49 days after starting the drug (50). Jaundice and itching were present in five, fever in two, rash in two, and arthralgia in one. Serum bilirubin, alanine transaminase, and alkaline phosphatase were increased in five, four, and six patients respectively. The type of hepatic injury was cholestatic in three, hepatocellular in one, and mixed in two. There were no differences in age, sex, drug dose, or serum thyroid hormone concentrations at time of diagnosis in those with hepatic injury compared with those without. Liver function normalized in all patients at 16–145 days after withdrawal of propylthiouracil. In addition to these cases of overt liver injury, 14% of the cohort had mild asymptomatic liver enzyme rises at a mean of 75 days after the start of treatment.

The reported incidence of liver injury in this report is higher (at 1.2%) than in previous reports, perhaps reflecting patient selection or ethnic differences in study populations. An association with propylthiouracil in the six cases described was supported by the temporal association with the start of therapy and recovery after withdrawal. This complication is likely to be a hypersusceptibility reaction, given the lack of dose association within the therapeutic range, the unpredictable occurrence, and an association with symptoms of hypersensitivity. The findings of this retrospective study do not indicate the need for regular monitoring of liver function tests in those taking propylthiouracil, but they do highlight the need to consider drug toxicity if overt hepatic injury develops, especially early in the course of propylthiouracil therapy.

Two cases of fatal fulminant hepatic failure have been described in previously healthy women aged 30 and 32 years who presented with jaundice 4 and 5 months respectively after starting to take propylthiouracil for Graves' hyperthyroidism (51). Another case of fatal fulminant liver failure with cholestatic jaundice 2 weeks after the start of treatment with propylthiouracil 100 mg tds has been described (52).

Pancreas

Acute pancreatitis and parotitis without antineutrophil cytoplasmic antibodies has been attributed to thiamazole (53).

- A 33-year-old woman developed acute pancreatitis together with mild cholestatic hepatitis and erythema nodosum 1 month after starting carbimazole for Graves' disease; rechallenge with a single dose of carbimazole (10 mg) 7 days after initial recovery led to a further episode of acute pancreatitis, from which she recovered (54).

The temporal association with carbimazole therapy, the response to rechallenge, and the absence of other causes of acute pancreatitis suggested that the drug was causative in this case.

Urinary tract

Chronic tubulointerstitial nephritis with renal insufficiency without antineutrophil cytoplasmic antibodies has been attributed to propylthiouracil (55).

Skin

The most common reaction to antithyroid drugs is a benign skin rash or pruritus without rash. Although such a reaction is usually not serious and can even disappear during continuous treatment, it nevertheless indicates an allergic reaction and requires withdrawal of therapy. Thiouracil can then be replaced by thioimidazoles, but allergy to both products can occasionally occur.

Sexual function

Sexual precocity associated with hypothyroidism has been reported after long-term treatment of children with propylthiouracil, and may reflect relative overdosage (56).

Immunologic

Hypersensitivity syndrome

Allergic reactions manifesting as fever, urticaria or other rashes, and arthralgia occur in 1–5% of patients taking antithyroid drugs. There has been a report of thiamazole-induced hypersensitivity syndrome associated with reactivation of human herpes virus 6 and cytomegalovirus (57).

Vasculitis

Antithyroid drugs, especially propylthiouracil, can be associated with the development of antineutrophil cytoplasmic antibody (ANCA)-positive vasculitis, often manifesting as renal disease. Atypical presentations, with pulmonary capillaritis (58) and lupus-like syndrome (59), have been described in individual cases. Furthermore, two cases of vasculitis have been associated with carbimazole, one presenting with eosinophilic granulomatous vasculitis localized to the stomach (60) and another with p-ANCA positive vasculitis causing simultaneous acute renal insufficiency and massive pulmonary hemorrhage (61).

The long-term effects of antithyroid drug treatment on the prevalence of ANCAs has been examined in 209 consecutive patients with hyperthyroidism who had been treated with antithyroid drugs, radioactive iodine, thyroidectomy, or a combination of these treatment options (62). Overall 12 patients who were taking antithyroid drugs were positive for antineutrophil cytoplasmic antibodies to myeloperoxidase, proteinase-3, or human leukocyte elastase; four of these had ANCA-associated vasculitis. When 77 of the 209 patients who were retested after 3–6 years (and antithyroid drug treatment had been withdrawn), ANCA could still be detected in three of six who had previously tested positive; in addition one patient who had not taken antithyroid drugs had developed a myeloperoxidase-associated ANCA. The presence of antithyroid drugs was highly associated with treatment with antithyroid drugs (OR = 12; 95% CI = 1.5, 93). This study highlights the fact that the presence of ANCA with or without vasculitis is associated with previous treatment with antithyroid drugs, possibly after years.

The mechanism of propylthiouracil-induced vasculitis has been investigated in two separate studies, suggesting that the avidity of myeloperoxidase-associated ANCA (63) or the presence of anti-endothelial cell antibodies (AECA) (64) may be associated with vasculitic disease activity.

The possible drug-induced causes of ANCA-positive vasculitis with high titers of antimyeloperoxidase antibodies in 30 new patients have been reviewed (65). The findings illustrated that this type of vasculitis is a predominantly drug-induced disorder. Only 12 of the 30 cases were not related to a drug. The most frequently implicated drug was hydralazine ($n = 10$); the remainder involved propylthiouracil ($n = 3$), penicillamine ($n = 2$), allopurinol ($n = 2$), and sulfasalazine ($n = 1$).

Cutaneous vasculitis is often a feature of such cases, although severe systemic manifestations often also occur. Two patients with propylthiouracil hypersensitivity presented with skin manifestations but also had renal, rheumatological, and hematological features (66). A review of the literature showed that the symptoms and signs in patients with ANCA-associated thionamide-induced vasculitis are diverse. Acral purpuric skin lesions are typically seen; recognition of these classical clinical features may allow early diagnosis and limit associated morbidity and the requirement for other therapies, particularly immunosuppression. Several other reports have described cases of MPO-ANCA-positive cases of vasculitis presenting in a variety of ways in both adults and children treated with propylthiouracil (67–70).

There have been reports of propylthiouracil-induced ANCA-associated small vessel vasculitis (71,72), crescentic glomerulonephritis (73), and Wegener's granulomatosis (74). More common, however, may be a condition termed "antithyroid arthritis syndrome," which is a transient migratory polyarthritis occurring within 2 months of starting thionamides and resolving within 4 weeks of stopping therapy (75).

ANCA-positive vasculitis in a patient with multinodular goiter has been described, together with a review of the clinical features in a further 26 cases (76). Renal involvement, typically with crescentic or necrotizing glomerulonephritis on biopsy, and arthralgia were the most common manifestations. A few cases of diffuse proliferative lupus nephritis associated with ANCAs have been reported (SEDA-20, 394). Other cases of ANCA-associated disease in patients have been reported, including subjects presenting with neutrophilic dermatosis (77), pyoderma gangrenosum, secondary sterile pyoarthrosis (78), and purpura fulminans (79). Small vessel vasculitis leading to pulmonary alveolar hemorrhage and crescentic glomerulonephritis has also been described (79).

In 61 patients with Graves' hyperthyroidism, 32 of whom were taking propylthiouracil and 29 methimazole, there was a higher prevalence of antimyeloperoxidase ANCAs in those taking propylthiouracil than in those taking thiamazole (25 versus 3.4%) (80). There were no significant differences in age, duration of therapy, or drug dosage in those who developed antimyeloperoxidase ANCAs compared with those who did not. Two ANCA-positive patients in this study developed rheumatoid arthritis or membranous glomerulonephritis, but none developed classical ANCA-associated vasculitis.

There have been reports of antimyeloperoxidase ANCAs associated with diffuse pulmonary alveolar hemorrhage (81), IgA nephropathy (82), and drug-induced neutropenia (83) in patients who had Graves' hyperthyroidism taking propylthiouracil. Investigation using serum from the last of these patients implicated a complement-mediated mechanism. In another case ANCAs developed in two of three monozygotic triplets, both of whom had Graves' disease treated with propylthiouracil, supporting a genetic role in the development of this drug complication (84).

Long-term outcomes in a series of seven children who developed myeloperoxidase-specific ANCA-positive necrotizing crescentic glomerulonephritis associated with propylthiouracil were studied in Japan (85). Three had nephritis alone and four had extrarenal vasculitis. All had taken glucocorticoids, some with additional drugs, and all had achieved remission. None had progressed to end-stage renal insufficiency or death during a mean period of follow-up of 58 months. This apparently benign course, albeit with a relatively short period of follow-up, is similar to that seen in adult patients with this drug complication and implies a better prognosis than in subjects with non-drug-induced ANCA-positive vasculitic disease.

The size of this problem has been addressed using serum samples from 117 patients with Graves' disease treated either with propylthiouracil or thiamazole, and from untreated patients (86). Myeloperoxidase ANCA and proteinase-3 antineutrophil cytoplasmic antibodies (PR3-ANCA) were tested by enzyme-linked immunosorbent assay. Myeloperoxidase ANCA was negative in all untreated patients and patients taking thiamazole, but positive in 21 of 56 patients taking propylthiouracil. In contrast, PR3-ANCA was not detected in any patient in the study. The proportion of patients who were positive for myeloperoxidase ANCA increased with the duration of propylthiouracil therapy. Of the 21 patients who were positive for myeloperoxidase ANCA, 12 had no symptoms, but nine complained of myalgia, arthralgia, or coryza-like symptoms after the appearance of the antibody; none had abnormal urinary findings. These findings suggest a specific association between propylthiouracil therapy and the development of myeloperoxidase ANCA in patients with Graves' disease.

ANCA-positive microscopic polyangiitis has been associated with propylthiouracil, with a fatal outcome despite treatment with glucocorticoids and cyclophosphamide (87). Another patient presented atypically with acute pericarditis 10 months after starting to take propylthiouracil 100 mg tds (88). Another patient developed ANCA-negative leukocytoclastic vasculitis of the skin (89).

Several cases of "collagen-like" or "lupus-like" disease have been reported (joint pain, skin rash, and positive antinuclear antibodies) during treatment with either propylthiouracil or thiamazole (SEDA-8, 372) (SEDA-10, 368). Some cases of general vasculitis can be fatal, although high-dose glucocorticoid therapy can be helpful (90).

Other reports have described serious immunological complications of propylthiouracil in the absence of ANCA, including interstitial nephritis and fatal Stevens–Johnson syndrome in a 90-year-old woman treated for 5 weeks (91) and disseminated intravascular coagulation and vasculitis 2 weeks after the introduction of propylthiouracil in a 42-year-old woman (92). The latter was treated successfully by drug withdrawal and intravenous methylprednisolone.

Second-Generation Effects

Pregnancy

Both the thiouracils and thioimidazoles readily cross the placenta and can cause fetal hypothyroidism, resulting in a slight delay in neurological or bone maturation. Various degrees of goiter have also been observed, even to the extent of severe tracheal compression and death. Antithyroid drug dosage should therefore be reduced to the minimum required to maintain a euthyroid state without supplementation of levothyroxine (93).

Teratogenicity

Aplasia cutis congenita has been attributed to carbimazole, or its active metabolite thiamazole, given during early pregnancy (SEDA-14, 367; 94), and a review revealed 16 cases of solitary skin defects associated with intrauterine exposure to thiamazole (94). The defects can be restricted to a region of the body or can be widespread. Several causes have been documented, including chromosomal abnormalities (for example trisomy 13) and single gene mutations, such as Goltz syndrome. A few cases are believed to result from in utero exposure to teratogens, including thionamides. To date, 16 cases of solitary skin defects associated with intrauterine exposure to thiamazole have been reported. Additional cases of aplasia cutis congenita in thionamide-exposed infants associated with other congenital abnormalities, such as bilateral atresia of the nasal choana, esophageal atresia, imperforate anus, and cardiovascular defects have also been reported (94).

Additional cases of aplasia cutis congenita in thionamide-exposed infants associated with other congenital abnormalities, such as choanal atresia, esophageal atresia, imperforate anus, and cardiovascular defects, were also reviewed. This pattern of abnormalities has previously led to the term "methimazole [thiamazole] embryopathy" (95).

- A 3-year-old child, whose mother had been treated for Graves' hyperthyroidism with thiamazole throughout pregnancy, had two scalp lesions and other abnormalities of tissues of ectodermal origin, including dystrophic nails and syndactyly.

The authors suggested that a history of in utero exposure to thiamazole should be sought in all children with aplasia cutis congenita, as well as other ectodermal tissue abnormalities, to allow better definition of the "methimazole embryopathy." However, cautious interpretation of the literature is required, given the small number of thiamazole-associated cases of aplasia cutis congenita compared with the widespread prescription of this drug in pregnant women with hyperthyroidism. On the other hand, the absence of an apparent association with the use of the alternative thionamide, propylthiouracil, argues in favor of using the latter in pregnant patients.

Aplasia cutis congenita and choanal atresia have been reported in association with maternal carbimazole therapy, suggesting a causative link either with the drug or with underlying hyperthyroidism.

- Choanal atresia with scalp aplasia cutis, umbilical hernia, sacral pilonidal sinus, limb hypertonia, and downslanting palpebral fissures affected the child of a woman who took methimazole 10 mg/day until the 8th week of gestation (96).
- Aplasia cutis affected one of twin boys born to a mother with Graves' disease, drug addiction, and psychosis, who had taken methimazole 40mg/day, propranolol, and haloperidol (with poor compliance) (96).
- Fatal gastroschisis occurred in a child born to a mother who had taken high-dose carbimazole (60 mg/day) during the first trimester of pregnancy (97).

These cases highlight a possible link between carbimazole, or its active metabolite methimazole, and congenital abnormalities, especially aplasia cutis and choanal atresia,

and suggest that propylthiouracil should be the drug of choice in early pregnancy.

Two other cases of choanal atresia in association with carbimazole treatment during the first trimester of pregnancy have been reported (98,99); in one case there were marked facial dysmorphic features and failure of breast development, thought to be secondary to maternal use of carbimazole during pregnancy (98). These cases continue to highlight a possible link between carbimazole, or its active metabolite methimazole, and congenital abnormalities, and they reinforce the view that propylthiouracil is the drug of choice in early pregnancy. However, it should be noted that one of the major hazards of antithyroid drug use in pregnancy is over-treatment, and hence induction of fetal hypothyroidism and goiter. It is therefore important to monitor maternal thyroid status carefully and to use the lowest possible dose of antithyroid drug sufficient to maintain maternal euthyroidism.

In a prospective study in 241 women referred to a teratology service because of exposure to thiamazole during pregnancy, congenital abnormalities were compared with those found in offspring of 1089 controls referred because of exposure to non-teratogenic drugs or radiography (95). There were no statistically significant differences between the two groups in terms of major abnormalities, gestational age at delivery, neonatal weight, or head circumference, but among the thiamazole-exposed infants two had a major malformation consistent with "methimazole embryopathy." One had choanal atresia (exposed at 4–7 gestational weeks) and the other had esophageal atresia (exposed at 0–16 gestational weeks) (100). These are very rare malformations, and the number of cases in the cohort was insufficient to reach statistical significance, so the possibility of a chance association with thiamazole exposure cannot be excluded. These cases do, however, lend support to the view that thiamazole may be teratogenic, although thyrotoxicosis itself may be the associated factor. Until further data are available, treatment of thyrotoxicosis with propylthiouracil may be preferable in women who are planning a pregnancy.

- Scalp atresia has been described in an infant whose mother had taken carbimazole in a high dose (60 mg/day) during the first 12 weeks of pregnancy and propylthiouracil thereafter (101). The infant had other dysmorphic features (a flat face, low-set ears, upper lip retraction, and a low-set fifth finger) in addition to transient hypothyroidism.
- Choanal atresia has been described in an infant whose mother presented in early pregnancy with Graves' hyperthyroidism and who took carbimazole in doses up to 60 mg/day in the first trimester (102). She was also clinically and biochemically severely hyperthyroid at this time.

Propylthiouracil crosses the placenta as readily as the thioimidazoles, but the rare and probably real association between thioimidazoles and fetal anomalies makes the thioimidazoles less attractive first-line alternatives (103–105). When propylthiouracil is used cautiously in minimal amounts and with frequent dose adjustments, it is probably the safest form of treatment of hyperthyroidism during pregnancy (SEDA-8, 373; SEDA-11, 357).

Fetotoxicity

Neonatal hypothyroidism has been reported after maternal use of antithyroid drugs (106,107). Transient neonatal hyperthyroidism in a female child born to a mother who had been treated with potassium iodide and carbimazole during pregnancy was followed by sexual precocity (108).

Lactation

The antithyroid drugs appear in human milk, and breast-feeding has therefore been considered contraindicated during such treatment. However, the amount of drug transferred in human milk is too small to affect thyroid function in the breastfed infant (109,110).

Susceptibility Factors

The antithyroid drugs should not be used in patients with a large intrathoracic goiter, which can further increase in size (111).

In severe hepatic disease, the dosages of antithyroid drugs should be very cautiously determined.

Drug Administration

Drug dosage regimens

There are two general patterns of use of antithyroid drugs: monotherapy with progressive reduction in dosage during recovery from hyperthyroidism and a higher dosage of antithyroid drugs complemented by thyroid replacement therapy to avoid hypothyroidism. There is no convincing evidence for a better short-term or long-term control of Graves' disease with either form of therapy, but combination therapy followed by monotherapy with levothyroxine increased the remission rate substantially. The administration of levothyroxine during antithyroid drug treatment reduces both the production of antibodies to TSH receptors and the frequency of recurrence of hyperthyroidism (112). During combination therapy with propylthiouracil and levothyroxine in normal therapeutic doses the inhibition of the conversion of T4 to T3 is of no importance. A single daily dose of antithyroid drugs cannot completely block iodine organification but can nevertheless control most cases of hyperthyroidism. Such therapy can therefore be used in some patients to improve compliance. The duration of therapy is also controversial, but a more prolonged duration of therapy is usually associated with a higher remission rate (SEDA-12, 354).

Drug overdose

Acute overdose of 13 g of propylthiouracil had no serious adverse effects, except for a temporary reduction in serum triiodothyronine (SEDA-5, 382).

Drug–Drug Interactions

Colestyramine

In a small randomized controlled study the combination of propylthiouracil 100 mg bd with colestyramine 4 g bd for 4 weeks led to a more rapid and complete fall in thyroid hormone concentrations in 30 patients with Graves' disease (113). The authors proposed that colestyramine reduced the total body pool of thyroid hormone by enhanced fecal loss, thus inducing a more rapid response to propylthiouracil.

Iodine

Since thionamides block the organification of iodine and incorporation of iodine into iodotyrosines, they inhibit the uptake of ^{131}I used therapeutically in hyperthyroidism. For this reason, thionamides are generally withdrawn for a period of up to a week before ^{131}I therapy is planned, and re-introduction is similarly delayed until several days after ^{131}I therapy. The effect of treatment with either thiamazole or propylthiouracil before ^{131}I has been studied retrospectively (114), the thionamide being withdrawn 5–55 days before ^{131}I administration. The findings confirmed the view that propylthiouracil, but not thiamazole, significantly reduced the cure rate after ^{131}I compared with that found in subjects not pretreated with propylthiouracil, and that discontinuation for 4 months was required for the cure rates to be similar. These findings highlight the fact that thionamides cause a relative "radio-resistance," and prolonged drug withdrawal or an increased dose of ^{131}I may be required to produce an acceptable cure rate.

References

1. Kampmann JP, Hansen JM. Clinical pharmacokinetics of antithyroid drugs. Clin Pharmacokinet 1981;6(6):401–28.
2. In: Langer P, Greer MA, editors. Antithyroid Substances and Naturally Occurring Goitrogens. Basel-Munchen-Paris-London-New York-Sidney: Karger, 1977:54.
3. Chopra IJ, Cody V. Triiodothyronines in health and disease. In: Gross F, editor. Monographs on Endocrinology 18. Berlin-Heidelberg-New York: Springer-Verlag, 1981:1.
4. Jansson R, Dahlberg PA, Johansson H, Lindstrom B. Intrathyroidal concentrations of methimazole in patients with Graves' disease. J Clin Endocrinol Metab 1983;57(1):129–32.
5. Marchant B, Lees JF, Alexander WD. Antithyroid drugs. Pharmacol Ther [B] 1978;3(3):305–48.
6. Reinwein D, Benker G, Lazarus JH, Alexander WD. A prospective randomized trial of antithyroid drug dose in Graves' disease therapy. European Multicenter Study Group on Antithyroid Drug Treatment. J Clin Endocrinol Metab 1993;76(6):1516–21.
7. Cooper DS. Antithyroid drugs. N Engl J Med 1984;311(21):1353–62.
8. Stege R. Antithyroid drug therapy in hyperthyroidism. Recurrence, hypothyroidism and thyroid antibodies. Acta Chir Scand Suppl 1980;501:1–130.
9. Roldan EC, Nigrin G. Peripheral neuritis after methimazole therapy. NY State J Med 1972;72(23):2898–900.

10. Sridama V, DeGroot LJ. Treatment of Graves' disease and the course of ophthalmopathy. Am J Med 1989;87(1):70–3.

11. Tallstedt L, Lundell G, Torring O, Wallin G, Ljunggren JG, Blomgren H, Taube AThe Thyroid Study Group. Occurrence of ophthalmopathy after treatment for Graves' hyperthyroidism. N Engl J Med 1992;326(26):1733–8.

12. Sponzilli T, Tarroni P, D'Amico A, Vinciguerra V, Lupinacci L. Neurite ottica retrobulbare in corso di terapia con metimazolo (contributo clinico). [Retrobulbar optic neuritis in the course of methimazole therapy (a clinical case).] Riv Neurobiol 1979;25(2):233–8.

13. Smith KE, Spaulding JS. Ototoxic reaction to propylthiouracil. Arch Otolaryngol 1972;96(4):368–70.

14. Sano M, Kitahara N, Kunikata R. Progressive bilateral sensorineural hearing loss induced by an antithyroid drug. ORL J Otorhinolaryngol Relat Spec 2004;66(5):281–5.

15. Brewer C. Psychosis due to acute hypothyroidism during the administration of carbimazole. Br J Psychiatry 1969;115(527):1181–3.

16. Messina M, Manieri C, Spagnuolo F, Sardi E, Allegramente L, Monaco A, Ciccarelli E. A case of methimazole-induced hypothyroidism in a patient with endemic goiter: effects of endogenous TSH hyperstimulation after discontinuation of the drug. Thyroidology 1989;1(1):53–7.

17. Polychronakos C, Ligier S. Resuspension of intermediate-acting insulin as a source of error in insulin dosing. Diabetes Care 1994;17(10):1234–5.

18. Bartalena L, Bogazzi F, Martino E. Adverse effects of thyroid hormone preparations and antithyroid drugs. Drug Saf 1996;15(1):53–63.

19. Tajiri J, Noguchi S, Murakami T, Murakami N. Antithyroid drug-induced agranulocytosis. The usefulness of routine white blood cell count monitoring. Arch Intern Med 1990;150(3):621–4.

20. Beebe RT, Propp S, McClintock JC, Versaci A. Fatal agranulocytosis during treatment of toxic goiter with propylthiouracil. Ann Intern Med 1951;34(4):1035–40.

21. Tait GB. Fatal agranulocytosis during carbimazole therapy. Lancet 1957;272(6963):303.

22. Roeloffzen WW, Verhaegh JJ, van Poelgeest AE, Gansevoort RT. Fever or a soar throat after start of antithyroidal drugs? A medical emergency. Neth J Med 1998;53(3):113–7.

23. Retsagi G, Kelly JP, Kaufman DW. Risk of agranulocytosis and aplastic anaemia in relation to use of antithyroid drugs. International Agranulocytosis and Aplastic Anaemia Study. BMJ 1988;297(6643):262–5.

24. Cooper DS, Goldminz D, Levin AA, Ladenson PW, Daniels GH, Molitch ME, Ridgway EC. Agranulocytosis associated with antithyroid drugs. Effects of patient age and drug dose. Ann Intern Med 1983;98(1):26–9.

25. Kaaja R, Ebeling P, Lamberg BA. Tyreostaathioidon aiheuttama agranulosystoos. [Agranulocytosis induced by antithyroid drugs.] Duodecim 1986;102(13):872–8.

26. Ohtsu F, Yano R, Inagaki K, Sakakibara J. [Estimation of adverse drug reactions by the evaluation scores of subjective symptoms (complaints) and background of patients. III. Drug-induced leucopenia.]Yakugaku Zasshi 2000;120(4):397–407.

27. Van Staa TP, Boulton F, Cooper C, Hagenbeek A, Inskip H, Leufkens HG. Neutropenia and agranulocytosis in England and Wales: incidence and risk factors. Am J Hematol 2003;72(4):248–54.

28. Pearce SH. Spontaneous reporting of adverse reactions to carbimazole and propylthiouracil in the UK. Clin Endocrinol (Oxf) 2004;61(5):589–94.

29. Tajiri J, Noguchi S. Antithyroid drug-induced agranulocytosis: special reference to normal white blood cell count agranulocytosis. Thyroid 2004;14(6):459–62.

30. Kroll H, Sun QH, Santoso S. Platelet endothelial cell adhesion molecule-1 (PECAM-1) is a target glycoprotein in drug-induced thrombocytopenia. Blood 2000;96(4):1409–14.

31. Bux J, Ernst-Schlegel M, Rothe B, Panzer C. Neutropenia and anaemia due to carbimazole-dependent antibodies. Br J Haematol 2000;109(1):243–7.

32. Tamai H, Sudo T, Kimura A, Mukuta T, Matsubayashi S, Kuma K, Nagataki S, Sasazuki T. Association between the DRB1*08032 histocompatibility antigen and methimazole-induced agranulocytosis in Japanese patients with Graves disease. Ann Intern Med 1996;124(5):490–4.

33. Dai WX, Zhang JD, Zhan SW, Xu BZ, Jin H, Yao Y, Xin WC, Bai Y. Retrospective analysis of 18 cases of antithyroid drug (ATD)-induced agranulocytosis. Endocr J 2002;49(1):29–33.

34. Maloisel F, Andres E, Kaltenbach G, Noel E, Koumarianou A. Prognostic factors of hematologic recovery in nonchemotherapy drug-induced agranulocytosis. Haematologica 2003;88:470–1.

35. Hirsch D, Luboshitz J, Blum I. Treatment of antithyroid drug-induced agranulocytosis by granulocyte colony-stimulating factor: a case of primum non nocere. Thyroid 1999;9(10):1033–5.

36. Tajiri J, Noguchi S, Okamura S, Morita M, Tamura M, Murakami M, Niho Y. Granulocyte colony-stimulating factor treatment of antithyroid drug-induced granulocytopenia. Arch Intern Med 1993;153(4):509–14.

37. Tamai H, Mukuta T, Matsubayashi S, Fukata S, Komaki G, Kuma K, Kumagai LF, Nagataki S. Treatment of methimazole-induced agranulocytosis using recombinant human granulocyte colony-stimulating factor (rhG-CSF). J Clin Endocrinol Metab 1993;77(5):1356–60.

38. Tajiri J, Noguchi S. Antithyroid drug-induced agranulocytosis: how has granulocyte colony-stimulating factor changed therapy? Thyroid 2005;15(3):292–7.

39. Fukata S, Kuma K, Sugawara M. Granulocyte colony-stimulating factor (G-CSF) does not improve recovery from antithyroid drug-induced agranulocytosis: a prospective study. Thyroid 1999;9(1):29–31.

40. Andres E, Maloisel F, Ruellan A. Use of colony-stimulating factors for the treatment of antithyroid drug-induced agranulocytosis: a retrospective study in twelve patients. Thyroid 2000;10(1):103.

41. Andres E, Maloisel F, Kurtz JE, Kaltenbach G, Alt M, Weber JC, Sibilia J, Schlienger JL, Blickle JF, Brogard JM, Dufour P. Modern management of non-chemotherapy drug-induced agranulocytosis: a monocentric cohort study of 90 cases and review of the literature. Eur J Intern Med 2002;13(5):324–8.

42. Mezquita P, Luna V, Munoz-Torres M, Torres-Vela E, Lopez-Rodriguez F, Callejas JL, Escobar-Jimenez F. Methimazole-induced aplastic anemia in third exposure: successful treatment with recombinant human granulocyte colony-stimulating factor. Thyroid 1998;8(9):791–4.

43. Breier DV, Rendo P, Gonzalez J, Shilton G, Stivel M, Goldztein S. Massive plasmocytosis due to methimazole-induced bone marrow toxicity. Am J Hematol 2001;67(4):259–61.

44. Yamamoto A, Katayama Y, Tomiyama K, Hosoai H, Hirata F, Kimura F, Fujita K, Yasuda H. Methimazole-induced aplastic anemia caused by hypocellular bone marrow with plasmacytosis. Thyroid 2004;14(3):231–5.

45. Calabro L, Alonci A, Bellomo G, D'Angelo A, Di Giacomo V, Musolino C. Methimazole-induced agranulocytosis and quick recovery with G-CSF: case report. Hepatology 2001;5:479–82.

46. Andres E, Kurtz JE, Perrin AE, Dufour P, Schlienger JL, Maloisel F. Haematopoietic growth factor in antithyroid-drug-induced agranulocytosis. QJM 2001;94(8):423–8.

47. Liaw YF, Huang MJ, Fan KD, Li KL, Wu SS, Chen TJ. Hepatic injury during propylthiouracil therapy in patients with hyperthyroidism. A cohort study. Ann Intern Med 1993;118(6):424–8.

48. Hartleb M, Biernat L, Kochel A. Drug-induced liver damage—a three-year study of patients from one gastroenterological department. Med Sci Monit 2002;8(4):CR292–6.

49. Hung YT, Yu WK, Chow E. Delayed cholestatic hepatitis due to methimazole. Hong Kong Med J 1999;5(2):200–1.

50. Kim HJ, Kim BH, Han YS, Yang I, Kim KJ, Dong SH, Kim HJ, Chang YW, Lee JI, Chang R. The incidence and clinical characteristics of symptomatic propylthiouracil-induced hepatic injury in patients with hyperthyroidism: a single-center retrospective study. Am J Gastroenterol 2001;96(1):165–9.

51. Ruiz JK, Rossi GV, Vallejos HA, Brenet RW, Lopez IB, Escribano AA. Fulminant hepatic failure associated with propylthiouracil. Ann Pharmacother 2003;37:224–8.

52. Chan AO, Ng IO, Lam CM, Shek TW, Lai CL. Cholestatic jaundice caused by sequential carbimazole and propylthiouracil treatment for thyrotoxicosis. Hong Kong Med J 2003;9:377–80.

53. Taguchi M, Yokota M, Koyano H, Endo Y, Ozawa Y. Acute pancreatitis and parotitis induced by methimazole in a patient with Graves' disease. Clin Endocrinol (Oxf) 1999;51(5):667–70.

54. Marazuela M, Sanchez de Paco G, Jimenez I, Carraro R, Fernandez-Herrera J, Pajares JM, Gomez-Pan A. Acute pancreatitis, hepatic cholestasis, and erythema nodosum induced by carbimazole treatment for Graves' disease. Endocr J 2002;49(3):315–8.

55. Nakahama H, Nakamura H, Kitada O, Sugita M. Chronic drug-induced tubulointerstitial nephritis with renal failure associated with propylthiouracil therapy. Nephrol Dial Transplant 1999;14(5):1263–5.

56. Sadeghi-Nejad A, Senior B. Sexual precocity: an unusual complication of propylthiouracil therapy. J Pediatr 1971;79(5):833–7.

57. Ozaki N, Miura Y, Sakakibara A, Oiso Y. A case of hypersensitivity syndrome induced by methimazole for Graves' disease. Thyroid 2005;15(12):1333–6.

58. Pirot AL, Goldsmith D, Pascasio J, Beck SE. Pulmonary capillaritis with hemorrhage due to propylthiouracil therapy in a child. Pediatr Pulmonol 2005;39(1):88–92.

59. Ozkan HA, Ozkalemkas F, Ali R, Ozkocaman V, Ozcelik T. Propylthiouracil-induced lupus-like syndrome: successful management with oral corticosteroids. Thyroid 2005;15(10):1203–4.

60. Seve P, Stankovic K, Michalet V, Vial T, Scoazec JY, Broussolle C. Carbimazole induced eosinophilic granulomatous vasculitis localized to the stomach. J Intern Med 2005;258(2):191–5.

61. Calanas-Continente A, Espinosa M, Manzano-Garcia G, Santamaria R, Lopez-Rubio F, Aljama P. Necrotizing glomerulonephritis and pulmonary hemorrhage associated with carbimazole therapy. Thyroid 2005;15(3):286–8.

62. Slot MC, Links TP, Stegeman CA, Tervaert JW. Occurrence of antineutrophil cytoplasmic antibodies and associated vasculitis in patients with hyperthyroidism treated with antithyroid drugs: a long-term followup study. Arthritis Rheum 2005;53(1):108–13.

63. Gao Y, Ye H, Yu F, Guo XH, Zhao MH. Anti-myeloperoxidase IgG subclass distribution and avidity in sera from patients with propylthiouracil-induced antineutrophil cytoplasmic antibodies associated vasculitis. Clin Immunol 2005;117(1):87–93.

64. Yu F, Zhao MH, Zhang YK, Zhang Y, Wang HY. Anti-endothelial cell antibodies (AECA) in patients with propylthiouracil (PTU)-induced ANCA positive vasculitis are associated with disease activity. Clin Exp Immunol 2005;139(3):569–74.

65. Choi HK, Merkel PA, Walker AM, Niles JL. Drug-associated antineutrophil cytoplasmic antibody-positive vasculitis: prevalence among patients with high titers of antimyeloperoxidase antibodies. Arthritis Rheum 2000;43(2):405–13.

66. Chastain MA, Russo GG, Boh EE, Chastain JB, Falabella A, Millikan LE. Propylthiouracil hypersensitivity: report of two patients with vasculitis and review of the literature. J Am Acad Dermatol 1999;41(5 Pt 1): 757–764.

67. Morita S, Ueda Y, Eguchi K. Anti-thyroid drug-induced ANCA-associated vasculitis: a case report and review of the literature. Endocr J 2000;47(4):467–70.

68. Sera N, Yokoyama N, Abe Y, Ide A, Usa T, Tominaga T, Ejima E, Kawakami A, Ashizawa K, Eguchi K. Antineutrophil cytoplasmic antibody-associated vasculitis complicating Graves' disease: report of two adult cases. Acta Med Nagasaki 2000;45:33–6.

69. Otsuka S, Kinebuchi A, Tabata H, Yamakage A, Yamazaki S. Myeloperoxidase–antineutrophil cytoplasmic antibody-associated vasculitis following propylthiouracil therapy. Br J Dermatol 2000;142(4):828–30.

70. Matsubara K, Nigami H, Harigaya H, Osaki M, Baba K. Myeloperoxidase antineutrophil cytoplasmic antibody positive vasculitis during propylthiouracil treatment: successful management with oral corticosteroids. Pediatr Int 2000;42(2):170–3.

71. Harper L, Cockwell P, Savage CO. Case of propylthiouracil-induced ANCA associated small vessel vasculitis. Nephrol Dial Transplant 1998;13(2):455–8.

72. Miller RM, Savige J, Nassis L, Cominos BI. Antineutrophil cytoplasmic antibody (ANCA)-positive cutaneous leucocytoclastic vasculitis associated with antithyroid therapy in Graves' disease. Australas J Dermatol 1998;39(2):96–9.

73. Fujieda M, Nagata M, Akioka Y, Hattori M, Kawaguchi H, Ito K. Antineutrophil cytoplasmic antibody-positive crescentic glomerulonephritis associated with propylthiouracil therapy. Acta Paediatr Jpn 1998;40(3):286–9.

74. Pillinger M, Staud R. Wegener's granulomatosis in a patient receiving propylthiouracil for Graves' disease. Semin Arthritis Rheum 1998;28(2):124–9.

75. Bajaj S, Bell MJ, Shumak S, Briones-Urbina R. Antithyroid arthritis syndrome. J Rheumatol 1998;25(6):1235–9.

76. Gunton JE, Stiel J, Caterson RJ, McElduff A. Clinical case seminar: anti-thyroid drugs and antineutrophil cytoplasmic antibody positive vasculitis. A case report and

review of the literature. J Clin Endocrinol Metab 1999;84(1):13–6.

77. Miller RM, Darben TA, Nedwich J, Savige J. Propylthiouracil-induced antineutrophil cytoplasmic antibodies in a patient with Graves' disease and a neutrophilic dermatosis. Br J Dermatol 1999;141(5):943–4.

78. Darben T, Savige J, Prentice R, Paspaliaris B, Chick J. Pyoderma gangrenosum with secondary pyarthrosis following propylthiouracil. Australas J Dermatol 1999;40(3):144–6.

79. Park KE, Chipps DR, Benson EM. Necrotizing vasculitis secondary to propylthiouracil presenting as purpura fulminans. Rheumatology (Oxford) 1999;38(8):790–2.

80. Wada N, Mukai M, Kohno M, Notoya A, Ito T, Yoshioka N. Prevalence of serum anti-myeloperoxidase antineutrophil cytoplasmic antibodies (MPO-ANCA) in patients with Graves' disease treated with propylthiouracil and thiamazole. Endocr J 2002;49(3):329–34.

81. Katayama K, Hata C, Kagawa K, Noda M, Nakamura K, Shimizu H, Fujimoto M. Diffuse alveolar hemorrhage associated with myeloperoxidase–antineutrophil cytoplasmic antibody induced by propylthiouracil therapy. Respiration 2002;69(5):473.

82. Winters MJ, Hurley RM, Lirenman DS. ANCA-positive glomerulonephritis and IgA nephropathy in a patient on propylthiouracil. Pediatr Nephrol 2002;17(4):257–60.

83. Akamizu T, Ozaki S, Hiratani H, Uesugi H, Sobajima J, Hataya Y, Kanamoto N, Saijo M, Hattori Y, Moriyama K, Ohmori K, Nakao K. Drug-induced neutropenia associated with anti-neutrophil cytoplasmic antibodies (ANCA): possible involvement of complement in granulocyte cytotoxicity. Clin Exp Immunol 2002;127(1):92–8.

84. Herlin T, Birkebaek NH, Wolthers OD, Heegaard NH, Wiik A. Anti-neutrophil cytoplasmic autoantibody (ANCA) profiles in propylthiouracil-induced lupus-like manifestations in monozygotic triplets with hyperthyroidism. Scand J Rheumatol 2002;31(1):46–9.

85. Fujieda M, Hattori M, Kurayama H, Koitabashi Y. Members and Coworkers of the Japanese Society for Pediatric Nephrology. Clinical features and outcomes in children with antineutrophil cytoplasmic autoantibody-positive glomerulonephritis associated with propylthiouracil treatment. J Am Soc Nephrol 2002;13(2):437–45.

86. Sera N, Ashizawa K, Ando T, Abe Y, Ide A, Usa T, Tominaga T, Ejima E, Yokoyama N, Eguchi K. Treatment with propylthiouracil is associated with appearance of antineutrophil cytoplasmic antibodies in some patients with Graves' disease. Thyroid 2000;10(7):595–9.

87. Seligman VA, Bolton PB, Sanchez HC, Fye KH. Propylthiouracil-induced microscopic polyangiitis. J Clin Rheumatol 2001;7:170–4.

88. Colakovski H, Lorber DL. Propylthiouracil-induced perinuclear-staining antineutrophil cytoplasmic autoantibody-positive vasculitis in conjunction with pericarditis. Endocr Pract 2001;7(1):37–9.

89. Meister LH, Guerra IR, Carvalho GD. Images in thyroidology. Vasculitis secondary to treatment with propylthiouracil. Thyroid 2001;11(2):199–200.

90. Wing SS, Fantus IG. Adverse immunologic effects of antithyroid drugs. CMAJ 1987;136(2):121–7.

91. Dysseleer A, Buysschaert M, Fonck C, Van Ginder Deuren K, Jadoul M, Tennstedt D, Cosyns JP, Daumerie C. Acute interstitial nephritis and fatal Stevens–Johnson syndrome after propylthiouracil therapy. Thyroid 2000;10(8):713–6.

92. Khurshid I, Sher J. Disseminated intravascular coagulation and vasculitis during propylthiouracil therapy. Postgrad Med J 2000;76(893):185–6.

93. Hamburger JI. Diagnosis and management of Graves' disease in pregnancy. Thyroid 1992;2(3):219–24.

94. Martin-Denavit T, Edery P, Plauchu H, Attia-Sobol J, Raudrant D, Aurand JM, Thomas L. Ectodermal abnormalities associated with methimazole intrauterine exposure. Am J Med Genet 2000;94(4):338–40.

95. Clementi M, Di Gianantonio E, Pelo E, Mammi I, Basile RT, Tenconi R. Methimazole embryopathy: delineation of the phenotype. Am J Med Genet 1999;83(1):43–6.

96. Ferraris S, Valenzise M, Lerone M, Divizia MT, Rosaia L, Blaid D, Nemelka O, Ferrero GB, Silengo M. Malformations following methimazole exposure in utero: an open issue. Birth Defects Res A Clin Mol Teratol 2003;67:989–92.

97. Guignon AM, Mallaret MP, Jouk PS. Carbimazole-related gastroschisis. Ann Pharmacother 2003;37:829–31.

98. Foulds N, Walpole I, Elmslie F, Mansour S. Carbimazole embryopathy: an emerging phenotype. Am J Med Genet A 2005;132(2):130–5.

99. Myers AK, Reardon W. Choanal atresia—a recurrent feature of foetal carbimazole syndrome. Clin Otolaryngol 2005;30(4):375–7.

100. Di Gianantonio E, Schaefer C, Mastroiacovo PP, Cournot MP, Benedicenti F, Reuvers M, Occupati B, Robert E, Bellemin B, Addis A, Arnon J, Clementi M. Adverse effects of prenatal methimazole exposure. Teratology 2001;64(5):262–6.

101. Bihan H, Vazquez MP, Krivitzky A, Cohen R. Aplasia cutis congenita and dysmorphic syndrome after antithyroid therapy during pregnancy. Endocrinologist 2002;12:87–91.

102. Barwell J, Fox GF, Round J, Berg J. Choanal atresia: the result of maternal thyrotoxicosis or fetal carbimazole? Am J Med Genet 2002;111(1):55–6.

103. Mandel SJ, Cooper DS. The use of antithyroid drugs in pregnancy and lactation. J Clin Endocrinol Metab 2001;86(6):2354–9.

104. Burrow GN. The management of thyrotoxicosis in pregnancy. N Engl J Med 1985;313(9):562–5.

105. Momotani N, Noh J, Oyanagi H, Ishikawa N, Ito K. Antithyroid drug therapy for Graves' disease during pregnancy. Optimal regimen for fetal thyroid status. N Engl J Med 1986;315(1):24–8.

106. Refetoff S, Ochi Y, Selenkow HA, Rosenfield RL. Neonatal hypothyroidism and goiter in one infant of each of two sets of twins due to maternal therapy with antithyroid drugs. J Pediatr 1974;85(2):240–4.

107. Low LC, Ratcliffe WA, Alexander WD. Intrauterine hypothyroidism due to antithyroid-drug therapy for thyrotoxicosis during pregnancy. Lancet 1978;2(8085):370–1.

108. Domenech E, Santisteban M, Moya M, Gonzalez C, Cortabarria C, Mendez A, Alvarez J, Rodriguez-Luis JC. Hipertiroidismo neonatal transitorio e hijo de madre hipertiroidea tratada. Posterior aparicion de precocidad sexual. [Transient neonatal hyperthyroidism in the child of a treated hyperthyroid mother. Subsequent appearance of sexual precocity.] An Esp Pediatr 1985;22(4):281–7.

109. Johansen K, Kampmann JP, Hansen JM, Andersen AN, Helweg J. Udskillelsen af antityreoide stoffer i modermaelk. [Excretion of antithyroid drugs in maternal milk.] Ugeskr Laeger 1982;144(22):1635–7.

110. Cooper DS, Bode HH, Nath B, Saxe V, Maloof F, Ridgway EC. Methimazole pharmacology in man: studies using a newly developed radioimmunoassay for methimazole. J Clin Endocrinol Metab 1984;58(3):473–9.

111. Hershey CO, McVeigh RC, Miller RP. Transient superior vena cava syndrome due to propylthiouracil therapy in intrathoracic goiter. Chest 1981;79(3):356–7.

112. Hashizume K, Ichikawa K, Sakurai A, Suzuki S, Takeda T, Kobayashi M, Miyamoto T, Arai M, Nagasawa T. Administration of thyroxine in treated Graves' disease. Effects on the level of antibodies to thyroid-stimulating hormone receptors and on the risk of recurrence of hyperthyroidism. N Engl J Med 1991;324(14):947–53.

113. Tsai WC, Pei D, Wang TF Wu DA, Li JC, Wei CL, Lee CH, Chen SP, Kuo SW. The effect of combination therapy with propylthiouracil and cholestyramine in the treatment of Graves' hyperthyroidism. Clin Endocrinol (Oxf) 2005;62(5):521–4.

114. Imseis RE, Vanmiddlesworth L, Massie JD, Bush AJ, Vanmiddlesworth NR. Pretreatment with propylthiouracil but not methimazole reduces the therapeutic efficacy of iodine-131 in hyperthyroidism. J Clin Endocrinol Metab 1998;83(2):685–7.

Thyroid hormones

General Information

Nomenclature

In this monograph the following terms are used:

- thyroxine (T4): the endogenous hormone;
- triiodothyronine (T3): the endogenous hormone;
- levothyroxine (rINN) and dextrothyroxine (rINN): the stereoisomers of thyroxine, as used therapeutically;
- liothyronine (rINN): triiodothyronine, as used therapeutically.

Physiology

The normal adult thyroid gland secretes about 90 micrograms of thyroxine (T4) and less than 10 micrograms of liothyronine (triiodothyronine, T3) per day. Somewhat less than half of the T4 is converted to T3 by several tissues (especially the liver). Most of the daily production of T3 thus comes from peripheral 5'-deiodination of T4 and not by direct glandular secretion. The thyroid hormones are tightly bound (T4 even more than T3) to plasma transport proteins; this explains their prolonged half-lives (about 8 days for T4 and about 1 day for T3). Nuclear receptors for thyroid hormones bind T3 much more efficiently than T4, explaining the more rapid onset of action and greater biological potency of T3. The intestinal absorption and hepatic clearance of orally ingested thyroid hormones also differ. T3 has higher systematic availability than T4, only about 60% of which appears in the peripheral circulation after oral administration (1). However, some formulations provide higher

intestinal absorption of T4 (80%) (2). These basic data form the background of optimal thyroid substitution. Thyroid hormones are used either to replace the failing function of the thyroid gland (spontaneous or drug-induced) or to suppress the endocrine function of abnormal thyroid tissues (especially non-toxic struma or goiter or after thyroidectomy for thyroid neoplasms). Although there are abnormalities of the peripheral metabolism of thyroid hormones in some forms of undernutrition or overnutrition, thyroid drug therapy cannot be considered a safe way of treating obesity.

Treatment with thyroid hormones therefore poses only a few essential questions: which dosage should be used, which formulation should be chosen, and how can therapy best be monitored so as to avoid short-term and long-term risks.

Uses

Thyroid hormones are among the most commonly prescribed drugs in the developed world, with a prevalence of prescription of 5–10% in the over 60 age group (3,4). Since about 25% of those who use thyroxine (T4) take doses sufficient to suppress serum TSH (4,5), much attention has focussed on potential adverse effects of this degree of over-treatment.

Levothyroxine is used as replacement therapy in hypothyroidism and to suppress the production of thyrotrophin (thyroid-stimulating hormone) in patients with thyroid carcinoma.

Dextrothyroxine has been used as a lipid-lowering agent. It significantly lowers the serum cholesterol (6) as does levothyroxine; however, dextrothyroxine has a much smaller hormonal effect on body tissues than levothyroxine. The literature is confusing, since older formulations of dextrothyroxine contained considerable amounts of levothyroxine.

Liothyronine can be used for thyroid substitution, but it has the disadvantage of having a short-lived action and its intestinal absorption can give rise to unusually high post-absorption peaks, causing tachycardia. Moreover, the dosage necessary to obtain euthyroidism is more difficult to evaluate, owing to fluctuations in serum T3 concentrations; furthermore, in patients taking liothyronine, measurements of thyrotrophin are also probably less reliable, since its secretion by the pituitary gland depends more on the extracellular T4 concentration than on the T3 concentration. Therapeutic use of liothyronine is therefore generally only recommended when a more rapid onset of action is necessary, for example when thyroid therapy needs to be interrupted for the administration of ^{131}I in the treatment of thyroid cancer. In myxedematous coma it is controversial whether the therapeutic choice should be liothyronine, or levothyroxine, or a combination (7). Moreover, long-term therapy with liothyronine is more likely to cause secondary osteoporosis than T4.

The drug of choice for thyroid replacement therapy is therefore levothyroxine since it is the natural secretory product of the thyroid, has a long half-life, and is metabolized to T3 in the peripheral tissues.

Doses

The optimal dosage of levothyroxine should be based on repeated measurements of T3 and TSH serum concentrations. The daily recommended dose depends on the aim of the therapy. Thyroid replacement therapy for control of spontaneous or iatrogenic hypothyroidism should aim at a dosage of levothyroxine that maintains TSH concentrations within the low reference range. This will usually be associated with a free T4 concentration in the high reference range and a T3 concentration within the reference range. The mean requirement for such patients is 112 micrograms/day (2) or 1.57 micrograms/kg per day (8). This dose is lower than that recommended previously because of better knowledge of the real production rate of T4, the availability of better pharmaceutical formulations allowing better availability, and especially because of better methods for drug monitoring (SEDA-12, 353; SEDA-15, 444; 9–11). Patients stabilized on one pharmaceutical formulation should not be switched to another without proper monitoring of thyroid hormones.

When thyroid therapy is used not only to replace deficiency but also to prevent the growth of remnants of a differentiated thyroid carcinoma, a suppressive dosage is used, aiming at T4 concentrations in the high reference range and an undetectable TSH concentration or at least one that is below the lower end of the reference range, as measured by two-sided assays. Such therapy is warranted because of its long-term safety, efficacy, and tolerance, but some additional therapy for osteoporosis prevention should be considered.

As with all forms of long-term therapy, adherence to the prescribed dosage of levothyroxine is not always optimal, and an unwarranted fear of thyroid-induced osteoporosis can add to this lack of adherence. Inadequacy of thyroxine replacement therapy is not always easily recognized. Several patients were reported with clearly inadequate or excessive consumption of levothyroxine despite a correct prescription. All patients had depression, which could be an additional susceptibility factor by promoting lack of adherence, and the resulting hypothyroidism or hyperthyroidism could further aggravate the depression (12).

When replacement therapy is with levothyroxine only, the T4/T3 ratio is increased compared with healthy subjects, suggesting that thyroid secretion of T3 is physiologically important. Animal studies have shown that euthyroidism is not restored in all tissues by levothyroxine alone (13). Mood and neuropsychological function improved in hypothyroid patients when 50 micrograms of thyroxine was replaced by 12.5 micrograms of liothyronine (14).

Several studies have failed to confirm the benefits of combined levothyroxine and liothyronine therapy. Liothyronine given once a day results in non-physiological peak serum concentrations of T3. Modified-release triiodothyronine plus thyroxine can normalize serum biochemistry, but it is not known whether this formulation is superior to levothyroxine alone (15).

In contrast to other protein-bound drugs for which a loading dose is given to achieve rapid steady-state concentrations, a slow and stepwise increase in thyroid hormone replacement therapy is advisable. This is preferred mainly to avoid sudden cardiac adverse effects, especially in older patients with long-standing myxedema. Moreover, since thyroid hormone substitution can change the metabolic clearance of this drug, steady-state concentrations are obtained only after several months (SEDA-6, 363).

General adverse effects

Ingestion of excessive amounts of thyroid hormones can cause symptoms and signs similar to those that result from endogenous overproduction. However, the symptoms and signs are generally relatively trivial in those who take standard doses of levothyroxine replacement therapy, although abnormalities have been evident in detailed studies of those who take levothyroxine in doses sufficient to suppress serum TSH (16). The adverse effects can therefore largely be avoided by adjusting the dosage according to the appropriately selected laboratory tests.

The adverse effects essentially comprise the symptoms of hyperthyroidism and include weight loss despite a normal or increased appetite, increased nervousness, tachycardia or dysrhythmias of various types, and increased general metabolism and its symptoms (hyperactivity, sweating, fever, etc.). Allergic reactions to pure thyroid formulations are rare and were first reported as late as 1986. Tumor-inducing effects have been investigated but not confirmed.

Organs and Systems

Cardiovascular

Overdosage of thyroid hormones causes tachycardia or palpitation but can also cause several types of dysrhythmia, for example atrial fibrillation. Evidence from the Framingham population that suppression of serum TSH is a susceptibility factor for atrial fibrillation has heightened concern that subclinical hyperthyroidism secondary to levothyroxine can also cause atrial fibrillation (17). Five women who reported frequent bouts of palpitation were investigated while taking levothyroxine and again after levothyroxine withdrawal (18). There was a clear increase in mean 24-hour heart rate during levothyroxine treatment, as well as an increase in atrial extra beats and the number of episodes of re-entrant atrioventricular nodal tachycardia. Four of these patients had evidence of abnormal conduction pathways, even when they were not taking levothyroxine, as evidenced by a short PR interval, but exacerbation of atrial dysrhythmias in these predisposed subjects is consistent with the view that thyroid hormones increase atrial excitability and may increase the risk of cardiac morbidity, especially if given in doses sufficient to suppress serum TSH.

Pre-existing cardiac disease, always to be suspected in elderly people or after long-standing hypothyroidism, can be severely aggravated by sudden thyroid substitution, resulting in severe angina pectoris, myocardial infarction, or sudden cardiac death (SEDA-13, 375). In such patients, the initial dosage should be low and the stepwise increase should be spaced out over a prolonged period and with careful clinical and cardiographic monitoring (19). In some circumstances, for example three-vessel disease, substitution should be postponed until after coronary bypass surgery (SEDA-6, 363). Cardiac decompensation can also result from the increased circulatory demand induced by thyroid hormone substitution or overtreatment. Long-term treatment with levothyroxine in doses that suppress thyrotrophin can have significant effects on cardiac function and structure, especially in patients with hyperthyroid symptoms (16,20), but large prospective studies are needed to assess cardiovascular risk in these patients.

In two cases of hypothyroidism myocardial infarction occurred at the start of thyroxine therapy in the absence of evidence of significant coronary artery disease (21).

- A 58-year-old man with a previous smoking history and a history of hypertension was severely biochemically hypothyroid (serum TSH 221 mU/l) and was given thyroxine, initially in a low dose (25 micrograms/day), increasing to 100 micrograms/day after 2 weeks. A month later he sustained a subendocardial myocardial infarction associated with only minor abnormalities on coronary angiography.
- A 61-year-old woman with severe hypothyroidism (serum TSH 115 mU/l) had an acute myocardial infarction (but no demonstrable abnormality on coronary angiography) 1 month after a thyroxine dosage increase from 50 to 100 micrograms/day.

Cautious introduction of thyroxine, especially in elderly people and those with severe or long-standing hypothyroidism, is prudent.

Myocardial infarction can also occur during long-term use of levothyroxine.

- A 71-year-old woman who had undergone total thyroidectomy with subsequent irradiation because of follicular carcinoma 3 years before (22). Since then, she had taken oral levothyroxine 0.15 mg and 0.2 mg on alternate days. When latent hypothyroidism became evident despite replacement therapy, the dose of levothyroxine was increased to 0.3 mg/day. Three weeks later, she had formed an acute posterior myocardial infarction, although she had no previous history of coronary artery disease. Subsequent coronary arteriograms revealed no evidence of disease of the major vessels. Myocardial scintigraphy 3 weeks after infarction still showed a persistent perfusion defect.

In the US Coronary Drug Project (23) a formulation of dextrothyroxine with a so-called low levothyroxine content was used. The study had to be terminated because of an excessive number of cardiac deaths and non-fatal infarcts.

Nervous system

Insomnia, psychic stimulation, general nervousness, and tremor are among the hyperthyroid symptoms that result from relative overdosage. Pseudotumor cerebri has incidentally been observed shortly after levothyroxine was

given for juvenile hypothyroidism. The headache and bilateral papilledema without focal neurological defects subsequently disappeared even when levothyroxine was continued (24).

Psychiatric

There is a well recognized association between hypothyroidism and psychiatric illness, and previous case reports have suggested that psychosis and mania can be the result of starting thyroid hormone replacement at too high a dosage (25). Two cases of mania associated with levothyroxine have suggested that caution should be exercised when prescribing levothyroxine, especially in elderly people (26,27). Several cases of mania have been reported even after dosages of levothyroxine that are usually considered safe (28).

Musculoskeletal

A slipped capital femoral epiphysis has been described during the treatment of hypothyroidism (SEDA-3, 340). Since slipping occurs more often during the pubertal growth spurt, it is advisable to check for the occurrence of this complication during the pubertal period in children taking thyroid treatment.

Prolonged overtreatment with levothyroxine can result in osteopenia (29). Thyroid hormones have a direct effect on bone cells, thereby increasing both bone resorption and formation with subsequent mild adaptation of the systemic calciotrophic hormones (30). Increased bone turnover can result in a small deficit during each cycle and therefore finally result in mild osteoporosis. There are no good data regarding the incidence of fracture, but the bone mineral content of several areas known to be at risk of fracture (lumbar spine, forearm, femur) has been measured, mainly in cross-sectional studies, but also in a few prospective studies. During replacement therapy for hypothyroidism a small bone deficit was associated with a prior history of Graves' disease and/or later therapy with dosages of liothyronine or levothyroxine that suppress TSH concentrations (SEDA-16, 471). Since overt hyperthyroidism is associated with bone loss, it is possible that the reduction in bone density reported in some studies of levothyroxine treatment reflects an adverse effect of previous thyrotoxicosis rather than levothyroxine therapy itself (SEDA-17, 473).

In 50 women taking levothyroxine either for primary thyroid failure or for hypothyroidism secondary to radioiodine treatment for hyperthyroidism, there was no difference between the two groups in terms of bone density at the hip or spine and no difference from the reference population (31). In addition, there was no correlation between bone density and circulating thyroid hormone concentrations or duration of levothyroxine replacement. These findings are reassuring, although large studies of fracture risk are required, in view of previous evidence of an adverse effect of levothyroxine on bone mineral density, especially in post-menopausal women (32).

In a meta-analysis of cross-sectional studies suppressive levothyroxine was associated with mild but significant

Table 1 Summary of studies on the effects of thyroid hormones on bone mineralization

Ref	Number and sex (age in years)	Disease	Follow-up period (years)	Femur	Spine	Radius
(33)	7 F1 M	Primary hypothyroidism; levothyroxine 125 micrograms/day	1	–	–9% per year	
(34)	6 F4 M	Hypothyroidism (50 years); levothyroxine135 micrograms/day	1	–7%	–5%	–
(35)	24 M (50)	Primary hypothyroidism (8 years) after ^{131}I	3	NS	NS	NS
(36)	18 F (60)	Hypothyroidism treated for 14 years	2			
		(a) low TSH (levothyroxine 170 micrograms/day)		–1.4% per year	–2.9% per year	–1.2% per year
		(b) normal TSH		–0.3% per year	–1.1% per year	–0.13% per year

bone loss in postmenopausal women (SEDA-20, 394). The best measure of the effects of prolonged levothyroxine therapy can probably be obtained from bone mineral content in patients treated with suppressive doses of levothyroxine for thyroid carcinoma (Table 1).

Postmenopausal women with intact parathyroid glands on prolonged suppressive levothyroxine therapy may be more susceptible to osteoporosis and should have their bone mineral density measured and/or take preventive osteoporosis therapy. Cautious use of levothyroxine, avoiding overdosage and unnecessary use, is probably safe for bone.

Data from more than 30 studies of the effect of thyroid hormone on bone have been reviewed (37). The results have supported the view, expressed before (38), that there is a small, but statistically significant, adverse effect on bone mineral density, especially in postmenopausal women.

A meta-analysis of studies of the effect of thyroxine in TSH-suppressive doses on measurements of bone mineral density has suggested a small but statistically significant adverse effect on bone mineral density, especially in post-menopausal women (39).

Large meta-analyses (40,41) have shown that levothyroxine in TSH-suppressive doses is associated with a minor but statistically significant reduction in bone mineral density. However, the evidence that suppressive doses of levothyroxine represent a risk factor for clinically relevant end points, such as the incidence of fractures and mortality, is scanty (42). A case-control study has examined the association between the use of thyroid hormone and hip fractures in women aged 65 years and over: 501 women with hip fractures in Northern California and 533 age-matched controls without hip fractures (43). There was no difference in the ever use or duration of use of exogenous thyroid hormone between cases and controls (OR = 1.1, 95% CI = 0.8, 1.6), although hip fractures were associated with visual impairment, prior use of glucocorticoids, and falls, as might be expected. These findings are in agreement with the results of another study of hip fracture rates in a large number of subjects in the UK taking thyroxine with those not taking thyroxine (44). There was no association between the use of thyroxine and the occurrence of fractures in women, although there

was an independent association in the smaller number of men taking thyroxine. Overall, these data are reassuring, given the prevalence of thyroxine prescription, especially among women.

Two small studies have shown that low doses of levothyroxine have no adverse effects on bone mass and do not lead to a higher prevalence of vertebral fractures, even if the serum TSH is fully suppressed (45,46).

Immunologic

Fever, liver dysfunction, and eosinophilia occurred during liothyronine or levothyroxine treatment of a hypothyroid patient and disappeared after withdrawal of therapy (47). In vitro lymphocyte testing confirmed sensitization for thyroid hormones.

Progressive re-institution of liothyronine subsequently proved possible in this patient without recurrence of hypersensitivity. Liothyronine was considered preferable because of the shorter biological half-life.

- A patient with a history of an immediate, severe, hypersensitivity reaction at the start of thyroxine therapy subsequently developed a systemic reaction after open challenge with thyroxine (48). Later blinded challenges with both intravenous and oral thyroxine were uneventful, and the final diagnosis was psychogenic vocal cord dysfunction.

This case illustrates the need to verify apparently severe reactions to thyroxine, since such reactions are physiologically unlikely, given that exogenous thyroxine is structurally identical to that produced endogenously.

It is well recognized that antithyroid drugs, and especially propylthiouracil, can be associated with development of anti-neutrophil cytoplasmic antibody (ANCA)-positive vasculitis, often manifesting as renal disease. Atypical presentations, with pyoderma gangrenosum (49) and progressive bilateral sensorineural hearing loss (50), have been described in separate case reports of subjects taking propylthiouracil.

The prevalence of ANCAs and their relation to drug therapy have been examined in a consecutive series of 407 patients with Graves' disease compared with 200 cases of autoimmune hypothyroidism and 649 controls (51).

The prevalence of ANCA, as measured by immunofluorescence, was significantly increased in those with Graves' disease (20%) compared with euthyroid controls (4.6%), as was the prevalence of specific myeloperoxidase (MPO)-ANCA, measured by ELISA. The prevalence of ANCA was more strongly associated with propylthiouracil (RR = 7.3; CI = 4.2, 12.9) than carbimazole (RR = 2.2; CI = 1.8, 2.8) when compared with controls, although there was still a positive association with carbimazole. ANCA positivity was not increased in patients with autoimmune thyroiditis. These findings suggest that the altered immune environment associated with autoimmune thyroid disease is not itself sufficient to increase the risk of development of ANCAs, but that thionamide therapy is required; the risk is higher with propylthiouracil than with carbimazole.

Anti-MPO antibodies have been studied in subjects with propylthiouracil-induced vasculitis or primary systemic vasculitis; there was a potential difference in epitope recognition (52).

Long-Term Effects

Drug abuse

Abuse of thyroid hormones, causing factitious hyperthyroidism, can have adverse effects (53,54), including sudden death, attributed to ventricular fibrillation (55).

Partial empty sella syndrome (pituitary atrophy) has been described in an elite body builder who had abused various hormones, including testosterone, growth hormone, and triiodothyronine 25 micrograms qds for many years (56). He presented with infertility, and investigations showed suppression of serum TSH, a raised serum T3, and a partially empty pituitary sella.

It is likely that in this case long-standing suppression of pituitary function secondary to negative feedback from exogenous hormone ingestion (including liothyronine) resulted in pituitary atrophy.

Tumorigenicity

A possible link between breast cancer in women and thyroid hormone therapy was suggested on the basis of a retrospective study of patients with breast cancer (SEDA-3, 340). A subsequent statistical re-analysis of the original data failed, as did later studies, to confirm such a relation (SEDA-3, 340; SEDA-4, 294; 57).

Second-Generation Effects

Pregnancy

The transplacental passage of maternal iodothyronines is quantitatively modest, although it might be sufficient to ensure adequate fetal development. Maternal thyroid hormone secretion is markedly increased during pregnancy (by 25–50%); thyroid therapy should therefore be carefully adjusted during pregnancy (58).

Teratogenicity

The issue of whether antithyroid drug administration in early pregnancy is associated with congenital abnormalities remains unclear. Aplasia cutis congenita and choanal atresia have been reported in association with maternal carbimazole therapy, suggesting a causative link either with the drug or with underlying hyperthyroidism. A further case of aplasia cutis has been described in an infant of a mother with Graves' disease exposed to methimazole (40 mg/day) for the first 6 weeks of gestation (59). Three further cases of choanal atresia have also been described in association with methimazole exposure in early fetal life (60). These cases continue to highlight a possible link between carbimazole, or its active metabolite methimazole, and congenital abnormalities, and they reinforce the view that propylthiouracil is the drug of choice in early pregnancy. However, it should be noted that one of the major hazards of antithyroid drug use in pregnancy is over-treatment, and hence induction of fetal hypothyroidism and goiter.

- Fetal hydrops and goiter occurred at 29 weeks of gestation after the mother had taken propylthiouracil 200 mg/day for Graves' disease (61). Although the mother was biochemically euthyroid, fetal blood sampling showed hypothyroidism, with a raised serum TSH. Both the fetal hydrops and goiter regressed after withdrawal of maternal propylthiouracil and intra-amniotic administration of levothyroxine.

It is important to monitor maternal thyroid status carefully and to use the lowest possible dose of antithyroid drug sufficient to maintain maternal euthyroidism.

Susceptibility Factors

Pre-existing cardiac disease and long-standing hypothyroidism carry serious risks.

Adrenal insufficiency can be associated with hypothyroidism (either by autoimmune destruction or due to hypophyseal disease) and carries the risk of acute Addisonian crisis if thyroid substitution precedes glucocorticoid therapy. The diagnostic problem presented by the fact that a few patients with central hypothyroidism have a moderately increased serum TSH should be kept in mind (62).

Some goitrous patients have autonomous thyroid hormone secretion, which is still within the reference range, but they become hyperthyroid even with relatively small amounts of exogenous thyroid hormones, since the latter accumulate with the endogenous autonomous thyroid secretion.

Rarely severe gastrointestinal disease can reduce the absorption of levothyroxine.

Since levothyroxine is occasionally used in supraphysiological doses to treat euthyroid people with refractory depression, adverse effects in healthy controls (n = 13) and patients with refractory depression also taking antidepressants (n = 13) have been studied in an 8-week, non-blind study (63). There was a higher rate of discontinuation of levothyroxine in the control subjects than in the patients, because of perceived adverse effects (38% versus 0%), together with a more marked rise in serum free T4 and free T3 in the controls. This suggests that the influence of supraphysiological doses of thyroxine is greater in healthy subjects than in those with psychiatric illness, perhaps reflecting the influence of the illness, or its therapy, on thyroid hormone metabolism in the latter.

Drug Administration

Drug overdose

Inadvertent excessive use of thyroid hormones (for example, by eating ground beef contaminated with thyroid hormones (64), the incorrect use of these drugs for the treatment of obesity (65), excessive thyroid substitution therapy, and factitious use of thyroid hormones for psychiatric reasons (66)) result in mild hyperthyroidism, but serious short-term adverse effects are rare.

Overdosage of levothyroxine causes increased metabolism resulting in increased heat production, with increased sweating and weight loss despite normal or even increased appetite. Accidental or suicidal injection of large amounts of thyroid hormones is exceptional (67). Clinical symptoms do not necessarily correlate well with plasma T4 concentrations and range from anxiety, confusion, or coma to tachycardia, atrial fibrillation, and angina. At least three lethal cases have been reported (SEDA-8, 371).

- A 34-year-old man took 900 tablets of veterinary levothyroxine, a total of 720 mg, and was given 60 g of activated charcoal (68). He became lethargic on days 2 and 3; on day 4 he had vomiting, sweating, and insomnia; on day 5 he became agitated and aggressive and stopped speaking intelligibly; and on day 6 he became combative and confused. He was sweating, mydriatic, hyper-reflexive, and tremulous, with clear lungs and active bowel sounds. He was given activated charcoal, haloperidol, diazepam, and phenobarbital, and had an endotracheal tube inserted. He was rehydrated and given propranolol and diazepam, but remained continuously tachycardic. On day 12 he became afebrile and his tachycardia resolved. Free T4 concentrations ranged from over 130 ng/l on day 6 to 12 ng/l on day 12. By discharge on day 15 he had lost 20 kg in weight, but was clinically euthyroid 2 weeks later.
- Self-induced thyrotoxicosis was associated with a marked rise in circulating free T4 and free T3 concentrations in a pregnant woman with an eating disorder who was abusing both levothyroxine and furosemide (69).

Treatment of thyroid overdosage is not standardized and can include gastric lavage, sedatives, beta-blockers, hydrocortisone, and specific antidysrhythmic drugs. Plasmapheresis (70) and exchange transfusion (71) have been used successfully to treat life-threatening cases. Iodine-containing organic radiographic agents (ipodate) can be effective, since they are potent inhibitors of the peripheral conversion of T4 to T3, but rebound effects can occur (67).

Drug–Drug Interactions

Antacids

Two patients with hypothyroidism taking a fixed dosage of levothyroxine took aluminium hydroxide and magnesium oxide (72). In both cases there was a marked increase in the serum concentration of TSH and low serum T4. After withdrawal of the antacids, TSH again fell. In vitro studies showed a dose-related adsorption of levothyroxine by a combination of aluminium hydroxide, magnesium hydroxide, and magnesium carbonate, but no effect of magnesium oxide alone.

Calcium carbonate

Calcium carbonate can reduce levothyroxine absorption (73).

- A 49-year-old woman, taking levothyroxine 150 micrograms/day and calcium carbonate (three tablets daily) for prevention of osteoporosis, developed symptoms of hypothyroidism and had a raised serum TSH concentration (22 mU/l). She was advised to continue taking the same dose of levothyroxine but to separate her medications. Repeat biochemical testing 8 months later showed a normal serum TSH (3.3 mU/l).
- A 61-year-old woman with hypothyroidism had celiac disease and a history of bowel resection for pancreatic cancer, was euthyroid taking thyroxine 175–188 micrograms/day (74). However, when she simultaneously took calcium carbonate (1250 mg/day) she had a raised serum thyrotropin (TSH) concentration of 41 mU/l. Delaying calcium carbonate ingestion by 4 hours returned her serum TSH concentration to high normal (5.7 mU/l) within a month.

Because of the possibility that calcium carbonate might impair levothyroxine absorption, another group carried out a prospective study in 20 patients taking stable long-term levothyroxine for hypothyroidism, who were given elemental calcium as calcium carbonate 1200 mg/day, taken with their levothyroxine for 3 months (75). Mean serum concentrations of free thyroxine and total thyroxine were significantly reduced during the calcium treatment period and rose after withdrawal. Mean concentrations of T3 did not change, but serum TSH rose during the calcium period, and 20% of the subjects had a serum TSH concentration above the reference range. The authors also reported the results of an in vitro study of thyroxine binding to calcium, which showed that there is adsorption of thyroxine to calcium at acidic pH. These findings show that calcium salts can have a modest put potentially clinically significant effect on levothyroxine treatment, probably by binding it and reducing its absorption; patients should be advised to separate their medications.

Colestyramine

Colestyramine can reduce thyroxine absorption (76).

Estrogens and selective estrogen receptor modulators

Estrogens and selective estrogen receptor modulators, such as tamoxifen citrate and raloxifene hydrochloride, can affect tests of thyroid function by their ability to increase the serum concentration of thyroxine binding globulin, leading to a rise in serum concentrations of total thyroxine and triiodothyronine (T3), although serum free T4, free T3, and TSH concentrations remain unchanged. These effects do not occur with transdermal estrogens (77). Thus, oral estrogens increase levothyroxine dosage requirements in women with primary hypothyroidism, at least during the first few months after the start of therapy.

In subjects with treated hypothyroidism it has been reported that exogenous estrogen, given as hormone replacement therapy, can lead to increased thyroxine dosage requirements (78).

- A 79 year old woman taking long-term thyroxine 150 micrograms/day developed a raised TSH and symptoms of hypothyroidism after the introduction of raloxifene hydrochloride 60 mg/day for osteopenia (79). Ingestion of thyroxine and raloxifene at the same time resulted in biochemical hypothyroidism, but not if ingestion they were separated by 12 hours. A 6-hour absorption test showed blunting of the rise in serum total thyroxine after ingestion of 100 micrograms of thyroxine co-administered with raloxifene.

While an effect of raloxifene on circulating thyroxine-binding globulin is well recognized, this case suggests an additional effect on thyroxine absorption.

Ferrous sulfate

Iron binds thyroxine in vitro (80) and ferrous sulfate can reduce thyroxine absorption (81). This can result in hypothyroidism (80,81). A similar interaction with ferrous fumarate has been described in a patient who took both medications simultaneously (83). Separation of thyroxine from iron may be prudent, since this interaction may reflect the formation of a non-absorbable complex in the gut (80).

Imatinib

In a small study, imatinib, a tyrosine kinase inhibitor used in the treatment of a number of neoplastic diseases, increased the doses of levothyroxine necessary for adequate replacement therapy (84).

Indinavir

Levothyroxine is metabolized in part through the action of glucuronyl transferase, which can be inhibited by some antiretroviral drugs, such as indinavir.

- Clinical and biochemical hyperthyroidism occurred in a 36-year-old woman, after previously stable levothyroxine replacement therapy, when antiretroviral drugs for HIV infection were introduced (85). She was reported to be taking a very large dose of levothyroxine (750 micrograms/day) after partial thyroidectomy for Graves' hyperthyroidism some 6 years before. One month after starting antiretroviral treatment she developed symptoms and signs suggestive of thyroid hormone excess and had markedly raised serum free T4 and free T3 concentrations, with suppression of TSH. The dose of levothyroxine was reduced progressively to 120 micrograms/day, and after about 2 months her thyroid function tests returned to normal.

While this pattern of biochemistry does not exclude transient relapse of Graves' hyperthyroidism (despite the finding of negative TSH receptor antibodies), or a transient thyroiditis, the authors speculated that indinavir (prescribed in this patient together with stavudine and lamivudine) had inhibited the glucuronidation of thyroxine and hence caused a rise in serum thyroid hormone concentrations.

Orlistat

There has been a report that orlistat, used in the management of obesity, reduced the systemic availability of levothyroxine (86).

Rifampicin

There was a modest rise in serum TSH concentration when rifampicin was given to a patient previously stabilized on thyroxine replacement (87). Rifampicin is believed to increase the metabolic clearance of both thyroxine and the inactive compound reverse triiodothyronine and in healthy volunteers it reduces circulating concentrations of total and free thyroxine, although in subjects without thyroid disease it has no effect on serum TSH (86).

Tricyclic antidepressants

Spurious hyperthyroidism occurred in a child taking thyroid hormone and imipramine for enuresis (89). The ability of thyroid hormone to increase receptor sensitivity to catecholamines has long been known, and has been used to enhance the clinical response in some refractory patients, especially women.

Monitoring Therapy

Some diseases (liver disease, kidney disease, and malnutrition) interfere with the transport or metabolism of thyroid hormones and thereby alter thyroid function tests.

Several drugs (for example amiodarone, androgens, glucocorticoids, phenytoin, and salicylates) interfere with the transport or metabolism of thyroid hormones and thereby alter thyroid function tests. These have been reviewed (90). In patients taking levothyroxine serum TSH rises after treatment with sertraline (91) and antimalarial prophylaxis with chloroquine and proguanil (SEDA-22, 469).

References

1. Chopra IJ, Cody V. Triiodothyronines in health and disease. In: Gross F, editor. Monographs on Endocrinology 18. Berlin–Heidelberg–New York: Springer-Verlag, 1981:1.

2. Fish LH, Schwartz HL, Cavanaugh J, Steffes MW, Bantle JP, Oppenheimer JH. Replacement dose, metabolism, and bioavailability of levothyroxine in the treatment of hypothyroidism. Role of triiodothyronine in pituitary feedback in humans. N Engl J Med 1987;316(13):764–70.

3. Kaufman SC, Gross TP, Kennedy DL. Thyroid hormone use: trends in the United States from 1960 through 1988. Thyroid 1991;1:285–91.

4. Parle JV, Franklyn JA, Cross KW, Jones SR, Sheppard MC. Thyroxine prescription in the community: serum thyroid stimulating hormone level assays as an indicator of undertreatment or overtreatment. Br J Gen Pract 1993;43:107–9.

5. Canaris GJ, Manowitz NR, Mayor G, Ridgway EC. The Colorado thyroid disease prevalence study. Arch Intern Med 2000;160:526–34.

6. Pristautz H, Leb G, Raber J, Goebel R, Steinberger R, Borkenstein J. Beeinflussung laborchemischer und nuklearmedizinischer Schilddrüsenparameter unter der Behandlung mit einem hochgereinigten D-Thyroxin-Präparat. [Influence of a highly purified D-thyroxine medication on thyroid iodine uptake and in vitro tests of thyroid function.] MMW Munch Med Wochenschr 1980;122(6):199–202.

7. Wartofsky L. Myxedema coma. In: Braverman LE, Utiger RD, editors. Werner and Ingbar's The Thyroid. 6th ed. Philadelphia: J.B. Lippincott, 1991:1089.

8. Carr D, McLeod DT, Parry G, Thornes HM. Fine adjustment of thyroxine replacement dosage: comparison of the thyrotrophin releasing hormone test using a sensitive thyrotrophin assay with measurement of free thyroid hormones and clinical assessment. Clin Endocrinol (Oxf) 1988;28(3):325–33.

9. Paul TL, Kerrigan J, Kelly AM, Braverman LE, Baran DT. Long-term L-thyroxine therapy is associated with decreased hip bone density in premenopausal women. JAMA 1988;259(21):3137–41.

10. Hiasa Y, Ishida T, Aihara T, Bando M, Nakai Y, Kataoka Y, Mori H. Acute myocardial infarction due to coronary spasm associated with L-thyroxine therapy. Clin Cardiol 1989;12(3):161–3.

11. Kologlu S, Baskal N, Kologlu LB, Laleli Y, Tuccar E. Hirsutism due to the treatment with L-thyroxine in patients with thyroid pathology. Endocrinologie 1988;26(3):179–85.

12. Exley A, O'Malley BP. Depression in primary hypothyroidism masquerading as inadequate or excessive L-thyroxine consumption. Q J Med 1989;72(269):867–70.

13. Escobar-Morreale HF, Obregon MJ, Escobar del Rey F, Morreale de Escobar G. Replacement therapy for hypothyroidism with thyroxine alone does not ensure euthyroidism in all tissues, as studied in thyroidectomized rats. J Clin Invest 1995;96(6):2828–38.

14. Bunevicius R, Kazanavicius G, Zalinkevicius R, Prange AJ Jr. Effects of thyroxine as compared with thyroxine plus triiodothyronine in patients with hypothyroidism. N Engl J Med 1999;340(6):424–9.

15. Hennemann G, Docter R, Visser TJ, Postema PT, Krenning EP. Thyroxine plus low-dose, slow-release triiodothyronine replacement in hypothyroidism: proof of principle. Thyroid 2004;14(4):271–5.

16. Biondi B, Fazio S, Cuocolo A, Sabatini D, Nicolai E, Lombardi G, Salvatore M, Sacca L. Impaired cardiac reserve and exercise capacity in patients receiving long-term thyrotropin suppressive therapy with levothyroxine. J Clin Endocrinol Metab 1996;81(12):4224–8.

17. Sawin CT, Geller A, Wolf PA, Belanger AJ, Baker E, Bacharach P, Wilson PW, Benjamin EJ, D'Agostino RB. Low serum thyrotropin concentrations as a risk factor for atrial fibrillation in older persons. N Engl J Med 1994;331(19):1249–52.

18. Biondi B, Fazio S, Coltorti F, Palmieri EA, Carella C, Lombardi G, Sacca L. Clinical case seminar. Reentrant atrioventricular nodal tachycardia induced by levothyroxine. J Clin Endocrinol Metab 1998;83(8):2643–5.

19. Toft AD, Boon NA. Thyroid disease and the heart. Heart 2000;84(4):455–60.

20. Ching GW, Franklyn JA, Stallard TJ, Daykin J, Sheppard MC, Gammage MD. Cardiac hypertrophy as a result of long-term thyroxine therapy and thyrotoxicosis. Heart 1996;75(4):363–8.

21. Kohno A, Hara Y. Severe myocardial ischemia following hormone replacement in two cases of hypothyroidism with normal coronary arteriogram. Endocr J 2001;48(5):565–72.

22. Locker GJ, Kotzmann H, Frey B, Messina FC, Strez FR, Weissel M, Laggner AN. Factitious hyperthyroidism causing acute myocardial infarction. Thyroid 1995;5(6):465–7.

23. The Coronary Drug Project Research Group. The coronary drug project. Findings leading to further modifications of its protocol with respect to dextrothyroxine. JAMA 1972;220(7):996–1008.

24. Van Dop C, Conte FA, Koch TK, Clark SJ, Wilson-Davis SL, Grumbach MM. Pseudotumor cerebri associated with initiation of levothyroxine therapy for juvenile hypothyroidism. N Engl J Med 1983;308(18):1076–80.

25. Josephson AM, Mackenzie TB. Thyroid-induced mania in hypothyroid patients. Br J Psychiatry 1980;137:222–8.

26. El Kaissi S, Kotowicz MA, Berk M, Wall JR. Acute delirium in the setting of primary hypothyroidism: the role of thyroid hormone replacement therapy. Thyroid 2005;15(9):1099–101.

27. Goldstein BI, Levitt AJ. Thyroxine-associated hypomania. J Am Acad Child Adolesc Psychiatry 2005;44(3):211.

28. Evans DL, Strawn SK, Haggerty JJ Jr, Garbutt JC, Burnett GB, Pedersen CA. Appearance of mania in drug-resistant bipolar depressed patients after treatment with L-triiodothyronine. J Clin Psychiatry 1986;47(10):521–2.

29. Medeiros-Neto GA. Osteopenia e tratamento com L-tiroxina. [Osteopenia and treatment with L-thyroxine.] Rev Assoc Med Bras 1995;41(1):34–6.

30. Auwerx J, Bouillon R. Mineral and bone metabolism in thyroid disease: a review. Q J Med 1986;60(232):737–52.

31. Hanna FW, Pettit RJ, Ammari F, Evans WD, Sandeman D, Lazarus JH. Effect of replacement doses of thyroxine on bone mineral density. Clin Endocrinol (Oxf) 1998;48(2):229–34.

32. Uzzan B, Campos J, Cucherat M, Nony P, Boissel JP, Perret GY. Effects on bone mass of long term treatment with thyroid hormones: a meta-analysis. J Clin Endocrinol Metab 1996;81(12):4278–89.

33. Krolner B, Jorgensen JV, Nielsen SP. Spinal bone mineral content in myxoedema and thyrotoxicosis. Effects of thyroid hormone(s) and antithyroid treatment. Clin Endocrinol (Oxf) 1983;18(5):439–46.

34. Ribot C, Tremollieres F, Pouilles JM, Louvet JP. Bone mineral density and thyroid hormone therapy. Clin Endocrinol (Oxf) 1990;33(2):143–53.

35. Toh SH, Brown PH. Bone mineral content in hypothyroid male patients with hormone replacement: a 3-year study. J Bone Miner Res 1990;5(5):463–7.

36. Stall GM, Harris S, Sokoll LJ, Dawson-Hughes B. Accelerated bone loss in hypothyroid patients overtreated with L-thyroxine. Ann Intern Med 1990;113(4):265–9.

37. Stathatos NWL. Effects of thyroid hormone on bone. Clin Rev Bone Mineral Metab 2005;2:135–50.

38. Uzzan B, Campos J, Cucherat M, Nony P, Boissel JP, Perret GY. Effects on bone mass of long term treatment with thyroid hormones: a meta-analysis. J Clin Endocrinol Metab 1996;81(12):4278–89.

39. Uzzan B, Campos J, Cucherat M, Nony P, Boissel JP, Perret GY. Effects on bone mass of long term treatment with thyroid hormones: a meta-analysis. J Clin Endocrinol Metab 1996;81:4278–89.

40. Faber J, Galloe AM. Changes in bone mass during prolonged subclinical hyperthyroidism due to L-thyroxine treatment: a meta-analysis. Eur J Endocrinol 1994;130(4):350–6.

41. Uzzan B, Campos J, Cucherat M, Nony P, Boissel JP, Perret GY. Effects on bone mass of long term treatment with thyroid hormones: a meta-analysis. J Clin Endocrinol Metab 1996;81(12):4278–89.

42. Boelaert K, Franklyn JA. Thyroid hormone in health and disease. J Endocrinol 2005; 187(1): 1–15.

43. Van Den Eeden SK, Barzilay JI, Ettinger B, Minkoff J. Thyroid hormone use and the risk of hip fracture in women > or = 65 years: a case-control study. J Womens Health (Larchmt) 2003;12:27–31.

44. Sheppard MC, Holder R, Franklyn JA. Levothyroxine treatment and occurrence of fracture of the hip. Arch Intern Med 2002;162:338–43.

45. Appetecchia M. Effects on bone mineral density by treatment of benign nodular goiter with mildly suppressive doses of L-thyroxine in a cohort women study. Horm Res 2005; 64(6):293–8.

46. Heijckmann AC, Huijberts MS, Geusens P, de Vries J, Menheere PP, Wolffenbuttel BH. Hip bone mineral density, bone turnover and risk of fracture in patients on long-term suppressive L-thyroxine therapy for differentiated thyroid carcinoma. Eur J Endocrinol 2005;153(1):23–9.

47. Shibata H, Hayakawa H, Hirukawa M, Tadokoro K, Ogata E. Hypersensitivity caused by synthetic thyroid hormones in a hypothyroid patient with Hashimoto's thyroiditis. Arch Intern Med 1986;146(8):1624–5.

48. Nugent JS, Nugent AL, Whisman BA, White K, Hagan LL. Levothyroxine anaphylaxis? Vocal cord dysfunction mimicking an anaphylactic drug reaction. Ann Allergy Asthma Immunol 2003;91:337–41.

49. Hong SB, Lee MH. A case of propylthiouracil-induced pyoderma gangrenosum associated with antineutrophil cytoplasmic antibody. Dermatology 2004;208(4):339–41.

50. Sano M, Kitahara N, Kunikata R. Progressive bilateral sensorineural hearing loss induced by an antithyroid drug. ORL J Otorhinolaryngol Relat Spec 2004;66(5):281–5.

51. Harper L, Chin L, Daykin J, Allahabadia A, Heward J, Gough SC, Savage CO, Franklyn JA. Propylthiouracil and carbimazole associated-antineutrophil cytoplasmic antibodies (ANCA) in patients with Graves' disease. Clin Endocrinol (Oxf) 2004;60(6):671–5.

52. Ye H, Zhao MH, Gao Y, Guo XH, Wang HY. Anti-myeloperoxidase antibodies in sera from patients with propylthiouracil-induced vasculitis might recognize restricted epitopes on myeloperoxidase molecule. Clin Exp Immunol 2004;138(1):179–82.

53. Keck FS, Loos U, Duntas L, Pfeiffer EF. Hyperthyreosis factitia acuta—Geringe klinische Symptome bei drei Fallen unter beta-Blocker-Behandlung. [Acute factitious hyperthyroidism—moderate clinical symptoms in 3 cases under beta-blocker treatment.] Klin Wochenschr 1986;64(7):319–26.

54. Galvan G. Hyperthyreosis factitia durch L-Thyroxinabusus: ein Fallbericht. [Factitious hyperthyroidism caused by L-thyroxin abuse. Case report.] Acta Med Austriaca 1983;10(2–3):79–81.

55. Bhasin S, Wallace W, Lawrence JB, Lesch M. Sudden death associated with thyroid hormone abuse. Am J Med 1981;71(5):887–90.

56. Dickerman RD, Jaikumar S. Secondary partial empty sella syndrome in an elite bodybuilder. Neurol Res 2001;23(4):336–8.

57. Gorman CA, Becker DV, Greenspan FS, Levy RP, Oppenheimer JH, Rivlin RS, Robbins J, Vanderlaan WP. Breast cancer and thyroid therapy. Statement by the American Thyroid Association. JAMA 1977;237(14):1459–60.

58. Glinoer D. Thyroid disease during pregnancy. In: Braverman LE, Utiger R, editors. Werner and Ingbar's The Thyroid. A Fundamental and Clinical Text. 8th ed.. Philadelphia: J.B. Lippincott, 2000:1013–27.

59. Barbero P, Ricagni C, Mercado G, Bronberg R, Torrado M. Choanal atresia associated with prenatal methimazole exposure: three new patients. Am J Med Genet A 2004;129(1):83–6.

60. Karg E, Bereg E, Gaspar L, Katona M, Turi S. Aplasia cutis congenita after methimazole exposure in utero. Pediatr Dermatol 2004;21(4):491–4.

61. Yanai N, Shveiky D. Fetal hydrops, associated with maternal propylthiouracil exposure, reversed by intrauterine therapy. Ultrasound Obstet Gynecol 2004;23(2):198–201.

62. Martino E, Bambini G, Bartalena L, Mammoli C, Aghini-Lombardi F, Baschieri L, Pinchera A. Human serum thyrotrophin measurement by ultrasensitive immunoradiometric assay as a first-line test in the evaluation of thyroid function. Clin Endocrinol (Oxf) 1986;24(2):141–8.

63. Bauer M, Baur H, Berghofer A, Strohle A, Hellweg R, Muller-Oerlinghausen B, Baumgartner A. Effects of supraphysiological thyroxine administration in healthy controls and patients with depressive disorders. J Affect Disord 2002;68(2–3):285–94.

64. Hedberg CW, Fishbein DB, Janssen RS, Meyers B, McMillen JM, MacDonald KL, White KE, Huss LJ, Hurwitz ES, Farhie JR, et al. An outbreak of thyrotoxicosis caused by the consumption of bovine thyroid gland in ground beef. N Engl J Med 1987;316(16):993–8.

65. Krotkiewski M. Thyroid hormones in the pathogenesis and treatment of obesity. Eur J Pharmacol 2002; 440(2–3):85–98.

66. Fuessl HS. Verwirrende Schilddruse. Hyperthyreosis factitia. [The confusing thyroid gland. Factitious hyperthyroidism.] MMW Fortschr Med 1999;141(36):53–4.

67. Cohen JH 3rd, Ingbar SH, Braverman LE. Thyrotoxicosis due to ingestion of excess thyroid hormone. Endocr Rev 1989;10(2):113–24.

68. Hack JB, Leviss JA, Nelson LS, Hoffman RS. Severe symptoms following a massive intentional L-thyroxine ingestion. Vet Hum Toxicol 1999;41(5):323–6.

69. Wark H, Wallace EM, Wigg S, Tippett C. Thyroxine abuse: an unusual case of thyrotoxicosis in pregnancy. Aust NZ J Obstet Gynaecol 1998;38(2):221–3.

70. May ME, Mintz PD, Lowry P, Geller R, Curnow RT. Plasmapheresis in thyroxine overdose: a case report. J Toxicol Clin Toxicol 1983;20(5):517–20.

71. Gerard P, Malvaux P, De Visscher M. Accidental poisoning with thyroid extract treated by exchange transfusion. Arch Dis Child 1972;47(256):981–982.

72. Mersebach H, Rasmussen AK, Kirkegaard L, Feldt-Rasmussen U. Intestinal adsorption of levothyroxine by antacids and laxatives: case stories and in vitro experiments. Pharmacol Toxicol 1999;84(3):107–9.

73. Butner LE, Fulco PP, Feldman G. Calcium carbonate-induced hypothyroidism. Ann Intern Med 2000;132(7):595.
74. Csako G, McGriff NJ, Rotman-Pikielny P, Sarlis NJ, Pucino F. Exaggerated levothyroxine malabsorption due to calcium carbonate supplementation in gastrointestinal disorders. Ann Pharmacother 2001;35(12):1578–83.
75. Singh N, Singh PN, Hershman JM. Effect of calcium carbonate on the absorption of levothyroxine. JAMA 2000;283(21):2822–5.
76. Farmer JA, Gotto AM Jr. Antihyperlipidaemic agents. Drug interactions of clinical significance. Drug Saf 1994;11(5):301–9.
77. Mazer NA. Interaction of estrogen therapy and thyroid hormone replacement in postmenopausal women. Thyroid 2004;14(Suppl 1):S27–34.
78. Arafah BM. Increased need for thyroxine in women with hypothyroidism during estrogen therapy. New Engl J Med 2001;344:1743–9.
79. Siraj ES, Gupta MK, Reddy SS. Raloxifene causing malabsorption of levothyroxine. Arch Intern Med 2003;163:1367–70.
80. Campbell NR, Hasinoff BB, Stalts H, Rao B, Wong NC. Ferrous sulfate reduces thyroxine efficacy in patients with hypothyroidism. Ann Intern Med 1992;117(12):1010–3.
81. Schlienger JL. Accroissement des besoins en thyroxine par le sulfate de fer. [Increased need for thyroxine induced by iron sulfate.] Presse Méd 1994;23(10):492.
82. Shakir KM, Chute JP, Aprill BS, Lazarus AA. Ferrous sulfate-induced increase in requirement for thyroxine in a patient with primary hypothyroidism. South Med J 1997;90(6):637–9.
83. Leger CS, Chye T. Ferrous fumarate-induced malabsorption of thyroxine. Endocrinologist 1999;9:493–5.
84. de Groot JW, Zonnenberg BA, Plukker JT, Der Graaf WT, Links TP. Imatinib induces hypothyroidism in patients receiving levothyroxine. Clin Pharmacol Ther 2005;78(4):433–8.
85. Lanzafame M, Trevenzoli M, Faggian F, Marcati P, Gatti F, Carolo G, Concia E. Interaction between levothyroxine and indinavir in a patient with HIV infection. Infection 2002;30(1):54–5.
86. Madhava K, Hartley A. Hypothyroidism in thyroid carcinoma follow-up: orlistat may inhibit the absorption of thyroxine. Clin Oncol (R Coll Radiol) 2005;17(6):492.
87. Nolan SR, Self TH, Norwood JM. Interaction between rifampin and levothyroxine. South Med J 1999;92(5):529–31.
88. Ohnhaus EE, Studer H. A link between liver microsomal enzyme activity and thyroid hormone metabolism in man. Br J Clin Pharmacol 1983;15(1):71–6.
89. Colantonio L, Orson J. Hyperthyroidism with normal T4-induction by imipramine. Clin Pharmacol Ther 1975;15:203.
90. Davies PH, Franklyn JA. The effects of drugs on tests of thyroid function. Eur J Clin Pharmacol 1991;40(5):439–51.
91. McCowen KC, Garber JR, Spark R. Elevated serum thyrotropin in thyroxine-treated patients with hypothyroidism given sertraline. N Engl J Med 1997;337(14):1010–1.

Thyrotrophin and thyrotropin

General Information

Thyrotrophin is native thyroid-stimulating hormone. Recombinant human thyrotrophin is called thyrotropin.

Thyrotropin stimulates iodine uptake, and this facilitates the diagnosis and treatment of recurrent disease or metastases in the follow-up of differentiated thyroid cancer. It is used as an alternative to thyroid hormone withdrawal, to avoid symptomatic hypothyroidism (1). Headache and nausea occur in 6–40% of patients after intramuscular administration, but are usually mild and transient (2,3).

The adverse effects of thyrotropin have been reviewed (4).

Organs and Systems

Immunologic

Many years ago bovine thyrotrophin was used for diagnostic purposes and to increase ^{131}I uptake. However, for diagnostic purposes it has been replaced by sensitive TSH assays, and because of antibody development and hypersensitivity reactions it is not used therapeutically. There is no evidence that thyrotropin causes allergic reactions, even after multiple injections (4).

Rapid tumor expansion has been occasionally reported after thyrotropin, including four of 55 patients with central nervous system metastases enrolled in a compassionate use protocol (5). Two patients with locally recurrent papillary carcinoma had tumor growth 12–48 hours after their second injection of recombinant thyrotropin (rTSH); rapid improvement in neck pain, stridor, and dysphonia after glucocorticoids suggested an inflammatory etiology (5). There were no features to suggest an allergic reaction; only one such case has been reported and there are no reports of antibody formation even after repeated dosing (1).

References

1. McDougall IR, Weigel RJ. Recombinant human thyrotropin in the management of thyroid cancer. Curr Opin Oncol 2001;13(1):39–43.
2. Haugen BR, Pacini F, Reiners C, Schlumberger M, Ladenson PW, Sherman SI, Cooper DS, Graham KE, Braverman LE, Skarulis MC, Davies TF, DeGroot LJ, Mazzaferri EL, Daniels GH, Ross DS, Luster M, Samuels MH, Becker DV, Maxon HR 3rd, Cavalieri RR, Spencer CA, McEllin K, Weintraub BD, Ridgway EC. A comparison of recombinant human thyrotropin and thyroid hormone withdrawal for the detection of thyroid remnant or cancer. J Clin Endocrinol Metab 1999;84(11):3877–85.
3. Durski JM, Weigel RJ, McDougall IR. Recombinant human thyrotropin (rhTSH) in the management of differentiated thyroid cancer. Nucl Med Commun 2000;21(6):521–8.
4. Robbins RJ, Robbins AK. Clinical review 156: Recombinant human thyrotropin and thyroid cancer management. J Clin Endocrinol Metab 2003;88(5):1933–8.
5. Braga M, Ringel MD, Cooper DS. Sudden enlargement of local recurrent thyroid tumor after recombinant human TSH administration. J Clin Endocrinol Metab 2001;86(11):5148–51.

INSULINS AND OTHER HYPOGLYCEMIC DRUGS

Aldose reductase inhibitors

General Information

Aldose reductase inhibitors (SEDA-19, 397; SEDA-20, 399; SEDA-21, 447; SEDA-22, 477) have been developed for the treatment of secondary complications in diabetes (1,2). They include alrestatin, benurestat, epalrestat, fidarestat, imirestat, lidorestat, minalrestat, ponalrestat, ranirestat, risarestat, sorbinil, tolrestat, zenarestat, and zopolrestat (all rINNs).

The aldose reductase inhibitors inhibit or reduce secondary complications induced by diabetes, specifically in tissues in which glucose uptake is not insulin-dependent (probably neural tissue, the lens, and glomeruli). Many of them (including alrestatin, imirestat, ponalrestat, and sorbinil) have been used in clinical trials, but have been withdrawn because of adverse effects or lack of effect (2). Their main adverse effects include fever, nausea, diarrhea, increases in liver enzymes, skin rashes, including toxic epidermal necrolysis and Stevens–Johnson syndrome, marked thrombocytopenia, lymphadenopathy, splenomegaly, and adult respiratory distress syndrome.

Tolrestat was withdrawn because of deaths from fatal hepatic necrosis (3) and poor efficacy in clinical trials. Sorbinil was withdrawn because of hypersensitivity reactions in more than 10% of patients.

Organs and Systems

Gastrointestinal

Nausea, vomiting, abdominal fullness, and diarrhea are reported with aldose reductase inhibitors (1).

References

1. Tsai SC, Burnakis TG. Aldose reductase inhibitors: an update. Ann Pharmacother 1993;27(6):751–4.
2. Krans HM. Recent clinical experience with aldose reductase inhibitors. Diabet Med 1993;10(Suppl 2):S44–8.
3. Foppiano M, Lombardo G. Worldwide pharmacovigilance systems and tolrestat withdrawal. Lancet 1997;349(9049):399–400.

Alpha-glucosidase inhibitors

General Information

Alpha-glucosidase inhibitors are competitive inhibitors of 1α-glucosidases, enzymes that are located in the brush border of epithelial cells, mainly in the upper half of the small intestine. The enzymes degrade complex carbohydrates into monosaccharides, which are absorbed. The alpha-glucosidase inhibitors bind reversibly in a dose-dependent manner to the oligosaccharide binding site of these enzymes and delay the degradation of polysaccharides and starch to glucose. They slow down food digestion in the gut, reducing peak blood glucose concentrations after meals. They also prevent reactive hypoglycemia, as can be seen after gastric operations, in dumping syndrome, and in idiopathic forms. When carbohydrates appear in the colon, bacterial fermentation can occur, leading to gastrointestinal adverse effects, of which flatulence and loose stools are the most frequent. During long-term treatment the colonic bacterial mass can increase. In elderly patients acarbose increases insulin sensitivity but not insulin release (1). Acarbose may reduce the incidence of colon cancer, the risk of which is 30% higher in people with diabetes than in the non-diabetic population (2).

The alpha-glucosidase inhibitors (polyhexose mimickers) in use are acarbose (rINN) (2–4), miglitol (rINN) (5–7), and voglibose (rINN), which is 20 times more potent (8). They have been reviewed (9).

Acarbose is not well absorbed and is mostly excreted in the feces. Miglitol is well absorbed from the gut and is almost completely excreted unchanged in the urine (10).

Observational studies

In a 2-year study of the tolerability and safety of acarbose in 2035 patients the incidence of adverse effects was 7.5% and of withdrawals 2.5% (11). Of 1907 patients, 444 (23%) reported one or more adverse events. In 143 patients the physician considered that there was a probable or possible relation between the adverse event (all gastrointestinal) and acarbose. There were 77 deaths, but none was considered to be related to acarbose; 52 stopped taking acarbose because of an adverse event and 45 were considered to be related to acarbose. Laboratory analyses were all within the reference ranges. HbA_{1c} fell by 1.92%.

The addition of metformin to acarbose in 49 patients produced a synergistic effect (12).

Of 1027 patients, 283 used acarbose as the treatment of choice (13). In 250 cases the physician was not sure of the benefit; 124 of these patients took acarbose and 126 patients took placebo besides regular therapy. In those taking acarbose HbA_{1c} fell. The adverse effects were bloating, flatulence, abdominal cramps, and diarrhea; there were moderate increases in serum transaminases.

In a post-marketing surveillance study in 27 803 patients with diabetes mellitus (94% type 2), data were reported after 12 weeks. The doses of acarbose were low: 4.1% took less than 100 mg/day, 64% 100–250 mg/day, 32% 250–300 mg/day, and 0.1% more than 300 mg/day. Only 2.1% stopped therapy, mainly because of gastrointestinal adverse events. Tolerability appeared to be good and independent of age. Abnormal liver function was reported in 0.01%. The difference between these results and those of many controlled trials may in part be explained by the fact that higher doses have been used in most trials (14).

Reduction of insulin resistance in impaired glucose tolerance, as found in a Chinese multicenter study (15), can be another incentive to start treatment with alpha-glucosidase inhibitors. Various studies of the effects of alpha-glucosidase inhibitors on hyperglycemia and insulin resistance in type 2 diabetes and impaired glucose tolerance have been reviewed (16).

Comparative studies

Voglibose and acarbose have been compared in 32 patients insufficiently treated by diet in an open crossover study (17). The metabolic results were identical. There were fewer adverse reactions in those who took voglibose. There was increased flatulence with acarbose in 96% and with voglibose in 57%; abdominal distension was reported in 17 and 10% respectively.

In a comparison of voglibose and acarbose in 21 in-patients with type 2 diabetes who took part in a randomized crossover study of acarbose 150 mg/day and voglibose 0.9 mg/day, there was marked interindividual variation in response (18). For both drugs efficacy was better in those with gastrointestinal adverse effects, such as abdominal distention and flatulence.

In an open study in 57 patients acarbose and gliclazide had the same effects on HbA$_{1c}$, blood glucose, and lipids, but the ratio of HDL to LDL cholesterol increased with acarbose (19). Acarbose caused flatulence in 30% and diarrhea in 3% and gliclazide caused at least one mild attack of hypoglycemia in 10%.

Placebo-controlled studies

The effect of adding acarbose (maximum 100 mg tds) or placebo to insulin (20) or metformin (21) has been investigated in 1946 patients with type 2 diabetes. The results were comparable with the results of the UK Prospective Diabetes Study (22). After 3 years, 39% were still using acarbose compared with 58% using placebo. The main reasons for stopping were flatulence (30 versus 12%) or diarrhea (16 versus 8%). After 3 years the HbA$_{1c}$ concentration was 0.5% lower (median 8.1 versus 8.6%). Acarbose was equally effective when added to diet, sulfonylurea, metformin, or insulin.

When acarbose or placebo was given to patients with type 1 diabetes taking insulin, acarbose reduced postprandial blood glucose but there was no difference in HbA$_{1c}$; the only adverse effects were gastrointestinal (23).

In a double-blind, placebo-controlled study in 74 patients for 2 years, acarbose 100 mg tds, after a stepwise increase in dosage over 5 weeks, improved HbA$_{1c}$ (−1.71%) more than placebo (24). Two patients taking acarbose withdrew with drug-related adverse effects.

In a randomized, double-blind, placebo-controlled, crossover study 12 healthy subjects took acarbose 100 mg or voglibose 0.3 mg tds (25). Postprandial glucose, the rise in plasma immunoreactive insulin, and urinary immunoreactive C-peptide were higher with acarbose than voglibose. The flatus score was higher with acarbose than voglibose, but the stool score was not different and was higher than with placebo. Voglibose before the evening meal may improve nocturnal hypoglycemia during intensive insulin therapy (26).

Acarbose reduced insulin resistance in 192 patients over 65 years of age (mean age 70) in a double-blind, placebo-controlled study (27). HbA$_{1c}$ was significantly but modestly reduced. The most frequent adverse effect was flatulence, which caused 12 patients (9 taking acarbose and 3 taking placebo) to withdraw.

In a multicenter, double-blind, placebo-controlled study, 81 patients, in whom treatment with metformin was inadequate, received extra acarbose or placebo during 24 weeks after a 4-week run-in period to establish the optimal dose of acarbose (28). HbA$_{1c}$ was reduced by 1.02% and fasting blood glucose by 1.13 mmol/l. Gastrointestinal adverse effects were more common in the acarbose group.

In a placebo-controlled study of 154 patients taking glibenclamide or metformin, miglitol (starting at 25 mg tds and increasing to 50 or 100 mg tds for 24 weeks) caused more meteorism, flatulence, and diarrhea (29). When miglitol was added to metformin, HbA$_{1c}$ improved and there was weight loss. In another study in 318 patients, more of the patients taking miglitol only or miglitol plus metformin withdrew because of flatulence and diarrhea than in the other groups (30).

The effects of miglitol 25 or 50 mg tds have been compared with placebo and various doses of glibenclamide in 411 patients aged over 60 years (mean 68 years) with mild type 2 diabetes insufficiently controlled by diet for 56 weeks (31). HbA$_{1c}$ fell after 1 year by 0.92% (glibenclamide), 0.49% (miglitol 25 mg), and 0.40% (miglitol 50 mg). Gastrointestinal events were most common in patients taking miglitol. Most (88%) of the hypoglycemic events were minor and occurred in the patients taking glibenclamide. Mean body weight increased continuously and significantly in those taking glibenclamide. In the other groups weight fell by more than 1 kg. The rate of withdrawal was the same in all groups; withdrawal was mostly occasioned by cardiovascular effects in those taking glibenclamide and by hyperglycemia, flatulence, or diarrhea in those taking miglitol.

When patients with inadequately controlled type 2 diabetes used glibenclamide plus metformin, miglitol, or placebo for 24 weeks in addition to their earlier therapy, fasting blood glucose concentrations improved with miglitol (29). Flatulence and diarrhea were significantly more common with miglitol. No patient stopped taking miglitol because of adverse effects.

General adverse effects

Acarbose and miglitol have been reviewed (17,32,33). Their major adverse effects are flatulence, abdominal discomfort, diarrhea, and bloating, particularly at the start of therapy, which sometimes prevent further use. They should not be given to patients with intestinal obstruction, malabsorption, inflammatory bowel disease, or hepatic impairment.

Organs and Systems

Sensory systems

Acarbose can cause altered taste sensation (34).

Metabolism

When acarbose is combined with insulin, the greatest effects are seen with regimens that involve only once- or twice-daily administration. The alpha-glucosidase inhibitors seem to be less effective when they are combined with intensive insulin therapy (35). In combination with insulin or oral hypoglycemic drugs the frequency of hypoglycemic episodes can increase; sucrose or higher carbohydrates are reported to be less effective, which can be understood from the mechanism of action.

Extreme weight loss has been attributed to acarbose (36).

- A 47-year-old woman weighing 59 kg took acarbose 50 mg tds. Her blood glucose improved but she lost about 1 kg/month. She had a sore tongue without oral ulcers and no evidence of malabsorption. Later she developed general weakness and iron deficiency anemia but no other evidence of malabsorption. After she had lost 7 kg in 5 months, acarbose was withdrawn. Her complaints disappeared, her weight normalized, and she had no signs of iron deficiency anemia, even without iron therapy.

Extreme weight loss due to acarbose is rare. In this case the mechanism was unclear.

In 36 Japanese patients who were relatively lean but had excess abdominal fat, glibenclamide and voglibose caused loss of weight and abdominal fat (37). The loss of abdominal fat was related to glycemic control. The ratio of subcutaneous to abdominal fat shifted toward subcutaneous fat only in those who took voglibose. Both voglibose and glibenclamide improved insulin sensitivity and the acute response to insulin.

Nutrition

In a 56-week study there was an association between the use of acarbose and low vitamin B_6 concentrations, which occurred in 33% of 240 patients taking acarbose compared with 23% of 119 patients taking placebo (38). Calcium concentrations fell more often in those who took acarbose (28% versus 16%) but returned to normal by the end. These findings have not been reported elsewhere and do not appear to be clinically significant.

Gastrointestinal

Abdominal pain and diarrhea with malabsorption have been described in patients taking acarbose, which can also cause carbohydrate malabsorption (39).

A review of miglitol included data on adverse effects in 3585 patients in well-designed clinical trials (40). Only the adverse effects in the gastrointestinal tract occurred with a significantly greater incidence with miglitol 50 or 100 mg tds. The adverse effects were the same as with other drugs in this class: flatulence, diarrhea, dyspepsia, and abdominal pain. There were no differences with monotherapy or combination therapy or in relation to age or ethnicity. There were more episodes of hypoglycemia when miglitol was combined with insulin but not with oral agents. The incidence of cardiovascular events was the same as with placebo.

Long-term acarbose had a good effect on late dumping syndrome in six patients with type 2 diabetes; one patient complained of increased flatulence (41).

In 33 patients with type 2 diabetes treated with sulfonylureas and insulin who took miglitol 50 mg bd for 1 week and then over the next month increased the dose to 50 mg tds, 15% developed adverse effects (6% diarrhea, 6% abdominal distension), which disappeared within 3 weeks of continuing therapy (42).

In the STOP-NIDDM trial of acarbose cardiovascular risk and hypertension were reduced; however, almost a quarter of the participants withdrew early, and the main cause of early withdrawal was gastrointestinal adverse effects (43).

The author of a review of the use of acarbose concluded that acarbose is safe in both monotherapy and combination therapy (44). The most common adverse effects are: mild to moderate gastrointestinal symptoms, such as flatulence, meteorism, diarrhea, soft stools, abdominal discomfort, and pain. As glucose oxidase increases in the small intestine during therapy, it is advisable to start with a low dose so that the gut can adapt to acarbose.

In a post-marketing surveillance study of 1142 patients in whom acarbose was added to insulin therapy for type 2 diabetes mellitus, HbA_{1c} improved by 0.9% and there were 108 adverse effects in 6.9% of the patients (45). Most of the complaints were gastrointestinal (flatulence, abdominal pain, diarrhea) and more than half were reported in the first week of acarbose therapy.

A meta-analysis of seven double-blind, randomized, placebo-controlled studies in which acarbose was used for a minimum of 52 weeks for the management of type 2 diabetes has shown that the frequency of the most common adverse events of flatulence, diarrhea, and abdominal pain varied from country to country: 53% of those taking acarbose reported symptoms in Germany compared with 73% in Canada (46). The frequency of adverse effects with placebo was also higher in Canada (39%) than in Germany (29%).

Although acarbose often causes abdominal complaints, dietary manipulation has not been used to reduce the complaints (47).

In 120 patients with type 1 diabetes, acarbose lowered postprandial glucose but did not reduce HbA_{1c} (22). Four patients taking acarbose withdrew because of gastrointestinal effects, which improved after withdrawal. One of the placebo group withdrew because of gastrointestinal problems and one other patient taking acarbose withdrew with a Bell's palsy, which was not considered to be related to acarbose.

Ileus has also been reported with acarbose (48–51).

Paralytic ileus with intestinal pneumatosis cystoides has been reported (50).

- An 87-year-old woman, who took acarbose, glibenclamide, and mannitol (for constipation), developed abdominal distention and loss of appetite. An X-ray showed distention of the small intestine, with pockets of small gas bubbles in the submucosal When her drugs were withdrawn, her symptoms subsided and the radiological evidence of ileus disappeared by 5 days. Although she had an atonic bladder, there were no signs of neuropathy. She was also hypothyroid, which could have contributed.

Acarbose may also have caused pneumatosis cystoides intestinalis in a 55-year-old woman with pemphigus vulgaris (52).

Most cases of ileus with acarbose have been reported in Japan.

- A 73-year-old man with diabetic gangrene who had used insulin and acarbose 300 mg/day for 15 months developed ileus with abdominal pain and vomiting after he took PL granules (containing salicylamide, paracetamol, anhydrous caffeine, and promethazine methylene disalicylate) for a common cold (51). The ileus subsided after acarbose and the other drugs were withdrawn.

Although the ileus in this case was not clearly related to the use of acarbose, the combination of acarbose, which can cause ileus, with the other drugs that the patient was taking, may have caused it. The anticholinergic effect of promethazine methylene disalicylate may have contributed.

Lymphocytic colitis activated by acarbose has been reported (53).

- A 52-year-old man developed watery diarrhea 6–8 times a day 2 weeks after he had started to take acarbose 100 mg. In 3 weeks he lost 3 kg. Duodenal biopsies were normal; colon biopsies showed a large increase in intraepithelial lymphocytes. The mononuclear cells expressed CD-25, and HLA-DR antigen was increased in epithelial cells. Within 4 days of acarbose withdrawal the diarrhea had disappeared, and biopsies 4 months later showed that CD-25 expression in the cells of the lamina propria was improved and HLA-DR was no longer expressed by the epithelial cells. On rechallenge the diarrhea recurred within 3 days. Biopsies showed pronounced HLA-DR in the epithelial cells and CD-25 expression in some mononuclear cells in the lamina propria.

Non-digestable sugar substitutes and alpha-glucosidase inhibitors should probably not be used in combination.

Liver

Liver damage with raised liver enzymes has been described (16,54). Four case of liver damage by acarbose have been described in women aged 52–57, three established (55) and one probable (56) All had signs of liver impairment within 2–8 months after starting to take acarbose and the changes subsidized within a month after withdrawal. The first patient was given acarbose again; her liver enzymes increased after 3 days and normalized within 10 days after withdrawal. The second and third patients had liver biopsies, which confirmed hepatic changes.

- A 45-year-old man took acarbose 50 mg tds for a year and developed an aspartate transaminase of 62 U/l and an alanine transaminase of 127 /l, with negative

serology; 3 months later the alanine transaminase was 153 U/l. After withdrawal of acarbose his liver enzymes normalized (57).

- A 54-year-old woman had fatigue and dark urine after taking acarbose 50 mg tds for 5 months (57). Her aspartate transaminase was 2436 U/l, alanine transaminase 2556 U/l, γ-glutamyl transpeptidase 601 U/l, and alkaline phosphatase 174 U/l; serology was negative and she had a normal liver and gall bladder on ultrasound. Her liver enzymes normalized 5 months after withdrawal.
- A 58-year-old man taking gliclazide 80 mg/day, atenolol 100 mg/day, and pravastatin 10 mg/day started to take acarbose 150 mg/day and benazepril 10 mg/day (58). After 2 weeks he developed weakness and myalgia and 1 week later his alanine transaminase was 22 times higher and aspartate transaminase 9 times higher than the upper limits of the reference ranges. Benazepril and pravastatin were withdrawn and his hypoglycemic therapy was changed to insulin. No viral or other antibodies related to liver disease were found. He improved and was given glibenclamide and acarbose instead of insulin. His enzymes increased 3 weeks later without subjective signs and he had an eosinophilia. A liver biopsy showed intralobular and periportal necrosis of liver cells and mononuclear infiltrates. Acarbose was withdrawn and he improved.
- A 57-year-old woman developed hepatitis 2 months after starting to take acarbose 100 mg tds (59). No other causes of hepatitis were found. Liver function tests normalized 3 months after withdrawal. Acarbose was reintroduced 3 years later and she again developed acute hepatitis. Liver function tests became normal 2 months after withdrawal.
- A 74-year-old woman who had used acarbose for 3 months developed progressive weakness and jaundice (60). Her bilirubin was 152 µmol/l (direct bilirubin 96 µmol/l). All of her liver enzymes were substantially raised. All other investigations were normal, except that she was positive for hepatitis C antigen. After withdrawal of acarbose everything became normal within 1 month.
- A 73-year-old woman who had taken acarbose 450 mg/day for 3 months became very tired and icteric (61). Her total bilirubin was 427 µmol/l (direct bilirubin 335 µmol/l) and her liver enzymes were very high. Liver biopsy showed cholestasis and cytolysis without eosinophils. Acarbose was continued for 3 days and her condition did not change. When the acarbose was withdrawn she improved rapidly.
- Another patient taking acarbose also had a serum alanine transaminase three times the upper limit of the reference range, but she had positive serology for hepatitis A (21).

Comparable reports have prompted a questionnaire investigation of 770 patients with type 2 diabetes at the start of acarbose therapy (62). Patients with one or more susceptibility factors for liver damage underwent ultrasonography and autoantibody assays. There was silent liver disease in 13% and 20 patients had a fatty liver without hepatic disease. In 15% of these patients there were slight reversible changes in transaminase activity after acarbose.

This supports the supposition that severe hepatotoxic reactions to acarbose are idiosyncratic.

In a 78-week double-blind single center study 139 patients with type 2 diabetes were randomized to acarbose or placebo in addition to their usual therapy (63). The mean dose of acarbose at the end of the study was 680 mg. Two patients taking 600 mg or more developed raised liver enzymes, to more than three times the upper limit of normal.

In a 56-week study there was an association between the dose of acarbose in the range 50–300 mg tds and the development of abnormal liver function in 359 patients with type 1 (21%) and type 2 diabetes (38). The patients took the maximum tolerated dose, and 30% took doses of 100 mg or less. Of the patents who were randomized to acarbose ($n = 240$), 8% developed abnormal liver function tests (alanine transaminase activity more than three times the upper limit of normal) compared with 1% of those who took placebo ($n = 119$). The dose of acarbose was 200–300 mg tds in those who developed abnormal liver function. Liver function recovered promptly on withdrawal.

However, in a double-blind study in 100 patients with compensated non-alcoholic liver cirrhosis and type 2 diabetes, acarbose for 28 weeks did not alter liver function (64). The number of hypoglycemic episodes was reduced.

Skin

Erythema multiforme and generalized pastulosis have been attributed to acarbose (65).

- A skin biopsy from a 58-year-old man showed necrosis of keratinocytes with lymphocytic and eosinophilic infiltration. Liver enzymes were normal. After withdrawal the rash disappeared. After 3 weeks, rechallenge with acarbose 50 mg caused the skin changes to reappear.
- A 43-year-old man developed generalized exanthema pustulosis 48 hours after the start of acarbose therapy (66). The lesions disappeared within 1 week after stopping acarbose. He was not retested.

Second-Generation Effects

Pregnancy

In six women with gestational diabetes, acarbose 50 mg before meals normalized fasting and postprandial glucose concentrations (67). The pregnancies were uneventful and the neonates were healthy. Internal discomfort persisted during the whole pregnancy.

Drug–Drug Interactions

Biguanides

Metformin can be effectively combined with miglitol (SEDA-25, 514) but metformin may accumulate in the gastrointestinal wall, and the combination of metformin

with acarbose or miglitol may reduce the absorption of metformin (68,69).

Colestyramine

Acarbose increases bowel motility, which reduces the effect of colestyramine.

Digoxin

Acarbose can reduce plasma concentrations of digoxin by impairing its absorption (70).

- An 82-year-old man with type 2 diabetes, taking digoxin and voglibose 0.9 mg/day, had digoxin serum concentrations in the target range (71). He was given acarbose 300 mg/day instead of voglibose and his digoxin concentrations fell from 0.8–2.0 ng/ml to 0.2–0.4 ng/ml. One month after restarting voglibose the digoxin concentrations were again in the target range.
- A 69-year-old woman with diabetes mellitus and heart failure repeatedly had unusual subtherapeutic plasma digoxin concentrations (72). When acarbose was withdrawn the plasma digoxin concentration rose.

In a randomized, crossover study in healthy men, acarbose 100–200 mg reduced the AUC and C_{max} of digoxin and prolonged its t_{max}, consistent with reduced absorption (73). However, in another study acarbose 50 mg tds for 12 days had no significant effect on the pharmacokinetics of a single oral dose of digoxin 0.75 mg (74).

In one study there was no interaction of voglibose with digoxin (75).

Glibenclamide

In a placebo-controlled study in six patients with type 2 diabetes, acarbose 300 mg/day for 7 days had no significant effect on the pharmacokinetics of a single dose of glibenclamide 5 mg (76).

Miglitol did not reduce the t_{max} or C_{max} of glibenclamide, but the 9-hour AUC was significantly reduced (77).

In a double-blind, crossover study in 12 healthy men, voglibose 5 mg tds for 8 days had no significant effect on the pharmacokinetics of a single dose of glibenclamide 1.75 mg (78).

Metformin

Acarbose reduces the absorption of metformin (79), as does miglitol (77).

Thioctic acid

In 24 healthy volunteers thioctic acid 600 mg orally had no significant effect on the actions of acarbose 50 mg and acarbose did not alter the pharmacokinetics of thioctic acid (80).

Warfarin

Acarbose may increase the availability of warfarin (81). However, neither miglitol (82) nor voglibose (83) has any effect.

References

1. Meneilly GS, Ryan EA, Radziuk J, Lau DC, Yale JF, Morais J, Chiasson JL, Rabasa-Lhoret R, Maheux P, Tessier D, Wolever T, Josse RG, Elahi D. Effect of acarbose on insulin sensitivity in elderly patients with diabetes. Diabetes Care 2000;23(8):1162–7.

2. Laube H. Acarbose: an update of its therapeutic use in diabetes treatment. Clin Drug Invest 2002;22:141–56.

3. Coniff R, Krol A. Acarbose: a review of US clinical experience. Clin Ther 1997;19(1):16–26.

4. Sels JP, Verdonk HE, Wolffenbuttel BH. Effects of acarbose (Glucobay) in persons with type 1 diabetes: a multicentre study. Diabetes Res Clin Pract 1998;41(2):139–45.

5. Johnston PS, Feig PU, Coniff RF, Krol A, Davidson JA, Haffner SM. Long-term titrated-dose alpha-glucosidase inhibition in non-insulin-requiring Hispanic NIDDM patients. Diabetes Care 1998;21(3):409–15.

6. Johnston PS, Feig PU, Coniff RF, Krol A, Kelley DE, Mooradian AD. Chronic treatment of African-American type 2 diabetic patients with alpha-glucosidase inhibition. Diabetes Care 1998;21(3):416–22.

7. Mitrakou A, Tountas N, Raptis AE, Bauer RJ, Schulz H, Raptis SA. Long-term effectiveness of a new alpha-glucosidase inhibitor (BAY m1099—miglitol) in insulin-treated type 2 diabetes mellitus. Diabet Med 1998;15(8):657–60.

8. Matsumoto K, Yano M, Miyake S, Ueki Y, Yamaguchi Y, Akazawa S, Tominaga Y. Effects of voglibose on glycemic excursions, insulin secretion, and insulin sensitivity in non-insulin-treated NIDDM patients. Diabetes Care 1998;21(2):256–60.

9. Delorme S, Chiasson J-L. Acarbose in the prevention of cardiovascular disease in subjects with impaired glucose tolerance and type 2 diabetes mellitus. Curr Opinion Pharmacol 2005;5:184–9.

10. Clissold SP, Edwards C. Acarbose. A preliminary review of its pharmacodynamic and pharmacokinetic properties, and therapeutic potential. Drugs 1988;35(3):214–43.

11. Mertes G. Efficacy and safety of acarbose in the treatment of type 2 diabetes: data from a 2-year surveillance study. Diabetes Res Clin Pract 1998;40(1):63–70.

12. Hanefeld M, Bar K. Efficacy and safety of combined treatment of type 2 diabetes with acarbose and metformin. Diabetes Stoffwechsel 1998;7:186–90.

13. Scorpiglione N, Belfiglio M, Carinci F, Cavaliere D, De Curtis A, Franciosi M, Mari E, Sacco M, Tognoni G, Nicolucci A. The effectiveness, safety and epidemiology of the use of acarbose in the treatment of patients with type II diabetes mellitus. A model of medicine-based evidence. Eur J Clin Pharmacol 1999;55(4):239–49.

14. Spengler M, Schmitz H, Landen H. Evaluation of the efficacy and tolerability of acarbose in patients with diabetes mellitus. A post marketing surveillance study Clin Drug Invest 2005;25:651–9.

15. Pan C-Y, Gao Y, Chen J-W, Luo B-Y, Fu Z-Z, Lu J-M, Guo X-H, Cheng H. Efficacy of acarbose in Chinese subjects with impaired glucose tolerance. Diabetes Res Clin Pract 2003;61:183–90.

16. cheen AJ. Is there a role for alpha-glucosidase inhibitors in the prevention of type 2 diabetes mellitus? Drugs 2003;63:933–51.

17. Vichayanrat A, Ploybutr S, Tunlakit M, Watanakejorn P. Efficacy and safety of voglibose in comparison with acarbose in type 2 diabetic patients. Diabetes Res Clin Pract 2002;55(2):99–103.

18. Fujisawa T, Ikegami H, Inoue K, Kawabata Y, Ogihara T. Effect of two α-glucosidase inhibitors, voglibose and acarbose, on postprandial hyperglycemia correlates with subjective abdominal symptoms. Metabolism 2005;54:387–90.

19. Salman S, Salman F, Satman I, Yilmaz Y, Ozer E, Sengul A, Demirel HO, Karsidag K, Dinccag N, Yilmaz MT. Comparison of acarbose and gliclazide as first-line agents in patients with type 2 diabetes. Curr Med Res Opin 2001;16(4):296–306.

20. Kelley DE, Bidot P, Freedman Z, Haag B, Podlecki D, Rendell M, Schimel D, Weiss S, Taylor T, Krol A, Magner J. Efficacy and safety of acarbose in insulin-treated patients with type 2 diabetes. Diabetes Care 1998;21(12):2056–61.

21. Rosenstock J, Brown A, Fischer J, Jain A, Littlejohn T, Nadeau D, Sussman A, Taylor T, Krol A, Magner J. Efficacy and safety of acarbose in metformin-treated patients with type 2 diabetes. Diabetes Care 1998;21(12):2050–5.

22. Holman RR, Cull CA, Turner RC. A randomized double-blind trial of acarbose in type 2 diabetes shows improved glycemic control over 3 years (U.K. Prospective Diabetes Study 44) Diabetes Care 1999;22(6):960–4.

23. Riccardi G, Giacco R, Parillo M, Turco S, Rivellese AA, Ventura MR, Contadini S, Marra G, Monteduro M, Santeusanio F, Brunetti P, Librenti MC, Pontiroli AE, Vedani P, Pozza G, Bergamini L, Bianchi C. Efficacy and safety of acarbose in the treatment of Type 1 diabetes mellitus: a placebo-controlled, double-blind, multicentre study. Diabet Med 1999;16(3):228–32.

24. Hasche H, Mertes G, Bruns C, Englert R, Genthner P, Heim D, Heyen P, Mahla G, Schmidt C, Schulze-Schleppinghof B, Steger-Johannsen G. Effects of acarbose treatment in type 2 diabetic patients under dietary training: a multicentre, double-blind, placebo-controlled, 2-year study. Diabetes Nutr Metab 1999;12(4):277–85.

25. Kageyama S, Nakamichi N, Sekino H, Fujita H, Nakano S. Comparison of the effects of acarbose and voglibose on plasma glucose, endogenous insulin sparing, and gastrointestinal adverse events in obese subjects: a randomized, placebo-controlled, double-blind, three-way crossover study. Curr Ther Res Clin Exp 2000;61:630–45.

26. Taira M, Takasu N, Komiya I, Taira T, Tanaka H. Voglibose administration before the evening meal improves nocturnal hypoglycemia in insulin-dependent diabetic patients with intensive insulin therapy. Metabolism 2000;49(4):440–3.

27. Josse RG, Chiasson JL, Ryan EA, Lau DC, Ross SA, Yale JF, Leiter LA, Maheux P, Tessier D, Wolever TM, Gerstein H, Rodger NW, Dornan JM, Murphy LJ, Rabasa-Lhoret R, Meneilly GS. Acarbose in the treatment of elderly patients with type 2 diabetes. Diabetes Res Clin Pract 2003;59(1):37–42.

28. Phillips P, Karrasch J, Scott R, Wilson D, Moses R. Acarbose improves glycemic control in overweight type 2 diabetic patients insufficiently treated with metformin. Diabetes Care 2003;26(2):269–73.

29. Standl E, Schernthaner G, Rybka J, Hanefeld M, Raptis SA, Naditch L. Improved glycaemic control with miglitol in inadequately-controlled type 2 diabetics. Diabetes Res Clin Pract 2001;51(3):205–13.

30. Chiasson JL, Naditch LMiglitol Canadian University Investigator Group. The synergistic effect of miglitol plus metformin combination therapy in the treatment of type 2 diabetes. Diabetes Care 2001;24(6):989–94.

31. Johnston PS, Lebovitz HE, Coniff RF, Simonson DC, Raskin P, Munera CL. Advantages of alpha-glucosidase

inhibition as monotherapy in elderly type 2 diabetic patients. J Clin Endocrinol Metab 1998;83(5):1515–22.

32. Lebovitz HE. Alpha-glucosidase inhibitors as agents in the treatment of diabetes. Diabetes Rev 1998;6:132–45.

33. Johnston PS, Coniff RF, Hoogwerf BJ, Santiago JV, Pi-Sunyer FX, Krol A. Effects of the carbohydrase inhibitor miglitol in sulfonylurea-treated NIDDM patients. Diabetes Care 1994;17(1):20–9.

34. Ruiz M, Matrone A, Alvari-as J, Burlando G, Jadzinsky M, Tesone P, Joge A, Bueno R, Castelli F, Fuente G, Gallego L, Garcia A, Del Hoyo N, Garcia S, Gianaula C, Maggiolo S, Marcello S, Mainetti H, Ortensi G, Righi S, Salzberg S, Traversa M, Vasta A, Vasquez V, Lemme L, Wendik A. Estudio multicentrico para determinar la eficacia y tolerancia de acarbose (Bay g 5421) en pacientes DMNID. Prensa Med Argent 1996;83:392–8.

35. Liebl A, Renner R, Hepp KD. Acarbose bei insulinbehandelten Diabetikern. Ein kritischer Überblick. Akt Endokrinol 1993;14:42–7.

36. Yoo WH, Park TS, Baek HS. Marked weight loss in a type 2 diabetic patient treated with acarbose. Diabetes Care 1999;22(4):645–6.

37. Takami K, Takeda N, Nakashima K, Takami R, Hayashi M, Ozeki S, Yamada A, Kokubo Y, Sato M, Kawachi S, Sasaki A, Yasuda K. Effects of dietary treatment alone or diet with voglibose or glyburide on abdominal adipose tissue and metabolic abnormalities in patients with newly diagnosed type 2 diabetes. Diabetes Care 2002;25(4):658–62.

38. Neuser D, Benson A, Brückner A, Goldberg RB, Hoogwerf BJ, Petzinna D. Safety and tolerability of acarbose in the treatment of type 1 and type 2 diabetes mellitus. Clin Drug Invest 2005;25:579–87.

39. Sobajima H, Mori M, Niwa T, Muramatsu M, Sugimoto Y, Kato K, Naruse S, Kondo T, Hayakawa T. Carbohydrate malabsorption following acarbose administration. Diabet Med 1998;15(5):393–7.

40. Scott LJ, Spencer CM. Miglitol: a review of its therapeutic potential in type 2 diabetes mellitus. Drugs 2000;59(3):521–49.

41. Hasegawa T, Yoneda M, Nakamura K, Ohnishi K, Harada H, Kyouda T, Yoshida Y, Makino I. Long-term effect of alpha-glucosidase inhibitor on late dumping syndrome. J Gastroenterol Hepatol 1998;13(12):1201–6.

42. de Luis Roman DA, del Pozo Garcia E, Aller R, Romero Bobillo E, Conde Valentin R. Utildad del miglitol en pacientes con diabetes mellitus tipo 2 y mal contrl glucenmico. Rev Clin Esp 2004;204:32–4.

43. Chiasson J-L, Josse RG, Gomis R, Hanefeld M, Karasik A, Laakso M. Acarbose treatment and the risk of cardiovascular disease and hypertension in patients with impaired glucose tolerance. J Am Med Assoc 2003;290:486–94.

44. Breuer H-WM. Review of acarbose therapeutic strategies in the long-term treatment and in the prevention of type 2 diabetes. Int J Clin Pharmacol Ther 2003;41:421–40.

45. Klocke KR, Stauch K, Landen H. Effect of add-on acarbose to insulin therapy in routine clinical practice. Clin Drug Invest 2003;23:621–7.

46. Hanefeld M, Cagatay M, Petrowitsch T, Neuser D, petzinna D, Rupp M. Acarbose reduces the risk for myocardial infarction in type 2 diabetic patients: meta-analysis of seven long-term studies. Eur Heart J 2004;25:10–16.

47. Lindstrom J, Tuomilehto J, Spengler MThe Finnish Acargbos Study Group. Acarbose treatment does not change the habitual diet of patients with type 2 diabetes mellitus. Diabet Med 2000;17(1):20–5.

48. Nishii Y, Aizawa T, Hashizume K. Ileus: a rare side effect of acarbose. Diabetes Care 1996;19(9):1033.

49. Odawara M, Bannai C, Saitoh T, Kawakami Y, Yamashita K. Potentially lethal ileus associated with acarbose treatment for NIDDM. Diabetes Care 1997;20(7):1210–1.

50. Azami Y. Paralytic ileus accompanied by pneumatosis cystoides intestinalis after acarbose treatment in an elderly diabetic patient with a history of heavy intake of maltitol. Intern Med 2000;39(10):826–9.

51. Oba K, Kudo R, Yano M, Watanabe K, Ajiro Y, Okazaki K, Suzuki T, Nakano H, Metori S. Ileus after administration of cold remedy in an elderly diabetic patient treated with acarbose. J Nippon Med Sch 2001;68(1):61–4.

52. Maeda A, Yokoi S, Kunou T, Murata T. [A case of pneumatosis cystoides intestinalis assumed to be induced by acarbose administration for diabetes mellitus and pemphigus vulgaris.]Nippon Shokakibyo Gakkai Zasshi 2002;99(11):1345–9.

53. Piche T, Raimondi V, Schneider S, Hebuterne X, Rampal P. Acarbose and lymphocytic colitis. Lancet 2000;356(9237):1246.

54. Carrascosa M, Pascual F, Aresti S. Acarbose-induced acute severe hepatotoxicity. Lancet 1997;349(9053):698–9.

55. Fujimoto Y, Ohhira M, Miyokawa N, Kitamori S, Kohgo Y. Acarbose-induced hepatic injury. Lancet 1998;351(9099):340.

56. Diaz-Gutierrez FL, Ladero JM, Diaz-Rubio M. Acarbose-induced acute hepatitis. Am J Gastroenterol 1998;93(3):481.

57. Andrade RJ, Lucena M, Vega JL, Torres M, Salmeron FJ, Bellot V, Garcia-Escano MD, Moreno P. Acarbose-associated hepatotoxicity. Diabetes Care 1998;21(11):2029–30.

58. Mennecier D, Zafrani ES, Dhumeaux D, Mallat A. Hépatite aiguë induite par l'acarbose. [Acarbose-induced acute hepatitis.] Gastroenterol Clin Biol 1999;23(12):1398–9.

59. de la Vega J, Crespo M, Escudero JM, Sanchez L, Rivas LL. Hepatitis aguda por acarbosa. Descripcion de 2 episodios en una misma paciente. [Acarbose-induced acute hepatitis. Report of two events in the same patient.] Gastroenterol Hepatol 2000;23(6):282–4.

60. Madonia S, Pietrosi G, Pagliaro L. Acarbose-induced liver injury in an anti-hepatitis C virus positive patient. Dig Liver Dis 2001;33(7):615–6.

61. Fernandez AB, Gacia AM, Fabuel AT, Merino AB. Hepatitis aguda inducida por acarbosa. Med Clin 2001;117:317–8.

62. Gentile S, Turco S, Guarino G, Sasso FC, Torella R. Aminotransferase activity and acarbose treatment in patients with type 2 diabetes. Diabetes Care 1999;22(7):1217–8.

63. Segal P, Eliahou HE, Petzinna D, Neuser D, Brückner A, Spengler M. Long-term efficacy and tolerability of acarbose treatment in patients with type 2 diabetes mellitus. Clin Drug Invest 2005;25:589–95.

64. Gentile S, Turco S, Guarino G, Oliviero B, Annunziata S, Cozzolino D, Sasso FC, Turco A, Salvatore T, Torella R. Effect of treatment with acarbose and insulin in patients with non-insulin-dependent diabetes mellitus associated with non-alcoholic liver cirrhosis. Diabetes Obes Metab 2001;3(1):33–40.

65. Kono T, Hayami M, Kobayashi H, Ishii M, Taniguchi S. Acarbose-induced generalised erythema multiforme. Lancet 1999;354(9176):396–7.

66. Poszepczynska-Guigné E, Viguier M, Assier H, Pinquier L, Hochedez P, Dubertret L. Acute generalized exanthema pustulosis induced by drugs with low-digestive absorption:

acarbose and nystatin. Ann Dermatol Venereol 2003; 130:439–42.

67. Zarate A, Ochoa R, Hernandez M, Basurto L. Eficacia de la acarbose para controlar el deterioro de la tolerancia a la glucosa durante la gestacion. [Effectiveness of acarbose in the control of glucose tolerance worsening in pregnancy.] Ginecol Obstet Mex 2000;68:42–5.

68. Dachman AH. New contraindication to intravascular iodinated contrast material. Radiology 1995;197(2):545.

69. Scheen AJ, Lefebvre PJ. Potential pharmacokinetics interference between alpha-glucosidase inhibitors and other oral antidiabetic agents. Diabetes Care 2002; 25(1):247–8.

70. Ben-Ami H, Krivoy N, Nagachandran P, Roguin A, Edoute Y. An interaction between digoxin and acarbose. Diabetes Care 1999;22(5):860–1.

71. Nagai Y, Hayakawa T, Abe T, Nomura G. Are there different effects of acarbose and voglibose on serum levels of digoxin in a diabetic patient with congestive heart failure? Diabetes Care 2000;23(11):1703.

72. Serrano JS, Jimenez CM, Serrano MI, Balboa B. A possible interaction of potential clinical interest between digoxin and acarbose. Clin Pharmacol Ther 1996;60(5):589–92.

73. Miura T, Ueno K, Tanaka K, Sugiura Y, Mizutani M, Takatsu F, Takano Y, Shibakawa M. Impairment of absorption of digoxin by acarbose. J Clin Pharmacol 1998;38(7):654–7.

74. Cohen E, Almog S, Staruvin D, Garty M. Do therapeutic doses of acarbose alter the pharmacokinetics of digoxin? Isr Med Assoc J 2002;4(10):772–5.

75. Kusumoto M, Ueno K, Fujimura Y, Kameda T, Mashimo K, Takeda K, Tatami R, Shibakawa M. Lack of kinetic interaction between digoxin and voglibose. Eur J Clin Pharmacol 1999;55(1):79–80.

76. Gerard J, Lefebvre PJ, Luyckx AS. Glibenclamide pharmacokinetics in acarbose-treated type 2 diabetics. Eur J Clin Pharmacol 1984;27(2):233–6.

77. Scheen AJ, Lefebvre PJ. Potential pharmacokinetics interference between alpha-glucosidase inhibitors and other oral antidiabetic agents. Diabetes Care 2002;25(1):247–8.

78. Kleist P, Ehrlich A, Suzuki Y, Timmer W, Wetzelsberger N, Lucker PW, Fuder H. Concomitant administration of the alpha-glucosidase inhibitor voglibose (AO-128) does not alter the pharmacokinetics of glibenclamide. Eur J Clin Pharmacol 1997;53(2):149–52.

79. Dachman AH. New contraindication to intravascular iodinated contrast material. Radiology 1995;197(2):545.

80. Gleiter CH, Schreeb KH, Freudenthaler S, Thomas M, Elze M, Fieger-Buschges H, Potthast H, Schneider E, Schug BS, Blume HH, Hermann R. Lack of interaction between thioctic acid, glibenclamide and acarbose. Br J Clin Pharmacol 1999;48(6):819–25.

81. Morreale AP, Janetzky K. Probable interaction of warfarin and acarbose. Am J Health Syst Pharm 1997;54(13):1551–2.

82. Schall R, Muller FO, Hundt HK, Duursema L, Groenewoud G, Middle MV. Study of the effect of miglitol on the pharmacokinetics and pharmacodynamics of warfarin in healthy males. Arzneimittelforschung 1996;46(1):41–6.

83. Fuder H, Kleist P, Birkel M, Ehrlich A, Emeklibas S, Maslak W, Stridde E, Wetzelsberger N, Wieckhorst G, Lucker PW. The alpha-glucosidase inhibitor voglibose (AO-128) does not change pharmacodynamics or pharmacokinetics of warfarin. Eur J Clin Pharmacol 1997;53(2):153–7.

Amylin analogues

General Information

Amylin is a peptide hormone produced in the beta-cells of the islets of Langerhans and co-secreted with insulin. It has glucoregulatory effects that may complement the actions of insulin.

Pramlintide (rINN) is an amyloid analogue (1). It is administered subcutaneously, but it precipitates above pH 5.5 and therefore cannot be co-administered with insulin. It received FDA approval in 2005 for both type 1 and type 2 diabetes. It reduces postprandial glucose excursions, probably by reducing stomach emptying, not by stimulating the release of glucagon-like peptide (GLP-1) (2). It can only be given by injection.

The most common adverse effect of pramlintide is nausea. Hypoglycemia can occur if the dose of insulin is not reduced when pramlintide is added. In no studies was there evidence of cardiac, hepatic, or renal toxicity or hypersensitivity reactions.

Pramlintide has been studied in a double-blind, placebo-controlled, multicenter study in 480 patients with type 1 diabetes for 1 year, followed by an 1-year open extension (3). Glucose control improved with pramlintide. Hypoglycemia was less frequent with pramlintide, but nausea and anorexia doubled in frequency and constituted the most common reason for withdrawal.

In a comparable study, 656 patients with type 2 diabetes took preprandial pramlintide 60 micrograms tds, 90 micrograms bd, or 120 micrograms bd (4). Only 120 micrograms bd gave a sustained reduction in HbA$_{1c}$. In the first 4 weeks there was an increase in the risk of hypoglycemia, but not thereafter. Mild to moderate nausea and headache were the most frequent adverse effects; nausea abated during treatment.

Observational studies

In 19 patients with type 1 diabetes using regular insulin and 21 using insulin lispro, who injected pramlintide 60 micrograms or placebo before a standardized breakfast in addition to their normal insulin treatment, there was a marked reduction in the postprandial blood glucose excursion; mild hypoglycemia (25%) and mild nausea (18%) were the most frequent adverse events (5).

Pramlintide 30 micrograms was given to 16 patients using insulin pumps as an injection at meal times (6). Mealtime insulin was reduced by 17%. Serum fructosamine improved. Nausea was the most common adverse effect. There was no hypoglycemia.

Placebo-controlled studies

In 18 subjects with type 1 diabetes, mean age 37 years, who received in random order on separate days pramlintide 60 micrograms or placebo plus their usual doses of regular insulin, hypoglycemia (pramlintide 28% versus 16%) and mild nausea (17% versus 11%) were the most common adverse effects (7). Nausea has also occurred in other long-term studies (1). Weight loss rather than weight gain has been reported in association with reductions in HB_{A1c} concentrations in patients with type 2 diabetes. Whether this relates to a reduction in insulin dose while using pramlintide, especially in those who are more obese, is uncertain.

In three studies in 477 patients with type 1 diabetes, pramlintide 30 or 60 micrograms three or four times a day ($n = 281$) was compared with placebo ($n = 196$) (8). The patients continued to take insulin in a mean daily dose of 50 units/day (pramlintide) or 48 units/day (placebo). After 26 weeks 43% of those using pramlintide had problems with nausea and 16% had *anorexia* compared with 10% and 2% of those who used placebo (9). A review of other studies showed that the rate of mild to moderate nausea was 9.5–59%, and that severe nausea was 0.7–8.5%. Most studies suggested that the nausea was transient (2–8 weeks) although most did not document the reduction in nausea.

Organs and Systems

Gastrointestinal

Pramlintide slows gastric emptying and it should not be used in those with gastroparesis. The manufacturer also recommends that analgesics should not be taken less than 1 hour before or 2 hours after pramlintide.

Drug-drug interactions

Insulin

Pramlintide buffers to a pH of 4.0 and precipitates at a pH at above 5.5 and would not be expected to be compatible with insulin, which is buffered at pH 7.8. In an open study of 51 patients with type 1 diabetes, pramlintide was mixed in the same syringe as insulin (regular insulin and isophane insulin) (10). The pharmacokinetics of insulin and pramlintide were not significantly altered. However, mixing pramlintide and insulin is not recommended.

References

1. Schmitz O, Brock B, Rungby J. Amylin agonists: a novel approach in the treatment of diabetes. Diabetes 2004; 53:S233–8.
2. Ahren B, Adner N, Svartberg J, Petrella E, Holst JJ, Gutniak MK. Anti-diabetogenic effect of the human amylin analogue, pramlintide, in Type 1 diabetes is not mediated by GLP-1. Diabet Med 2002;19(9):790–2.
3. Whitehouse F, Kruger DF, Fineman M, Shen L, Ruggles JA, Maggs DG, Weyer C, Kolterman OG. A randomized study and open-label extension evaluating the long-term efficacy of pramlintide as an adjunct to insulin therapy in type 1 diabetes. Diabetes Care 2002;25(4):724–30.
4. Hollander PA, Levy P, Fineman MS, Maggs DG, Shen LZ, Strobel SA, Weyer C, Kolterman OG. Pramlintide as an adjunct to insulin therapy improves long-term glycemic and

weight control in patients with type 2 diabetes: a 1-year randomized controlled trial. Diabetes Care 2003;26(3):784–90.
5. Weyer C, Gottlieb A, Kim DD, Lutz K, Schwartz S, Gutierrez M, Wang Y, Ruggles JA, Kolterman OG, Maggs DG. Pramlintide reduces postprandial glucose excursions when added to regular insulin or insulin lispro in subjects with type 1 diabetes. Diabetes Care 2003;26:1074–9.
6. Levetan C, Want LL, Weyer C, Strobel SA, Crean J, Wang Y, Maggs DG, Kolterman OG, Chandran M, Mudaliar SR, Henry RR. Impact of pramlintide on glucose fluctuations and postprandial glucose, glucagon, and triglyceride excursions among patients with type 1 diabetes intensively treated with insulin pumps. Diabetes Care 2003;26(1):1–8.
7. Ceriello A, Piconi L, Quagliaro L, Wang Y, Schnabel CA, Ruggles JA, Gloster MA, Maggs DG, Weyer C. Effects of pramlintide on postprrandial glucose excursions and measures of oxidative stress in patients with type 1 diabetes. Diabetes Care 2005;28:632–7.
8. Ryan GJ, Jobe LJ, Martin R. Pramlintide in the treatment of type 1 and type 2 diabetes mellitus. Clin Ther 2005; 27:1500–12.
9. Ratner R, Whitehouse F, Fineman MS, Strobel S, Shen L, Maggs DG, Kolterman OG, Weyer C. Adjunctive therapy with pramlintide lowers HbA1c without concomitant weight gain and increased risk of severe hypoglycemia in patients with type 1 diabetes approaching glycemic targets. Exp Clin Endocrinol Diabetes 2005;113:199–204.
10. Weyer C, Fineman MS, Strobel S, Shen L, Data J, Kolterman OG, Sylvestri MF. Properties of pramlintide and insulin upon mixing. Am J Health-Syst Pharm 2005;62:816–22.

Biguanides

General Information

Biguanides (1) and metformin (2–4) have been reviewed. Metformin (rINN) is the only biguanide commonly used; buformin (rINN) and phenformin (rINN) have been withdrawn in many countries (SEDA-4, 306) because of dangerous adverse effects. However, they are still available in a few countries, and with increasing travel, adverse effects of drugs no longer available in one country can occur if the drug is obtained elsewhere.

The biguanides have a special affinity for the mitochondrial membrane, which causes an alteration in electron transport and results in reduced oxygen consumption. Inhibition of the active transport of glucose in the intestinal mucosa, absent activation of glucose transporters, inhibition of gluconeogenesis, and inhibition of fatty acid oxidation and of lipid synthesis are the effects that are considered to cause lowering of the blood glucose and improving blood lipids in diabetes mellitus. The blood glucose lowering effect of metformin was comparable to that of sulfonylureas, according to a meta-analysis, but body weight increases with sulfonylureas and falls with metformin, leading to a mean weight change difference of 2.9 kg (5).

Most (70–90%) of a dose of metformin is eliminated via the kidneys with a half-life of 9 hours (6). In contrast, phenformin is mostly eliminated by metabolism; its half-life is about 11 hours (7).

Observational studies

In a large American study in 3234 non-diabetic people with a raised fasting blood glucose and a raised blood glucose 2 hours after a glucose load, diabetes occurred in 7.8 cases per 100 participants per year after a mean treatment period of 2.8 years with metformin 850 mg bd; there were 11 cases per 100 participants per year after placebo and 4.8 cases per 100 participants per year after a life-style intervention program (8). Gastrointestinal symptoms were most frequent in those who took metformin. In a later study, glucose tolerance tests were performed after a 14-day washout period of metformin and placebo in the patients who had not developed diabetes (9). Diabetes was more frequently diagnosed in the metformin group, but when the diabetes conversions during treatment and washout were combined, diabetes was still significantly less common in the metformin group.

Comparative studies

Metformin and troglitazone have been compared in 21 patients with type 2 diabetes unresponsive to glibenclamide 10 mg bd (10). Metformin stabilized weight and reduced adipocyte size, leptin concentrations, and glucose transport. GLUT1 and GLUT4 in isolated adipocytes were not changed. Insulin-stimulated whole-body glucose disposal rate increased by 20%. Troglitazone caused increases in body weight, adipocyte size, leptin concentrations, and basal and insulin-stimulated glucose transport. GLUT4 protein expression was increased two-fold and insulin-stimulated whole-body glucose disposal rate increased by 44%.

Placebo-controlled studies

In a placebo-controlled study in 40 patients with impaired glucose tolerance metformin 500 mg bd for 6 months increased insulin-stimulated glucose metabolism by 20% with minimal improvement in glucose tolerance; this effect was maintained after 12 months (11).

In 82 children aged 10–16 years with type 2 diabetes, metformin lowered HbA_{1c} and fasting blood glucose compared with placebo (12). More patients who took placebo had to drop out because more medication was necessary. Most of the adverse events (abdominal pain, diarrhea, nausea, vomiting) occurred during metformin treatment.

Combinations of oral hypoglycemic drugs

The different mechanisms of action of the various classes of hypoglycemic drugs makes combined therapy feasible: the sulfonylureas and meglitinides stimulate insulin production by different mechanisms, the biguanides reduce glucose production by the liver and excretion from the liver, acarbose reduces the absorption of glucose from the gut, and the thiazolidinediones reduce insulin resistance in fat. It is not necessary to wait until the maximal dose of one drug has been reached before starting another. However, sulfonylureas and meglitinides should no longer be used when endogenous insulin production is minimal. Combinations of insulin with sulfonylureas or meglitinides should only be used while the patient is changing to insulin, except when long-acting insulin is given at night in order to give the islets a rest and to stimulate daytime insulin secretion.

This subject has been reviewed in relation to combined oral therapy. In a systematic review of 63 studies with a duration of at least 3 months and involving at least 10 patients at the end of the study, and in which HbA_{1c} was reported, five different classes of oral drugs were almost equally effective in lowering blood glucose concentrations (13). HbA_{1c} was reduced by about 1–2% in all cases. Combination therapy gave additive effects. However, long-term vascular risk reduction was demonstrated only with sulfonylureas and metformin.

In a placebo-controlled study in 116 patients who responded insufficiently to metformin 2.5 g/day, rosiglitazone 2 or 4 mg bd was added for 26 weeks (14). HbA_{1c} and fasting plasma glucose improved and hemoglobin fell. Edema was reported in 5.2% of the patients who took rosiglitazone and two patients withdrew because of headache.

Metformin has been reviewed, with special attention to therapy in combination with other hypoglycemic drugs (15). The general conclusions were that it can effectively lower HbA_{1c} concentrations, improve lipid profiles, and improve vascular and hemodynamic indices.

Biguanides plus glitazones

The combination of metformin + thiazolidinediones (glitazones) is contraindicated or not recommended in patients taking therapy for cardiac failure. In a retrospective study of 12 505 and 13 158 patients with cardiac failure and diabetes in two different years (1998/9 and 2000/1) (16), 7.1% (later 11%) had a prescription for metformin, 7.2% (16%) for thiazolidinediones and 14% (24%) for both drugs added to cardiac drugs. This suggests that many patients with heart failure are taking hypoglycemic drugs, notwithstanding contraindications.

Biguanides + glitazones + sulfonylureas

Glibenclamide 2.5 mg/day + metformin 500 mg/day in a combination tablet was increased to a maximum of 10 mg/day + 2000 mg/day in patients with type 2 diabetes, mean age 57 years and weight 93 kg; 181 patients also took rosiglitazone and 184 took placebo for 24 weeks (17). Rosiglitazone was added to a maximum of 8 mg/day aiming to reduce the HB_{A1c} concentration to less than 7.0%. There was *hypoglycemia* in 140 patients; 95 (53%) of those who took rosiglitazone reported hypoglycemia compared with 45 (25%) of those who took placebo. One patient taking rosiglitazone withdrew owing to hypoglycemia. HB_{A1c} concentrations were less than 7% in 42% of those taking rosiglitazone compared with 14% of those taking placebo. Weight gain was greater in those taking rosiglitazone, 3 kg compared with 0.03 kg.

Biguanides + meglitinides

Patients with type 2 diabetes with unsatisfactory control after taking metformin for 6 months were randomized to metformin alone, repaglinide alone, or metformin + repaglinide (each 27 patients) (18). Combined therapy reduced HbA_{1c} after 3 months by 1.4% and fasting glucose by 2.2 mmol/l. Repaglinide alone or in combination with metformin increased insulin concentrations. The most common adverse effects were hypoglycemia, diarrhea, and headache. Gastrointestinal adverse effects were common in those taking metformin alone, and body weight increased in both groups taking repaglinide.

In 12 patients with type 2 diabetes, a combination of nateglinide 120 mg or placebo with metformin 500 mg before each meal on two separate days was well tolerated (19). One patient taking nateglinide had a headache. One patient was withdrawn because of a myocardial infarction and had multivessel coronary artery disease on catheterization.

In a prospective, randomized, double-blind, placebo-controlled study for 24 weeks, 701 patients took nateglinide 120 mg before the three main meals, or metformin 500 mg tds, or the combination of the two, or placebo (20). The most frequent adverse effect was hypoglycemia, and it was most common in the combination group. There were no differences between those who took nateglinide only or metformin only and there were no episodes of serious hypoglycemia. Diarrhea was more frequent in those taking metformin or the combination, but infection, nausea, headache, and abdominal pain were comparable in the two groups.

Of 82 patients insufficiently controlled by metformin, 27 continued to take metformin with placebo, 28 took titrated repaglinide with placebo, and 27 took metformin with titrated repaglinide for 4–5 months (21). There were no serious adverse effects. Nine patients taking metformin + repaglinide reported 30 hypoglycemic events and three patients taking repaglinide reported 9 events.

The combination of nateglinide + metformin for 3–4 months reported caused mild adverse events in 2.9% of patients, the most common being gastrointestinal complaints (22).

Biguanides plus sulfonylureas

The combination of metformin with various sulfonylurea derivatives has been extensively reviewed (15). When metformin or pioglitazone were added to sulfonylureas in patients with type 2 diabetes who were poorly controlled, those with reduced pancreatic beta cell function responded better to metformin, while those with greater insulin resistance responded better to pioglitazone (23).

Combination tablets containing metformin + glibenclamide (250 + 1.25 mg) were compared with monotherapy with metformin 500 mg/day or glibenclamide 2.5 mg/day for 16 weeks in 486 patients (24). The total daily doses were adjusted depending on fasting plasma glucose. The final mean doses with combined therapy were lower than with monotherapy. Gastrointestinal symptoms, such as diarrhea, nausea, vomiting, and abdominal pain, were significantly more frequent with metformin monotherapy than with either combined therapy or glibenclamide monotherapy. Hypoglycemia was most frequent in those who took combination therapy and least with metformin monotherapy, but

finger-stick glucose concentrations under 2.8 mmol/l were rare with metformin monotherapy and equally common with glibenclamide monotherapy and combination therapy.

In the United Kingdom Prospective Diabetes Study a subgroup of patients taking sulfonylurea therapy to which metformin was added appeared to have had excess mortality. Data from 263 general practices in the UK were analysed; 8488 patients took a sulfonylurea initially, to which metformin was added in 1868 (25). The crude mortality rates per 1000 person years were 59 and 40 respectively. Metformin was used initially in 3099 patients and a sulfonylurea was added in 867. The crude mortality rates per 1000 person years were 25 and 20 respectively. These results suggest there is no increased mortality risk with a combination of a sulfonylurea and metformin.

Insulin + biguanides

Metformin was given as an adjunct to insulin in a double-blind, placebo-controlled study in 28 adolescents needing more than 1 U/kg/day (26). The dose of metformin was 1000 mg/day when body weight was under 50 kg, 1500 mg/day when it was 50–75 kg, and 2000 mg/day when it was over 75 kg. Metformin lowered insulin requirements. The number of episodes of hypoglycemia increased compared with placebo. There was gastrointestinal discomfort in six patients taking metformin and five taking placebo.

A comparable placebo-controlled study was reported in 353 patients with type 2 diabetes for 48 weeks. All were taking insulin, and HbA_{1c} fell in those who also took metformin. Body weight was reduced by 0.4 kg by metformin and increased by 1.2 kg by placebo. Symptomatic episodes of hypoglycemia were more common with metformin. There were mild transient gastrointestinal complaints in 56 and 13% respectively (27).

Insulin plus metformin (27 patients, 2000 mg/day) or troglitazone (30 patients, 600 mg/day) in patients with type 2 diabetes using at least 30 U/day was compared with insulin alone (30 patients) for 4 months (28). Body weight increased in the insulin and the insulin plus troglitazone groups. In the insulin plus metformin group there were significantly more gastrointestinal adverse effects but less hypoglycemia than the other groups.

In 80 patients taking metformin 850 or 1000 mg tds plus NPH insulin at bedtime, metformin was withdrawn and repaglinide 4 mg tds added in half of the patients for 16 weeks (29). In the repaglinide group the dose of insulin increased slightly and weight gain was 1.8 kg more. Mild hypoglycemia occurred more often in the metformin group; nightly episodes of hypoglycemia occurred only with repaglinide. One patient taking repaglinide had a myocardial infarction, and one had three separate hospitalizations for chest pain (myocardial infarction was excluded). No specific data were presented about gastrointestinal adverse effects or infections.

Contraindications

Contraindications to treatment with biguanides are:

1. impaired renal function (serum creatinine may not be a sufficient indicator; creatinine clearance must be estimated)

2. an increased risk of impaired renal function in inter-current diseases with fever, congestive heart failure, or infections of the urinary tract, during treatment with diuretics, intravenous pyelography, or severe dieting
3. states associated with tissue hypoxia (respiratory insufficiency, heart insufficiency, anemia, and peripheral vascular disease)
4. hepatitis and hepatic cirrhosis
5. excessive use of alcohol
6. wasting diseases
7. preoperatively and postoperatively.

In general, biguanides should not be used in people aged over 75 years (30).

Of 308 patients 73% had contraindications, risk factors, or intercurrent illnesses necessitating withdrawal of metformin (31): 19% had renal impairment, 25% heart failure, 6.5% respiratory insufficiency, and 1.3% hepatic impairment; 51% had advanced coronary heart disease, 9.8% atrial fibrillation, 3.3% chronic alcohol abuse, 2% advanced peripheral arterial disease, and 0.7% were pregnant.

Four fatal cases in 18 months in a community hospital were reported; three had clear contraindications (32): a 45-year-old woman with liver cirrhosis, a 64-year-old man with coronary artery disease, and a 65-year-old man with peripheral arterial disease and asthma; a 74-year-old man had renal insufficiency.

In a retrospective study of 1874 patients with type 2 diabetes taking metformin, 25% had contraindications, including acute myocardial infarction, cardiac failure, renal impairment, and chronic liver disease (33). However, contraindications often did not lead to withdrawal of metformin: in 621 episodes, only 10% stopped taking it. Only 25 and 18% stopped taking metformin when they developed renal impairment or myocardial infarction, respectively. One patient developed lactic acidosis, but this may have been a consequence of myocardial infarction.

Contraindications to the use of metformin have been debated (34), in relation to the reduced number of cardiovascular events seen in the obese patients treated with metformin in the UK prospective diabetes study (UKPDS) (35). The authors stated inter alia that lactic acidosis is rare (1–5 cases per 100 000) and that in the absence of renal insufficiency accumulation of metformin is rare. Moreover, the authors of a Cochrane systematic review concluded that treatment with metformin was not associated with an increased risk of lactic acidosis (36). Tissue hypoxia is often the trigger for metformin accumulation. Many physicians do not comply with the official British contraindications. The author suggested the following necessary precautionary measures:

- withdraw the drug during periods of suspected tissue hypoxia (myocardial infarction and sepsis);
- withdraw 3 days after the administration of an iodine-containing contrast medium and 2 days before general anesthesia;
- check renal function in both cases before metformin is restarted;
- serum creatinine over 150 μmol/l is a contraindication.

To this one could add that drugs that compromise renal function should not be combined with metformin.

Others have stated that metformin is contraindicated when serum creatinine concentrations are over 133 μmol/l (1.5 mg/dl) in men or 124 μmol/l (1.4 mg/dl) in women (15).

However, creatinine is sometimes a poor predictor of renal function. For example, it must be related to muscular mass and the "normal" serum creatinine may be too high in a person of 50 kg and little muscle. It is therefore better to use creatinine clearance below 60 ml/min as a criterion.

For some reactions the usefulness of withdrawing metformin before operations, except in emergency, cardiac, and vascular surgery and in operations requiring deliberate hypotension, has been discussed (37) and the creatinine threshold value has been discussed (38).

Reconsideration of contraindications has also been proposed in a prospective study in patients with serum creatinine concentrations of 130–220 μmol/l and coronary heart disease ($n = 226$), congestive heart failure ($n = 94$) and chronic obstructive pulmonary disease ($n = 91$). Half of the patients continued to take metformin and the other half stopped (39). Bodyweight and HbA_{1c} increased over 4 years in those who stopped taking metformin. Lactic acid concentrations were similar in the two groups. Deaths were similar in the two groups (62 and 64 respectively). The incidences of myocardial infarction, all cardiovascular events, and cardiovascular mortality were the same. Changes in additional therapy were only significant for insulin (30% versus 45% respectively) and diet (25% versus 0% respectively).

Organs and Systems

Cardiovascular

The cardiovascular effects of metformin have been reviewed (40). Metformin reduces blood pressure and has a beneficial effect on blood lipid concentrations.

In a retrospective study, cardiovascular deaths in patients using a sulfonylurea only ($n = 741$) were compared with deaths in patients taking a sulfonylurea + metformin ($n = 169$) (41). In patients taking the combination the adjusted odds ratios (95% CI) were:

- overall mortality 1.63 (1.27, 2.09);
- mortality from ischemic heart disease 1.73 (1.17, 2.55);
- stroke 2.33 (1.17, 4.63).

The patients taking the combination were younger, had had diabetes for longer, were more obese, and had higher blood glucose concentrations.

Nervous system

Two cases of encephalopathy, which improved after metformin was withdrawn, have been reported (42).

- One week after starting to take metformin 850 mg in divided dose a 74-year-old man became confused and disoriented and had speech abnormalities and bilateral horizontal gaze-evoked nystagmus. Electroencephalography suggested a toxic-metabolic encephalopathy. Metformin was withdrawn, he became alert and oriented, and the electroencephalogram normalized.

- A 67-year-old man took metformin for 4 years after which repaglinide 3 mg/day was added. After 3 weeks he became confused and had general diffuse myoclonic jerks and bilateral asterixis. The electroencephalogram showed a general slowing. He improved after stopping both hypoglycemic drugs and became asymptomatic within 3 days. Metformin was reinstituted, as repaglinide was considered to have caused the changes. However, within 2 days the same clinical picture evolved. After withdrawal of metformin he normalized progressively and he had no confusion over the next year.

Sensory systems

Altered vision has been attributed to metformin (43).

- A 62-year-old man with diabetes was given metformin 750 mg bd and his blood glucose concentration fell from 22 to 15 mmol/l within 4 days. The dose of metformin was increased to 850 mg bd and the blood glucose concentration fell to 8.7 mmol/l over the next week. Within 2 days of starting therapy his vision became blurred. Slit lamp examination 2 weeks later showed cracked shaped lines on the lens. The cracks resolved spontaneously by 3 months.

Although the timing made metformin a possible candidate in this case, it is much more likely that the problem was caused by rapid changes in blood glucose concentration and the associated fluid shifts.

Metabolism

Hypoglycemia

Biguanides cause hypoglycemia in 0.24 cases per 100 patient-years and it is more common when they are used in combination with a sulfonylurea (44). In 102 consecutive patients with drug-induced hospital-related hypoglycemic coma, 13 were taking metformin + glibenclamide and 3 were taking metformin + insulin (45).

When hypoglycemia occurs it should lead to a search for other potential problems.

- A 72-year-old man taking metformin 1 g bd for type 2 diabetes began to have episodes of hypoglycemia, which resolved on stopping the metformin; he also had anterior pituitary failure (46).

Lactic acidosis

DoTS classification
Adverse effect: Lactic acidosis due to biguanides
Dose-relation: toxic effect
Time-course: time-independent
Susceptibility factors: genetic (slow phenformin metabolizers); age; disease (impaired liver, kidney, or cardiac function, alcoholism)

Biguanides can cause lactic acidosis, which is fatal in 50% of cases (47).

- A 65-year-old man with a creatinine clearance of 67 ml/minute taking metformin 850 mg bd developed lactic acidosis (lactate 25 mmol/l, pH 7.13, bicarbonate 5 mmol/l) (48). Despite the relatively small dosage of metformin, he had unexplained very high metformin concentrations (61 μg/ml).

A possible explanation for the high metformin concentration in this case was that an unknown substance related to intestinal inclusion inhibited its tubular excretion. Other cases involving metformin have included the following:

- a 62-year-old woman: pH 6.60, blood lactate 45 mmol/l, creatinine 133 μmol/l (49);
- a 72-year-old woman: pH 6.84, creatinine 125 μmol/l (50);
- a 75-year-old woman: pH 6.73, lactate 18 mmol/l (50);
- a patient with creatinine 91 μmol/l, creatinine clearance 52 ml/minute, metformin concentration 61 μg/ml (target under 5 μg/ml) (51);
- a 52-year-old woman, a chronic alcohol user: pH 6.74, lactate over 30 mmol/l, creatinine 710 μmol/l (52);
- an 83-year-old woman with mild renal insufficiency (53).

All survived, but all needed hemodialysis. In all cases there were contraindications to metformin.

- An 82-year-old man and a 76-year-old man with normal renal function developed increased lactate concentrations (3.6 mmol/l and 3.2 mmol/l respectively) a few weeks after starting to take metformin (54). Both had a low bicarbonate concentration and high anion gap. The second patient was also taking ciprofloxacin for a urinary tract infection. In both patients lactate reached normal values after metformin was withdrawn.
- A 40-year-old man taking metformin 850 mg bd developed severe metabolic acidosis (pH 6.62, base deficit 31 mmol/l, anion gap 37 mmol/l, lactate over 20 mmol/l) and hypoglycemia (1.9 mmol/l) (55).
- A 42-year-old man developed nausea and vomiting and felt suicidal. He had type 2 diabetes and was taking metformin (56). His blood lactate concentration was 8.9 mmol/l, bicarbonate 16 mmol/l, and pH 7.2. Severe hypotension required intensive care. The lactate concentration rose to 22 mmol/l and the bicarbonate fell to 6.7 mmol/l and the pH to 6.89. The metformin concentration was high at 191 mg/l. He survived, having been treated with intermittent hemodialysis.
- A 61-year-old woman developed a bradydysrhythmia after a cardiac arrest (57). Her lactate concentration was 18 mmol/l, pH 6.60, blood glucose 19 mmol/l, and creatinine 1136 μmol/l. She had a 5-year history of type 2 diabetes treated with glimepiride 3 mg/day and metformin 850 mg tds, and 4 months before admission had had a serum creatinine concentration of 1.1 mg/dl. In the few days before admission she had had abdominal pain, nausea, and a speech disorder. She was treated with hemodialysis, and 6 weeks later the creatinine was 0.54 mg/dl. Further information about events leading to the acute renal insufficiency was not given, but a diagnosis of metformin-associated lactic acidosis was made.

There is no doubt from reports such as this in people who take overdoses that metformin can cause lactic acidosis. In a review of enquires to a poison center relating to metformin between 1995 and 2003 there were 109 enquires, of which 62 were for attempted suicide and 47 for adverse effects; 14 patients had had lactic acidosis (57). Eight were taking metformin as regular therapy, of whom one died; of six who had attempted suicide, three died.

Five patients with metformin-associated severe lactic acidosis, seen between 1 September 1998 and 31 May 2001, have been reported (58). Two had attempted suicide. All had severe metabolic acidosis with a high anion gap and raised blood lactate concentrations. Four developed profound hypotension and three had acute respiratory failure. Three had normal preceding renal function. Three required conventional hemodialysis and two continuous renal replacement therapy.

Cases also continue to be reported with buformin and phenformin (59).

- A 67-year-old man who had taken phenformin and glibenclamide for 2 years became lethargic and confused (60). His pH was 6.91, serum lactate 25 mmol/l and later 30 mmol/l, and blood glucose very low (0.5 mmol/l), possibly because of vomiting, anorexia, and glibenclamide. Hemodialysis was advised but not performed, since he recovered spontaneously.
- In Spain a 69-year-old woman with a dilated cardiomyopathy and poor inferior ventricular function developed lactic acidosis after an increase in the dose of buformin (pH 7.1, lactate 18 mmol/l). After withdrawal of buformin and infusion of sodium bicarbonate her renal function and electrolyte disturbances were corrected (61).
- Two other cases were reported in Japan. One developed in a patient with type 2 diabetes without any underlying disease (62). The other case was caused by suicide (63).

Buformin is no longer registered in many countries.

Incidence
In patients taking metformin, lactic acidosis is rare (3 per 100 000 patient-years) and is most often seen when contraindications to metformin (impaired kidney or liver function, alcoholism, circulatory problems, old age) are neglected or not detected (64). Although the relative risk of lactic acidosis with metformin is significantly lower than with phenformin or buformin (65), it has been repeatedly reported (SEDA-6, 371) (66), even in the absence of known contraindications (67).

Experience with metformin in a large American health organization in 9875 patients has been presented (68). There was one probable case of lactic acidosis in an 82-year-old woman who developed renal impairment while taking metformin 500 mg/day.

In 11 797 patients (22 296 person-years) in Saskatchewan who took metformin from 1980–95 there were 9 cases of lactic acidosis per 100 000 patient-years (69), a much lower incidence than the estimated rate of 40–64 cases for phenformin.

The lower frequency of lactic acidosis during treatment with metformin compared with other biguanides may be caused by its short non-polar hydrophobic side chains substituted with two CH_3 groups. This has a lower affinity for hydrophobic structures, such as phospholipids in mitochondrial and cellular membranes, than the longer monosubstituted side-chains of the other biguanides (64).

Mechanism and susceptibility factors
Biguanides in high doses inhibit the oxidation of carbohydrate substrates by affecting mitochondrial function. Anoxidative carbohydrate metabolism stimulates the production of lactate. High lactate production leads to lactic acidosis (type B) with a low pH (<6.95). Hyperlactatemia was common in patients taking buformin, even without alcoholism or impaired liver, kidney, or cardiac function (70).

In reaction to a report of lactic acidosis at a therapeutic metformin concentration (SEDA-22, 476), in which a mitochondrial defect was supposed to have increased susceptibility to metformin, it has been observed that diabetes itself may dispose to hyperlactatemia (71). Others (72) have taken issue with the opinion (SEDA-22, 476) that the association of lactic acidosis with metformin may be coincidental, as lactic acidosis can also emerge during critical illnesses (type A lactic acidosis, caused by circulatory insufficiency). However, patients with type B lactic acidosis, with high biguanide concentrations, will also develop circulatory insufficiency after some hours.

The main susceptibility factor for lactic acidosis due to metformin is renal insufficiency (49). In patients taking phenformin, poor oxidative metabolism may contribute (73).

All patients admitted to a hospital during 6 months who had taken at least one dose of metformin were retrospectively evaluated for susceptibility factors for metformin-associated lactic acidosis (8). There were 263 hospitalizations in 204 patients. In 71 admissions there was at least one contraindication, such as renal or liver disease, renal dysfunction, congestive cardiac failure, metabolic acidosis, or an intravenous iodinated contrast medium given within 48 hours of metformin. In 29 (41%) metformin was continued despite the contraindication. The most frequent contraindication was a raised serum creatinine, but in only eight of the 32 admissions was metformin withdrawn. Of nine patients using metformin who died (not necessarily directly related to metformin), six had an absolute contraindication. In two patients who died and in one who survived, blood lactate was increased and this was temporally related to the use of metformin.

Whether metformin in therapeutic doses can cause lactic acidosis in the absence of renal insufficiency has been investigated by studying case histories of metformin-associated lactic acidosis in various databases published from May 1995 to January 2000 (74). Overdoses and lactic acidosis caused by contrast media were excluded. There were 21 reports of 26 cases, of which five did not comply with the criteria (lactate over 5 mmol/l, pH 7.35 or less). Plasma metformin concentration was measured in only four cases. The authors distinguished between lactic acidosis precipitated by metformin, which was defined as occurring without accumulation of metformin, and lactic acidosis that occurred during primary acute or chronic renal insufficiency, with accumulation of metformin. In the first group, six of the eight patients died. In the second group, notwithstanding a mean lactate concentration of nearly 15 mmol/l, only one of the 12 patients died, having refused dialysis. They concluded that there is no relation between the use of metformin and lactic acidosis, except when metformin accumulates. This has been illustrated by the case of a 76-year-old woman taking 850 mg metformin bd who developed lactic acidosis due to metformin accumulation during deteriorating kidney function (75).

Drugs that can precipitate lactic acidosis in patients taking metformin include ACE inhibitors, thiazide diuretics, NSAIDs, and drugs such as furosemide, nifedipine, cimetidine, amiloride, triamterene, trimethoprim, and digoxin, which are all secreted in the renal tubules, compete with metformin, and can contribute to increased plasma metformin concentrations (76).

The need to follow recommended guidelines strictly in order to avoid lactic acidosis in patients taking metformin has been emphasized (77).

Presentation

The early symptoms of lactic acidosis are nausea, vomiting, and diarrhea; since these are common adverse effects of biguanides, a careful watch should be kept for their sudden onset or aggravation, which might point to lactic acidosis (78).

In retrospective studies, neither the degree of hyperlactatemia nor accumulation of metformin had prognostic significance, but mortality was linked to the underlying disease (79,80).

Management

The best therapy of metformin-induced lactic acidosis is immediate hemodialysis, but metformin in the tissues continues to produce lactate while the drug is being removed during dialysis. Sodium bicarbonate is not very effective and can paradoxically lower the pH and cause hypernatremia and fluid overload. Tracheal intubation and mechanical ventilation may be necessary (76). Theophylline and dichloroacetate have also been used. Theophylline stimulates oxygen exchange in the lungs. Dichloroacetate activates pyruvate dehydrogenase, inhibiting lactate formation, but it is neurotoxic, can cause cataract, and is mutagenic (SEDA-7, 410).

The results of hemodialysis in biguanide-induced lactic acidosis are variable. Metformin and buformin are dialysable, but phenformin is poorly eliminated. Successful continuous venovenous hemofiltration has been reported (81).

- A 68-year-old woman with type 2 diabetes and hypertension took phenformin 90 mg/day and glibenclamide 6 mg/day. She developed a urinary tract infection and oliguria followed by respiratory distress and mental confusion without neurological defects. Her pH was 6.84, serum lactate 28 mmol/l, creatinine 186 μmol/l, and glucose 10.4 mmol/l, and there were no ketone bodies. She received assisted ventilation, bicarbonate, dopamine + obutamine, glucose + insulin, and antibiotics. Her

serum lactate increased to 44 mmol/l and continuous venovenous hemofiltration was started. After 5 days her lactate concentration was in the reference range (0.5–2.2 mmol/l). The serum phenformin concentration was almost 600 ng/ml (10 times the therapeutic value).

Reviews

The questions "Does metformin cause lactic acidosis?" (82) and "What is the risk of lactic acidosis accompanying metformin therapy for patients with type 2 diabetes?" (83) have been posed and answered using data from a Cochrane review.

In contrast to the numerous reports of lactic acidosis in patients taking metformin, a systematic review has shown no evidence of an association (36). This highlights a problem of comparing randomized controlled trials with anecdotal reports from real-life therapy. An effect that occurs only in people with a particular susceptibility may be missed in even very large randomized trials and may therefore only be reported anecdotally. Absence of evidence from a meta-analysis in such circumstances is not evidence against an effect in susceptible individuals.

In another review it was suggested that the risk of lactic acidosis when metformin is used as recommended is close to zero (84). The author discussed the COSMIC study, which compared metformin treatment for 1 year ($n = 7227$) with usual care with other antidiabetic agents ($n = 1505$). There were no cases of lactic acidosis. The findings in controlled trials contrast with case reports of lactic acidosis. About one million patients have received metformin in the USA and the FDA has received 47 reports of lactic acidosis (20 fatal). Of these, 43 patients had renal insufficiency or susceptibility factors for lactic acidosis, such as congestive cardiac failure. Only four cases appeared to have no other susceptibility factors, one of which may have been precipitated by urinary sepsis; none of these four died.

Six experts in intensive care or metabolic disease reviewed all case reports of lactic acidosis from 1957 to 1999—37 articles reporting 80 cases (85). To be assessed the reports had to meet strict criteria, including: a diagnosis of type 2 diabetes, metformin therapy before lactic acidosis, a pH of 7.35 or less, or a plasma bicarbonate concentration below 22 mmol/l and a lactic acid concentration of at least 5 mmol/l. Because of lack of information, 33 cases were excluded. There were other susceptibility factors for lactic acidosis besides metformin in 46 of 47 cases. Only 13 of the 47 cases were classified as probably due to metformin by at least three experts. The authors suggested a rethink about the relation between lactic acidosis and metformin. However, they still recommended withdrawing therapy in acute renal insufficiency and when contrast dyes are used for radiological investigation.

In a review of reports to the Australian Adverse Drugs Reactions Advisory Committee between 1985 and 2001 there were 48 cases of lactic acidosis with metformin (86). In 35 of the 48 cases known susceptibility factors were identified. The estimated frequency was one case of lactic acidosis in 30 000 patients taking metformin. The authors discussed the arbitrary cut-off point of a creatinine concentration of 150 µmol/l often set for withdrawal of metformin. They suggest that the concentration should be individualized and that age, muscle mass, and protein turnover should also be considered. They recommended using the Cockcroft–Gault equation to estimate creatinine clearance, and an absolute cut-off point of 30 ml/minute, below which metformin should be withdrawn. In patients with a creatinine clearance of 30–50 ml/minute there should be caution. Metformin should be withdrawn during significant intercurrent illnesses and when using iodinated contrast agents.

Nutrition

Metformin can cause reduced vitamin B_{12} absorption, reducing serum B_{12} concentrations and causing megaloblastic anemia (87), the prevalence of which was 9% in 600 patients with type 2 diabetes taking biguanides (phenformin or metformin) for a mean of 12 years (88). In 353 patients with type 2 diabetes, treated with insulin, who took metformin for 16 weeks in a placebo-controlled study, metformin increased serum homocysteine concentrations by 4% and reduced serum folate by 7% and vitamin B_{12} by 14% (89).

- A 63-year-old man with type 2 diabetes, who had taken metformin for at least 5 years, had a low serum vitamin B_{12} concentration (110 pg/ml; reference range 200–230) and a normal serum folate (90). There were no autoantibodies. A Schilling test showed malabsorption of vitamin B_{12}. Metformin was withdrawn and 2 months later a Schilling test showed no malabsorption.
- This case prompted a report of 10 metformin- associated patients with cobalamin deficiency among 162 patients with vitamin B_{12} concentrations below 200 pg/ml (91). They had taken a mean dose of metformin of 2015 mg/day for an average of 8.9 years. The mean vitamin B_{12} concentration was 140 pg/ml. All had normal serum folate and creatinine concentrations and no antibodies to intrinsic factor. In one patient there was malabsorption.

Hematologic

Megaloblastic anemia is rare with metformin, but vitamin B_{12} concentrations can be reduced by metformin and phenformin (92) because of reduced absorption, and pre-existing deficiency can be exacerbated (64).

Metformin can occasionally cause a hemolytic anemia.

- A 68-year-old woman of North African Jewish descent with a raised HbA_{1c} was given metformin 850 mg tds and repaglinide 1 mg tds, and 14 days later developed extreme weakness and anemia, her hemoglobin having fallen from 12 to 8 g/dl within 1 week (93). Her reticulocyte count was 11%, with polychromasia. The bilirubin rose to 35 µmol/l (27 µmol/l direct). The haptoglobin concentration was low and a direct Coombs' test was negative. Metformin was withdrawn. Two units of erythrocytes were transfused and the hemoglobin rose to 11 g/dl and remained stable. Glucose-6-phosphate dehydrogenase (G6PD) activity was significantly reduced. There were no other precipitating factors for hemolysis due to G6PD deficiency.

It is unclear whether metformin caused hemolysis directly in this case or via G6PD deficiency. Two other patients have been reported with normal G6PD activity (94,95); one had a positive Coombs' test (95).

Gastrointestinal

At the start of therapy watery diarrhea, nausea, abdominal bloating, flatulence, anorexia and dyspepsia are common, but they resolve mostly within a few weeks (15). Phenformin can cause hemorrhagic gastritis (96).

The gastrointestinal adverse effects of metformin can be reduced by giving the metformin during or immediately after meals, starting with a low dose and increasing it gradually (64).

In 43 patients with poorly controlled type 2 diabetes using insulin, the addition of metformin improved HbA_{1c} and reduced the dose of insulin (97). Seven patients in the metformin group and four in the placebo group had nausea; nine versus four had diarrhea.

- Three patients who had taken metformin for more than 2 years developed diarrhea (98). After withdrawal of metformin the diarrhea resolved within 1 month. A fourth patient developed diarrhea after taking metformin for 4 months, which stopped after withdrawal; rechallenge with metformin 8 months later led to recurrence. Three of these patients had bowel disease (diverticulosis, irritable bowel syndrome, and diabetic neuropathy).
- A 49-year-old woman developed chronic diarrhea after using metformin 850 mg tds and insulin for 5 years (99). After 5 months, metformin was withdrawn and the diarrhea resolved within 3 days. On rechallenge the diarrhea returned.
- A 44-year-old non-diabetic man took metformin 1700 mg/day for some weeks for obesity (100). He developed severe gastrointestinal hemorrhage needing blood transfusion. A bleeding Meckel's diverticulum was removed and he had no further hemorrhage. Coagulation studies, to investigate whether reduced platelet aggregation or altered coagulation factors (increased tissue plasminogen activator (tPA) or reduced tPA-Ag, or PAI-1) could have contributed, were not done.

The use of metformin in polycystic ovarian syndrome, which is often accompanied by insulin resistance or other aspects of the metabolic syndrome, has been systematically reviewed (101). Metformin was therapeutically less effective than weight loss. Adverse effects were nausea, vomiting, and gastrointestinal disturbances.

Liver

Metformin can cause hepatitis (102).

- A 52-year-old woman took glipizide and enalapril and then, because of persistent hyperglycemia, metformin 1000 mg/day (103). Her liver enzymes were normal, and after 2 weeks the dosage of metformin was increased to 2000 mg/day. Two weeks later she became icteric and her bilirubin and liver enzymes were increased. Serological studies were negative. All drugs were withdrawn. A liver biopsy was consistent with toxic hepatitis. She had normal liver enzymes after a month.

Hepatitis after sulfonylureas is known, and this patient had taken glipizide for several years. The combination of glipizide and metformin may have been to blame.

- A 75-year-old man taking insulin about 40 U/day was given metformin 500 mg bd (104). He also used enteric-coated aspirin, diltiazem XR, ibuprofen, and lovastatin. Two months later his liver enzymes were raised, but he felt well. Hepatitis antibodies were negative. After withdrawal of metformin his liver enzymes became normal. He agreed to restart metformin. His liver enzymes remained normal, but he finally preferred insulin monotherapy.

It is not clear what caused the hepatitis in this case, although it seems that metformin was not to blame.

- A 73 year old Japanese woman, weight 33.5 kg, took nateglinide 270 mg/day and pioglitazone 15 mg/day for 6 months (105). Her Hb_{A1c} concentration was 8.6% and fasting glucose 11.4 mmol/l. Metformin 250 mg bd was added and 3 weeks later she developed jaundice and fatigue. A few months before her liver function tests had been normal. Aspartate transaminase activity was 689 IU/l, alanine transaminase 772 IU/l, alkaline phosphatase 639 IU/l, and bilirubin 6.5 mg/dl. All oral therapy was withdrawn and insulin started. Her liver function improved over the next few weeks.
- A 64-year-old man developed cholestatic jaundice 2 weeks after starting to take metformin 500 mg bd (106). It resolved slowly over several months after withdrawal.

Pancreas

Phenformin can cause pancreatitis (107).

Skin

Urticaria and rashes are seen occasionally with metformin. Lichen ruber planus has been reported (108).

- Erythema multiforme has been attributed to metformin after 4 days of therapy in a 58-year-old man with type 2 diabetes; the rash resolved within 2 weeks of stopping the drug (109).

Immunologic

Leukocytoclastic vasculitis and pneumonitis have been attributed to metformin (110,111).

Death

In 2275 diabetic patients aged 45–74 years compared with 9047 non-diabetics with proven coronary artery disease, 32% of those taking metformin and 44% of those taking combined metformin and glibenclamide died during 7.7 years (112). After 4 years the risks of death with metformin alone and combined therapy were equal, but after 7 years combined therapy had a worse prognosis.

Second-Generation Effects

Pregnancy

Metformin crosses the placenta, and although there is no evidence that it is not safe in pregnancy there are insufficient data to say that it is (113). A trial of metformin in pregnancy has been announced (114), although its safety in pregnancy has not been established.

In an audit in Auckland there was no increase in perinatal mortality or pre-eclampsia (115). The MIG prospective randomized comparison of metformin and insulin aims to recruit 750 women; 70 have been recruited so far without serious adverse events in the metformin arm.

In a review of 60 publications on metformin and pregnancy malabsorption of vitamin B_{12}, which occurs in non-pregnant women, was thought to be a potential problem (116). The data did not suggest an increased risk of teratogenesis.

Teratogenicity

Fetuses are exposed to therapeutic concentrations of metformin, which for part of the day may be higher than those found in the mother (117). Although many women have become pregnant while taking metformin, until recently most have stopped taking it during pregnancy. A review of the safety of metformin therapy for the management of polycystic ovary syndrome has shown an increased frequency of malformations in children born to mothers who took metformin during pregnancy. This was a personal communication and no information was given about the malformations, the numbers, or how the data were collected. It was also not stated who gave the communication. Animal studies with excessive doses have shown anophthalamia, anencephaly, and delayed blastocyst development (118).

In 126 infants born to 109 mothers with polycystic ovary syndrome who conceived while taking metformin and continued to take it during pregnancy, there were no differences in infant growth up to 18 months of age or in motor and social development (119). The doses during pregnancy were 2.55 g/day ($n = 74$), 1.5–2 g/day ($n = 43$), and 1 g/day ($n = 5$). In 18 pregnancies the metformin was stopped at a median of 12 weeks because the obstetrician did not want it to continue. Pre-eclampsia occurred in five of 122 pregnancies (4.1%), which was no different to community controls (nine of 252 (3.6%)).

Lactation

Metformin is increasingly being used in the polycystic ovarian syndrome and therefore in lactating women. In seven breastfeeding mothers taking a median dose of 1500 mg/day, the mean relative infant dose transferred in the milk was 0.28% (120). Serum metformin concentrations were very low or undetectable in infants and they appeared to be healthy. A specific warning was given for children with impaired renal function (prematurity, renal insufficiency).

Susceptibility Factors

Age

The effect of age on the response to metformin has been studied in 174 patients aged over 70 years, not well-controlled on glibenclamide 7.5 mg/day or gliclazide 120 mg/day (121). They were given either maximal doses of a sulfonylurea (glibenclamide 15 mg/day or gliclazide 240 mg/day) or a sulfonylurea + metformin (1700 mg/day). Renal function and liver function were normal. There were nine cases of non-severe hypoglycemia in the first group. In the second group there were two cases of hypoglycemia after delayed meals and 35% had transient mild gastrointestinal discomfort. There were no increases in lactic acid. Lipid concentrations were a little lower in the second group. The authors concluded that age as such is not a contraindication to metformin, provided that contraindications, such as renal impairment, are absent and that blood glucose is measured regularly.

Renal disease

When to stop metformin in people with diabetes mellitus and abnormal renal function continues to be debated. It has been suggested that it should not be used in those with an eGFR (MDRD) of less than 60 ml/minute (122). However, this would exclude many people who have been taking metformin for many years without apparent ill effect. Others have recommended using the Cockcroft–Gault equation (SEDA-29, 527), which is preferable.

Liver disease

The use of metformin in patients with non-alcoholic fatty liver disease has been reported in two trials (123,124). Patients had abnormal liver function tests, which improved during the studies. No-one withdrew because of worsening of liver function tests or lactic acidosis.

Drug Administration

Drug formulations

Modified-release formulations of metformin allow once daily dosage. In a double-blind, parallel-group comparison of an immediate-release and an extended-release formulation in 191 patients for 24 weeks adverse events did not differ between the groups (125).

Adverse effects are more likely to occur with metformin at the start of therapy. In retrospective case note review comparison of modified-release and immediate-release metformin 9.2% of those newly started on modified-release metformin ($n = 65$) had gastrointestinal adverse effects compared with 20% of those who started on immediate-release metformin ($n = 363$) (126). The main gastrointestinal adverse effect was diarrhea. The mean doses were 1258 mg/day for modified-release metformin and 1282 mg/day for immediate-release metformin.

Metformin XR uses a modified-release system to allow once-daily dosing. In 16 healthy volunteers aged 18–40 years, 1-week regimens of metformin XR 500, 1000, and 1500 mg/day, followed by either metformin XR 2000 mg/day or metformin IR 1000 mg bd during weeks 4 and 5, produced 137 adverse events (127). These were mainly gastrointestinal, including abdominal pain, reduced appetite, diarrhea, nausea, and vomiting. There were similar adverse effects with metformin XR and IR. There was no relation between the dose of metformin XR and the number of events.

Drug overdose

The regional poison centers certified by the American Association of Poison Control have reported 55 cases of metformin ingestion by children (128). Unintentional ingestion of 1700 mg of metformin did not pose health risks. In 21 children tested for blood glucose, lactate, or electrolytes, there was no evidence of lactic acidosis. Plasma metformin concentrations were not determined.

- A 37-year-old woman purposely took metformin 10 g (129). She did not develop hypoglycemia, but the serum lactate increased to 3.2 mmol/l (reference range under 2.1 mmol/l) and she became nauseated. She recovered.
- A healthy 21-year-old woman took metformin 45 g (53×850 mg) in a suicide attempt and developed acute pancreatitis with metabolic acidosis (pH 6.96), hypoglycemia (1.3 mmol/l), and an anion gap of 37 mmol/l (130). She was given 290 g of dextrose, and her blood glucose rose to 25 mmol/l. Other laboratory tests were normal. When later measured, serum amylase was 121 U/l, urinary amylase 97 U/l (both twice the upper limit of the reference range), and serum lipase 724 U/l (5–6 times raised). A CT scan with contrast showed stage B acute pancreatitis. Serum amylase and serum lipase rose to 368 and 1900 U/l respectively. She recovered after 8 days. A CT scan 1 month later was normal. Lactic acid and metformin were not determined. The use of alcohol or other drugs that can cause pancreatitis could not be established. Gallstones and hyperlipidemia were not present. The initial hypoglycemia could have been a direct effect of metformin; hyperglycemia is more often seen during lactic acidosis.
- A non-diabetic 25-year-old woman died after 2 days of lactic acidosis and multiple organ failure, having taken an unknown amount of her father's metformin (58,131).
- A 58-year-old woman with type 2 diabetes took an overdose of metform in 55 g plus 100 mg of glibenclamide and 3.1 g of acarbose (58,131). She developed lactic acidosis and survived with hemodialysis.
- A 70-year-old man survived a suicidal attempt with metformin 63 g (132). His serum lactate concentration was 24 mmol/l and creatinine 216 µmol/l. He received bicarbonate hemodialysis, blood pressure support, and active warming for hypothermia. After 6 hours lactate and creatinine normalized.
- A 48-year-old man successfully committed suicide with metformin and alcohol (133). The authors used a simplified, rapid, and sensitive HPLC assay, with no interference from other drugs or toxic substances,

which determined metformin extracted from blood and various tissues both ante-mortem and post- mortem. The serum metformin concentration on admission was 141 µg/ml.

- A 40-kg 14-year-old girl was thought to have taken up to 63 g of metformin, 1050 mg of diclofenac, and 1400 mg of atenolol (134). She had a Glasgow coma scale score of 5, a blood glucose concentration of 1.9 mmol/l, a pH of 7.1, a bicarbonate concentration of 10.6 mmol/l, and a base excess of –18.6mmol/l. The peak lactate concentration was 38 mmol/l.
- A 15-year-old girl took 38 g of metformin (135). Her pH was 7.29, bicarbonate 17 mmol/l, base excess –10 mmol/l, and blood glucose 9.2 mmol/l after receiving glucose from the rescue team. Her condition worsened—the bicarbonate fell to 15 mmol/l, the pH to 7.2, and the blood glucose to 2.7 mmol/l; the lactate rose to 8.7 mmol/l. The lactate concentration subsequently peaked at 21 mmol/l.

These two cases show that although metfomin at recommended doses is not usually associated with hypoglycemia, severe hypoglycemia can occur at higher doses. Overdosage is also associated with lactic acidosis in people with normal renal function. Metformin interferes with the production and clearance of lactate by a variety of mechanisms, including a shift in intracellular redox potential from aerobic to anaerobic metabolism, increasing lactate production. In both of these cases lactate concentrations peaked several hours after ingestion of metformin. This needs to be considered when managing metformin overdose.

When a patient in coma has an unexplained anion gap, a suicide attempt with metformin should be considered.

Drug–Drug Interactions

Alpha-glucosidase inhibitors

Metformin can be effectively combined with miglitol (SEDA-25, 514) but metformin may accumulate in the gastrointestinal wall, and the combination of metformin with acarbose or miglitol may reduce the absorption of metformin (136,137).

Cephalexin

In a double-blind, randomized, crossover study in 12 healthy volunteers, cefalexin 500 mg increased the C_{max} and AUC of a single dose of metformin 500 mg by 34 and 24% respectively and reduced its renal clearance to 14% (138). The authors suggested that cefalexin inhibits the renal tubular secretion of metformin.

Contrast media for radiological investigations

Radiocontrast media can induce acute renal insufficiency in patients taking metformin (139,140). Metformin should be withdrawn 2 days before an iodinated contrast medium is given (SEDA-21, 445) and the following protocol has been suggested (141):

- take a blood sample for creatinine baseline estimation before giving a contrast medium;

- withdraw metformin 48 hours before the investigation;
- if the urine output is normal for 48 hours after the radiological procedure the patient can resume metformin;
- when it is discovered after a procedure that the pre-investigation creatinine was raised (since the procedure may be carried out before the creatinine is known), the patient's physician should be contacted and the creatinine must be measured again within 48 hours.

Since January 1998 the package insert approved by the FDA has stated: "Glucophage (metformin) should be discontinued at the time of or prior to the procedure and withheld for 48 hours subsequent to the procedure and reinstituted only after renal function has been re-evaluated and found to be normal" (142).

Multiple hypoglycemic drugs

The combination of metformin with other drugs that can lower the blood glucose concentration can result in severe hypoglycemia.

- A 79-year-old woman was admitted to hospital stuporose and unresponsive (143). She had taken metformin 850 mg bd for 14 days, during which time she complained of loss of appetite and consumed little starch. On that morning she had had nausea and dizziness. Her blood glucose was 2.0 mmol/l and her serum potassium 3.3 mmol/l. A CT scan of the head was normal.

The combination of metformin, which itself does not cause hypoglycemia, with an ACE inhibitor, nitrofurantoin, and an NSAID, which all have glucose-lowering effects, and poor food intake may have led to hypoglycemia in this case.

NSAIDs

Drug interactions can precipitate metformin-induced lactic acidosis, as has been reported after the addition of indometacin (144).

- A 57-year-old woman, who had taken metformin 500 mg bd for 15 years, took indometacin 50 mg qds for 2 months. She developed oliguria and acidosis (pH 6.82, serum lactate 21 mmol/l, creatinine 480 µmol/l). After stopping metformin and indometacin she improved and left hospital with stable impaired kidney function.

The authors reported that two other cases of metformin-associated lactic acidosis with concurrent NSAID therapy have been reported to the Committee on Safety of Medicines in the UK. Indometacin can impair kidney function and may have done so in this case. Phenformin can cause tubular damage and oliguria in animals (145) and so it is conceivable that metformin-induced renal damage may also have contributed.

Nucleoside analogue reverse transcriptase inhibitors

Nucleoside analogue reverse transcriptase inhibitors can rarely cause lactic acidosis with hepatic steatosis and might potentiate the effect of metformin.

- A 52-year-old man with advanced HIV infection taking many medicines took metformin 500 mg bd for 6 days (146). He became increasingly unwell, with nausea, vomiting, abdominal pain, lethargy, and jaundice. His pH was 7.28 and lactic acid 15 mmol/l. Antiviral drugs and metformin were withdrawn, but he died after 30 hours.

Orlistat

A possible interaction of orlistat with metformin has been reported.

- A 59-year-old obese woman with normal renal function, taking metformin 500 mg tds, took orlistat 120 mg tds for 3 months (147). She developed abdominal pain and diarrhea, for which she was given cimetidine, and became weak and dizzy, with blurred vision, reduced consciousness, agitation, and confusion. Her pH was 6.5, bicarbonate 2 mmol/l, base deficit 38 mmol/l, and lactate 21 mmol/l. She required rehydration, bicarbonate, inotropic support and renal replacement therapy.

The authors suggested that chronic diarrhea induced by orlistat could have led to impaired renal function or that orlistat could have increased the absorption of metformin by reducing fat absorption.

Phenprocoumon

The clearance of phenprocoumon was increased by metformin, perhaps because of increased liver blood flow (148).

Rofecoxib

Lactic acidosis in a patient taking metformin and rofecoxib has been attributed to renal damage by the latter.

- A 58-year-old woman with type 2 diabetes taking metformin 500 mg bd took rofecoxib for 1 month for osteoarthritis of the knees and developed lactic acidosis (149).

Rosiglitazone

In 16 male volunteers aged 22–55 years, rosiglitazone 2 mg bd had no effect on the steady-state pharmacokinetics of oral metformin 500 mg bd; there were no clinically significant episodes of hypoglycemia and blood lactic acid concentrations did not increase (150).

Warfarin

Potentiation of the anticoagulant action of warfarin by phenformin has been reported (151).

In one case a complication of warfarin therapy contributed to lactic acidosis.

- A 73-year-old woman taking metformin 1000 mg bd and warfarin 5 mg/day developed epistaxis, hematuria, gingival bleeding, a retroperitoneal hematoma, and bilateral perinephric blood with obstruction of both collecting systems (152). She received fresh frozen plasma, vitamin K_1 10 mg, and packed erythrocytes. In the next 8 hours she developed a metabolic acidosis

(pH 7.06, lactate 16.5 mmol/l). She had a cardiopulmonary arrest, was resuscitated, and recovered with sodium bicarbonate, additional fresh frozen plasma, vitamin K_1, and hemodialysis. Serum metformin was 7.3 µg/ml (usual target range 1–2).

Interference with warfarin by metformin has been described before (SED-14, 1513).

References

1. Bailey CJ. Biguanides and NIDDM. Diabetes Care 1992;15(6):755–72.
2. Bailey CJ, Turner RC. Metformin. N Engl J Med 1996;334(9):574–9.
3. Pugh J. Metformin monotherapy for type II diabetes. Adv Ther 1997;14:338–47.
4. Scheen AJ. Clinical pharmacokinetics of metformin. Clin Pharmacokinet 1996;30(5):359–71.
5. Johansen K. Efficacy of metformin in the treatment of NIDDM. Meta-analysis. Diabetes Care 1999;22(1):33–7.
6. Pentikainen PJ, Neuvonen PJ, Penttila A. Pharmacokinetics of metformin after intravenous and oral administration to man. Eur J Clin Pharmacol 1979;16(3):195–202.
7. Alkalay D, Khemani L, Wagner WE, Bartlett MF. Pharmacokinetics of phenformin in man. J Clin Pharmacol 1975;15(5-6):446–8.
8. Knowler WC, Barrett-Connor E, Fowler SE, Hamman RF, Lachin JM, Walker EA, Nathan DM. Diabetes Prevention Program Research Group. Reduction in the incidence of type 2 diabetes with lifestyle intervention or metformin. N Engl J Med 2002;346(6):393–403.
9. Diabetes Prevention Program Research Group. Effects of withdrawal from metformin on the development of diabetes in the diabetes prevention program. Diabetes Care 2003;26(4):977–80.
10. Ciaraldi TP, Kong AP, Chu NV, Kim DD, Baxi S, Loviscach M, Plodkowski R, Reitz R, Caulfield M, Mudaliar S, Henry RR. Regulation of glucose transport and insulin signaling by troglitazone or metformin in adipose tissue of type 2 diabetic subjects. Diabetes 2002;51(1):30–6.
11. Lehtovirta M, Forsen B, Gullstrom M, Haggblom M, Eriksson JG, Taskinen MR, Groop L. Metabolic effects of metformin in patients with impaired glucose tolerance. Diabet Med 2001;18(7):578–83.
12. Jones KL, Arslanian S, Peterokova VA, Park JS, Tomlinson MJ. Effect of metformin in pediatric patients with type 2 diabetes: a randomized controlled trial. Diabetes Care 2002;25(1):89–94.
13. Van Gaal LF, De Leeuw IH. Rationale and options for combination therapy in the treatment of Type 2 diabetes. Diabetologia 2003;46(Suppl 1):M44–50.
14. Gomez-Perez FJ, Fanghanel-Salmon G, Antonio Barbosa J, Montes-Villarreal J, Berry RA, Warsi G, Gould EM. Efficacy and safety of rosiglitazone plus metformin in Mexicans with type 2 diabetes. Diabetes Metab Res Rev 2002;18(2):127–34.
15. Setter SM, Iltz JL, Thams J, Campbell RK. Metformin hydrochloride in the treatment of type 2 diabetes mellitus: a clinical review with a focus on dual therapy. Clin Ther 2003;25:2991–306.
16. Masoudi FA, Wang Y, Inzucchi SE, Setaro JF, Havranek EP, Foody JM, Krumholz HM. Metformin and thiazolidinedione use in Medicare patients with heart failure. J Am Med Assoc 2003;290:81–5.

17. Dailey GE III, Noor MA, Park J-S, Bruce S, Fiedorek FT. Glycemic control with glyburide/metformin tablets in combination with rosiglitazone in patients with type 2 diabetes: a randomised double-blind trial. Am J Med 2004;116:223–9.

18. Moses R, Slobodniuk R, Boyages S, Colagiuri S, Kidson W, Carter J, Donnelly T, Moffitt P, Hopkins H. Effect of repaglinide addition to metformin monotherapy on glycemic control in patients with type 2 diabetes. Diabetes Care 1999;22(1):119–24.

19. Hirschberg Y, Karara AH, Pietri AO, McLeod JF. Improved control of mealtime glucose excursions with coadministration of nateglinide and metformin. Diabetes Care 2000;23(3):349–53.

20. Horton ES, Clinkingbeard C, Gatlin M, Foley J, Mallows S, Shen S. Nateglinide alone and in combination with metformin improves glycemic control by reducing mealtime glucose levels in type 2 diabetes. Diabetes Care 2000;23(11):1660–5.

21. Moses R. Repaglinide in combination therapy with metformin in Type 2 diabetes. Exp Clin Endocrinol Diabetes 1999;107(Suppl 4):S136–9.

22. Schatz H, Schoppel K, Lehwalder D, Schandry R. Efficacy, tolerability and safety of nateglinide in combination with metformin. Results from a study under general practice conditions. Exp Clin Endocrinol Diabetes 2003;111:262–6.

23. Nagasaka S, Aiso Y, Yoshiwaza K, Ishibashi S. Comparison of pioglitazone and metformin efficacy using homeostasis model assessment. Diabetic Med 2004;21:136–4.

24. Garber AJ, Donovan Jr DS, Dandona P, Bruce S, Park J-S. Efficacy of glyburide/metformin tablets compared with initial monotherapy in type 2 diabetes. J Clin Endocrinol Metab 2003;88:3598–604.

25. Gulliford M, Latinovic R. Mortality in type 2 diabetic subjects prescribed metformin and sulphonylurea drugs in combination: cohort study. Diabetes Metab Res Rev 2004;20:239–45.

26. Hamilton J, Cummings E, Zdravkovic V, Finegood D, Daneman D. Metformin as an adjunct therapy in adolescents with type 1 diabetes and insulin resistance: a randomized controlled trial. Diabetes Care 2003;26(1):138–43.

27. Wulffele MG, Kooy A, Lehert P, Bets D, Ogterop JC, Borger van der Burg B, Donker AJ, Stehouwer CD. Combination of insulin and metformin in the treatment of type 2 diabetes. Diabetes Care 2002;25(12):2133–40.

28. Strowig SM, Aviles-Santa ML, Raskin P. Comparison of insulin monotherapy and combination therapy with insulin and metformin or insulin and troglitazone in type 2 diabetes. Diabetes Care 2002;25(10):1691–8.

29. Furlong NJ, Hulme SA, O'Brien SV, Hardy KJ. Repaglinide versus metformin in combination with bedtime NPH insulin in patients with type 2 diabetes established on insulin/metformin combination therapy. Diabetes Care 2002;25(10):1685–90.

30. Sulkin TV, Bosman D, Krentz AJ. Contraindications to metformin therapy in patients with NIDDM. Diabetes Care 1997;20(6):925–8.

31. Holstein A, Nahrwold D, Hinze S, Egberts EH. Contraindications to metformin therapy are largely disregarded. Diabet Med 1999;16(8):692–6.

32. Beis SJ, Goshman LM, Newkirk GL. Risk factors for metformin-associated lactic acidosis. WMJ 1999;98(4):56–7.

33. Emslie-Smith AM, Boyle DI, Evans JM, Sullivan F, Morris AD. DARTS/MEMO Collaboration. Contraindications to metformin therapy in patients with Type 2 diabetes—a population-based study of adherence to prescribing guidelines. Diabet Med 2001;18(6):483–8.

34. Jones GC, Macklin JP, Alexander WD. Contraindications to the use of metformin. Br Med J 2003;326:4–5.

35. UK Prospective Diabetes Study Group. Effect of intensive blood-glucose control with metformin on complications in overweight patients with type 2 diabetes (UKPDS 34). Lancet 1998;352:854–65.

36. Salpeter S, Greyber E, Pasternak G, Salpeter E. Risk of fatal and nonfatal lactic acidosis with metformin use in type 2 diabetes mellitus. Cochrane Database Syst Rev 2003;(2):CD002967.

37. Jones P, Yate P. Blanket banning of metformin two days before surgery may not be a good idea. Br Med J 2003;326:5.

38. Elder AT. Age and creatinine clearance need to be taken in consideration. Br Med J 2003;326:4.

39. Rachmani R, Slavachevski I, Levi Z, Zadok B-S, Kedar Y, Ravid M. Metformin in patients with type 2 diabetes mellitus: reconsideration of traditional contraindications. Eur J Int Med 2002;13:428–33.

40. Howes LG, Sundaresan P, Lykos D. Cardiovascular effects of oral hypoglycaemic drugs. Clin Exp Pharmacol Physiol 1996;23(3):201–6.

41. Olsson J, Lindberg G, Gottsater M, Lindwall K, Sjostrand A, Tisell A, Melander A. Increased mortality in Type II diabetic patients using sulphonylurea and metformin in combination: a population-based observational study. Diabetologia 2000;43(5):558–60.

42. Vander T, Hallevy H, Ifergane G, Herishanu YO. Metformin-induced encephalopathy without lactic acidosis. Diabetic Med 2003;21:194–5.

43. Tangelder GJM, Dubbleman M, Ringens PJ. Sudden reversible osmotic lens damage ("sugar cracks") after initiation of metformin. N Engl J Med 2005;353:2621–2.

44. Guariglia A, Gonzi GL, Regolisti G, Vinci S. Treatment of biguanide-induced lactic acidosis: reproposal of the "physiological" approach and review of the literature. Ann Ital Med Int 1994;9(1):35–9.

45. Ben-Ami H, Nagachandran P, Mendelson A, Edoute Y. Drug-induced hypoglycemic coma in 102 diabetic patients. Arch Intern Med 1999;159(3):281–4.

46. Newey PJ, Abousleiman Y, Jamieson A. Pituitary failure, metformin and hypoglycaemia in type 2 diabetes. Br J Diabetes Vasc Dis 2004;4:128–30.

47. Cohen RD, Woods HF. Lactic acidosis revisited. Diabetes 1983;32(2):181–91.

48. Lalau JD, Race JM, Brinquin L. Lactic acidosis in metformin therapy. Relationship between plasma metformin concentration and renal function. Diabetes Care 1998;21(8):1366–7.

49. Reeker W, Schneider G, Felgenhauer N, Tempel G, Kochs E. Metformin-induzierte Laktatazidose. [Metformin-induced lactic acidosis.] Dtsch Med Wochenschr 2000;125(9):249–51.

50. Lovas K, Fadnes DJ, Dale A. Metforminassosiert laktacidose–pasienteksempel og litteraturgjennomgang. [Metformin associated lactic acidosis—case reports and literature review.] Tidsskr Nor Laegeforen 2000;120(13):1539–41.

51. Soomers AJ, Tack CJ. Ernstige lactaatacidose bij metforminegebruik bij een patient met contra-indicaties voor metformine. [Severe lactic acidosis due to metformin ingestion in a patient with contra-indication for metformin.] Ned Tijdschr Geneeskd 2001;145(2):104–5.

52. Houwerzijl EJ, Snoek WJ, van Haastert M, Holman ND. Ernstige lactaatacidose bij metforminegebruik bij een patient met contra-indicates voor metformine. [Severe

lactic acidosis due to metformin therapy in a patient with contra-indications for metformin.] Ned Tijdschr Geneeskd 2000;144(40):1923–6.

53. Berner B, Hummel KM, Strutz F, Ritzel U, Ramadori G, Hagenlocher S, Kleine P, Muller GA. Metformin-assoziierte Lactatazidose mit akutem Nierenversagen bei Diabetes mellitus Typ 2. [Metformin-associated lactic acidosis with acute renal failure in type 2 diabetes mellitus.] Med Klin (Munich) 2002;97(2):99–103.

54. Khan JK, Pallaki M, Tolbert SR, Hornick TR. Lactic acidemia associated with metformin. Ann Pharmacother 2003;37:66–9.

55. Edwards CMB, Barton MA, Snook J, David M, Mak VHF, Chowdhury TA. Metformin-associated lactic acidosis in a patient with liver disease. Quart J Med 2003;96:315–8.

56. Panzer U, Kluge S, Kreymann G, Wolf G. Combination of intermittent haemodialysis and high-volume continous haemofiltration for the treatment of severe metformin-induced lactic acidosis. Nephrol Dial Transplant 2004;19:2157–8.

57. von Mach M-A, Sauer O, Weilemann LS. Experiences of a poison centre with metformin-associated lactic acidosis. Exp Clin Endocrinol Diabetes. 2004;112:187–90.

58. Chang CT, Chen YC, Fang JT, Huang CC. Metformin-associated lactic acidosis: case reports and literature review. J Nephrol 2002;15(4):398–402.

59. Irsigler K, Kritz H, Kaspar L, Lageder H, Regal H. Vier todliche Laktazidosen unter Biguanidtherapie. [Four cases of fatal lactic acidosis during biguanide therapy (author's transl).] Wien Klin Wochenschr 1978;90(6):201–6.

60. Kwong SC, Brubacher J. Phenformin and lactic acidosis: a case report and review. J Emerg Med 1998;16(6):881–6.

61. Montero Alonso M, Salvador Cervelló G, Perelló Rosso A, Roig Osca MA. Acidosis láctica asociada al uso de buformina. Rev Clin Esp 2003;203:216.

62. Tamura Y, Tsukamoto K, Yakamoto N, Ishibashi S, Kadowaki T, Kimura S. A case of buformin treated type 2 diabetes mellitus without any other underlying disease complicated by acute renal failure, lactic acidosis, subsequent diarrhea and vomiting [Japanese]. Tonyobyo 2003;46:325–7.

63. Kurita S, Muramoto S, Okabe G. A case of lactic acidosis acute renal failure caused by taking a lot of buformin for suicide [Japanese]. Tonyobyo 2003;46:329–31.

64. Cusi K, DeFronzo RA. Metformin: a review of its metabolic effects. Diabetes Rev 1998;6:89–131.

65. Berger W. Zur Problematik der Biguanidbehandlung. Pharma-Kritik (Bern) 1979;1:9.

66. Hermann LS. Metformin: a review of its pharmacological properties and therapeutic use. Diabete Metab 1979;5(3):233–45.

67. Tymms DJ, Leatherdale BA. Lactic acidosis due to metformin therapy in a low risk patient. Postgrad Med J 1988;64(749):230–1.

68. Selby JV, Ettinger B, Swain BE, Brown JB. First 20 months' experience with use of metformin for type 2 diabetes in a large health maintenance organization. Diabetes Care 1999;22(1):38–44.

69. Stang M, Wysowski DK, Butler-Jones D. Incidence of lactic acidosis in metformin users. Diabetes Care 1999;22(6):925–7.

70. Perusicova J, Skrha J, Hodinar A, Bernovska A, Cacakova V, Richtrova A. Hladiny kyseliny mlecne u diabetiku II. Typu lecenych buforminem. [Levels of lactic acid in type II diabetics treated with buformin.] Vnitr Lek 1996;42(1):7–11.

71. Chan NN, Darko D, O'Shea D. Lactic acidosis with therapeutic metformin blood level in a low-risk diabetic patient. Diabetes Care 1999;22(1):178.

72. Cohen RD, Woods HF. Metformin and lactic acidosis. Diabetes Care 1999;22(6):1010–1.

73. Oates NS, Shah RR, Idle JR, Smith RL. Influence of oxidation polymorphism on phenformin kinetics and dynamics. Clin Pharmacol Ther 1983;34(6):827–34.

74. Lalau JD, Race JM. Lactic acidosis in metformin therapy: searching for a link with metformin in reports of "metformin-associated lactic acidosis". Diabetes Obes Metab 2001;3(3):195–201.

75. Kruse JA. Metformin-associated lactic acidosis. J Emerg Med 2001;20(3):267–72.

76. Lothholz H, Rahn A, Thurman P. Metformin-assoziierte Lactatazidose mit akutem Nierenversagen bei Diabetes mellitus Typ 2. [Metformin-associated lactic acidosis with acute renal failure in type 2 diabetes mellitus.] Med Klin (Munich) 2002;97(7):434–5.

77. Chan NN, Brain HP, Feher MD. Metformin-associated lactic acidosis: a rare or very rare clinical entity? Diabet Med 1999;16(4):273–81.

78. Vigneri R, Goldfine ID. Role of metformin in treatment of diabetes mellitus. Diabetes Care 1987;10(1):118–22.

79. Lalau JD, Race JM. Lactic acidosis in metformin therapy. Drugs 1999;58(Suppl 1):55–60.

80. Lalau JD, Race JM. Lactic acidosis in metformin-treated patients. Prognostic value of arterial lactate levels and plasma metformin concentrations. Drug Saf 1999;20(4):377–84.

81. Mariano F, Benzi L, Cecchetti P, Rosatello A, Merante D, Goia F, Capra L, Lanza G, Curto V, Cavalli PL. Efficacy of continuous venovenous haemofiltration (CVVH) in the treatment of severe phenformin-induced lactic acidosis. Nephrol Dial Transplant 1998;13(4):1012–5.

82. Ebell M. Link between metformin and lactic acidosis? Am Fam Phys 2004;70:2109–10.

83. Anonymous. POEMs. Metformin-induced lactic acidosis extremely rare. J Fam Pract 2004;53:261.

84. Misbin RI. The phantom of lactic acidosis due to metformin in patients with diabetes. Diabetes Care 2004;27:1791–2.

85. Stades AME, Heikens JT, Erkelens DW, Holleman F, Hoekstra JBL. Metformin and lactic acidosis: cause or coincidence? A review of case reports. J Int Med 2004;255:179–87.

86. Nisbet JC, Sturtevant JM, Prins JB. Metformin and serious adverse effects. Med J Aust 2004;180:53–4.

87. Fujita H, Narita T, Yoshioka N, Hosoba M, Ito S. A case of megaloblastic anemia due to vitamin B12 deficiency precipitated in a totally gastrectomized type II diabetic patient following the introduction of metformin therapy. Endocr J 2003;50:483–4.

88. Filioussi K, Bonovas S, Katsaros T. Should we screen diabetic patients using biguanides for megaloblastic anaemia? Aust Fam Physician 2003;32:383–4.

89. Wulffelé MG, Kooy A, Lehert P, Bets D, Ogterop JC, Borger van den Burg B, Donker AJM, Stehouwer CDA. Effects of short-term treatment with metformin on serum concentrations of homocysteine, folate and vitamin B12 in type 2 diabetes mellitus: a randomized, placebo- controlled trial. J Intern Med 2003;254:455–63.

90. Gilligan MA. Metformin and vitamin B12 deficiency. Arch Intern Med 2002;162(4):484–5.

91. Andres E, Noel E, Goichot B. Metformin-associated vitamin B12 deficiency. Arch Intern Med 2002;162(19):2251–2.

92. Adams JF, Clark JS, Ireland JT, Kesson CM, Watson WS. Malabsorption of vitamin B12 and intrinsic factor secretion during biguanide therapy. Diabetologia 1983; 24(1):16–8.

93. Meir A, Kleinman Y, Rund D, Da'as N. Metformin-induced hemolytic anemia in a patient with glucose-6-phosphate dehydrogenase deficiency. Diabetes Care 2003;26(3):956–7.

94. Lin KD, Lin JD, Juang JH. Metformin-induced hemolysis with jaundice. N Engl J Med 1998;339(25):1860–1.

95. Kashyap AS, Kashyap S. Haemolytic anaemia due to metformin. Postgrad Med J 2000;76(892):125–6.

96. Florianello F, Gatti C, Marinoni M, Bagni CM. Gastrite emorragica da antidiabetici. Acta Chir Ital 1978;34:597.

97. Aviles-Santa L, Sinding J, Raskin P. Effects of metformin in patients with poorly controlled, insulin-treated type 2 diabetes mellitus. A randomized, double-blind, placebo-controlled trial. Ann Intern Med 1999;131(3):182–8.

98. Raju B, Resta C, Tibaldi JT. Metformin and late gastrointestinal complications. Am J Med 2000;109(3):260–1.

99. Foss MT, Clement KD. Metformin as a cause of late-onset chronic diarrhea. Pharmacotherapy 2001;21(11):1422–4.

100. Burrull-Madero MA, Del-Villar-Ruiz A, Grau-Cerrato S, Andreu-Garcia M, Goday-Arno A. Digestive hemorrhage caused by a Meckel's diverticulum in a metformin-treated patient: is there any connection? Pharm World Sci 2001;23(3):120–1.

101. Lord JM, Flight IHK, Norman RJ. Metformin in polycystic ovary syndrome: systematic review and meta-analysis. Br Med J 2003;327:351–5.

102. Cubukcu A, Yilmaz MT, Satman I, Buyukdevrim AS. Metformin kullanimina bag_li bir akut hepatit vakasi. [Metformin-induced hepatitis.] Istanb Tip Fak Mecm 1991;54:447–52.

103. Babich MM, Pike I, Shiffman ML. Metformin-induced acute hepatitis. Am J Med 1998;104(5):490–2.

104. Swislocki AL, Noth R. Pseudohepatotoxicity of metformin. Diabetes Care 1998;21(4):677–8.

105. Kutoh E. Possible metformin-induced hepatotoxicity. Am J Geriatr Pharmacother 2005;3:270–3.

106. Desilets DJ, Shorr AF, Moran KA, Holtzmuller KC. Cholestatic jaundice associated with the use of metformin. Am J Gastroenterol 2001;96(7):2257–8.

107. Graeber GM, Marmor BM, Hendel RC, Gregg RO. Pancreatitis and severe metabolic abnormalities due to phenformin therapy. Arch Surg 1976;111(9):1014–6.

108. Azzam H, Bergman R, Friedman-Birnbaum R. Lichen planus associated with metformin therapy. Dermatology 1997;194(4):376.

109. Burger DE, Goyal S. Erythema multiforme from metformin. Ann Pharmacother 2004;38:1537.

110. Klapholz L, Leitersdorf E, Weinrauch L. Leucocytoclastic vasculitis and pneumonitis induced by metformin. BMJ (Clin Res Ed) 1986;293(6545):483.

111. Dore P, Perault MC, Recart D, Dejean C, Meurice JC, Fougere MC, Vandel B, Patte F. Pneumopathie medicamenteuse a la metformine?. [Pulmonary diseases induced by metformin?.] Therapie 1994;49(5):472–3.

112. Fisman EZ, Tenenbaum A, Boyko V, Benderly M, Adler Y, Friedensohn A, Kohanovski M, Rotzak R, Schneider H, Behar S, Motro M. Oral antidiabetic treatment in patients with coronary disease: time-related increased mortality on combined glyburide/metformin therapy over a 7.7-year follow-up Clin Cardiol 2001;24(2):151–8.

113. Simmons D, Walters BNJ, Rowan JA, McIntryre HD. Metformin therapy and diabetes in pregnancy. Med J Aust 2004;180:462–4.

114. Hague WM, Davoren P, Oliver J, Rowan J. Metformin may be useful in gestational diabetes. Br Med J 2003;236:762–3.

115. Hughes R Rowan J. Metformin in pregnancy: an audit. Proceedings of the Medicine and Pregnancy Meeting, October 2003. Australasian Diabetes in Pregnancy Society Newsletter, December 2003.

116. McGarthy EA, Walker SP, McLachlan K, Boyle J, Permezel M. Metformin in obstetric and gynaecologic practice: a review. Obstet Gynaecol Surv 2004;59:118–27.

117. Vanky E, Zahlsen K, Spigset O, Carlsen SM. Placental passage of metformin in women with polycysitc ovary syndrome. Fertil Steril 2005;83:1575–8.

118. Brock B, Smidt K, Ovesen P, Schmitz O, Rungby J. Is metformin therapy for polycystic ovary syndrome safe during pregnancy? Basic Clin Pharmacol Toxicol 2005;96:410–2.

119. Glueck CJ, Goldenberg N, Pranikoff J, Loftspring M, Sieve l, Wang P. Height, weight and motor-social development during the first 18 months of life in 126 infants born to 109 mothers with polycystic ovary syndrome who conceived on and continued metformin through pregnancy. Hum Reprod 2004;19:1323–30.

120. Hale TW, Kristensen JH, Hackett LP, Kohan R, Ilett KF. Transfer of metformin into human milk. Diabetologia 2002;45(11):1509–14.

121. Gregorio F, Ambrosi F, Manfrini S, Velussi M, Carle F, Testa R, Merante D, Filipponi P. Poorly controlled elderly Type 2 diabetic patients: the effects of increasing sulphonylurea dosages or adding metformin. Diabet Med 1999;16(12):1016–24.

122. Fall PJ, Szerlip HM. Lactic acidosis: from sour milk to septic shock. J Intens Care Med 2005;20:255–71.

123. Bugianesi E, Gentilcore E, Manini R, Natale S, Vanni E, Villanova N, David E, Rizzetto M, Marchesini G. A randomised controlled trial of metformin versus vitamin E or prescriptive diet in non-alcoholic fatty liver disease. Am J Gastroenterol 2005;100:1082–90.

124. Schwimmer JB, Middleton MS, Deutsch R, Lavine JE. A phase 2 clinical trial of metformin as a treatment for non-diabetic paediatric non-alcoholic steatohepatitis. Aliment Pharmacol Ther 2005;21:871–9.

125. Fujioka K, Pans M, Joyal S. Glycemic control in patients with type 2 diabetes mellitus switched from twice-daily immediate-release metformin to a once-daily extended-release formulation. Clin Ther 2003;25:515–29.

126. Blone L, Dailey GE, Jabbour SA, Reasner CA, Mills DJ. Gastrointestinal tolerability of extended-release metformin tablets compared to immediate-release metformin tablets: results of a retrospective cohort study. Curr Med Res Opin 2004;20:565–72.

127. Timmins P, Donahue S, Meeker J, Marathe P. Steady-state pharmacokinetics of a novel extended-release metformin formulation. Clin Pharmacokinet 2005;44:721–9.

128. Spiller HA, Weber JA, Winter ML, Klein-Schwartz W, Hofman M, Gorman SE, Stork CM, Krenzelok EP. Multicenter case series of pediatric metformin ingestion. Ann Pharmacother 2000;34(12):1385–8.

129. Bates D, Caton B. Metformin overdose. Can J Hosp Pharm 1999;52:173–5.

130. Ben MH, Thabet H, Zaghdoudi I, Amamou M. Metformin associated acute pancreatitis. Vet Hum Toxicol 2002;44(1):47–8.

131. Chang CT, Chen YC, Fang JT, Huang CC. High anion gap metabolic acidosis in suicide: don't forget metformin intoxication—two patients' experiences. Ren Fail 2002;24(5):671–5.

132. Gjedde S, Christiansen A, Pedersen SB, Rungby J. Survival following a metformin overdose of 63 g: a case report. Pharmacol Toxicol 2003;93:98–9.

133. Moore KA, Levine B, Titus JM, Fowler DR. Analysis of metformin in antemortem serum and postmortem specimens by a novel HPLC method and application to an intoxication case. J Anal Toxicol 2003;27:592–4.

134. Harvey B, Hickman C, Hinson G, Ralph T, Mayer A. Severe lactic acidosis complicating metformin overdose successfully treated with high-volume venovenous hemofiltration and aggressive alkalization. Pediatr Crit Care Med 2005;6:598–601.

135. Lacher M, Hermanns-Clausen M, Haeffner K, Brandis M, Pohl M. Severe metformin intoxication with lactic acidosis in an adolescent. Eur J Pediatr 2005;164:362–5.

136. Dachman AH. New contraindication to intravascular iodinated contrast material. Radiology 1995;197(2):545.

137. Scheen AJ, Lefebvre PJ. Potential pharmacokinetics interference between alpha-glucosidase inhibitors and other oral antidiabetic agents. Diabetes Care 2002;25(1):247–8.

138. Jayasagar G, Krishna Kumar M, Chandrasekhar K, Madhusudan Rao C, Madhusudan Rao Y. Effect of cephalexin on the pharmacokinetics of metformin in healthy human volunteers. Drug Metabol Drug Interact 2002;19(1):41–8.

139. Zandijk E, Demey HE, Bossaert LL. Lactic acidosis due to metformin. Tijdschr Geneeskd 1997;53:543–6.

140. Safadi R, Dranitzki-Elhalel M, Popovtzer M, Ben-Yehuda A. Metformin-induced lactic acidosis associated with acute renal failure. Am J Nephrol 1996;16(6):520–2.

141. Rasuli P, Hammond DI. Metformin and contrast media: where is the conflict? Can Assoc Radiol J 1998;49(3):161–6.

142. Hammond DI, Rasuli P. Metformin and contrast media. Clin Radiol 1998;53(12):933–4.

143. Zitzmann S, Reimann IR, Schmechel H. Severe hypoglycemia in an elderly patient treated with metformin. Int J Clin Pharmacol Ther 2002;40(3):108–1089.

144. Chan NN, Fauvel NJ, Feher MD. Non-steroidal anti-inflammatory drugs and metformin: a cause for concern? Lancet 1998;352(9123):201.

145. Schwarzbeck A. Non-steroidal anti-inflammatory drugs and metformin. Lancet 1998;352(9130):818.

146. Worth L, Elliott J, Anderson J, Sasadeusz J, Street A, Lewin S. A cautionary tale: fatal lactic acidosis complicating nucleoside analog and metformin therapy. Clin Infect Dis 2003;37:315–6.

147. Dawson D, Conlon C. Case study: metformin associated lactic acidosis: could orlistat be relevant? Diabetes Care 2003;26:2471–2.

148. Ohnhaus EE, Berger W, Duckert F, Oesch F. The influence of dimethylbiguanide on phenprocoumon elimination and its mode of action. A drug interaction study. Klin Wochenschr 1983;61(17):851–8.

149. Price G. Metformin lactic acidosis, acute renal failure and rofecoxib. Br J Anaesth 2003;91:909–10.

150. Di Cicco RA, Allen A, Carr A, Fowles S, Jorkasky DK, Freed MI. Rosiglitazone does not alter the pharmacokinetics of metformin. J Clin Pharmacol 2000;40(11):1280–5.

151. Hamblin TJ. Interaction between warfarin and phenformin. Lancet 1971;2(7737):1323.

152. Schier JG, Hoffman RS. Metformin acidosis due to a warfarin adverse drug event. Ann Pharmacother 2003;37:1145.

Blood glucose meters

General Information

There are various makes of meters used for measuring the blood glucose concentration. On occasion, some have been found to give false readings.

In early June 1998, the manufacturers of SureStep blood glucose meters (LifeScan) announced that they were going to replace some of the meters used by diabetics to test their blood sugar concentration because they were giving confusing error readings. SureStep home blood glucose meters manufactured before August 1997 may have been giving an error message ("Er-1") instead of "HI" (high) when a blood sugar concentration was very high—500 mg/dl (28 mmol/l) or greater. Such a concentration is potentially dangerous if not recognized and treated, and could result in hospitalization or death. The FDA had received reports of two deaths in people whose glucose was very high but who repeatedly got error message readings from the SureStep blood glucose meters and delayed seeking medical care. The FDA was concerned that some diabetics, wholesalers, and distributors who purchase these meters might not realize that this product replacement procedure concerns a potentially serious malfunction (1). The FDA classified LifeScan's recall as a Class I recall, that is a situation in which there is a reasonable probability that the use of the product will cause serious adverse health consequences or death.

People using the affected SureStep meters needed to know that an "Er-1" message might actually mean a very high concentration of blood glucose instead of an error. If users got an "Er-1" message, they needed to use the visual color change indicator to see if their blood glucose was too high. They had to compare the blue dot on the test strip to the color chart on the test strip bottle. If the dot on the strip was as dark as or darker than the color chart, it indicated a very high blood glucose, and they were advised to contact a health professional immediately.

People with diabetes who use the SureStep brand glucose meters were advised not to stop testing their blood glucose concentrations. They could continue to test with these meters as long as they knew that an "Er-1" message could actually mean a very high concentration. It was considered far more dangerous not to check blood glucose than to use a blood glucose meter that might give an unclear error message at high glucose concentrations.

Factors that alter measurements

High altitude

Sports like hiking and skiing at moderate high altitude make glucose estimation mandatory for people with diabetes. Changes in temperature, PaO$_2$, and humidity can result in errors in blood glucose determination. When tested at 3000 m (10 000 feet) the glucose meter Elite (Bayer Diagnostics) had a tendency to overestimate glucose concentrations, while the Life Scan One Touch II had a tendency to underestimate them (2). The bias was not clinically meaningful, although some care may be necessary when low or intermediate blood glucose concentrations are measured with the Glucometer Elite.

Icodextrin

Icodextrin in the dialysis fluid in continuous ambulatory peritoneal dialysis can contribute to overestimation of blood glucose (SEDA-26, 461). In a comparison of a meter using the glucose oxidation method and a meter using the glucose dehydrogenase method, only the former gave results that were comparable with the laboratory method (3). The authors concluded that meters must be cross-checked with the laboratory before they can be used to measure blood glucose in patients in contact with icodextrin.

Site of blood withdrawal

The site of blood withdrawal can give different values during acute monitoring of glucose (SEDA-26, 461). Blood was tested before and 60, 90, 120, 150, and 180 minutes after a meal from the finger tips, the arms, and the thighs with the One-Touch Ultra Blood Glucose Monitoring System (LifeScan) and an extra finger prick using a blood monitoring system. When the blood glucose concentration was rising, only the finger prick gave accurate results; the readings from the other sites were lower (even after extensive rubbing) (4).

In patients with diabetes given a 75 g oral glucose load followed by a rapid-acting insulin, producing a wide range of blood glucose concentrations, of three different devices for blood glucose estimation, only finger-prick estimations followed the changes in blood glucose (5), although patients preferred other sites for testing (6).

A subcutaneous continuous glucose monitoring system was used for 24 hours in seven strictly regulated adolescents and young adults. For comparison, blood was drawn from an intravenous cannula and determined in the laboratory, and capillary samples were measured on a glucose meter. During the night-time the readings on the continuous glucose monitoring system were on average 38% lower than the other measurements, indicating a high number of false (asymptomatic) attacks of hypoglycemia (7).

Organs and Systems

Immunologic

Finger sepsis aggressive enough to cause osteomyelitis has been reported in two women, one aged 61 years with *Staphylococcus aureus*, *Staphylococcus agalactiae*, and *Enterococcus faecalis*, and another aged 57 years with a beta-hemolytic staphylococcus, *Candida non-albicans*, and unidentified anaerobic bacteria. Antibiotic treatment and local drainage were unsuccessful and the third phalanx had to be amputated. Both patients had poorly controlled diabetes (HbA$_{1c}$ 14% and 12% respectively); they had estimated their blood glucose six times a week using an automatic lancet without changing their disposable needle (8).

References

1. Anonymous. Blood glucose meters-recalled because of error reading. WHO Newsletter 1998;9/10:16.
2. Pecchio O, Maule S, Migliardi M, Trento M, Veglio M. Effects of exposure at an altitude of 3000 m on performance of glucose meters. Diabetes Care 2000;23(1):129–31.
3. Oyibo SO, Pritchard GM, McLay L, James E, Laing I, Gokal R, Boulton AJ. Blood glucose overestimation in diabetic patients on continuous ambulatory peritoneal dialysis for end-stage renal disease. Diabet Med 2002;19(8):693–6.
4. Ellison JM, Stegmann JM, Colner SL, Michael RH, Sharma MK, Ervin KR, Horwitz DL. Rapid changes in postprandial blood glucose produce concentration differences at finger, forearm, and thigh sampling sites. Diabetes Care 2002;25(6):961–4.
5. Jungheim K, Koschinsky T. Glucose monitoring at the arm: risky delays of hypoglycemia and hyperglycemia detection. Diabetes Care 2002;25(6):956–60.
6. Tieszen KL, New JP. Alternate site blood glucose testing: do patients prefer it? Diabet Med 2003;20(4):325–8.
7. McGowan K, Thomas W, Moran A. Spurious reporting of nocturnal hypoglycemia by CGMS in patients with tightly controlled type 1 diabetes. Diabetes Care 2002;25(9):1499–503.
8. Monami M, Mannucci E, Masotti G. Finger sepsis in two poorly controlled diabetic patients with reuse of lancets. Diabetes Care 2002;25(6):1103.

Dipeptidyl peptidase IV inhibitors

General information

Dipeptidyl peptidase IV (DPP IV) is an enzyme that is involved in the rapid metabolism of incretins, such as glucagon-like peptide. Inhibitors of DPP IV therefore extend the action of incretins. The incretins increase glucose-dependent insulin secretion from the pancreas, and so inhibition of DPP IV is a new therapeutic approach in the treatment of type 2 diabetes. Unlike the incretin mimetic analogues of glucagon-like peptide, which are given subcutaneously, inhibitors of DPP IV can be given orally.

Sitagliptin ([2R]-4-oxo-4-[3-(trifluoromethyl)-5,6-dihydro(1,2,4)triazolo(4,3-a)pyrazin-7(8H)-yl]-1-[2,4,5-trifluorophenyl]butan-2-amine) (1) is the first inhibitor of DPP IV to have received a licence in the UK (in 2007).

There are other closely related DPP enzymes, such as DPP 8 and DPP 9. When these enzymes are inhibited in experimental animals multiorgan toxicity occurs. Sitagliptin appears to be highly selective for DPP IV and has 2600 times selectivity for DPP IV compared with DPP 8 and DPP9. Compared with placebo, sitagliptin produces an approximately two-fold increase in postprandial active glucagon-like peptide 1 concentrations (2).

Pharmacokinetics

Sitagliptin is well absorbed and about 80% is excreted unchanged in the urine; the half-life is 8–14 hours (2).

Renal clearance averages 388 ml/minute and is largely uninfluenced by dose. The AUC is dose-dependent and is not affected by food. The pharmacokinetics are not affected by obesity (3).

Observational studies

In 34 healthy men, mean age 33 years, weight 77 kg, single doses of sitagliptin 1.5–600 mg resulted in 79 adverse events, of which 19 were thought to be drug related; 14 occurred in those taking sitagliptin and five in those taking placebo (1). Adverse events were reported to be mild to moderate and resolved without treatment. The study was designed to investigate the single-dose pharmacokinetics and pharmacodynamics of sitagliptin, and data on the nature of the adverse events were not given. However, it was reported that there were no cases of hypoglycemia, and blood counts and liver and renal function tests were reported as unaffected.

Placebo-controlled studies

In a placebo-controlled study in 521 patients with type 2 diabetes mellitus aged 27–76 years, sitagliptin 100 or 200 mg/day for 18 weeks significantly improved glycemic control (4). Hypoglycemia and gastrointestinal adverse events were not significantly different between sitagliptin and placebo.

Organs and Systems

Metabolism

In a randomized, double-blind, placebo-controlled study in 741 patients sitagliptin 100 or 200 mg for 24 weeks caused no changes in body weight, although those who took placebo lost 1.1 kg (5). However, in other similar studies, body weight fell similarly with sitagliptin and placebo (4,6).

Drug-drug interactions

Metformin

In a placebo-controlled, multiple-dose, crossover study in 13 patients with type 2 diabetes, sitagliptin 50 mg bd and metformin 1000 mg bd did not alter the pharmacokinetics of each other (7).

References

1. Herman GA, Stevens C, Van Dyck K, Bergman A, Yi B, De Smet M, Snyder K, Hilliard D, Tanen M, Tanaka W, Wang AQ, Zeng W, Musson D, Winchell G, Davies MJ, Ramael S, Gottesdiener KM, Wagner JA. Pharmacokinetics and pharmacodynamics of sitagliptin, an inhibitor of dipeptidyl peptidase IV, in healthy subjects: results from two randomized, double-blind, placebo-controlled studies with single oral doses. Clin Pharmacol Ther 2005;78(6):675–88.
2. Miller S, St Onge EL. Sitagliptin: a dipeptidyl peptidase IV inhibitor for the treatment of type 2 diabetes. Ann Pharmacother 2006;40(7-8):1336–43.
3. Herman GA, Bergman A, Liu F, Stevens C, Wang AQ, Zeng W, Chen L, Snyder K, Hilliard D, Tanen M, Tanaka W, Meehan AG, Lasseter K, Dilzer S, Blum R, Wagner JA. Pharmacokinetics and pharmacodynamic effects of the oral DPP-4 inhibitor sitagliptin in middle-aged obese subjects. J Clin Pharmacol 2006;46(8):876–86.
4. Raz I, Hanefeld M, Xu L, Caria C, Williams-Herman D, Khatami H; Sitagliptin Study 023 Group. Efficacy and safety of the dipeptidyl peptidase-4 inhibitor sitagliptin as monotherapy in patients with type 2 diabetes mellitus. Diabetologia 2006;49(11):2564–71.
5. Aschner P, Kipnes MS, Lunceford JK, Sanchez M, Mickel C, Williams-Herman DE; Sitagliptin Study 021 Group. Effect of the dipeptidyl peptidase-4 inhibitor sitagliptin as monotherapy on glycemic control in patients with type 2 diabetes. Diabetes Care 2006;29(12):2632–7.
6. Charbonnel B, Karasik A, Liu J, Wu M, Meininger G; Sitagliptin Study 020 Group. Efficacy and safety of the dipeptidyl peptidase-4 inhibitor sitagliptin added to ongoing metformin therapy in patients with type 2 diabetes inadequately controlled with metformin alone. Diabetes Care 2006;29(12):2638–43.
7. Herman GA, Bergman A, Yi B, Kipnes M; The Sitagliptin Study 012 Group. Tolerability and pharmacokinetics of metformin and the dipeptidyl peptidase-4 inhibitor sitagliptin when co-administered in patients with type 2 diabetes. Curr Med Res Opin 2006;22(10):1939–47.

Glucagon

General Information

Glucagon, which is produced in the alpha cells of the islets of Langerhans, is used in diabetes mellitus type 1 to stimulate glucose output from the liver during hypoglycemia (1 mg subcutaneously, repeated once or twice) when glucose cannot be given intravenously. In some countries it is often used by personnel, such as family members, who are not medically qualified, as the first action when the patient cannot take sugar orally. The antihypoglycemic effect of an intramuscular injection is longer lasting and more potent than that of intravenous glucagon (1). It is sometimes given by infusion to treat chronic hypoglycemia. However, when there is insulin reserve in the pancreas, glucagon induces hypoglycemia by stimulating insulin release (2).

Glucagon has also been used to stimulate insulin and C-peptide secretion, to see whether the islets still produce insulin, as a stimulatory test during pheochromocytoma, hyperinsulinism, and Zollinger–Ellison syndrome, or as an additive in upper gastrointestinal X-ray investigations (0.5–1 mg). It has been used in myocardial infarction, although its inotropic effects may present a risk. It has also been used to treat overdoses with beta-blockers (3) and calcium channel blockers (4), although its efficacy in such cases has only been demonstrated in animals (5) and to treat overdose with tricyclic antidepressants (6,7).

During long-term administration glucagon can cause the same effects as a glucagonoma: hyperglycemia, necrolytic migratory erythema, weight loss, anemia, angular cheilitis, and venous thrombosis (8).

Organs and Systems

Cardiovascular

Glucagon has been reported to have caused myocardial ischemia (9).

Endocrine

Glucagon infusions in the treatment of tumor-induced hypoglycemia can cause adverse effects comparable to the effects of a glucagonoma (hyperglycemia, necrolytic migratory erythema, weight loss, anemia, angular cheilitis, and venous thrombosis), as reported in three patients (10).

- A 38-year-old woman developed erythematous dermatitis, in a skin biopsy consistent with necrolytic migratory erythema, and angular cheilitis, which disappeared after withdrawal of glucagon infusion after 2 months.
- After 5 months of glucagon treatment a 38-year-old man developed an erythematous scaly rash and angular cheilitis, which subsided dramatically after withdrawal of the glucagon.
- A 57-year-old man who was given glucagon developed massive thrombosis, which resolved after removal of glucagon infusion and medical therapy.

Metabolism

When there is insulin reserve in the pancreas, glucagon can cause hypoglycemia by stimulating insulin secretion.

Electrolyte balance

Hyponatremia can occur during long-term administration of glucagon (11).

Hyponatremia and thrombocytopenia during glucagon infusion [SEDA-25, 466] prompted a retrospective investigation in 2045 preterm infants (before 37 weeks of gestation), of whom 28 had received glucagon infusion (12). One had severe hyponatremia but it was easily corrected and it was considered to be dilutional. There were no cases of thrombocytopenia.

Hematologic

Thrombocytopenia can occur during long-term administration of glucagon (11).

Gastrointestinal

Glucagon can cause nausea, vomiting, and diarrhea (13).

Skin

Chronic administration of glucagon can cause an eczema-like maculopapular scaly rash, which can progress to necrolytic migratory erythema, as in glucagonoma (8,14,15). Erythema multiforme has also been reported (16).

Glucagon, used to treat persistent hyperinsulinemic hypoglycemia of infancy, caused erythema necrolyticum migrans in two neonates (17).

- In the first child, a monozygotic twin girl, delivered at 30 weeks, diazoxide, chlorothiazide, and nifedipine did not alter glucose requirements, but octreotide halved the need, and intravenous glucagon lowered it further. However, the child then developed a maculopapular rash on the face and trunk. After 4 weeks the lesions worsened, increased in size, and became superficially necrosed with thick-caked scales. The rash also involved the limbs and mucous membranes, making feeding almost impossible. When glucagon was withdrawn the skin lesions resolved from the center within 2 days and disappeared without scarring in 10 days.
- The second child, who was delivered at term, had a blood glucose of 0.8 mmol/l 6 hours after birth and suffered a seizure that was treated with subcutaneous glucagon, octreotide, and other drugs. It was impossible to give sufficient feeding, and notwithstanding subcutaneous glucagon 11 micrograms/kg/hour and octreotide 4.3 micrograms/kg/hour, she had a generalized seizure when the blood glucose was 1.4 mmol/l. At 6 months, subtotal pancreatectomy was performed. During glucagon therapy she had seborrheic skin with silvery scales and on the thoracic skin an area of pale lichenification with mild hyperkeratosis. Within 2 weeks after surgery (and withdrawal of glucagon) the skin became totally normal.

Susceptibility Factors

Age

Hypoglycemia often occurs in premature children and can usually be treated by intravenous glucose. For intractable hypoglycemia an infusion of glucagon can be used. However, it can cause thrombocytopenia and hyponatremia with convulsions (11).

- A female triplet was born at 35 weeks by cesarean section after a normal pregnancy, during which her mother had had normal glucose tolerance. At 2 hours the baby's serum glucose was 1.0 mmol/l. Intravenous glucose was not effective. At 36 hours, dexamethasone was added, but 24 hours later her blood glucose was below 2.0 mmol/l. Dexamethasone was withdrawn and glucagon 1 mg/day was added to the infusion. After 4 hours the blood glucose became stable at 4.0 mmol/l. Her serum sodium fell from 138 to 116 mmol/l at about 120 hours, her potassium rose to 7.6 mmol/l, and her platelet count fell to 13×10^9/l. The glucagon infusion was stopped and within 24 hours her sodium and platelets normalized.

Glucagon infusion in premature babies is risky; more information is necessary.

References

1. Namba M, Hanafusa T, Kono N, Tarui SThe GL-G Hypoglycemia Study Group. Clinical evaluation of biosynthetic glucagon treatment for recovery from hypoglycemia developed in diabetic patients. Diabetes Res Clin Pract 1993;19(2):133–8.

2. Thoma ME, Glauser J, Genuth S. Persistent hypoglycemia and hyperinsulinemia: caution in using glucagon. Am J Emerg Med 1996;14(1):99–101.

3. Hazouard E, Ferrandiere M, Lesire V, Joye F, Perrotin D, de Toffol B. Peduncular hallucinosis related to propranolol self-poisoning: efficacy of intravenous glucagon. Intensive Care Med 1999;25(3):336–7.

4. Salhanick SD, Shannon MW. Management of calcium channel antagonist overdose. Drug Saf 2003;26(2):65–79.

5. Bailey B. Glucagon in beta-blocker and calcium channel blocker overdoses: a systematic review. J Toxicol Clin Toxicol 2003;41(5):595–602.

6. Sensky PR, Olczak SA. High-dose intravenous glucagon in severe tricyclic poisoning. Postgrad Med J 1999;75(888):611–2.

7. Teece S, Hogg K. Towards evidence based emergency medicine: best BETs from the Manchester Royal Infirmary. Glucagon in tricyclic overdose. Emerg Med J 2003;20(3):264–5.

8. Wermers RA, Fatourechi V, Wynne AG, Kvols LK, Lloyd RV. The glucagonoma syndrome. Clinical and pathologic features in 21 patients. Medicine (Baltimore) 1996;75(2):53–63.

9. Chin DT. Myocardial ischemia induced by glucagon. Ann Pharmacother 1996;30(1):84–5.

10. Case CC, Vassilopoulou R. Reproduction of features of the glucagonoma syndrome with continuous intravenous glucagon infusion as therapy for tumor-induced hypoglycemia. Endocrine Pract 2003;9:22–5.

11. Belik J, Musey J, Trussell RA. Continuous infusion of glucagon induces severe hyponatremia and thrombocytopenia in a premature neonate. Pediatrics 2001;107(3):595–7.

12. Chrasha DS, McKinley PS, Whitfield JM. Glucagon infusion for treatment of hypoglycemia: efficacy and safety in sick, premature infants. Pediatrics 2003;111:220–1.

13. Ranganath L, Schaper F, Gama R, Morgan L. Mechanism of glucagon-induced nausea. Clin Endocrinol (Oxf) 1999;51(2):260–1.

14. Beltzer-Garelli E, Cesarini JP, Cywiner-Golenzer C, Eskenazi A, Grupper C. Lesions cutanées révélatrices d'un glucagonome. [Skin lesions revealing a glucagonoma.] Sem Hop 1980;56(11–12):579–82.

15. Dai W, Shi Y, Cai L. [Report of a case of glucagonoma misdiagnosed as "eczema" and "hepatic angioma" for three years and review of literature.]Zhonghua Nei Ke Za Zhi 1995;34(3):190–2.

16. Edell SL. Erythema multiforme secondary to intravenous glucagon. AJR Am J Roentgenol 1980;134(2):385–6.

17. Wald M, Lawrenz K, Luckner D, Seimann R, Mohnike K, Schober E. Glucagon therapy as a possible cause of erythema necrolyticum migrans in two neonates with persistent hyperinsulinaemic hypoglycaemia. Eur J Pediatr 2002;161(11):600–3.

Glucagon-like peptide-1

General Information

Glucagon-like peptide-1 is an intestinal hormone that increases insulin secretion and biosynthesis, has a trophic effect on beta cells, suppresses glucagon secretion, delays gastric emptying, increases satiety, and reduces food intake (1). Its effects are glucose-dependent and it should not cause hypoglycemia. However, in healthy subjects hypoglycemia can occur after high doses or after fasting.

Although it is a candidate for the treatment of type 2 diabetes, it has to be injected subcutaneously and is extremely rapidly degraded by dipeptidyl peptidase IV. Analogues that are resistant to degradation and inhibitors of the degrading enzyme are being investigated.

In a randomized, crossover study with glucagon-like peptide-1, metformin, or the combination, there were no differences between the monotherapies (2). The combination had additive effects in lowering blood glucose and tended to reduce appetite.

In a crossover study, 20 patients with type 2 diabetes were treated for 6 weeks with glucagon-like peptide-1 or saline added to continuous subcutaneous insulin infusion; glucagon-like peptide-1 reduced appetite and caused nausea and reduced well-being (3).

In healthy volunteers, a fatty acid derivative of glucagon-like peptide-1, NN2211, which binds to albumin and has a half-life of about 12 hours, caused more dizziness, headache, nausea, and vomiting than placebo (4,5).

Glucagon-like peptide-1 is quickly degraded and therefore long-acting glucagon-like peptide receptor agonists and oral inhibitors of dipeptidyl peptidase IV (DPP-IV), which inhibit the degradation of glucagon-like peptide-1, and glucose-dependent insulinotropic peptide (GIP) have been developed and reviewed (6). The agonists can cause nausea and vomiting, but have more potency for glucose lowering than DPP-IV inhibitors. No hypoglycemia was seen when glucagon-like peptide-1 was given to lean people with type 2 diabetes (7). When glucagon-like peptide-1 was given as a continuous subcutaneous infusion for 12 weeks to patients who stopped taking oral therapy or without withdrawing oral therapy, one patient had fatigue and dry eyes during the study and two had nausea during the first week (8). There were no episodes of hypoglycemia.

Organs and Systems

Metabolism

In a double-blind, randomized, crossover study in 10 healthy subjects, subcutaneous glucagon-like peptide-1 after a 16-hour fast caused a near five-fold rise in plasma insulin concentration and circulating plasma glucose concentrations fell below the reference range in all subjects

(9). One subject had symptoms of hypoglycemia. A rise in pulse rate correlated with the fall in plasma glucose concentration and there was an increase in blood pressure.

In eight patients with type 2 diabetes and seven matched non-diabetics, subcutaneous glucagon-like peptide-1 and intravenous glucose caused reactive hypoglycemia in five controls but not in the patients (10). Glucagon was suppressed.

References

1. Holst JJ. Therapy of type 2 diabetes mellitus based on the actions of glucagon-like peptide-1. Diabetes Metab Res Rev 2002;18(6):430–41.
2. Zander M, Taskiran M, Toft-Nielsen MB, Madsbad S, Holst JJ. Additive glucose-lowering effects of glucagon-like peptide-1 and metformin in type 2 diabetes. Diabetes Care 2001;24(4):720–5.
3. Zander M, Madsbad S, Madsen JL, Holst JJ. Effect of 6-week course of glucagon-like peptide 1 on glycaemic control, insulin sensitivity, and beta-cell function in type 2 diabetes: a parallel-group study. Lancet 2002;359(9309):824–30.
4. Elbrond B, Jakobsen G, Larsen S, Agerso H, Jensen LB, Rolan P, Sturis J, Hatorp V, Zdravkovic M. Pharmacokinetics, pharmacodynamics, safety, and tolerability of a single-dose of NN2211, a long-acting glucagon-like peptide 1 derivative, in healthy male subjects. Diabetes Care 2002;25(8):1398–404.
5. Agerso H, Jensen LB, Elbrond B, Rolan P, Zdravkovic M. The pharmacokinetics, pharmacodynamics, safety and tolerability of NN2211, a new long-acting GLP-1 derivative, in healthy men. Diabetologia 2002;45(2):195–202.
6. Drucker DJ. Enhancing incretin action for the treatment of type 2 diabetes. Diabetes Care 2003;26:2929–40.
7. Knop FK, Vilsbøll T, Larsen S, Madsbad S, Holst JJ, Krarup T. No hypoglycemia after subcutaneous administration of glucagon-like peptide-1 in lean type 2 diabetic patients and in patients with diabetes secondary to chronic pancreatitis. Diabetes Care 2003;26:2581–7.
8. Meneilly GS, Greig N, Tildesley H, Habener JF, Egan JM, Elahi D. Effects of 3 months of continuous subcutaneous administration of glucagon-like peptide 1 in elderly patients with type 2 diabetes. Diabetes Care 2003;26:2835–41.
9. Edwards CM, Todd JF, Ghatei MA, Bloom SR. Subcutaneous glucagon-like peptide-1 (7-36) amide is insulinotropic and can cause hypoglycaemia in fasted healthy subjects. Clin Sci (Lond) 1998;95(6):719–24.
10. Vilsboll T, Krarup T, Madsbad S, Holst JJ. No reactive hypoglycaemia in Type 2 diabetic patients after subcutaneous administration of GLP-1 and intravenous glucose. Diabet Med 2001;18(2):144–9.

Guar gum

General Information

Guar gum is a low-viscosity water-soluble dietary fiber that has been used to treat diabetes because it slows the absorption of glucose from the gut. However, adverse effects such as regurgitation, obstipation, abdominal cramps, diarrhea, and itching are common (1). Partially hydrolysed guar gum has been added to enteral formulas and food products as a source of dietary fiber; it can reduce laxative use, diarrhea in septic patients receiving total enteral nutrition, and symptoms of irritable bowel syndrome (2).

In a systematic review of 11 trials of the use of guar gum to treat obesity, the most common adverse events were abdominal pain, flatulence, diarrhea, and cramps; 11 patients (3%) dropped out owing to adverse events (3).

Organs and Systems

Gastrointestinal

Of 26 reports of suspected adverse reactions to a diet formulation containing guar gum (Cal-Ban 3000), there were 18 cases of esophageal obstruction and seven of small bowel obstruction (4). There were pre-existing esophageal or gastric disorders in 50% of those with esophageal obstruction, including peptic stricture, pyrosis, hiatus hernia, esophagitis, gastric stapling, Schatzki ring, and muscular dystrophy. Fourteen patients with esophageal obstruction were treated successfully by endoscopy, although the tenacious gel-like material was often difficult to remove. One patient who developed a pulmonary embolism after surgical repair of an intraoperative esophageal tear died.

Immunologic

Guar gum can cause occupational rhinitis (5) and asthma (6). Of 162 employees at a carpet-manufacturing plant where guar gum was used to adhere dye to the fiber, 37 (23%) had a history suggestive of occupational asthma and 59 (36%) occupational rhinitis (7). Eight (5%) had immediate skin reactivity to guar gum and 11 (8.3%) had serum IgE antibodies to guar gum.

An employee of a pet food plant developed a severe cough, rhinitis, and conjunctivitis, and skin tests confirmed guar allergy. The symptoms resulted in obstructive sleep apnea which resolved after absence from work and recurred after rechallenge with guar gum dust (8).

References

1. Chuang LM, Jou TS, Yang WS, Wu HP, Huang SH, Tai TY, Lin BJ. Therapeutic effect of guar gum in patients with non-insulin-dependent diabetes mellitus. J Formos Med Assoc 1992;91(1):15–9.
2. Slavin JL, Greenberg NA. Partially hydrolyzed guar gum: clinical nutrition uses. Nutrition 2003;19(6):549–52.
3. Pittler MH, Ernst E. Guar gum for body weight reduction: meta-analysis of randomized trials. Am J Med 2001;110(9):724–30.
4. Lewis JH. Esophageal and small bowel obstruction from guar gum-containing "diet pills": analysis of 26 cases reported to the Food and Drug Administration. Am J Gastroenterol 1992;87(10):1424–8.
5. Kanerva L, Tupasela O, Jolanki R, Vaheri E, Estlander T, Keskinen H. Occupational allergic rhinitis from guar gum. Clin Allergy 1988;18(3):245–52.

6. Lagier F, Cartier A, Somer J, Dolovich J, Malo JL. Occupational asthma caused by guar gum. J Allergy Clin Immunol 1990;85(4):785–90.
7. Malo JL, Cartier A, L'Archeveque J, Ghezzo H, Soucy F, Somers J, Dolovich J. Prevalence of occupational asthma and immunologic sensitization to guar gum among employees at a carpet-manufacturing plant. J Allergy Clin Immunol 1990;86(4 Pt 1):562–9.
8. Leznoff A, Haight JS, Hoffstein V. Reversible obstructive sleep apnea caused by occupational exposure to guar gum dust. Am Rev Respir Dis 1986;133(5):935–6.

Incretin mimetics

General Information

Incretins are compounds that increase insulin secretion from the pancreas in a glucose-dependent manner; they are therefore potential therapies for the treatment of diabetes mellitus. Glucagon-like peptide-1 (GLP-1) (30 amino acids) is a naturally occurring incretin. It is largely produced in the distal ileum and colon in response to food that contains carbohydrate and fat. Other incretins include gastric inhibitory polypeptide (GIP). The half life of GLP-1 is only minutes, as it is rapidly metabolized by dipeptidyl peptidase type IV, which is another therapeutic target. Other actions of GLP-1 include delayed gastric emptying, appetite suppression, and increased beta cell mass. There is suppression of raised glucagon concentrations, but the counter-regulatory response remains intact.

Subcutaneous GLP-1 also has a short half-life (about 30 minutes) and so longer-acting GLP-1 receptor agonists are being developed. These drugs are known as incretin mimetics. Exenatide (39 amino acids) is the first to have received FDA approval. Liraglutide (32 amino acids) is undergoing trials. Exenatide is injected subcutaneously into the thigh, abdomen, or upper arm. It is administered twice daily. The pharmacokinetics of exenatide 10 micrograms subcutaneously are: C_{max} 211 pg/ml, t_{max} median 2.1 hours, apparent volume of distribution 28 liters, clearance 9.1 l/hour, terminal half-life 2.4 hours. Elimination is by glomerular filtration followed by proteolytic degradation. The clearance is not affected by mild or moderate renal impairment. However, clearance is reduced in end-stage renal insufficiency and dialysis. It is recommended that exenatide should not be used in such patients.

Exenatide (synthetic exendin-4, from the saliva from a lizard), which has a 53% overlap with glucagon-like peptide-1 and which also binds to the glucagon-like peptide-1 receptor, has been investigated in a placebo-controlled study for 28 days in 116 patients with type 2 diabetes in addition to a sulfonylurea or metformin (1). The most common adverse effects were nausea (mostly only in the first week) and mild to moderate hypoglycemia, for which no treatment was needed.

Liraglutide is also injected subcutaneously, but once daily because of its longer half-life.

Incretin mimetics are an exciting development, because when used alone they do not promote hypoglycemia, as their actions on insulin and glucagon are strictly glucose dependent. They are accompanied by weight loss, and they may preserve beta cell mass.

Reviews of incretin mimetics (2,3) have suggested that nausea and vomiting are adverse effects common to all those currently in clinical trials. The adverse effects occur transiently and in association with peak plasma concentrations of glucagon-like peptide (GLP)-1. The doses of both exenatide and liraglutide that have maximum glucose lowering effects are similar to the doses that are associated with these adverse effects. Liraglutide is a long-acting incretin mimetic designed for once-daily subcutaneous injection.

Observational studies

In 190 patients, mean age 57 years, randomized to different doses of liraglutide (0.045–0.75 mg/day) for 12 weeks, gastrointestinal events increased with increasing doses; 10 of 135 patients exposed to liguratide reported nausea (five in the highest dose group), compared with 1 of 29 who took placebo (4). Diarrhea, vomiting, and constipation also occurred. Most (two-thirds) of the gastrointestinal symptoms resolved within 3 days. Headache was also reported.

Placebo-controlled studies

Patients with type 2 diabetes treated with a sulfonylurea alone, aged 22–76 years, were randomized to placebo ($n = 123$) or subcutaneous exenatide 5 micrograms bd ($n = 254$); after 4 weeks 129 patients increased their dose to 10 micrograms bd (5). During the 30 weeks of the study 12 subjects had mild to moderate transient abnormalities of creatine kinase. Serious adverse events were no more frequent with exenatide (4% with 10 micrograms and 3% with 5 micrograms) than with placebo (8%). The adverse events that were related to treatment included nausea, which occurred in 49 patients (39%) of those who used 5 micrograms and 66 (51%) of those who used 10 micrograms, compared with 9 (7%) of those who used placebo. The nausea was worst during the first 8 weeks then abated. Other adverse effects included hypoglycemia, dizziness, and a jittery feeling. There was hypoglycemia in 36% of those taking 10 micrograms, 14% of those taking 5 micrograms, and 3% of those using placebo. One subject withdrew owing to hypoglycemia. Weight loss was progressive over 30 weeks and was most apparent in those taking 10 micrograms (–1.6 kg). Those who did not report nausea also lost weight.

Organs and Systems

Metabolism

Hypoglycemia

Hypoglycemia is more common when incretin mimetics are taken with sulfonylureas but not metformin. Many of the actions of GLP-1 and incretin mimetics are glucose dependent and do not on their own provoke hypoglycemia. However, it is thought that because of the ability of sulfonylureas to open K_{ATP} channels at low blood glucose concentrations, GLP-1 can augment insulin secretory responses at lower concentrations than it would normally. The same problem may occur when incretin mimetics are combined with meglitinides.

Mild or moderate hypoglycemia occurred with a similar frequency in patients with type 2 diabetes who took exenatide or placebo: 5.3% in those who took 10 micrograms bd, 4.5% in those who took 5 micrograms bd, and 5.3% in those who took placebo (6). However, in a study in which exenatide was combined with metformin and a sulfonylurea in 733 subjects the incidence of hypoglycemia was greater in those who took exenatide (13% placebo, 19% 5 micrograms bd, and 28% 10 micrograms bd) (7). The incidence of hypoglycemia was lowest in those who were taking the lowest dose of sulfonylurea. The effect of exenatide to stimulate insulin production is glucose dependent, and it is likely that the hypoglycemia observed in this study related to the non-glucose-dependent actions of sulfonylureas superimposed on the effect of exenatide. It is therefore appropriate in patients whose HB_{A1c} concentration is close to target to reduce their dose of sulfonylurea when they start to take exenatide and to make further adjustments depending on response.

Weight loss

Weight loss has been reported with exenatide. It occurs regardless of initial weight and does not relate to the degree of nausea (see below), but exenatide reduces food intake (8). In a 30-week study those who took 10 micrograms bd lost 2.8 kg and those who took 5 micrograms bd lost 1.6 kg compared with 0.3 kg in those who took placebo.

Gastrointestinal

Both exenatide and liraglutide slow gastric emptying; this may have an effect on the speed of absorption of other drugs (2) and partly contributes to nausea.

DoTS classification:
Reaction: Nausea due to exenatide
Dose-relation: Collateral
Time-course: Intermediate
Susceptibility factors: None known.

The mechanism is not fully established, but possible mechanisms include delay in gastric emptying, activation of afferent nerves, and or central effects of GLP-1 receptor activation (9). It is dose related in the therapeutic range of doses and is more likely to occur in the first eight weeks (10,11).Increasing the dose of exenatide gradually may be helpful (12).

During continuous subcutaneous infusion of exenatide at different doses in 12 patients with type 2 diabetes nausea was the most common adverse effect (13). The dose of exenatide appears to be important. In a placebo-controlled study in 156 patients (mean age 52 years, BMI 33–36 kg/m^2) with type 2 diabetes who received exenatide for 28 days, nausea varied with dose 23% of those who took 2.5 micrograms bd, 26% of those who took 5 micrograms bd, 61% of those who took 7.5 micrograms bd, and 52% of those who took 10 micrograms bd (14). The nausea was maximal during the first week (33%), falling to 6% by the end of the study.

In another placebo-controlled study, the incidence of nausea also fell with time (7). Patients with type 2 diabetes (mean age 55 years; $n = 733$) taking metformin and a sulfonylurea took either exenatide 5 micrograms bd or placebo for 4 weeks. Those taking exenatide were then randomized to either 5 micrograms bd or 10 micrograms bd for 30 weeks. Nausea, the most frequent severe adverse event, occurred at similar rates in both groups— 5% of those taking 5 micrograms bd and 3% of those taking 10 micrograms bd. The overall incidence of nausea was slightly higher at all times in those who took 10 micrograms bd, about 31% at the start of the study falling to about 10% compared with about 24% in those who took 5 micrograms bd, falling to 7%.

Of 210 patients with type 2 diabetes, 179 completed a randomized study of the effects of five different doses (0.045, 0.225, 0.45, 0.6, and 0.75 mg) or metformin 100 mg bd for 12 weeks after a 4-week metformin run-in phase. The numbers of people who reported nausea and vomiting were small (4%) and comparable to the incidence with metformin (6%) (15). Careful upwards titration allows higher doses (2 mg/day) to be tolerated (2).

In 336 patients with type 2 diabetes who took metformin, 36% of those who were randomized to exenatide 5 micrograms bd and 45% of those who took 10 micrograms bd had nausea compared with 23% of those who took placebo (6). The frequency of nausea fell during the study in all groups.

Immunologic

Antibodies to exenatide have been found in several studies, with an incidence of 43% and 49% (6, 7). The development of antibodies did not appear to alter glycemic control or adverse events. The titers of antibodies were low (1/125). The long-term effects of these antibodies are unknown, but could include a reduced response to exenatide. There appears to be no cross-reaction between exenatide antibodies and native human GLP-1 (16).

After the end of 12 weeks no antibodies to liraglutide were detected (15).

Long-Term Effects

Tumorigenicity

GLP-1 increases beta-cell mass in animals. Thus, exenatide has the potential to cause increased beta-cell mass through augmented differentiation of precursor cells and inhibition of apoptosis (9). No malignant islet cell tumors were found in 130 mice and rats who received the equivalent human dose of 20 micrograms/day for 2 years (17). Long-term follow-up is required to ensure safety.

Drug administration

Drug administration route

The concentration versus time profiles after subcutaneous injection of 10 micrograms of exenatide into the abdomen, arm, and thigh were similar in 28 people with type 2 diabetes, mean age 56 years (18). Long-term injection of insulin can cause local problems such as lipohypertrophy, and so rotation of injection sites is recommended. Similar problems have also been reported with growth hormone. It would therefore be wise to vary the injection site of exenatide, as systemic availability is comparable.

Drug-Drug Interactions

Digoxin

In 21 healthy Asian men who took *digoxin* and exenatide there was no important change in digoxin exposure; C_{max} fell by 17% and t_{max} was prolonged by a median of 2.5 hours. No digoxin concentrations increased to more than 2.0 mg/l (19). The summary of product characteristics (SPC) for exenatide specifies that dosage adjustment is not required for paracetamol or digoxin.

Paracetamol

In 40 healthy people aged 18–65 years the absorption of exenatide 10 micrograms was unaffected by paracetamol 1000 mg (20). However, the absorption of paracetamol was reduced, depending on the timing of ingestion in relation to the injection of exenatide. When paracetamol was taken 1 hour before exenatide there was no change in plasma paracetamol concentrations. However, when it was taken at the same time as the injection or 1 or 2 hours after there was up to a 56% reduction in C_{max} and the t_{max} was prolonged from 0.6 hours to a maximum of 4.2 hours. Exenatide reduces the rate of gastric emptying.

References

1. Fineman MS, Bicsak TA, Shen LZ, Taylor K, Gaines E, Varns A, Kim D, Baron AD. Effect of glycemic control of exenatide (synthetic exendine-4) additive to existing metformin and/or sulfonylurea treatment in patients with type 2 diabetes. Diabetes Care 2003;26:2370–7.
2. Nauck MA. Glucagon-like peptide 1 (GLP-1) and incretin mimetics for the treatment of diabetes. Pract Diabetes Int 2005;22:171–9.
3. Gryskiewicz K, Coleman CI. Exenatide. A novel incretin mimetic hormone for the treatment of type 2 diabetes. Formulary 2005;40:86–90.
4. Madsbad S, Schmitz O, Ranstam J, Jakobsen G, Matthews DR, on behalf of the NN2211-1310 International Study Group. Improved glycemic control with no weight increase in patients with type 2 diabetes after once daily treatment with the long acting glucagons like peptide 1 analog liraglutide (NN2211). Diabetes Care 2004;27:1335–42.
5. Buse JB, Henry RR, Han J, Kim DD, Fineman MS, Baron AD, for the Exenatide-113 Clinical Study Group. Effects of exenatide (exendin-4) on glycemic control over 30 weeks in sulfonylurea-treated patients with type 2 diabetes. Diabetes Care 2004;27:2628–35.
6. DeFronzo RA, Ratner RE, Han J, Kim DD, Fineman MS, Baron AD. Effects of exenatide (exendin-4) on glycemic control and weight over 30 weeks in metformin-treated patients with type 2 diabetes. Diabetes Care 2005;28:1092–100.
7. Kendall DM, Riddle MC, Rosenstock J, Zhuang D, Kim DD, Fineman MS, Baron AD. Effects of exenatide (exendin-4) on glycemic control over 30 weeks in patients with type 2 diabetes treated with metformin and a sulfonylurea. Diabetes Care 2005;28:1083–91.
8. Edwards CMB, Stanley SA, Davis R, Brynes AE, Frost GS, Seal LJ, Ghatei MA, Bloom SR. Exendin-4 reduces fasting and postprandial glucose and decreases energy intake in healthy volunteers. Am J Physiol Endocrinol Metab 2001;281:E155–61.
9. Ahren B. Exenatide: a novel treatment of type 2 diabetes. Therapy 2005;2:207–22.
10. Barnett AH. Exenatide. Drugs Today 2005;41:563–78.
11. Keating GM. Exenatide. Drugs 2005;65:1681–92.
12. Sinclair EM, Drucker DJ. Glucagon-like peptide 1 receptor agonists and dipeptidyl peptidase IV inhibitors: new therapeutic agents for the treatment of type 2 diabetes. Curr Opin Endocrinol Diabetes 2005;12:146–51.
13. Taylor K, Kim D, Nielsen LL, Aisporna M, Baron AD, Fineman MS. Day-long subcutaneous infusion of exenatide lowers glycemia in patients with type 2 diabetes. Horm Metabol Res 2005;37:627–32.
14. Poon T, Nelson P, Shen L, Mihm M, Taylor K, Fineman M, Kim D. Exenatide improves glycemic control and reduces body weight in subjects with type 2 diabetes: a dose-ranging study. Diabetes Technol Ther 2005;7:467–72.
15. Feinglos MN, Saad MF, Pi-Sunyert FX, An B, Santiago O; on behalf of Lirglutide Dose-response Study Group. Effects of liraglutide (NN2211) a long acting GLP-1 analogue, on glycemic control and bodyweight in subjects with type 2 diabetes. Diabetic Med 2005;22:1016–23.
16. Nauck MA, Meier JJ. Glucagon-like peptide 1 and its derivatives in the treatment of diabetes. Regulatory Peptides 2005;128:135–48.
17. Hiles R, Carpenter T, Serota D, Schafer K, Ross P, Nelson D, Rebelatto M. Exenatide does not cause pancreatic islet cell proliferative lesions in rats and mice following 2-year exposure. Diabetes 2004;53 (Suppl 2):A380.
18. Calara F, Taylor K, Han J, Zabala E, Carr EM, Wintle M, Fineman M. A randomized, open-label, crossover study examining the effect of injection site on bioavailability of exenatide (synthetic exendin-4). Clin Ther 2005;27:210–5.
19. Kothare PA, Soon DKW, Linnebjerg H, Park S, Chan C, Yeo A, Lim M, Mace KF, Wise SD. Effect of exenatide on the steady-state pharmacokinetics on digoxin. J Clin Pharmacol 2005;45:1032–7.
20. Blase E, Taylor K, Gao H, Wintle M, Fineman M. Pharmacokinetics of an oral drug (acetaminophen) administered at various times in relation to subcutaneous injection of exenatide (exendin-4) in healthy subjects. J Clin Pharmacol 2005;45:570–7.

Insulin

General Information

Insulin is used for substitution therapy in patients with an absolute or relative deficiency of insulin. Most of the insulins now prescribed are either human or highly purified insulins of animal origin or synthetic insulins closely related to human insulin. The use of insulin of lesser purity is declining, but it is still used in considerable quantities in Eastern and Central Europe and in less developed countries. In some countries, both highly purified insulins of Western origin in concentrations of 100 U/ml, and locally produced less pure insulins in concentrations of 20, 40, or 80 U/ml are available at the same time, creating confusion. Patients have to realize that the syringe used for injection has to be concordant with the specific strength of insulin for which it has been made. The manner and the site of administration, the variation in duration of action of the various insulin formulations, the grade of purification, and differences in concentration cause specific problems.

The effects of insulin are modified by various factors. The speed and extent of absorption of insulin depends, for example, on the site of injection (1), the depth of the subcutaneous injection, skin temperature (2), the presence of lipodystrophy, and variation in the extent of inactivation of injected insulin. The disposal of insulin depends on many factors. Exercise and hard work lower the blood glucose and thereby increase the effect of insulin. Infections and obesity reduce its effect. The timing of food intake and the composition of meals are also related to the action of insulin. A thin layer of fat, as sometimes occurs in the upper arm or in the thighs of thin men, can result in intramuscular injection, leading to faster absorption of long-acting insulins. This can reduce the absorption time by half (3). The major factors that affect the fate of injected insulin (and thereby also its risks) are listed in Table 1 (4).

Insulin has a half-life of only a few minutes when injected intravenously. It is therefore prepared in different formulations for subcutaneous injection, with different half-lives of absorption, giving different durations of action. The main formulations, with their approximate durations of action are given in Table 2.

An alternative method of altering the duration of action of insulin is to use analogues in which there are amino acid substitutions. Analogues are listed in Table 3. Insulin aspart, insulin detemir, insulin glargine, and insulin lispro are all covered in separate monographs.

Combination studies

Insulin + amylin analogues
Pramlintide 30 micrograms was given to 16 patients using insulin pumps as an injection at meal times (5). Meal time insulin was reduced by 17%. Serum fructosamine improved. Nausea was the most common adverse effect. There was no hypoglycemia.

Insulin + biguanides
In a multicenter, open, parallel-group study in USA, 188 patients responded insufficiently to two oral hypoglycemic drugs (HbA$_{1c}$ over 8.0%) and received either a third oral drug or metformin with insulin 70/30 mix twice a day (6). HbA$_{1c}$ and fasting plasma glucose did not differ between the groups and neither did minor episodes of hypoglycemia. Weight gain was 3.5 and 2.9 kg respectively. Lack of efficacy or adverse effects prompted withdrawal in 13 % of those taking triple therapy and 2% of those taking insulin + metformin. In those taking insulin + metformin cholesterol and triglycerides fell and the mean cost was $10.40 for the triple group and $3.20 for the insulin + metformin group.

Metformin was given as an adjunct to insulin in a double-blind, placebo-controlled study in 28 adolescents needing more than 1 unit/kg/day (7). The dose of metformin was 1000 mg/day when body weight was under 50 kg, 1500 mg/day when it was 50–75 kg, and 2000 mg/day when it was over 75 kg. Metformin lowered insulin

Table 1 The major factors that affect the fate of injected insulin

Variable	Clinical relevance
Insulin formulation	Ultra-short-acting insulin (half-life 0.5–2 hours)
	Regular insulin (half-life 2–4 hours)
	Intermediate-acting insulin (half-life 16–20 hours)
	Prolonged-acting insulin (half-life 36 hours and over)
	Intraindividual variation in absorption up to 50%
	Interindividual variation from day-to-day up to 25%
Insulin species	Of minimal importance
Injection technique	Contributes to variance
Injected region	Absorption faster from abdominal region than from femoral and gluteal regions; exercising the injected limb speeds up absorption (applies especially to regular insulin)
Subcutaneous blood flow	A major determinant of absorption rate and clinically significant for regular insulin (influenced by smoking, ambient temperature, exercise, and local massage)
Subcutaneous degradation of insulin	Usually of no clinical significance; in rare cases after insulin need exceeds 120 IU/day it might explain brittleness
Insulin antibodies	Increase unpredictably the circulating fraction of insulin and prolong its half-life; a rare cause of insulin resistance

Table 2 Formulations of human insulin (all rINNs) and their durations of action

Type of insulin	Onset of action (hours)	Maximum action (hours)	Duration of action (hours)
Ultra-short-acting			
Insulin aspart, insulin lispro	0.05–2	0.5–1.5	4
Short-acting			
Neutral insulin injection	0.3–0.5	1–3	5–8
Intermediate-acting			
Insulin zinc suspension (amorphous) (semilente)	1–2	6–10	12–16
Isophane insulin (Neutral Protamine Hagedorn, NPH)	1–2	4–6	11–20
Globin zinc insulin suspension	1–2	6–10	10–18
Compound insulin zinc suspension (lente)	2–4	3–12	14–24
Long-acting			
Protamine zinc insulin injection	4–6	16–24	24–36
Insulin zinc suspension (crystalline) (ultralente)	4–6	16–24	24–36
Insulin glargine, insulin detemir	0.5–1	1–24	22–28
Combined formulations			
Diphasic insulin injection	0.7–1	3–18	12–24

Table 3 Insulin analogs

Analogue	Comments
Insulin aspart	Rapid-acting, short-acting; the proline at site 28 of the B chain is replaced by aspartate (B28Asp)
Insulin defalan	Prepared from insulin by removal of the terminal phenylalanine
Insulin detemir	Long-acting; the threonine is deleted at B30 and the lysine at B28 is acylated with a miristoyl side-chain (B29Lys (ϵ-tetradecanoyl)desB30)
Insulin glargine	Long-acting; the asparagine at A21 is replaced by glycine and two arginines are added to the C terminus of the B chain (A21Gly,B31Arg,B32Arg)
Insulin glulisine	Rapid-acting, short-acting; the asparagine at B3 is replaced by lysine and the lysine at B29 is replaced by glutamic acid (B3Lys,B29Glu)
Insulin lispro	Rapid-acting, short-acting (2–4 hours); the lysine at site 29 and the proline at site 28 of the B chain are interchanged (B28Lys,B29Pro)

requirements. The number of episodes of hypoglycemia increased compared with placebo. There was gastrointestinal discomfort in six patients taking metformin and five taking placebo.

A comparable placebo-controlled study was reported in 353 patients with type 2 diabetes for 48 weeks. All were taking insulin, and HbA$_{1c}$ fell in those who also took metformin. Body weight was reduced by 0.4 kg by metformin and increased by 1.2 kg by placebo. Symptomatic episodes of hypoglycemia were more common with metformin. There were mild transient gastrointestinal complaints in 56% and 13% respectively (8).

Insulin plus metformin (27 patients, 2000 mg/day) or troglitazone (30 patients, 600 mg/day) in patients with type 2 diabetes using at least 30 units/day was compared with insulin alone (30 patients) for 4 months (9). Body weight increased in the insulin and the insulin plus troglitazone groups. In the insulin plus metformin group there were significantly more gastrointestinal adverse effects but less hypoglycemia than the other groups.

Insulin + meglitinides
In 80 patients taking metformin 850 or 1000 mg tds plus NPH insulin at bedtime, metformin was withdrawn and repaglinide 4 mg tds added in half of the patients for 16 weeks (10). In the repaglinide group the dose of insulin increased slightly and weight gain was 1.8 kg more. Mild hypoglycemia occurred more often in the metformin group; nightly episodes of hypoglycemia occurred only with repaglinide. One patient taking repaglinide had a myocardial infarction, and one had three separate hospitalizations for chest pain (myocardial infarction was excluded). No specific data were presented about gastrointestinal adverse effects or infections.

Insulin + meglitinides + sulfonylureas
When repaglinide 4 mg tds and glimepiride 160 mg bd in combination with bedtime NPH insulin were compared for 13 weeks in 80 patients, there were no differences in improvement of glycemic control, hypoglycemia, or weight gain, except in one patient taking gliclazide + NPH, who needed third party help for hypoglycemia (11).

Insulin + thiazolidinediones
Insulin plus metformin (27 patients, 2000 mg/day) or troglitazone (30 patients, 600 mg/day) in patients with type 2 diabetes using at least 30 units/day was compared with insulin alone (30 patients) for 4 months (307). Body

weight increased in the insulin and the insulin plus troglitazone groups. In the insulin plus metformin group there were significantly more gastrointestinal adverse effects but less hypoglycemia than the other groups.

The addition of rosiglitazone to insulin for 26 weeks in a double-blind study in 315 patients with inadequately controlled type 2 diabetes improved glycemic control and was well tolerated (12). There was a significant fall in hemoglobin, and some patients in both the rosiglitazone and placebo groups developed edema.

General adverse effects

The major adverse effect of insulin is hypoglycemia, which is specifically dangerous when the patient's awareness of hypoglycemia is reduced or when long-acting formulations are used. Allergic reactions, although less common with newer formulations, regularly occur (13). Rare complications are lipoatrophy or hypertrophy and insulin edema. Insulin has to be given by injection, with pumps or specific devices for intensive therapy, which all generate specific problems. Other ways of administrating insulin are still experimental.

Additives introduced as preservatives or to change the duration of action of insulin can also cause adverse effects.

Organs and Systems

Cardiovascular

In 215 subjects with type 1 diabetes atherosclerosis was assessed using carotid intima media thickness (14). There was a positive correlation with cumulative short-acting insulin exposure but no correlation with intermediate-acting insulin. There was no power to distinguish between analogues and regular insulin. A review of insulin therapy has suggested that hyperglycemia is important, based on the results of the DCCT study, in which the intensive control group had less progression of atherosclerosis than the conventional group. Most studies have shown a beneficial or neutral effect of exogenous insulin on cardiovascular disease and atherosclerosis, which is different to the epidemiological data on endogenous insulin, which show an increased cardiovascular risk with increasing insulin concentrations (15).

Respiratory

Pulmonary edema secondary to hypoglycemia was reported particularly in the 1930s when insulin shock treatment was used for schizophrenia. It is less common nowadays, but has been reported after insulin overdose (16).

Nervous system

Cerebral edema has been described during therapy of diabetic ketoacidosis with a large volume of fluid, resulting in rapid changes in plasma osmolality, mostly in young patients (SEDA-26, 462). However, in 10 adults with

ketoacidosis, no signs of cerebral edema (supported by CT scans) were found (17).

Susceptibility factors for cerebral edema during ketoacidosis in children have been investigated in 61 cases of cerebral edema during 6977 hospital admissions (18). They were matched with two types of controls for each case: three children with ketoacidosis randomly selected and three children matched for age (within 2 years), onset of diabetes, blood pH, and serum glucose at entry. The results suggested that high initial serum urea concentrations and a low $PaCO_2$ are associated with an increased probability of cerebral edema. Children with these abnormalities should be monitored for signs of neurological deterioration, and hyperosmolar therapy should be immediately available. Treatment with bicarbonate was associated with an increased risk and should be avoided. In an accompanying editorial it was stated that high doses of insulin, hypotonic fluids, and bicarbonate are often seen as culprits, but it is also possible that it is an idiosyncratic response to diabetic ketoacidosis; there is no proof of either theory (19).

Sensory systems

Acute angle closure glaucoma has been reported as rare complication of rapid insulin therapy for hyperglycemic non-ketotic coma (20). It was postulated that raised glucose concentrations in the lens leads to increased sorbitol and water influx. The osmotic changes in the lens are not immediately corrected when the glucose concentration in aqueous humor is lowered, and this can lead to obstruction of the canal of Schlemm and increased intraocular pressure.

Metabolism

Hypoglycemia

The most frequent complication of insulin therapy is inadvertent hypoglycemia (21–23). Over 5% of deaths in diabetes can be attributed to hypoglycemia. The frequency increases with rigorous maintenance of normoglycemia (24,25). In the Diabetes Control and Complications Trial (DCCT) (26) the frequency of serious hypoglycemia was more than three times increased in the intensively treated group, and the frequency of the attacks was related to the concentration of HbA_{1c} (27). The UK Prospective Diabetes Study in patients with type 2 diabetes also showed an increased risk of hypoglycemia with more intensive treatment (28).

Attacks of hypoglycemia are often preceded by less marked attacks, which are unnoticed or not reported to the family or physician. Attacks can be caused by reduced resistance to insulin or switch to a type of insulin with a different duration of action. The reasons for hypoglycemia can be inaccurate or excessive insulin injections, heavy physical exercise, or omission of meals. The action of highly purified insulins and some new analogues, even when in long-acting form, is somewhat faster and shorter compared with less pure formulations. Errors in injection techniques, such as superficial subcutaneous injections, forming nodules or causing bleeding, can introduce variation in the absorption of insulin, resulting in an increase in the mean administered dose and in inadvertent hypoglycemia. Twice-daily isophane insulin for 6 months has been compared with once-daily ultralente insulin in 60 patients (29). Isophane was associated with fewer attacks of hypoglycemia, lower HbA_{1c}, lower evening glucose concentrations, and greater patient satisfaction.

The Somogyi effect, unnoticed hypoglycemia during sleep, causes a rebound increase in morning blood glucose with accompanying glycosuria. When, in response to this, the evening dose of long-acting insulin is increased, the risk of nocturnal hypoglycemia also increases, creating a vicious cycle. Blood glucose monitoring late at night helps to establish the diagnosis. Of 39 poorly controlled patients with insulin-treated diabetes aged 9–66 years, 22 had recurrent nocturnal hypoglycaemia, the best clinical clue to which was intermittent symptoms, however mild and infrequent they appeared to be (30).

Hypoglycemia can also be induced by concomitant diseases, for example renal disease, hepatic disease (cirrhosis), hypopituitarism, hypoadrenocorticalism, hypoglucagonism, hypothyroidism, malnutrition, anorexia nervosa, pregnancy, termination of pregnancy, recovery from infections, operations, or stress.

In a 12-month open study of 64 patients with type 2 diabetes (mean age 58 years) who used either once-daily bedtime NPH insulin + tablets or twice-daily 30% soluble + 70% NPH, there was less hypoglycemia in the former (2.7 hypoglycemic events per person compared with 4.3); the improvement in HB_{A1c} was similar (31). Weight gain was also less in those who used once-daily NPH (1.3 kg compared with 4.2 kg).

Frequency

In a review of 102 consecutive drug-induced, hospital-related cases of coma, 23 were caused by insulin only, 14 by insulin + glibenclamide, and 3 by insulin + metformin (32). The likelihood of readmission for hypoglycemia after a previous admission was 2.9 times greater.

Of 546 Spanish diabetic children and teenagers, 14% had one period of hypoglycemia and 21% had more than one episode (33). The highest incidence was in the morning, possibly related to the frugal Spanish breakfast and abundant food intake in the evening.

Hypoglycemia was retrospectively monitored in 1055 patients who had had type 2 diabetes for more than 2 months, and who visited the clinic at least twice in 6 months (34). They all received aggressive treatment to reach near-normal blood glucose concentrations. Symptoms of hypoglycemia were mentioned by 12% of those treated with diet alone, 16% of those using oral agents, and 30% of those using any form of insulin. In only five patients, all using insulin, was there severe hypoglycemia. A low HbA_{1c} concentration at follow-up, symptoms of hypoglycemia at the initial visit, and younger age were independently associated with an increased incidence of symptoms.

During 12 months, 244 episodes of severe hypoglycemia in 166 patients were recorded in a district with a population of 367 051 people (8655 with diabetes); there were 69 (7.1%) episodes in people with type 1 diabetes, 66 (7.3%) in people with type 2 diabetes using insulin, and 23 (0.8%) in those taking a sulfonylurea. Age, duration of diabetes, and lower social class were risk factors. The total cost of emergency treatment was estimated to be no more than $92 078 per year (35). In a German study in a comparable group of 200 000 people, there were 92 cases in those with type 1 diabetes and 146 cases in those with type 2 diabetes during 3 years (36). The estimated costs were lower: $88 676 per year for type 2 diabetes and $16 258 for type 1 diabetes.

In 28 children aged 3.1–8.3 years using twice- or thrice-daily insulin, blood glucose was measured with a subcutaneous continuous glucose monitoring system on 3 consecutive days and nights (37). Hypoglycemia was defined as a blood glucose concentration below 3.3 mmol/l for longer than 15 minutes. The prevalence of hypoglycemia was 10% and it was more common at night than during the day (19 versus 4.4%). Hypoglycemia at night had a longer duration (median 3.3 hours) and was asymptomatic in 91% of the episodes. The highest prevalence occurred at between 04.00 and 07.30. On a thrice-daily insulin injection regimen, nightly hypoglycemia was less frequent, but the frequency was higher on the following morning. With increasing age there was less hypoglycemia.

The frequency and nature of episodes of hypoglycemia have been quantified in a retrospective survey of 215 patients with type 2 diabetes treated with insulin (38). More than 90% used a mixture of short-acting or rapid-acting insulin plus an intermediate acting insulin twice daily, six used NPH insulin twice daily, and 13 used three or more injections per day. In the preceding year 32 of them had 60 periods of severe hypoglycemia (requiring assistance), 0.28 episodes/patient/year. One patient with 13 episodes had impaired awareness. The frequency increased with age, duration of insulin therapy, and duration of diabetes, but not with a lower concentration of HbA_{1c} or a higher dose of insulin. There was mild hypoglycemia in 64%. In those with mainly autonomic symptoms the occurrence of symptoms was inversely related to age. The neuroglycopenic symptoms were more frequent with increasing duration of insulin therapy.

In 1500 patients in intensive care, there was hypoglycemia (4 mmol/l and less) in 5.2% of the intensively treated group and 0.8% of those who received conventional therapy (93). It has been reported that 11% of drug errors are from insulin administration errors and it has been recommended that frequent checks be made of infusion systems (93).

In a systematic review of short-acting analogues, 42 randomized controlled trials in 7933 patients with type 1, type 2, and gestational diabetes showed only minor differences in overall hypoglycemia (39). The standardized mean differences of episodes per patient per month were –0.05 and –0.04 in adults with type 1 and type 2 diabetes respectively, comparing short-acting analogues with regular insulin. There were no differences between children and pregnant women with type 1 diabetes and women with gestational diabetes. The change in Hb_{A1c} was small. Hypoglycemia remains a clinical problem whether analogue or regular insulin is used.

Mechanisms

The concentrations of the counter-regulatory hormones adrenaline and glucagon were higher before treatment of coma in insulin-treated persons admitted to hospital for hypoglycemia than in the fasting state. However, concentrations of adrenaline, glucagon, cortisol, and growth hormone are lower during a hypoglycemic episode in a diabetic than when these hormones are measured during induced hypoglycemia in non-diabetics (40). There was an inverse correlation between glucose and adrenaline in hypoglycemia, but no direct relation between the other hormones and blood glucose concentrations. The addition of intramuscular glucagon during intravenous glucose therapy did not result in different glucose concentrations at any time (40). In type 2 diabetes counter-regulatory hormones are reduced compared with controls, but the patients release the hormones at higher blood glucose concentrations than type 1 diabetics, and the glucagon response is not blunted (41,42).

- Low responses of counter-regulatory hormones during induced hypoglycemia in a 27-year-old woman with poorly controlled diabetes (HbA$_{1c}$ 11%), with frequent hypoglycemic instances of which she was not aware, improved dramatically after 3 months of good regulation (43); only growth hormone showed no reaction.

Hypoglycemia increased beta-adrenoceptor sensitivity in healthy subjects but reduced it in type 1 diabetes (44).

In 20 insulin-treated diabetic patients with episodes of severe hypoglycemia in 1982–84, re-evaluated in 1992–94, emergency visits were reduced from 1.05/year to 0.42/year between 1984 and 1994 (45). There were no cases of fatal hypoglycemia. There was no association with HbA$_{1c}$. Multiple daily insulin doses reduced the frequency of hypoglycemia to one-third. In 1984, unawareness was a predisposing factor and most of the patients had deficient counter-regulation (adrenaline). Most patients had a long history of insulin injections (mean 29 years). In 1994, six patients were partly and eight patients totally retested and compared with 10 matched control patients with type 1 diabetes. When hypoglycemia was induced by insulin the patients with frequent hypoglycemia reached values under 3.0 mmol much faster, and in six patients the test had to be stopped before the normal duration of 3 hours for hypoglycemia; this never happened in the control patients. Counter-regulation was deficient in both 1984 and 1994, indicating that reduced counter-regulation can be permanent and does not only depend on specific circumstances.

In 86 intensively treated patients with type 1 diabetes aged 7–18 years, the incidence of severe hypoglycemia correlated with the serum activity of acetylcholine esterase. Patients with acetylcholine esterase activity at the median or above reported 3.0 events/year and those with acetylcholine esterase activity below the median reported 0.5 events/year, suggesting that a genetic factor may play a role in the emergence of severe hypoglycemia (46).

Autoimmune insulin hypoglycemia is rare, and is most often seen in East Asia. Patients have low concentrations of insulin and C-peptides, but insulin can be released from the insulin antibody complex or receptor antibodies can stimulate the message in the receptor.

- A 72-year-old woman with type 2 diabetes was treated with insulin but developed repeated attacks of hypoglycemia, with blood glucose concentrations below 2.2 mmol/l (47). She stopped taking insulin, but the attacks continued, causing disorientation, loss of consciousness, palpitation, and sweating. Her HbA$_{1c}$ concentration was raised at 6.3%. There were insulin antibodies 58% and also insulin receptor antibodies. Treatment with prednisone and glucose tablets resolved the hypoglycemic episodes within 48 hours.

Presentation

Symptoms of hypoglycemia have to be expected when the blood glucose concentration is below 2.6 mmol/l. The effects of hypoglycemia vary from patient to patient and can vary in the same patient. The symptoms and signs are of two types: adrenergic effects, due to release of catecholamines, and neuroglycopenic effects, due to the effects of hypoglycemia on the nervous system.

- *Adrenergic effects* Hunger, restlessness, profuse sweating, palor, tachycardia, and palpitation.
- *Neuroglycopenic effects* Headache, confusion, drowsiness, fatigue, difficulties in finding words, frequent yawning, anxiety, blurred vision, diplopia, and numbness of the nose, lip, and fingers.

Some patients do not experience the noradrenergic symptoms of hypoglycemia. They are taken by surprise, may lose consciousness and have hypoglycemic blood glucose concentrations without any preceding symptoms. After frequent episodes of hypoglycemia, there is altered awareness of hypoglycemia (30,48,49). It is difficult to substantiate altered awareness. Neuroendocrine responses and symptoms of hypoglycemia, but not cognitive dysfunction, are shifted to lower plasma glucose concentrations after recent hypoglycemia (50). Repeated episodes of hypoglycemia reduce the awareness of symptoms of hypoglycemia. This is accompanied by a lower blood glucose concentration, to elicit the response of counter-regulatory hormones (51). Beta-blockers also suppress the adrenergic symptoms, apart from sweating, which is mediated by sympathetic cholinergic transmission. Training increases awareness (52). Intensively treated patients may have reduced preservation of higher brain functions (53). Some groups, mainly in the UK, have suggested that transfer from animal to human insulin increases unawareness (SEDA-15, 452) (54), but this was not substantiated in other studies (55–57).

Every patient treated with insulin (or with hypoglycemic agents) who develops a neurological or psychiatric disorder has to be considered to be hypoglycemic until proven otherwise.

A rapid fall in blood glucose in a diabetic patient can cause symptoms of hypoglycemia, even when blood glucose concentrations are still normal or above normal. Experience with pumps has shown that many patients continue to feel hypoglycemic for a long time after normoglycemia has been restored. After an attack of hypoglycemia, patients often felt less well for a period of up to 48 hours. Headache, tiredness, and lack of initiative may disappear only gradually. These symptoms in the morning may indicate unnoticed hypoglycemic periods during sleep. Wet pyjamas or sheets may also indicate unnoticed hypoglycemia. During anesthesia, profuse sweating may indicate hypoglycemia.

A rise in C reactive protein has been observed during spontaneous attacks of hypoglycemia in diabetics and after experimental hypoglycemia in healthy controls (58).

Cardiovascular effects of hypoglycemia
The cardiovascular effects of hypoglycemia include angina pectoris, dysrhythmias, electrocardiographic changes, and coronary thrombosis. Raised concentrations of catecholamines and reduced concentrations of potassium contribute to cardiac damage during hypoglycemia.

Respiratory effects of hypoglycemia
• A 19-year-old woman with diabetes developed hypoglycemia with pulmonary edema (59). This has previously been seen as a complication of insulin shock therapy for psychiatric illnesses.

Nervous system effects of hypoglycemia
When hypoglycemia does not resolve spontaneously or is not terminated, cerebral dysfunction becomes manifest as confusion or reduced consciousness. Lethargy and depression or obstructive behavior develop and are accompanied by loss of consciousness, snoring, deep respiration, and facial paralysis. Neurological involvement can appear as cramps, paralysis, hemiplegia, or paraplegia. Epileptic seizures can accompany attacks of hypoglycemia. In deep coma the pupils are dilated, but they may react to light. Coma can develop very rapidly.

In a teaching hospital in Edinburgh, 56 admissions of 51 patients for hypoglycemia were registered during 12 months; 41 patients had diabetes mellitus and 33 were using insulin (60). There was a high incidence of neurological effects. Psychiatric illness or alcoholism was common. Four patients died but only one as a direct consequence of hypoglycemia. A further six patients died within 15 months, not related to hypoglycemia.

In 37 drivers with type 1 diabetes, fewer corrective actions were taken when the blood glucose was below 2.8 mmol/l (61). This was related to increased neuroglycopenic symptoms and increased electroencephalographic theta-wave activity. The authors suggested that diabetics should not begin to drive when the blood glucose concentration is in the 4.0–4.5 mmol/l range. In two editorials, the possibility of further restricting driving licenses in people with diabetes has been discussed (62,63). However, there is no evidence of higher accident rates in drivers with diabetes.

A retrospective questionnaire was sent to 195 consecutive patients addressing questions of severe hypoglycemia, coma, awareness of hypoglycemia, and fear of hypoglycemia (64). The mean duration of diabetes was 20 years and 82% had received intensive therapy. Coma was reported in 19% and severe hypoglycemia in 41%.

Coma was independently related to neuropathy, beta-blockers, and alcohol.

In reaction to a report of pulmonary edema and hypoglycemia (SEDA-24, 488) it has been noted that in many cases, one or more seizures precede pulmonary edema (acute respiratory distress syndrome), suggesting a neurogenic mechanism (65).

In 304 insulin-treated patients, 8.2% of those with type 1 diabetes and 2.2% of those with type 2 diabetes had blood glucose concentrations below 4 mmol/l on arrival in the clinic (66). None had complained of symptoms of hypoglycemia or had taken glucose, but when questioned, 59% had autonomic symptoms and 12% had neuroglycopenic symptoms; 29% were asymptomatic.

Autonomic failure can occur as a result of hypoglycemia, since antecedent hypoglycemia causes both defective glucose counter-regulation and lack of awareness of hypoglycemia. The role of the brain in lack of awareness of hypoglycemia and the question of whether the brain is the primary site for sensing hypoglycemia has been discussed (67). In older people, markedly fewer autonomic symptoms are reported and there is greater slowing of psychomotor performance. In young children, hypoglycemia can lead to more mood and behavioral disturbances than in adults, although they also occur in the latter. It may be that the cortical responses to recurrent hypoglycemia are less plastic and reversible than the hypothalamic and glucose-sensing functions (68).

Hypoglycemic neuropathy has been described in association with an insulinoma (69).

Hypoglycemia can cause dysesthesia.

• A 26-year-old woman had numbness and tingling in her hands and feet on awakening (70). They were most pronounced in the hands and resolved within minutes. Her insulin regimen had recently been changed from NPH 50 U in the morning to 35 NPH and 5 regular in the morning and 8 NPH and 5 regular before dinner. The morning glucose concentrations averaged 3.3 mmol/l. One month after reducing the dose of insulin the symptoms of hypoglycemic neuropathy had disappeared and low morning glucose concentrations were rare.

Psychological and psychiatric effects of hypoglycemia
Using evidence from auditory-evoked brain potentials and hypoglycemic clamps, it has been argued that antecedent hypoglycemia not only reduces awareness, but also that several aspects of cognitive function are attenuated during subsequent hypoglycemia 18–24 hours later (71). However, there were no effects of repeated hypoglycemia on cognitive function in patients included in the DCCT, a large American study that included more than 1400 patients, which showed that normalization of blood glucose prevents or delays the development of secondary (microvascular) complications in type 1 diabetes (72).

Nevertheless, long periods of hypoglycemia can cause permanent brain damage. There is concern that frequent attacks of hypoglycemia impair brain function but there are few hard data.

Hypoglycemic coma due to insulin with extensive mental changes has been reported, including a review of six comparable cases in patients aged 37–56 years, whose coma lasted from 36 hours to 31 days (73).

- A 37-year-old man could not be wakened in the morning. He had injected insulin without eating. His blood glucose was 1.5 mmol/l and he did not improve with intravenous glucose 16 g. In hospital he remained unconscious with a blood glucose of 12.2 mmol/l. There was no alcohol in the blood, his pH was 7.35, and he had a normal anion gap (18 mmol/l). His serum creatinine concentration was 288 µmol/l and his creatine kinase activity was high, suggesting rhabdomyolysis. A brain CT scan was normal and repeated electroencephalography showed slow waves with reduced voltages but no focal changes or irritation. He gradually recovered and was discharged after 6 days. Because of the dissociation between physical and mental improvement he was checked after 6 months and still had antegrade memory loss and problems with memory, complaining that he needed reminders on paper, and had less vitality and reduced emotionality.

Of the six reviewed patients, two died in coma; the other four had neuropsychological problems that did not improve after 6 months and up to 2 years. They had comparable electroencephalographic changes. During coma there was hypokalemia and hypocalcemia combined with increased lipolysis; this may have accounted for the permanent cerebral changes.

Of 20 patients with severe hypoglycemic coma and 20 with no or light coma, those with hypoglycemia had chronic depression and anxiety and performed persistently more poorly in several cognitive tests (74).

In 42 patients with at least two episodes of severe hypoglycemia in the previous 2 years and 51 patients with no episodes, low blood glucose, hypoglycemia-impaired ability to do mental subtractions, and awareness of neuroglycopenia and hypoglycemia predicted future severe attacks of hypoglycemia (75). In another study, blood glucose awareness training increased adrenaline responses to hypoglycemia (76). However, in a reanalysis of data from the Diabetes Control and Complications Study, a large study relating the development of secondary complications to less strict control of blood glucose (26), there was no effect of repeated hypoglycemia (72).

The effect of hypoglycemia on cognitive function has been investigated in 142 children aged 6–15 years with type 1 diabetes intensively treated for 18 months; 58 had 111 periods of treatment. There were no effects on cognitive functions (77). In 29 prepubertal children, with diabetes for at least 12 months and using twice-daily mixed insulin, observed for two nights, asymptomatic hypoglycemia occurred in 13 children on the first night and in 11 children on the second night; cognitive performance was not altered, but mood was reduced (78).

In healthy volunteers hypoglycemia caused significant deterioration in short-term attention, whereas sustained attention and intelligence scores did not deteriorate (79).

Sensory effects of hypoglycemia
Temporary blindness after severe coma (80,81) and retinal damage by gazing in the sun during hypoglycemia (82) have been reported.

Differential diagnosis
When a patient does not react rapidly to sufficient therapy, other diagnoses have to be considered during suspected attacks of hypoglycemia.

Alcohol can confuse the diagnosis of hypoglycemia (SEDA-5, 386). Alcohol inhibits gluconeogenesis. It makes the patient more susceptible to hypoglycemia and can even cause hypoglycemia in healthy individuals. The symptoms of alcohol abuse and hypoglycemia are almost identical. If hypoglycemia is predominant, glucose administration will help. In attacks of hypoglycemia, the symptoms disappear rapidly after glucose intake.

Vascular episodes in older diabetics can mimic attacks of hypoglycemia. True epilepsy or strokes can cause comparable symptoms or accompany hypoglycemia.

Differentiation of hypoglycemia from hyperglycemic coma is usually not difficult. The development of hyperglycemic coma takes a longer time and the blood glucose concentration is high. However, urine testing may show positive glycosuria, if urine produced before the hypoglycemic period is still in the bladder. Even ketonuria may be present if a patient has been fasting for a long period.

Timing
The emergence of attacks of hypoglycemia depends on the times and amounts of food eaten and the duration of action of the insulin used (see Table 2). When only one type of insulin is used, the symptoms of hypoglycemia mostly occur at the end of the period of maximal insulin activity. Modern insulin therapy involves using a combination of long-acting and short-acting insulins. Long-acting insulins are given once or twice a day in combination with and/or in addition to short-acting insulins, which are given 2–4 times a day. Hypoglycemia can then develop at times when the combined effects are most prominent. Hypoglycemia in the mid-morning can be a consequence of the action of the long-acting insulin of the previous day and the short-acting insulin given earlier in the same morning. Hypoglycemia during the night or in the early morning can be caused by too much long-acting insulin or by short-acting insulin late at night without sufficient food. Repeated symptoms of hypoglycemia at the same time of the day indicate that the timing of the insulin injection or the relative proportions of long-acting and short-acting insulins have to be changed. If the interval between insulin injection and the subsequent meal is very short, the effective insulin concentration in the blood will still be low when glucose is absorbed from the gut. This will cause very high postprandial glucose concentrations. An increase in the dose of insulin will then cause hypoglycemia at a later time. It is therefore advisable to try first to increase the interval between the injection and start of the meal. New synthetic insulins, like lispro insulin, give a more rapid increase and fall of insulin

concentrations than regular insulin; in that case, postprandial hypoglycemia can occur 1–3 hours after the injection (83).

Susceptibility factors

Hypoglycemia is an important problem in children (84–86). Children do not always establish the connection between the symptoms of threatening hypoglycemia and the danger involved. Overdosage of insulin is relatively common (SEDA-7, 406).

Older patients are particularly susceptible to hypoglycemia (87). Factors such as cerebral blood flow, blood PO_2 and PCO_2, permeability of the blood–brain barrier, and the presence of underlying neurological defects influence the hypoglycemic effects.

Hypoglycemic periods are often seen in "brittle diabetics," many of whom are overtreated with insulin. Changes in the insulin regimen (reduced use of long-acting insulin, frequent small injections of short-acting insulin) or the use of continuous infusion pumps can often lead to better results, but not everyone with brittle diabetes responds in that way (SEDA-7, 405). Apparently brittle diabetes may in fact be due to factitious hypoglycemia, the hypoglycemic periods of which are caused by surreptitious self-injection of insulin, Munchausen syndrome by proxy (SEDA-18, 413), or manipulation of the prescribed doses. In factitious hypoglycemia, low blood glucose concentrations are accompanied by high insulin concentrations but low concentrations of C peptide (88). Suicide attempts with insulin may be less uncommon than is often thought. A Medline search between 1966 and 1999 identified 46 papers containing 69 cases of factitious hypoglycemia; 46 were women, 52 were not diabetic, 29 had no close links with diabetes in their environment (89). In 47 the hypoglycemia was induced by insulin. Two patients died and one had severe impairment of intellectual function and short-term memory. In 32 cases unnecessary surgical procedures were performed.

Impaired hypoglycemic awareness was associated with an increased rate of severe hypoglycemia in 130 children and adolescents (aged 3–17 years) (90). One-third of the severe episodes developed without warning symptoms. Impaired awareness, young age, and recent attacks of hypoglycemia were independent susceptibility factors.

The authors of a systematic review of whether there is a difference in the frequency and awareness of hypoglycemia induced by human or animal insulins identified 52 randomized, controlled trials; 37 were double-blind (91). They found no support for the supposition that human insulin per se affects the frequency, severity, or symptoms of hypoglycemia. In a few studies, mainly of less rigorous design, there was an effect when people were transferred from animal to human insulin, indicating increased frequency or reduced awareness of hypoglycemia.

A questionnaire about the prevalence of severe hypoglycemia in relation to susceptibility factors was answered by 387 patients in 1984 and by 641 patients in 1998; 178 patients answered both questionnaires (92). The following changed significantly from 1984 to 1998: multiple injection therapy increased from 71 to 98%, daily self-

monitoring from 17 to 48%, episodes of nocturnal hypoglycemia from 76 to 83%, and lack of awareness from 40 to 55%; HbA_{1c} fell from 7.6 to 7.4%.

The use of insulin during intensive therapy for critically ill patients has been reviewed (93). In a safety study from the GIST (post-stroke hyperglycemic management) trial in 25 patients using a GKI (glucose, potassium, insulin) infusion one patient required therapy for symptomatic hypoglycemia (94). Of 452 patients, mean age 75 years, 20 had blood glucose concentrations below 4 mmol/l within 30 minutes of stopping the GKI infusion and required intravenous dextrose. The patients had been randomized to GKI infusion or saline to maintain blood glucose concentrations at 4–7 mmol/l, and only 69 of the 452 had type 2 diabetes.

Awareness of hypoglycemia

Avoidance of hypoglycemia for 3 months can improve hypoglycemic awareness for a period of over 3 years (95). In contrast, supervised induction of brief hypoglycemia twice weekly reduced clinical awareness of hypoglycemia by 33% and reduced the important adrenaline response, so reducing the behavioral and physiological defences against hypoglycemia (96).

Management

Patients have to be instructed to have a rapidly absorbed form of carbohydrate (for example dextrose tablets) available at all times and to use it when the first symptoms of hypoglycemia are felt. Often they fail to do so (97). If patients are used to self-monitoring, it is advisable that they monitor blood glucose first, although they should be told that a rapid drop in blood glucose concentration without reaching hypoglycemic values can cause a hypoglycemic reaction. Hypoglycemic reactions are sometimes difficult to discriminate from other feelings of malaise. Carbohydrate will always give rapid relief if the diagnosis is hypoglycemia and it is always safe to try taking it.

The conscious patient should take oral glucose at once. The treatment of choice in hypoglycemic coma is immediate intravenous injection of 20–50 g of dextrose. The patient may try to resist the injection, and help with the immobilization of the arm may therefore be needed. Injection of concentrated glucose solution outside a blood vessel leads to inflammatory and necrotic reactions. If intravenous injection of glucose is impossible, 1 mg of glucagon can be injected subcutaneously. However, in patients with residual insulin secretion (type 2 diabetes) glucagon may elicit extra insulin secretion and perpetuate hypoglycemia (98). The Epipen (a pen filled with a solution of adrenaline) is not a good substitute for the glucagon pen (in which glucagon must be dissolved before it can be used) in the treatment of hypoglycemia (99).

When the patient has taken high doses of long-acting insulin, hypoglycemia may relapse after a single dose of glucose has provided temporary relief, and monitoring should continue for a longer period. After hypoglycemic reactions elicited by long-acting insulins or oral hypoglycemic drugs the patient should be observed for possible recurrence during the next few days (100). The longer the duration of coma, the poorer the prognosis. Persistent posthypoglycemic coma can be due to cerebral edema. Fever can accompany this severe form of coma, which requires treatment with intravenous mannitol and glucocorticoids. Severe coma can last for several days and require intensive management. Encephalopathy with neurological symptoms can be the consequence.

Infusion of too much glucose over an extended period in the treatment of hypoglycemia is dangerous (101). Glucose utilization in the postabsorptive state is 2 mg/kg/minute and can increase, if insulin concentrations are high, to 6 mg/kg/minute (about 600 g/day in a 70 kg individual). It is better to infuse glucose in concentrations of 10 or 20% rather than 40%.

The opinion of experts about when and how to treat asymptomatic hypoglycemia in children varies greatly (102). Hypoglycemia in children is often undetected. Using a subcutaneous continuous glucose monitoring system (103) or the non-invasive Glucowatch biographer (104), hypoglycemic periods were more frequent and prolonged than when only fingerprick testing was available. For treating hypoglycemia in children, small doses of glucagon are suggested. The contents of a 1 mg/ml ampoule can be drawn into a 1 ml U100 syringe. For children under 2 years, 20 micrograms should be given initially; 10 micrograms is added for every year, up to 150 micrograms at age 15. When the effect is insufficient, the dose can be repeated once or twice (105).

Fat metabolism

- A 14-year-old adolescent girl, who had only used regular insulin developed lipoatrophy (106). Histology showed lipoblastoma-like cells, a possible sign of dedifferentiation. Skin tests showed no signs of allergy. The concentrations of immunoglobulins and TNF-alfa were normal.

Body weight

The DCCT Research Group has reported that patients in the intensive treatment group had substantial excess weight gain (107). In the first 9 months a group of patients who received intensive treatment gained 3.3 kg, compared with 1.2 kg in the control group; the percentage of people who gained more than 5 kg/m^2 was consistently higher with intensive therapy. This weight gain was related to both lean body mass and fat.

Electrolyte balance

Hypokalemia occurred in 29 children undergoing insulin tolerance tests; the mean serum potassium concentration at the start was 4.1 mmol/l, falling to a mean of 3 mmol/l at 30 minutes (108). Ten children had a serum potassium concentration below 2.9 mmol/l and one had a concentration of 2.2 mmol/l. There were no cardiac events.

- An 8-year-old girl had an insulin tolerance test with 0.05IU/kg to assess growth hormone concentrations. The blood glucose concentration fell to 0.9 mmol/l and she was given intravenous dextrose. She had a generalized seizure and developed ventricular flutter.

The serum potassium concentration was 2.6 mmol/l. Catecholaminergic polymorphous ventricular tachycardia was later diagnosed.

Fluid balance

Insulin edema is a rare syndrome of unidentified origin that occurs in patients with either type 1 or type 2 diabetes, most often in the early years after the introduction or intensification of insulin treatment; it has been reviewed (109). It is mostly seen when dysregulated patients with progressive weight loss are treated with relatively high amounts of insulin. Reduced sodium excretion (110), sodium reabsorption, and water retention by a possible direct action of insulin on the kidney may be involved (111). The role of aldosterone or of inhibition of the renin–angiotensin–aldosterone system in insulin edema is unclear. Insulin edema is a specific adverse effect, but it can aggravate pulmonary edema, congestive heart failure, and hypertension. Treatment consists of reduction of the insulin dose, after which the edema resolves within 3–4 days.

In studies in the 1970s peripheral edema developed in 15 of 86 middle-aged insulin-treated patients (112) and between 4 and 10% of intensively treated people with type I diabetes (113). In later studies of patients with type 2 diabetes, 5.4% of 408 patients treated with insulin developed edema compared with 15% of those who received insulin and a glitazone. In a further study edema occurred in 4.8% of patients who used rosiglitazone alone (114). Insulin can cause edema that can become clinically significant, particularly when it is combined with other therapies that cause edema.

- A 39-year-old man developed type 1 diabetes and lost 9 kg over 6 months (115). He was treated with intravenous fluids and insulin. Within 1 month he developed bilateral edema to the knees. The jugular venous pressure was not raised.

Insulin edema has been described in children with newly discovered diabetes (116).

- A 13-year-old girl with diabetes was given insulin 2 U/kg/day. She developed generalized edema and gained 20 kg over 2 weeks. With less insulin, furosemide, and later ephedrine the edema disappeared within 1 month.
- A 14-year-old girl with diabetes was given insulin up to 1.5 U/kg/day and gradually developed edema and gained 8.5 kg over 9 days. With furosemide, the edema gradually disappeared in 1 month.

Both of these children received rather high doses of insulin and they lacked the extreme acidosis that often occurs in young people when diabetes first appears.

Liver

When giving insulin for diabetic ketoacidosis an increase in liver enzymes can occur. These patients have often higher concentrations of HbA$_{1c}$, glucose, and triglycerides, need more insulin, and have more fat disposition in the liver during treatment of the acute phase (117).

- A 45-year-old man, who drank alcohol 60 g/day until diabetes was diagnosed, had mild liver function test abnormalities 6 months earlier, but only the gamma-glutamyl transpeptidase was raised (167 IU/l) (118). When insulin was given, the transaminases also increased. Liver function normalized after withdrawal of insulin. Reinstitution of insulin and a switch to another human insulin formulation again increased the liver enzymes. He was managed with glibenclamide and liver biopsy was not performed. Lymphocyte stimulation tests gave negative results to all insulin formulations. All hepatitis-related virus markers were negative.

As the changes in this case were seen with different types of insulin, it is improbable that additions to the formulation were responsible. It is possible that the use of alcohol made the liver more sensitive to the damaging effects of exogenous insulin.

Hepatic dysfunction can contribute to insulin edema.

- A 68-year-old woman developed marked insulin insensitivity during acute liver dysfunction due to autoimmune hepatitis treated with prednisolone 40 mg/day (119). Her recently diagnosed diabetes had been treated with diet only and her HbA_{1c} was 6.2%. Prednisolone reversed her anorexia and general malaise and improved her liver function tests. However, even 112 units of insulin per day could not control her blood glucose adequately, notwithstanding the fact that she was producing a substantial amount of her own insulin (C peptide excretion in the urine was 70 µg/day). She gained 8.5 kg in weight and developed pitting edema, pleural infusions, and ascites. Diuretic therapy and salt restriction eliminated fluid retention and restored insulin sensitivity in 4 weeks.

Four girls aged 11–14 years with poorly controlled type 1 diabetes had hepatomegaly and raised transaminase activities up to 30 times the upper limit of the reference range (120). Their diabetes was poorly controlled (HB_{A1c} 9.2–15%) despite high doses of insulin (1.3–2.2 units/kg/day). After admission for diabetes control their insulin requirements fell to 0.9–1.2 units/day and their liver function normalized within days. A biopsy in one case showed abundant deposits of glycogen. In these patients diabetes was poorly controlled, as shown by the HbA_{1c}, but the doses of insulin were high. Because insulin promotes glycogenesis, the authors suggested that when high blood glucose concentrations are treated intermittently with high doses of insulin, glucose is driven into the liver, which then promotes abnormal liver function. When insulin is used regularly, less insulin is needed and the liver problem resolves. This is in contrast to non-alcoholic steatohepatitis (NASH), which does not resolve promptly.

Skin

Hypertrophy of the subcutaneous tissues after insulin injections leads to delayed and variable insulin absorption. Of 282 children (160 boys and 122 girls, median age

12 years) prospectively evaluated for 3 months, 29% had mild skin hypertrophy and 18% had massive hypertrophy (121). The latter had higher HbA_{1c} concentrations and longer durations of diabetes and required more daily injections. There was no relation to the length of the needles used.

Amyloid-like deposition in the skin has been reported in a patient using porcine insulin (122).

- A 34-year-old man with a 17-year history of type 1 diabetes developed a 7 cm firm mass, distinct from adjacent areas of lipohypertrophy, and numerous smaller lesions of the same consistency. The lump consisted of acellular waxy material that appeared to be amyloid, formed by insulin. He had used porcine insulin for a long time.

This complication has been described before (SEDA-14, 373).

Musculoskeletal

A specific complication of the use of large amounts of insulin during hyperosmolar diabetic coma is rhabdomyolysis (123). Low intramuscular phosphate and potassium concentrations, often masked by relatively high blood glucose concentrations, may be important contributory factors.

Immunologic

Insulin allergy is quite common (SEDA-7, 403; 124–126). Allergy has been reported to human insulin and protamine (127) and to human insulin (128,129).

- A 41-year-old woman became allergic to all types of insulin (beef, pork, human, lente, etc.). She had used insulin for the first time during pregnancy and was intermittently treated unsatisfactorily with oral agents. She used lispro insulin for more than 6 months without an allergic reaction.
- A 54-year-old woman with gestational diabetes was later found to be allergic to chromium, pollen, dust, penicillin, acarbose, and metformin (130). She was treated with diet and glibenclamide, but later required insulin. With Humulin N insulin she developed a wheal of 15 mm immediately after the injection, which resolved in a few hours. However, a painful itchy induration appeared 2–3 hours after the injection and lasted a few days. She had an immediate reaction to isophane insulin, with induration, but insulin lispro was well-tolerated.
- A 5-year-old child with diabetes, Pierre Robin syndrome, cleft palate, allergic rhinitis, recurrent sinusitis, and obstructive sleep apnea, who had previously had skin rashes after penicillin, sulfonamides, and clindamycin, was given soluble and isophane human insulins (131). Three years later she developed local reactions, 2–5 cm areas, 30–120 minutes after injection. Skin-prick tests were negative for the diluent, isophane, and soluble insulin, but intradermal testing was positive with both insulins. Cetirizine and dexamethasone added to the insulin gave temporary relief. She was

then given insulin lispro by pump. After about 8 months, she started to develop local reactions again but with cetirizine and the pump her reactions were manageable.

- A 6-year-old boy developed recurrent generalized urticaria 1 year after he started to use human Mixtard insulin (132). The rash started 10 minutes after injections in the arms, thighs, and buttocks, at sites where earlier injections had been given, and disappeared within 12 hours. When he was changed to insulin lispro he had three urticarial reactions in the first 2 weeks and then sporadically. The reactions were treated with chlorphenamine for 2 years.

Presentation

Although serious systemic reactions are rare, local reactions at the site of injection are not infrequent. They appear as reddening, swelling, heat, burning, and itching, with or without frankly painful sensations. They can set in immediately or after some hours. The lesion can extend gradually and persist for variable periods. Some immediate reactions are related to IgE (or IgE/IgG) concentrations (133), but a direct relation between allergic reactions and a specific IgG fraction cannot be established (134).

- A 45-year-old woman who had used insulin for 4 years had a biphasic hypersensitivity reaction to human insulin (or another component of the injection fluid) (135). Within 20 minutes after the injection a swelling developed and in a later phase papular lesions with lichenoid features and post-inflammatory hyperpigmentation emerged. Histologically, there was neutrophilic infiltration with erythrocyte extravasation and eosinophilic amorphous material, surrounded by neutrophilic infiltrate. Saline injection did not elicit an effect. IgE anti-insulin antibodies were not found. There was no Arthus reaction (type IV allergy).

Other reactions are of the tuberculin granulomatous type or of the local vasculitis Arthus type. The local reactions can be accompanied, preceded, or followed by a generalized reaction, such as urticaria, nausea, vomiting, diarrhea, angioedema, wheezing, or anaphylactic shock. The last of these is rare, but sometimes fatal.

Insulin can induce local, painful lumps at injection sites. Sclerosing granulomata are occasionally seen (136) perhaps due to zinc (137). Such reactions are most commonly a consequence of an incorrect injection technique, generally the use of too short a needle or too superficial an injection. General edema (SEDA-11, 364) or abscesses (SEDA-7, 406) generated by insulin injections are extremely rare.

- A 21-year-old woman with a history of allergy, in whom coconuts and penicillin had caused laryngeal edema, had uncontrolled diabetes and subcutaneous allergy for insulin (138). Treatment with an antihistamine was not effective. Intradermal tests with animal and human insulins, regular and NPH insulins, and protamine were all positive. No rapid-acting analogues were tested. Gradual desensitization with small doses

of insulin was impossible, as she needed larger doses for metabolic control. When she was given a pump with insulin lispro, used food with a low glycemic index, and temporarily increased basal infusion rates in stead of pre-meal boluses, no reactions were seen. HbA_{1c} fell from 13.5% to 8.2% after 3 months and 7.5–8.0% after 6 months. She had only two minor episodes of hypoglycemia.

- A 64-year-old man with type 2 diabetes used premixed regular and NPH insulin and after 14 months noticed local wheal-and-flare reactions accompanied by sweating and slight dyspnea for 1 hour (139). Notwithstanding treatment with an antihistamine his symptoms became worse. Glibenclamide and metformin caused abnormal liver function tests. Rapid-acting analogues, regular insulin, NPH insulin, and insulin-like growth factor-I gave positive reactions on intradermal testing. Crystalline zinc insulin (Novolin® U), which contains no monomeric insulin, gave no reaction. However, the first subcutaneous injection of zinc insulin provoked an itchy wheal-and-flare reaction within 10 minutes and lasted for 1 hour. The addition of prednisolone 0.07 mg per unit of insulin, starting with a low dose and increasing the dose every other day, produced improvement. When a dose of 34 U/day was reached regulation was still not optimal. Glimepiride 6 mg/day improved HbA_{1c} to below 7.0% and the prednisolone was tapered. With insulin 30 U/day and glimepiride 6 mg/day he remained well regulated.

It may be that the exposure time to monomeric insulin plays a role in allergic effects. Pumps with extra short acting insulin give a short contact of monomeric insulin with the body. The same may be true for zinc insulin; the released monomers are only for a short period in the circulation.

Lipodystrophy, lipoatrophy, or lipohypertrophy can be a consequence of chronic local insulin reactions that can be elicited by less pure as well as by highly purified preparations (140), but such reactions can also develop at sites distant to the injection.

Leukocytoclastic vasculitis has been attributed to human insulin.

- A 48-year-old woman with type 1 diabetes developed tender induration within 2–6 hours and persisting for 1–3 days after injection of both isophane and regular insulins (141). This was followed by intense itching and redness, but no wheal-and-flare reaction. Switching to semisynthetic insulin and other insulin analogues or continuous subcutaneous insulin infusion had no effect. After 3 years the condition became incapacitating. Humalog 5–6 times a day, including an injection at 0300 hours was the best tolerated regimen. Intradermal tests showed allergy to human, porcine, and bovine insulins, but no reaction to protamine or other additives. Skin biopsies showed a leukocytoclastic vasculitis. Prednisolone 10 mg/day plus azathioprine 50 mg/day, later replaced by methotrexate 7–15 mg/week, produced complete resolution within 8 weeks.

Pathogenesis

Allergic reactions to insulin were originally thought to be caused by impurities present in the formulation. However, after the introduction of monocomponent insulins and human synthetic insulins, these reactions continued to be seen, even in patients without a history of treatment with other insulins (142). Switching from animal to human insulin can paradoxically cause allergic reactions, which subside when treatment with animal insulin is re-introduced (143). In patients who have never used other types of insulin, allergic reactions can be seen when human insulin is used and anti-insulin antibodies can be demonstrated (144). Antibodies against human insulin have also been found in sera collected from patients before human insulin was available (145). However, insulin antibodies can be found during or before the emergence of type 1 diabetes. Circulating insulin-binding antibodies can increase insulin resistance (146) and extend insulin action by slowing release. The titers of antibodies fall when purified insulins or human insulin are used, but they can be demonstrated even when modern insulins of high purity have been used exclusively. Anti-receptor antibodies are seldom seen.

In India, insulin antibodies have been investigated in 25 patients with type 1 diabetes, 19 patients with so-called malnutrition-related diabetes, and eight patients with fibrocalculous pancreatopathy, who used bovine insulin because it was cheaper (147). Antibodies appeared within 3 months of treatment. The development of antibodies was not related to the type of diabetes. There was a fall in antibody titer with increased duration of treatment. There was no correlation between daily insulin requirement and antibody titers.

Allergic reactions can also be elicited by excipients in insulin formulations, such as Surfen (aminoquinuride) (148), zinc (149), and protamine (150,151). Remnants of fluids used for cleansing the skin can be co-injected in micro-amounts and elicit allergic reactions (152). Allergy to latex in vial tops or syringes can become manifest during insulin treatment (153). In excised (infected) lumps, amyloid fibrils, proteins containing intact insulin, were demonstrable (154). Plastic syringes can release silicone particles, which can diminish the effect of insulin (155) or themselves induce granulomatous reactions (156).

It has been suggested that increased concentrations of corticotropin-releasing hormone, which has an immunomodulatory effect and causes vasodilatation and mast cell degranulation, could play a role in urticaria that develops during hypoglycemic periods in type 1 diabetes (SEDA-13, 381). Adrenal hyperandrogenemia is found in many diseases with hypersensitivity (157).

Susceptibility factors

Intermittent insulin administration seems to favor the development of allergic reactions to insulin (SEDA-6, 369).

Continuous intraperitoneal infusion of insulin causes increased insulin immunogenicity, but it is not known if this is accompanied by an increased frequency of autoimmune diseases. Antibodies against insulin, thyroglobulin, thyroperoxidase, gastric parietal cells, smooth muscle, mitochondria, liver and kidney microsomes, endomysium, and gliadin, and antinuclear antibodies were determined before and yearly after transfer to continuous intraperitoneal infusion of insulin in 28 patients; 19 remained negative for all investigated antibodies and in the other 9 the anti-insulin titer increased but other antibody titers remained constant or fluctuated (158). The authors concluded that during continuous intraperitoneal infusion of insulin in type 1 diabetes the frequency of other autoimmune diseases like hyperthyroidism was not increased. However, this conclusion was criticized, as the small numbers did not allow a positive or negative conclusion (159).

Treatment

In 95% of cases the local reactions disappear spontaneously. A switch to less immunogenic, highly purified insulin, or insulin lispro (160), is necessary if the reactions persist. For local allergic reactions, antihistamines or the addition of hydrocortisone 2 mg along with the insulin are seldom needed. Hydrocortisone suppresses local allergic reactions. For generalized reactions, skin testing is often necessary to establish allergic desensitization. One should start with low intradermal doses and, if necessary, add hydrocortisone.

For therapy of local lumps, extravasation, etc., one should first seek to improve the injection technique. Substitution with highly purified insulin is recommended. Injection with purified insulin into the affected area may speed up resorption of the lumps. Lipodystrophy or lipoatrophy improve after switching to highly purified human or insulin lispro. Lipohypertrophy, on the other hand, often fails to respond to changes in the insulin regimen (161). Varying the injection site may help, but differences in absorption rate then have to be taken into account.

Insulin resistance is said to be present when more than 200 U/day have to be injected; it is generally due to insulin antibodies. In general, antibody titers fall when highly purified insulins are used, but they sometimes persist after the switch. Some diseases, such as infections, endocrine hyperfunctional states (acromegaly, Cushing's syndrome, thyrotoxicosis), leukemia, or stress, can contribute to insulin resistance. Recombinant IGF-I (insulin-like growth factor I), which has a structure comparable to insulin, may help to overcome insulin resistance (162); adverse effects are burning at the injection site, hypoglycemia, fluid retention, facial edema, increased heart rate, arthralgia, myalgia, parotid gland tenderness, and dyspnea.

Continuous subcutaneous insulin infusion with fast-acting insulin has been used in two cases.

- A 43-year-old man with type 1 diabetes developed local pruritus, redness, and swelling 4–5 times a week, 15–20 minutes after an injection, subsiding within 1–2 hours (163). Later he had a generalized urticarial reaction 5 minutes after an injection. Insulin lispro did not help. When checked for allergens, he was positive for all types of insulin and negative for additives. With oral mizolastine the local reactions abated for a week, but then reappeared with every injection. Generalized urticaria recurred later. With continuous subcutaneous insulin infusion the local reactions immediately disappeared and metabolic control was improved.

- A 79-year-old man used mixed insulin for 2 months and developed swelling at injection sites, lasting 48 hours (164). The lesions persisted despite switching to various types of insulin. He was allergic to insulin, as shown by a raised eosinophil count, a markedly increased IgE concentration, and antibodies to human, bovine, and porcine insulins in the RAST test. He was not allergic to needles or additives. With subcutaneous bolus doses of insulin lispro and Humulin he developed induration and wheal-and-flare reactions. When hydrocortisone 10 mg was added to each injection, the allergic reactions disappeared, but they recurred after 2 months. With continuous subcutaneous insulin infusion there were no allergic responses for 3 months. His raised IgE concentrations fell.

Infection risk

The risk of infection from insulin injection sites is small, but infections can give problems in diagnosis and treatment, especially when they are atypical.

- A 43-year-old woman with a 23-year history of poorly controlled diabetes (HbA$_{1c}$ 14%) developed abscesses at injection sites on the thighs and abdomen (165). Repeated treatment with flucloxacillin had no effect and cultures were sterile. From aspirated pus, cultured for 6 weeks, *Mycobacterium chelonae* was isolated and clarithromycin and ciprofloxacin were effective.

Repeated episodes of catheter obstruction by fibrin clots or omental encapsulation can be a problem during continuous peritoneal insulin infusion from implanted pumps (SEDA 20, 397). In the encapsulated tissue, collagen fibrosis, inflammatory reactions with lymphocytes, and amyloid-like deposits reacting to anti-insulin antibodies can occur; higher macrophage chemotaxis may also promote these processes.

- A 54-year-old woman and a 62-year-old man with catheter blockages both developed aseptic peritonitis (166). In both cases clots had earlier been removed by laparoscopy, which also showed diffuse thickening around the tip and in the peritoneal fat, with fluid accumulation or inflammation and whitish urticaria-like plaques. The tissue was granulomatous, with histiocytes, fibrosis, and pseudo-amyloid material that could not be labeled by anti-insulin antibodies. The peritoneal fluid contained a lot of fibrin, monocytes, lymphocytes, and macrophages, but no bacteria or cancer cells.

Long-Term Effects

Drug misuse

Some body-builders misuse insulin to manipulate the effects of diet.

- A 31-year-old healthy man who used insulin as an adjunct for body-building became unconscious (167).

His blood glucose was 0.6 mmol/l and he had a respiratory acidosis and dehydration. He recovered with 50 ml of intravenous dextrose 50%. He admitted that he used insulin three times per week and glucocorticoids to support his diet before competitions. This time he had used a fast-acting insulin.

Drug tolerance

Insulin resistance has been reported with continuous subcutaneous infusion.

- Diabetes mellitus in a 36-year-old man with acute pancreatitis could not be controlled with continuous subcutaneous insulin infusion, even with doses up to 1800 U/day, because of insulin resistance (168). Intravenous insulin by pump had to be stopped because of a catheter infection. The continuous subcutaneous infusion of freeze-dried insulin and the addition of aprotinin, a protease inhibitor, soluble dexamethasone or prednisolone, and intravenous immunoglobulin was ineffective. An implantable pump for intraperitoneal delivery established good regulation at a dosage of 30 U/day.
- A 23-year-old diabetic woman had severe subcutaneous insulin resistance for 11 years (169). Continuous subcutaneous insulin infusion with regular or insulin lispro did not prevent periods of fluctuating responses to insulin. The addition of heparin to insulin lispro in the pump improved serum insulin concentrations and metabolic control. The addition of heparin to regular insulin gave no improvement.

Heparin may improve the transport of insulin lispro but not of regular insulin.

Insulin-induced lipohypertrophy can cause reduced efficacy of insulin, which should prompt review of injection technique and injection sites (170).

Second-Generation Effects

Pregnancy

In a longitudinal cohort survey of 278 pregnant women with type 1 diabetes, the frequency of severe hypoglycemia increased two to three times compared with the last 4 months before pregnancy (25%, including 9% with hypoglycemic coma, before pregnancy and 41%, including 19% with coma, during pregnancy) (171). A history of severe hypoglycemia before pregnancy, a longer duration of diabetes, an HbA$_{1c}$ concentration of 6.5% or less, and a daily insulin dose of over 0.1 U/kg were indicators of increased risk.

Continuous subcutaneous insulin infusion in pregnancy has been studied retrospectively in a nested case-control study (172). Those who used the pump had higher fasting blood glucose concentrations at the start, came sooner to the pregnancy clinic, used more insulin, put on more weight, and were more likely to have the baby admitted to the special baby care unit. Birth weights and neonatal hypoglycemia were similar.

- A 37-year-old nurse with type 1 diabetes was adequately treated with lispro and isophane insulin during her first pregnancy (173). In her second pregnancy, 3 years later, she had frequent episodes of hypoglycemia with the same regimen, for which she sometimes needed an injection of glucagon during the night. When the isophane in the evening was changed to glargine she had no more serious episodes of hypoglycemia.

Teratogenicity

In animals, teratogenicity of insulin during pregnancy has been observed (SEDA-8, 908) (174). No proof has been given that this also holds good in humans. A statistical significant relation found between insulin use for or during pregnancy and musculoskeletal anomalies (175) may also be caused by increased blood glucose or other to diabetes related factors.

Susceptibility Factors

Age

In 3805 children and adolescents with type 1 diabetes in 21 pediatric centers in 17 countries, feedback was given on the overall mean HbA_{1c} concentration in all the centers (176). After 3 years insulin therapy was more intensive, but glycemic control improved in only three centers. The relative risk of severe hypoglycemia was lowest in the center with the best glycemic control.

The incidence of hypoglycemia has been assessed in 6309 children with type 1 diabetes living in Germany and Austria (177). Despite modern care, young children aged 0–5 years had frequent episodes of severe hypoglycemic (31/100 patient-years), significantly more than in children aged 5–7 and 7–9 years (20/100 and 22/100 patient-years respectively). The youngest children also had higher rates of severe hypoglycemia, regardless of treatment regimen. Of children under 5 years 71% were using three or more injections per day or a pump.

Renal disease

In renal insufficiency the renal metabolism of insulin is impaired and generation of glucose reduced (178).

- A 64-year-old man who had had type 2 diabetes for 15 years used insulin 35 units/day without problematic hypoglycemia, but within 2 weeks had three episodes. He was found to have developed renal insufficiency secondary to diclofenac and his serum creatinine concentration had increased to 440 μmol/l.

Drug Administration

Drug formulations

The formulation of insulin differs in various countries. A strength of 100 U/ml (U100) is increasingly used in many countries, but in other countries strengths of 20, 40, or 80 U/ml (U20, U40, and U80) are still in use. The increased frequency of travelling and tourism has increased the importance of the problem. In some countries in various parts of the world, both U40 insulin of variable purity and highly purified U100 insulin are available at the same time. U100 insulin used in U40 syringes causes severe unexpected hypoglycemia and the reverse induces apparent insulin resistance (SEDA-6, 367).

Stability of insulin solutions

Two patients, who measured their blood glucose concentration four times a day and used glargine (Lantus®) insulin bottles for 2 months and 40 days respectively, observed that in the last 25% of the bottles the activity of the insulin was reduced (179). This prompted an enquiry by the manufacturers about the stability of their products. Insulin loses up to 1% of its potency over 30 days when stored at room temperature but only up to 0.03% when refrigerated. No insulin should ever be frozen; it must than be discarded. Unopened vials can be kept for at least 24 months when stored at 2–8°C. When kept in an open vial, of which some insulin was taken out every day and kept at 5 or 25°C, insulin met all stability criteria after 28 days. After that time it is recommended that insulin be discarded. Prefilled syringes kept at 5°C became turbid in 2–3 days depending on the type of syringe. Lantus® (Aventis) should always be kept out of the light. Other manufacturers, such as Lilly and NovoNordisk advise keeping unopened vials and cartridges refrigerated (at 2–8°). They can than be used until the expiry date. Vials and pens in use should be kept at room temperature to prevent local injection site reactions to cold insulin. The maximum-use period for opened vials and pen syringes is 28–30 days. For the mix Flex pen, which contains 70% insulin aspart protamine and 30% insulin aspart, the maximal period is 14 days. The 2003 guidelines of the American Diabetes Association state that if uncertain over the potency of insulin in a vial, that vial should be replaced with another of the same type (180).

Drug contamination

A skin reaction to latex in rubber associated with an insulin formulation has been reported (181).

- In a 35-year-old woman, pruritic, erythematous, urticated plaques occurred at insulin injection sites, and persisted for 48 hours, after the use of a prefilled cartridge pen containing Humulin (Lilly) and Human Monotard (Novo Nordisk) aspirated from a punctured vial, but not when the insulin was taken directly from the vial. She had positive skin-prick tests to latex solutions. Both the cartridge bungs and the vial bungs contain butyl rubber with added natural rubber latex. Switching to latex-free vials alleviated the problem.

Drug administration route

The American Diabetes Association has published revised guidelines on insulin administration, including storage of insulin, use and reuse of needles, alternatives to syringes, injection techniques, and patient management related to dosing of insulin, self-monitoring, and hypoglycemia (182).

Developments in the administration of insulin through the skin, the mouth, the nose, and the lung have been reviewed (183). Methods of absorption other than subcutaneous, such as nasal insulin, buccal insulin, rectal insulin, and insulin in enteric-coated capsules, are still experimental. A problem in nasal administration is still how to get a daily reproducible dose (184). The frequency of hypoglycemia is comparable to the frequency with subcutaneous insulin (185). Nasal irritation, sometimes with congestion, and dyspnea (186) can occur. Pulmonary insulin, delivered by aerosol inhalation, is another experimental method. No lung obstruction was reported, but the uptake varied considerably (187).

Single subcutaneous injection

Injection of insulin into abnormal subcutaneous tissues can result in poor control of blood glucose (188).

- A 42-year-old man who had had type 1 diabetes for 24 years had deteriorating blood glucose control despite increasing insulin doses (HB_{A1c} increased from 11% to 17%). He was injecting into two areas that contained 4 cm hard woody nodules. Biopsy showed collagen with fibroblasts and necrosis. When he avoided the areas his blood glucose improved with reduced insulin doses.

The authors went on to audit 73 consecutive patients; 32 had clinical lipohypertrophy and a further two had hard nodular lumps.

Continuous subcutaneous insulin infusion

Continuous subcutaneous insulin infusion (CSII) often gives a better quality of life (189).

There has been a systematic review of 11 studies of at least 10 weeks duration, comparing soluble insulin with the analogues lispro and, in one case, aspart in pumps (190). The analogue produced a small, significant improvement in HbA_{1c}. There were no differences in hypoglycemia. Ketosis, hyperglycemia, and clogging were not common.

In 132 patients with type 2 diabetes using insulin randomly assigned to continuous subcutaneous insulin infusion (with insulin aspart) or multiple daily injections of insulin aspart and NPH insulin) for 16 weeks, after 8 weeks training to establish optimal dosages (191) there were more episodes of hyperglycemia (blood glucose over 19.4 mmol/l) with multiple daily injections. HbA_{1c} was identical. Most of the patients who expressed a view (93%) wanted to stay on the pump.

In 40 patients aged 4–25 years with type 1 diabetes who were given continuous subcutaneous insulin infusion for 6 months the number of episodes of hypoglycemia was reduced by a half (192). There were two episodes of diabetic ketoacidosis. In 10 patients lipohypertrophy developed at the insertion site and three patients had signs of skin redness, which improved with local antibiotic treatment.

Continuous subcutaneous insulin infusion in 23 children, aged 9.4–13.9 years, was compared with multiple daily insulin injections in a randomized crossover study of two periods of 3.5 months (193). Insulin dosage requirements fell during continuous infusion and increased with multiple injections. Episodes of mild diurnal and nocturnal hypoglycemia were the same. There was one severe episode of nocturnal hypoglycemia during continuous infusion and three (two nocturnal) during multiple injections. Diabetic ketoacidosis did not occur; episodes of mild ketosis were related to problems with infusion sets. There were 12 minor infections at infusion sites, 16 blockages, and 42 dislodgements. Three patients developed intercurrent infections, two during continuous infusion and one during injection therapy.

- A 56-year-old man was given a continuous subcutaneous insulin infusion because of frequent episodes of hypoglycemia of which he was unaware and he had four separate episodes of profound ketoacidosis (194). Multiple daily injections produced less flexibility in his mealtimes, more episodes of hypoglycemia, and the need for more injections. However, injecting 60% of his basal needs as insulin glargine once daily in combination with continuous subcutaneous infusion prevented further episodes of diabetic ketoacidosis.

Continuous subcutaneous insulin infusion (CSII)

Continuous subcutaneous insulin infusion (CSII) has been compared with multiple daily injections of insulin in a randomized study in 32 patients, mean age 13 years, over 16 weeks (195). Of the 16 patients who used CSII one returned the pump twice and one returned the pump once, in both cases for pump software errors. Medtronic MiniMed 508 or Paradigm 511 pumps were used in the study.

In two randomized crossover trials metabolic deterioration occurred earlier and was of greater amplitude with insulin lispro than with regular insulin when a pump was discontinued (196). However, when the pump was restarted, insulin lispro was more effective than regular insulin in correcting metabolic deterioration.

CSII is associated with infections at the site of infusion, about 40 episodes per 100 patient years (196). One-third required oral antibiotics. Surgical drainage was very rarely needed (197).

Lipoatrophy, although rare, has been reported in patients using both regular and lispro insulin in CSII pumps (198,199).

Continuous subcutaneous insulin infusion (CSII)

The use of CSII for 6 or more months has been reported in 70 children aged 2–12 (mean 9.1) years (200). A retrospective review of charts compared with the year before CSII showed a non-significant reduction in severe hypoglycemia associated with a slight fall in Hb_{A1c}. There were two episodes of diabetic ketoacidosis, compared with none during the control period. There were no practical problems; the children did not play with the pumps.

In 100 children aged 1.6 to 18 years who had used a pump for 6 or more months data were obtained from the insulin pump memory: 10% missed meal-time boluses and 7% had programming and adjusting errors (201). One child aged 16 years had an episode of severe hypoglycemia due to overdosing on meal boluses. There were no episodes of diabetic ketoacidosis.

Children under the age of 10 years often do well, as the pumps are under the control of their carers. The use of pumps in 10 preschool children aged 6 years and under appeared to be safe (202). Hypoglycemia appeared to be reduced compared with twice-daily mixed insulin. The use of pumps in children appears to be safe with appropriate commitment from the patients and their carers.

Insulin syringes

Disposable syringes can release silicon particles into the insulin vials, reducing the effectiveness of insulin (203). This can happen when insulin is injected back into the vial, during correction for the desired dose, and is specifically seen when low doses are used for long periods. Flocculation of insulin, found before the expiry date, may be related to this problem (SEDA-12, 360).

Insulin pens

Insulin pens are being increasingly used for intensive insulin therapy. For low doses, pens are more accurate than syringes (204). In 48 children and adolescents pen devices were more accurate than syringes when under 5 U of insulin had to be injected; for higher doses pens and syringes were comparable (205).

Long-acting isophane insulin in pens can be insufficiently resuspended before an injection, resulting in a great variation in the dose of insulin per injection; in one study isophane content ranged from 5 to 214% (205). Only 10% of 109 patients tipped and rolled the pen more than 10 times. There was no relation between inadequate suspension and the number of attacks of hypoglycemia. It was mechanically proven that 20 cycles are necessary for good suspension. After education, suspension errors were less common in 80% of the patients. They had fewer attacks of hypoglycemia, but HbA_{1c} did not change.

A warning has been given that over 0.3 µl of blood (and viruses) can reflux in insulin cartridges in pen-like injectors. Reflux was measured using a rubber tube containing a dye solution. A questionnaire study in 193 patients using cartridges showed that 20 patients sometimes noted a reddish cartridge and that two patients shared their cartridges with other patients (206).

After injecting insulin, the pen has to be kept in place for some time. Many pens leak from the tip of the needle when the pen is removed from the injection site 7 seconds after the injection is finished. In one study only the Novopen 1.5 ml and Novolet 1.5 ml showed no leakage; eight of twenty 3 ml BD pens and Novo pens, 16 of 20 Novolets 3 ml and 19 of 20 Saline pens 3 ml (Lilly) leaked 4.0, 4.7, 5.9, and 9.2 mg respectively (207). It is necessary to keep the needle in place for 10–30 seconds after injection. Measured by ultrasonography, 86% of injections with needles of 12.7 mm and 38% of injections with needles of 8 mm in diabetic children with a BMI below the 60

percentile were intramuscular instead of subcutaneous (208). The injection changed from intramuscular to subcutaneous in half of the injections in the arm and in two-thirds of injections in the thigh when 8 mm needles were used. Nowadays, 6 mm needles are available in many countries.

In general, intensive therapy produces lower blood glucose concentrations and HbA_{1c} concentrations. This may result in worsening of proliferative retinopathy (209), or weight gain M14.42.9]. Pens can develop inaccuracies in rare instances, which may be unnoticed by the patient (210). Clogging of the system is often the cause. The result is diabetic coma or ketoacidosis, but this is not more frequent than with other systems. When needles are not regularly renewed, infections may emerge.

Insulin pumps

The usefulness of devices for constant subcutaneous, intravenous, or intraperitoneal insulin administration is well established. To establish feedback systems reliable, constantly functioning insulin sensors are essential, but they have been in a developmental phase for more than 25 years, and no long-acting glucose sensors for non-experimental use are yet available (211). Experience with pumps in large groups of patients has been reported (212–214). When starting intensive therapy, temporary worsening of secondary complications, mostly retinopathy, but sometimes nephropathy, has been reported (SEDA-14, 374). Weight gain is also a complication. The major candidates for insulin pump therapy include patients with type 1 diabetes, pregnant women, some types of brittle diabetics, patients wanting to become pregnant, and children.

Most pumps deliver insulin subcutaneously. Implantable pumps delivering insulin intraperitoneally with remote control devices are increasingly used (215,216). Pumps provide signals to alert users to malfunction, but leakage of connections often does not activate the alarm. Since the patient has no natural reserve of insulin, breakdown of the pump, leakage, or intercurrent infection without adjustment of the dose rapidly leads to ketoacidosis. The sudden release of insulin from a "runaway" pump is an exceptional event. Hypoglycemic deaths, infections (for example with *Mycobacterium fortuitum*) (217), local allergic reactions and infections, thrombosis in intravenous systems, allergy to nickel in needles (218), skin infections (219), needle breakage (SEDA-13, 382), problems with bad batteries, breakdown of the pump, leakage in delivery systems, or wrong insertion of the needle have all been described (SEDA-7, 405) (220). Pumps with sealed reservoirs (waterproof) can expel more insulin when used at high altitudes (skiing, mountaineering, pressurized cabins in airplanes) inducing serious hypoglycemia (SEDA-16, 486) (221); adapters that allow pressure equilibrium obviate this. Pumps that deliver insulin intravenously are almost obsolete, since they can cause thrombosis, vasculitis, and septicemia.

Efficacy

Continuous subcutaneous insulin infusion has been reviewed (222,223). Probably more than 100 000 patients in the USA are using it. Some studies have shown no difference in mean glucose concentration or HbA$_{1c}$ compared with intensive treatment, but most have shown a slight difference favoring continuous subcutaneous infusion. With fast-acting analogues the postprandial glucose peaks are lower. In one study, when insulin delivery was intentionally interrupted, the increase in glucose concentrations or the development of ketonuria was later with regular insulin, but in another study there was no difference in the development of hyperglycemia or beta-hydroxybutyric acid between fast-acting analogues and regular insulin. Patients preferred to continue treatment with pumps.

Insulin delivery by a pump may be superior to glargine insulin. Continuous subcutaneous insulin infusion was compared with intensive therapy with insulin glargine plus insulin lispro in 19 patients (224). The patients who received insulin glargine were exposed to glucose concentrations under 3.9 mmol/l overnight for three times as long as those who used continuous subcutaneous insulin infusion.

In a meta-analysis of the metabolic and psychosocial impact of pumps, 52 studies were found; 22 were published before 1987 and 13 after 1993, the year in which the results of the DCCT were published (225). The authors stated that therefore conclusions about efficacy are not definitive. All pump malfunctions were reported before 1988. All types of changes were reported when the frequency and severity of hypoglycemia were compared with prepump times. Infection and skin irritation were expressed in different ways in the various studies. The risk of diabetic ketoacidosis fell after 1993. Most users preferred to continue pump treatment, mainly because of more flexibility, greater freedom, and improved glycemic control.

When continuous subcutaneous insulin infusion and sulfonylureas were compared in nine normolipidemic patients with type 2 diabetes, HbA$_{1c}$ was not different but triglycerides and small LDL particles were reduced by the continuous infusion (226).

Continuous subcutaneous insulin infusion treatment is feasible in obese patients (BMI over 30 kg/m^2) with type 2 diabetes and severe insulin resistance, as has been shown in a study in 10 patients over 40 weeks (227). HbA$_{1c}$ improved from 12 to 9.6% and weight was reduced by 2.5 kg. There were no adverse effects.

Use in children

In a randomized, crossover study in 10 children aged 7–10 years who used subcutaneous insulin pumps only in the evening and at nighttime, fasting, and 0300 hours, concentrations of blood glucose and fructosamine were improved (228). There was a better quality of life and a reduced fear of hypoglycemia. Children of this age may not be capable of handling a pump during the day.

In 95 patients aged 4–18 years with a median follow-up of 28 months, continuous subcutaneous insulin infusion produced no change in medical complications (diabetic ketoacidosis, visit to the emergency department), but there was a reduction in the number of episodes of hypoglycemia (229). HbA$_{1c}$ was significantly lower than prepump values, but gradually increased in the first year and then remained stable.

In 118 children aged 1.5–18 years treated with continuous subcutaneous insulin infusion, HbA$_{1c}$ in preschool children fell from 7.1 to 6.5%, in school children from 7.8 to 7.3%, and in adolescents from 8.1 to 7.4% (230). Daily insulin consumption did not increase and the frequency of severe episodes of hypoglycemia fell.

General adverse effects

Continuous intraperitoneal insulin infusion with implantable pumps has been assessed in 34 patients with poorly controlled diabetes (231). In two patients, the pump was explanted: in one patient with Werner's syndrome (no subcutaneous fat) the pump was explanted because of infection in the pocket, and one pump was explanted because the patient had local complaints and psychological problems. One patient refused to be included. Patients were followed for 58 months. HbA$_{1c}$ fell from 10.0 to 9.0% in the first year and remained there. Median days in hospital fell from 45 to 13 after 1 year. The quality of life was relatively low and many had psychiatric problems. Although long-term glycemic control improved and lengths of hospital stay were reduced, normal glucose control and normal quality of life could not be achieved.

Local adverse effects

Implantable insulin infusion pumps have been reviewed (232,233), as has the use of pumps in children (234). In 31 centers, 914 pumps were implanted, representing 2121 patient-years. Some commonly reported pump complications were (233):

- hematoma or seroma, usually resolved by needle aspiration;
- pump migration, the frequency lessening with experience; surgical intervention is necessary;
- rare pump pocket infections; the causes were difficult to determine, but in two patients, coagulase-negative staphylococci were found, suggesting contamination with skin flora during refill;
- progressive thinning of the skin, 1–30 months after implantation in 2 per 100 patient-years; pain and skin erosion often followed; the cause is unclear; only a correlation with physical activity could be found.

Catheter malfunction was the most frequent event (obstruction, total occlusion, and peritoneal adhesions: 13, 10, and 3.1 events per 100 patient-years respectively). Flushing sometimes prevented occlusion. Better tip design had a big effect. Adhesion formation decreased with daily injections of heparin. The frequency of ketoacidosis was comparable to that reported with continuous subcutaneous insulin infusion and was usually related to catheter obstruction. It diminished during the review period. Episodes of severe hypoglycemia were fewer than during intensive subcutaneous therapy.

The tendency of insulin molecules to aggregate in concentrated solutions sometimes requires specific insulin or insulin lispro for pumps. There is a difference of opinion about whether insulin absorption kinetics change (improve) during placement of the catheter (SEDA-16, 488) (SEDA-18, 412). Changing the injection site and renewing the infusion system every 2–4 days is important in preventing clogging, local allergy, and infection at the insertion site.

In implanted pumps, catheters for continuous intraperitoneal insulin infusion can be obstructed by deposits of fibrin on the catheter tip. They mostly reappear after the plug is blown out, necessitating replacement (235). Hematoma, skin erosions, infections (236), pain, pump migration, and pocket complications are not rare (SEDA-20, 397) (237). Erosion of the cecum, mimicking appendicitis, is reported (238). During the start of pump therapy, some patients feel as if they are constantly hypoglycemic, even though low blood glucose concentrations cannot be objectified.

There was no macrophage activation in 10 patients with obstructed ($n = 3$) or non-obstructed ($n = 7$) catheters in implantable pumps (239).

When insulin delivery stops during continuous subcutaneous insulin infusion, ketoacidosis can develop rapidly, but it can be easily corrected if ketoacidosis has developed recently, although exceptions occur (240).

- A 32-year-old woman with well-regulated diabetes, using about 35 U/day of insulin by continuous subcutaneous infusion, tried a sauna for the first time when her blood glucose was 7 mmol/l. She stayed for about 45 minutes and the temperature reached 70°C for 10 minutes. The blood glucose concentration rose to 11 and 17 mmol/l, despite a bolus of insulin 6 units. She felt sick and vomited during the night; the next morning her blood glucose was 21 mmol/l and she had ketonuria, abdominal cramps, and extreme fatigue. Insulin 25 units by pump produced no improvement, but after opening a new vial, the situation improved; within 6 hours she was normoglycemic, and her ketonuria disappeared within 16 hours.

It is not clear in this case whether insulin had formed aggregates and fibrils due to the high temperature or if the action of counter-regulatory hormones induced by hyperthermia was increased, or both.

Problems with insulin delivery in implanted pumps are difficult to correct. A change in Hoechst 21 pH-neutral semisynthetic insulin 400 U/ml in accordance with regulations of the European Pharmacopoeia (SEDA-20, 397) resulted in more frequent clogging when this insulin was used in the Minimed 2001 implantable pump (MIP 2001). From October 1995 to October 1996, 17 pumps were implanted (241). The refilling period was reduced from 90 to 30–45 days and the reservoirs were washed with insulin-free buffer before each refill. Backflow was seen in 13 pumps after a mean period of 7.2 months. Modification of the manufacturing process produced 21PH ETP insulin (human semisynthetic insulin, Genapol-stabilized) 400 U/ml, Hoechst, with improved stability since July 1997. All pumps were specifically cleaned before the new insulin was used for refill. The refill period was increased from 38 to 78 days. In 16 pumps, only one backflow was seen after 14 months.

The incidence of catheter blockage did not change. The better stability of this insulin for implantable pumps has been confirmed in a study in which 88 pumps were refilled every 45 days and 108 pumps every 90 days (242).

Pump failure

Almost all pumps are programmable and pump failure is rare (2 per 100 patient-years) (233).

Risk of hypoglycemia

Continuous subcutaneous insulin infusion in 75 youths aged 12–20 years has been compared with multiple daily injections over 12 months (243). HbA$_{1c}$ was lower, and the number of attacks of hypoglycemia in the pump group was 50% less. Ketoacidosis seldom occurred: once during intensive therapy and twice during pump therapy. Weight increased more during pump treatment. Coping with diabetes was less difficult with pump therapy.

In 103 patients who used continuous subcutaneous insulin infusion for 2 years, the incidence of severe hypoglycemia fell from 0.70 cases/patient/year before treatment to 0.06 cases/patient/year during treatment, and HbA$_{1c}$ improved from 7.7 to 7.2% (244). The incidence of abscesses was 0.1 cases/patient/year and of ketoacidosis 0.01 cases/patient/year. The patients with HbA$_{1c}$ concentrations above 8.5% had a higher incidence of serious hypoglycemia and abscesses. Quality of life assessments showed great improvements. The reasons for continuous subcutaneous insulin infusion were optimization of metabolic control, greater flexibility, or prevention of severe hypoglycemia.

In 138 patients treated with continuous subcutaneous insulin infusion for 7 years, there was a fall in the incidence of episodes of serious hypoglycemia (from 0.31 to 0.09 cases/patient/year) and ketoacidosis (from 0.41 to 0.11 cases/patient/year); the number of infections was unchanged (0.2 infections/patient/year) (245).

When continuous subcutaneous insulin infusion was instituted in patients with long-standing poor glycemic control during a crossover study in 79 patients for 32 weeks, 17 dropped out after the first crossover, making it impossible to use the second arm. HbA$_{1c}$ and quality of life both improved. There were more episodes of mild hypoglycemia with continuous subcutaneous insulin infusion (246). The authors of an editorial concluded that continuous subcutaneous insulin infusion can anticipate changes in insulin need, which is important for diabetics with a variable lifestyle or an exaggerated dawn phenomenon (247). For a large group the increase in cost and the hassle of continuous subcutaneous insulin infusion do not offset that, and multiple daily injections with glargine as basal insulin (see below) can be equally effective.

Continuous subcutaneous insulin infusion was found to be feasible in 56 children and adolescents (aged 7–23 years) (248). HbA$_{1c}$ improved in 36 and deteriorated in 6. The rate of severe attacks of hypoglycemia fell, but not significantly. Hypoglycemia and seizure frequency were less overall in the group, with better HbA$_{1c}$ concentrations. One patient had a catheter infection and was treated with local antibiotics and a new infusion system at another site.

Suitable types of insulin

Short-acting neutral buffered insulin by pump is sometimes ineffective. Treatment with non-buffered insulin can make things worse, but short-acting acidified insulin can improve HbA$_{1c}$. This type of insulin is well tolerated for over 3 years. The acid insulin may contain more monomers than neutral insulin, which may act less rapidly, as it contains more polymers (249).

Insulin lispro is sometimes less beneficial in continuous subcutaneous insulin infusion (250).

- A 58-year-old man with diabetes and unawareness of hypoglycemia had 53 emergency hospital admissions in 2 years before he started regular continuous subcutaneous insulin infusion. His attacks of hypoglycemia were reduced to one every 2–3 weeks. His mean blood glucose was 7.0 mmol/l. When insulin lispro was introduced in the pump he had an attack every 2–3 days for 68 days and hospital admission was required seven times. The mean blood glucose was 6.3 mmol/l. After he used soluble insulin instead of insulin lispro, the number of attacks of hypoglycemia fell substantially. The mean blood glucose was 6.4 mmol/l.

It may be that the more rapid diffusion and absorption of insulin lispro in diabetics who achieve tight metabolic control and have hypoglycemia unawareness destabilizes glycemic control.

Continuous subcutaneous insulin infusion with insulin lispro has been reported to give variable control (251).

- A 12-year-old boy with type 1 diabetes had problems with insulin lispro in his pump. After multiple daily injections, he started continuous subcutaneous insulin infusion with insulin lispro and could freely adjust his eating schedule; he had fewer episodes of hypoglycemia and his HbA$_{1c}$ was 5.4%. Later, he developed a pattern of variable responsiveness to insulin, starting with increased responsiveness on the day on which he changed his subcutaneous needle, followed by reduced sensitivity and hyperglycemia on the third day. The infusion site was changed and Velosulin was added to insulin lispro, making it possible for him to use his injection site for 3 days consistently; the HbA$_{1c}$ was 7.2%. After 2.5 years he started using insulin aspart. It then became possible to change the infusion site every 4–5 days, when the cartridge was empty. The HbA$_{1c}$ fell to 6.2%.

Continuous subcutaneous insulin infusion has been compared with short-acting insulins plus glargine or isophane as long-acting insulins for 1 year in 32 patients with poor control (252). Four of them had serious attacks of hypoglycemia. There were no differences in HbA$_{1c}$ or other metabolic parameters (including lipids). In those treated with continuous subcutaneous insulin infusion, the reduction in the amount of insulin required was larger.

Hoechst 21 pH-neutral insulin in intraperitoneal pumps increases the production of antibodies to insulin, in contrast to the same insulin in subcutaneous pumps (253). It is not clear whether the intraperitoneal route or modification of insulin during storage in the implanted reservoir causes greater antigenicity. When a newly designed side-port catheter on the Minimed pump was used in 40 patients for 450 days per patient, there was one catheter encapsulation, one clogging, and six cases of catheter/pump related underdelivery (254). This was comparable to the position before 1994, when the formula of the Hoechst 21 pH-neutral insulin was changed for the first time.

Other devices

Other devices, such as long-term subcutaneous catheters (255,256), which have to be renewed every 4 days (257), or intraperitoneal catheters (258) for pumps, pose the same types of problems as subcutaneous catheters for pumps, except that the catheters are indwelling for longer periods. The jet-stream injector, introduced as an alternative for people who are afraid of injections, has given problems with delayed pain and bleeding. The advantages of these methods are questionable.

Oral administration

Metabolism of insulin and the lack of a specific carrier to transport insulin through the gut made the oral route impossible (183).

Inhaled insulin

In the lungs, insulin has to be absorbed from the alveoli (183). Enhancers to give the particles the right size and constituency to reach the alveoli improve systemic availability (259). The relative potency of inhaled insulin is about 10%, which means that a 10-fold increase in dose is necessary. The effects of inhaled insulin are comparable to those of injected regular or fast-acting insulins or even faster. However, it is difficult to get a good action profile. The anatomy of the pharynx affects the transport of the particles. In smokers, the permeability of the lung epithelium is much greater and absorption from the alveoli is faster and higher than in non-smokers; during actual smoking, uptake is reduced. In the short term the excipients in the sprays have no adverse effects. More participants in a study of inhaled human insulin were satisfied with inhaled insulin than they were with subcutaneous insulin (260).

Ten severely hyperglycemic patients with type 2 diabetes taking oral agents were treated at random with two injections of isophane daily or with lyophilized nasal insulin before each meal, with an added injection of subcutaneous isophane when necessary (261). The periods were separated by 2 months. Nasal insulin produced control of diabetes comparable to isophane, except in three patients. Adverse effects included transient pruritus, sneezing and rhinorrhea, and chronic nasal crusts. One patient was withdrawn because of cough and dizziness after each nasal dose.

Inhaled insulin has been studied in 72 patients in an open, parallel-group, randomized trial for 12 weeks; 35 used inhaled insulin (206). The inhaled insulin was given three times before meals with isophane insulin at bedtime. Controls used their regular insulin two or three times a day with a long-acting insulin at bedtime. HbA$_{1c}$ did not differ between the groups and there was no difference in the frequency or severity of attacks of hypoglycemia. Pulmonary function tests were stable and showed no differences between the groups. There were no serious or major adverse effects.

The dose of inhaled insulin is about 10 times higher than the subcutaneous dose that produces the same hypoglycemic effect. In an open, randomized, crossover study subcutaneous insulin was compared with a 10 times higher dose of inhaled insulin in 15 non-smoking patients with type 2 diabetes (262). The peak action of inhaled insulin was earlier. Apart from that, the effects were similar. There were no differences in FEV$_1$ at baseline or at 4 or 8 hours after treatment. Absorption of inhaled insulin is significantly higher in smokers (263). In non-diabetics, absorption is reduced in asthma (264). Inhaled insulin may increase the titer of insulin antibodies (265).

Non-injection routes
Non-invasive insulin delivery is still experimental. The various methods (transdermal, nasal, lungs, oral) have been reviewed, with special attention to the various techniques and administration of inhaled insulin, which seems the most promising alternative to injection (266,267).

Inhalation
In the AERx® insulin diabetes management system liquid insulin droplets are delivered from an insulin strip to the deep lung only during precise predefined inspiratory flow and volume. In 107 patients with type 2 diabetes randomly assigned during 12 weeks to inhaled fast-acting insulin or subcutaneous fast-acting insulin before meals, both with evening NPH insulin the change in HbA$_{1c}$ was identical (268). Inhaled insulin caused hypoglycemia in three cases, compared with no episodes in those using injections. Pulmonary function tests were not consistently altered. Breath holding after inhalation for 0, 3, or 10 seconds had no effect on the pharmacokinetics or pharmacodynamics of inhaled insulin (269).

Insulin-binding IgG antibodies are found in about 75% of patients with type 2 diabetes using inhaled insulin (270). This is more than one would expect from the use of subcutaneous insulin. The antibodies appear to plateau after 1 year. There are no obvious clinical effects.

In an open study of 107 patients with type 2 diabetes using the AERx insulin diabetes management system ($n = 54$) or subcutaneous insulin ($n = 53$), the number of people with insulin antibodies increased from 6% to 35% in those who used the AERx insulin diabetes management system (271). The number of patients with antibodies remained stable at about 10% in those who used subcutaneous insulin. There were no obvious clinical consequences. Similar results were found in a study of patients with type 1 diabetes: 29% of those who used inhaled insulin compared with 3% of those who used subcutaneous insulin (272).

Most trials of inhaled insulin exclude smokers and patients with severe asthma or chronic obstructive pulmonary disease. Mild to moderate cough is a common adverse effect (270). Smoking can reduce the dosage requirements of inhaled insulin, because of increased permeability of the alveolar capillary barrier (273). A reduction in carbon monoxide diffusion capacity has been reported in phase III trials with an insulin aerosol delivery system, Exubera. In further studies to investigate this, the changes in lung function were transient or reversible. In patients who used AERx for 12 weeks there were no changes in lung function (274).

The risk of hypoglycemia with inhaled insulin has been reported to be similar to that with subcutaneous insulin (273). In an open study of 107 patients with type 2 diabetes, mean age 58 years, using liquid insulin aerosol droplets + subcutaneous NPH insulin ($n = 54$) compared with Actrapid + NPH ($n = 53$) for 24 weeks, there were three major episodes of hypoglycemia in two patients using inhaled insulin and none in the other group (268).

Of 335 patients with type 1 diabetes randomized to receive preprandial inhaled insulin as a dry powder formulation via an aerosol delivery system (Exubera) plus bedtime subcutaneous Ultralente insulin, or to continue NPH and regular insulins subcutaneously, 170 received inhaled insulin (mean age 33 years) (272). Six discontinued inhaled insulin, one because of mild cough, two because of hypoglycemia, and three because of insufficient responses. The risk of hypoglycemia was slightly lower in those who used inhaled insulin, at 8.6 events per month compared with 9.0 events per month in the conventional insulin group.

Both powdered insulin formulations and liquid inhaled insulin formulations are being developed. There have been no direct comparisons of these formulations, and it is therefore difficult to make definitive statements about whether one is superior to the other (274).

Further information will need to be obtained about the possible long-term adverse effects of inhaled insulin.

Exubera, an insulin powder with a particle size of < 7.5 μm combined with a dry powder carrier, is commercially available in the UK. Other inhaled formulations are in development, including AERx, which is a liquid, and ProMaxx, which uses proprietary technology to produce microspheres of 1–5 μm. Regardless of the system used for delivery systemic availability is low (under 20%), and so high dosages are required. There is also variation in absorption and the intraindividual coefficient of variation can be about 34%, although the absorption of subcutaneously administered insulin is also variable. Smoking can increase the absorption rate by as much as 50%; this is reversed on stopping smoking but will recur when smoking is restarted (275).

In this and other reviews the lack of long-term data, which is particularly important for understanding the management of a chronic disease that requires many years of therapy for an individual, has been discussed. Data from 4-year open studies suggest that lung function does not deteriorate compared with subcutaneous insulin. However, patients with lung disease have usually been excluded from such studies (276,277).

In a single-dose comparison of healthy individuals with those with asthma the latter had reduced insulin absorption and greater intra-subject variation in insulin concentrations (277).

Antibodies to inhaled insulin continue to be a concern, although there has been no correlation with antibody titer and insulin dosage or the development of hypoglycemia. Presensitization may be important. Patients with type 2 diabetes who had not used insulin before starting to use inhaled insulin had a lower antibody response, despite the addition of subcutaneous insulin in 32% of participants by the end of the study (278).

In 10 non-diabetic volunteers with upper respiratory tract infections there were no differences in insulin pharmacokinetics after a single dose of inhaled insulin (AERx) given during the infection compared with recovery (279). The authors suggested that this shows that AERx can be continued safely in patients with upper respiratory tract infections. The dose used was small (equivalent to 6 units of short-acting insulin). Insulin dosage often increases substantially during illness and further experience in patients with diabetes would be required before establishing safety.

Oral administration

When variable amounts of insulin (50, 100, 135, or 150 units) were given to healthy volunteers in capsules containing SNAC (sodium N-(8-(2-hydroxybenzoyl)amino)-caprylate) 700 mg insulin was absorbed in the proximal part of the gut (280). SNAC had no adverse effects in animals and a single dose of 2800 mg in was not problematic in healthy volunteers during follow-up for 8 weeks.

In a phase I trial of oral modified insulin (HIM 2), 16 patients (mean age 37 years) with type 1 diabetes using CSII over 2 separate days used basal CSII on one day and basal CSII and oral insulin on another (281). There were 58 adverse events in 15 patients, although it was not clear whether they were drug-related. Weakness, headache, ataxia, thirst, dry mouth, and nausea were reported, among other symptoms.

Nasal administration

Insulin is rapidly absorbed after nasal administration, but even with absorption enhancers its systemic availability is low and its metabolic effect very short (183).

Gelified nasal insulin has been compared with twice daily isophane insulin and three times daily subcutaneous regular insulin in 16 patients with type 1 diabetes (261). Three patients had to withdraw because of nasal burning and one because of persistent sinusitis. One patient had purulent sinusitis after 6 months. The efficacy of gelified insulin was comparable to that of regular insulin.

Transdermal administration

Application to the skin, a highly efficient general barrier, did not result in sufficient and reproducible absorption (183).

Drug overdose

- Insulin overdose has been reported in patients without diabetes (282) and in a 25-year-old man with Munchausen's syndrome (283).
- Suicide by insulin has been reported in a 68-year-old, non-diabetic physician who had also taken metoprolol and alcohol. The blood metoprolol concentration was 0.4 microgram/ml (usual target range 0.035–0.5 microgram/ml) and alcohol 122 mg/dl (27 mmol/l). C-peptide could not be detected, serum insulin was 1849 µU/ml (normal fasting concentration below 16 µU/ml) (284).

Hypokalemia, hypophosphatemia, and hypomagnesemia can occur after insulin overdose (285).

- A 47-year-old man with type 2 diabetes attempted suicide by taking a bottle of wine, triazolam 2 mg, zoplicone 75 mg, and subcutaneous insulin (soluble 300 U and isophane 1800 U). His blood glucose was 1.5 mmol/l, potassium 2.4 mmol/l, phosphate 0.74 mmol/l, and magnesium 1.06 mmol/l. After 80 ml of 50% glucose and gastric lavage he needed a glucose infusion 6.6 mg/kg/minute for 24 hours to keep his blood glucose at 5.5–11.1 mmol/l. There was no brain damage on neurological examination or CT scan.

Acute liver damage has been attributed to insulin overdose followed by excessive glucose administration (99).

- In a suicide attempt, a 48-year-old woman took clomipramine 225 mg, diazepam 50 mg, oxazepam 150 mg, flurazepam 120 mg, and aspirin 10 g and injected insulin subcutaneously (1000 U short-acting and 1000 U long-acting). Her blood glucose was undetectable. She was intubated and given 40% glucose 20 ml and an infusion of 20% glucose (total 100 g over 2 hours). She continued to receive intravenous glucose 40% with potassium chloride for 36 hours (total 4430 g) in spite of high glucose concentrations. Her aspartate and alanine transaminase activities rose to 420 and 610 U/l respectively, the total bilirubin to 147 µmol/l (mainly unconjugated), the alkaline phosphatase to 178 U/l, and the serum lactate to 6.8 mmol/l. An ultrasound scan of the liver was normal. When the glucose infusion was stopped, everything normalized rapidly.

Acute steatosis of the liver may have explained this presentation. In insulin overdose, the combination of greatly increased hepatic production of triglycerides from glucose and reduced production of apolipoprotein B 100 results in an insufficient increase in the transport of triglycerides in VLDL particles from liver to muscle and adipose tissue and contributes to the steatosis.

Drug–Drug Interactions

ACE inhibitors

Whether ACE inhibitors aggravate or generate hypoglycemia is debated (286). In a case-control study of 404 cases and 1375 controls, the risk of hypoglycemia was

5.5 times greater (95% CI = 4.0, 7.6) in insulin versus sulfonylurea users and was not influenced by use of ACE inhibitors overall (288). However, the use of enalapril was associated with an increased risk of hypoglycemia (OR = 2.4; 95% CI = 1.1, 5.3).

Alcohol

Alcohol and hypoglycemia have additive effects on cognitive performance. This makes it even more important that people with type 1 diabetes refrain from alcohol when driving (287).

Beta-blockers

Beta-blockers have various effects on glucose metabolism, but these are usually too small to be of clinical significance (288,289). However, beta-blockers can block the adrenergic symptoms of hypoglycemia.

- A 68-year-old woman with diabetes and hypertension using 42 units of isophane insulin and propranolol 20 mg qds died with a blood glucose concentration below 1.4 mmol/l without any symptoms of hypoglycemia (290).

Chloroquine and hydroxychloroquine

There may be an interaction of chloroquine with insulin. An oral glucose load given to healthy subjects and to patients with non-insulin-dependent diabetes mellitus, before and during a short course of chloroquine, showed a small but significant reduction in fasting blood glucose concentration in the control group and improvement in glucose tolerance in the patients (SEDA-12, 240). The response seems to reflect reduced degradation of insulin rather than increased pancreatic output.

Ciprofloxacin

Hypoglycemia occurred in a patient treated with insulin and ciprofloxacin 500 mg bd (291).

Clozapine

Severe insulin resistance with ketoacidosis (pH 6.9) has been reported with clozapine (292). After withdrawal, insulin requirements fell. Reinstitution of clozapine induced an identical increase in insulin need.

Glucocorticoids

Glucocorticoids are counter-regulatory and can cause increased insulin requirements. Conversely, reducing the dose of a glucocorticoid, without changing the dosage of insulin, can cause hypoglycemia.

Maprotiline

- Maprotiline, a tetracyclic antidepressant, repeatedly induced hypoglycemia in a 39-year-old woman with type 1 diabetes, even when the insulin dosage was reduced from 20 U/day to 4–10 U/day. Maprotiline seems to prolong the half-life of insulin. A glucagon

stimulation test showed a maximum C-peptide concentration of only 0.22 nmol/l (293).

Olanzapine

Olanzapine has been reported to have precipitated diabetes (294).

- A 31-year-old man with a treatment-refractory psychiatric disorder without prior diabetes was given olanzapine 10 mg/day. After 3 months he developed hyperglycemia and an acidosis (pH 7.11). After treatment he needed at least 64 U/day of insulin, but 15 days after stopping olanzapine his insulin requirements fell and 15 days later insulin was withdrawn.

Recreational drugs

In London an anonymous confidential postal questionnaire was sent to 158 young adults (15–30 years) attending an urban diabetes clinic (295). Of 85 respondents 25 admitted using street drugs; 12 told their friends or performed extra blood tests. Only 23% of the users and non-users were aware of effects of recreational drugs on diabetes. Two had become hypoglycemic after cannabis and two had developed ketoacidosis after using ecstasy and cannabis. Street drugs affect diabetes in various ways. Amphetamines stimulate catecholamine release. Ecstasy creates a syndrome of inappropriate antidiuretic hormone release (hyponatremia and cerebral edema). Cocaine causes hyperglycemia via α-adrenoceptors. Withdrawal of opiates can cause ketoacidosis.

Thiazolidinediones

When thiazolidinediones are combined with insulin, edema can develop if there is cardiac dysfunction (296).

Interference with Diagnostic Tests

Blood glucose measurement

Three diabetic patients on chronic ambulatory peritoneal dialysis (CAPD) had symptoms of hypoglycemia when glucose readings on strips were higher than 4 mmol/l (297). Venous testing showed glucose concentrations as low as 1.8 mmol/l. Large amounts of glucose are used in CAPD, which not only affects the regulation of diabetes but can also affect the peritoneal wall. Since 1999, icodextrin has been used in dialysis fluids. Icodextrin is glucose-free and reduces the need for insulin. However, it is also absorbed systematically and can be metabolized to maltose and maltotriose. Paper systems that use either glucose oxidase or glucose dehydrogenase overestimate glucose readings when icodextrin is used, and patients and their carers are not able to measure low blood glucose concentrations. Another factor is that during end-stage renal insufficiency, insulin catabolism is reduced. This contributes to the problems when CAPD is changed to automated (overnight) peritoneal dialysis, in which daytime hypoglycemia can be prevented by reducing the amount of insulin used during the day.

Management of adverse drug reactions

Secondary growth hormone insensitivity syndrome is thought to develop when chronic insulin deficiency and poor metabolic control occur in people with type 1 diabetes. High growth hormone concentrations are found in conjunction with low concentrations of IGF1.

Intensifying insulin therapy in people with poor metabolic control exacerbates retinopathy. In three cases progressive retinopathy followed intensified insulin therapy, and the authors suggested that subcutaneous octreotide may be of benefit in management (298). The cases were managed concurrently with standard therapy, including laser photocoagulation. Octreotide reduced IGF1 concentrations and reduced insulin requirements. However its role in managing retinopathy was unclear. There was speculation that it may be helpful for macular edema.

Training for patients in diabetes management to allow for dietary flexibility improves glycemic control without increasing the risk of severe hypoglycemia. In an analysis of data from 96 hospitals in Germany a low concentration of Hb_{A1c} was associated with a high risk of hypoglycemia before treatment (299). After treatment hypoglycemia did not correlate with HB_{A1c}; there were 0.11 episodes of severe hypoglycemia per patient per year in the highest quintile of Hb_{A1c} compared with 0.16 in the lowest. Before treatment the figures were 0.18 and 0.54 respectively.

Monitoring Therapy

Frequent self-control by pricking the fingertips can cause anemia (300) or pyoderma gangrenosum and fingertip ulceration (301).

Problems with the use of blood glucose measurement systems are reported from time to time. For example, it is easy to read glucose meters wrongly (SEDA-25, 508). Hypoglycemia was missed when a patient inadvertently switched the glucose meter from mmol/l to mg/dl and read 266 mg/dl as 26.6 mmol/l and 158 mg/dl as 15.8 mmol/l (302).

- An 89-year-old man wrongly read the glucose concentrations in his home glucose meter (303). The meter read 561 mg/dl and 591 mg/dl but testing in the clinic 2 hours later showed concentrations of 175 mg/dl and 188 mg/dl. He had read the digital display upside down: 591 instead of 165 and 561 instead of 195.

Patients should be instructed about the correct orientation of digital meters.

In Raynaud's phenomenon, blood glucose concentrations measured by finger prick are often lower than the real values (66). The arm reacts more slowly to rapid changes in glucose concentrations. When glucose is monitored in the arm, changes in glucose concentrations are later seen than when monitored by finger prick (304). Rubbing the arm reduces the differences (305).

The development of glucose sensor systems has been reviewed (306). An automated device for sampling in the arm (307) and a microdialysis-based glucose sensor system (308) have been developed.

References

1. Koivisto VA, Felig P. Alterations in insulin absorption and in blood glucose control associated with varying insulin injection sites in diabetic patients. Ann Intern Med 1980;92(1):59–61.
2. Sindelka G, Heinemann L, Berger M, Frenck W, Chantelau E. Effect of insulin concentration, subcutaneous fat thickness and skin temperature on subcutaneous insulin absorption in healthy subjects. Diabetologia 1994;37(4):377–80.
3. Vaag A, Handberg A, Lauritzen M, Henriksen JE, Pedersen KD, Beck-Nielsen H. Variation in absorption of NPH insulin due to intramuscular injection. Diabetes Care 1990;13(1):74–6.
4. Binder C, Lauritzen T, Faber O, Pramming S. Insulin pharmacokinetics. Diabetes Care 1984;7(2):188–99.
5. Levetan C, Want LL, Weyer C, Strobel SA, Crean J, Wang Y, Maggs DG, Kolterman OG, Chandran M, Mudaliar SR, Henry RR. Impact of pramlintide on glucose fluctuations and postprandial glucose, glucagon, and triglyceride excursions among patients with type 1 diabetes intensively treated with insulin pumps. Diabetes Care 2003;26:1–8.
6. Schwartz S, Sievers R, Strange P, Lyness WH, Hollander P. Insulin 70/30 mix plus metformin versus triple oral therapy in the treatment of type 2 diabetes after failure of two oral drugs. Diabetes Care 2003;26:2238–43.
7. Hamilton J, Cummings E, Zdravkovic V, Finegood D, Danemen D. Metformin as an adjunct therapy in adolescents with type 1 diabetes and insulin resistance. Diabetes Care 2003;26:138–43.
8. Wulffelé MG, Kooy A, Lehert P, Bets D, Ogterop JC, Borger Van Den Burg B, Donker AJM, Stehouwer CDA. Combination of insulin and metformin in the treatment of type 2 diabetes. Diabetes Care 2002;25:2133–40.
9. Strowig SM, Avilés-Santa ML, Raskin P. Comparison of insulin monotherapy and combination therapy with insulin and metformin or insulin and troglitazone in type 2 diabetes. Diabetes Care 2002;25:1691–8.
10. Furlong NJ, Hulme SA, O'Brien SV, Hardy KJ. Repaglinide versus metformin in combination with bedtime NPH insulin in patients with type 2 diabetes established on insulin/metformin combination therapy. Diabetes Care 2002;25:1685–90.
11. Furlong NJ, Hulme SA, O'Brien SV, Hardy KJ. Comparison of repaglinide vs gliclazide in combination with bedtime NPH insulin in patients with type 2 diabetes inadequately controlled with oral hypoglycaemic agents. Diabetic Med 2003;20:935–41.
12. Raskin P, Rendell M, Riddle MC, Dole JF, Freed MI, Rosenstock J. A randomized trial of rosiglitazone therapy in patients with inadequately controlled insulin-treated type 2 diabetes. Diabetes Care 2001;24:1226–32.
13. Burge MR, Schade DS. Insulins. Endocrinol Metab Clin North Am 1997;26(3):575–98.
14. Muis MJ, Bots ML, Bilo HJG, Hoogma RPLM, Hoekstra JBL, Grobbee DE, Stolk RP. High cumulative insulin exposure: a risk factor of atherosclerosis in type 1 diabetes? Atherosclerosis 2005;181:185–92.
15. Gerstein HC, Rosenstock J. Insulin therapy in people who have dysglycemia and type 2 diabetes mellitus: can it offer both cardiovascular protection and beta-cell preservation? Endocrinol Metab Clin N Am 2005;34:137–54.
16. Uchida D, Ohigashi S, Hikita S, Kitamura N, Motoyoshi M, Tatasuno I. Acute pulmonary edema caused by hypoglycaemia due to insulin overdose. Int Med 2004;43:1056–9.

17. Azzopardi J, Gatt A, Zammit A, Alberti G. Lack of evidence of cerebral oedema in adults treated for diabetic ketoacidosis with fluids of different tonicity. Diabetes Res Clin Pract 2002;57(2):87–92.

18. Glaser N, Barnett P, McCaslin I, Nelson D, Trainor J, Louie J, Kaufman F, Quayle K, Roback M, Malley R, Kuppermann N. Pediatric Emergency Medicine Collaborative Research Committee of the American Academy of Pediatrics. Risk factors for cerebral edema in children with diabetic ketoacidosis. The Pediatric Emergency Medicine Collaborative Research Committee of the American Academy of Pediatrics. N Engl J Med 2001;344(4):264–9.

19. Dunger DB, Edge JA. Predicting cerebral edema during diabetic ketoacidosis. N Engl J Med 2001;344(4):302–3.

20. Blake DR, Nathan DM. Acute angle closure glaucoma following rapid correction of hyperglycemia. Diabetes Care 2003;26:3197–8.

21. Auzepy P, Caquet R. Hypoglycémies graves dues a l'insuline. Risques et accidents des médicaments antidiabétiques. [Severe hypoglycemia due to insulin. Risks and adverse effects of antidiabetic drugs.] Sem Hop 1983;59(10):697–705.

22. Seltzer HS. Severe drug-induced hypoglycemia: a review. Compr Ther 1979;5(4):21–9.

23. McAulay V, Deary IJ, Frier BM. Symptoms of hypoglycaemia in people with diabetes. Diabet Med 2001;18(9):690–705.

24. Gold AE, Deary IJ, Frier BM. Recurrent severe hypoglycaemia and cognitive function in type 1 diabetes. Diabet Med 1993;10(6):503–8.

25. Egger M, Davey Smith G, Stettler C, Diem P. Risk of adverse effects of intensified treatment in insulin-dependent diabetes mellitus: a meta-analysis. Diabet Med 1997;14(11):919–28.

26. The Diabetes Control and Complications Trial Research Group. The effect of intensive treatment of diabetes on the development and progression of long-term complications in insulin-dependent diabetes mellitus. N Engl J Med 1993;329(14):977–86.

27. The Diabetes Control and Complications Trial Research Group. Hypoglycemia in the Diabetes Control and Complications Trial. Diabetes 1997;46(2):271–86.

28. UK Prospective Diabetes Study (UKPDS) Group. Intensive blood-glucose control with sulphonylureas or insulin compared with conventional treatment and risk of complications in patients with type 2 diabetes (UKPDS 33). Lancet 1998;352(9131):837–53.

29. Taylor R, Davies R, Fox C, Sampson M, Weaver JU, Wood L. Appropriate insulin regimes for type 2 diabetes: a multicenter randomized crossover study. Diabetes Care 2000;23(11):1612–8.

30. Gale EA, Tattersall RB. Unrecognised nocturnal hypoglycaemia in insulin-treated diabetics. Lancet 1979;1(8125):1049–52.

31. Goudswaard AN, Stolk RP, de Zuithoff P, Valk HW, Rutten GE. Starting insulin in type 2 diabetes: continue oral hypoglycaemic agents? J Fam Pract 2004;53:393–9.

32. Ben-Ami H, Nagachandran P, Mendelson A, Edoute Y. Drug-induced hypoglycemic coma in 102 diabetic patients. Arch Intern Med 1999;159(3):281–4.

33. Lopez MJ, Oyarzabal M, Rodriguez M, Barrio R, Hermoso F, Blasco L. Severe hypoglycemia in Spanish diabetic children and adolescents. Study Group of Infantile Diabetes of the Spanish Paediatric Endocrinology Society. J Pediatr Endocrinol Metab 1999;12(1):85–7.

34. Miller CD, Phillips LS, Ziemer DC, Gallina DL, Cook CB, El-Kebbi IM. Hypoglycemia in patients with type 2 diabetes mellitus. Arch Intern Med 2001;161(13):1653–9.

35. Leese GP, Wang J, Broomhall J, Kelly P, Marsden A, Morrison W, Frier BM, Morris AD. DARTS/MEMO Collaboration. Frequency of severe hypoglycemia requiring emergency treatment in type 1 and type 2 diabetes: a population-based study of health service resource use. Diabetes Care 2003;26(4):1176–80.

36. Holstein A, Plaschke A, Egberts EH. Incidence and costs of severe hypoglycemia. Diabetes Care 2002;25(11):2109–10.

37. Amin R, Ross K, Acerini CL, Edge JA, Warner J, Dunger DB. Hypoglycemia prevalence in prepubertal children with type 1 diabetes on standard insulin regimen: use of continuous glucose monitoring system. Diabetes Care 2003;26(3):662–7.

38. Henderson JN, Allen KV, Deary IJ, Frier BM. Hypoglycaemia in insulin-treated type 2 diabetes: frequency, symptoms and impaired awareness. Diabetic Med 2003;20:1016–21.

39. Plank J, Siebenhofer A, Berghold A, Jeitler K, Horvath K, Mrak P, Pieber TR. Systematic review and meta-analysis of short-acting insulin analogues in patients with diabetes mellitus. Arch Intern Med 2005;165:1337–44.

40. Hvidberg A, Christensen NJ, Hilsted J. Counterregulatory hormones in insulin-treated diabetic patients admitted to an accident and emergency department with hypoglycaemia. Diabet Med 1998;15(3):199–204.

41. Levy CJ, Kinsley BT, Bajaj M, Simonson DC. Effect of glycemic control on glucose counterregulation during hypoglycemia in NIDDM. Diabetes Care 1998;21(8):1330–8.

42. Burge MR, Schmitz-Fiorentino K, Fischette C, Qualls CR, Schade DS. A prospective trial of risk factors for sulfonylurea-induced hypoglycemia in type 2 diabetes mellitus. JAMA 1998;279(2):137–43.

43. Kaneto H, Ikeda M, Kishimoto M, Iida M, Hoshi A, Watarai T, Kubota M, Kajimoto Y, Yamasaki Y, Hori M. Dramatic recovery of counter-regulatory hormone response to hypoglycaemia after intensive insulin therapy in poorly controlled type I diabetes mellitus. Diabetologia 1998;41(8):982–3.

44. Fritsche A, Stumvoll M, Grub M, Sieslack S, Renn W, Schmulling RM, Haring HU, Gerich JE. Effect of hypoglycemia on beta-adrenergic sensitivity in normal and type 1 diabetic subjects. Diabetes Care 1998;21(9):1505–10.

45. Oskarsson P, Adamson U, Sjobom NC, Lins PE. Long-term follow-up of insulin-dependent diabetes mellitus patients with recurrent episodes of severe hypoglycaemia. Diabetes Res Clin Pract 1999;44(3):165–74.

46. Nordfeldt S, Samuelsson U. Serum ACE predicts severe hypoglycemia in children and adolescents with type 1 diabetes. Diabetes Care 2003;26(2):274–8.

47. Kim CH, Park JH, Park TS, Baek HS. Autoimmune hypoglycemia in a type 2 diabetic patient with anti-insulin and insulin receptor antibodies. Diabetes Care 2004;27:228–9.

48. Gerich JE, Mokan M, Veneman T, Korytkowski M, Mitrakou A. Hypoglycemia unawareness. Endocr Rev 1991;12(4):356–71.

49. Amiel SA. R.D. Lawrence Lecture 1994. Limits of normality: the mechanisms of hypoglycaemia unawareness Diabet Med 1994;11(10):918–24.

50. Hvidberg A, Fanelli CG, Hershey T, Terkamp C, Craft S, Cryer PE. Impact of recent antecedent hypoglycemia on hypoglycemic cognitive dysfunction in nondiabetic humans. Diabetes 1996;45(8):1030–6.

51. Hepburn DA, MacLeod KM, Frier BM. Physiological, symptomatic and hormonal responses to acute hypoglycaemia in type 1 diabetic patients with autonomic neuropathy. Diabet Med 1993;10(10):940–9.

52. Pohl J, Frohnau G, Kerner W, Fehm-Wolfsdorf G. Symptom awareness is affected by the subjects' expectations during insulin-induced hypoglycemia. Diabetes Care 1997;20(5):796–802.

53. Maran A, Lomas J, Macdonald IA, Amiel SA. Lack of preservation of higher brain function during hypoglycaemia in patients with intensively-treated IDDM. Diabetologia 1995;38(12):1412–8.

54. Teuscher A, Berger WG. Hypoglycaemia unawareness in diabetics transferred from beef/porcine insulin to human insulin. Lancet 1987;2(8555):382–5.

55. Colagiuri S, Miller JJ, Petocz P. Double-blind crossover comparison of human and porcine insulins in patients reporting lack of hypoglycaemia awareness. Lancet 1992;339(8807):1432–5.

56. George E, Bedford C, Peacey SR, Hardisty CA, Heller SR. Further evidence for a high incidence of nocturnal hypoglycaemia in IDDM: no effect of dose for dose transfer between human and porcine insulins. Diabet Med 1997;14(6):442–8.

57. Klein BE, Klein R, Moss SE. Risk of hypoglycemia in users of human insulin. The Wisconsin Epidemiologic study of Diabetic Retinopathy. Diabetes Care 1997;20(3):336–9.

58. Galloway PJ, Thomson GA, Fisher BM, Semple CG. Insulin-induced hypoglycemia induces a rise in C-reactive protein. Diabetes Care 2000;23(6):861–2.

59. Ortega E, Wagner A, Caixas A, Barcons M, Corcoy R. Hypoglycemia and pulmonary edema: a forgotten association. Diabetes Care 2000;23(7):1023–4.

60. Hart SP, Frier BM. Causes, management and morbidity of acute hypoglycaemia in adults requiring hospital admission. QJM 1998;91(7):505–10.

61. Cox DJ, Gonder-Frederick LA, Kovatchev BP, Julian DM, Clarke WL. Progressive hypoglycemia's impact on driving simulation performance. Occurrence, awareness and correction. Diabetes Care 2000;23(2):163–70.

62. Marrero D, Edelman S. Hypoglycemia and driving performance: a flashing yellow light? Diabetes Care 2000;23(2):146–7.

63. Frier BM. Hypoglycemia and driving performance. Diabetes Care 2000;23(2):148–50.

64. ter Braak EW, Appelman AM, van de Laak M, Stolk RP, van Haeften TW, Erkelens DW. Clinical characteristics of type 1 diabetic patients with and without severe hypoglycemia. Diabetes Care 2000;23(10):1467–71.

65. Matz R. Hypoglycemia, seizures, and pulmonary edema. Diabetes Care 2000;23(11):1715.

66. Bradley KJ, Paton RC. Silent hypoglycaemia at the diabetic clinic. Diabet Med 2001;18(5):425–6.

67. Cryer PE. Hypoglycaemia: the limiting factor in the glycaemic management of Type I and Type II diabetes. Diabetologia 2002;45(7):937–48.

68. Smith D, Amiel SA. Hypoglycaemia unawareness and the brain. Diabetologia 2002;45(7):949–58.

69. Jaspan JB, Wollman RL, Bernstein L, Rubenstein AH. Hypoglycemic peripheral neuropathy in association with insulinoma: implication of glucopenia rather than hyperinsulinism. Medicine 1982;61:33–44.

70. Tesfaye N, Seaquist ER. Silent hypoglycemia presenting as dysesthesias. Diabetes Care 2004;27:628–9.

71. Fruehwald-Schultes B, Born J, Kern W, Peters A, Fehm HL. Adaptation of cognitive function to hypoglycemia in healthy men. Diabetes Care 2000;23(8):1059–66.

72. Austin EJ, Deary IJ. Effects of repeated hypoglycemia on cognitive function: a psychometrically validated reanalysis of the Diabetes Control and Complications Trial data. Diabetes Care 1999;22(8):1273–7.

73. Berger A, Croisier M, Jacot E, Kehtari R. Coma hypoglycémique de longue durée. [Hypoglycemic coma of long duration.] Rev Med Suisse Romande 1999;119(1):49–53.

74. Strachan MW, Deary IJ, Ewing FM, Frier BM. Recovery of cognitive function and mood after severe hypoglycemia in adults with insulin-treated diabetes. Diabetes Care 2000;23(3):305–12.

75. Cox DJ, Gonder-Frederick LA, Kovatchev BP, Young-Hyman DL, Donner TW, Julian DM, Clarke WL. Biopsychobehavioral model of severe hypoglycemia. II. Understanding the risk of severe hypoglycemia. Diabetes Care 1999;22(12):2018–25.

76. Kinsley BT, Weinger K, Bajaj M, Levy CJ, Simonson DC, Quigley M, Cox DJ, Jacobson AM. Blood glucose awareness training and epinephrine responses to hypoglycemia during intensive treatment in type 1 diabetes. Diabetes Care 1999;22(7):1022–8.

77. Wysocki T, Harris MA, Mauras N, Fox L, Taylor A, Jackson SC, White NH. Absence of adverse effects of severe hypoglycemia on cognitive function in school-aged children with diabetes over 18 months. Diabetes Care 2003;26(4):1100–5.

78. Matyka KA, Wigg L, Pramming S, Stores G, Dunger DB. Cognitive function and mood after profound nocturnal hypoglycaemia in prepubertal children with conventional insulin treatment for diabetes. Arch Dis Child 1999;81(2):138–42.

79. McAulay V, Deary IJ, Ferguson SC, Frier BM. Acute hypoglycemia in humans causes attentional dysfunction while nonverbal intelligence is preserved. Diabetes Care 2001;24(10):1745–50.

80. Gold AE, Marshall SM. Cortical blindness and cerebral infarction associated with severe hypoglycemia. Diabetes Care 1996;19(9):1001–3.

81. Odeh M, Oliven A. Hypoglycemia and bilateral cortical blindness. Diabetes Care 1996;19(3):272–3.

82. Aiello LP, Arrigg PG, Shah ST, Murtha TJ, Aiello LM. Solar retinopathy associated with hypoglycemic insulin reaction. Arch Ophthalmol 1994;112(7):982–3.

83. Burge MR, Castillo KR, Schade DS. Meal composition is a determinant of lispro-induced hypoglycemia in IDDM. Diabetes Care 1997;20(2):152–5.

84. Daneman D, Frank M, Perlman K, Tamm J, Ehrlich R. Severe hypoglycemia in children with insulin-dependent diabetes mellitus: frequency and predisposing factors. J Pediatr 1989;115(5 Pt 1):681–5.

85. Amiel SA. Studies in hypoglycaemia in children with insulin-dependent diabetes mellitus. Horm Res 1996;45(6):285–90.

86. Tupola S, Rajantie J. Documented symptomatic hypoglycaemia in children and adolescents using multiple daily insulin injection therapy. Diabet Med 1998;15(6):492–6.

87. Jaap AJ, Jones GC, McCrimmon RJ, Deary IJ, Frier BM. Perceived symptoms of hypoglycaemia in elderly type 2

diabetic patients treated with insulin. Diabet Med 1998;15(5):398–401.

88. Arem R, Zoghbi W. Insulin overdose in eight patients: insulin pharmacokinetics and review of the literature. Medicine (Baltimore) 1985;64(5):323–32.

89. Charlton R, Smith G, Day A. Munchausen's syndrome manifesting as factitious hypoglycaemia. Diabetologia 2001;44(6):784–5.

90. Barkai L, Vamosi I, Lukacs K. Prospective assessment of severe hypoglycaemia in diabetic children and adolescents with impaired and normal awareness of hypoglycaemia. Diabetologia 1998;41(8):898–903.

91. Airey CM, Williams DR, Martin PG, Bennett CM, Spoor PA. Hypoglycaemia induced by exogenous insulin—"human" and animal insulin compared. Diabet Med 2000;17(6):416–32.

92. Bragd J, Adamson U, Lins PE, Wredling R, Oskarsson P. A repeated cross-sectional survey of severe hypoglycaemia in 178 Type 1 diabetes mellitus patients performed in 1984 and 1998. Diabet Med 2003;20(3):216–9.

93. Lewis KS, Kane-Gill SL, Bobek MB, Dasta JF. Intensive insulin therapy for critically ill patients. Crit Care 2004;38:1243–51.

94. Gray CS, Hildreth AJ, Alberti GKMM, O'Connell JE, on behalf of the GIST collaboration. Poststroke hyperglycaemia natural history and immediate management. Stroke 2004;35:122–6.

95. Dagogo-Jack S, Fanelli CG, Cryer PE. Durable reversal of hypoglycemia unawareness in type 1 diabetes. Diabetes Care 1999;22(5):866–7.

96. Ovalle F, Fanelli CG, Paramore DS, Hershey T, Craft S, Cryer PE. Brief twice-weekly episodes of hypoglycemia reduce detection of clinical hypoglycemia in type 1 diabetes mellitus. Diabetes 1998;47(9):1472–9.

97. Clarke B, Ward JD, Enoch BA. Hypoglycaemia in insulin-dependent diabetic drivers. BMJ 1980;281(6240):586.

98. Thoma ME, Glauser J, Genuth S. Persistent hypoglycemia and hyperinsulinemia: caution in using glucagon. Am J Emerg Med 1996;14(1):99–101.

99. Monsod TP, Tamborlane WV, Coraluzzi L, Bronson M, Yong-Zhan T, Ahern JA. Epipen as an alternative to glucagon in the treatment of hypoglycemia in children with diabetes. Diabetes Care 2001;24(4):701–4.

100. Torres Marti A, Font J, Cano F, Rodriguez de Castro L, Camp J, Borras A, Milla J. Estudio epidemiologico del sindrome hipoglucemico en un servicio de urgencias. Analisis sobre 71 cases. [Epidemiologic study of hypoglycemic syndrome in an emergency unit. Study of 71 cases.] Med Clin (Barc) 1981;77(10):405–9.

101. Jolliet P, Leverve X, Pichard C. Acute hepatic steatosis complicating massive insulin overdose and excessive glucose administration. Intensive Care Med 2001;27(1):313–6.

102. Tupola S, Sipila I, Huttunen NP, Salo S, Nuuja A, Akerblom HK. Management of asymptomatic hypoglycaemia in children and adolescents with Type 1 diabetes mellitus. Diabet Med 2000;17(10):752–3.

103. Deiss D, Kordonouri O, Meyer K, Danne T. Long hypoglycaemic periods detected by subcutaneous continuous glucose monitoring in toddlers and pre-school children with diabetes mellitus. Diabet Med 2001;18(4):337–8.

104. Pitzer KR, Desai S, Dunn T, Edelman S, Jayalakshmi Y, Kennedy J, Tamada JA, Potts RO. Detection of hypoglycemia with the GlucoWatch biographer. Diabetes Care 2001;24(5):881–5.

105. Haymond MW, Schreiner B. Mini-dose glucagon rescue for hypoglycemia in children with type 1 diabetes. Diabetes Care 2001;24(4):643–5.

106. Jermendy G, Nadas J, Sapi Z. "Lipoblastoma-like" lipoatrophy induced by human insulin: morphological evidence for local dedifferentiation of adipocytes? Diabetologia 2000;43(7):955–6.

107. The Diabetes Control and Complications Trial Research Group. Influence of intensive diabetes treatment on body weight and composition of adults with type 1 diabetes in the Diabetes Control and Complications Trial. Diabetes Care 2001;24(10):1711–21.

108. Binder G, Bosk A, Gass M, Ranke MB, Heidemann PH. Insulin tolerance test causes hypokalaemia and can provoke cardiac arrhythmias. Hormone Res 2004;62:84–7.

109. Kalambokis GN, Tsatsoulils AA, Tsianos EV. The edematogenic properties of insulin. Am J Kidney Dis 2004;44:575–90.

110. Saule H. Insulin-induzierte Ödeme bei Adoleszenten mit Diabetes mellitus Typ I. [Insulin-induced edema in adolescents with type 1 diabetes mellitus.] Dtsch Med Wochenschr 1991;116(31–32):1191–4.

111. DeFronzo RA. The effect of insulin on renal sodium metabolism. A review with clinical implications. Diabetologia 1981;21(3):165–71.

112. Lawrence JR, Dunnigan MG. Diabetic (insulin) oedema. Br Med J 1979;2(6187):445.

113. Rosenbloom AL Giordano B. Chronic overtreatment with insulin in children and adolescents. Am J Dis Child 1977;131:881–5.

114. Actos Prescribing Information. Lincolnshire IL: Takeda Pharmaceuticals North America Inc, 2001.

115. Chelliah A, Burge MR. Insulin edema in the twenty-first century: review of the existing literature. J Invest Med 2004;52:104–8.

116. Juliusson PB, Bjerknes R, Sovik O, Kvistad PH. Generaliserte odemer ved insulinbehandling av nyoppdaget diabetes mellitus. [Generalized edema following insulin treatment of newly diagnosed diabetes mellitus.] Tidsskr Nor Laegeforen 2001;121(8):919–20.

117. Takaike H, Uchigata Y, Iwasaki N, Iwamoto Y. Transient elevation of liver transaminase after starting insulin therapy for diabetic acidosis or ketoacidosis in newly diagnosed type 1 diabetes mellitus. Diabetes Res Clin Pract 2004;64:27–32.

118. Tawata M, Ikeda M, Kodama Y, Aida K, Onaya T. A type 2 diabetic patient with liver dysfunction due to human insulin. Diabetes Res Clin Pract 2000;49(1):17–21.

119. Zenda T, Murase Y, Yoshida I, Muramoto H, Okada T, Yagi K. Does the use of insulin in a patient with liver dysfunction increase water retention in the body, i.e. cause insulin oedema? Eur J Gastroenterol Hepatol 2003;15:545–9.

120. Yu YM, Howard CP. Improper insulin compliance may lead to hepatomegaly and elevated hepatic enzymes in type 1 diabetic patients. Diabetic Care 2004;27:619–20.

121. Kordonouri O, Lauterborn R, Deiss D. Lipohypertrophy in young patients with type 1 diabetes. Diabetes Care 2002;25(3):634.

122. Swift B. Examination of insulin injection sites: an unexpected finding of localized amyloidosis. Diabet Med 2002;19(10):881–2.

123. Singhal PC, Abramovici M, Venkatesan J. Rhabdomyolysis in the hyperosmolal state. Am J Med 1990;88(1):9–12.

124. Kahn CR, Rosenthal AS. Immunologic reactions to insulin: insulin allergy, insulin resistance, and the autoimmune insulin syndrome. Diabetes Care 1979;2(3):283–95.

125. deShazo RD, Boehm TM, Kumar D, Galloway JA, Dvorak HF. Dermal hypersensitivity reactions to insulin: correlations of three patterns to their histopathology. J Allergy Clin Immunol 1982;69(2):229–37.

126. Ross JM. Allergy to insulin. Pediatr Clin North Am 1984;31(3):675–87.

127. Yoshino K, Takeda N, Muramatsu M, Morita H, Mune T, Ishizuka T, Yasuda K. [A case of generalized allergy to both human insulin and protamine in insulin preparation]. J Jpn Diabetes Soc 1999;42:927–30.

128. Warita E, Shimuzi H, Ubukata T, Mori M. [A case of human insulin allergy.] J Jpn Diabetes Soc 1999;42:1013–5.

129. Abraham MR, al-Sharafi BA, Saavedra GA, Khardori R. Lispro in the treatment of insulin allergy. Diabetes Care 1999;22(11):1916–7.

130. Panczel P, Hosszufalusi N, Horvath MM, Horvath A. Advantage of insulin lispro in suspected insulin allergy. Allergy 2000;55(4):409–10.

131. Eapen SS, Connor EL, Gern JE. Insulin desensitization with insulin lispro and an insulin pump in a 5-year-old child. Ann Allergy Asthma Immunol 2000;85(5):395–7.

132. Sackey AH. Recurrent generalised urticaria at insulin injection sites. BMJ 2000;321(7274):1449.

133. Kumar D. Insulin allergy: differences in the binding of porcine, bovine, and human insulins with anti-insulin IgE. Diabetes Care 1981;4(1):104–7.

134. Soto-Aguilar MC, deShazo RD, Morgan JE, Mather P, Ibrahim G, Frentz JM, Lauritano AA. Total IgG and IgG subclass specific antibody responses to insulin in diabetic patients. Ann Allergy 1991;67(5):499–503.

135. Al-Sheik OA. Unusual local cutaneous reactions to insulin injections: a case report. Saudi Med J 1998;19:199–201.

136. Elte JW, van der Schroeff JG, van Leeuwen AW, Radder JK. Sclerosing granuloma after short-term administration of depot-insulin Hoechst. Case report and a review of the literature. Klin Wochenschr 1982;60(23):1461–4.

137. Jordaan HF, Sandler M. Zinc-induced granuloma—a unique complication of insulin therapy. Clin Exp Dermatol 1989;14(3):227–9.

138. Sola-Gazagnes A, Pecquet C, Radermecker R, Piétri L, Elgrably F, Slama G, Sélam J-L. Successful treatment of insulin allergy in a type 1 diabetic patient by means of constant subcutaneous pump infusion of insulin. Diabetes Care 2003;26:2961–2.

139. Yokoyama H, Fukumoto S, Koyama H, Emoto M, Kitagawa Y, Nishizawa Y. Insulin allergy: desensitization with crystalline zinc-insulin and steroid tapering. Diabetes Res Clin Pract 2003;61:161–6.

140. Young RJ, Steel JM, Frier BM, Duncan LJ. Insulin injection sites in diabetes—a neglected area? BMJ (Clin Res Ed) 1981;283(6287):349.

141. Mandrup-Poulsen T, Molvig J, Pildal J, Rasmussen AK, Andersen L, Skov BG, Petersen J. Leukocytoclastic vasculitis induced by subcutaneous injection of human insulin in a patient with type 1 diabetes and essential thrombocytemia. Diabetes Care 2002;25(1):242–3.

142. Jones GR, Statham B, Owens DR, Jones MK, Hayes TM. Lipoatrophy and monocomponent porcine insulin. BMJ (Clin Res Ed) 1981;282(6259):190.

143. Silverstone P. Generalised allergic reaction to human insulin. BMJ (Clin Res Ed) 1986;292(6525):933–4.

144. Ganz MA, Unterman T, Roberts M, Uy R, Sahgal S, Samter M, Grammer LC. Resistance and allergy to recombinant human insulin. J Allergy Clin Immunol 1990;86(1):45–51.

145. Patterson R, Roberts M, Grammer LC. Insulin allergy: re-evaluation after two decades. Ann Allergy 1990;64(5):459–62.

146. Kurtz AB, Nabarro JD. Circulating insulin-binding antibodies. Diabetologia 1980;19(4):329–34.

147. Goswami R, Jaleel A, Kochupillai NP. Insulin antibody response to bovine insulin therapy: functional significance among insulin requiring young diabetics in India. Diabetes Res Clin Pract 2000;49(1):7–15.

148. Goerz G, Ruzicka T, Hofmann N, Drost H, Gruneklee D. Granulomatöse allergische Reaktion vom verzögerten Typ auf Surfen. [Granulomatous allergic reaction of the delayed type to Surfen.] Hautarzt 1981;32(4):187–90.

149. Feinglos MN, Jegasothy BV. "Insulin" allergy due to zinc. Lancet 1979;1(8108):122–4.

150. Bruni S, Barolo P, Gamba S, Grassi G, Blatto A. Case of generalized allergy due to zinc and protamine in insulin preparation. Diabetes Care 1986;9(5):552.

151. Gin H, Aubertin J. Generalized allergy due to zinc and protamine in insulin preparation treated with insulin pump. Diabetes Care 1987;10(6):789–90.

152. Diem P. Allergy to insulin. BMJ 1980;281(6247):1068–9.

153. MacCracken J, Stenger P, Jackson T. Latex allergy in diabetic patients: a call for latex-free insulin tops. Diabetes Care 1996;19(2):184.

154. Dische FE, Wernstedt C, Westermark GT, Westermark P, Pepys MB, Rennie JA, Gilbey SG, Watkins PJ. Insulin as an amyloid–fibril protein at sites of repeated insulin injections in a diabetic patient. Diabetologia 1988;31(3):158–61.

155. Chantelau EA, Berger M. Pollution of insulin with silicone oil, a hazard of disposable plastic syringes. Lancet 1985;1(8443):1459.

156. Lapiere CM, Pierard GE, Hermanns JF, Lefebvre P. Unusual extensive granulomatosis after long-term use of plastic syringes for insulin injections. Dermatologica 1982;165(6):580–90.

157. Sacerdote AS. Hypoglycemic urticaria revisited. Diabetes Care 1999;22(5):861.

158. Lassmann-Vague V, SanMarco M, LeJeune PJ, Alessis C, Vague P, Belicar P. Autoimmunity and intraperitoneal insulin treatment by programmable pumps: lack of relationship. Diabetes Care 1998;21(11):2041–4.

159. Charles MA. Autoimmunity and intraperitoneal insulin. Diabetes Care 1998;21:2043–4.

160. Frigerio C, Aubry M, Gomez F, Graf L, Dayer E, de Kalbermatten N, Gaillard RC, Spertini F. Desensitization-resistant insulin allergy. Allergy 1997;52(2):238–9.

161. Valenta LJ, Elias AN. Insulin-induced lipodystrophy in diabetic patients resolved by treatment with human insulin. Ann Intern Med 1985;102(6):790–1.

162. Cusi K, DeFronzo RA. Treatment of NIDDM IDDM, and other insulin-resistant states with IGF-I. Diabetes Rev 1995;3:206–36.

163. Naf S, Esmatjes E, Recasens M, Valero A, Halperin I, Levy I, Gomis R. Continuous subcutaneous insulin infusion to resolve an allergy to human insulin. Diabetes Care 2002;25(3):634–5.

164. Pratt EJ, Miles P, Kerr D. Localized insulin allergy treated with continuous subcutaneous insulin. Diabet Med 2001;18(6):515–6.

165. Finucane K, Ambey P, Narayan S, Archer CB, Dayan C. Insulin injection abscesses caused by Mycobacterium chelonae. Diabetes Care 2003;26:2483–4.
166. Renard E, Raingeard I, Costalat G, Apostol D, Lauton D, Boulet F, Bringer J. Aseptic peritonitis revealed through recurrent catheter obstructions in type 1 diabetic patients treated with continuous peritoneal insulin infusion. Diabetes Care 2004;27:276–7.
167. Evans PJ, Lynch RM. Insulin as a drug of abuse in body building. Br J Sports Med 2003;37:356–7.
168. Riveline JP, Capeau J, Robert JJ, Varroud-Vial M, Cerf-Baron I, Deburge A, Charpentier G. Extreme subcutaneous insulin resistance successfully treated by an implantable pump. Diabetes Care 2001;24(12):2155–6.
169. Tokuyama Y, Nozaki O, Kanatsuka A. A patient with subcutaneous-insulin resistance treated by insulin lispro plus heparin. Diabetes Res Clin Pract 2001;54(3):209–12.
170. Chowdhury TA, Escudier V. Poor glycaemic control caused by insulin induced lipohypertrophy. Br Med J 2003;327:383–4.
171. Evers IM, ter Braak EW, de Valk HW, van Der Schoot B, Janssen N, Visser GH. Risk indicators predictive for severe hypoglycemia during the first trimester of type 1 diabetic pregnancy. Diabetes Care 2002;25(3):554–9.
172. Simmons D, Thompson CF, Conroy C, Scott DJ. Use of insulin pumps in pregnancies complicated by type 2 diabetes and gestational diabetes in a multiethnic community. Diabetes Care 2001;24(12):2078–82.
173. Devlin JT, Hothersall L, Wilkis JL. Use of insulin glargine during pregnancy in a type 1 diabetic woman. Diabetes Care 2002;25(6):1095–6.
174. Landauer W. Is insulin a teratogen? Teratology 1972;5(2):129–35.
175. Queisser-Luft A, Eggers I, Stolz G, Kieninger-Baum D, Schlaefer K. Serial examination of 20,248 newborn fetuses and infants: correlations between drug exposure and major malformations. Am J Med Genet 1996;63(1):268–76.
176. Danne T, Mortensen HB, Hougaard P, Lynggaard H, Aanstoot HJ, Chiarelli F, Daneman D, Dorchy H, Garandeau P, Greene SA, Hoey H, Holl RW, Kaprio EA, Kocova M, Martul P, Matsuura N, Robertson KJ, Schoenle EJ, Sovik O, Swift PG, Tsou RM, Vanelli M, Aman JFor the Hvidore Study Group on Childhood Diabetes. Persistent differences among centers over 3 years in glycemic control and hypoglycemia in a study of 3,805 children and adolescents with type 1 diabetes from the Hvidore Study Group. Diabetes Care 2001;24(8):1342–7.
177. Wagner VM, Grabert M, Holl RW. Severe hypoglcyemia, metabolic control and diabetes management in children with type 1 diabetes in the decade after the diabetes control and complications trial – a large scale multicentre study. Eur J Pediatr 2005;164:73–9.
178. Parmar MS. Recurrent hypoglycaemia in a diabetic patient as a result of unexpected renal failure. BMJ 2004;328:883–4.
179. Grajower MM, Fraser CG, Holcombe JH, Daugherty ML, Harris WC, De Felippis MR, Santiago OM, Clark NG. How long should insulin be used once a vial is started? Diabetes Care 2003;26:2665–9.
180. ADA Clinical Practice Recommendations. Insulin administration. Diabetes Care 2003;26 Suppl 1:S121–4.
181. Roest MA, Shaw S, Orton DI. Insulin-injection-site reactions associated with type I latex allergy. N Engl J Med 2003;348(3):265–6.
182. American Diabetes Association. Insulin administration. Diabetes Care 2001;24(11):1984–7.
183. Heinemann L, Pfutzner A, Heise T. Alternative routes of administration as an approach to improve insulin therapy: update on dermal, oral, nasal and pulmonary insulin delivery. Curr Pharm Des 2001;7(14):1327–51.
184. Gizurarson S, Bechgaard E. Intranasal administration of insulin to humans. Diabetes Res Clin Pract 1991;12(2):71–84.
185. Hilsted J, Madsbad S, Hvidberg A, Rasmussen MH, Krarup T, Ipsen H, Hansen B, Pedersen M, Djurup R, Oxenboll B. Intranasal insulin therapy: the clinical realities. Diabetologia 1995;38(6):680–4.
186. Heinemann L, Traut T, Heise T. Time-action profile of inhaled insulin. Diabet Med 1997;14(1):63–72.
187. Laube BL, Georgopoulos A, Adams GK 3rd. Preliminary study of the efficacy of insulin aerosol delivered by oral inhalation in diabetic patients. JAMA 1993;269(16):2106–2109.
188. Wallymahmed ME, Littler P, Clegg C, Haqqani MT, Macfarlane IA. Nodules of fibrocollagenous scar tissue induced by subcutaneous insulin injections: a cause of poor diabetic control. Postgrad Med J 2004;80:732–3.
189. Kamoi K, Miyakoshi M, Maruyama R. A quality-of-life assessment of intensive insulin therapy using insulin lispro switched from short-acting insulin and measured by an ITR-QOL questionnaire: a prospective comparison of multiple daily insulin injections and continuous insulin infusion. Diabetes Res Clin Pract 2004;64:19–25.
190. Colquitt J, Royle P, Waugh N. Are analogue insulins better than soluble in continuous subcutaneous insulin infusion? Results of a meta-analysis. Diabetic Med 2003;20:863–6.
191. Raskin P, Bode BW, Marks JB, Hirsch IB, Weinstein RL, McGill JB, Peterson GE, Mudaliar SR, Reinhardt RR. Continuous subcutaneous insulin infusion treatment and multiple daily injection therapy are equally effective in type 2 diabetes. Diabetes Care 2003;26:2598–603.
192. Sulli N, Shashaj B. Continuous subcutaneous insulin infusion in children and adolescents with diabetes mellitus: decreased HbA1c with low risk of hypoglycemia. J Pediatr Endocrinol Metab 2003;16:393–9.
193. Weintrob N, Benzaquen H, Galatzer A, Shalitin S, Lazar L, Fayman G, Lilos P, Dickerman Z, Phillip M. Comparison of continuous subcutaneous insulin infusion and multiple daily injection regimens in children with type 1 diabetes: a randomized open crossover trial. Pediatrics 2003;112:559–64.
194. Phillips BD, Aurand LA, Bedwell MM, Levy JR. A novel approach to preventing diabetic ketoacidosis in a patient treated with an insulin pump. Diabetes Care 2003;26:2960–1.
195. Doyle EA, Weinzimer SA, Steffen AT, Ahern JH, Vincent M, Tamborlane WV. A randomised prospective trial comparing the efficacy of continuous subcutaneous insulin infusion with multiple daily injections using insulin glargine. Diabetes Care 2004;27:1554–8.
196. Radermecker RP, Scheen AJ. Continuous subcutaneous insulin infusion with short-acting insulin analogues or human regular insulin: efficacy, safety, quality of life, and cost-effectiveness. Diabetes Metab Res Rev 2004;20:178–88.
197. Hammond P. Continuous subcutaneous insulin infusion: short-term benefits apparent, long-term benefits speculative. Br J Diabetes Vasc Dis 2004;4:104–8.

198. Griffin ME, Feder A, Tamborlane WV. Lipoatrophy associated with lispro in insulin pump therapy. Diabetes Care 2001;24:174.

199. Ampudia-Biasco FJ, Hasbrum B, Carneba R. A new case of lipoatrophy with lispro insulin in insulin pump therapy. Diabetes Care 2003;26:953–4.

200. Mack-Fogg JE, Orlowski CC, Jospe N. Continuous subcutaneous insulin infusion in toddlers and children with type 1 diabetes is safe and effective. Pediatr Diabetes 2005; 6:17–21.

201. Pankowska E, Skorka A, Szypowska A, Lipka M. Memory of insulin pumps and their record as a source of information about insulin therapy in children and adolescents with type 1 diabetes. Diabetes Technol Ther 2005;7:308–14.

202. Jeha GS, Karaviti LP, Anderson B, O'Brian Smith E, Donaldson S, McGirk TS, Haymond MW. Insulin pump therapy in preschool children with type 1 diabetes mellitus improves glycemic control and decreases glucose excursions and the risk of hypoglycemia. Diabetes Technol Ther 2005;7:876–84.

203. Chantelau E, Berger M, Bohlken B. Silicone oil released from disposable insulin syringes. Diabetes Care 1986;9(6):672–3.

204. Lteif AN, Schwenk WF. Accuracy of pen injectors versus insulin syringes in children with type 1 diabetes. Diabetes Care 1999;22(1):137–40.

205. Jehle PM, Micheler C, Jehle DR, Breitig D, Boehm BO. Inadequate suspension of neutral protamine Hagendorn (NPH) insulin in pens. Lancet 1999;354(9190):1604–7.

206. Skyler JS, Cefalu WT, Kourides IA, Landschulz WH, Balagtas CC, Cheng SL, Gelfand RA. Efficacy of inhaled human insulin in type 1 diabetes mellitus: a randomised proof-of-concept study. Lancet 2001;357(9253):331–5.

207. Annersten M, Frid A. Insulin pens dribble from the tip of the needle after injection. Pract Diabetes Int 2000;17:109–11.

208. Tubiana-Rufi N, Belarbi N, Du Pasquier-Fediaevsky L, Polak M, Kakou B, Leridon L, Hassan M, Czernichow P. Short needles (8 mm) reduce the risk of intramuscular injections in children with type 1 diabetes Diabetes Care 1999;22(10):1621–5.

209. Rosenlund EF, Haakens K, Brinchmann-Hansen O, Dahl-Jorgensen K, Hanssen KF. Transient proliferative diabetic retinopathy during intensified insulin treatment. Am J Ophthalmol 1988;105(6):618–25.

210. Hardy K, Gill G. Bubble ketoacidosis. Lancet 1988;1(8598):1336–7.

211. Fischer U. Fundamentals of glucose sensors. Diabet Med 1991;8(4):309–21.

212. Mecklenburg RS, Benson EA, Benson JW Jr, Blumenstein BA, Fredlund PN, Guinn TS, Metz RJ, Nielsen RL. Long-term metabolic control with insulin pump therapy. Report of experience with 127 patients. N Engl J Med 1985;313(8):465–8.

213. Mecklenburg RS, Guinn TS, Sannar CA, Blumenstein BA. Malfunction of continuous subcutaneous insulin infusion systems: a one-year prospective study of 127 patients. Diabetes Care 1986;9(4):351–5.

214. Chantelau E, Spraul M, Muhlhauser I, Gause R, Berger M. Long-term safety, efficacy and side-effects of continuous subcutaneous insulin infusion treatment for type 1 (insulin-dependent) diabetes mellitus: a one centre experience. Diabetologia 1989;32(7):421–6.

215. Saudek CD. Implantable insulin pumps: a current look. Diabetes Res Clin Pract 1990;10(2):109–14.

216. Belicar P, Lassmann-Vague V. Local adverse events associated with long-term treatment by implantable insulin pumps. The French EVADIAC Study Group experience. Evaluation dans le Diabete du Traitement par Implants Actifs. Diabétes Care 1998;21(2):325–6.

217. Toth EL, Boychuk LR, Kirkland PA. Recurrent infection of continuous subcutaneous insulin infusion sites with *Mycobacterium fortuitum*. Diabetes Care 1995;18(9):1284–5.

218. Morton C. Nickel allergy: a complication of CSII. Pract Diabetes 1990;7:179.

219. Chantelau E, Lange G, Sonnenberg GE, Berger M. Acute cutaneous complications and catheter needle colonization during insulin-pump treatment. Diabetes Care 1987;10(4):478–82.

220. Fishman V, Fishman M. Practical problems with insulin pumps. N Engl J Med 1982;306(22):1369–70.

221. Wredling R, Lin PE, Adamson U. Pump "run-away" causing severe hypoglycaemia. Lancet 1989;2(8657):273.

222. Zinman B. Insulin pump therapy and rapid acting insulin: what have we learned? Int J Clin Pract Suppl 2001;(123):47–50.

223. Pickup J, Keen H. Continuous subcutaneous insulin infusion at 25 years: evidence base for the expanding use of insulin pump therapy in type 1 diabetes. Diabetes Care 2002;25(3):593–8.

224. King AB, Armstrong D. A comparison of basal insulin delivery: continuous subcutaneous insulin infusion versus glargine. Diabetes Care 2003;26(4):1322.

225. Weissberg-Benchell J, Antisdel-Lomaglio J, Seshadri R. Insulin pump therapy: a meta-analysis. Diabetes Care 2003;26(4):1079–87.

226. Rivellese AA, Patti L, Romano G, Innelli F, Di Marino L, Annuzzi G, Iavicoli M, Coronel GA, Riccardi G. Effect of insulin and sulfonylurea therapy, at the same level of blood glucose control, on low density lipoprotein subfractions in type 2 diabetic patients. J Clin Endocrinol Metab 2000;85(11):4188–92.

227. Wainstein J, Metzger M, Wexler ID, Cohen J, Raz I. The use of continuous insulin delivery systems in severely insulin-resistant patients. Diabetes Care 2001;24(7):1299.

228. Kaufman FR, Halvorson M, Kim C, Pitukcheewanont P. Use of insulin pump therapy at nighttime only for children 7–10 years of age with type 1 diabetes. Diabetes Care 2000;23(5):579–82.

229. Plotnick LP, Clark LM, Brancati FL, Erlinger T. Safety and effectiveness of insulin pump therapy in children and adolescents with type 1 diabetes. Diabetes Care 2003;26(4):1142–6.

230. Ahern JA, Boland EA, Doane R, Ahern JJ, Rose P, Vincent M, Tamborlane WV. Insulin pump therapy in pediatrics: a therapeutic alternative to safely lower HbA1c levels across all age groups. Pediatr Diabetes 2002;3(1):10–5.

231. DeVries JH, Eskes SA, Snoek FJ, Pouwer F, Van Ballegooie E, Spijker AJ, Kostense PJ, Seubert M, Heine RJ. Continuous intraperitoneal insulin infusion in patients with "brittle" diabetes: favourable effects on glycaemic control and hospital stay. Diabet Med 2002;19(6):496–501.

232. Pinget M, Jeandidier N. Long term safety and efficacy of intraperitoneal insulin infusion by means of implantable pumps. Horm Metab Res 1998;30(8):475–86.

233. Jeandidier N, Boivin S. Current status and future prospects of parenteral insulin regimens, strategies and delivery systems for diabetes treatment. Adv Drug Deliv Rev 1999;35(2–3):179–98.

234. Kaufman FR, Halvorson M, Miller D, Mackenzie M, Fisher LK, Pitukcheewanont P. Insulin pump therapy in

type 1 pediatric patients: now and into the year 2000. Diabetes Metab Res Rev 1999;15(5):338–52.

235. Bousquet-Rouaud R, Castex F, Costalat G, Bastide M, Hedon B, Bouanani M, Jouvert S, Mirouze J. Factors involved in catheter obstruction during long-term peritoneal insulin infusion. Diabetes Care 1993;16(5):801–5.

236. Levy RP, Borchelt MD, Kremer RM, Francis SJ, O'Connor CA. *Hemophilus influenza* infection of an implantable insulin-pump pocket. Diabetes Care 1992;15(11):1449–50.

237. Scavini M, Cristallo M, Sarmiento M, Dunn FL. Pump-pocket complications during long-term insulin delivery using an implanted programmable pump. Diabetes Care 1996;19(4):384–5.

238. Renard E, Taourel P, Quenet F, Domergue J, Bruel JM, Bringer J. Cecum erosion: unusual but serious complication of an implanted catheter for peritoneal insulin delivery. Diabetes Care 1995;18(3):408–9.

239. Kessler L, Tritschler S, Bohbot A, Sigrist S, Karsten V, Boivin S, Dufour P, Belcourt A, Pinget M. Macrophage activation in type 1 diabetic patients with catheter obstruction during peritoneal insulin delivery with an implantable pump. Diabetes Care 2001;24(2):302–7.

240. Bienvenu B, Timsit J. Sauna-induced diabetic ketoacidosis. Diabetes Care 1999;22(9):1584.

241. Renard E, Souche C, Jacques-Apostol D, Lauton D, Gibert-Boulet F, Costalat G, Bringer J, Jaffiol C. Improved stability of insulin delivery from implanted pumps using a new preparation process for infused insulin. Diabetes Care 1999;22(8):1371–2.

242. Boivin S, Belicar P, Melki V. Assessment of in vivo stability of a new insulin preparation for implantable insulin pumps. A randomized multicenter prospective trial. EVADIAC Group. Evaluation Dans le Diabéte du Traitement par Implants Actifs. Diabetes Care 1999;22(12):2089–90.

243. Boland EA, Grey M, Oesterle A, Fredrickson L, Tamborlane WV. Continuous subcutaneous insulin infusion. A new way to lower risk of severe hypoglycemia, improve metabolic control, and enhance coping in adolescents with type 1 diabetes. Diabetes Care 1999;22(11):1779–84.

244. Linkeschova R, Raoul M, Bott U, Berger M, Spraul M. Less severe hypoglycaemia, better metabolic control, and improved quality of life in type 1 diabetes mellitus with continuous subcutaneous insulin infusion (CSII) therapy; an observational study of 100 consecutive patients followed for a mean of 2 years. Diabet Med 2002;19(9):746–51.

245. Bruttomesso D, Pianta A, Crazzolara D, Scaldaferri E, Lora L, Guarneri G, Mongillo A, Gennaro R, Miola M, Moretti M, Confortin L, Beltramello GP, Pais M, Baritussio A, Casiglia E, Tiengo A. Continuous subcutaneous insulin infusion (CSII) in the Veneto region: efficacy, acceptability and quality of life. Diabet Med 2002;19(8):628–34.

246. DeVries JH, Snoek FJ, Kostense PJ, Masurel N, Heine RJDutch Insulin Pump Study Group. A randomized trial of continuous subcutaneous insulin infusion and intensive injection therapy in type 1 diabetes for patients with long-standing poor glycemic control. Diabetes Care 2002;25(11):2074–80.

247. Schade DS, Valentine V. To pump or not to pump. Diabetes Care 2002;25(11):2100–2.

248. Maniatis AK, Klingensmith GJ, Slover RH, Mowry CJ, Chase HP. Continuous subcutaneous insulin infusion ther-

apy for children and adolescents: an option for routine diabetes care. Pediatrics 2001;107(2):351–6.

249. Kamoi K, Sasaki H, Kobayashi T. Effect on glycemic control of short-acting acidified insulin administered three years in patients treated by continuous subcutaneous insulin infusion. J Jpn Diabetes Soc 2000;43:847–52.

250. Ooi C, Mullen P, Williams G. Insulin lispro: the ideal pump insulin for patients with severe hypoglycemic unawareness? Diabetes Care 1999;22(9):1598–9.

251. Becker DI. Pediatric use of insulin pumps: longer infusion site lifetime with NovoLog. Diabetes Care 2002;25(9):1663.

252. Lepore G, Dodesini AR, Nosari I, Trevisan R. Both continuous subcutaneous insulin infusion and a multiple daily insulin injection regimen with glargine as basal insulin are equally better than traditional multiple daily insulin injection treatment. Diabetes Care 2003;26(4):1321–2.

253. Jeandidier N, Boullu S, Busch-Brafin MS, Chabrier G, Sapin R, Gasser F, Pinget M. Comparison of antigenicity of Hoechst 21PH insulin using either implantable intraperitoneal pump or subcutaneous external pump infusion in type 1 diabetic patients. Diabetes Care 2002;25(1):84–8.

254. Gin H, Melki V, Guerci B, Catargi BEvaluation dans le Diabé du Traitement par Implants Actifs Study Group. Clinical evaluation of a newly designed compliant side port catheter for an insulin implantable pump: the EVADIAC experience. Evaluation dans le Diabéte du Traitement par Implants Actifs. Diabetes Care 2001;24(1):175.

255. Hanas R, Ludvigsson J. Side effects and indwelling times of subcutaneous catheters for insulin injections: a new device for injecting insulin with a minimum of pain in the treatment of insulin-dependent diabetes mellitus. Diabetes Res Clin Pract 1990;10(1):73–83.

256. Käär ML, Mäenpää J, Knip M. Insulin administration via a subcutaneous catheter. Effects on absorption. Diabetes Care 1993;16(10):1412–3.

257. Hanas SR, Carlsson S, Frid A, Ludvigsson J. Unchanged insulin absorption after 4 days' use of subcutaneous indwelling catheters for insulin injections. Diabetes Care 1997;20(4):487–90.

258. Wredling R, Adamson U, Lins PE, Backman L, Lundgren D. Experience of long-term intraperitoneal insulin treatment using a new percutaneous access device. Diabet Med 1991;8(6):597–600.

259. Heinemann L, Klappoth W, Rave K, Hompesch B, Linkeschowa R, Heise T. Intra-individual variability of the metabolic effect of inhaled insulin together with an absorption enhancer. Diabetes Care 2000;23(9):1343–7.

260. Gerber RA, Cappelleri JC, Kourides IA, Gelfand RA. Treatment satisfaction with inhaled insulin in patients with type 1 diabetes: a randomized controlled trial. Diabetes Care 2001;24(9):1556–9.

261. Lalej-Bennis D, Boillot J, Bardin C, Zirinis P, Coste A, Escudier E, Chast F, Peynegre R, Selam JL, Slama G. Efficacy and tolerance of intranasal insulin administered during 4 months in severely hyperglycaemic Type 2 diabetic patients with oral drug failure: a cross-over study. Diabet Med 2001;18(8):614–8.

262. Perera AD, Kapitza C, Nosek L, Fishman RS, Shapiro DA, Heise T, Heinemann L. Absorption and metabolic effect of inhaled insulin: intrapatient variability after inhalation via the Aerodose insulin inhaler in patients with type 2 diabetes. Diabetes Care 2002;25(12):2276–81.

263. Himmelmann A, Jendle J, Mellen A, Petersen AH, Dahl UL, Wollmer P. The impact of smoking on inhaled insulin. Diabetes Care 2003;26(3):677–82.

264. Henry RR, Mudaliar SR, Howland WC 3rd, Chu N, Kim D, An B, Reinhardt RR. Inhaled insulin using the AERx Insulin Diabetes Management System in healthy and asthmatic subjects. Diabetes Care 2003;26(3):764–9.

265. Stoever JA, Palmer JP. Inhaled insulin and insulin antibodies: a new twist to an old debate. Diabetes Technol Ther 2002;4(2):157–61.

266. Owens DR, Zinman B, Bolli G. Alternative routes of insulin delivery. Diabetic Med 2003;20:886–98.

267. Cefalu WT. Concepts, strategies, and feasibility of noninvasive insulin delivery. Diabetes Care 2004;27:239–46.

268. Hermansen K, Rönnemaa T, Petersen AH, Bellaire S, Adamson U. Intensive therapy with inhaled insulin via the AERx insulin diabetes management system. Diabetes Care 2004;27:162–7.

269. An B, Reinhardt RR. Effects of different duration of breath holding after inhalation of insulin using the AERx® insulin diabetes management system. Clin Ther 2003;25:2233–44.

270. Schatz H. Inhaled insulin and the dream of a needle-free insulin application. Exp Clin Endocrinol Diabetes 2004;112:285–7.

271. Hermansen K, Ronnemaa T, Petersen AH, Bellaire S, Adamson U. Intensive therapy with inhaled insulin via the AERx insulin diabetes management system. Diabetes Care 2004;27:162–7.

272. Quattrin T, Belanger A, Bohannon NJV, Schwartz SL, Efficacy and safety of inhaled insulin (Exubera) compared with subcutaneous insulin therapy in patients with type 1 diabetes. Diabetes Care 2004;27:2622–7.

273. Barnett AH. Exubera inhaled insulin: a review. Int J Clin Pract 2004;5:394–401.

274. Heinemann L, Heise T. Current status of the development of inhaled insulin. Br J Diabetes Vasc Dis 2004;4:295–301.

275. Mandal TK. Inhaled insulin for diabetes mellitus. Am J Health-Syst Pharm 2005;62:1359–64.

276. Odegard PS, Capoccia KL. Inhaled insulin: Exubera. Ann Pharmacother 2005;39:843–53.

277. Harsch IA, Inhaled insulins: their potential in the treatment of diabetes mellitus. Treat Endocrinol 2005;4:131–8.

278. Fineberg SE, Kawabata T, Finco-Kent D, Liu C, Krasner A. Antibody response to inhaled insulin in patients with type 1 or type 2 diabetes. An analysis of initial phase II and III inhaled insulin (Exubera) trials and a two year extension trial. J Clin Endocrinol Metab 2005;90:3287–94.

279. McElduff A, Mather LE, Kam PC, Clauson P. Influence of acute respiratory tract infection on the absorption of inhaled insulin using the AERx insulin diabetes management system. Br J Clin Pharmacol 2005;59:546–51.

280. Kidron M, Dinh S, Menachem Y, Abbas R, Variano B, Goldberg M, Arbit E, Bar-On H. A novel per-oral insulin formulation: proof of concept study in non-diabetic subjects. Diabetic Med 2004;21:354–7.

281. Clement S, Dandona P, Still JG, Kosutic G. Oral modified insulin (HIM2) in patients with type 1 diabetes mellitus: results from a phaseI/II clinical trial. Metabolism 2004;53:54–8.

282. Winston DC. Suicide via insulin overdose in nondiabetics: the New Mexico experience. Am J Forensic Med Pathol 2000;21(3):237–40.

283. Bretz SW, Richards JR. Munchausen syndrome presenting acutely in the emergency department. J Emerg Med 2000;18(4):417–20.

284. Junge M, Tsokos M, Puschel K. Suicide by insulin injection in combination with beta-blocker application. Forensic Sci Int 2000;113(1–3):457–60.

285. Matsumura M, Nakashima A, Tofuku Y. Electrolyte disorders following massive insulin overdose in a patient with type 2 diabetes. Intern Med 2000;39(1):55–7.

286. Morris AD, Boyle DI, McMahon AD, Pearce H, Evans JM, Newton RW, Jung RT, MacDonald TM. ACE inhibitor use is associated with hospitalization for severe hypoglycemia in patients with diabetes. DARTS/MEMO Collaboration. Diabetes Audit and Research in Tayside, Scotland. Medicines Monitoring Unit. Diabetes Care 1997;20(9):1363–7.

287. Cheyne EH, Sherwin RS, Lunt MJ, Cavan DA, Thomas PW, Kerr D. Influence of alcohol on cognitive performance during mild hypoglycemia: implications for type 1 diabetes. Diabetic Med 2004;21:230–7.

288. Thamer M, Ray NF, Taylor T. Association between antihypertensive drug use and hypoglycemia: a case-control study of diabetic users of insulin or sulfonylureas. Clin Ther 1999;21(8):1387–400.

289. Wicklmayr M, Rett K, Dietze G, Mehnert H. Effects of beta-blocking agents on insulin secretion and glucose disposal. Horm Metab Res Suppl 1990;22:29–33.

290. Cooper JW. Fatal asymptomatic hypoglycemia in an elderly insulin-dependent diabetic patient taking an oral beta-blocking medication. Diabetes Care 1998;21(12):2197–8.

291. Kljucar S, Rost KL, Landen H. Ciprofloxacin in der Therapie des nosobomialen pneumonie: Eine Anwendungs beobachtung bei 676 patienten. [Ciprofloxacin in the treatment of hospital-acquired pneumonia: a surveillance study in 676 patients.] Pneumologie 2002;56(10):599–604.

292. Colli A, Cocciolo M, Francobandiera F, Rogantin F, Cattalini N. Diabetic ketoacidosis associated with clozapine treatment. Diabetes Care 1999;22(1):176–7.

293. Isotani H, Kameoka K. Hypoglycemia associated with maprotiline in a patient with type 1 diabetes. Diabetes Care 1999;22(5):862–3.

294. Gatta B, Rigalleau V, Gin H. Diabetic ketoacidosis with olanzapine treatment. Diabetes Care 1999;22(6):1002–3.

295. Ng RSH, Darko DA, Hillson RM. Street drug use among young patients with type 1 diabetes in the UK. Diabetic Med 2004;21:295–6.

296. Nesto RW, Bell D, Bonow RO, Fonseca V, Grundy SM, Horton ES, Winter ML, Porte D, Semenkovich CF, Smith S, Young LH, Kahn R. Thiazolidinedione use, fluid retention and congestive heart failure. Diabetes Care 2004;27:256–63.

297. Mehmet S, Quan G, Thomas S, Goldsmith D. Important causes of hypoglycaemia in patients with diabetes on peritoneal dialysis. Diabet Med 2001;18(8):679–82.

299. Frystyk J, Chantelau E. Progression of diabetic retinopathy during improved metabolic control may be treated with reduced insulin dosage and /or somatostatin analogue administration – a case report. Growth Horm IGF Res 2005;15:130–5.

299. Sämann A, Mühlhauser I, Bender R, Kloos Ch, Müller UA. Glycaemic control and severe hypoglycaemia following training in flexible, intensive insulin therapy to enable dietary freedom in people with type 1 diabetes: a prospective implementation study. Diabetologia 2005;48:1965–70.

300. Cordray JP, Merceron RE, Guillerd X, Nys P. Baisse du fer sérique due à l'auto-surveillance glycémique chez le

diabétique. [Low serum iron level caused by self-monitoring of blood glucose in the diabetic patient.] Presse Méd 1991;20(7):310.

301. Cox NH, Dufton PA. Pyoderma gangrenosum and fingertip ulceration in a diabetic patient. Pract Diabetes 1987;4:236.

302. Prakash PK, Banerjee M, Harlow J, Hanna FW. An unusual case of hypoglycaemia. Diabet Med 2001;18(9):769–70.

303. Steward DE, Khardori R. An avoidable cause of false home glucose measurements. Diabetes Care 2001;24(4):794.

304. Jungheim K, Koschinsky T. Risky delay of hypoglycemia detection by glucose monitoring at the arm. Diabetes Care 2001;24(7):1303–6.

305. McGarraugh G. Glucose monitoring at the arm. Diabetes Care 2001;24:1304–6.

306. Koschinsky T, Heinemann L. Sensors for glucose monitoring: technical and clinical aspects. Diabetes Metab Res Rev 2001;17(2):113–23.

307. Fineberg SE, Bergenstal RM, Bernstein RM, Laffel LM, Schwartz SL. Use of an automated device for alternative site blood glucose monitoring. Diabetes Care 2001;24(7):1217–20.

308. Jungheim K, Wientjes KJ, Heinemann L, Lodwig V, Koschinsky T, Schoonen AJGlucose Monitoring Study Group. Subcutaneous continuous glucose monitoring: feasibility of a new microdialysis-based glucose sensor system. Diabetes Care 2001;24(9):1696–7.

Insulin aspart

See also Insulin

General Information

Insulin aspart is a rapid-acting synthetic insulin in which proline is replaced by aspartate at position 28 in the B chain. Insulin aspart has been reviewed (1). Its adverse effects do not differ from those of soluble human insulin and it has a similar effect on the blood glucose concentration (2).

A new development is the binding of two 9-fluorenyl-methoxy-carbonyl moieties to two amino acids in the structure of aspart insulin, phenylalanine and lysine (3). This compound has no biological activity but gradually releases its groups and keeps diabetic animals in a good metabolic state over 2–3 days. Experiments in humans have not yet been reported.

Aspart insulin and biphasic insulin aspart (30% soluble rapid-acting insulin and 70% protamine-bound aspart insulin) have been reviewed (4).

Comparative studies

In a double-blind, crossover study of insulin aspart or soluble human insulin before meals and protamine zinc insulin before bedtime, 90 of 104 patients with type 1 diabetes completed the trial (5). Insulin aspart improved postprandial control by reducing hyperglycemic and hypoglycemic variations, but night-time control was inferior. There were 547 hypoglycemic episodes in the aspart period compared with 615 in the regular insulin period (no significant difference). However, there were only 20 major hypoglycemic events in 16 patients using aspart versus 44 events in 24 patients using human insulin. One patient was withdrawn with fatigue and anorexia during aspart. Convulsions during hypoglycemia occurred once in each group.

Insulin aspart had an increased maximal effect compared with regular insulin in euglycemic clamps in non-diabetics (6).

In an open comparison of insulin aspart and regular human insulin for 6 months in 882 patients with type 1 diabetes and extended to 714 patients for another 6 months, postprandial glucose concentrations were lower with insulin aspart (7). HbA$_{1c}$ was slightly but significantly lower (7.78 versus 7.93%). There were no differences in hypoglycemic periods or adverse events.

Insulin aspart has been compared with regular insulin in 1065 patients for 26 weeks (8). HbA$_{1c}$ improved significantly with aspart. The number of major attacks of hypoglycemia fell in the aspart group from 11 to 8%; there were no other differences.

Insulin aspart has been compared with buffered regular insulin by continuous subcutaneous infusion (9). There was some crystal formation with both formulations, but less with insulin aspart. Patients who used aspart required a slightly higher basal dose of insulin but had fewer unexplained attacks of hypoglycemia.

Frequent addition of isophane to a regimen of insulin aspart is unnecessary, as has been shown in a multicenter, multinational, randomized, open study in 368 patients followed for 64 weeks (10). Frequent addition of isophane up to four times daily to insulin aspart did not improve HbA$_{1c}$ or change the number of episodes of hypoglycemia compared with regular insulin combined with isophane. Only postprandial blood glucose concentrations were reduced.

When insulin lispro and insulin aspart were compared in a single-blind, randomized, crossover study in 14 patients with type 1 diabetes, insulin lispro had a faster onset of action but a shorter duration (11). However, in another study the pharmacokinetic and the pharmacodynamic profiles of insulin aspart compared with human insulin were the same in 24 healthy Japanese as in non-Japanese (12). Insulin aspart and insulin lispro were equally effective in another 24 patients with type 1 diabetes (13).

Combination with long-acting insulin

In a multinational study for 6 months in 448 patients with type 1 diabetes, two-thirds were given the long-acting insulin detemir and one-third received isophane, both in addition to premeal rapid-acting insulin aspart (14). HbA$_{1c}$ concentrations were comparable, but in the detemir group the risk of hypoglycemia was 22% less and the risk of nocturnal hypoglycemia was 34% lower. There were two cases of severe hypoglycemia with detemir and one with isophane. Three patients who used detemir developed reactions at the injection site (pain, myalgia, redness, or lipodystrophy) compared with one who used isophane (itching). One potentially allergic reaction was possibly related to detemir.

The new, short-acting insulins can be bound to protamine, allowing the preparation of mixed formulations. In an open, randomized, single-dose, three-way, crossover trial biphasic insulin aspart 30 (30% aspart plus 70% protaminated aspart, BIAsp 30), biphasic insulin lispro 25 (25% lispro plus 75% protaminated lispro, Mix 25), and biphasic human insulin 30 (30% regular plus 70% isophane insulin, BHI 30) were compared in 45 patients (15). Biphasic insulin aspart improved postprandial control better. There were 23 episodes of hypoglycemia with BIAsp 30, 19 with Mix 25, and 11 with BHI 30; two episodes with BIAsp 30, five with Mix 25, and two with BHI 30 required third-party intervention.

When 30% insulin aspart plus 70% protamine aspart was compared with the same mixture of regular plus isophane insulins, both injected twice-daily for 12 weeks, in 294 patients with type 1 and type 2 diabetes, control was better with the aspart mixture (16). There were fewer episodes of major hypoglycemia (20 versus 42) but the same number of minor episodes (362) with aspart.

Placebo-controlled studies

In a double-blind, crossover study with insulin aspart and human insulin in type 1 diabetes, human insulin was given 30 minutes before a meal with placebo immediately before the meal, or placebo was given 30 minutes before the meal with aspart insulin or human insulin immediately before the meal (17). On average, insulin aspart was absorbed twice as fast as human insulin. Postprandial glucose control improved on aspart. There were no episodes of serious hypoglycemia.

Organs and Systems

Immunologic

When short-acting insulins are given to patients who are allergic to regular insulin the allergic reactions can disappear. Although the short-acting insulins often have the same immunogenic epitopes, rapid dissociation of the fast-acting insulins into monomers can reduce their antigenic effects. Insulin lispro is known to be beneficial, and this has also been reported for aspart insulin (18).

- A 45-year-old man with type 2 diabetes treated with glibenclamide and metformin received combined chemotherapy for non-Hodgkin's lymphoma and was given premixed insulin. He developed local wheal-and-flare reactions immediately after the injections. Skin prick tests were positive for various types of insulin but weakly positive for lispro and negative for insulin aspart. He tolerated aspart insulin without any allergic reactions.

A few patients treated with insulin aspart developed antibodies, which cross-reacted with antibodies against human insulin and fell after 3 months (19). In lipodystrophy with lipoatrophic diabetes high insulin resistance is often found, for which leptin deficiency is one contributory factor.

Allergic reactions have been described with insulin aspart.

- A 53-year-old woman had type 2 diabetes that was not well controlled with diet and oral hypoglycemic drugs (20). She took intermediate-acting insulins, and after 2 months noticed redness and itching at injection sites. When she used insulin aspart and insulin lispro successively, the local reactions continued. She had a high serum concentration of total IgE (748 IU/ml; reference range below 400) and insulin-specific IgE (20 IU/ml; reference range below 0.34), positive insulin antibodies, and positive prick tests for insulin lispro, insulin aspart, human insulin, porcine insulin, and protamine. With intensive nutrition therapy and oral drugs her HbA_{1c} fell to 5.5%.
- A 29-year-old woman with raised insulin concentrations during therapy had lipodystrophy and high insulin antibody titers with high binding capacity and high affinity (21).

Insulin antibodies are rarely found in patients with lipodystrophy.

References

1. Lindholm A, Jacobsen LV. Clinical pharmacokinetics and pharmacodynamics of insulin aspart. Clin Pharmacokinet 2001;40(9):641–59.
2. Heinemann L, Weyer C, Rauhaus M, Heinrichs S, Heise T. Variability of the metabolic effect of soluble insulin and the rapid-acting insulin analogue insulin aspart. Diabetes Care 1998;21(11):1910–4.
3. Gershonov E, Shechter Y, Fridkin M. New concept for long-acting insulin: spontaneous conversion of an inactive modified insulin to the active hormone in circulation: 9-fluorenylmethoxycarbonyl derivative of insulin. Diabetes 1999;48(7):1437–42.
4. Chapman TM, Noble S, Goa KL. Insulin aspart: a review of its use in the management of type 1 and 2 diabetes mellitus. Drugs 2002;62(13):1945–81.
5. Home PD, Lindholm A, Hylleberg B, Round PUK Insulin Aspart Study Group. Improved glycemic control with insulin aspart: a multicenter randomized double-blind crossover trial in type 1 diabetic patients. Diabetes Care 1998;21(11):1904–9.
6. Mudaliar SR, Lindberg FA, Joyce M, Beerdsen P, Strange P, Lin A, Henry RR. Insulin aspart (B28 asp-insulin): a fast-acting analogue of human insulin: absorption kinetics and action profile compared with regular human insulin in healthy nondiabetic subjects. Diabetes Care 1999;22(9):1501–6.
7. Raskin P, Guthrie RA, Leiter L, Riis A, Jovanovic L. Use of insulin aspart, a fast-acting insulin analogue, as the mealtime insulin in the management of patients with type 1 diabetes. Diabetes Care 2000;23(5):583–8.
8. Home PD, Lindholm A, Riis AEuropean Insulin Aspart Study Group. Insulin aspart vs. human insulin in the management of long-term blood glucose control in type 1

diabetes mellitus: a randomized controlled trial. Diabet Med 2000;17(11):762–70.

9. Bode BW, Strange P. Efficacy, safety, and pump compatibility of insulin aspart used in continuous subcutaneous insulin infusion therapy in patients with type 1 diabetes. Diabetes Care 2001;24(1):69–72.

10. DeVries JH, Lindholm A, Jacobsen JL, Heine RJ, Home PDTri-Continental Insulin Aspart Study Group. A randomized trial of insulin aspart with intensified basal NPH insulin supplementation in people with Type 1 diabetes. Diabet Med 2003;20(4):312–8.

11. Hedman CA, Lindstrom T, Arnqvist HJ. Direct comparison of insulin lispro and aspart shows small differences in plasma insulin profiles after subcutaneous injection in type 1 diabetes. Diabetes Care 2001;24(6):1120–1.

12. Kaku K, Matsuda M, Urae A, Irie S. Pharmacokinetics and pharmacodynamics of insulin aspart, a rapid-acting analogue of human insulin, in healthy Japanese volunteers. Diabetes Res Clin Pract 2000;49(2-3):119–26.

13. Plank J, Wutte A, Brunner G, Siebenhofer A, Semlitsch B, Sommer R, Hirschberger S, Pieber TR. A direct comparison of insulin aspart and insulin lispro in patients with type 1 diabetes. Diabetes Care 2002;25(11):2053–7.

14. Vague P, Selam JL, Skeie S, De Leeuw I, Elte JW, Haahr H, Kristensen A, Draeger E. Insulin detemir is associated with more predictable glycemic control and reduced risk of hypoglycemia than NPH insulin in patients with type 1 diabetes on a basal-bolus regimen with premeal insulin aspart. Diabetes Care 2003;26(3):590–6.

15. Hermansen K, Colombo M, Storgaard H, O'Stergaard A, Kolendorf K, Madsbad S. Improved postprandial glycemic control with biphasic insulin aspart relative to biphasic insulin lispro and biphasic human insulin in patients with type 2 diabetes. Diabetes Care 2002;25(5):883–8.

16. Boehm BO, Home PD, Behrend C, Kamp NM, Lindholm A. Premixed insulin aspart 30 vs. premixed human insulin 30/70 twice daily: a randomized trial in Type 1 and Type 2 diabetic patients. Diabet Med 2002;19(5):393–9.

17. Lindholm A, McEwen J, Riis AP. Improved postprandial glycemic control with insulin aspart. A randomized double-blind cross-over trial in type 1 diabetes. Diabetes Care 1999;22(5):801–5.

18. Airaghi L, Lorini M, Tedeschi A. The insulin analogue aspart: a safe alternative in insulin allergy. Diabetes Care 2001;24(11):2000.

19. Lindholm A, Jensen LB, Home PD, Raskin P, Boehm BO, Rastam J. Immune responses to insulin aspart and biphasic insulin aspart in people with type 1 and type 2 diabetes. Diabetes Care 2002;25(5):876–82.

20. Takata H, Kumon Y, Osaki F, Kumagai C, Arii K, Ikeda Y, Suehiro T, Hashimoto K. The human insulin analogue aspart is not the almighty solution for insulin allergy. Diabetes Care 2003;26(1):253–4.

21. Usui H, Makino H, Shikata K, Sugimoto T, Wada J, Yamana J, Matsuda M, Yoneda M, Koshima I. A case of congenital generalized lipodystrophy with lipoatrophic diabetes developing anti-insulin antibodies. Diabet Med 2002;19(9):794–5.

Insulin detemir

See also Insulin

General Information

Insulin detemir is a long-acting insulin analogue that lacks threonine at the B30 position and is acylated with a 14-carbon myristoyl fatty acid side-chain at the epsilon-amino group of the lysine in the B28 position. This stimulates binding to albumin and increases the half-life, extending its duration of action.

The pharmacokinetic profile of detemir does not differ in various age groups, including children. The profile is less variable than that of NPH insulin (1).

Comparative studies

In healthy volunteers, there was a dose-related increase in blood insulin concentrations after the administration of insulin detemir (2). However, there was no clear dose-response metabolic effect and individual variability was high.

Insulin detemir has been compared with protamine zinc insulin in 59 patients with type 1 diabetes (3). All used insulin detemir for 6 weeks and protamine zinc insulin for 6 weeks in a randomized order. About 2.35 times higher doses of detemir were necessary than protamine zinc insulin. Fasting blood glucose concentrations were lower at the end of the detemir period and there were fewer attacks of hypoglycemia.

In a 6-month, multinational, open, parallel-group comparison of insulin detemir and protamine zinc insulin in 448 patients with type 1 diabetes, the two treatments produced comparable HbA_{1c} concentrations and fasting plasma glucose concentrations with less within-subject variation in fasting blood glucose with insulin detemir (4). The risk of hypoglycemia was 22% lower with insulin detemir and 34% lower for nocturnal hypoglycemia.

Combination with short-acting insulin

In a multinational study for 6 months in 448 patients with type 1 diabetes, two-thirds were given insulin detemir and one-third received isophane, both in addition to premeal rapid-acting insulin aspart (4). HbA_{1c} concentrations were comparable, but in the detemir group the risk of hypoglycemia was 22% less and the risk of nocturnal hypoglycemia was 34% lower. There were two cases of severe hypoglycemia with detemir and one with isophane. Three patients who used detemir developed reactions at the injection site (pain, myalgia, redness, or lipodystrophy) compared with one who used isophane (itching). One potentially allergic reaction was possibly related to detemir.

Organs and Systems

Metabolism

Phase 3 trials have suggested that insulin detemir is associated with less weight gain (0.4 kg) than NPH insulin (1.3 kg); the mechanism is uncertain (5).

Immunologic

An unspecified allergic reaction to insulin detemir has been reported (4).

References

1. Danne T, Lüpke K, Walte K, Von Schuetz W, Gall M-A. Insulin detemir is characterized by a consistent pharmacokinetic profile across age-groups in children, adolescents, and adults with type 1 diabetes. Diabetes Care 2003;26:3087–92.
2. Heinemann L, Sinha K, Weyer C, Loftager M, Hirschberger S, Heise T. Time-action profile of the soluble, fatty acid acylated, long-acting insulin analogue NN304. Diabet Med 1999;16(4):332–8.
3. Hermansen K, Madsbad S, Perrild H, Kristensen A, Axelsen M. Comparison of the soluble basal insulin analogue insulin detemir with NPH insulin: a randomized open crossover trial in type 1 diabetic subjects on basal-bolus therapy. Diabetes Care 2001;24(2):296–301.
4. Vague P, Selam JL, Skeie S, De Leeuw I, Elte JW, Haahr H, Kristensen A, Draeger E. Insulin detemir is associated with more predictable glycemic control and reduced risk of hypoglycemia than NPH insulin in patients with type 1 diabetes on a basal-bolus regimen with premeal insulin aspart. Diabetes Care 2003;26(3):590–6.
5. Khan R. Weight gain and insulin therapy. Br J Diabetes Vasc Dis 2004;4:264–7.

Insulin glargine

See also Insulin

General Information

Insulin glargine is a new long-acting human insulin analogue, in which phenylalanine is removed from site 30 of the C terminal of the B chain and two arginine molecules replace it, adding two positive charges; asparagine on site 21 of the A chain is replaced by the more stable glycine to avoid deamination. Older long-acting insulins, such as protamine zinc insulin and insulin zinc suspension (crystalline) (ultralente), had a maximal hypoglycemic effect after about 20 hours (in the middle of the night), and the glucose-lowering action then abated gradually. The newer analogues have a more constant profile of action (1–3).

The binding of insulin analogues to insulin and IGF-I receptors and their metabolic and mitogenic properties have been evaluated in vitro (4). In general the metabolic potencies correlated with insulin receptor binding and the mitogenic properties correlated with IGF-I receptor binding. The rapid-acting analogues resembled insulin, except that the binding of insulin lispro to the IGF-I receptor was slightly increased. Insulin glargine had a 6- to 8-fold greater affinity for IGF-I and mitogenic potency than human insulin (suggesting greater growth-stimulating potential). In insulin detemir the balance between the metabolic and mitogenic potency was not changed, but receptor affinity was reduced, which may explain its lower efficacy on a molar base in humans.

Insulin glargine has been reviewed (5,6). The general conclusion was that it is an effective long-acting insulin with no pronounced peaks of action. Patients using insulin glargine have a reduced risk of hypoglycemia. Insulin glargine, which is metabolically active for at least 24 hours, could have an overlapping effect after a second injection. However, there was no evidence of accumulation when insulin glargine, mean dose 24 U/day, was used in combination with insulin lispro for 11 days (7). In reaction to comments, and discussing whether fluctuations in insulin concentrations still occur during the administration of insulin glargine, the authors agreed that the dose should be constant for at least 2 days before a change is made. It is also not clear whether higher doses of insulin glargine could accumulate because of slower inactivation (8).

Clinical studies of new long-acting insulins, have been reviewed, mainly with reference to insulin glargine (9). The author concluded that these new analogues have efficacy and safety advantages over NPH insulin.

Observational studies

In 82 patients transferred from once or twice daily NPH to insulin glargine once daily (and unchanged usual short-acting insulin) to reduce nocturnal hypoglycemia and to improve fasting glucose the first effect was a reduction in HbA_{1c} of about 0.3% (10). Patients with a high HbA_{1c} or pre-supper glucose concentrations were given insulin glargine twice daily (n = 20). The 62 patients who took a single dose of insulin glargine had an improved HbA_{1c} of 0.6% and the patients who used a split regimen had a final mean HbA_{1c} 0.5% lower than the starting value.

Comparative studies

The absorption of insulin glargine was delayed compared with protamine zinc insulin in a study using radioactive tracers (11).

In single-dose, double-blind, euglycemic clamp studies, insulin glargine had a smoother metabolic effect with a peakless profile of action starting at 2–4 hours and continuing over 24 hours than protamine zinc insulin, whose peak occurred at 4 hours and whose activity subsequently fell (12).

In a randomized, parallel-group study, there were fewer episodes of nocturnal and serious hypoglycemia when insulin glargine was compared with once- or twice-daily protamine zinc insulin (13,14). Other adverse reactions and reactions at the injection sites were identical.

Insulin glargine did not cause a peak in blood insulin concentration, compared with protamine zinc insulin and crystalline insulin zinc suspension (ultralente); the effect lasted 24 hours, almost comparable to continuous subcutaneous infusion of a short-acting insulin (15).

In general, one daily injection of insulin glargine gives more constant insulin concentrations and fewer nightly attacks of hypoglycemia than protamine zinc insulin. Treatment satisfaction was constantly better with insulin glargine in 517 patients (16). There was a consistent mean reduction in the perceived frequency of attacks of hypoglycemia. Other adverse effects were not mentioned.

- A 60-year-old man with type 2 diabetes received radiation therapy for a carcinoma of the esophagus and needed continuous enteric tube feeding (17). One daily injection of glargine controlled his diabetes well: his HbA_{1c} concentration was 6.1% and he had no episodes of hypoglycemia for almost 4 months. This made continuous infusion of a short-acting insulin unnecessary.

However, control can be inadequate with a once-daily injection.

- A 53-year-old man with type 1 diabetes needed tube feeding after a stroke and received glargine insulin once daily (18). He had marked hyperglycemia after 22 hours and when the dose was divided into two equal doses every 12 hours, the hyperglycemia was reduced.

Insulin glargine and protamine zinc insulin have been compared in 349 children and adolescents in a multicenter, open, randomized study (19). Besides the usual thrice-daily regimen of regular insulin they took either insulin glargine at bedtime or protamine zinc insulin at bedtime or twice daily. HbA_{1c} did not differ. The target for fasting blood glucose was 4.4–8.8 mmol/l, and 5% more patients who used insulin glargine reached the target (44% compared with 39% of the patients who used protamine zinc insulin). Symptomatic hypoglycemia was similar with the two treatments.

Six children were treated with insulin glargine and six with protamine zinc insulin as the long-acting insulin component (20). After 3 months, unbound insulin concentrations were lower during the night with insulin glargine. There were three cases of hypoglycemia with protamine zinc insulin and one with insulin glargine.

In a 24-week, randomized, open, multicenter study NPH insulin + insulin glargine was compared with oral hypoglycemic drugs alone in 764 overweight patients with type 2 diabetes; HbA_{1c} and fasting plasma glucose were reduced to the same extent (21). The target HbA_{1c} was 7.0% or less. When this goal was reached, nocturnal hypoglycemia was less frequent with insulin glargine (33 versus 27%) and other categories of symptomatic hypoglycemia (such as symptomatic events or confirmed events at various glucose concentrations) were 21–48% less frequent with insulin glargine.

In a comparison of combinations of glimepiride (3 mg/day) and NPH insulin at bedtime or insulin glargine in the morning or at bedtime in 695 patients for 24 weeks both morning and bedtime insulin glargine reduced nocturnal

hypoglycemia and morning insulin glargine provided better glycemic control than bedtime NPH and bedtime insulin glargine (22).

Combination with short-acting insulin

Insulin glargine plus a short-acting insulin has been compared with isophane insulin for 4 weeks in a double-blind study in 256 patients with type 1 diabetes (23). The patients were all taking once- or twice-daily isophane insulin and continued to do so or switched to insulin glargine with added zinc 30 or 80 micrograms/ml at bedtime. The patients who used insulin glargine had more attacks of hypoglycemia at the start of the study than those who used isophane insulin, but this tended to equalize during the 4 weeks. Fasting plasma glucose was lower in those who used insulin glargine. HbA_{1c} concentrations were not reported.

The combinations insulin lispro + insulin glargine and regular + isophane have been compared in a randomized, crossover study for 32 weeks in 25 patients (24). HbA_{1c} was not different, but the total insulin dose was lower with insulin lispro + insulin glargine and there were fewer episodes of nocturnal hypoglycemia.

Organs and Systems

Metabolism

In 619 patients with type 1 diabetes treated with protamine zinc insulin and insulin lispro, randomized to once-daily insulin glargine or to once-daily or twice-daily protamine zinc insulin for 16 weeks in an open study, there was no difference in the frequency of hypoglycemic episodes, severe hypoglycemia, or HbA_{1c} (25). Fasting plasma glucose concentrations were lower with insulin glargine.

In 518 patients with type 2 diabetes using protamine zinc insulin, with or without short-acting insulin, randomized to insulin glargine or protamine zinc insulin, there was less nocturnal hypoglycemia with insulin glargine (26). HbA_{1c} and mild symptomatic hypoglycemia was the same in both groups.

In 426 patients with type 2 diabetes poorly controlled with oral therapy, randomized to protamine zinc insulin or insulin glargine, glucose concentrations after dinner were lower with insulin glargine and there were significantly fewer attacks of hypoglycemia (27). HbA_{1c} was 8.2 and 8.1% with insulin glargine and protamine zinc insulin respectively.

Immunologic

Insulin glargine solved a problem in a man with type 1 diabetes after pork, beef, and human insulins had elicited allergic reactions (28). Antihistamines ameliorated the reactions but did not resolve them. Insulin glargine elicited no reactions, even when regular insulin was given. This case suggests that the A chain, which is modified in insulin glargine, is part of the allergic epitope. Tolerance to insulin glargine appeared to suppress allergy to regular insulin.

Drug Administration

Drug formulations

In contrast to most medium- and long-acting formulations, insulin glargine is a clear solution. In two cases, patients gave themselves rapid-acting insulin instead of glargine.

- A 25-year-old woman and a 52-year-old woman injected lispro instead of insulin glargine (29). The first realized her mistake and managed to prevent severe hypoglycemia by eating continuously, despite a fall in blood glucose to 3.7 mmol/l. The other had a blood glucose of 3.1 mmol/l and recovered after intravenous dextrose.

Four other mistakes have been reported (30,31). The authors advised the use of pens for injection of short-acting insulins, as all the mistakes were made by patients who used vials and syringes to administer both types of insulin.

References

1. Bolli GB, Di Marchi RD, Park GD, Pramming S, Koivisto VA. Insulin analogues and their potential in the management of diabetes mellitus. Diabetologia 1999;42(10):1151–67.
2. Bolli GB, Owens DR. Insulin glargine. Lancet 2000;356(9228):443–5.
3. McKeage K, Goa KL. Insulin glargine: a review of its therapeutic use as a long-acting agent for the management of type 1 and 2 diabetes mellitus. Drugs 2001;61(11):1599–624.
4. Kurtzhals P, Schaffer L, Sorensen A, Kristensen C, Jonassen I, Schmid C, Trub T. Correlations of receptor binding and metabolic and mitogenic potencies of insulin analogues designed for clinical use. Diabetes 2000;49(6):999–1005.
5. Campbell RK, White JR, Levien T, Baker D. Insulin glargine. Clin Ther 2001;23(12):1938–57.
6. Home PD, Ashwell SG. An overview of insulin glargine. Diabetes Metab Res Rev 2002;18(Suppl 3):S57–63.
7. Heise T, Bott S, Rave K, Dressler A, Rosskamp R, Heinemann L. No evidence for accumulation of insulin glargine (LANTUS): a multiple injection study in patients with Type 1 diabetes. Diabet Med 2002;19(6):490–5.
8. Biermann E. No evidence for accumulation of insulin glargine (LANTUS). Diabet Med 2003;20(4):333–5.
9. Barnett AH. A review of basal insulins. Diabetic Med 2003;20:873–85.
10. Albright ES, Desmond R, Bell DSH. Efficacy of conversion from bedtime NPH insulin injection to once- or twice-daily injections of insulin glargine in type 1 diabetic patients using basal/bolus therapy. Diabetes Care 2004;27:632–3.
11. Owens DR, Coates PA, Luzio SD, Tinbergen JP, Kurzhals R. Pharmacokinetics of ^{125}I-labeled insulin glargine (HOE 901) in healthy men: comparison with NPH insulin and the influence of different subcutaneous injection sites. Diabetes Care 2000;23(6):813–9.
12. Heinemann L, Linkeschova R, Rave K, Hompesch B, Sedlak M, Heise T. Time-action profile of the long-acting insulin analogue insulin glargine (HOE901) in comparison with those of NPH insulin and placebo. Diabetes Care 2000;23(5):644–9.
13. Pieber TR, Eugene-Jolchine I, Derobert E. Efficacy and safety of HOE 901 versus NPH insulin in patients with type 1 diabetes. The European Study Group of HOE 901 in type 1 diabetes. Diabetes Care 2000;23(2):157–62.
14. Ratner RE, Hirsch IB, Neifing JL, Garg SK, Mecca TE, Wilson CAU.S. Study Group of Insulin Glargine in Type 1 Diabetes. Less hypoglycemia with insulin glargine in intensive insulin therapy for type 1 diabetes. Diabetes Care 2000;23(5):639–43.
15. Lepore M, Pampanelli S, Fanelli C, Porcellati F, Bartocci L, Di Vincenzo A, Cordoni C, Costa E, Brunetti P, Bolli GB. Pharmacokinetics and pharmacodynamics of subcutaneous injection of long-acting human insulin analogue glargine, NPH insulin, and ultralente human insulin and continuous subcutaneous infusion of insulin lispro. Diabetes 2000;49(12):2142–8.
16. Ooi C, Mullen P, Williams G. Insulin lispro: the ideal pump insulin for patients with severe hypoglycemic unawareness? Diabetes Care 1999;22(9):1598–9.
17. Putz D, Kabadi UM. Insulin glargine in continuous enteric tube feeding. Diabetes Care 2002;25(10):1889–90.
18. Clement S, Bowen-Wright H. Twenty-four hour action of insulin glargine (Lantus) may be too short for once-daily dosing: a case report. Diabetes Care 2002;25(8):1479–80.
19. Schober E, Schoenle E, Van Dyk J, Wernicke-Panten KPediatric Study Group of Insulin Glargine. Comparative trial between insulin glargine and NPH insulin in children and adolescents with type 1 diabetes. Diabetes Care 2001;24(11):2005–8.
20. Mohn A, Strang S, Wernicke-Panten K, Lang AM, Edge JA, Dunger DB. Nocturnal glucose control and free insulin levels in children with type 1 diabetes by use of the long-acting insulin HOE 901 as part of a three-injection regimen. Diabetes Care 2000;23(4):557–9.
21. Riddle MC, Rosenstock J, Gerich J. The treat to target trial: randomized addition of glargine or human NPH insulin to oral therapy of type 2 diabetic patients. Diabetes Care 2003;26:3080–6.
22. Fritsche A, Schweitzer MA, Häring H-U, 4001 Study group. Glimepiride, combined with morning insulin glargine, bedtime neutral protamine Hagedorn insulin, or bedtime insulin glargine in patients with type 2 diabetes. Ann Intern Med 2003;138:952–9.
23. Rosenstock J, Park G, Zimmerman J. U.S. Insulin Glargine (HOE 901) Type 1 Diabetes Investigator Group. Basal insulin glargine (HOE 901) versus NPH insulin in patients with type 1 diabetes on multiple daily insulin regimens. U.S. Insulin Glargine (HOE 901) Type 1 Diabetes Investigator Group Diabetes Care 2000;23(8):1137–42.
24. Murphy NP, Keane SM, Ong KK, Ford-Adams M, Edge JA, Acerini CL, Dunger DB. Randomized crossover trial of insulin glargine plus lispro or NPH insulin plus regular human insulin in adolescents with type 1 diabetes on intensive insulin regimens. Diabetes Care 2003;26(3):799–804.
25. Raskin P, Klaff L, Bergenstal R, Halle JP, Donley D, Mecca T. A 16-week comparison of the novel insulin analogue insulin glargine (HOE 901) and NPH human insulin used with insulin lispro in patients with type 1 diabetes. Diabetes Care 2000;23(11):1666–71.
26. Rosenstock J, Schwartz SL, Clark CM Jr, Park GD, Donley DW, Edwards MB. Basal insulin therapy in type 2 diabetes: 28-week comparison of insulin glargine (HOE 901) and NPH insulin. Diabetes Care 2001;24(4):631–6.
27. Yki-Jarvinen H, Dressler A, Ziemen MHOE 901/300s Study Group. Less nocturnal hypoglycemia and better

post-dinner glucose control with bedtime insulin glargine compared with bedtime NPH insulin during insulin combination therapy in type 2 diabetes. HOE 901/3002 Study Group. Diabetes Care 2000;23(8):1130–6.

28. Moriyama H, Nagata M, Fujihira K, Yamada K, Chowdhury SA, Chakrabarty S, Jin Z, Yasuda H, Ueda H, Yokono K. Treatment with human analogue (GlyA21, ArgB31, ArgB32) insulin glargine (HOE901) resolves a generalized allergy to human insulin in type 1 diabetes. Diabetes Care 2001;24(2):411–2.

29. Adlersberg MA, Fernando S, Spollett GR, Inzucchi SE. Glargine and lispro: two cases of mistaken identity. Diabetes Care 2002;25(2):404–5.

30. Schutta MH. Reducing mistakes in patient administration of glargine and lispro. Diabetes Care 2002;25(6):1098–9.

31. Phillips W, Lando H. Insulin confusion: an observation. Diabetes Care 2002;25(6):1103–4.

Insulin lispro

See also Insulin

General Information

Insulin lispro induces more rapid and constant release of insulin from the injection site, since it consists of monomeric insulin. The change of one or more amino acids in the insulin molecule prevents insulin from forming dimers or hexamers. More rapid absorption, rapid availability, and rapid inactivation make the action better than that of endogenously secreted insulin. When the interval between meals is long, the premeal blood glucose concentration increases rapidly.

After the administration of insulin lispro it is not necessary to delay a meal until sufficient insulin is absorbed. Insulin lispro can be given immediately before or during a meal and can be used when rapid action is important, as in outpatient treatment of ketonuria (1) or in continuous subcutaneous insulin infusion (2). Insulin lispro can be successful in patients with subcutaneous insulin resistance (3).

Observational studies

During Ramadan, insulin lispro reduced the number of attacks of hypoglycemia and reduced postprandial blood glucose (4). It also reduced post-snack raised blood glucose concentrations when sugar-rich snacks were used (5).

Combination with long-acting insulin

The combinations insulin lispro + insulin glargine and regular + NPH have been compared in a randomized, crossover study for 32 weeks in 25 patients (6). HbA$_{1c}$ was not different, but the total insulin dose was lower with insulin lispro + insulin glargine and there were fewer episodes of nocturnal hypoglycemia.

The new short-acting insulins can be bound to protamine, allowing the preparation of mixed formulations. In a randomized, open, crossover study for 24 weeks, a 50% mixture of insulin lispro and protamine lispro injected immediately before each meal plus NPH in the evening gave a comparable profile to regular insulin injected 30 minutes before each meal plus NPH in the evening (7). There were no differences in HbA$_{1c}$ or episodes of hypoglycemia. When Mix25TM (25% insulin lispro plus 75% protamine lispro) was compared with 30/70 human insulin in an open, randomized, crossover study during Ramadan, the daily average blood glucose concentration was better with the insulin lispro combination. The number of hypoglycemic episodes was the same with the two formulations (8).

In an open, randomized, single-dose, three-way, crossover trial, biphasic insulin aspart 30 (30% aspart plus 70% protaminated aspart, BIAsp 30), biphasic insulin lispro 25 (25% lispro plus 75% protaminated lispro, Mix 25), and biphasic human insulin 30 (30% regular plus 70% NPH insulin, BHI 30) were compared in 45 patients (9). Biphasic insulin aspart improved postprandial control better. There were 23 episodes of hypoglycemia with BIAsp 30, 19 with Mix 25, and 11 with BHI 30; two episodes with BIAsp 30, five with Mix 25, and two with BHI 30 required third-party intervention.

Comparative studies

In an open, randomized, crossover study, 113 patients with at least 6 months of continuous subcutaneous insulin infusion before the study were treated with regular insulin or insulin lispro (2). Postprandial blood glucose was lower and HbA$_{1c}$ fell more with insulin lispro. There were no differences in catheter obstruction, hypoglycemic episodes, or other adverse effects. Satisfaction with treatment was better with insulin lispro.

There were no differences between human protamine zinc insulin and human ultralente insulin when either was added once or twice daily to insulin lispro (10).

When either insulin lispro or regular insulin was given during the evening meal in a randomized, double-blind study in insulin-using adolescents, insulin lispro reduced the number of hypoglycemic episodes at night but redistribution of evening carbohydrate might be necessary to reduce postprandial hypoglycemia (11).

Premeal hyperglycemia is common. The short action of insulin lispro can then be extended by the addition of protamine zinc insulin. In a 3-month study in addition to a once-daily injection of protamine zinc insulin, at each meal insulin lispro or insulin lispro + protamine zinc insulin was injected; the postprandial blood glucose concentration was lower, but the post-absorptive glucose concentration was higher in the insulin lispro-only group; there was no difference in HbA$_{1c}$. The addition of protamine zinc insulin (30% at breakfast, 40% at lunch, and 10% at dinner) improved post-absorptive glucose and HbA$_{1c}$ (12).

Insulin Mix 25 (25% insulin lispro and 75% neutral protamine zinc insulin) reduced the glucose response to a standardized breakfast meal better than premixed 30% regular + 70% protamine zinc insulin when 22 patients with type 2 diabetes were studied three times in a double-blind fashion (13). Protamine zinc insulin mixed with insulin lispro has the same action profile of insulin lispro, with the continuing action of the long-acting component (14). The same mixture given three or four times daily provides acceptable control (15), but gives no possibility of adjusting the short-acting insulin regularly. Protamine zinc insulin must be mixed with insulin lispro in the syringe immediately before the meal (16). The mixture is not stable for longer as there is partial exchange of the rapid-acting analogue and the protamine-bound human insulin. Instant mixing is no solution when pens are used.

The use of insulin lispro instead of regular insulin reduced the frequency of nocturnal attacks of hypoglycemia but did not change HbA_{1c} (17). This was confirmed by the UK Prospective Diabetes Study (18), which also found a fall in postprandial glucose with an increase in fasting and preprandial glucose.

In an open, crossover, randomized study in 33 patients with type 1 diabetes who used regular or insulin lispro, the latter was associated with a lower incidence of severe hypoglycemia, mostly due to reduced nocturnal hypoglycemia; HbA_{1c} was not different (19).

A crossover comparison of regular insulin + protamine zinc insulin at bedtime with insulin lispro + multiple protamine zinc insulin showed no effect on overall hypoglycemia but there was less frequent severe hypoglycemia with the second treatment (20). The reduction in HbA_{1c} was small and not significant. Insulin doses were the same. Patients preferred the second treatment.

In an open, randomized, multicenter study, 33 women with type 1 diabetes for at least 2 years were randomized to preprandial lispro or regular insulin in week 15 of their pregnancy; both groups used NPH insulin as well (21). HbA_{1c} concentrations fell at the same rate. One patient in the regular group had one episode of severe hypoglycemia and one had three episodes. Biochemical hypoglycemia (under 3.0 mmol/l) was significantly more frequent in the lispro group (5.5 versus 3.9%). Retinopathy progressed during pregnancy in three of the 16 who used lispro and six of the 17 who used regular insulin; retinal aneurysms were seen at the beginning of the study in 10/16 and 5/17 patients respectively. There were no differences in the neonates.

When insulin lispro and insulin aspart were compared in a single-blind, randomized crossover study in 14 patients with type 1 diabetes, insulin lispro had a faster onset of action but a shorter duration (22). However, in another study, the pharmacokinetic and pharmacodynamic profiles of insulin aspart compared with human insulin in 24 healthy Japanese were the same as those in non-Japanese subjects (23).

Insulin aspart, insulin lispro, and buffered regular insulin in continuous subcutaneous insulin infusion have been compared in an open, randomized, parallel-group study in 146 patients (24). HbA_{1c}, hypoglycemic episodes, and blockages of pumps or infusion sets did not differ.

Insulin lispro and insulin aspart were equally effective in 24 patients with type 1 diabetes (25).

Insulin lispro and repaglinide were given to seven patients with diabetes related to cystic fibrosis (26). They had normal fasting blood glucose and insulin concentrations, but postprandial glucose concentrations were substantially raised. Insulin lispro had a larger and more sustained effect in lowering postprandial glucose than repaglinide. However, the doses of insulin lispro (0.1 U/kg) and repaglinide (1 mg) may not have been comparable.

Organs and Systems

Metabolism

Hypoglycemia
Hypoglycemic events in 24 controlled trials of rapid-acting insulin analogues have been analysed (27). In 22 trials, insulin lispro was used, 19 studies were open and unblinded, and five were double-blind. In five of 22 studies there was a significant reduction in mild hypoglycemia, but there were no changes in the frequency of severe hypoglycemia in 10 of 12 studies that reported these events; there was a fall in nocturnal hypoglycemia in 6 studies, but in 18 studies there was no fall. The author stated that rapid-acting insulins are only appropriate in intensive therapy, which involves well-educated and well-motivated patients.

In a comparison of insulin lispro and soluble insulin during a crossover study over 24 weeks in prepubertal children (7–11 years), there were no differences in HbA_{1c} or mean insulin doses (28). Insulin lispro produced a lower mean blood glucose concentration in the evening (0018–0022 hours), higher blood glucose in the early night (0022–0040 hours), and later identical concentrations. Episodes of hypoglycemia were most frequent in the afternoon and less than half occurred at night. They were less frequent with insulin lispro, but this was not statistically significant.

In 42 children (aged 6–12 years) and 34 adolescents (aged 13–17 years) in two crossover periods of 6 weeks there was no difference in fructosamine or HbA_{1c} concentrations; only blood glucose 2 hours after breakfast was significantly lower in the postprandial period (29). The risk of hypoglycemia was not different and there were no differences between the age groups.

In a 6-month comparison of three times daily regular insulin + NPH at night versus premeal insulin lispro + NPH at lunch and at night, HbA_{1c} fell more in the second group and glucose concentrations 2 hours after a meal were lower (30). The frequencies of episodes of hypoglycemia were not significantly different.

- A 42-year-old woman and a 39-year-old woman who were transferred from preprandial regular insulin to insulin lispro, without a reduction in the total dose of insulin, developed postprandial hypoglycemia (31).

This has been reported before [SEDA 22, 475].

Lipodystrophy
Lipoatrophy due to insulin lispro during pump therapy has been reported before [SEDA-25, 510; SEDA-27, 449].

- A 35-year-old woman transferred from regular insulin to insulin lispro, as she had developed unawareness of hypoglycemia (32). After 23 months she developed a circumscribed area of lipoatrophy about 3 cm in diameter at an injection site on the right thigh. Her anti-insulin antibodies were high (50%). Six months later incipient lipoatrophy was seen in the same area in the contralateral thigh and the first lesion remained unchanged, although no more insulin had been injected there. She was transferred to insulin aspart, which caused no changes over 6 months. The anti-insulin antibodies were then 31%.

Skin

Lipoatrophy has previously been reported with lispro (SEDA-27, 449).

- A 35-year-old woman with type 1 diabetes was transferred after 7 years to lispro subcutaneously tds and NPH twice daily (33). Within 2 years she developed lipoatrophy and further lipoatrophy at another site 6 months later.

Immunologic

Switching from ordinary insulin to insulin lispro can reduce the production of insulin antibodies.

- A 54-year-old woman with type 2 diabetes had poor metabolic control, despite using 60–80 units of short-acting and long-acting human insulins for 10 years (34). Transfer to insulin lispro reduced the daily amount of insulin to 28 units. Insulin specific antibodies fell from 2.7 to 0.3% and cross-reactive antibodies, binding both human insulin and insulin lispro, fell from 44 to 16%. Specific insulin lispro antibodies rose from 0 to 0.3%. HbA$_{1c}$ fell from 9.1% to 6.8% and body mass index from 30 to 27, probably because of the reduced dose of insulin.

Pregnancy

Maternal and fetal outcomes have been investigated when insulin lispro has been used during pregnancy [Radermecker 178]. Insulin lispro is unlikely to cross the placenta when used in a single standard dose. Lispro was not found in the cord blood of neonates whose mothers had received a continuous intravenous infusion of lispro. These data and data from controlled studies showing similar outcomes in women treated with conventional insulin are reassuring.

In a prospective comparison in 69 pregnant women of lispro (n = 36) with conventional insulin (n = 33), there was no adverse impact on the progression of diabetic retinopathy [Radermecker 178].

Drug dosage regimens

It is still a matter of debate what the optimal timing is for injecting insulin lispro, specifically when postprandial glucose is taken into account. Insulin lispro acts so rapid that it must be injected just before a meal, which is more convenient for the patient. Some physicians advise injecting the new short-acting insulins after a meal. However, when insulin lispro was injected postprandially in 31 patients in a random crossover design during two alternating periods of 3 months, mean HbA$_{1c}$ increased, mean postprandial blood glucose was higher, and mean pre-prandial blood glucose was lower in those who injected

postprandially (35). There was no difference in episodes of hypoglycemia.

Two cases of lipoatrophy induced by insulin lispro during continuous subcutaneous insulin infusion have been reported (28).

- An 8-year-old girl was switched to continuous subcutaneous insulin infusion using insulin lispro for better regulation after 4 years of diabetes. After 12 months she developed lipoatrophy of the abdominal wall, which progressed during the next months. When she changed to neutral buffered regular human insulin, no further lipoatrophy developed, but the existing atrophy did not improve either.
- A 51-year-old woman started to use continuous subcutaneous insulin and after 2 years the insulin was changed to insulin lispro. She developed lipoatrophy in the abdomen and buttocks 1 year later and there was an increase in the time before the bolus started to peak. Buffered regular human insulin stopped progression of the lipoatrophy.
- A 35-year-old woman transferred from regular insulin to insulin lispro, as she had developed unawareness of hypoglycemia (36). After 23 months she developed a circumscribed area of lipoatrophy about 3 cm in diameter at an injection site on the right thigh. Her anti-insulin antibodies were high (50%). Six months later incipient lipoatrophy was seen in the same area in the contralateral thigh and the first lesion remained unchanged, although no more insulin had been injected there. She was transferred to insulin aspart, which caused no changes over 6 months. The anti-insulin antibodies were then 31%.

Skin

Insulin lispro can cause lipoatrophy, but it was less extensive in a case in which it had occurred with regular insulin, perhaps because of the greater solubility of insulin lispro.

- Several combinations of regular and NPH insulin reduced the risk of hypoglycemia and optimized blood glucose in a 29-year-old woman who had had type 1 diabetes for 6 years (37). Continuous subcutaneous insulin infusion with regular insulin reduced the risk of hypoglycemia, but after 7 months she developed lipoatrophy. Changing the site of the cannula did not help. She was given insulin lispro instead and after 11 months a new, less extensive area of lipoatrophy emerged, which did not disappear.
- A 35-year-old woman with type 1 diabetes was transferred after 7 years to lispro subcutaneously tds and NPH twice daily (38). Within 2 years she developed lipoatrophy and further lipoatrophy at another site 6 months later.

Immunologic

The long-term antigenicity of insulin lispro and cross-reactivity with human insulin antibodies over 4 years has been investigated in 1221 patients with both type 1 and type 2 diabetes, either insulin-naïve or with prior insulin treatment, in a multicenter combination of controlled and non-controlled open studies (39). Like recombinant human insulin, insulin lispro elicited a low immunogenic response. The reversal of amino acids in B28 and B29 is in a relatively non-immunogenic area. Moreover, antigenicity often correlates with residence of insulin in subcutaneous tissues, and insulin lispro has a short residence time. The patients did not develop increased dosage requirements. Intermittent treatment did not increase specific or cross-reactive responses. The antibody responses were slightly higher in type 1 than in type 2 diabetes. In lipodystrophy with lipoatrophic diabetes, high insulin resistance is often found, for which leptin deficiency is one contributory factor.

Switching from ordinary insulin to insulin lispro can reduce the production of insulin antibodies.

- A 54-year-old woman with type 2 diabetes had poor metabolic control, despite using 6080 units of short-acting and long-acting human insulins for 10 years (40). Transfer to insulin lispro reduced the daily amount of insulin to 28 units. Insulin specific antibodies fell from 2.7 to 0.3% and cross-reactive antibodies, binding both human insulin and insulin lispro, fell from 44 to 16%. Specific insulin lispro antibodies rose from 0 to 0.3%. HbA1c fell from 9.1% to 6.8% and body mass index from 30 to 27, probably because of the reduced dose of insulin.

Second-Generation Effects

Pregnancy

Rapid improvement of regulation by insulin lispro during pregnancy causes proliferative diabetic retinopathy more often. In 14 patients treated with insulin lispro to improve control before or at the beginning of pregnancy, six of the 10 patients with normal optic fundi remained negative. However, three patients developed bilateral progressive retinopathy with marked vision impairment, in two cases with vitreous hemorrhage; one patient with a negative examination 6 months before pregnancy, but with minimal lesions 18 months earlier, developed progressive retinopathy with vitreous hemorrhages in spite of multiple coagulations (41). The authors advised care when starting insulin lispro in patients with a history of retinal lesions and to look for those at risk by performing fluorescein angiography, which distinguishes incipient changes better.

In a comparison of premeal regular insulin and premeal insulin lispro in gestational diabetes there were fewer attacks of hypoglycemia, but fasting glucose, postprandial glucose, and HbA$_{1c}$ were similar in the two groups (42). There were no fetal or neonatal abnormalities.

Maternal and fetal outcomes have been investigated when insulin lispro has been used during pregnancy (43). Insulin lispro is unlikely to cross the placenta when used in a single standard dose. Lispro was not found in the cord blood of neonates whose mothers had received a continuous intravenous infusion of lispro. These data and data from controlled studies showing similar outcomes in women treated with conventional insulin are reassuring.

In a prospective comparison in 69 pregnant women of lispro (n = 36) with conventional insulin (n = 33), there was no adverse impact on the progression of diabetic retinopathy (44).

Susceptibility Factors

Age

The newer insulins are not registered for use in children in many countries. A report of the use of postprandial insulin lispro versus preprandial regular insulin in an open, crossover, randomized study in 24 prepubertal children showed no large differences (45). Fasting blood glucose was higher with insulin lispro. The number of hypoglycemic episodes was almost the same with both insulins. There was one case of severe hypoglycemia.

Renal disease

The pharmacodynamic and pharmacokinetic properties of regular soluble insulin and insulin lispro have been investigated in 12 patients with and without nephropathy in a double-blind, crossover study with euglycemic glucose clamping (46). Insulin clearance was reduced by 30–40% in patients with nephropathy, but in both groups the time to reach the maximal effect was shorter with insulin lispro. The overall metabolic effect of regular soluble insulin, but not of insulin lispro, was lower in nephropathy, in which a 50% higher dose of regular insulin may be necessary.

Drug Administration

Drug dosage regimens

It is still a matter of debate what the optimal timing is for injecting insulin lispro, specifically when postprandial glucose is taken into account. Insulin lispro acts so rapid that it must be injected just before a meal, which is more convenient for the patient. Some physicians advise injecting the new short-acting insulins after a meal. However, when insulin lispro was injected postprandially in 31 patients in a random crossover design during two alternating periods of 3 months, mean HbA$_{1c}$ increased, mean postprandial blood glucose was higher, and mean preprandial blood glucose was lower in those who injected postprandially (47). There was no difference in episodes of hypoglycemia.

Drug administration route

Insulin lispro by repeated injection has been compared with insulin lispro by continuous subcutaneous infusion in 41 patients who were C-peptide negative (48). HbA$_{1c}$, mean blood glucose concentrations, and mean insulin doses were significantly lower during continuous subcutaneous infusion; the frequency of attacks of hypoglycemia was the same.

References

1. Travaglini MT, Garg SK, Chase HP. Use of insulin lispro in the outpatient management of ketonuria. Arch Pediatr Adolesc Med 1998;152(7):672–5.

2. Renner R, Pfutzner A, Trautmann M, Harzer O, Sauter K, Landgraf RGerman Humalog-CSII Study Group. Use of insulin lispro in continuous subcutaneous insulin infusion treatment. Results of a multicenter trial. Diabetes Care 1999;22(5):784–8.

3. Darmon P, Curtillet C, Boullu S, Laugier A, Dutour A, Oliver C. Insulin analogue lispro decreases insulin resistance and improves glycemic control in an obese patient with insulin-requiring type 2 diabetes. Diabetes Care 1998;21(9):1575.

4. Akram J, De Verga VRamadan Study Group. Insulin lispro (Lys(B28), Pro(B29) in the treatment of diabetes during the fasting month of Ramadan. Diabet Med 1999;16(10):861–6.

5. Kong N, Kitchen MM, Ryder RE. The use of lispro for high sugar content snacks between meals in intensive insulin regimens. Diabet Med 2000;17(4):331–2.

6. Murphy NP, Keane SM, Ong KK, Ford-Adams M, Edge JA, Acerini CL, Dunger DB. Randomized crossover trial of insulin glargine plus lispro or NPH insulin plus regular human insulin in adolescents with type 1 diabetes on intensive insulin regimens. Diabetes Care 2003;26(3):799–804.

7. Herz M, Arora V, Sun B, Ferguson SC, Bolli GB, Frier BM. Basal-bolus insulin therapy in Type 1 diabetes: comparative study of pre-meal administration of a fixed mixture of insulin lispro (50%) and neutral protamine lispro (50%) with human soluble insulin. Diabet Med 2002;19(11):917–23.

8. Mattoo V, Milicevic Z, Malone JK, Schwarzenhofer M, Ekangaki A, Levitt LK, Liong LH, Rais N, Tounsi HRamadan Study Group. A comparison of insulin lispro Mix25 and human insulin 30/70 in the treatment of type 2 diabetes during Ramadan. Diabetes Res Clin Pract 2003;59(2):137–43.

9. Hermansen K, Colombo M, Storgaard H, OStergaard A, Kolendorf K, Madsbad S. Improved postprandial glycemic control with biphasic insulin aspart relative to biphasic insulin lispro and biphasic human insulin in patients with type 2 diabetes. Diabetes Care 2002;25(5):883–8.

10. Zinman B, Ross S, Campos RV, Strack TThe Canadian Lispro Study Group. Effectiveness of human ultralente versus NPH insulin in providing basal insulin replacement for an insulin lispro multiple daily injection regimen. A double-blind randomized prospective trial. Diabetes Care 1999;22(4):603–8.

11. Mohn A, Matyka KA, Harris DA, Ross KM, Edge JA, Dunger DB. Lispro or regular insulin for multiple injection therapy in adolescence. Differences in free insulin and glucose levels overnight. Diabetes Care 1999;22(1):27–32.

12. Ciofetta M, Lalli C, Del Sindaco P, Torlone E, Pampanelli S, Mauro L, Chiara DL, Brunetti P, Bolli GB. Contribution of postprandial versus interprandial blood glucose to HbA1c in type 1 diabetes on physiologic intensive therapy with lispro insulin at mealtime. Diabetes Care 1999;22(5):795–800.

13. Koivisto VA, Tuominen JA, Ebeling P. Lispro Mix25 insulin as premeal therapy in type 2 diabetic patients. Diabetes Care 1999;22(3):459–62.

14. Rave K, Heinemann L, Puhl L, Gudat U, Woodworth JR, Weyer C, Heise T. Premixed formulations of insulin lispro. Activity profiles in type 1 diabetic patients. Diabetes Care 1999;22(5):865–6.

15. Lalli C, Ciofetta M, Del Sindaco P, Torlone E, Pampanelli S, Compagnucci P, Cartechini MG, Bartocci L, Brunetti P, Bolli GB. Long-term intensive treatment of type 1 diabetes with the short-acting insulin analogue lispro in variable combination with NPH insulin at mealtime. Diabetes Care 1999;22(3):468–77.

16. Joseph SE, Korzon-Burakowska A, Woodworth JR, Evans M, Hopkins D, Janes JM, Amiel SA. The action profile of lispro is not blunted by mixing in the syringe with NPH insulin. Diabetes Care 1998;21(12):2098–102.

17. Heller SR, Amiel SA, Mansell PU.K. Lispro Study Group. Effect of the fast-acting insulin analogue lispro on the risk of nocturnal hypoglycemia during intensified insulin therapy. Diabetes Care 1999;22(10):1607–11.

18. Gale EA. A randomized, controlled trial comparing insulin lispro with human soluble insulin in patients with Type 1 diabetes on intensified insulin therapy. The UK Trial Group. Diabet Med 2000;17(3):209–14.

19. Ferguson SC, Strachan MW, Janes JM, Frier BM. Severe hypoglycaemia in patients with type 1 diabetes and impaired awareness of hypoglycaemia: a comparative study of insulin lispro and regular human insulin. Diabetes Metab Res Rev 2001;17(4):285–91.

20. Colombel A, Murat A, Krempf M, Kuchly-Anton B, Charbonnel B. Improvement of blood glucose control in Type 1 diabetic patients treated with lispro and multiple NPH injections. Diabet Med 1999;16(4):319–24.

21. Persson B, Swahn ML, Hjertberg R, Hanson U, Nord E, Nordlander E, Hansson LO. Insulin lispro therapy in pregnancies complicated by type 1 diabetes mellitus. Diabetes Res Clin Pract 2002;58(2):115–21.

22. Hedman CA, Lindstrom T, Arnqvist HJ. Direct comparison of insulin lispro and aspart shows small differences in plasma insulin profiles after subcutaneous injection in type 1 diabetes. Diabetes Care 2001;24(6):1120–1.

23. Kaku K, Matsuda M, Urae A, Irie S. Pharmacokinetics and pharmacodynamics of insulin aspart, a rapid-acting analogue of human insulin, in healthy Japanese volunteers. Diabetes Res Clin Pract 2000;49(2–3):119–26.

24. Bode B, Weinstein R, Bell D, McGill J, Nadeau D, Raskin P, Davidson J, Henry R, Huang WC, Reinhardt RR. Comparison of insulin aspart with buffered regular insulin and insulin lispro in continuous subcutaneous insulin infusion: a randomized study in type 1 diabetes. Diabetes Care 2002;25(3):439–44.

25. Plank J, Wutte A, Brunner G, Siebenhofer A, Semlitsch B, Sommer R, Hirschberger S, Pieber TR. A direct comparison of insulin aspart and insulin lispro in patients with type 1 diabetes. Diabetes Care 2002;25(11):2053–7.

26. Moran A, Phillips J, Milla C. Insulin and glucose excursion following premeal insulin lispro or repaglinide in cystic fibrosis-related diabetes. Diabetes Care 2001;24(10):1706–1710.

27. Heinemann L. Hypoglycemia and insulin analogues: is there a reduction in the incidence? J Diabetes Complications 1999;13(2):105–14.

28. Ford-Adams ME, Murphy NP, Moore EJ, Edge JA, Ong KL, Watts AP, Acerini CL, Dunger DB. Insulin lispro: a potential role in preventing nocturnal hypoglycaemia in young children with diabetes mellitus. Diabetic Med 2003;20:656–60.

29. Danne T, Amna J, Schober E, Deiss D, Jacobsen JL, Friberg HH, Jensen LH. A comparison of postprandial administration of insulin aspart in children and adolescents with type 1 diabetes. Diabetes Care 2003;26:2359–64.

30. Sargin H, Sargin M, Altuntas Y, Sengul AM, Orbay E, Seber S, Ucak S, Yayla A. Comparison of lunch and bedtime NPH insulin plus mealtime insulin lispro therapy with premeal regular insulin plus bedtime NPH insulin therapy in type 2 diabetes. Diabetes Res Clin Pract 2003;62:79–86.

31. Fujiwara M, Baba T, Neugebauer S, Hasegawa K, Hosoya E, Tanaka K, Shimada K, Yamada D, Watanabe T. Postprandial hypoglycaemia due to insulin lispro. Diabetic Med 2004;21:297–8.

32. Arranz A, Andia V, López-Gúzman A. A case of lipoatrophy with lispro insulin without insulin pump therapy. Diabetes Care 2004;27:625–6.

33. Arranz AA, Andia V, Lopez-Guzman A. A case of lipoatrophy with lispro insulin without insulin pump therapy. Diabetes Care 2004;27:625–6.

34. Asai M, Kodera T, Ishizeki K, Uebori S, Kashiwaya T, Itoh H, Makino. Insulin lispro reduces insulin antibodies in a patient with type 2 diabetes with immunological insulin resistance. Diabetes Res Clin Pract 2003;61:89–92.

35. Schenthaner G, Wein W, Shnawa N, Bates PC, Birkett MA. Preprandial vs. postprandial lispro—a comparative crossover trial in patients with type 1 diabetes. Diabetic Med 2004;21:279–84.

36. Griffin ME, Feder A, Tamborlane WV. Lipoatrophy associated with lispro insulin in insulin pump therapy: an old complication, a new cause? Diabetes Care 2001;24(1):174.

37. Arranz A, Andia V, López-Gúzman A. A case of lipoatrophy with lispro insulin without insulin pump therapy. Diabetes Care 2004;27:625–6.

38. Ampudia-Blasco FJ, Hasbum B, Carmena R. A new case of lipoatrophy with lispro insulin in insulin pump therapy: is there any insulin preparation free of complications? Diabetes Care 2003;26(3):953–4.

39. Arranz AA, Andia V, Lopez-Guzman A. A case of lipoatrophy with lispro insulin without insulin pump therapy. Diabetes Care 2004;27:625–6.

40. Fineberg SE, Huang J, Brunelle R, Gulliya KS, Anderson JH Jr. Effect of long-term exposure to insulin lispro on the induction of antibody response in patients with type 1 or type 2 diabetes. Diabetes Care 2003;26(1):89–96.

41. Asai M, Kodera T, Ishizeki K, Uebori S, Kashiwaya T, Itoh H, Makino. Insulin lispro reduces insulin antibodies in a patient with type 2 diabetes with immunological insulin resistance. Diabetes Res Clin Pract 2003;61:89–92.

42. Kitzmiller JL, Main E, Ward B, Theiss T, Peterson DL. Insulin lispro and the development of proliferative diabetic retinopathy during pregnancy. Diabetes Care 1999;22(5):874–6.

43. Jovanovic L, Ilic S, Pettitt DJ, Hugo K, Gutierrez M, Bowsher RR, Bastyr EJ 3rd. Metabolic and immunologic effects of insulin lispro in gestational diabetes. Diabetes Care 1999;22(9):1422–7.

44. Radermecker RP, Scheen AJ. Continuous subcutaneous insulin infusion with short-acting insulin analogues or human regular insulin: efficacy, safety, quality of life, and cost-effectiveness. Diabetes Metab Res Rev 2004;20:178–88.

45. Schenthaner G, Wein W, Shnawa N, Bates PC, Birkett MA. Preprandial vs. postprandial lispro—a comparative crossover trial in patients with type 1 diabetes. Diabetic Med 2004;21:279–84.

46. Tupola S, Komulainen J, Jaaskelainen J, Sipila I. Post-prandial insulin lispro vs. human regular insulin in prepubertal children with Type 1 diabetes mellitus. Diabet Med 2001;18(8):654–8.

47. Rave K, Heise T, Pfutzner A, Heinemann L, Sawicki PT. Impact of diabetic nephropathy on pharmacodynamic and Pharmacokinetic properties of insulin in type 1 diabetic patients. Diabetes Care 2001;24(5):886–90.

48. Hanaire-Broutin H, Melki V, Bessieres-Lacombe S, Tauber JP. Comparison of continuous subcutaneous insulin infusion and multiple daily injection regimens using insulin lispro in type 1 diabetic patients on intensified treatment: a randomized study. The Study Group for the Development of Pump Therapy in Diabetes. Diabetes Care 2000;23(9):1232–5.

Insulin-like growth factor (IGF-I)

General Information

Insulin growth factor (IGF) and the IGF-I receptor are structurally comparable to insulin and the insulin receptor. Recombinant human IGF-I has 54% identity to proinsulin. Insulin and IGF-I can bind to both receptors, but insulin can only transfer 1% of the IGF message on the IGF receptor and IGF-I only 1% of the insulin message on the insulin receptor.

Recombinant human IGF-I is used as an adjunct to insulin therapy in patients with large daily variations in insulin effect. It is sometimes given in insulin resistance syndromes caused by changes in the insulin receptor or in type B insulin resistance syndrome caused by antibodies to the insulin receptor.

In 14 adolescents, the addition of IGF-I to diabetic treatment for 12 weeks did not change leptin concentrations (1).

IGF-I was given as co-therapy with insulin in 223 patients for 12 weeks twice-daily (2). The doses of IGF-I were 40/40, 80/40, or 80/60 micrograms/kg. Patients who received co-therapy were able to reduce their daily doses of insulin. The number of episodes of hypoglycemia was the same, but glucose regulation was tighter during IGF-I co-therapy. The fall in HbA$_{1c}$ concentration was greater with co-therapy (–1.2%) than with intensive therapy only (–0.7%). The dosage regimen of 40/40 micrograms/kg was well tolerated. Higher doses had no greater effect but were associated with edema, jaw pain, headache, palpitation, tachycardia, syncope, or early worsening of retinopathy.

Organs and Systems

Sensory systems

Of 199 patients, 16 developed significant worsening of retinopathy, including neovascularization, over 12 weeks; 12 of the 16 had optic disc swelling, which necessitated laser therapy in three of them (3). This was mostly seen in patients using a high dose of IGF-I, but a long-term effect of low-dose IGF-I could not be excluded either.

Immunologic

IGF-I can cause allergic reactions (4).

- A 75-year-old man with glucose intolerance, severe hyperinsulinemia, and extreme insulin resistance with anti-insulin receptor antibodies had immunosuppressive therapy and plasmapheresis to remove the antibodies, without lasting success. Treatment with hrIGF-I, 0.4 mg/kg/day, reduced HbA_{1c} from 13.8% to 8.0%. After 5 months he developed a generalized skin eruption 20 minutes after the injection. When IGF-I was withdrawn the HbA_{1c} rose again. After careful desensitization with hrIGF-I, 0.1 mg three times a week, IGF-I was continued, with good effect on HbA_{1c}.

Long-Term Effects

Tumorigenicity

A non-Hodgkin's lymphoma developed in the right femur of a 58-year-old man who had used IGF-I 40 micrograms bd (5) in a study of the effect of adding IGF to insulin therapy (SEDA-23, 457).

References

1. Thrailkill KM, Fowlkes JL, Hyde JF, Litton JC. The effects of co-therapy with recombinant human insulin-like growth factor I and insulin on serum leptin levels in adolescents with type 1 diabetes mellitus. Pediatr Diabetes 2001;2(1):25–9.
2. Thrailkill KM, Quattrin T, Baker L, Kuntze JE, Compton PG, Martha PM Jr. Cotherapy with recombinant human insulin-like growth factor I and insulin improves glycemic control in type 1 diabetes. RhIGF-I in IDDM Study Group. Diabetes Care 1999;22(4):585–92.
3. Lanzetta P, Malara C. Cotherapy with recombinant human IGF-I and insulin improves glycemic control in type 1 diabetes. Diabetes Care 2000;23(3):436–7.
4. Yamamoto T, Sato T, Mori T, Yamakita T, Hasegawa T, Miyamoto M, Hosoi M, Ishii T, Yoshioka K, Tanaka S, Fujii S. Clinical efficacy of insulin-like growth factor-1 in a patient with autoantibodies to insulin receptors: a case report. Diabetes Res Clin Pract 2000;49(1):65–9.
5. Mayer-Davis EJ. Cancer in a patient receiving IGF-I therapy. Diabetes Care 2000;23:433–4.

Meglitinides

General Information

The meglitinides bind with high affinity to a site, distinct from the sulfonylurea receptor site, on the ATP-sensitive potassium channels in pancreatic beta cells and stimulate insulin secretion. After binding, the ATP-dependent potassium channels are closed, reducing potassium efflux and depolarizing the cell membrane. The meglitinides do not have to be internalized in the membrane, in contrast to the sulfonylureas. This may explain their rapid onset of the action and the end of that action when glucose concentrations are falling. MgADP potentiates the effect in beta cells but not in cardiac cells (1), which may explain the reduced cardiovascular adverse effects of repaglinide in vivo. Meglitinide-stimulated insulin secretion depends on the glucose concentration; insulin secretion is not stimulated in vitro or in fasted animals. Nateglinide (and perhaps repaglinide) reduces the secretion of glycated insulin, which has poor activity, from islet cells; this may contribute to its hypoglycemic action (2).

Repaglinide (rINN) is a carbamoylmethyl benzoic acid derivative, which contains the non-sulfonylurea moiety of glibenclamide, and nateglinide (rINN) is a phenylalanine derivative. Nateglinide acts more quickly than repaglinide, and both act more quickly than sulfonylureas, which stimulate insulin secretion independent of blood glucose concentrations (3). It has been stated (4) that earlier studies (SEDA-22, 478) (SEDA-23, 462) (5) showed that the efficacy in lowering HbA_{1c} is almost equivalent for sulfonylureas and repaglinide and is slightly lower for nateglinide. When a lunch-time meal was omitted (SEDA-23, 462) patients taking glibenclamide had the lowest blood glucose concentrations, often within the hypoglycemic range, in contrast to patients taking repaglinide. Both drugs can cause hypoglycemia.

Repaglinide has been reviewed (6–8). It stimulates glucose-dependent insulin secretion, amplifying insulin bursts without changing burst frequency, but it does not restore disrupted pulsatile secretion in type 2 diabetes (9). It is rapidly absorbed. It is metabolized by CYP3A4 in the liver and is 90% excreted in the feces. It has a half-life of 32 minutes. Its pharmacokinetics do not differ in young or older healthy persons (10). It can be given as monotherapy (11), and the effective dose is 0.5–8 mg/day, starting with 0.5 mg/day. It has to be given before each meal and can be adapted to irregular food intake or missed meals (12). When given preprandially it improves glucose control without increasing the risk of adverse effects (13). There were no differences in action in healthy younger or older volunteers (14). Repaglinide is short-acting and seems to be associated with significantly fewer episodes of serious hypoglycemia (15). In a short review of a number of clinical studies the following contraindications were reported (16):

- known hypersensitivity to repaglinide or one of the constituents of Novonorm®;
- type 1 diabetes;
- renal or hepatic impairment.

Nateglinide (and perhaps repaglinide) reduces the excretion of glycated insulin, which has impaired biological activity, from the islets (17). This may contribute to the anti-hyperglycemic action of nateglinide.

Observational studies

In eight patients with type 2 diabetes, nateglinide given 5 minutes before a meal reduced the postprandial blood glucose excursion by 64% (18). There were no attacks of hypoglycemia even with a dosage of 180 mg/day; other adverse effects were not mentioned.

Comparative studies

In 424 patients in a European multicenter, randomized, double-blind study for 1 year, two-thirds of the patients used repaglinide (0.5–4 mg tds) and the others glibenclamide (1.75–10.5 mg/day) (19). HbA$_{1c}$ first fell but later increased. The same trends were seen in fasting blood glucose. There were no differences in hypoglycemia. A comparable American study of 576 patients (20) showed essentially the same result.

In a 14-week, double-blind, multicenter, randomized, parallel-group trial of repaglinide and glibenclamide in 118 patients with type 2 diabetes with borderline or poor control but still responsive to oral hypoglycemic drugs, HbA$_{1c}$ fell at the same rate in both groups (21). The 2-hour postprandial blood glucose concentration was lower with repaglinide, but fasting and mean glucose concentrations did not differ. Repaglinide was associated with 20 hypoglycemic episodes in nine patients and glibenclamide with 15 episodes in nine patients. There were no serious adverse effects.

The effects of repaglinide and glibenclamide have been compared in 235 patients during Ramadan, when people eat two meals a day (22). Before Ramadan, they were adjusted to optimal treatment with thrice-daily repaglinide or once- or twice-daily glibenclamide. During Ramadan they took twice-daily repaglinide or glibenclamide. After Ramadan they continued to take the pre-Ramadan regimen for 4 weeks. Mid-day hypoglycemia (blood glucose below 4.5 mmol/l) occurred in 2.8% of those who took repaglinide and 7.9% of those who took glibenclamide. There were 19 events reported by 15 patients in the repaglinide group and 35 by 19 patients in the glibenclamide group. During Ramadan the numbers were nine events in seven patients and 12 events in nine patients respectively. Mean serum fructosamine concentrations fell by 17 and 7 μmol/l during Ramadan in those taking repaglinide and glibenclamide respectively.

Insulin lispro and repaglinide were given to seven patients with diabetes related to cystic fibrosis (23). They had normal fasting blood glucose and insulin concentrations, but postprandial glucose concentrations were substantially raised. Insulin lispro had a larger and more sustained effect in lowering postprandial glucose than repaglinide. However, the doses of lispro (0.1 U/kg) and repaglinide (1 mg) may not have been comparable.

Repaglinide has been compared with nateglinide in an open 16-week study (24). Repaglinide was started in a dose of 0.5 mg per meal and increased up to 4 mg per meal if necessary. Nateglinide was started in a dose of 60 mg per meal and increased up to 120 mg per meal. Of those who used repaglinide, 54% achieved an HB$_{A1c}$ concentration of less than 7%, compared with 42% of those who used nateglinide. There were 0.016 *hypoglycemic events* per patient in those who used repaglinide compared with none in those who used nateglinide. Weight gain was 1.8 kg with repaglinide and 0.7 kg with nateglinide. There were no noticeable differences in the pattern of adverse events, which included constipation, arthralgia, and headache.

Placebo-controlled studies

In a randomized, double-blind, placebo-controlled, multicenter study, 289 patients took nateglinide in doses of 30 mg ($n = 51$), 60 mg ($n = 58$), 120 mg ($n = 63$), and 180 mg ($n = 57$), or placebo ($n = 60$) before main meals (25). Meal-time insulin increased rapidly and meal-time glucose excursions were reduced. HbA$_{1c}$ concentrations were significantly reduced after 12 weeks in those taking 60 mg and more. Fasting plasma glucose was only significantly reduced in those taking 120 mg. The drug was withdrawn in one patient taking 180 mg because of increased liver enzymes; at the next visit the enzymes were normal. There were mild symptoms of hypoglycemia, such as increased sweating, tremor, dizziness, weakness, and increased appetite. Blood glucose concentrations were between 2.7 and 3.3 mmol/l in three patients taking 120 mg/day.

Single doses of nateglinide 120 mg, repaglinide 0.5 and 2 mg, and placebo 10 minutes preprandially or 2 mg repaglinide 1 minute preprandially have been compared in 15 healthy volunteers (26). Nateglinide stimulated early insulin secretion more than repaglinide, and insulin concentrations returned more promptly to the preprandial values. The highest but slowest rise was seen with placebo. There were no episodes of hypoglycemia.

In a randomized, double-blind, placebo-controlled comparison of glibenclamide and nateglinide for 8 weeks in 152 patients, nateglinide produced higher postprandial insulin concentrations (27). Hypoglycemia and low blood glucose concentrations were more common with glibenclamide.

In a multicenter, double-blind, randomized, fixed-dose trial of placebo and repaglinide 1 mg and 4 mg for 24 weeks in 361 patients there were no episodes of severe hypoglycemia (28). Most patients withdrew from the placebo group because of hyperglycemia, hypoglycemia, erythematous rash, headache, diarrhea, fatigue, or abnormal vision. Adverse effects had about the same frequencies in the two groups.

Combinations of oral hypoglycemic drugs

The different mechanisms of action of the various classes of hypoglycemic drugs makes combined therapy feasible: the sulfonylureas and meglitinides stimulate insulin production by different mechanisms, the biguanides reduce glucose production by the liver and excretion from the liver, acarbose reduces the absorption of glucose from the gut, and the thiazolidinediones reduce insulin resistance in fat. It is not necessary to wait until the maximal dose of one drug has been reached before starting another. However, sulfonylureas and meglitinides should no longer be used when endogenous insulin production is minimal. Combinations of insulin with sulfonylureas or meglitinides should only be used while the patient is changing to insulin, except when long-acting insulin is given at night in order to give the islets a rest and to stimulate daytime insulin secretion.

Large studies of the effects of lifestyle changes, the effects of drugs in preventing or postponing the complications of diabetes, or the usefulness of various combinations are regularly published. The different mechanisms of action of the various classes give different metabolic effects and different adverse effects profiles (29). Comparative costs of the various therapies in the USA have been presented (30).

This subject has been reviewed in relation to combined oral therapy. In a systematic review of 63 studies with a duration of at least 3 months and involving at least 10 patients at the end of the study, and in which HbA_{1c} was reported, five different classes of oral drugs were almost equally effective in lowering blood glucose concentrations (31). HbA_{1c} was reduced by about 1–2% in all cases. Combination therapy gave additive effects. However, long-term vascular risk reduction was demonstrated only with sulfonylureas and metformin.

The adverse effects of combined drug therapy are attributable to the adverse effects of the single drugs. Increased adverse effects or new adverse effects in patients taking combinations have not been reported.

Meglitinides + biguanides

Patients with type 2 diabetes, with unsatisfactory control after taking metformin for 6 months, were randomized to metformin alone, repaglinide alone, or metformin + repaglinide (each 27 patients) (32). Combined therapy reduced HbA_{1c} after 3 months by 1.4% and fasting glucose by 2.2 mmol/l. Repaglinide alone or in combination with metformin increased insulin concentrations. The most common adverse effects were hypoglycemia, diarrhea, and headache. Gastrointestinal adverse effects were common in those taking metformin alone and body weight increased in both groups taking repaglinide.

In 12 patients with type 2 diabetes, a combination of nateglinide 120 mg or placebo with metformin 500 mg before each meal on two separate days was well tolerated (33). One patient taking nateglinide had a headache. One patient was withdrawn because of a myocardial infarction and had multivessel coronary artery disease on catheterization.

In a prospective, randomized, double-blind, placebo-controlled study for 24 weeks, 701 patients took nateglinide 120 mg before the three main meals, or metformin 500 mg tds, or the combination of the two, or placebo (34). The most frequent adverse effect was hypoglycemia, and it was most common in the combination group. There were no differences between those who took nateglinide only or metformin only and there were no episodes of serious hypoglycemia. Diarrhea was more frequent in those taking metformin or the combination, but infection, nausea, headache, and abdominal pain were comparable in the two groups.

Of 82 patients insufficiently controlled by metformin, 27 continued to take metformin with placebo, 28 took titrated repaglinide with placebo, and 27 took metformin with titrated repaglinide for 4–5 months (35). There were no serious adverse effects. Nine patients taking metformin + repaglinide reported 30 hypoglycemic events and three patients taking repaglinide reported nine events.

The combination of nateglinide + metformin for 3–4 months reported caused mild adverse events in 2.9% of patients, the most common being gastrointestinal complaints (36).

Meglitinides plus glitazones

In 246 patients pioglitazone 30 mg/day, repaglinide (optimal dosage), or pioglitazone + repaglinide were compared over 12 weeks after an initial 12 weeks to establish dosages in an open study (37). There were no episodes of major hypoglycemia or raised transaminases. HbA_{1c} changed in the three groups by −0.18%, + 0.32%, and −1.76% respectively. Fasting glucose improved most in the combined group. There were minor episodes of hypoglycemia in 8%, 3%, and 5% respectively. There were weight gains of 0.3, 2.0, and 5.5 kg respectively. The main reason for discontinuation before the end of the trial (41%, 58% and 15%) respectively was insufficient effect.

The combination of rosiglitazone + repaglinide during 24 weeks (38) in 252 patients with HbA_{1c} over 7.0% produced one major episode of hypoglycemia. Minor episodes occurred in 9% of those taking combined therapy, 6% of those taking repaglinide, and 2% of those taking rosiglitazone. There was peripheral edema in 4% of those taking combined therapy and 3 % of those taking rosiglitazone. Weight gain was + 4.4 kg in those taking combined therapy, 2.3 kg in those taking rosiglitazone, and 1.6 kg in those taking repaglinide.

Meglitinides + sulfonylureas

Glipizide, nateglinide, and their combination have been compared in a double-blind, randomized, placebo-controlled study in 20 patients with type 2 diabetes not requiring insulin (39). Before a standardized breakfast, they took glipizide 10 mg, nateglinide 120 mg, both, or placebo; 4 hours after the meal, blood glucose concentrations were significantly higher after nateglinide, but peak and integrated glucose concentrations did not differ. Integrated insulin concentrations were higher with glipizide. There were three episodes of hypoglycemia in the glipizide alone group and three in the combined group; three required treatment with glucose.

Meglitinides + thiazolidinediones

In 585 patients in a double-blind, randomized, placebo-controlled, multicenter study lasting 16 weeks nateglinide 40 mg tds alone, troglitazone 200 mg/day alone, and the combination were compared (40). The combination was most effective in lowering HbA_{1c}. The most frequent adverse effects were mild hypoglycemia, most often in the combination group. Three patients (two in the combination group and one in the troglitazone alone group) withdrew because of hypoglycemia. Most of the withdrawals were related to increased liver enzymes and weight gain, known adverse effects of troglitazone. Twelve patients withdrew because of predefined changes from baseline (transaminases more than 200% and alkaline phosphatase and bilirubin more than 100% over baseline); seven were taking troglitazone alone, four combined therapy, and one placebo.

In an open trial, 256 patients with type 2 diabetes with inadequate hypoglycemic control (HbA$_{1c}$ over 7.0% during previous therapy) took repaglinide (0.5–4 mg at meals), troglitazone (200–600 mg/day), or a combination of the two for 22 weeks (41). Combination therapy was most effective. Repaglinide only was more effective than troglitazone only. Mean body weight increased in both groups. Serious adverse events were chest pain, cerebrovascular disorders, malignancies, dysrhythmias, electrocardiographic changes suggesting myocardial infarction, and increased aspartate transaminase activity (in one patient taking troglitazone). The serious adverse effects were similar in the different groups. Hypoglycemia occurred in 4% of the patients taking combined therapy, in 16% of those taking troglitazone only, and in 27% of those taking repaglinide only; none needed assistance. There were changes in liver function tests in three patients in the combined group and in one patient each in the two other groups; the drugs were withdrawn in the affected patients and liver function normalized. There were no differences in adverse effects in the different groups. Hypoglycemia occurred in 11 patients taking repaglinide, in seven taking combination therapy, and in one taking troglitazone. Anemia occurred in four patients taking combined therapy and in two taking troglitazone only.

Insulin + meglitinides

In 80 patients taking metformin 850 or 1000 mg tds plus NPH insulin at bedtime, metformin was withdrawn and repaglinide 4 mg tds added in half of the patients for 16 weeks (42). In the repaglinide group the dose of insulin increased slightly and weight gain was 1.8 kg more. Mild hypoglycemia occurred more often in the metformin group; nightly episodes of hypoglycemia occurred only with repaglinide. One patient taking repaglinide had a myocardial infarction, and one had three separate hospitalizations for chest pain (myocardial infarction was excluded). No specific data were presented about gastrointestinal adverse effects or infections.

General adverse effects

The most frequent adverse effect of meglitinides is hypoglycemia. The overall incidence of hypoglycemia with repaglinide is similar to that reported with sulfonylureas, but the incidence of serious hypoglycemia is lower. Other adverse effects are respiratory tract infections and headache. Cardiovascular events and cardiovascular mortality are not different from those in users of sulfonylureas. In Europe, repaglinide is contraindicated in patients with severe liver dysfunction and it is not recommended in people over 75 years old; in America the advice is to use repaglinide cautiously in patients with impaired liver function and there is no restriction on its use in elderly patients. In renal impairment, the half-life of repaglinide is prolonged. Reasons for withdrawal are hyperglycemia, hypoglycemia, and myocardial infarction (43).

Organs and Systems

Metabolism

Repaglinide has a short duration of action and improves postprandial hyperglycemia, a potential risk factor for cardiovascular changes (44). In a double-blind, multiple-dose, parallel-group study repaglinide stimulated mealtime insulin secretion (45). Bouts of hypoglycemia were equally frequent with placebo and repaglinide. When repaglinide was added to NPH monotherapy in patients with HbA$_{1c}$ over 7.1% for 3 months, 38% of the patients had an HbA$_{1c}$ below 7.1% (46). The incidence of hypoglycemia did not change.

When glipizide was compared with repaglinide in 75 patients there were no major hypoglycemic events; minor events were the same in both groups, but after the start of therapy the events occurred much later with repaglinide than glipizide (47).

The effect of a missed meal during repaglinide and glibenclamide therapy has been compared in 83 randomized patients (48). During two meals there were six separate hypoglycemic events in those taking glibenclamide. Blood glucose fell from 4.3 mmol/l to 3.4 mmol/l in those taking glibenclamide when lunch was omitted. There were no changes in blood glucose in those taking repaglinide.

Factitious hypoglycemia has been attributed to repaglinide in an 18-year-old man who had bouts of hypoglycemia for 2 months (49). After glucose administration he recovered promptly and was sent home, but the next night his glucose was 1 mmol/l with high concentrations of insulin (395 pmol/l), C-peptide (2966 pmol/l), and proinsulin (81 pmol/l). The plasma concentrations of repaglinide in three specimens were 4.8–21 ng/ml. Metformin was below the detection limit. He finally admitted to taking repaglinide 4 mg regularly.

Gastrointestinal

When repaglinide 4 mg tds and glimepiride 160 mg bd were used in combination with bedtime NPH insulin for 13 weeks in 80 patients, one patient had severe diarrhea and fecal incontinence which subsided after stopping repaglinide (50).

Liver

Hepatotoxicity has been attributed to repaglinide (51).

- A 70-year-old man developed diabetes and started to take repaglinide 1 mg tds. After 2 weeks he developed malaise, anorexia, and jaundice. Liver function tests, including bilirubin, were raised. Repaglinide was withdrawn and the liver function tests returned to normal. There were no other obvious causes.

Another patient developed abnormal liver function tests, which normalized after withdrawal of repaglinide; he was not retested (50).

Immunologic

- A 62-year-old woman with type 2 diabetes, hypertension, and chronic hepatitis C virus infection developed palpable purpura over her legs and buttocks 3 weeks after starting to take repaglinide 500 mg qds (52). The purpura ulcerated and became infected. Repaglinide was withdrawn and the purpura resolved. A biopsy showed leukocytoclastic vasculitis.

Repaglinide, which is metabolized in the liver, is cleared more slowly in people with liver disease, and hepatitis C may have played a part in this case. Although hepatitis C can cause a leukocytoclastic vasculitis, the clinical correlation and the rapid disappearance of the purpura after the withdrawal of repaglinide makes it likely that this was an adverse effect of the drug. Caution with repaglinide in liver disease is important.

Susceptibility Factors

Genetic

When the pharmacokinetics of repaglinide 0.5, 1.0, and 2.0 mg were studied in healthy men, 15 Caucasians and 12 Japanese, AUC and C_{max} were higher in the Japanese (53).

Hypoglycemic reactions were more common at the highest dose, and were more common in the Japanese men.

Age

Of 358 patients aged 35–84 years who were given nateglinide over 12 weeks, 115 took 120 mg before main meals (group 1) and 214 took metformin and nateglinide in combination (group 2) (54). There were no differences in rates of hypoglycemia. Three patients in group 2 had serious adverse events, one of which was thought to be related to the study drug (details not given). Adverse events included nausea, vomiting, and headache. There was no information about how these events related to age.

Renal disease

In renal impairment the half-life of repaglinide is prolonged. Patients with severe renal impairment (creatinine clearance 20–40 ml/minute) had excess accumulation of the drug after taking multiple doses for 5 days (55).

In 235 patients with normal renal function or moderate to severe renal impairment switched from their original therapy to repaglinide (titrated to 0.5–4 mg tds within 4 weeks and continued for 3 months), the number of episodes of hypoglycemia increased with increasing severity of renal impairment during the run-in period but not during treatment (56). The final dose tended to be lower in patients with severe renal impairment. Although the concentrations of repaglinide in the patients with renal impairment were higher, they did not exceed the effective concentrations in people without renal impairment.

Patients with mild to moderate impairment can be treated with repaglinide. However, patients with severe renal impairment have other problems, and it is wise not to use repaglinide in patients with severe renal disease, or at least to adjust the dosage (55).

Hepatic disease

The clearance of repaglinide is reduced and the half-life prolonged (2.5-fold) in patients with chronic liver disease (57).

Drug–Drug Interactions

Numerous drugs have been reported not to interact with repaglinide, including cimetidine, theophylline, and warfarin (58).

Clarithromycin

Clarithromycin, an inhibitor of CYP3A4, increases the plasma concentrations and the effect of repaglinide; this can enhance the blood glucose lowering effect and increase the risk of hypoglycemia (59).

Digoxin

In 12 healthy volunteers aged 19–36 years nateglinide had no effects on the pharmacokinetics of a single dose of digoxin (60). Similarly, in 14 healthy adults, repaglinide 2 mg three times had no effect on the steady-state pharmacokinetics of digoxin (61). These results suggest that the meglitinides do not affect P glycoprotein.

Fibrates

In 12 healthy subjects gemfibrozil raised the AUC of repaglinide 8-fold and itraconazole raised it 1.4-fold; however, the combination increased it nearly 20-fold (62).

However, in a formal study bezafibrate and fenofibrate did not affect the pharmacokinetics or pharmacodynamics of a single dose of repaglinide 0.25 mg (63).

Ketoconazole

In healthy subjects, ketoconazole increased mean AUC of repaglinide by 15% and mean C_{max} by 7% (64).

Nifedipine

Concomitant treatment with the CYP3A4 substrate nifedipine altered the mean AUC and mean C_{max} of repaglinide by 11 and 3% respectively (64).

Oral contraceptives

Concomitant treatment with ethinylestradiol + levonorgestrel altered the mean AUC and mean C_{max} of repaglinide by 1 and 17% respectively (64).

Rifampicin

Studies involving rifampicin and repaglinide have yielded conflicting results, perhaps because of timing and dosages. In one study rifampicin had no effect on the pharmacokinetics and pharmacodynamics of a single dose repaglinide given after 7 days of rifampicin (65). In contrast, rifampicin 600 mg reduced the AUC of repaglinide by 57% and shortened its half-life from 1.5 to 1.1 hours in nine healthy volunteers after 5 days (66). The effect may even be greater when rifampicin is used for a longer period. In another study in healthy volunteers, rifampicin reduced the mean AUC of repaglinide by 31% and the mean C_{max} by 26%. These studies differed in timing and doses.

In a more recent study, 12 male volunteers took rifampicin 600 mg/day for 7 days followed by two doses of repaglinide 4 mg 24 hours apart; the AUC for repaglinide was reduced by 50% on day 7, and by 80% on day 8 (67). Timing of the drugs may alter the clinical effects.

Simvastatin

Concomitant treatment with the CYP3A4 substrate simvastatin altered the mean AUC and mean C_{max} of repaglinide by 2 and 27% respectively (64).

Trimethoprim

CYP2C8 and CYP3A4 are involved in the metabolism of repaglinide (68). Trimethoprim is a selective inhibitor of CYP2C8. When nine healthy volunteers aged 19–23 years, 8 men) took placebo or trimethoprim 160 mg bd for 3 days followed by 0.25 mg of repaglinide 1 hour after the last dose of trimethoprim, the AUC of repaglinide increased by 61% and the C_{max} increased by 41% compared with placebo.

References

1. Dabrowski M, Wahl P, Holmes WE, Ashcroft FM. Effect of repaglinide on cloned beta cell, cardiac and smooth muscle types of ATP-sensitive potassium channels. Diabetologia 2001;44(6):747–56.
2. Lindsay JR, McKillop AM, Mooney MH, O'Harte FP, Flatt PR, Bell PM. Effects of nateglinide on the secretion of glycated insulin and glucose tolerance in type 2 diabetes. Diabetes Res Clin Pract 2003;61(3):167–73.
3. Hu S, Boettcher BR, Dunning BE. The mechanisms underlying the unique pharmacodynamics of nateglinide. Diabetologia 2003;46(Suppl 1):M37–43.
4. Cohen RM, Ramlo-Halsted BA. How do the new insulin secretagogues compare? Diabetes Care 2002;25(8):1472–3.
5. Kahn SE, Montgomery B, Howell W, Ligueros-Saylan M, Hsu CH, Devineni D, McLeod JF, Horowitz A, Foley JE. Importance of early phase insulin secretion to intravenous glucose tolerance in subjects with type 2 diabetes mellitus. J Clin Endocrinol Metab 2001;86(12):5824–9.
6. Parulkar AA, Fonseca VA. Recent advances in pharmacological treatment of type 2 diabetes mellitus. Compr Ther 1999;25(8–10):418–26.
7. Ratner RE. Repaglinide therapy in the treatment of type 2 diabetes. Today's Ther Trends 1999;17:57–66.
8. Culy CR, Jarvis B. Repaglinide: a review of its therapeutic use in type 2 diabetes mellitus. Drugs 2001;61(11):1625–60.
9. Juhl CB, Porksen N, Hollingdal M, Sturis J, Pincus S, Veldhuis JD, Dejgaard A, Schmitz O. Repaglinide acutely amplifies pulsatile insulin secretion by augmentation of burst mass with no effect on burst frequency. Diabetes Care 2000;23(5):675–81.

10. Hatorp V, Huang WC, Strange P. Repaglinide pharmacokinetics in healthy young adult and elderly subjects. Clin Ther 1999;21(4):702–10.
11. Gomis R. Repaglinide as monotherapy in Type 2 diabetes. Exp Clin Endocrinol Diabetes 1999;107(Suppl 4):S133–5.
12. Damsbo P, Marbury TC, Hatorp V, Clauson P, Muller PG. Flexible prandial glucose regulation with repaglinide in patients with type 2 diabetes. Diabetes Res Clin Pract 1999;45(1):31–9.
13. Moses RG, Gomis R, Frandsen KB, Schlienger JL, Dedov I. Flexible meal-related dosing with repaglinide facilitates glycemic control in therapy-naive type 2 diabetes. Diabetes Care 2001;24(1):11–5.
14. Hatorp V, Huang WC, Strange P. Pharmacokinetic profiles of repaglinide in elderly subjects with type 2 diabetes. J Clin Endocrinol Metab 1999;84(4):1475–8.
15. Massi-Benedetti M, Damsbo P. Pharmacology and clinical experience with repaglinide. Expert Opin Investig Drugs 2000;9(4):885–98.
16. Bouhanick B, Barbosa SS. Repaglinide: Novonorm, une alternative chez le diabétique de type 2. [Rapaglinide: Novonorm, an alternative in type 2 diabetes.] Presse Méd 2000;29(19):1059–61.
17. Lindsay JR, McKillop AM, Mooney MH, O'Harte FPM, Flatt PR, Bell PM. Effect of nateglinide on the secretion of glycated insulin and glucose tolerance in type 2 diabetes. Diab Res Clin Pract 2003;61:167–73.
18. Gribble FM, Manley SE, Levy JC. Randomized dose ranging study of the reduction of fasting and postprandial glucose in type 2 diabetes by nateglinide (A-4166). Diabetes Care 2001;24(7):1221–5.
19. Wolffenbuttel BH, Landgraf RDutch and German Repaglinide Study Group. A 1-year multicenter randomized double-blind comparison of repaglinide and glyburide for the treatment of type 2 diabetes. Diabetes Care 1999;22(3):463–7.
20. Marbury T, Huang WC, Strange P, Lebovitz H. Repaglinide versus glyburide: a one-year comparison trial. Diabetes Res Clin Pract 1999;43(3):155–66.
21. Landgraf R, Bilo HJ, Muller PG. A comparison of repaglinide and glibenclamide in the treatment of type 2 diabetic patients previously treated with sulphonylureas. Eur J Clin Pharmacol 1999;55(3):165–71.
22. Mafauzy M. Repaglinide versus glibenclamide treatment of type 2 diabetes during Ramadan fasting. Diabetes Res Clin Pract 2002;58(1):45–53.
23. Moran A, Phillips J, Milla C. Insulin and glucose excursion following premeal insulin lispro or repaglinide in cystic fibrosis-related diabetes. Diabetes Care 2001;24(10):1706–10.
24. Rosenstock J, Hassman DR, Maddere RD, Brazinsky SA, Farrell J, Khutoryansky N, Hale PM, for the Repaglinide Versus Nateglinide Comparison Study Group. Repaglinide versus nateglinide monotherapy. Diabetes Care 2004;27:1265–70.
25. Hanefeld M, Bouter KP, Dickinson S, Guitard C. Rapid and short-acting mealtime insulin secretion with nateglinide controls both prandial and mean glycemia. Diabetes Care 2000;23(2):202–7.
26. Kalbag JB, Walter YH, Nedelman JR, McLeod JF. Mealtime glucose regulation with nateglinide in healthy volunteers: comparison with repaglinide and placebo. Diabetes Care 2001;24(1):73–7.
27. Hollander PA, Schwartz SL, Gatlin MR, Haas SJ, Zheng H, Foley JE, Dunning BE. Importance of early insulin secretion: comparison of nateglinide and glyburide in previously

diet-treated patients with type 2 diabetes. Diabetes Care 2001;24(6):983–8.

28. Jovanovic L, Dailey G 3rd, Huang WC, Strange P, Goldstein BJ. Repaglinide in type 2 diabetes: a 24-week, fixed-dose efficacy and safety study. J Clin Pharmacol 2000;40(1):49–57.

29. Inzucchi SE. Oral antihyperglycemic therapy for type 2 diabetes: scientific review. JAMA 2002;287(3):360–72.

30. Holmboe ES. Oral antihyperglycemic therapy for type 2 diabetes: clinical applications. JAMA 2002;287(3):373–6.

31. Van Gaal LF, De Leeuw IH. Rationale and options for combination therapy in the treatment of Type 2 diabetes. Diabetologia 2003;46(Suppl 1):M44–50.

32. Moses R, Slobodniuk R, Boyages S, Colagiuri S, Kidson W, Carter J, Donnelly T, Moffitt P, Hopkins H. Effect of repaglinide addition to metformin monotherapy on glycemic control in patients with type 2 diabetes. Diabetes Care 1999;22(1):119–24.

33. Hirschberg Y, Karara AH, Pietri AO, McLeod JF. Improved control of mealtime glucose excursions with coadministration of nateglinide and metformin. Diabetes Care 2000;23(3):349–53.

34. Horton ES, Clinkingbeard C, Gatlin M, Foley J, Mallows S, Shen S. Nateglinide alone and in combination with metformin improves glycemic control by reducing mealtime glucose levels in type 2 diabetes. Diabetes Care 2000;23(11):1660–5.

35. Moses R. Repaglinide in combination therapy with metformin in Type 2 diabetes. Exp Clin Endocrinol Diabetes 1999;107(Suppl 4):S136–9.

36. Schatz H, Schoppel K, Lehwalder D, Schandry R. Efficacy, tolerability and safety of nateglinide in combination with metformin. Results from a study under general practice conditions. Exp Clin Endocrinol Diabetes 2003;111:262–6.

37. Javanovic L, Hassman DR, Gooch B, Jain R, Greco S, Khutoryansky N, Hale PM. Treatment of type 2 diabetes with a combination regimen of repaglinide plus pioglitazone. Diabetes Res Clin Pract 2004;63:127–34.

38. Raskin P, McGill J, Saad MF, Cappleman JM, Kaye W, Khutoryansky N, Hale PM. Combination therapy for type 2 diabetes: repaglinide plus rosiglitazone. Diabetic Med 2004;21:329–35.

39. Carroll MF, Izard A, Riboni K, Burge MR, Schade DS. Control of postprandial hyperglycemia: optimal use of short-acting insulin secretagogues. Diabetes Care 2002;25(12):2147–52.

40. Rosenstock J, Shen SG, Gatlin MR, Foley JE. Combination therapy with nateglinide and a thiazolidinedione improves glycemic control in type 2 diabetes. Diabetes Care 2002;25(9):1529–33.

41. Raskin P, Jovanovic L, Berger S, Schwartz S, Woo V, Ratner R. Repaglinide/troglitazone combination therapy: improved glycemic control in type 2 diabetes. Diabetes Care 2000;23(7):979–83.

42. Furlong NJ, Hulme SA, O'Brien SV, Hardy KJ. Repaglinide versus metformin in combination with bedtime NPH insulin in patients with type 2 diabetes established on insulin/metformin combination therapy. Diabetes Care 2002;25(10):1685–90.

43. Schatz H. Preclinical and clinical studies on safety and tolerability of repaglinide. Exp Clin Endocrinol Diabetes 1999;107(Suppl 4):S144–8.

44. Schmitz O, Lund S, Andersen PH, Jonler M, Porksen N. Optimizing insulin secretagogue therapy in patients with type 2 diabetes: a randomized double-blind study with repaglinide. Diabetes Care 2002;25(2):342–6.

45. Van Gaal LF, Van Acker KL, De Leeuw IH. Repaglinide improves blood glucose control in sulphonylurea-naive type 2 diabetes. Diabetes Res Clin Pract 2001;53(3):141–8.

46. de Luis DA, Aller R, Cuellar L, Terroba C, Ovalle H, Izaola O, Romero E. Effect of repaglinide addition to NPH insulin monotherapy on glycemic control in patients with type 2 diabetes. Diabetes Care 2001;24(10):1844–5.

47. Madsbad S, Kilhovd B, Lager I, Mustajoki P, Dejgaard A. Scandinavian Repaglinide Group. Comparison between repaglinide and glipizide in Type 2 diabetes mellitus: a 1-year multicentre study. Diabet Med 2001;18(5):395–401.

48. Damsbo P, Clauson P, Marbury TC, Windfeld K. A double-blind randomized comparison of meal-related glycemic control by repaglinide and glyburide in well-controlled type 2 diabetic patients. Diabetes Care 1999;22(5):789–94.

49. Hirshberg B, Skarulis MC, Pucino F, Csako G, Brennan R, Gorden P. Repaglinide-induced factitious hypoglycemia. J Clin Endocrinol Metab 2001;86(2):475–7.

50. Furlong NJ, Hulme SA, O'Brien SV, Hardy KJ. Comparison of repaglinide vs gliclazide in combination with bedtime NPH insulin in patients with type 2 diabetes inadequately controlled with oral hypoglycaemic agents. Diabetic Med 2003;20:935–41.

51. Nan DN, Hernandez JL, Fernandez-Ayala M, Carrascosa M. Acute hepatoxicity caused by repaglinide. Ann Intern Med 2004;141:823.

52. Margolin N. Severe leucocytoclastic vasculitis induced by repaglinide in a patient with chronic hepatitis C. Clin Drug Invest 2002;22:795–6.

53. Thomsen MS, Chassard D, Evène E, Nielsen KK, Jørgensen M. Pharmacokinetics of repaglinide in healthy Caucasian and Japanese subjects. J Clin Pharmacol 2003;43:23–8.

54. Weaver JU, Robertson D, Atkin SL, on behalf of the Nateglinide Glycaemic Control Investigators. Nateglinide alone or with metformin safely improves glycaemia to target in patients up to an age of 84. Diabetes Obesity Metab 2004;6:344–52.

55. Schumacher S, Abbasi I, Weise D, Hatorp V, Sattler K, Sieber J, Hasslacher C. Single- and multiple-dose pharmacokinetics of repaglinide in patients with type 2 diabetes and renal impairment. Eur J Clin Pharmacol 2001;57(2):147–52.

56. Hasslacher CMultinational Repaglinide Renal Study Group. Safety and efficacy of repaglinide in type 2 diabetic patients with and without impaired renal function. Diabetes Care 2003;26(3):886–91.

57. Anonymous. Clinical news. Interactions and pharmacokinetics of repaglinide. Pharm J 2000;264:503.

58. Plosker GL, Figgitt DP. Repaglinide: a pharmacoeconomic review of its use in type 2 diabetes mellitus. Pharmacoeconomics 2004;22(6):389–411.

59. Niemi M, Neuvonen PJ, Kivisto KT. The cytochrome P4503A4 inhibitor clarithromycin increases the plasma concentrations and effects of repaglinide. Clin Pharmacol Ther 2001;70(1):58–65.

60. Zhou H, Walter YH, Smith H, Devineni D, McLeod JF. Nateglinide, a new mealtime glucose regulator. Lack of pharmacokinetic interaction with digoxin in healthy volunteers. Clin Drug Invest 2000;19:465–71.

61. Hatorp V, Thomsen MS. Drug interaction studies with repaglinide: repaglinide on digoxin or theophylline pharmacokinetics and cimetidine on repaglinide pharmacokinetics. J Clin Pharmacol 2000;40(2):184–92.

62. Niemi M, Backman JT, Neuvonen M, Neuvonen PJ. Effects of gemfibrozil, itraconazole, and their combination on the pharmacokinetics and pharmacodynamics of repaglinide: potentially hazardous interaction between gemfibrozil and repaglinide. Diabetologia 2003;46(3):347–51.

63. Kajosaari LI, Backman JT, Neuvonen M, Laitila J, Neuvonen PJ. Lack of effect of bezafibrate and fenofibrate on the pharmacokinetics and pharmacodynamics of repaglinide. Br J Clin Pharmacol 2004;58:390–6.

64. Hatorp V, Hansen KT, Thomsen MS. Influence of drugs interacting with CYP3A4 on the pharmacokinetics, pharmacodynamics, and safety of the prandial glucose regulator repaglinide. J Clin Pharmacol 2003;43(6):649–60.

65. Hartop V, Hansen KT, Thomsen MK. Influence of drugs interacting with CYP3A4 on the pharmacokinetics, pharmacodynamics and safety of the prandial glucose regulator repaglinide. J Clin Pharmacol 2003;43:649–60.

66. Neimi M, Kajosaari LI, Neuvonen M, Backman JT, Neuvonen PJ. The CYP2C8 inhibitor trimethoprim increases the plasma concentrations of repaglinide in healthy subjects. Br J Clin Pharmacol 2004;57:441–7.

67. Bidstrup TB, Stilling N, Damkier P, Scharling B, Thomsen MS, Brøsen K. Rifampicin seems to act as both an inducer and inhibitor of the metabolism of repaglinide. Eur J Clin Pharmacol 2004;60:109–14.

68. Niemi M, Backman JT, Neuvonen M, Neuvonen PJ, Kivisto KT. Rifampin decreases the plasma concentrations and effects of repaglinide. Clin Pharmacol Ther 2000;68(5):495–500.

Sulfonylureas

General Information

Sulfonylureas act by inhibiting ATP-sensitive potassium channels (K_{ATP} channels) in pancreatic beta cells, increasing the amount of insulin released. The beta cells of patients taking these drugs are chronically stimulated. Changes in the pattern of insulin secretion and increased peripheral resistance to insulin both result in increased output of glucose from the liver. A rise in the number of insulin receptors, amelioration of the postbinding defect, and inhibition of the increased glucose output from the liver have been described (SEDA-5, 391), mostly in in vitro or animal experiments of short duration. The K_{ATP} channels in the beta cells and other tissues have been reviewed, including a discussion of the effects of various sulfonylureas (1). Enhanced action on beta cells by the addition of ADP suggests that the action of sulfonylureas varies with the metabolic state of the islet. Chlorpropamide and glibenclamide have high islet-binding specificity, while glibenclamide also binds with high affinity to extra-pancreatic binding sites.

Increased insulin release reduces blood glucose and glycosuria and contributes to a reduction in energy loss. This leads to increased storage of body fat when more is eaten than is necessary to meet daily energy needs and provokes feelings of hunger. Traditionally therefore, the sulfonylureas have been regarded as being unsuitable for overweight diabetics, who primarily need to lose weight. However, the results of the Diabetes Control and Complications Trial (DCCT) (2) and the UK Prospective Diabetes Study (UKPDS) (3) have shown that a sustained increase in the blood glucose concentration accelerates the development of secondary complications of diabetes mellitus. Being overweight may therefore be the price to be paid for normalization of blood glucose. However, not all secondary changes, such as macroangiopathy, seem to depend directly on the blood glucose concentration.

The potencies and the durations of action of oral hypoglycemic drugs vary (see Table 1). Oral drugs may make the cell more sensitive to insulin, and it is difficult to predict how long the hypoglycemic effect will last. The blood concentration does not always determine the

Table 1 Doses, durations of action, and half-lives of sulfonylureas

| RINN | Dose (mg) | | Duration of action (hours) | Half-life (hours) | |
| | Mean/day | Maximum/day | | Renal function | |
				Normal	Anuric
Acetohexamide	250–1000	1500	12–24	16	48
Carbutamide[a]	500–1500	2500			
Chlorpropamide	100–500	1000	20–60	35	200
Glibenclamide (glyburide)	2.5–10	20	12–18	5–8	11
Glibornuride	12.5–100		10–15		
Gliclazide	40–240	240	12–18	8–11	
Glimepiride	1–4	6	12–20	5–8	
Glipizide	2.5–20	30	6–12	3–5	Unchanged[b]
Gliquidone	15–90	120	6–12	6–10	Unchanged[b]
Glisoxepide	2–12	15	5–10		
Glymidine (glycodiazine)	500–1500	3000	6–12		
Tolazamide	100–500	1000	12–16	8–10	
Tolbutamide	500–2000	3000	6–12	3–5	48

[a]Obsolete
[b]Hypoglycemia occurs despite the unchanged half-life

duration of action. When the concentration is falling, stimulation of insulin secretion can continue for some time.

There have been reviews of oral hypoglycemic drugs (4–8).

Maturity-onset diabetes of the young (MODY) is characterized by type 2 diabetes at or before adolescence. It is a genetically heterogeneous disease, for which at least five different genes have been identified. MODY3, one of the most common forms, is characterized by a mutation in the hepatocyte nuclear factor (HNF)-1α gene. MODY3 can be very sensitive to sulfonylureas (SEDA-22, 475) (9,10). Three new cases have been presented, all with a mutation in the HNF-1α gene; low-dose glibenclamide was the best treatment in all cases (11).

The UK Prospective Diabetes Study (3) has shown that timely treatment, by reducing blood glucose concentrations before subjective complaints develop, reduces secondary complications in type 2 diabetes mellitus.

Combinations of oral hypoglycemic drugs

The different mechanisms of action of the various classes of hypoglycemic drugs makes combined therapy feasible: the sulfonylureas and meglitinides stimulate insulin production by different mechanisms, the biguanides reduce glucose production by the liver and excretion from the liver, acarbose reduces the absorption of glucose from the gut, and the thiazolidinediones reduce insulin resistance in fat. It is not necessary to wait until the maximal dose of one drug has been reached before starting another. However, sulfonylureas and meglitinides should no longer be used when endogenous insulin production is minimal. Combinations of insulin with sulfonylureas or meglitinides should only be used while the patient is changing to insulin, except when long-acting insulin is given at night in order to give the islets a rest and to stimulate daytime insulin secretion.

Large studies of the effects of lifestyle changes, the effects of drugs in preventing or postponing the complications of diabetes, or the usefulness of various combinations are regularly published. The different mechanisms of action of the various classes give different metabolic effects and different adverse effects profiles (12). Comparative costs of the various therapies in the USA have been presented (13).

This subject has been reviewed in relation to combined oral therapy. In a systematic review of 63 studies with a duration of at least 3 months and involving at least 10 patients at the end of the study, and in which HbA_{1c} was reported, five different classes of oral drugs were almost equally effective in lowering blood glucose concentrations (14). HbA_{1c} was reduced by about 1–2% in all cases. Combination therapy gave additive effects. However, long-term vascular risk reduction was demonstrated only with sulfonylureas and metformin.

The adverse effects of combined drug therapy are attributable to adverse effects of the individual drugs. Increased adverse effects or new adverse effects in patients taking combinations have not been reported.

Sulfonylureas plus biguanides

The combination of metformin with various sulfonylurea derivatives has been extensively reviewed (15). When metformin or pioglitazone were added to sulfonylureas in patients with type 2 diabetes who were poorly controlled, those with reduced pancreatic beta cell function responded better to metformin, while those with greater insulin resistance responded better to pioglitazone (16).

Combination tablets containing metformin + glibenclamide (250 + 1.25 mg) were compared with monotherapy with metformin 500 mg/day or glibenclamide 2.5 mg/day for 16 weeks in 486 patients (17). The total daily doses were adjusted depending on fasting plasma glucose. The final mean doses with combined therapy were lower than with monotherapy. Gastrointestinal symptoms, such as diarrhea, nausea, vomiting, and abdominal pain, were significantly more frequent with metformin monotherapy than with either combined therapy or glibenclamide monotherapy. Hypoglycemia was most frequent in those who took combination therapy and least with metformin monotherapy, but finger-stick glucose concentrations under 2.8 mmol/l were rare with metformin monotherapy and equally common with glibenclamide monotherapy and combination therapy.

In the United Kingdom Prospective Diabetes Study a subgroup of patients taking sulfonylurea therapy to which metformin was added appeared to have had excess mortality. Data from 263 general practices in the UK were analysed; 8488 patients took a sulfonylurea initially, to which metformin was added in 1868 (18). The crude mortality rates per 1000 person years were 59 and 40 respectively. Metformin was used initially in 3099 patients and a sulfonylurea was added in 867. The crude mortality rates per 1000 person years were 25 and 20 respectively. These results suggest there is no increased mortality risk with a combination of a sulfonylurea and metformin.

Sulfonylureas + biguanides + glitazones

Glibenclamide 2.5 mg/day + metformin 500 mg/day in a combination tablet was increased to a maximum of 10 mg/day + 2000 mg/day in patients with type 2 diabetes, mean age 57 years and weight 93 kg; 181 patients also took rosiglitazone and 184 took placebo for 24 weeks (19). Rosiglitazone was added to a maximum of 8 mg/day aiming to reduce the HB_{A1c} concentration to less than 7.0%. There was *hypoglycemia* in 140 patients; 95 (53%) of those who took rosiglitazone reported hypoglycemia compared with 45 (25%) of those who took placebo. One patient taking rosiglitazone withdrew owing to hypoglycemia. HB_{A1c} concentrations were less than 7% in 42% of those taking rosiglitazone compared with 14% of those taking placebo. Weight gain was greater in those taking rosiglitazone, 3 kg compared with 0.03 kg.

Sulfonylureas plus glitazones

Rosiglitazone 8 mg/day + glibenclamide 7.5 mg/day were compared with glibenclamide alone (maximum 15 mg/day) in 335 patients over 26 weeks (20). HbA_{1c} fell by 0.81% with combination therapy. One patient taking combination therapy had a single episode of serious hypoglycemia; mild to moderate hypoglycemia was reported in 19% of the patients taking combination therapy and 4.1% in those taking glibenclamide alone. There was edema in 9.5% versus 2.9%, weight gain of 3.1 kg versus 0.14 kg, and reduced hemoglobin in those taking combination therapy.

Sulfonylureas + meglitinides

Glipizide, nateglinide, and their combination have been compared in a double-blind, randomized, placebo-controlled study in 20 patients with type 2 diabetes not requiring insulin (21). Before a standardized breakfast they took glipizide 10 mg, nateglinide 120 mg, both, or placebo; 4 hours after the meal blood glucose concentrations were significantly higher after nateglinide, but peak and integrated glucose concentrations did not differ. Integrated insulin concentrations were higher with glipizide. There were three episodes of hypoglycemia in the glipizide alone group and three in the combined group; three required treatment with glucose.

Sulfonylureas + thiazolidinediones

Troglitazone 100 or 200 mg/day or placebo was given for 16 weeks to 259 patients already taking sulfonylurea therapy (22). HbA_{1c} was 0.4 and 0.7% lower and blood glucose concentrations fell. The most common event was hypoglycemia, but this did not occur more often when troglitazone was added. Liver enzymes increased to the same extent in the three groups and never rose above normal. No patients withdrew because of drug-related effects.

Sulfonylureas plus insulin

When 51 recently diagnosed patients with type 2 diabetes were treated with mixed insulin (30% soluble + 70% NPH) twice daily or glibenclamide in doses that kept HbA_{1c} no more than 1% above the upper normal concentration for 1 year, early insulin treatment prolonged endogenous insulin secretion and improved metabolic control. Adverse effects and quality of life were not different (23). This differs from the UKPDS, in which early institution of insulin made no difference in metabolic control.

Organs and Systems

Cardiovascular

Early studies suggested that tolbutamide caused excessive cardiovascular deaths (24) as reported in the University Group Diabetes Program (UGDP) (SEDA-4, 301), but the UK Prospective Diabetes Study did not find different mortality in patients treated with insulin, glibenclamide, or chlorpropamide (3). The results of the UGDP study are now widely regarded as impossible to be unanimously interpreted, but the question of whether sulfonylureas have a negative effect during myocardial infarction and survival during infarction has lingered.

This effect of tolbutamide, if it occurs, has been attributed to prevention of ischemic preconditioning, a protective manoeuvre that reduces myocardial damage after temporary stoppage of coronary blood flow (25).

Transient myocardial ischemia augments post-ischemic myocardial function and prevents dysrhythmias. K_{ATP} channels play a role in this so-called ischemic preconditioning. In 48 atrial trabeculae, obtained during catheterization, the recovery of the developed muscle force in patients treated with a sulfonylurea was only half of what was found in non-diabetics or diabetics treated with insulin. This suggests that inhibition of K_{ATP} channels by oral sulfonylureas might contribute to increased cardiovascular mortality (26). The question of whether the findings obtained mainly with glibenclamide can be generalized to all sulfonylureas has been discussed, since sulfonylureas differ greatly in their ability to interfere with vascular or cardiac K_{ATP} channels (27). Both glimepiride and glibenclamide (28) improved glycemia in 29 patients in a randomized, double-blind, placebo-controlled, crossover study of a number of susceptibility factors for ischemic heart disease (plasminogen activator inhibitor activity, plasminogen activator inhibitor antigen, LDL cholesterol, C peptide, proinsulin, des-31,32 proinsulin, etc.), but K_{ATP} channels were not investigated.

New data on the sulfonylurea receptor as part of the ATP-dependent potassium channel (SUR-1 in the beta pancreatic cells, involved in insulin secretion, and SUR-2 in the myocardium, involved in cardiac adaptation during ischemia) has still not yielded a definitive answer. The available experimental and clinical data have been systematically reviewed (29). The conclusion was that experimentally the effects of sulfonylureas on heart muscle are both deleterious and protective for glibenclamide while tolbutamide, glimepiride, and gliclazide have no effects. There seem to be no adverse cardiac consequences of chronic treatment with sulfonylureas.

In a randomized study of 48 patients with type 2 diabetes, mean age 58 years, those who took glibenclamide for 8 weeks had a mean increase in systolic blood pressure of 3.1 mmHg (30). In the same study the systolic and diastolic blood pressures fell in those who took rosiglitazone. The authors speculated whether changes in insulin concentrations and sympathetic activity were responsible.

Glibenclamide prevented the increase in tolerance to myocardial ischemia normally observed during the second of two sequential exercise tests (31).

Respiratory

- A 76-year-old man who had taken glibenclamide for 2 weeks, having switched from voglibose, developed pneumonitis; a lymphocyte stimulation test was positive for glibenclamide (32).

Sensory systems

A change in taste sensation has been reported with glipizide (33).

Metabolism

In 36 Japanese patients who were relatively lean but had excess abdominal fat, glibenclamide and voglibose caused loss of weight and abdominal fat (34). The loss of abdominal fat was related to glycemic control. The ratio of subcutaneous to abdominal fat shifted toward subcutaneous fat only in those who took voglibose. Both voglibose and glibenclamide improved insulin sensitivity and the acute response to insulin.

In a meta-analysis of 1444 patients who took glimepiride for a year there was no change in weight (35).

Hypoglycemia

DoTS classification (BMJ 2003;327:1222–5)
Adverse effect: Hypoglycemia due to sulfonylureas
Dose-relation: toxic effect
Time-course: time-independent
Susceptibility factors: disease (impaired liver or kidney function, alcoholism); drug interactions; reduced food intake; exercise

Hypoglycemia is the most frequent complication in patients with diabetes taking oral hypoglycemic drugs (36–38).

Presentation

In general, hypoglycemia caused by oral hypoglycemic drugs is more dangerous and of longer duration than hypoglycemia caused by insulin (39), and the most dangerous hypoglycemic attacks are those that result from long-acting drugs, such as chlorpropamide, and later sulfonylureas, such as glibenclamide (SEDA-4, 303). Sulfonylureas are mostly used by elderly people, and the characteristic warning symptoms of hypoglycemia (dizziness, breathlessness, sweating, and a feeling of hunger) are often absent or not well-interpreted.

Neurological symptoms are common and hypoglycemia can cause hemiplegia, which can be confused with neurological symptoms of other origin (transient ischemic attack, stroke, etc.). A bilateral case has been reported (40).

- A 68-year-old man started to take glibenclamide and 1 week later developed a blurred voice andsided hemiplegia with a blood glucose of 1.4 mmol/l. Ten minutes after intravenous glucose 50 g his motor function returned to normal. Six hours later he developed slurred speech and left-sided hemiplegia; his blood glucose was 1.9 mmol/l. During glucose administration his deficit resolved.
- A 75-year-old man taking gliclazide 80 mg bd and metformin 850 mg tds became hypoglycemic and was treated successfully (41). All hypoglycemic drugs were withdrawn, but he received more through his doctor's prescription computer and again became hypoglycemic on two occasions. On the second he became unconscious for 4.5 hours and his plasma glucose was 1.2 mmol/l. After resuscitation his abbreviated mental test was 5/10 and did not improve. He later became very aggressive and died of bronchopneumonia.

Three patients became comatose due to hypoglycemia (42):

- an 83-year-old woman who took two times 5 mg glibenclamide bd;
- a 61-year-old man who took 2 mg glimepiride bd and 500 mg metformin bd;
- a 79-year-old woman who took 5 mg glibenclamide tds and metformin 850 mg bd.

All of these patients had general malaise, reduced food intake, and vomiting; glucose had to be given for a long time and one patient died with pneumonia.

Frequent attacks of hypoglycemia can result in encephalopathy, and after withdrawal of the hypoglycemic drug cerebral injury can persist. It is not exceptional for prolonged hypoglycemic coma to end fatally (43,44). In 494 cases of severe hypoglycemia, 10% of the patients died and 9% had permanent sequelae (45).

Factitious hypoglycemia can take a long time to diagnose.

- A 20-year-old woman with unexplained hypoglycemia had an exploratory laparotomy with pancreatic biopsy, which showed a histological picture compatible with hyperplasia (46). Glipizide was detected in the blood at a concentration of 0.72 (usual target range 0.1–0.49) µg/ml. The diagnosis was factitious hypoglycemia.
- A 33-year-old nurse with unexplained hypoglycemia had only small increases in insulin and C-peptide, and glibenclamide was found in her serum (47). However, she denied using it and did not want psychiatric therapy.

Reported cases again illustrate that hypoglycemia induced by tablets tends to relapse and that long-term observation after normalizing the blood glucose concentration is necessary.

Hypoglycemia has been reported in a worker, not wearing a mask, working with a machine preparing ultrafine sulfonylurea powder (48).

In a retrospective study 400 doctors in Germany were asked to compare the characteristics of severe hypoglycemia in patients in acute care induced by glimepiride and glibenclamide (49). Only 24 responded (6%). There were no differences in clinical characteristics or time course.

Incidence

In 13 963 sulfonylurea users over 65 years of age, there were 255 severe attacks of hypoglycemia during 20 715 patient-years of use (50).

In an open comparative study in 57 patients acarbose and gliclazide had the same effects on HbA$_{1c}$, blood glucose, and lipids, although the ratio of HDL:LDL cholesterol increased during acarbose therapy (51). Of those who took gliclazide 10% reported at least one mild hypoglycemic reaction.

In an 8-week, non-interventional cohort study in 22 045 patients with type 2 diabetes, of whom 4.9% discontinued therapy, adverse advents occurred in 2.3% (52). There were attacks of hypoglycemia in 0.3%. Of the 6547 patients taking glimepiride, 2.5% had adverse reactions and 0.4% had hypoglycemic reactions.

In an open, multicenter study, 849 patients with poorly controlled diabetes were treated with glimepiride monotherapy for 6 months in doses that were titrated from 1 to 6 mg (53). The authors tried to identify factors that could predict the response to glimepiride. Patients who achieved a fasting blood glucose below 7.7 mmol/l and HbA_{1c} below 7.5% or a reduction in fasting blood glucose of over 20% and/or in HbA_{1c} of at least 10% were defined as responders (57% of the 849 patients). Earlier treatment with other oral hypoglycemic drugs or long-standing diabetes increased the rate of non-responders. In 9.2% of the patients there were episodes of hypoglycemia, 1.4 per patient, and third-party or medical assistance was required five times as often. A family history of type 2 diabetes doubled the risk; a high HbA_{1c} reduced the risk.

In a retrospective study in Hong Kong, drug-induced hypoglycemia accounted for 0.5% of admissions; 50% of the episodes were related to sulfonylureas (54). These patients were older, predominantly female, in poorer general health, and needing assistance in daily activities, including feeding. Co-morbidities, such as macrovascular complications, renal insufficiency, and concurrent infections, were common. Low plasma albumin concentrations probably reflected poor nutritional status. Of those who had recurrent admissions, 67% lived in old peoples' homes, compared with 22% in those without previous admissions. The prognosis in this group was poor: 23% died within 1 year. Patients taking gliclazide ($n = 13$) or glipizide ($n = 10$) accounted for 37% of the episodes. They had more vascular complications than patients who used glibenclamide or chlorpropamide. They had a higher frequency of previous admissions (47 versus 19%) and a higher mortality rate (1 year, 47 versus 10%; 5 years, 72 versus 34%).

In a period of 12 months 23 episodes of severe hypoglycemia were recorded in those taking a sulfonylurea in a district with a population of 367 051 (8655 with diabetes) (55). The total cost of emergency treatment was estimated to be up to $92 078/year.

In a 2-year study in 507 patients, mean age 61 years, the incidence of symptoms suggestive of hypoglycemia was 4.8 per 100 patient years (56). Seven patients withdrew after 1 year because of adverse events, which were thought to be unrelated to the gliclazide.

Causes and susceptibility factors

Most sulfonylureas are at least partly metabolized in the liver (SEDA-9, 709) (57), and hence liver insufficiency, liver disease, and liver enzyme inhibition (alcohol) or induction (drugs) can alter the half-life of the drug and its duration of action.

Renal dysfunction is another cause of hypoglycemia (58). Some sulfonylureas, such as chlorpropamide (30%) and tolbutamide (50%), are excreted by the kidney. Other drugs, such as acetohexamide, glibenclamide (glyburide), glibornuride, and glymidine, are mainly metabolized, but some of their metabolites also have a hypoglycemic effect and are excreted by the kidneys, so that renal insufficiency can prolong their hypoglycemic actions. The reduction in insulin metabolism in diseased

kidneys (nephropathy) can contribute to hypoglycemia, since it increases the half-life of insulin.

Hypoglycemia can also result from drug interactions, with the simultaneous use of drugs that have glucose-lowering effects or that inhibit the clearance of oral hypoglycemic drugs.

The conclusion (SEDA-22, 475) (59) that fasting is well tolerated and that old age is no contraindication to sulfonylurea therapy has not been accepted by others (60,61), as the previous study included only a small number of relatively healthy patients with type 2 diabetes.

Hypoglycemia can result from overdosage of sulfonylureas (62,63). Factitious hypoglycemia induced by tablets is difficult to diagnose, since C peptide concentrations will be high and not suppressed. Reduced intake of food or alcohol can also play a role (64).

Severe hypoglycemia induced by long-acting and short-acting sulfonylureas in Basel, Switzerland (200 000 inhabitants), has been analysed in a retrospective study in 28 patients (median age 73 years) (65); 11 men and 5 women (2.24 per 1000 person-years) were taking long-acting sulfonylureas (15 glibenclamide, 1 chlorpropamide) and 2 men and 10 women (0.75 per 1000 person-years) short-acting sulfonylureas (10 glibornuride, 2 gliclazide). Metformin was only involved when combined with a sulfonylurea. There were no deaths. Reduced food intake ($n = 9$), increased activity ($n = 2$), impaired renal function ($n = 2$), alcohol ($n = 2$), too many tablets ($n = 3$), and no obvious factor ($n = 10$) were the causes.

Drug-induced hypoglycemia in 102 non-alcoholic, non-epileptic patients has been reviewed (66). There were susceptibility factors for hypoglycemia in 94; 84 were over 60 years old, of whom 70 were over 70 years; 66 had renal impairment, of whom 28 also had reduced energy intake, 10 had reduced energy intake, 30 had infections, 5 had liver cirrhosis, and 10 had malignant neoplasia; 14 had used hypoglycemia-potentiating drugs, such as beta-blockers ($n = 8$), cimetidine ($n = 2$), co-trimoxazole ($n = 2$), and aspirin ($n = 2$). Forty patients had protracted hypoglycemia lasting 12–72 hours. Head trauma ($n = 4$), skeletal injury ($n = 3$), seizures ($n = 8$), transient asymptomatic myocardial ischemia ($n = 2$), and transient right hemiplegia ($n = 1$) were seen. Five patients died. Ten used glibenclamide + metformin, 14 used glibenclamide + insulin, and 53 used only glibenclamide.

To study the impact of Munchausen's syndrome, 129 patients with unexplained hypoglycemia in France had blood tests for sulfonylureas, which were found in 22 cases—glibenclamide in 19 patients and gliclazide in 3 (67). The concentrations were usually higher than the usual target concentration: in seven cases they were five times higher and the highest value was 18 times higher. In most cases an insulinoma was suggested and pancreatectomy was planned.

Hypoglycemia appears to be less of a problem with glimepiride than with other sulfonylurea drugs. In nine patients who had severe hypoglycemia associated with glimepiride the hydroxylated metabolite was detectable 4–8 hours longer than glimepiride itself.

This may be useful in suspected poisoning. The clinical relevance of the hydroxylated metabolite is uncertain (68).

Management

Treatment of sulfonylurea-induced hypoglycemia and of overdose with sulfonylureas has been reviewed (69). If intravenous dextrose is insufficient, octreotide is recommended (70) but not diazoxide. In patients with insulin reserve, dextrose can stimulate insulin secretion and paradoxically worsen the condition. Patients with drug-induced hypoglycemia should not be given glucagon, since it will stimulate insulin secretion. Hypoglycemia can last for up to 5 days. Continued observation is important, because recurrence after temporary recovery is common.

Nutrition

In patients taking maximal doses of sulfonylureas, plasma homocysteine concentrations were raised during secondary failure with poor metabolic control, which may indicate increased vascular risk (71). The concentrations correlated inversely with endogenous insulin concentrations.

Electrolyte balance

Mild hyponatremia has been reported with sulfonylureas, most commonly with chlorpropamide (72,73). The mechanism with chlorpropamide is secretion of ADH (74).

In 70 non-insulin-dependent patients with diabetes, taking one of five different oral hypoglycemic drugs, 21% of prescriptions were associated with a low plasma sodium concentration, but it was lower than 129 mmol/l in only 8% (75). Every oral hypoglycemic agent was associated with a low plasma sodium concentration, which normalized on withdrawal. Extreme hyponatremia was only seen with chlorpropamide and, in one case, with glibenclamide.

Fluid balance

Water retention with oliguria, uremia, and edema has been reported with gliclazide (76). Resistance to diuretics can be caused by chlorpropamide (77) or, to a lesser extent, tolbutamide. Changing to a sulfonylurea without an antidiuretic effect (glibenclamide) or to one that enhances water excretion (acetohexamide, glipizide, or tolazamide) (78) may be advisable.

Hematologic

The most dangerous adverse reaction of sulfonylureas is agranulocytosis. Aplastic anemia (79), red cell aplasia (80), pure white cell aplasia (81), bone marrow aplasia, and hemolytic anemia have been described during treatment with chlorpropamide (82), glibenclamide (83), or tolbutamide (84).

Thrombocytopenia has been described with chlorpropamide (85), tolbutamide (86), glibenclamide (87), and glimepiride (88).

- A 68-year-old man, who had taken pipotiazine and trihexyphenidyl for 12 years for chronic psychosis, took glimepiride for hyperglycemia. No platelet counts were performed before or during this. He had no symptoms of bleeding. He developed a petechial rash and hematomas on his trunk, legs, and face, hemorrhagic bullae in his mouth, and gingival bleeding. There was thrombocytopenia ($1 \times 10^9/l$), with no malignant cells in a bone marrow aspirate and no serological evidence of recent viral infection. All medications were withdrawn and he was given prednisone and human immunoglobulin. After 7 days the hemorrhagic syndrome abated, although his platelet count was still $2 \times 10^9/l$. After four weeks the platelet count was $23 \times 10^9/l$ and the prednisone was gradually withdrawn. After 6 months the platelet count was normal ($346 \times 10^9/l$).

Glibenclamide can cause hemolysis by a non-immune mechanism (89).

- A 68-year-old man with a long history of type 2 diabetes and a slowly progressive myelodysplastic syndrome for 2 years took glibenclamide 5 mg/day for more than a year, buformin 150 mg/day, and voglibose 0.6 mg/day. His hemoglobin was 8.4 g/dl. No other cause of hemolysis was found and glibenclamide was withdrawn. His hemoglobin rose to 11.1 g/dl.

Eosinophilic infiltrations have been described with tolbutamide (SEDA-8, 917; 90), and chronic eosinophilic pneumonia has been described with chlorpropamide (91) and tolazamide (92).

Anemia has been attributed to glibenclamide (93).

- After taking metformin 850 mg tds and glibenclamide 5 mg bd for 5 days, a 58-year-old woman of Burkina Faso origin became anemic. The hemoglobin concentration was 9.4 g/dl, the reticulocyte count was 6.6%, and the glucose-6-phsophate dehydrogenase (G6PD) activity was low (0.4 UI/g Hb, reference range 4.0–6.8). Glibenclamide was withdrawn and metformin continued. The hemoglobin rose to 11.5 g/dl.

There have been rare reports of autoimmune hemolytic anemia attributed to glibenclamide and the manufacturer's product leaflet also mentions reports of pancytopenia.

Gastrointestinal

Gastrointestinal tract disturbances are frequent with sulfonylureas. They comprise nausea, vomiting, heartburn, dyspepsia, a metallic taste, and abdominal pain (94). They are less troublesome when the drug is taken after meals.

Liver

The risk of hepatotoxicity with the sulfonylureas varies with both the drug and the dosage. It has been described with chlorpropamide (95), tolazamide (96), tolbutamide (97), glipizide (98), and glibenclamide (99). Anicteric, cytolytic hepatitis has been described after glibenclamide (100).

Hepatic granulomas have been reported as a hypersensitivity reaction to chlorpropamide (101). Cholestatic jaundice from sulfonylureas is also probably of allergic origin; it is rare and has been described with glibenclamide (102), also in combination with hepatorenal syndrome (103), acetohexamide (104), chlorpropamide (105), gliclazide (106), and tolazamide (107).

- A 64-year-old man who had taken glibenclamide 10 mg/day for 4 years developed cholestasis (108). There was no extrahepatic obstruction on ERCP and serological tests for hepatitis A, B, and C, *Helicobacter pylori*, and antimitochondrial or antinuclear antibodies were all negative. Liver biopsy showed portal and periportal inflammation, edema, and prominent centrilobular hepatocanalicular cholestasis. When glibenclamide was withdrawn and insulin given, the laboratory values normalized within 8 weeks. Rechallenge was considered unethical.

Hepatitis has been described with glibenclamide (109) and gliclazide (110).

- A 60-year-old woman with normal liver function tests developed acute hepatitis 6 weeks after starting to take gliclazide. No viruses, autoimmune factors, or metabolic factors that could have caused hepatitis could be found. A lymphocyte transformation test was not performed. A liver biopsy was compatible with drug-related acute hepatitis. When gliclazide was withdrawn she improved. She took glibenclamide and recovered fully within 6 weeks.
- A 64-year-old man who took gliclazide 160 mg bd for 3 months developed hepatitis (111). No other cause could be detected. Gliclazide was withdrawn. A liver biopsy after 2 weeks showed resolving acute hepatitis, consistent with a drug reaction, and 3 months later the liver profile was normal.
- A 42-year-old woman with newly diagnosed diabetes and no other known diseases developed a slightly abnormal liver profile (112). Good glycemic control was obtained with metformin 850 mg bd and gliclazide 80 mg bd. After 4 weeks she developed a pruritic skin rash, which resolved after 4 days of treatment with fexofenadine. A liver profile 2 weeks later was abnormal. Metformin was withdrawn, but 3 days later she was icteric and gliclazide was withdrawn. A liver biopsy was consistent with cirrhosis and there were moderate inflammatory infiltrates. The liver function tests improved and after 3 weeks she was rechallenged with metformin without exacerbation.

In the last case cirrhosis may have contributed to the adverse effect of gliclazide.

- After increasing his dose of glibenclamide from 2.5 to 5 mg/day for 1 month a 55-year-old man developed jaundice and liver dysfunction, which improved after withdrawal for 2 months (113). Re-treatment caused an exacerbation. Liver function became normal after complete withdrawal.
- A 65-year-old man developed jaundice 2 weeks after presenting with type 2 diabetes. He had been given

glimepiride 2 mg/day (114). There was a stone in the common bile duct, which was treated with sphincterotomy. However, his liver function tests remained abnormal. Glimepiride was withdrawn, his liver function gradually normalized, and glimepiride was restarted. Liver function became abnormal once more and returned to normal within 1 month of withdrawal of glimepiride.

- A 50-year-old obese woman taking glipizide 5 mg/day who had been drinking a bottle of rum daily for 2 months developed an acute hepatitis and died (115). The viral hepatitis profile was negative. At autopsy the liver weighed 1800 g and there was focal necrosis without evidence of autoimmune or alcoholic hepatitis. There was no brain edema.

In the last case the picture was characteristic of subfulminant hepatic failure, possibly caused by glipizide and potentiated by excessive alcohol consumption.

Pancreas

A possible relation between 2 years of treatment with a sulfonylurea and damage to the islets of Langerhans has been reported (116). A fatal case of pancreatitis has been attributed to glibenclamide (117).

In a case-control study in 1.4 million people in Sweden, 462 who were hospitalized for pancreatitis without gallbladder disease were compared with 1781 randomly selected controls; 6% of the cases and 3% of the controls had diabetes (118). Diet and insulin therapy were not associated with an increased risk, but the risk of pancreatitis with glibenclamide had a crude odds ratio of 3.2 and was higher in people aged over 70 years and in those taking beta-blockers.

Urinary tract

Nephrotic syndrome and immune complex glomerulonephritis have been attributed to chlorpropamide (119).

Skin

Photosensitization has been described with carbutamide (120), tolbutamide (121), chlorpropamide (122), and glibenclamide (123), sometimes combined with porphyrinuria.

Allergic skin reactions have been described with all sulfonylureas. They include pruritic rashes, erythema nodosum, urticaria, blisters (100), erythema multiforme, exfoliative dermatitis, Quincke's edema, erythroderma, and itching, while lichenoid drug reactions with ulceration have occurred after chlorpropamide and tolazamide (124). More generalized hypersensitivity reactions may prove fatal, but rarely.

Erythema multiforme has been attributed to glibenclamide (125).

- A 69-year-old woman, who had taken gliclazide 40 mg/day for 3 months, was switched to glibenclamide 2.5 mg/day. She had malaise for 2 days, followed by anorexia, fever, and 2 days later erythema multiforme over her whole body. She also had liver dysfunction, renal impairment, and rhabdomyolysis. A lymphocyte stimulation test was positive for glibenclamide, which was withdrawn; the rash improved and the laboratory tests normalized within 4 days.

Pigmented purpuric dermatosis has been attributed to glipizide (126).

- A 66-year-old man took glipizide for 4 weeks and developed brownish, non-pruritic, purpuric, scaling patches on his upper legs and buttocks. Biopsy showed dilated capillaries with surrounding extravasated erythrocytes, perivascular lymphocytic infiltrates, and areas of hemosiderin deposition. After withdrawal of glipizide the rash cleared.

Immunologic

Hypersensitivity vasculitis has been described with glibenclamide (127). Glibenclamide contains a sulfa moiety and can cause allergic reactions in someone who is allergic to sulfonamides.

- A 57-year-old man with a previously undocumented sulfa allergy used atenolol 100 mg/day, hydrochlorothiazide 25 mg/day, docusate sodium 100 mg/day, and ranitidine 300 mg bd for several months (128). He started to take celecoxib 200 mg/day, and 1 month later developed erythema multiforme and difficulty in breathing caused by swelling of the throat. He improved after withdrawal of his drugs and further treatment. He was then instructed to reintroduce his previous drugs one a day. One day later, after taking glibenclamide 5 mg, he developed new lesions and dyspnea. After 3 weeks he had another relapse when he reintroduced hydrochlorothiazide. He omitted glibenclamide, celecoxib, and hydrochlorothiazide, but continued to use insulin, metformin, ranitidine, and psyllium. The urticarial lesions disappeared.

Celecoxib and hydrochlorothiazide also have sulfa moieties and could have contributed in this case.

- A 67-year-old man developed Stevens–Johnson syndrome after taking glibenclamide 20 mg/day for 4 weeks, having previously used insulin. He died from hemorrhagic bronchopneumonia. Post mortem examination also showed features of granulomatous arteritis and cholestatic interface hepatitis, suggestive of a hypersensitivity reaction (129).

Death

Of 2275 diabetic patients aged 45–74 years with proven coronary artery disease, followed for 7.7 years, 990 were treated with diet alone, 79 with metformin, 953 with glibenclamide, and 253 with a combination of metformin and glibenclamide (130). They were compared with 9047 non-diabetics. Mortality was lowest in the non-diabetics; death rates in the others were: diet alone 26%, metformin 32%, glibenclamide 34%, and combined therapy 44%.

Second-Generation Effects

Pregnancy

Sulfonylureas ($n = 68$) and metformin ($n = 50$) have been compared retrospectively with insulin ($n = 42$) in pregnancy (131). There were no severe attacks of hypoglycemia, no jaundice, and no differences in neonatal morbidity. However, in those who took metformin, pre-eclampsia and perinatal deaths were more common. Since metformin was given to obese women, and since obesity contributes to pre-eclampsia and perinatal mortality, this may have been an effect of obesity.

In 404 pregnant women at 11–33 weeks of gestation, with a fasting blood glucose of 5.3–7.8 mmol/l, randomly assigned to insulin or glibenclamide, there were no differences in perinatal outcome (132). Glibenclamide was not found in cord blood. The data were analysed separately for women with mean glucose concentrations at home above and below 5.8 mmol/l. In the high blood glucose group there were large children for gestational age in 19% (insulin) and 17% (glibenclamide), compared with 10% (insulin) and 11% (glibenclamide) in the low glucose group; it is not clear whether these differences were significant. There were no other differences (for example macrosomia, insulin in cord blood) between the groups.

Of 197 patients with gestational diabetes, 73 took glibenclamide, and 59 (81%) achieved satisfactory blood glucose control (133). Of these 59, nine had adverse effects, including malaise and weakness ($n = 4$), nausea ($n = 2$), lightheadedness ($n = 1$), and hypoglycemia ($n = 2$). Glibenclamide was withdrawn in one patient because of adverse effects; 11 of the 59 had babies who weighed over 4 kg. No anomalies were identified, but glibenclamide was started at a mean of 30 weeks.

In 70 patients with gestational diabetes randomized to insulin ($n = 27$), glibenclamide ($n = 24$), or acarbose ($n = 19$) satisfactory blood glucose concentrations were not achieved in five of the women allocated to glibenclamide compared with eight of those allocated to acarbose (134). Babies who were large for gestational age were found in 3.7% (insulin), 25% (glibenclamide), and 10% (acarbose). Neonatal hypoglycemia occurred in eight of the babies whose mothers had taken glibenclamide compared with one each of those whose mothers had taken acarbose or insulin. There was therefore more macrosomia and hypoglycemia in the babies of women taking glibenclamide. However, glibenclamide is inexpensive and may be useful if other more appropriate therapies are unavailable during pregnancy.

Teratogenicity

There is anecdotal evidence of a risk of teratogenicity of sulfonylureas, and on theoretical grounds it is inadvisable to give sulfonylureas to women of fertile age. In women using self-administered hypoglycemic drugs during pregnancy, chlorpropamide, glibenclamide, and tolbutamide were associated with serious malformations, such as microtia, deafness, facial deformities, ventricular septal defect (with or without aortic rotation), atrial septal defect, and a single umbilical artery (135). Of 332 children of women using a sulfonylurea during the first week of pregnancy, 12% had major and 5% had minor abnormalities, related to the increase in HbA_{1c} (136). An effect of high blood glucose could not be excluded. Chromosomal damage is described with chlorpropamide (137), which may have contributed to the development of a cleft palate in another case (138). The choice for pregnant women with diabetes is between insulin given frequently in a short-acting form to avoid overdosage, or a continuous insulin infusion system, since overdosage of insulin can harm the developing fetus.

Fetotoxicity

Hypoglycemia has been reported in a neonate whose mother had taken tolbutamide (139).

- A woman with pre-existing hypertension took labetalol 600 mg/day and tolbutamide for gestational diabetes and had long-standing hypoglycemia. She had started to take tolbutamide 500 mg/day in week 23 and increased the dosage to 1500 mg/day in week 29. Her HbA_{1c} concentration was 5.0–5.8%. She felt no intrauterine movements during week 34 and an emergency cesarean section was performed. The baby had diabetic fetopathy (details not specified) and a blood glucose concentration of 0.8 mmol/l. Despite the administration of 20% glucose 10 ml as a bolus and then 8 ml/hour, the blood glucose remained below 1 mmol/l, and 10 hours after birth octreotide, a somatostatin analogue, was given. Intravenous glucose was discontinued after 3 days and octreotide on day 9. There were no signs of encephalopathy. C peptide, proinsulin, and insulin concentrations in the child were inappropriately high. Serum tolbutamide in the child was 141 µmol/l at 3 hours and the half-life was 46 hours.

The half-life of tolbutamide in this case was much longer than the reported half-life in adults of 7 hours, but the normal half-life in neonates is not known. The activity of CYP2C9, which metabolizes tolbutamide, may be reduced in the first 2 days of life.

Transient diabetes insipidus was seen in a child born to a mother who took chlorpropamide during pregnancy (140).

Neonatal thrombocytopenia and congenital malformations have been associated with administration of tolbutamide to the mother (141).

Susceptibility Factors

Age

Old age increases sensitivity to sulfonylureas and the frail elderly are at greatest risk (142). Chlorpropamide is no longer recommended for treatment of type 2 diabetes. However, in 1993 and 1994, of 3050 older Mexican Americans, 365 used inappropriate medicines, of whom 36 used chlorpropamide (143). In a comparable study of 5734 patients over 65 years old, hospitalized in 81 geriatric and internal medicine wards in Italy during 2 different months in 1997 and 1998, 17 patients (0.3%) were still using chlorpropamide (144).

Renal disease

Glimepiride (6), which is metabolized in the liver, was given for 3 months to two groups of diabetic patients with renal impairment: those with creatinine clearances of 30–60 ml and 10–30 ml (145). The goal was to reach a fasting blood glucose concentration below 10 mmol/l. There was recurrent hypoglycemia in one patient who did not need further drug therapy. There was one "silent" myocardial infarct. There were no other adverse effects. Serum insulin and C peptide concentrations did not change. There was increased clearance of glimepiride in the group with low creatinine clearances, probably caused by altered protein binding, increasing the unbound fraction available for hepatic metabolism. Glimepiride should be used with caution in patients with renal or liver disease (146,147,148).

Other features of the patient

Hypopituitarism, hypoadrenalism, and hypothyroidism all increase sensitivity to sulfonylureas because of reduced secretion of counter-regulatory hormones.

In insuloma, sensitivity to sulfonylureas is increased because insulin secretion from the tumor cells is greater than from normal islet cells.

Exercise training can force a reduction in the dose of various drugs in the treatment of diabetes (149). The hypoglycemic action of exercise in combination with sulfonylurea on postabsorptive glucose concentration is mainly caused by greater inhibition of glucose production in the liver (150).

Prolonged hypoglycemia in patients with end-stage renal disease prompted a search for predisposing factors in such patients with type 2 diabetes taking oral therapy only (151). Seven patients with and 31 without prolonged attacks of hypoglycemia, all on hemodialysis, were studied. All were using glibenclamide, except for three controls who took tolbutamide. The hypoglycemic episodes lasted 28–256 hours and glucose 83–2000 g was given for each episode. A recent fall in food intake, previous hypoglycemic episodes, longer duration of episodes, and a history of cerebrovascular disease were associated with prolonged hypoglycemia. There were no relations to age, sex, betablockers, ACE inhibitors, or drug doses. There were no cases of liver disease or alcohol abuse. Glibenclamide is seven times more highly concentrated in the pancreatic islets than other sulfonylureas, it has a long half-life, and its degradation products have hypoglycemic activity (SEDA-14, 1510).

Drug Administration

Drug formulations

New formulations of some sulfonylureas offer the possibility of once-daily therapy. They include gliclazide MR

(SEDA-25, 511) and glipizide GITS (SEDA-22, 444; SEDA-23, 475).

Gliclazide is available in various formulations with different kinetics in vivo and in vitro (152). Gliclazide MR is a modified-release formulation that allows once-a-day dosing. In a double-blind study 800 patients were randomized to gliclazide or gliclazide MR; there were no differences in adverse reactions or hypoglycemia (153). When comparing identical doses of Diamicron™ and Diabrezide™ in an open, crossover study, Diabrezide had a larger acute and mid-term hypoglycemic effect than Diamicron (154).

In a small study, gliclazide MR 30–120 mg/day had similar efficacy to 80–320 mg/day of the immediate-release formulation. The most commonly observed adverse events were arthralgia, arthritis, back pain, and bronchitis, which may not all have been directly related to the drug, as they also occurred with placebo. There was symptomatic hypoglycemia in about 5%.

Glipizide GITS was also studied in 19 patients with type 2 diabetes in an open, randomized, two-way, crossover study for 5 days, comparing 20 mg/day and 10 mg bd (155). Despite lower serum concentrations with glipizide GITS, the effects on serum concentrations of glucose, insulin, and C-peptide were the same. This may explain the low overall rate of hypoglycemia and lack of weight gain with glipizide GITS.

The effects of an immediate-release formulation of glipizide up to 20 mg bd, glipizide GITS up to 20 mg before breakfast, and nateglinide 120 mg tds on postprandial blood glucose have been compared during three admissions with intervals of 1 week (156). The three formulations gave equivalent control of postprandial hyperglycemia and there were no episodes of severe hypoglycemia. One person taking glipizide 10 mg had one episode of hypoglycemia before lunch and one taking glipizide GITS 15 mg had hypoglycemia 30 minutes before and 15 minutes after lunch.

A once-daily modified-release formulation of gliclazide has been reviewed (157). It has a low tendency to cause hypoglycemia in all patients, including the elderly and patients with mild renal insufficiency. Arthralgia, arthritis, back pain, and bronchitis are its most commonly reported adverse effects, although it is not clear whether they are all related to gliclazide.

From time to time, drug names are confused and the wrong drug is prescribed or dispensed instead of the one intended. Of all the errors that occur, sulfonylureas are often implicated (158). Examples include chlorpropamide instead of chlorpromazine, chloroquine or etodolac instead of chlorpropamide, glyburide instead of thyroxine, and oxybutynin hydrochloride or acetohexamide instead of acetazolamide (SEDA-16, 490; SEDA-17, 495; SEDA-18, 414; SEDA-19, 395; SEDA-21, 443).

Drug dosage regimens

There were no differences in episodes of hypoglycemia, concentrations of glucose, insulin, HbA1c, or lipids, or body weight when glibenclamide was given in one daily dose instead of divided doses (159).

Continuous exposure to high concentrations of sulfonylureas impairs rather than improves therapeutic efficacy (160). The authors suggested that the sulfonylurea receptor is desensitized during long-term therapy. This suggests either that the concentration–effect curve of sulfonylurea drugs is shifted to the right with time or that it is not sigmoidal but bell-shaped. The optimum dosage for a specific drug should not be exceeded. It has been suggested that this might be 10 mg/day for glipizide and 7–10 mg/day for glibenclamide. In a 3-month crossover study of placebo or glipizide 10, 20, or 40 mg in randomized order, glipizide 10 mg/day produced higher insulin concentrations and lower glucose concentrations than 20 or 40 mg/day (161).

Drug overdose

A suicide attempt with chlorpropamide has been reported (62).

- A 23-year-old woman took chlorpropamide 5–10 g. She needed assisted respiration and cardiac pacing for bradycardia (probably due to blockade of potassium channels), fluid infusion, and forced diuresis for 3 days. Notwithstanding continuous glucose infusion and glucose boluses she relapsed into severe hypoglycemia with convulsions. Only on day 27 was her urine free of chlorpropamide and her blood glucose normal.

Chlorpropamide is the longest-acting sulfonylurea. The high doses of glucose this patient was given may have stimulated further insulin secretion, thus contributing to the long period of fluctuating hypoglycemia. In the preceding 5 years 12 fatal cases of chlorpropamide poisoning with 3–15 g were seen in the same institution.

- Glibenclamide self-poisoning has been reported in a 48-year-old man with von Willebrand disease, Prinzmetal angina, hepatitis C, and depression (63). He had frequent hypoglycemic attacks, which were not reduced by reducing the dose of glibenclamide. Laparotomy for an insulinoma was considered until a glibenclamide concentration of 0.32 µg/ml was found, although glibenclamide was supposed to have been withdrawn.

Permanentsided hemiplegia, dysphasia, and hepatitis occurred after a suicide attempt with gliclazide (162).

- A 14-year-old non-diabetic girl took 15 tablets of gliclazide (1200 mg) and had gastric lavage 6 hours later. She developed lethargy, vomiting, and generalized tonic-clonic convulsions. Her blood glucose concentration was 0.8 mmol/l, aspartate transaminase 147 U/l (2.45 µkat/l), alanine transaminase 102 U/l (1.07 µkat/l), bilirubin 78 µmol/l (direct 31 µmol/l), and alkaline phosphatase 63 U/l. Electroencephalography showed voltage suppression in the left hemisphere and generalized slow-wave activity. A CT scan showed cerebral edema. Hypoglycemia was controlled within 24 hours with intravenous glucose. The convulsions could not be controlled with phenytoin, dexamethasone, or mannitol, given for cerebral edema, but they stopped on day 9. After 3.5 months of follow-up she could perceive words but could not speak and was severely hemiplegic.

Drug–Drug Interactions

General

Drugs that potentiate the actions of sulfonylureas and the mechanisms responsible have been reviewed (163). Mechanisms include:

- prolongation of the half-life by inhibition of metabolism or excretion (phenylbutazone, coumarins, chloramphenicol, doxycycline, bezafibrate, probenecid, sulfaphenazole, naproxen, fenyramidol);
- competition with plasma protein binding sites (NSAIDs, salicylates, and sulfonamides);
- potentiation of their hypoglycemic action by inhibition of gluconeogenesis, enhancement of oxidation of glucose, or stimulation of insulin secretion (beta-adrenoceptor antagonists, monoamine oxidase inhibitors, salicylates).

Examples are given in Table 2.

ACE inhibitors

In a retrospective case-control study, a primary diagnosis of hypoglycemia was identified in 413 patients registered as diabetic in 1993 (164). Five controls of the same age and sex, without hypoglycemia, were selected for each case from the same cohort. The relative risks of hypoglycemia with ACE inhibitors, beta-blockers, calcium antagonists, and salicylates were determined. There was an association between enalapril and sulfonylureas. However, other ACE inhibitors could not be identified as a risk factor. There was no interaction with beta-blockers, calcium channel blockers, or salicylates.

The interaction of ACE inhibitors with sulfonylureas has also been illustrated in case reports (165,166).

- A 67-year-old man using glucocorticoids for asthma, ranitidine 300 mg/day, and enalapril 5 mg/day developed a low blood glucose (1.2 mmol/l) within 48 hours of starting to take glibenclamide 5–10 mg/day.
- A 64-year-old man, who used, amongst other drugs, glibenclamide 2.5 mg/day and metformin 850 mg bd, lost consciousness after a week of dwindling appetite and loose stools. His blood glucose was 2.2 mmol/l. He had renal impairment (creatinine 362 µmol/l). He also used ranitidine and ramipril 2.5 mg/day, which could have contributed to both the hypoglycemic effect and renal insufficiency.

In the second case, renal insufficiency could have reduced the clearance of the active metabolites of glibenclamide.

Table 2 Drug interactions with oral hypoglycemic drugs

Interactions	Mechanisms
Enhanced hypoglycemia	
ACE inhibitors	7
Alcohol	3
Allopurinol	1 or 6
Azapropazone	2
Beta-adrenoceptor antagonists	3
Bezafibrate	7
Chloramphenicol	1
Cimetidine	7
Coumarin anticoagulants	7
Isoniazid	7
Levodopa	3
Naproxen	2
Perhexiline	3
Probenecid	1, 2, or 6
Pyrazolones	1, 2, or 6
Salicylates	2 or 6
Sulfonamides	1, 2 or 6
Reduced hypoglycemia	
Acetazolamide	7
Furosemide	7
Glucocorticoids	5
Oral contraceptives	5
Phenothiazines	7
Rifampicin	4
Sulfamethoxydiazine	7
Thiazide diuretics	5

Key to mechanisms:
[1]—Inhibition of drug-metabolizing enzymes
[2]—Displacement of drug from protein-binding sites
[3]—Impairment of glucose homeostatic mechanism
[4]—Induction of metabolizing enzymes
[5]—Increased insulin resistance
[6]—Reduced renal secretion
[7]—Unknown

Alcohol

A disulfiram-like effect after use of alcohol has been described with chlorpropamide, but also with gliclazide, glipizide, and acetohexamide. However, the hepatic effects of sulfonylureas include inhibition of the enzymatic degradation of ethanol, an effect that is only partly comparable with the action of disulfiram, which blocks the degradation of aldehyde but not that of ethanol itself. This interaction results in a vasomotor reaction, with giddiness, tachycardia, headache, angina pectoris, and skin reactions. The most prominent drug to elicit these effects is chlorpropamide, but tolbutamide and other drugs can also do it. The specific effect of alcohol and chlorpropamide has been propagated to be of use as a genetic marker, but this has not been confirmed (SEDA-7, 407).

Excessive use of alcohol, sometimes found in older persons living alone, may also contribute to changes in sensitivity to oral hypoglycemic drugs. Low doses of alcohol (4.35 mmol/l/kg, comparable to one or two drinks) in fasting diabetics taking glibenclamide 20 mg/day in a randomized, double-blind, placebo-controlled study caused a greater fall in blood glucose concentrations than saline and increased counter-regulatory hormone concentrations (167).

Clarithromycin

Two men aged 82 and 72 years with impaired renal function and taking glibenclamide 5 mg/day and glipizide 15 mg/day, respectively, became comatose due to hypoglycemia within 48 hours of starting to take clarithromycin (168). Clarithromycin inhibits cytochrome CYP3A4. It should be used carefully in patients with diabetes and reduced renal function taking oral drugs.

- Severe hypoglycemia occurred in two elderly men with type 2 diabetes mellitus and mild to moderate impaired renal function, who took clarithromycin 1000 mg/day for respiratory infections, in addition to a sulfonylurea (glibenclamide 5 mg/day in one case and glipizide 15 mg/day in the other) (168). Both developed severe hypoglycemia within 48 hours of starting clarithromycin.

Diltiazem

The interaction of tolbutamide with diltiazem has been studied in eight healthy men (169). Tolbutamide had no effect on diltiazem, but diltiazem increased the AUC of tolbutamide by 10% without an effect on blood glucose concentrations.

Fibrates

Fibrates are highly bound to albumin and displace other similarly bound drugs. This can affect treatment with sulfonylureas. Hypoglycemia occurred in a diabetic patient taking glibenclamide plus gemfibrozil (170).

In 10 healthy volunteers, gemfibrozil 600 mg bd increased the mean total AUC of a single dose of glimepiride 0.5 mg by 23% (range 6–56%) (171). The mean half-life of glimepiride was prolonged from 2.1 to 2.3 hours. This effect may have been caused by inhibition of CYP2C9. However, there were no statistically significant effects on serum insulin or blood glucose variables.

Fluconazole

The concurrent administration of fluconazole with tolbutamide resulted in increased tolbutamide concentrations (SED-12, 682; 172).

- A 56-year-old HIV-positive patient with diabetes mellitus taking gliclazide 160 mg/day developed severe hypoglycemia when treated with co-trimoxazole 480 mg/day and fluconazole 200 mg/day (173). The authors speculated that fluconazole might have inhibited gliclazide metabolism by inhibiting CYP2C9.

The effects of fluconazole and fluvoxamine on the pharmacokinetics and pharmacodynamics of glimepiride have been studied in a randomized, double-blind, crossover study in 12 healthy volunteers who took fluconazole 200 mg/day (400 mg on day 1), fluvoxamine 100 mg/day,

or placebo once daily for 4 days (174). On day 4 they took a single oral dose of glimepiride 0.5 mg. Fluconazole increased the mean total AUC of glimepiride to 238% and the peak plasma concentration to 151% of control values, and the half-life of glimepiride was prolonged from 2.0 to 3.3 hours. This was probably due to inhibition of CYP2C9-mediated biotransformation of glimepiride by fluconazole. However, fluconazole did not cause statistically significant changes in the effects of glimepiride on blood glucose concentrations.

Fluoroquinolones

Ciprofloxacin can precipitate hypoglycemia in patients taking glibenclamide.

- A 68-year-old man with type 2 diabetes, who was taking glibenclamide 1.25 mg bd, warfarin, furosemide 40 mg/day, fosinopril 10 mg/day, clopidogrel 75 mg/day, lovastatin 40 mg/day, and metoprolol XL 50 mg/day, took ciprofloxacin 250 mg bd for 1 day (175). He had renal impairment (creatinine 203 μmol/l). On admission he was hypoglycemic with a capillary blood glucose concentration of 1.1 mmol/l (20 mg/dl). The hypoglycemia continued for 24 hours.

There has been a previous report of hypoglycemia in a patient taking glibenclamide and ciprofloxacin (176).

A similar effect has been reported with another fluoroquinolone, gatifloxacin (177).

- A 79-year-old man with type 2 diabetes taking glibenclamide 10 mg/day and metformin 2.5 g/day became hypoglycemic after taking one dose of gatifloxacin 400 mg. The hypoglycemia continued for 24–48 hours.
- An 84-year-old woman taking glibenclamide 5 mg/day and metformin 2 g/day became hypoglycemic after taking gatifloxacin 400 mg. The hypoglycemia continued for 24–36 hours.

In 48 patients with type 2 diabetes on diet, gatifloxacin reduced blood glucose concentration by 1.1 mmol/l (20 mg/dl) (178). In Japan gatifloxacin is contraindicated in patients with diabetes. Low blood glucose concentrations were reported in 75 patients, 58 of who had diabetes (177).

Hydroxychloroquine

The addition of hydroxychloroquine to sulfonylureas has been investigated in a placebo-controlled study in 125 adipose patients whose diabetes was not well enough controlled with a sulfonylurea alone (179). During the first six months HbA$_{1c}$ was significantly reduced by 1.02%. There were no significant differences in adverse effects, but those who took hydroxychloroquine had a greater incidence of minor corneal changes.

Ibuprofen

Ibuprofen (150 mg, 3 doses) for arthralgias was associated with hypoglycemia in a 72-year-old man who was taking glibenclamide 2.5 mg/day for type 2 diabetes mellitus;

after the last dose he lost consciousness, and his blood glucose concentration was under 2.2 mmol/l (180).

Miconazole

Enhancement of the effects of hypoglycemic sulfonamides has been reported (SED-12, 679) (181).

Rifampicin

Reduced efficacy of gliclazide has been attributed to induction of CYP2C9 by rifampicin (182).

- A 65-year-old man who had taken gliclazide 80 mg/day for 2 years took rifampicin for an infection with *Mycobacterium gordonae*, after which the dose of gliclazide had to be increased to 120 mg/day and later to 160 mg/day. After 75 days of combined therapy, gliclazide 80 mg/day gave a plasma concentration of 1.4 μg/ml; 7 months after stopping rifampicin it increased to 4.7 μg/ml. Gliclazide was then reduced to 80 mg/day.

It is important to check the blood glucose concentration if rifampicin is given in combination with oral hypoglycemic drugs.

Sulfonamides

Tolbutamide is mainly metabolized by CYP2C9, which also has a role in the metabolism of sulfonamides. Of various sulfonamides, sulfaphenazole had the largest inhibitory effect on the metabolism of tolbutamide in vitro (183). This gives a theoretical basis for being careful when tolbutamide and sulfonamides are co-administered.

Hypoglycemia, often during the first hours of combining the two drugs, is the result of an important interaction between sulfonylureas and sulfonamides (184–187). For example, the half-life of tolbutamide was increased from 9.5 to 29 hours by chronic sulfaphenazole and from 9.2 to 26 hours by a single dose of sulfaphenazole (188). Interference by sulfonamides with the protein binding of sulfonylureas may contribute.

Most reports of this interaction have described hypoglycemia with tolbutamide in combination with sulfaphenazole (184,185,188,189), sulfafurazole (185), or co-trimoxazole (187,190). The inhibitory effect of sulfonamides on tolbutamide metabolism is mediated by CYP2C9 (191).

Chlorpropamide produces the same interaction (192).

The combination of gliclazide, fluconazole, and sulfamethoxazole can cause severe hypoglycemia (193).

Management of adverse drug reactions

Octreotide inhibits the secretion of various neuropeptides, including insulin. It thus helps reduce the hyperstimulation of endogenous insulin production by sulfonylureas. The use of octreotide to manage sulfonylurea-induced hypoglycemia has been reviewed (194). Intravenous or subcutaneous octreotide was used over a period of days as necessary in young children and adults. The authors suggested a management guideline based on

the use of intravenous glucose supplemented with octreotide either to treat or prevent relapse of hypoglycemia.

References

1. Ashcroft FM, Gribble FM. ATP-sensitive K+ channels and insulin secretion: their role in health and disease. Diabetologia 1999;42(8):903–19.
2. The Diabetes Control and Complications Trial Research Group. The effect of intensive treatment of diabetes on the development and progression of long-term complications in insulin-dependent diabetes mellitus. N Engl J Med 1993;329(14):977–86.
3. Turner RC, Holman RR, Cull CA, Stratton IM, Matthews DR, Frighi V, Manley E, Neil A, McElroy H, Wright D, Kohner E, Fox C, Hadden D. Intensive blood-glucose control with sulphonylureas or insulin compared with conventional treatment and risk of complications in patients with type 2 diabetes (UKPDS 33). UK Prospective Diabetes Study (UKPDS) Group. Lancet 1998;352(9131):837–53.
4. DeWitt DE, Evans TC. Perioperative management of oral antihyperglycemic agents: special consideration for metformin. Semin Anesth 1998;17:267–72.
5. Anonymous. New oral antihyperglycaemic agents expand armamentarium in the battle against type 2 diabetes mellitus. Drugs Ther Perspect 1998;12:6–9.
6. Parulkar AA, Fonseca VA. Recent advances in pharmacological treatment of type 2 diabetes mellitus. Compr Ther 1999;25(8–10):418–26.
7. DeFronzo RA. Pharmacologic therapy for type 2 diabetes mellitus. Ann Intern Med 1999;131(4):281–303.
8. Lebovitz HE. Insulin secretagogues: old and new. Diabetes Rev 1999;7:139–53.
9. Hathout EH, Cockburn BN, Mace JW, Sharkey J, Chen-Daniel J, Bell GI. A case of hepatocyte nuclear factor-1 alpha diabetes/MODY3 masquerading as type 1 diabetes in a Mexican–American adolescent and responsive to a low dose of sulfonylurea. Diabetes Care 1999;22(5):867–8.
10. Hansen T, Eiberg H, Rouard M, Vaxillaire M, Moller AM, Rasmussen SK, Fridberg M, Urhammer SA, Holst JJ, Almind K, Echwald SM, Hansen L, Bell GI, Pedersen O. Novel MODY3 mutations in the hepatocyte nuclear factor-1alpha gene: evidence for a hyperexcitability of pancreatic beta-cells to intravenous secretagogues in a glucose-tolerant carrier of a P447L mutation. Diabetes 1997;46(4):726–30.
11. Pearson ER, Liddell WG, Shepherd M, Corrall RJ, Hattersley AT. Sensitivity to sulphonylureas in patients with hepatocyte nuclear factor-1alpha gene mutations: evidence for pharmacogenetics in diabetes. Diabet Med 2000;17(7):543–5.
12. Inzucchi SE. Oral antihyperglycemic therapy for type 2 diabetes: scientific review. JAMA 2002;287(3):360–72.
13. Holmboe ES. Oral antihyperglycemic therapy for type 2 diabetes: clinical applications. JAMA 2002;287(3):373–6.
14. Van Gaal LF, De Leeuw IH. Rationale and options for combination therapy in the treatment of type 2 diabetes. Diabetologia 2003;46(Suppl 1):M44–50.
15. Setter SM, Iltz JL, Thams J, Campbell RK. Metformin hydrochloride in the treatment of type 2 diabetes mellitus: a clinical review with a focus on dual therapy. Clin Ther 2003;25:2991–306.
16. Nagasaka S, Aiso Y, Yoshiwaza K, Ishibashi S. Comparison of pioglitazone and metformin efficacy using homeostasis model assessment. Diabetic Med 2004;21:136–41.

17. Garber AJ, Donovan Jr DS, Dandona P, Bruce S, Park J-S. Efficacy of glyburide/metformin tablets compared with initial monotherapy in type 2 diabetes. J Clin Endocrinol Metab 2003;88:3598–604.

18. Gulliford M, Latinovic R. Mortality in type 2 diabetic subjects prescribed metformin and sulphonylurea drugs in combination: cohort study. Diabetes Metab Res Rev 2004;20:239–45.

19. Dailey GE III, Noor MA, Park J-S, Bruce S, Fiedorek FT. Glycemic control with glyburide/metformin tablets in combination with rosiglitazone in patients with type 2 diabetes: a randomised double-blind trial. Am J Med 2004;116:223–9.

20. Kerenyi Z, Samer H, James R, Yan Y Stewart M. Combination therapy with rosiglitazone and glibenclamide compared with upward titration of glibenclamide alone in patients with type 2 diabetes mellitus. Diabetes Res Clin Pract 2004;63:213–23.

21. Carroll MF, Izard A, Riboni K, Burge MR, Schade DS. Control of postprandial hyperglycemia: optimal use of short-acting insulin secretagogues. Diabetes Care 2002;25(12):2147–52.

22. Buysschaert M, Bobbioni E, Starkie M, Frith LTroglitazone Study Group. Troglitazone in combination with sulphonylurea improves glycaemic control in Type 2 diabetic patients inadequately controlled by sulphonylurea therapy alone. Diabet Med 1999;16(2):147–53.

23. Alvarsson M, Sundkvist G, Lager I, Henricsson M, Berntorp K, Fernqvist-Forbes E, Steen L, Westermark G, Westermark P, Örn T, Grill V. Beneficial effects of insulin versus sulphonylurea on insulin secretion and metabolic control in recently diagnosed type 2 diabetic patients. Diabetes Care 2003;26:2231–7.

24. Leibowitz G, Cerasi E. Sulphonylurea treatment of NIDDM patients with cardiovascular disease: a mixed blessing? Diabetologia 1996;39(5):503–14.

25. Schwartz TB, Meinert CL. The UGDP controversy: thirty-four years of contentious ambiguity laid to rest. Perspect Biol Med 2004;47(4):564–74.

26. Cleveland JC Jr, Meldrum DR, Cain BS, Banerjee A, Harken AH. Oral sulfonylurea hypoglycemic agents prevent ischemic preconditioning in human myocardium. Two paradoxes revisited Circulation 1997;96(1):29–32.

27. Wascher TC. Sulfonylureas and cardiovascular mortality in diabetes: a class effect? Circulation 1998;97(14):1427–8.

28. Britton ME, Denver AE, Mohamed-Ali V, Yudkin JS. Effects of glimepiride vs glibenclamide on ischaemic heart disease risk factors and glycaemic control in patients with type 2 diabetes mellitus. Clin Drug Invest 1998;16:303–17.

29. Riveline JP, Danchin N, Ledru F, Varroud-Vial M, Charpentier G. Sulfonylureas and cardiovascular effect: from experimental data to clinical use. Available data in humans and clinical applications. Diabetes Metab 2003;29:207–22.

30. Yosefy C, Magen E, Kiselevich A, Priluk R, London D, Volchek L, Viskoper JR. Rosiglitazone improves, while glibenclamide worsens blood pressure control in treated hypertensive diabetic and dyslipidemic subjects via modulation of insulin resistance and sympathetic activity. J Cardiovasc Pharmacol 2004;44:215–22.

31. Tomai F, Danesi A, Ghini AS, Crea F, Perino M, Gaspardone A, Ruggeri G, Chiariello L, Gioffre PA. Effects of K(ATP) channel blockade by glibenclamide

on the warm-up phenomenon. Eur Heart J 1999;20(3):196–202.

32. Ishibashi R, Takagi Y, Ozaki S. [A case with glibenclamide induced pneumonitis.]Jpn J Chest Dis 1999;58:758–62.

33. Feinglos MN, Lebovitz HE. Long-term safety and efficacy of glipizide. Am J Med 1983;75(5B):60–6.

34. Takami K, Takeda N, Nakashima K, Takami R, Hayashi M, Ozeki S, Yamada A, Kokubo Y, Sato M, Kawachi S, Sasaki A, Yasuda K. Effects of dietary treatment alone or diet with voglibose or glyburide on abdominal adipose tissue and metabolic abnormalities in patients with newly diagnosed type 2 diabetes. Diabetes Care 2002;25(4):658–62.

35. Bugos M, Austin T, Atherton T, Viereck C. Long-term treatment of type 2 diabetes mellitus with glimepiride is weight neutral: a meta-analysis. Diabetes Res Clin Pract 2000;50 (Suppl 1):S47.

36. Sulfonylurea drugs: basic and clinical considerations. Sydney, Australia, 20 November 1988Proceedings. Diabetes Care 1990;13(Suppl 3):1–58.

37. Berger W, Caduff F, Pasquel M, Rump A. Die relative Haufigkeit der schweren Sulfonylharnstoff-Hypoglykämie in den letzten 25 Jahren in der Schweiz. Resultät von zwei gesamtschweizerischen Umfragen in den Jahren 1969 und 1984. [The relatively frequent incidence of severe sulfonylurea-induced hypoglycemia in the last 25 years in Switzerland. Results of 2 surveys in Switzerland in 1969 and 1984.] Schweiz Med Wochenschr 1986;116(5):145–51.

38. Ohsawa K, Koike N, Takamura T, Nagai Y, Kobayashi K. Hypoglycemic attacks after administration of bezafibrate in three cases of non-insulin dependent diabetes mellitus. J Jpn Diabetes Soc 1994;37:295–300.

39. Colagiuri S, Miller JJ, Petocz P. Double-blind crossover comparison of human and porcine insulins in patients reporting lack of hypoglycaemia awareness. Lancet 1992;339(8807):1432–5.

40. Wattoo MA, Liu HH. Alternating transient dense hemiplegia due to episodes of hypoglycemia. West J Med 1999;170(3):170–1.

41. Croxson SC, McConvey R, Molodynski L. Profound hypoglycaemia and cognitive impairment. Pract Diabetes Int 2001;18:315–6.

42. van Vonderen MG, Thijs A. Hypoglykemie bij orale blood glucoseverlagende middelen: kans oprecidief na herstel van de glucosespiegel. [Hypoglycemia caused by oral hypoglycemic agents: risk of relapse after normalisation of blood glucose.] Ned Tijdschr Geneeskd 2002;146(7):289–92.

43. Auzepy P, Caquet R. Hypoglycémies gravesdues a l'insuline. Risques et accidents des médicaments antidiabétiques. [Severe hypoglycemia due to insulin. Risks and adverse effects of antidiabetic drugs.] Sem Hop 1983;59(10):697–705.

44. Asplund K, Wiholm BE, Lithner F. Glibenclamide-associated hypoglycaemia: a report on 57 cases. Diabetologia 1983;24(6):412–7.

45. Kennedy TD, Keat AC, Chester M, et al. Predisposing factors in fatal glibenclamide induced hypoglycaemia. Pract Diabetes 1988;5:217.

46. Gorgojo GG, Cancer E, Andreu M, Camblor M, Lajo T, Alvarez V, Moreno B. Hipoglucemia factitia induca por glipizida en una paciente con síndrome de Münchhausen. Endocrinologia 1998;45:38–42.

47. Meier JJ, Hucking K, Gruneklee D, Schmiegel W, Nauck MA. Unterschiede im Insulin-Sekretionsverhalten

erleichtern die Differentialdiagnose von Insulinom und Hypoglycaemia factitia. [Differences in insulin secretion facilitate the differential diagnosis of insulinoma and factitious hypoglycaemia.] Dtsch Med Wochenschr 2002;127(8):375–8.

48. Ludwig A. Akzidentelle Hypoglykämie durch Inhalation von Sulfonylharnstoffstaub. Arbeitsmed Sozialmed Praventivmed 1991;26:31–2.

49. Holstein A, Plaschke A, Hammer C, Egberts E-H. Characteristics and time course of severe glimiperide- versus glibenclamide-induced hypoglycemia. Eur J Clin Pharmacol 2003;59:91–7.

50. Anonymous. Sulfonylureas and hypoglycemia in the elderly. Hosp Practice 1996;31:28167.

51. Salman S, Salman F, Satman I, Yilmaz Y, Ozer E, Sengul A, Demirel HO, Karsidag K, Dinccag N, Yilmaz MT. Comparison of acarbose and gliclazide as first-line agents in patients with type 2 diabetes. Curr Med Res Opin 2001;16(4):296–306.

52. Scholz GH, Schneider K, Knirsch W, Becker G. Effect and tolerability of glimepiride in daily practice: a non-interventional observational cohort study. Clin Drug Invest 2001;21:597–604.

53. Charpentier G, Vaur L, Halimi S, Fleury F, Derobert E, Grimaldi A, Oriol V, Etienne S, Altman JJ. DIAMETRE. Predictors of response to glimepiride in patients with type 2 diabetes mellitus. Diabetes. Metab 2001;27(5 Pt 1): 563–571.

54. So WY, Chan JC, Yeung VT, Chow CC, Ko GT, Li JK, Cockram CS. Sulphonylurea-induced hypoglycaemia in institutionalized elderly in Hong Kong. Diabet Med 2002;19(11):966–8.

55. Leese GP, Wang J, Broomhall J, Kelly P, Marsden A, Morrison W, Frier BM, Morris AD. DARTS/MEMO Collaboration. Frequency of severe hypoglycemia requiring emergency treatment in type 1 and type 2 diabetes: a population-based study of health service resource use. Diabetes Care 2003;26(4):1176–80.

56. Drouin P, Standl E, for the diamicron MR study group. Gliclazide modified release: results of a 2 year study in patients with type 2 diabetes. Diabetes Obesity Metab 2004;6:414–21.

57. Tomizawa HH. Properties of glutathione insulin transhydrogenase from beef liver. J Biol Chem 1962;237:3393–6.

58. Pettipierre B, Fabre J. Effet de l'insuffisance rénale sur l'action hypoglycémiante des sylfonylurées. Cinétique de la chlorpropamide en cas de néphropathie. [The effect of renal insufficiency on the hypoglycemic action of sulfonylureas. Kinetics of chlorpropamide in a case of nephropathy.] Schweiz Med Wochenschr 1972;102(16):570–8.

59. Burge MR, Schmitz-Fiorentino K, Fischette C, Qualls CR, Schade DS. A prospective trial of risk factors for sulfonylurea-induced hypoglycemia in type 2 diabetes mellitus. JAMA 1998;279(2):137–43.

60. Shorr RI. Hypoglycemia from glipizide and glyburide. JAMA 1998;279(18):1441–2.

61. Gambassi G, Carbonin P, Bernabei R. Hypoglycemia from glipizide and glyburide. JAMA 1998;279(18):1442–3.

62. Ciechanowski K, Borowiak KS, Potocka BA, Nowacka M, Dutkiewicz G. Chlorpropamide toxicity with survival despite 27-day hypoglycemia. J Toxicol Clin Toxicol 1999;37(7):869–71.

63. Torello AL, Canonge RS, Pascual CH, Manteca JM. Occult ingestion of sulfonylureas: a diagnostic challenge. Endocrinol Nutr 2000;47:174–5.

64. Seltzer HS. Severe drug-induced hypoglycemia: a review. Compr Ther 1979;5(4):21–9.

65. Stahl M, Berger W. Higher incidence of severe hypoglycaemia leading to hospital admission in type 2 diabetic patients treated with long-acting versus short-acting sulphonylureas. Diabet Med 1999;16(7):586–90.

66. Ben-Ami H, Nagachandran P, Mendelson A, Edoute Y. Drug-induced hypoglycemic coma in 102 diabetic patients. Arch Intern Med 1999;159(3):281–4.

67. Trenque T, Hoizey G, Lamiable D. Serious hypoglycemia: Munchausen's syndrome? Diabetes Care 2001;24(4):792–3.

68. Holstein A, Plaschke A, Ptak M, Egberts E-H, Tenberken O, Maurer H. The diagnostic value of determining the hydroxymetabolite of glimepiride in the blood serum in cases of severe hypoglycaemia associated with glimepiride therapy. Diabetes Obesity Metab 2004;6:391–3.

69. Moore DF, Wood DF, Volans GN. Features, prevention and management of acute overdose due to antidiabetic drugs. Drug Saf 1993;9(3):218–29.

70. Boyle PJ, Justice K, Krentz AJ, Nagy RJ, Schade DS. Octreotide reverses hyperinsulinemia and prevents hypoglycemia induced by sulfonylurea overdoses. J Clin Endocrinol Metab 1993;76(3):752–6.

71. Drzewoski J, Czupryniak L, Chwatko G, Bald E. Total plasma homocysteine and insulin levels in type 2 diabetic patients with secondary failure to oral agents. Diabetes Care 1999;22(12):2097–9.

72. Hirokawa CA, Gray DR. Chlorpropamide-induced hyponatremia in the veteran population. Ann Pharmacother 1992;26(10):1243–4.

73. Kadowaki T, Hagura R, Kajinuma H, Kuzuya N, Yoshida S. Chlorpropamide-induced hyponatremia: incidence and risk factors. Diabetes Care 1983;6(5):468–71.

74. Chan TY. Drug-induced syndrome of inappropriate antidiuretic hormone secretion. Causes, diagnosis and management. Drugs Aging 1997;11(1):27–44.

75. Gin H, Lars I, Morlat P, Beauvieux JM, Aubertin J. Hyponatrémie induite par les sulfamides hypoglycémiants. [Hyponatremia induced by hypoglycemic sulfonamides: a study of 70 patients.] Ann Med Interne (Paris) 1988;139(7):455–9.

76. Tsumura K. Clinical evaluation of glimepiride (HOE490) in NIDDM, including a double blind comparative study versus gliclazide. Diabetes Res Clin Pract 1995;28(Suppl):S147–9.

77. Ravina A. Antidiuretic action of chlorpropamide. Lancet 1973;2(7822):203.

78. Moses AM, Howanitz J, Miller M. Diuretic action of three sulfonylurea drugs. Ann Intern Med 1973;78(4):541–4.

79. Traumann KJ, Grom E, Schwarzkopf H. Panzytopenie bei Diabetes-mellitus-Therapie mit Tolbutamid?. [Pancytopenia in diabetes mellitus treatment with tolbutamide?.] Dtsch Med Wochenschr 1975;100(6):250–1.

80. Gill MJ, Ratliff DA, Harding LK. Hypoglycemic coma, jaundice, and pure RBC aplasia following chlorpropamide therapy. Arch Intern Med 1980;140(5):714–5.

81. Levitt LJ. Chlorpropamide-induced pure white cell aplasia. Blood 1987;69(2):394–400.

82. Saffouri B, Cho JH, Felber N. Chlorpropamide-induced haemolytic anaemia. Postgrad Med J 1981;57(663):44–5.

83. Nataas OB, Nesthus I. Immune haemolytic anaemia induced by glibenclamide in selective IgA deficiency. BMJ (Clin Res Ed) 1987;295(6594):366–7.

84. Malacarne P, Castaldi G, Bertusi M, Zavagli G. Tolbutamide-induced hemolytic anemia. Diabetes 1977;26(2):156–8.

85. Cunliffe DJ, Gorst DW, Palmer HM. Chlorpropamide-induced thrombocytopenia. Postgrad Med J 1977;53(616):87–8.

86. Sauer H, Fischer K, Landbeck G. [Allergic thrombocytopenia in tolbutamide therapy of diabetes mellitus.]Med Welt 1962;36:1899–903.

87. Vaatainen N, Fraki JE, Hyvonen M, Neittaanmaki H. Purpura with a linear epidermo-dermal deposition of IgA. Acta Derm Venereol 1983;63(2):169–70.

88. Cartron G, Jonville-Bera AP, Autret-Leca E, Colombat P. Glimepiride-induced thrombocytopenic purpura. Ann Pharmacother 2000;34(1):120.

89. Noto H, Tsukamoto K, Kimura S. Glyburide-induced hemolysis in myelodysplastic syndrome. Diabetes Care 2000;23(1):129.

90. Bernhard H. Long-term observations on oral hypoglycemic agents in diabetes; The effect of carbutamide and tolbutamide. Diabetes 1965;14:59–70.

91. Bell RJ. Pulmonary infiltration with eosinophils caused by chlorpropamide. Lancet 1964;42:1249–50.

92. Bondi E, Slater S. Tolazamide-induced chronic eosinophilic pneumonia. Chest 1981;80(5):652.

93. Vinzio S, Andres E, Perrin A-E, Schlienger J-L, Goichot B. Glibenclamide-induced acute haemolytic anaemia revealing a G6PD-deficiency. Diabetes Res Clin Pract 2004;64:181–3.

94. Berger W, Constam GR, Siegenthaler W. Die Behandlungsmoglichkeiten des Diabetes mellitus mit Biguaniden. Klinische Erfahrungen bei 122 Diabetikern mit Dimethylbiguanid (Glucophage). [Therapeutic possibilities in diabetes mellitus with biguanides. Clinical experiences in 122 diabetics with dimethylbiguanide (Glucophage).] Schweiz Med Wochenschr 1966;96(40):1335–42.

95. Schneider HL, Hornbach KD, Kniaz JL, Efrusy ME. Chlorpropamide hepatotoxicity: report of a case and review of the literature. Am J Gastroenterol 1984;79(9):721–4.

96. Nakao NL, Gelb AM, Stenger RJ, Siegel JH. A case of chronic liver disease due to tolazamide. Gastroenterology 1985;89(1):192–5.

97. Rumboldt Z, Bota B. Favorable effects of glibenclamide in a patient exhibiting idiosyncratic hepatotoxic reactions to both chlorpropamide and tolbutamide. Acta Diabetol Lat 1984;21(4):387–91.

98. Clementsen P, Hansen CL, Hoegholm A. Glipizidinduceret toksisk hepatitis. [Glipizide induced toxic hepatitis.] Ugeskr Laeger 1986;148(13):771–2.

99. De Rosa G, Corsello SM, Pizzi C, et al. Epatopatia citolitica amitterica da glibenclamide. Epatologia 1980;26:73.

100. Wongpaitoon V, Mills PR, Russell RI, Patrick RS. Intrahepatic cholestasis and cutaneous bullae associated with glibenclamide therapy. Postgrad Med J 1981;57(666):244–6.

101. Rigberg LA, Robinson MJ, Espiritu CR. Chlorpropamide-induced granulomas. A probable hypersensitivity reaction in liver and bone marrow. JAMA 1976;235(4):409–10.

102. Lambert M, Geubel A, Rahier J, Branquinho F. Cholestatic hepatitis associated with glibenclamide therapy. Eur J Gastroenterol Hepatol 1990;2:389–91.

103. Krivoy N, Zaher A, Yaacov B, Alroy G. Fatal toxic intrahepatic cholestasis secondary to glibenclamide. Diabetes Care 1996;19(4):385–6.

104. Rank JM, Olson RC. Reversible cholestatic hepatitis caused by acetohexamide. Gastroenterology 1989;96(6):1607–8.

105. Gupta R, Sachar DB. Chlorpropamide-induced cholestatic jaundice and pseudomembranous colitis. Am J Gastroenterol 1985;80(5):381–3.

106. Dourakis SP, Tzemanakis E, Sinani C, Kafiri G, Hadziyannis SJ. Gliclazide-induced acute hepatitis. Arch Hell Med 1998;15:87–9.

107. Bridges ME, Pittman FE. Tolazamide-induced cholestasis. South Med J 1980;73(8):1072–4.

108. Tholakanahalli VN, Potti A, Heyworth MF. Glibenclamide-induced cholestasis. West J Med 1998;168(4):274–7.

109. Goodman RC, Dean PJ, Radparvar A, Kitabchi AE. Glyburide-induced hepatitis. Ann Intern Med 1987;106(6):837–9.

110. Dourakis SP, Tzemanakis E, Sinani C, Kafiri G, Hadziyannis SJ. Gliclazide-induced acute hepatitis. Eur J Gastroenterol Hepatol 2000;12(1):119–21.

111. Subramanian G, Walmsley D, Blewitt RW. Gliclazide-induced hepatitis. Pract Diabetes Int 2003;20:18–20.

112. Chitturi S, Le V, Kench J, Loh C, George J. Gliclazide-induced acute hepatitis with hypersensitivity features. Dig Dis Sci 2002;47(5):1107–10.

113. Ichimyya Y, Furuya K, Hasegawa A, Nishimura M. Dose related glibenclamide–induced hepatitis: a case report. J Japan Diab Soc 2003;46:241–5.

114. Chounta A, Zouridakis S, Ellinas C, Tsiodras S, Zoumpouli C, Kopanaks S, Giamoarellou H. Cholestatic liver injury after glimepiride therapy. J Hepatol 2005;42:944–6.

115. Ilario MJ-M, Turyan HV, Axiotis CA. Glipizide treatment with short-term alcohol abuse resulting in subfulminant hepatic failure. Virchows Arch 2003;443:104–5.

116. Tavani E, Giardini R. Alterazioni istopatologiche delle isole di Langerhans in un caso di diabete mellito trattato con sulfaniluree. [Histopathological changes in the islands of Langerhans in a case of diabetes mellitus treated with sulfonylurea.] Pathologica 1978;70(999–1000):105–8.

117. Roblin X, Abinader Y, Baziz A. Pancréatite aiguë sous gliclazide. [Acute pancreatitis induced by gliclazide.] Gastroenterol Clin Biol 1992;16(1):96.

118. Blomgren KB, Sundstrom A, Steineck G, Wiholm BE. Obesity and treatment of diabetes with glyburide may both be risk factors for acute pancreatitis. Diabetes Care 2002;25(2):298–302.

119. Appel GB, D'Agati V, Bergman M, Pirani CL. Nephrotic syndrome and immune complex glomerulonephritis associated with chlorpropamide therapy. Am J Med 1983;74(2):337–42.

120. Temime P, Oddoze L, Privat Y, Costes A, Maurin J. [Erythrodermia secondary to an intense photosenitization caused by carbutamide (BZ 55).]Bull Soc Fr Dermatol Syphiligr 1962;69:124–5.

121. Kar PK, Das Gupta SK, Das KD. Tolbutamide photosensitivity. J Indian Med Assoc 1984;82(8):289–91.

122. Feuerman E, Frumkin A. Photodermatitis induced by chlorpropamide. A report of five cases. Dermatologica 1973;146(1):25–9.

123. Fujii S, Nakashima T, Kaneko T. Glibenclamide-induced photosensitivity in a diabetic patient with erythropoietic protoporphyria. Am J Hematol 1995;50(3):223.

124. Barnett JH, Barnett SM. Lichenoid drug reactions to chlorpropamide and tolazamide. Cutis 1984;34(6):542–4.

125. Aoki T, Sobajima H, Suzuki Y, Sassa H. [A case of erythema multiforme and rhabdomyolysis induced by Daonil

(glibenclamide) 2.5 mg tablet.]J Jpn Diabetes Soc 1999;42:759–63.

126. Adams BB, Gadenne AS. Glipizide-induced pigmented purpuric dermatosis. J Am Acad Dermatol 1999;41(5 Pt 2):827–9.

127. Clarke BF, Campbell IW, Ewing DJ, Beveridge GW, MacDonald MK. Generalized hypersensitivity reaction and visceral arteritis with fatal outcome during glibenclamide therapy Diabetes 1974;23(9): 739–742.

128. Ernst EJ, Egge JA. Celecoxib-induced erythema multiforme with glyburide cross-reactivity. Pharmacotherapy 2002;22(5):637–40.

129. Duncan C, Sommerfield AJ, Nawroz I, Campbell IW. Stevens–Johnson syndrome with visceral arteritis due to sulphonylurea therapy. Pract Diabetes Int 2004;21:195–8.

130. Fisman EZ, Tenenbaum A, Boyko V, Benderly M, Adler Y, Friedensohn A, Kohanovski M, Rotzak R, Schneider H, Behar S, Motro M. Oral antidiabetic treatment in patients with coronary disease: time-related increased mortality on combined glyburide/metformin therapy over a 7.7-year follow-up Clin Cardiol 2001;24(2):151–8.

131. Hellmuth E, Damm P, Molsted-Pedersen L. Oral hypoglycaemic agents in 118 diabetic pregnancies. Diabet Med 2000;17(7):507–11.

132. Langer O, Conway DL, Berkus MD, Xenakis EM, Gonzales O. A comparison of glyburide and insulin in women with gestational diabetes mellitus. N Engl J Med 2000;343(16):1134–8.

133. Kremer CJ, Duff P. Glyburide for the treatment of gestational diabetes. Am J Obstet Gynecol 2004;190:1438–9.

134. Bertini AM, Silva JC, Taborda W, Becker F, Bebber FRL, Viesi JMZ, Aquim G, Ribeiro TE. Perinatal outcomes and the use of oral hypoglycaemic agents. J Perinat Med 2005;33:519–23.

135. Piacquadio K, Hollingsworth DR, Murphy H. Effects of in-utero exposure to oral hypoglycaemic drugs. Lancet 1991;338(8771):866–9.

136. Towner D, Kjos SL, Leung B, Montoro MM, Xiang A, Mestman JH, Buchanan TA. Congenital malformations in pregnancies complicated by NIDDM. Diabetes Care 1995;18(11):1446–51.

137. Berger W. Orale Antidiabetika 1977. [Oral antidiabetics 1977.] ZFA (Stuttgart) 1978;54(9):513–24.

138. Ansaldi E, Gilardi GB. Chlorpropamide and cleft palate. J Foetal Med 1984;4:50.

139. Christesen HB, Melander A. Prolonged elimination of tolbutamide in a premature newborn with hyperinsulinaemic hypoglycaemia. Eur J Endocrinol 1998;138(6):698–701.

140. Uhrig JD, Hurley RM. Chlorpropamide in pregnancy and transient neonatal diabetes insipidus. Can Med Assoc J 1983;128(4):368370–1.

141. Schiff D, Aranda JV, Stern L. Neonatal thrombocytopenia and congenital malformations associated with administration of tolbutamide to the mother. J Pediatr 1970;77(3):457–8.

142. Shorr RI, Ray WA, Daugherty JR, Griffin MR. Incidence and risk factors for serious hypoglycemia in older persons using insulin or sulfonylureas. Arch Intern Med 1997;157(15):1681–6.

143. Raji MA, Ostir GV, Markides KS, Espino DV, Goodwin JS. Potentially inappropriate medication use by elderly Mexican Americans. Ann Pharmacother 2003;37:1197–202.

144. Onder G, Landi F, Cesari M, Gambassi G, Carbonin P, Bernabei R. Inappropriate medication use among older adults in Italy: results from the Italian group of pharmacoepidemiology in the elderly. Eur J Clin Pharmacol 2003;59:157–62.

145. Profozic V, Mrzljac V, Nazar I, Metelko Z, Rosenkranz B, Lange C, Malerczyk V. Safety, efficacy, and pharmacokinetics of glimepiride in diabetic patients with renal impairment over a 3-month period. Diabetol Croat 1999;28:25–32.

146. Massi-Benedetti M. Glimiperide in type 2 diabetes mellitus: a review of the worldwide therapeutic experience. Clin Ther 2003;25:799–816.

147. Korytkowski MT. Sulfonylurea treatment of type 2 diabetes mellitus focus on glimepiride. Pharmacotherapy 2004;24:606–20.

148. Davis SN. The role of glimepiride in the effective management of type 2 diabetes. J Diabetes Comp 2004;18:367–76.

149. Valenta LJ, Elias AN. Insulin-induced lipodystrophy in diabetic patients resolved by treatment with human insulin. Ann Intern Med 1985;102(6):790–1.

150. Cusi K, DeFronzo RA. Treatment of NIDDM IDDM, and other insulin-resistant states with IGF-I. Diabetes Rev 1995;3:206–36.

151. Krepinsky J, Ingram AJ, Clase CM. Prolonged sulfonylurea-induced hypoglycemia in diabetic patients with end-stage renal disease. Am J Kidney Dis 2000;35(3):500–5.

152. McGavin JK, Perry CM, Goa KL. Gliclazide modified release. Drugs 2002;62(9):1357–64.

153. Drouin P. Diamicron MR once daily is effective and well tolerated in type 2 diabetes: a double-blind, randomized, multinational study. J Diabetes Complications 2000;14(4):185–91.

154. Galeone F, Fiore G, Mannucci E. Medium-term hypoglycaemic effects of two different oral formulations of gliclazide. Diabet Med 1999;16(7):618–9.

155. Chung M, Kourides I, Canovatchel W, Sutfin T, Messig M, Chaiken RL. Pharmacokinetics and pharmacodynamics of extended-release glipizide GITS compared with immediate-release glipizide in patients with type II diabetes mellitus. J Clin Pharmacol 2002;42(6):651–7.

156. Carroll MF, Gutierrez A, Castro M, Tsewang D, Schade DS. Targeting postprandial hyperglycemia: a comparative study of insulinotropic agents in type 2 diabetes. J Cin Endocrinol Metab 2003;88:S248–54.

157. Schernthaner G. Gliclazide modified release: a critical review of pharmacodynamic, metabolic, and vasoprotective effects. Metabolism 2003;52 Suppl 1:29–34.

158. Aronson JK. Confusion over similar drug names. Problems and solutions. Drug Saf 1995;12(3):155–60.

159. Wan Mohamad WB, Tun Fizi A, Ismail RB, Mafauzy M. Efficacy and safety of single versus multiple daily doses of glibenclamide in type 2 diabetes mellitus. Diabetes Res Clin Pract 2000;49(2–3):93–9.

160. Melander A. Kinetics-effect relations of insulin-releasing drugs in patients with type 2 diabetes. Diabetes 2004;53:S151-S155.

161. Stenman S, Melander A, Groop P-H, Groop L. What is the benefit of increasing the sulphonylurea dose? Ann Intern Med 1993;118:169–72.

162. Caksen H, Kendirci M, Tutus A, Uzum K, Kurtoglu S. Gliclazide-induced hepatitis, hemiplegia and dysphasia in a suicide attempt. J Pediatr Endocrinol Metab 2001;14(8):1157–9.

163. Chelliah A, Burge MR. Hypoglycaemia in elderly patients with diabetes mellitus causes and strategies for prevention. Drugs Aging 2004;21:511–30.

164. Thamer M, Ray NF, Taylor T. Association between antihypertensive drug use and hypoglycemia: a case-control

study of diabetic users of insulin or sulfonylureas. Clin Ther 1999;21(8):1387–400.

165. Parlapiano C, Paoletti V, Campana E, Giovanniello T, Pantone P. Increased risk of hypoglycemia from enalapril plus ranitidine with glibenclamide: a clinical case. Adv Ther 1999;16:130–2.

166. Collin M, Mucklow JC. Drug interactions, renal impairment and hypoglycaemia in a patient with type II diabetes. Br J Clin Pharmacol 1999;48(2):134–7.

167. Burge MR, Zeise TM, Sobhy TA, Rassam AG, Schade DS. Low-dose ethanol predisposes elderly fasted patients with type 2 diabetes to sulfonylurea-induced low blood glucose. Diabetes Care 1999;22(12):2037–43.

168. Bussing R, Gende A. Severe hypoglycemia from clarithromycin–sulfonylurea drug interaction. Diabetes Care 2002;25(9):1659–61.

169. Dixit AA, Rao YM. Pharmacokinetic interaction between diltiazem and tolbutamide. Drug Metabol Drug Interact 1999;15(4):269–77.

170. Ahmad S. Gemfibrozil: interaction with glyburide. South Med J 1991;84(1):102.

171. Niemi M, Backman JT, Neuvonen M, Laitila J, Neuvonen PJ, Kivisto KT. Effects of fluconazole and fluvoxamine on the pharmacokinetics and pharmacodynamics of glimepiride. Clin Pharmacol Ther 2001;69(4):194–200.

172. Pahls S, Schaffner A. Aspergillus fumigatus pneumonia in neutropenic patients receiving fluconazole for infection due to Candida species: is amphotericin B combined with fluconazole the appropriate answer? Clin Infect Dis 1994;18(3):484–6.

173. Abad S, Moachon L, Blanche P, Bavoux F, Sicard D, Salmon-Ceron D. Possible interaction between gliclazide, fluconazole and sulfamethoxazole resulting in severe hypoglycaemia. Br J Clin Pharmacol 2001;52(4):456–7.

174. Niemi M, Neuvonen PJ, Kivisto KT. Effect of gemfibrozil on the pharmacokinetics and pharmacodynamics of glimepiride. Clin Pharmacol Ther 2001;70(5):439–45.

175. Lin G, Hays DP, Spillane L. Refractory hypoglycaemia from ciprofloxacin and glyburide interaction. J Toxicol Clin Toxicol 2004;42:295–7.

176. Roberge RJ, Kaplan R, Frank R, Fore C. Glyburide–ciprofloxacin interaction with resistant hypoglycaemia. Ann Emerg Med 2000;36:160–3.

177. Leblanc M, Belanger C, Cossette P. Severe and resistant hypoglycaemia associated with concomitant gatifloxacin and glyburide therapy. Pharmacotherapy 2004;24:926–31.

178. Gajjar DA, LaCreta FP, Kollia GD Stolz RR, Berger S, Smith WB, Swingle M, Grasela DM. Effect of multiple-dose gatifloxacin or ciprofloxacin on glucose homeostasis and insulin production in patients with non-insulin-dependent diabetes mellitus maintained with diet and exercise. Pharmacotherapy 2000;20(6 pt 2):76S–86S.

179. Gerstein HC, Thorpe KE, Taylor DW, Haynes RB. The effectiveness of hydroxychloroquine in patients with type 2 diabetes mellitus who are refractory to sulfonylureas—a randomized trial. Diabetes Res Clin Pract 2002;55(3):209–19.

180. Sone H, Takahashi A, Yamada N. Ibuprofen-related hypoglycemia in a patient receiving sulfonylurea. Ann Intern Med 2001;134(4):344.

181. Drouhet E, Dupont B. Evolution of antifungal agents: past, present, and future. Rev Infect Dis 1987;9(Suppl 1):S4–S14.

182. Kihara Y, Otsuki M. Interaction of gliclazide and rifampicin. Diabetes Care 2000;23(8):1204–5.

183. Dische FE, Wernstedt C, Westermark GT, Westermark P, Pepys MB, Rennie JA, Gilbey SG, Watkins PJ. Insulin as an amyloid-fibril protein at sites of repeated insulin injections in a diabetic patient. Diabetologia 1988;31(3):158–61.

184. Christensen LK, Hansen JM, Kristensen M. Sulphaphenazole-induced hypoglycaemic attacks in tolbutamide-treated diabetic. Lancet 1963;41:1298–301.

185. Soeldner JS, Steinke J. Hypoglycemia in tolbutamide-treated diabetes; Report of two casses with measurement of serum insulin. JAMA 1965;193:398–9.

186. Dubach UC, Bückert A, Raaflaub J. Einfluss von Sulfonamiden auf die blutzuckersenkende Wirkung oraler Antidiabetica. Schweiz Med Wochenschr 1966;44:1483.

187. Wing LM, Miners JO. Cotrimoxazole as an inhibitor of oxidative drug metabolism: effects of trimethoprim and sulphamethoxazole separately and combined on tolbutamide disposition. Br J Clin Pharmacol 1985;20(5):482–5.

188. Pond SM, Birkett DJ, Wade DN. Mechanisms of inhibition of tolbutamide metabolism: phenylbutazone, oxyphenbutazone, sulfaphenazole. Clin Pharmacol Ther 1977;22(5 Pt 1):573–9.

189. Hansen JM, Christensen LK. Drug interactions with oral sulphonylurea hypoglycaemic drugs. Drugs 1977;13(1):24–34.

190. Schattner A, Rimon E, Green L, Coslovsky R, Bentwich Z. Hypoglycemia induced by co-trimoxazole in AIDS. BMJ 1988;297(6650):742.

191. Komatsu K, Ito K, Nakajima Y, Kanamitsu S, Imaoka S, Funae Y, Green CE, Tyson CA, Shimada N, Sugiyama Y. Prediction of in vivo drug–drug interactions between tolbutamide and various sulfonamides in humans based on in vitro experiments. Drug Metab Dispos 2000;28(4):475–81.

192. Baciewicz AM, Swafford WB Jr. Hypoglycemia induced by the interaction of chlorpropamide and co-trimoxazole. Drug Intell Clin Pharm 1984;18(4):309–10.

193. Abad S, Moachon L, Blanche P, Bavoux F, Sicard D, Salmon-Ceron D. Possible interaction between gliclazide, fluconazole and sulfamethoxazole resulting in severe hypoglycaemia. Br J Clin Pharmacol 2001;52(4):456–7.

194. Lheureux PER, Zahir S, Penaloza A, Gris M Bench-to-bench review: antidotal treatment of sulfonylurea-induced hypoglycemia with octreotide. Crit Care 2005;9:543–9.

Thiazolidinediones

General Information

The thiazolidinediones include pioglitazone and rosiglitazone; darglitazone is in development; ciglitazone, englitazone, and troglitazone have been withdrawn owing to adverse effects on the liver (all names are rINNs).

The thiazolidinediones reduce insulin resistance and are sometimes designated as insulin sensitizers. They promote glucose utilization in peripheral tissues by stimulating non-oxidative glucose metabolism and suppressing gluconeogenesis. They activate the so-called Peroxisome Proliferator Activated Receptor Gamma (PPARγ), a nuclear hormone receptor that enhances a number of genes encoding enzymes involved in glucose and fat metabolism. PPARγ is essential for normal insulin sensitivity

(1–3). They may also intervene directly in the fuel metabolism of skeletal muscle and liver, as suggested by in vitro experiments (4). They can reduce HbA_{1c}, the glucose AUC after a glucose tolerance test, and the glucose AUC after a meal in glucocorticoid-induced diabetes, as has been shown in seven patients taking troglitazone (5). They may ameliorate albuminuria in incipient diabetic nephropathy (6).

In some systems, troglitazone behaves as a partial agonist, but in fat cells it behaves as a full agonist. The transcriptional activities of troglitazone and rosiglitazone differ (7). The thiazolidinediones promote fat accumulation in subcutaneous tissue (8) rather than in the abdominal region, which plays such a bad role in the insulin resistance syndrome. Troglitazone lowers fasting glucose and postprandial glucose. Its effects persist for 2–3 weeks after withdrawal (9). It is also effective in insulin-resistant glucocorticoid-induced diabetes (10). It has a greater insulin-sparing effect than biguanides when given to patients on continuous subcutaneous insulin infusion (11).

The thiazolidinediones have been frequently reviewed (12–22). They can be prescribed as single drugs or in combination with other hypoglycemic drugs (23). In 12 healthy people, meals did not affect the absorption of rosiglitazone (24).

Observational studies

In 244 patients with type 2 diabetes who took pioglitazone 30 or 45 mg/day for 20 weeks or 30 mg/day for 12 weeks and then 45 mg/day for 8 weeks, blood pressure, liver enzymes, and lipid profile improved and HbA_{1c} fell by 1% (25). There was one serious adverse effect related to pioglitazone: severe headache and severe weight gain in a patient taking 30 mg/day, which required drug withdrawal.

In a post-marketing surveillance study in 8760 patients for 16 weeks the most common serious adverse effect was weight gain, followed by edema of the legs, nausea, headache, and dizziness (26).

When pioglitazone 30 mg/day was added to acarbose or acarbose with a sulfonylurea for 16 weeks in 20 patients, there were reductions in HbA_{1c}, fasting plasma glucose, and postprandial glucose (27). There were edema, mild hypoglycemia, and increases in lactate dehydrogenase and creatine kinase activities. Two patients, who had had angina pectoris before entry, had myocardial infarctions. They An almost identical study in 20 patients for 16 weeks gave the same results and adverse effects (28).

Comparative studies

In a parallel-group study in patients starting on hypoglycemic therapy with thiazolidinediones, 35 took troglitazone 600 mg/day, 36 took rosiglitazone 8 mg/day, and 30 took pioglitazone 45 mg/day (29). At 2 and 4 months, there was an equal effect on glucose lowering and greater weight gain with pioglitazone; pioglitazone had the largest beneficial effect on lipids and rosiglitazone the least.

In 203 patients, randomly assigned for 1 year to rosiglitazone 4 mg bd or glibenclamide to achieve optimal control, there was significant and sustained reduction in hyperglycemia and a significant reduction in diastolic blood pressure with rosiglitazone (30). There were no differences in adverse effects or in left ventricular mass index.

Placebo-controlled studies

Rosiglitazone monotherapy has been studied double-blind in 493 patients for 26 weeks (31). There was a dose-related fall in hemoglobin. Rosiglitazone caused more mild to moderate edema. One patient had a temporary rise in transaminases, which normalized spontaneously.

In a parallel-group, double-blind, placebo-controlled, dose-ranging study of rosiglitazone 4, 8, and 12 mg/day in 369 patients for 8 weeks after a run-in period, hematocrit and hemoglobin, C peptide, fasting blood glucose, and fructosamine all fell (32). Hepatotoxicity, significant cardiac events, or hypoglycemia were not different from placebo.

In 574 patients taking a sulfonylurea, twice-daily placebo ($n = 192$ patients) was compared with rosiglitazone 1 mg/day ($n = 199$ patients) or rosiglitazone 2 mg/day ($n = 183$ patients) for 26 weeks (33). Rosiglitazone improved HbA_{1c}. With the higher dose of rosiglitazone there were more cases of hypoglycemia and a small increase in mean body weight; some patients complained of headache and upper respiratory tract infections.

In a placebo-controlled study, 959 patients took placebo, rosiglitazone 4 mg od, 2 mg bd, 8 mg od, or 4 mg bd for 26 weeks (34). In the placebo group 38% withdrew and in the rosiglitazone groups 20%. Two patients (one in the placebo and one in the 4 mg bd group) had changes in alanine transaminase of more than three times the upper limit of the reference range. Other adverse events related to edema were seen in 1.6% of the placebo group and in 4.1% of those taking 2 mg bd and 6.6% in those taking 4 mg bd. There were small dose-dependent falls in hemoglobin and hematocrit.

In a multicenter, double-blind, placebo-controlled study, 408 patients took pioglitazone 7.5, 15, 30, or 45 mg/day (35). There was no hepatotoxicity and the overall adverse events profiles did not differ, except for edema in 12 of 329 patients who took pioglitazone. There was a significant fall in triglycerides and a small fall in LDL cholesterol. However, in another study in 150 patients, postprandial triglycerides were not reduced by pioglitazone (36).

In 561 patients with HbA_{1c} concentrations of at least 8.0% on stable treatment with a sulfonylurea, pioglitazone was added for 16 weeks in a double-blind study (37). The incidence of edema increased from 2% in the placebo group to 7%. With pioglitazone there were more episodes of hypoglycemia, a dose-related increase in body weight, and a dose-related fall in hemoglobin. The frequency of adverse cardiovascular effects was the same.

The addition of rosiglitazone 2 mg bd (n = 215), 4 mg bd (n = 210), or placebo (n = 105) to sulfonylurea therapy in Chinese patients, of whom 56% were seropositive for hepatitis B and/or C, caused a significant fall in HbA_{1c}

(38). There were more respiratory infections, weight gain, edema of the legs, hyperlipidemia, and episodes hypoglycemia in those who took rosiglitazone. In all groups there were a few cases of slight increases in transaminases, but no signs of hepatotoxicity.

Combinations of oral hypoglycemic drugs

The different mechanisms of action of the various classes of hypoglycemic drugs make combined therapy feasible: the sulfonylureas and meglitinides stimulate insulin production by different mechanisms, the biguanides reduce glucose production by the liver and excretion from the liver, acarbose reduces the absorption of glucose from the gut, and the thiazolidinediones reduce insulin resistance in fat. It is not necessary to wait until the maximal dose of one drug has been reached before starting another. However, sulfonylureas and meglitinides should no longer be used when endogenous insulin production is minimal. Combinations of insulin with sulfonylureas or meglitinides should only be used while the patient is changing to insulin, except when long-acting insulin is given at night in order to give the islets a rest and to stimulate daytime insulin secretion.

Large studies of the effects of lifestyle changes, the effects of drugs in preventing or postponing the complications of diabetes, or the usefulness of various combinations are regularly published. The different mechanisms of action of the various classes give different metabolic effects and different adverse effects profiles (39). Comparative costs of the various therapies in the USA have been presented (40).

This subject has been reviewed in relation to combined oral therapy. In a systematic review of 63 studies with a duration of at least 3 months and involving at least 10 patients at the end of the study, and in which HbA_{1c} was reported, five different classes of oral drugs were almost equally effective in lowering blood glucose concentrations (41). HbA_{1c} was reduced by about 1–2% in all cases. Combination therapy gave additive effects. However, long-term vascular risk reduction was demonstrated only with sulfonylureas and metformin.

The adverse effects of combined drug therapy are attributable to the adverse effects of the single drugs. Increased adverse effects or new adverse effects in patients taking combinations have not been reported.

Thiazolidinediones + biguanides
In a multicenter, randomized, double-blind study, 116 patients were treated for 26 weeks with metformin plus placebo, 119 with metformin plus rosiglitazone 4 mg/day, and 113 with metformin plus rosiglitazone 8 mg/day (42). In both rosiglitazone groups there were small but statistically significant falls in hemoglobin and hematocrit. Edema was rare but more common in the rosiglitazone groups (2.5% with 4 mg/day and 3.5% with 8 mg/day). Body weight fell by 1.2 kg from baseline with placebo but increased by 0.7 kg with rosiglitazone 4 mg/day and by 1.9 kg with 8 mg/day. No one taking rosiglitazone had an increase in alanine transaminase greater than three times the upper limit of the reference range.

In a placebo-controlled study in 116 patients who responded insufficiently to metformin 2.5 g/day, rosiglitazone 2 or 4 mg bd was added for 26 weeks (43). HbA_{1c} and fasting plasma glucose improved and hemoglobin fell. Edema was reported in 5.2% of the patients who took rosiglitazone and two patients withdrew because of headache.

The combination of metformin + thiazolidinediones (glitazones) is contraindicated or not recommended in patients taking therapy for cardiac failure. In a retrospective study of 12 505 and 13 158 patients with cardiac failure and diabetes in two different years (1998/9 and 2000/1) (44) 7.1% (later 11.%) had a prescription for metformin, 7.2% (16.%) for thiazolidinediones and 14% (24%) for both drugs added to cardiac drugs. This suggests that many patients with heart failure are taking hypoglycemic drugs, notwithstanding contraindications.

Thiazolidinediones + biguanides + sulfonylureas
Glibenclamide 2.5 mg/day + metformin 500 mg/day in a combination tablet was increased to a maximum of 10 mg/day + 2000 mg/day in patients with type 2 diabetes, mean age 57 years and weight 93 kg; 181 patients also took rosiglitazone and 184 took placebo for 24 weeks (45). Rosiglitazone was added to a maximum of 8 mg/day aiming to reduce the HbA_{1c} concentration to less than 7.0%. There was *hypoglycemia* in 140 patients; 95 (53%) of those who took rosiglitazone reported hypoglycemia compared with 45 (25%) of those who took placebo. One patient taking rosiglitazone withdrew owing to hypoglycemia. HbA_{1c} concentrations were less than 7% in 42% of those taking rosiglitazone compared with 14% of those taking placebo. Weight gain was greater in those taking rosiglitazone, 3 kg compared with 0.03 kg.

Thiazolidinediones + meglitinides
In 585 patients in a double-blind, randomized, placebo-controlled, multicenter study lasting 16 weeks, nateglinide 40 mg tds alone, troglitazone 200 mg/day alone, and the combination were compared (46). The combination was most effective in lowering HbA_{1c}. The most frequent adverse effects were mild hypoglycemia, most often in the combination group. Three patients (two in the combination group and one in the troglitazone alone group) withdrew because of hypoglycemia. Most of the withdrawals were related to increased liver enzymes and weight gain, known adverse effects of troglitazone. Twelve patients withdrew because of predefined changes from baseline (transaminases more than 200% and alkaline phosphatase and bilirubin more than 100% over baseline); seven were taking troglitazone alone, four combined therapy, and one placebo.

In an open trial, 256 patients with type 2 diabetes with inadequate hypoglycemic control (HbA_{1c} over 7.0% during previous therapy) took repaglinide (0.5–4 mg at meals), troglitazone (200–600 mg/day), or a combination of the two for 22 weeks (47). Combination therapy was most effective. Repaglinide only was more effective than troglitazone only. Mean body weight increased in both groups. Serious adverse events were chest pain, cerebrovascular disorders, malignancies, dysrhythmias, electrocardiographic changes suggesting myocardial infarction, and increased aspartate transaminase activity (in one patient taking troglitazone). The serious adverse effects were similar in the different groups. Hypoglycemia occurred in 4% of the patients taking combined therapy, in 16% of those taking troglitazone only, and in 27% of those taking repaglinide only; none needed assistance. There were changes in liver function tests in three patients in the combined group and in one patient each in the two other groups; the drugs were withdrawn in the affected patients and liver function normalized. There were no differences in adverse effects in the different groups. Hypoglycemia occurred in 11 patients taking repaglinide, in seven taking combination therapy, and in one taking troglitazone. Anemia occurred in four patients taking combined therapy and in two taking troglitazone only.

In 246 patients pioglitazone 30 mg/day, repaglinide (optimal dosage), or pioglitazone + repaglinide were compared over 12 weeks after an initial 12 weeks to establish dosages in an open study (48). There were no episodes of major hypoglycemia or raised transaminases. HbA$_{1c}$ changed in the three groups by –0.18%, + 0.32%, and –1.76% respectively. Fasting glucose improved most in the combined group. There were minor episodes of hypoglycemia in 8%, 3%, and 5% respectively. There were weight gains of 0.3, 2.0, and 5.5 kg respectively. The main reason for discontinuation before the end of the trial (41%, 58% and 15%) respectively was insufficient effect.

The combination of rosiglitazone + repaglinide during 24 weeks (49) in 252 patients with HbA$_{1c}$ over 7.0% produced one major episode of hypoglycemia. Minor episodes occurred in 9% of those taking combined therapy, 6% of those taking repaglinide, and 2% of those taking rosiglitazone. There was peripheral edema in 4% of those taking combined therapy and 3 % of those taking rosiglitazone. Weight gain was + 4.4 kg in those taking combined therapy, 2.3 kg in those taking rosiglitazone, and 1.6 kg in those taking repaglinide.

Thiazolidinediones + sulfonylureas
Troglitazone 100 or 200 mg/day or placebo was given for 16 weeks to 259 patients already taking sulfonylurea therapy (50). HbA$_{1c}$ was 0.4 and 0.7% lower and blood glucose concentrations fell. The most common event was hypoglycemia, but this did not occur more often when troglitazone was added. Liver enzymes increased to the same extent in the three groups and never rose above normal. No patients withdrew because of drug-related effects.

Rosiglitazone 8 mg/day + glibenclamide 7.5 mg/day were compared with glibenclamide alone (maximum 15 mg/day) in 335 patients over 26 weeks (51). HbA$_{1c}$ fell by 0.81% with combination therapy. One patient taking combination therapy had a single episode of serious hypoglycemia; mild to moderate hypoglycemia was reported in 19% of the patients taking combination therapy and 4.1% in those taking glibenclamide alone. There

was edema in 9.5% versus 2.9%, weight gain of 3.1 kg versus 0.14 kg, and reduced hemoglobin in those taking combination therapy.

Insulin + thiazolidinediones

Insulin plus metformin (27 patients, 2000 mg/day) or troglitazone (30 patients, 600 mg/day) in patients with type 2 diabetes using at least 30 U/day was compared with insulin alone (30 patients) for 4 months (52). Body weight increased in the insulin and the insulin plus troglitazone groups. In the insulin plus metformin group there were significantly more gastrointestinal adverse effects but less hypoglycemia than the other groups.

The addition of rosiglitazone to insulin for 26 weeks in a double-blind study in 315 patients with inadequately controlled type 2 diabetes improved glycemic control and was well tolerated (53). There was a significant fall in hemoglobin, and some patients in both the rosiglitazone and placebo groups developed edema.

General adverse effects

The adverse effects of the thiazolidinediones are comparable and include weight gain, upper respiratory tract infections, headache, and hypoglycemia (mostly in combination with other hypoglycemic drugs). Fluid retention sometimes occurs (19,21) and can lead to or exacerbate heart failure and pulmonary and general edema, which was reported in 1.5–12% of patients taking pioglitazone. Small clinically unimportant falls in hematocrit and hemoglobin occur because of hemodilution. Changes in liver enzymes and bilirubin have not been reported with rosiglitazone, and although there have been some reports of hepatic-related adverse effects, they have not been definitive (SEDA-25, 515). However, troglitazone causes liver complications, sometimes fatal, and this has led to its withdrawal from the market. There are no drug interactions with other hypoglycemic agents.

The use and safety of thiazolidinediones have been reviewed. Liver damage is rare, while weight gain and fluid retention are common. The mechanisms for fluid retention are suggested to be a change in intestinal ion transport resulting in an increased plasma volume, vasodilatation causing reflex sympathetic activity activation, and increased vascular permeability (54).

Organs and Systems

Cardiovascular

The American Heart Association and the American Diabetes Association have published a consensus statement in which they stated that in patients with signs or symptoms of NYHA class III or IV cardiac failure thiazolidinediones should not be used and in class I or II they should be used cautiously, starting with a very low dosage (rosiglitazone 2 mg or pioglitazone 15 mg) (55). Gradual dose escalation is warranted, with careful observation to identify weight gain, edema, or exacerbation of cardiac failure. Even if there are no signs of chronic heart failure, it can develop when thiazolidinediones are begun. When thiazolidinediones are combined with insulin, edema is more common.

- A 74-year-old man with long-standing type 2 diabetes and compensated systolic dysfunction taking glibenclamide was given rosiglitazone 4 mg/day, increasing to 8 mg/ml after 1 month (56). After 2 weeks he had weight gain of 5 kg, increased jugular venous pressure, shortness of breath, bibasal crackles, and a gallop rhythm. Subsequently he had a total weight gain of 17 kg and worse symptoms. When rosiglitazone was withdrawn his weight fell within 12 days to the pretreatment weight and the edema disappeared.

Cardiac dysfunction increases insulin resistance, suggesting that thiazolidinediones, which reduce insulin resistance might be a good choice in patients with diabetes and cardiac dysfunction. However, this case suggests that they can worsen fluid retention, perhaps by vasodilatation (57).

In a retrospective study in diabetic patients taking various oral hypoglycemic agents from January 1995 to March 2001 in a large insurance company there were 5441 thiazolidinedione users and 28 103 non-thiazolidinedione users (58). Those taking thiazolidinediones were younger but more likely to have coronary artery disease or complications of diabetes. The adjusted incidence of heart failure after 40 months was 8.2% in those taking thiazolidinediones and 5.3% in those not taking thiazolidinediones. The validity of the conclusion was discussed (59) but other commentators supported the need to be vigilant for heart failure when prescribing thiazolidinediones (60).

In 40 ambulatory hemodialysis patients, 25 of whom were taking pioglitazone and 15 rosiglitazone, there were no increases in intravascular volume, anemia, edema, or chronic heart failure in a retrospective study (61). It may be that dialysis obviates any increase in intravascular volume. The use of these drugs during dialysis seems to be safe, although there were reductions in systolic and diastolic blood pressures.

Of 143 patients (62) studied retrospectively, eight stopped taking treatment because of significant peripheral edema, one had an exacerbation of cardiac failure, and one reported myalgia. HbA$_{1c}$, lipid profiles, and blood pressure improved. In 38 patients taking pioglitazone brain natriuretic peptide, which may play a role in fluid retention, did not rise (63).

Respiratory

A single case of pleuropulmonary disease possibly induced by troglitazone has been reported (64).

Nervous system

Ataxia has been attributed to troglitazone in two patients aged about 80 years (a man and a woman) (65). The ataxia developed during treatment and disappeared in one case 2–3 days after withdrawal and in the other within 2 weeks. In one, the ataxia was accompanied by a dementia-like syndrome, which completely disappeared within 8 weeks. One of the patients was rechallenged and developed ataxia again.

Neuromuscular

A myopathy has been reported in a man taking rosiglitazone, fenofibrate, and metformin (66).

- A 75-year-old man with type 2 diabetes and no history of muscle injury or viral illness presented with a creatine kinase of 6897 (reference range 0–171) U/l, MB fraction 1%, myoglobin 902 (0–110) ng/ml, and creatinine 116 (30–70) μmol/l. He had had diabetes for 11 years and his creatine kinase had been 250–350 U/l during the previous 4 years. Simvastatin had been changed 15 weeks before to fenofibrate 200 mg/day for raised triglycerides, and rosiglitazone 2 mg bd had been added 3 weeks before. He was also taking metformin 1 g bd, phenprocoumon, valsartan, and inhaled sympathomimetics. The metformin was withdrawn because of the increased creatinine. Fenofibrate and rosiglitazone were withdrawn because of a suspected drug interaction.

It is possible that the combination of rosiglitazone with fenofibrate was responsible for the severe myopathy, although the possibility of a single drug cannot be excluded. Raised creatine kinase activity has been reported with troglitazone, and there has been a report of rhabdomyolysis in a patient with type 2 diabetes taking pioglitazone when fenofibrate was added.

Sensory systems

Macular edema has been associated with rosiglitazone (67).

- A 55-year-old man with diabetes, taking regular insulin, glargine, rosiglitazone, atorvastatin, amlodipine, quinapril, hydrochlorohiazide, and sertraline, had proliferative retinopathy, neuropathy, and nephropathy. His vision was 20/30 OD and 20/25 OS. The dose of rosiglitazone was increased from 2 to 8 mg bd and 1 month later his vision was 20/80 OD and 20/70 OS. At the same time he developed peripheral edema. The dose of rosiglitazone was reduced to 2 mg bd and his vision improved to 20/25 OU and the macular edema resolved over the next 3 weeks.

There have been several other reports of this rare adverse effect of rosiglitazone, which has been added to the SPC. Caution should be taken and appropriate follow-up should take place when rosiglitazone is added to the therapy of someone at risk of macular edema.

- A 53 year old Hispanic woman developed bilateral, painless, slowly progressive proptosis over 12 months (68). She had taken rosiglitazone 8 mg for 18 months. She had also noticed weight gain of 9 kg and an increase in abdominal girth of 4 inches. The dose of rosiglitazone was gradually educed, with no change in appearance. A CT scan of the orbits showed normal extraocular muscles. Thyroid function was normal.

The authors postulated that there had been an increase in orbital fat in parallel to the increase in abdominal fat. Rosiglitazone can reactivate thyroid inflammatory orbitopathy and treatment of orbital fibroblasts in culture with PPARγ agonists can stimulate thyrotropin hormone receptor expression and subsequently promote adipogenesis (69).

Endocrine

Exacerbation of thyroid eye disease, stable and inactive for more than 2 years, by pioglitazone in a 57-year-old man was explained by the effect of PPARγ agonists on preadipocytes from orbits in thyroid eye disease or from neck fat during Graves' disease in hormone/agonist induced models (70). The agonists increased adipogenesis 2–13 times and PPARγ antagonists reduced adipogenesis 2–7 times, suggesting that thiazolidinediones may have a direct effect of on fat proliferation in thyroid eye disease.

It has been suggested that thiazolidinediones may be novel candidates for redifferentiation therapy of various cancers. Five patients with papillary or follicular thyroid cancer took rosiglitazone 4 mg/day for 1 month and 8 mg/day for 2 months (71). There were increased thyroglobulin concentrations in four. The significance of this increase was uncertain. Although the authors suggested that redifferentiation might have been the cause, thyroglobulin concentrations also increase with increased tumor mass.

Metabolism

Weight
The thiazolidinediones increase body weight. With troglitazone the increase in body weight is accompanied by changed fat distribution, but central fat, in part responsible for the cardiovascular changes seen in diabetes, remains the same; weight gain is accompanied by increased subcutaneous fat (72).

In one study, troglitazone increased body weight, adipocyte size, leptin concentrations, GLUT4 protein expression, basal and insulin-stimulated glucose transport, and insulin-stimulated whole-body glucose disposal rate (73).

In a 24-week study, in which 40 patients taking troglitazone and glibenclamide were compared with patients taking glibenclamide, serum fasting insulin, serum triglycerides, and insulin resistance were reduced when troglitazone was added. Fat deposition in the liver and the visceral fat area were reduced, but deposition in skeletal muscle was not (74).

Thiazolidinediones cause recruitment and conversion of pre-adipocytes into adipocytes and are therefore adipogenic (75). In 18 patients without diabetes, mean age 46 years, who took pioglitazone 30 mg/day for 48 weeks for non-alcoholic steatohepatitis, there was a mean weight gain of 3.5 kg in 72% (76). Similarly, in 91 patients with type 2 diabetes who took pioglitazone 30 or 45 mg/day for 1 year there was a mean weight gain of 3 kg, compared with 1.1 kg in the 109 who took glibenclamide (77).

In a randomized placebo-controlled study in 48 people with type 2 diabetes, aged 35–75 years, who took pioglitazone 45 mg/day or placebo for 24 weeks, those taking pioglitazone gained 3.88 kg at 6 months, compared with a reduction of 0.79 kg in those who took placebo (78). Scans showed that this was mainly due to a generalized increase in subcutaneous fat. Visceral adipose tissue did not change significantly. Subjective ratings of hunger did not change and neither was there a change in metabolic rate. However, more sensitive measures are probably required, as the calorie change to cause this sort of weight gain is small (175 kcal/day).

Hypoglycemia
The thiazolidinediones can cause hypoglycemia both when used alone or in combination with other hypoglycemic drugs (79).

When patients taking troglitazone were switched to equivalent amounts of rosiglitazone ($n = 60$) or pioglitazone ($n = 60$) there were no changes in HbA_{1c} or other parameters, except that with pioglitazone there was a significant improvement in lipid profile, with an average fall in total cholesterol of 0.5 mmol/l (80).

However, in 23 patients who took pioglitazone for 16 weeks, in whom fasting and mean glucose concentrations and mean free fatty acid concentrations fell, weight gain of 3.6 kg was associated with an increase in peripheral fat without edema (81).

In 38 patients taking metformin 2550 mg/day and glimiperide 6 mg/day, rosiglitazone 4 or 8 mg/day was added for 20 weeks (82). HbA_{1c} and fasting blood glucose fell significantly. There was hypoglycemia in 19% of those who took 4 mg/day and 28% of those who took 8 mg/day, and body weight increased by 4.2 and 4.6 kg respectively. There were no signs or symptoms of liver disease and no changes in liver function tests.

Insulin resistance in type 2 diabetes contributes to reduced efficacy of both endogenous and exogenous insulin. When metformin and pioglitazone were compared in patients who had not taken previous drug therapy, they were equally efficacious in glycemic control, but parameters of insulin sensitivity increased much more with pioglitazone (83).

Highly active antiretroviral therapy (HAART) can increase insulin resistance and cause lipodystrophy (loss of subcutaneous fat and increased intra-abdominal fat). In patients with lipodystrophy associated with HAART, pioglitazone 30 mg/day was given for 3 months and than increased to 45 mg/day for another 3 months (84). There was a significant increase in total and leg fat mass. However, insulin resistance was prevented only partially or not at all. Cholesterol and triglycerides did not change. The serum leptin concentration was low and did not increase during treatment. There were no effects on liver function tests. The results on insulin resistance and lipid profiles were opposite to those found in a comparable study with rosiglitazone (85).

In 30 patients with lipodystrophy associated with HAART rosiglitazone 8 mg/day for 24 weeks had no effect on body weight, subcutaneous or intra-abdominal fat, total body fat, anthropometry, or serum leptin concentrations (84). However, it reduced percentage liver fat and serum insulin concentrations and normalized liver function tests. During the first 12 weeks serum triglycerides rose from 3.5 to 6.5 mmol/l and serum cholesterol from 6.0 to 7.8 mmol/l. The results on insulin resistance and lipid profiles were opposite to those found in a comparable study with pioglitazone (83).

Lipid abnormalities

Reductions in VLDL cholesterol, LDL cholesterol, and chylomicrons may contribute to a reduction in cardiac complications. Pioglitazone reduced both lipoprotein(a) and the remnant particles (cholesterol-rich particles after the release of triglycerides from the chylomicrons), whereas troglitazone caused increases in lipoprotein(a) (86).

Triglycerides have been reported to increase by a mean of 0.99 mmol/l in patients taking rosiglitazone, with no change in those taking pioglitazone (87). A more profound change in triglycerides has also been reported with rosiglitazone, although this is likely to be rare (88).

- A 64-year-old woman who had taken metformin for 3 years had a high-density lipoprotein concentration of 1.2 mmol/l, which fell to 0.26 mmol/l when she took rosiglitazone. The Hb_{A1c} fell from 10.1% to 7.9%. Fenofibrate was added and the HDL concentration fell further to 0.11 mmol/l. Triglycerides, 2.7 mmol/l before treatment, increased to 4.7 mmol/l. Apolipoprotein A1 concentrations were low at 0.14 g/l (reference range 1.1–2.05 g/l). On withdrawing both the rosiglitazone and the fenofibrate the HDL concentration rose to 0.95 mmol/l.
- A 64-year-old man took metformin and glipizide. The Hb_{A1c} concentration was 11.4%, HDL 0.99 mmol/l, and triglycerides 3.8 mmol/l. Bezafibrate was added and the Hb_{A1c} fell to 8.7%, HDL was unchanged at 0.98 mmol/l, and triglycerides fell to 1.9 mmol/l. After starting rosiglitazone 4 mg/day the HDL fell to 0.44 mmol/l, and on increasing the dose of rosiglitazone to 8 mg/day the HDL fell to 0.26 mmol/l, triglycerides rose to 5.2 mmol/l and apo-1 concentrations were 0.27 g/l. On withdrawal of rosiglitazone the HDL returned to 0.98 mmol/l.
- A 64-year-old man had rosiglitazone added to his therapy and the HDL concentration fell from 0.90 to 0.31 mmol/l. Triglycerides rose from 4.0 to 8.0 mmol/l. Apo-1 concentrations were reduced (0.57 g/l).

Hypolipoproteinemia is likely to be a rare adverse effect. The measurement of HDL cholesterol and triglycerides before and after staring thiazolidinedione therapy will allow its detection. On withdrawing therapy concentrations return to normal. This effect may be specific to rosiglitazone, as it is becoming apparent that the PPAR-γ agonists vary in their effects.

Lipoma formation has been attributed to rosiglitazone.

- A 58-year-old HIV-positive man with type 2 diabetes was given rosiglitazone and over the next 3 months developed several dozen lipomas measuring 1–4 cm in diameter. Biopsy showed well circumscribed tumors of normal appearing fat cells, beneath normal-looking skin. The rosiglitazone was withdrawn and the lipomas resolved (89).

In a placebo-controlled study in 108 non-diabetic adults with HIV-1 infection and lipoatrophy, rosiglitazone 4 mg/day for 48 weeks had no beneficial effect on the lipoatrophy (87). However 30 of those who took rosiglitazone developed hypertriglyceridemia, compared with 20 taking placebo, and 11 developed hypercholesterolemia, compared with four taking placebo.

Mineral balance

In 20 people with type 2 diabetes and hypertension taking glibenclamide 15 mg/day rosiglitazone 4 mg/day was added; serum calcium and magnesium concentration rose slightly at 26 weeks (90). The significance of this is unknown.

Fluid balance

Two cases of pulmonary and general edema have been reported with rosiglitazone (91).

- A 78-year-old man became short of breath. He had been taking rosiglitazone 8 mg/day for 6 months. He had renal insufficiency, atrial fibrillation, hypertension, and congestive heart failure, with pitting edema and bilateral pleural effusions. He was refractory to intravenous furosemide and metolazone. Withdrawal of rosiglitazone and administration of bumetanide gave a net fluid output of 9.5 litres and the edema resolved.
- A 67-year-old man, who had taken troglitazone 600 mg/day for 4 months and who had renal insufficiency, stroke, and cardiomyopathy, developed pitting edema, hepatomegaly, ascites, and a pleural effusion. The edema was resistant to treatment until troglitazone was changed to glipizide 10 mg/day, when he had a diuresis of 18 litres in 6 days. Later he took rosiglitazone 4 mg bd for 3 weeks and had weight gain of 5 kg and pitting edema. Diuretic therapy failed until rosiglitazone was withdrawn, after which he reached his baseline weight in 4 days.

Pioglitazone also causes fluid retention, possibly because of increased production of vascular endothelial growth factor (92). The safety profile of monotherapy and combined therapy with pioglitazone has been evaluated in 3500 patients over 2500 patient-years, and some data from post-marketing surveillance were included; peripheral edema and hemodilution were common (93).

In patients who had taken either rosiglitazone ($n = 96$) or pioglitazone ($n = 107$) for at least 2 months, adverse effects included peripheral edema (33% and 21% respectively), and 7% and 4% respectively had treatment withdrawn (94). The edema was not related to dose. Pulmonary edema occurred in two patients taking pioglitazone and three taking rosiglitazone.

In another study the combination of a thiazolidinedione with insulin increased the prevalence of edema and the dose of thiazolidinedione was important (95). Of 319 patients taking insulin, 13% developed edema when taking rosiglitazone 4 mg/day compared with 16% taking 8 mg/day and 4.7% taking placebo (96).

In 556 patients taking insulin, edema developed in 18% of those who took pioglitazone 30 mg/day, 13% of those who took 15 mg/day, and 7.0% of those who took placebo (97). The authors undertook a retrospective review of 79 subjects taking thiazolidinediones and insulin; 20 had developed edema. The mean dose of pioglitazone was 24 mg/day and rosiglitazone 6 mg/day. The mean time to edema was 135 days. They reported a 77% resolution rate with various interventions. Whether thiazolidinediones need to be withdrawn in patients with edema has been discussed in several papers.

- A 58-year-old man with type 2 diabetes and angina, weight 106 kg, taking metformin and insulin took rosiglitazone 2 mg bd, increased to 4 mg bd 4 months later (98). Hb_{A1c} improved from 9.6% to 8% after a further 2 months, although his weight had increased to 113 kg and he had developed ankle edema. Therapy was continued and furosemide 20 mg/day was added. After a further 2 months the edema had increased, his weight was 115 kg, and Hb_{A1c} had improved to 7.5%. The furosemide was increased to 20 mg bd. Two months later his weight had increased further to 117 kg and he was short of breath on exertion. Metformin was withdrawn, furosemide was increased to 80 mg bd, and irbesartan 75 mg bd was added. However, his symptoms worsened. Two weeks later the rosiglitazone was stopped and his symptoms gradually improved.
- A 73-year-old man with angina and hypertension had an Hb_{A1c} concentration of 16% while taking insulin (97). He weighed 114 kg. Since he was unable to take a sulfonylurea or metformin, he was given rosiglitazone 2 mg bd with an increased dose of insulin. Two months later his Hb_{A1c} had improved to 11%, his weight had risen to 120 kg, and there was a trace of edema. After 7 months he developed paroxysmal dyspnea and bilateral edema. The rosiglitazone was withdrawn and the dose of furosemide was increased. His symptoms improved within 3 months.

There have been other reports of resolution of edema while continuing therapy with thiazolidinediones (75).

- A 54-year-old obese woman with type 2 diabetes had rosiglitazone 4 mg bd added to insulin and metformin. Five months later she reported shortness of breath on exertion, paroxysmal nocturnal dyspnea, and peripheral edema. One month later a chest X-ray confirmed bilateral pulmonary edema. The dose of rosiglitazone was reduced to 4 mg/day and furosemide 20 mg/day was added. Her symptoms improved.
- Ten months after adding rosiglitazone 4 mg bd to insulin and metformin a 68-year-old woman developed

shortness of breath on exertion and edema. The rosiglitazone was continued in the same dosage, and her symptoms resolved.

- An 80-year-old man taking insulin developed edema 10 months after starting to take rosiglitazone. The rosiglitazone was withdrawn and pioglitazone 30 mg/day started instead. The edema initially improved but then worsened. Furosemide was given and the pioglitazone withdrawn.

These reports suggest that edema can improve with continued therapy of thiazolidinediones, but in some patients reducing or withdrawing therapy is necessary for resolution of symptoms. The time of onset of symptoms suggests that in some patients the edema can occur as part of the natural disease process and that the thiazolidinedione can exacerbate symptoms and impairs the response to diuretic therapy.

Fluid retention with thiazolidinediones may be dose-dependent and a class effect (99). There is little or no evidence to suggest a direct negative effect on cardiac performance. Because the symptoms may be due to increased permeability of the microcirculation, they may respond more quickly to drug withdrawal than to diuretic therapy.

In a retrospective cohort study of interventions for chronic heart failure before and after the use of rosiglitazone in 139 patients aged 66–75 years (mainly men), 20 had received treatment for heart failure before therapy with rosiglitazone and 50 needed it within 6 months of starting therapy (100).

The pre-treatment plasma concentration of natriuretic peptide type B may be a good marker for pioglitazone-induced congestive heart failure but this needs confirmation (99).

Hematologic

In 303 patients who took placebo or rosiglitazone for 8 weeks after a run-in period, rosiglitazone 4 mg bd had the same effect as 6 mg bd, but hemoglobin and hematocrit were lower with 6 mg bd (101). In another study troglitazone produced small reductions in hemoglobin, hematocrit, and erythrocyte counts and increases in lactate dehydrogenase and blood urea nitrogen (102).

Liver

The thiazolidinediones are hepatotoxic (103).

Pioglitazone

Hepatocellular damage has occasionally been attributed to pioglitazone.

- A 67-year-old man took pioglitazone 30 mg/day after having taken glibenclamide 2.5 mg/day for 10 years and voglibose 0.6 mg/day for 5 years (104). His liver function was normal before and during 6 months of pioglitazone therapy, but at 7 months he had abnormal liver function tests (total bilirubin 10 µmol/l, aspartate transaminase 1.95 µkat/l, alanine transaminase 5.65 µkat/l, alkaline phosphatase 17 µkat/l, gamma-glutamyl transferase 8 µkat/l). He was asymptomatic, with negative viral serology and normal liver ultrasonography. After withdrawal of pioglitazone his liver function normalized within a month.

- A 49-year-old man developed scleral icterus with raised bilirubin and transaminases after using pioglitazone 15-30 mg for 6 months and 45 mg for 1 week (105). No other cause for hepatitis was found. After withdrawal his liver function improved substantially within 14 days.

- A 49-year-old woman developed jaundice after taking pioglitazone 30 mg/day for 6 weeks, and after 3 weeks the alanine transaminase was 131 U/l and aspartate transaminase 79 U/l (106). Tests for viral hepatitis were negative. A liver biopsy showed marked portal edema, patchy chronic inflammation, a cellular infiltrate, and marked bile duct proliferation. There was no fibrosis. The laboratory results worsened after pioglitazone was withdrawn, and 1 month after withdrawal the bilirubin reached a peak of 585 µmol/l. Over the next 8 weeks the symptoms and laboratory tests improved, and after 6 months her condition was the same as when she had started to take pioglitazone.

- A 42-year-old man took pioglitazone 30 mg/day for 6 weeks and developed abnormal liver function tests, which returned to normal 1 month after withdrawal (107).

- A 63-year-old man was given pioglitazone instead of gliclazide and within 3 months developed jaundice and malaise (108). Liver function was deranged, with aspartate transaminase activity of 1984 IU/l, alanine transaminase 455 IU/l, alkaline phosphatase 1053 IU/l, and bilirubin 522 µmol/l. He died 9 days later. Histology showed parenchymal damage with steatohepatitis, including Mallory bodies superimposed on a severely fibrotic liver.

The authors of the second report speculated that this patient had pioglitazone-induced acute liver damage superimposed on chronic liver disease related to diabetes.

Rosiglitazone

The frequency of liver damage with rosiglitazone is much lower than with troglitazone and the reported cases seem to have been less serious. No deaths have been reported.

- A 61-year-old man developed hepatotoxicity 8 days after starting to take rosiglitazone 4 mg/day, and it was withdrawn (109). The alanine transaminase was 28 µkat/l, aspartate transaminase 23 µkat/l, alkaline phosphatase 8.7 µkat/l, total bilirubin 14 µmol/l, and direct bilirubin 13 µmol/l. All the tests were normal 5 months later. He had taken troglitazone for 1 week 8 months before this incident but had stopped because of nausea and an upset stomach.

- A 69-year-old man taking rosiglitazone 4 mg/day and metformin 500 mg/day developed hepatic failure within a week and both drugs were withdrawn (110). His alanine transaminase was 32 µkat/l, aspartate transaminase 47 µkat/l, total bilirubin 65 µmol/l, and direct bilirubin 41 µmol/l. He became comatose and the aspartate

transaminase rose to 185 µkat/l. The enzyme activities were normal 7 weeks after withdrawal.

- A 58-year-old woman started to feel ill 2 weeks after starting to take rosiglitazone 4 mg/day (111). One week later her peak aspartate transaminase was 5.2 µkat/l, alanine transaminase 4.2 µkat/l, and bilirubin 41 µmol/l. Four weeks later all the values had returned to normal.

- In a 47-year-old woman, who took rosiglitazone 4 mg/day for a short, unspecified time, the alkaline phosphatase increased (11 µkat/l) and returned to normal 2 weeks after withdrawal (112).

- An obese 37-year-old man with type 2 diabetes, who used rosiglitazone for 15 months, at first 4 mg/day then 8 mg/day for 6 months, developed granulomatous hepatitis (113). His liver enzymes were normal at 6 and 8 months. After 14 months he developed fatigue, abdominal discomfort, and weight loss and 3 weeks later chills, nausea, vomiting, and diarrhea. No hepatic viruses were found. A liver biopsy showed a periportal mixed cellular infiltrate and granulomas within the portal triad and the parenchyma. There was no evidence of sarcoidosis. After withdrawal of rosiglitazone he improved and the liver enzymes became normal within 2 months.

- A 49-year-old man with pre-existing hepatic pathology took rosiglitazone 4 mg/day for 2 months and 8 mg/day for 5 months (114). He developed a "bull" face and then edema of the eyelids and neck. He had anorexia and nausea. His serum sodium was 110 mmol/l, potassium 3.3 mmol/l, chloride 81 mmol/l, cholesterol 21 mmol/l, triglycerides 33 mmol/l, and his liver enzymes were raised. Rosiglitazone was withdrawn and he was given saline and potassium, acarbose for his diabetes, spironolactone 200 mg/day for edema, and atorvastatin 10 mg/day for hyperlipidemia. He improved over 3 weeks.

- Rosiglitazone 8 mg/day increased liver enzymes (115) in a very obese 41-year-old woman (body mass index 36), who had intractable diarrhea on metformin. She already had increased liver enzymes (alanine transaminase 60 IU/l, γ-glutamyl transpeptidase 299 IU/l, alkaline phosphatase 189 IU/l), supposedly related to hepatic steatosis. Eight weeks later she had severe malaise and the alanine transaminase was 12 times higher, γ-glutamyl transpeptidase three times higher, and alkaline phosphatase twofold higher. After withdrawal of rosiglitazone, the liver enzymes reached pretreatment concentrations in 30 days.

- A 52-year-old man with a history of heavy alcohol use took rosiglitazone for at least 30 days before developing jaundice (116). Liver histology showed cholestatic hepatitis with enlarged xanthomatous Kupffer cells and no evidence of cirrhosis.

In a review it has been suggested that hepatotoxicity with pioglitazone and rosiglitazone may not be causal but due to confounding medical factors (117). For example, hepatotoxicity has been attributed to rosiglitazone, secondary to cardiac failure (118).

- An 84-year-old man took rosiglitazone 4 mg/day for 11 months in combination with metformin 1 g bd and gliclazide 160 mg bd. He developed abnormal liver function tests, with alanine transaminase activity of 4336IU/l, which later increased to 7776 IU/l, alkaline phosphatase activity of 358 IU/l, and a normal bilirubin. Serum lactate was high at 8.59 mmol/l. Rosiglitazone was withdrawn and his diabetes was treated with insulin. His liver function normalized within 4 weeks, but he died after developing a chest infection.

The authors speculated about the role of rosiglitazone, suggesting that it may have precipitated congestive cardiac failure, which then led to ischemic hepatitis. A direct hepatotoxic effect was thought to be unlikely.

Liver function was monitored in patients aged 30–80 years with type 2 diabetes taking rosiglitazone (119). When a patient had transaminase or alkaline phosphatase activities higher than 2.5 times the upper limit of the reference range, they were not included in the studies. In 5006 patients taking rosiglitazone as monotherapy or combined therapy there were no hepatotoxic effects. At entry to the studies, 5.6% of the patients had values between 1.0 and 2.5 times the upper limit. Of the placebo-treated patients, 39% had a fall to normal values and 39% had an increase, but not over three times the upper limit. In 66% of the patients treated with a hypoglycemic drug the values fell (often with a fall in HbA$_{1c}$); in 13% they increased to below three times the upper limit and in 2.0% to over three times (four patients).

The incidence of drug-induced liver injury with rosiglitazone has been calculated at 0.02% for alanine transaminase activity 10 times the upper end of the reference range and 0.001% for jaundice (120). The above case report is unusual because, although liver damage is rare, hepatic necrosis occurs more commonly than cholestatic hepatitis.

Fertility

In a study of women with polycystic ovary syndrome, 23 of 25 women with oligomenorrhea, four of five with secondary amenorrhea, and two of three with polymenorrhea achieved regular menstrual cycles after taking rosiglitazone 4 mg/day for 24 weeks. It may be worth informing women that their fertility may increase (121).

Troglitazone

Troglitazone causes liver damage more often than the other members of the family. Hepatotoxicity delayed and finally prevented the registration of troglitazone in Europe. In the US, a patient with diabetes who used troglitazone in a study, developed hepatic failure necessitating liver transplantation and died. Troglitazone was withdrawn from a major National Institutes of Health evaluation of various regimens for preventing type 2 diabetes. In Japan the government recommended in December 1997 that liver function tests should be assessed every month in patients taking troglitazone. In 1998 there were 21 fatal cases of liver failure and three liver transplantations in patients taking troglitazone (122). Monitoring of liver function was intensified and in 1998 troglitazone was withdrawn for monotherapy. In 1999 the FDA received 61 reports of fatal hepatic toxicity and seven cases requiring liver

transplantation (123) and in spring 2000 troglitazone was withdrawn in America and in Japan.

- A 58-year-old man developed severe hepatitis after taking troglitazone 400 mg/day and glibenclamide 5 mg/day (124). Glibenclamide was stopped after 6 weeks as his HbA$_{1c}$ was 7.0%. About 2 weeks later he developed malaise and 1 week later jaundice. His bilirubin and transaminases were greatly raised and there was ascites. He had taken about 34 g of troglitazone. Drug-induced lymphocyte stimulation test was strongly positive for troglitazone and not for other drugs. Troglitazone was withdrawn and 3 days later the plasma concentration was below the limit of detection. Notwithstanding intensive therapy he died after 5 weeks. At autopsy, the liver showed yellow atrophy and massive hepatocellular coagulation necrosis with moderate neutrophil, monocyte, and eosinophil infiltration.

The positive lymphocyte stimulation test, the eosinophils, and the low blood concentrations 3 days after withdrawal suggest that hypersensitivity to troglitazone was the underlying cause. The authors reported that another patient with hepatitis after troglitazone had had a subacute course after withdrawal of the drug.

Late hepatic damage has also been reported.

- A 62-year-old woman with normal liver function tests took troglitazone 400 mg/day in combination with gliclazide 80 mg/day and pravastatin (125). After 9 months her transaminases were slightly above normal, but the HbA$_{1c}$ was 7.0% and treatment was continued. Her liver enzymes were measured monthly and after 19 months rose abruptly. Troglitazone was withdrawn immediately and she received insulin. Her liver enzymes improved rapidly. A biopsy showed hepatic necrosis round the central vein and a mild inflammatory infiltrate and fibrosis in the portal area compatible with protracted acute hepatitis. A lymphocyte stimulation test and a skin test were negative for troglitazone.
- A 76-year-old man took troglitazone 400 mg in addition to glimepiride 4 mg/day, metformin 1 g/day, aspirin, and pravastatin (126). After 18 months his liver function deteriorated and improved after withdrawal of troglitazone.

There are no differences in outcome between these two patterns of hepatotoxicity, "rapid risers," in whom liver failure takes only a few days to develop, and "slower risers." The estimated death rate is one in 100 000, but the estimate of the FDA advisory committee was one in 15 154 at 8 months of treatment. It is unclear whether hepatotoxicity is a class effect of thiazolidinediones or whether the lipophilic alpha-tocopherol moiety of troglitazone is responsible for this effect. The basic quinone structure of alpha-tocopherol is common to other drugs that can form hepatotoxic free radicals by CYP2E1-mediated oxidation.

The relation of liver disease to oral hypoglycemic drugs has been investigated in 44 406 patients, of whom 605 had liver disease (127). When 185 patients with mild and transient disorders, 249 with a predisposing condition, and 113 with another cause were excluded, 57 cases with possibly drug-induced liver changes were left. Of these, 11 could be attributed to other drugs and eight were attributed to fatty liver disease caused by diabetes. In 51 patients, oral drugs were continued without worsening of the liver enzymes. In two cases (a 58-year-old woman, whose liver function improved after discontinuing metformin, and an 86-year-old woman, who developed jaundice and died shortly after metformin and glibenclamide were prescribed) a causal relation could not be excluded.

There has been a report of hepatic injury with troglitazone but not with rosiglitazone (128).

- A 38-year-old woman was given insulin when glibenclamide and acarbose failed. Troglitazone 400 mg/day was added and increased to 800 mg/day 1 month later. After 2 months her liver function tests were normal, but she developed jaundice after 4 months. Total and direct bilirubin were 127 and 101 μmol/l and alanine transaminase was 34 μkat/l. After withdrawal of troglitazone her symptoms disappeared and her liver function tests normalized within several months. Metformin 1000 mg bd reduced her insulin requirement. Rosiglitazone 4 mg bd was added and her liver function tests remained normal for 10 months.

Musculoskeletal

Rhabdomyolysis has been attributed to troglitazone in combination with alcohol (129).

- A 59-year-old man took troglitazone 400 mg/day for 6 months and alcohol about 40 g/day. He developed weakness and muscle pain. He had mild liver damage. His HbA_{1c} concentration was 9.0%. All his muscles were tender, his creatine kinase activity was 10 570 IU/ml, and his myoglobin, aldolase, and aspartate transaminase were raised. Troglitazone was withdrawn. He improved biochemically and clinically.

There was an increase in creatine phosphokinase activity to over 10 times the upper limit of the reference range in seven of 1510 patients taking pioglitazone in the USA; four normalized during treatment, two normalized after withdrawal, and one had fallen but not normalized at follow-up (21).

Immunologic

- Angioedema has been reported in an obese woman after she had taken pioglitazone 30 mg/day for 7 days (130). She developed a sore throat followed by dyspnea and swelling of the lips and tongue. There was no rash. After intravenous glucocorticoids her symptoms rapidly abated.

Susceptibility Factors

Age

Pioglitazone was as effective in those aged over 65 years as in those under 65 years. Adverse events were also similar, with similar numbers of cardiovascular and hypoglycemic events in the studies reviewed (131).

Renal disease

A single dose of rosiglitazone or a single or repeated doses of pioglitazone reduced the glucose AUC in patients with moderate or severe renal impairment (132,133). Both drugs are primarily metabolized in the liver and their tolerability and adverse effects were the same in patients with normal renal function or with renal impairment. In a post-hoc analysis of three studies in which rosiglitazone or placebo was added for 6 months to a sulfonylurea regimen in 824 patients, 301 of whom had mild to moderate renal impairment (creatinine clearance 30–80 ml/minute) HbA_{1c} and fasting glucose improved to the same extent in those with renal impairment as in those without (134). Weight increase, edema (not serious), and mild hypoglycemia did not differ between the groups.

Dosage adjustment of rosiglitazone is not necessary when renal function is reduced (135).

Drug–Drug Interactions

Pioglitazone is metabolized in vitro by several cytochrome P450 isozymes, CYP2C8, CYP2C9, and CYP3A4 (136). The metabolites have about 40–60% of the hypoglycemic activity of pioglitazone and longer half-lives.

Fibrates

In 10 healthy volunteers gemfibrozil increased the plasma concentrations of rosiglitazone, (137). Gemfibrozil inhibits CYP2C8 and CYP2C9 in vitro, but in vivo it inhibits CYP2C8 but not CYP2C9. Itraconazole inhibits CYP3A4. In 12 volunteers aged 20–27 years weight 55–85 kg, who took gemfibrozil 600 mg, itraconazole 100 mg, both, or placebo at 0800 h and 2000 h for 4 days and a single dose of 15 mg of pioglitazone on day 3, gemfibrozil increased the mean AUC of unchanged pioglitazone about three-fold and the half-life from 8 to 23 hours (138). There was no change in those taking itraconazole. In those taking the combination the mean AUC of pioglitazone increased four-fold and the half-life from 8 to 40 hours. Gemfibrozil inhibited the oxidative metabolism of pioglitazone, whereas itraconazole appeared to have no effect. This suggests that in vivo CYP2C8 may be more important than CYP3A4 in the metabolism of pioglitazone. Gemfibrozil should be used cautiously when it is combined with pioglitazone.

Immunosuppressants

Rosiglitazone is not metabolized by CYP3A4 and interactions with drugs such as ciclosporin and tacrolimus are therefore not expected. Several studies have confirmed this.

Rosiglitazone 4 mg/day, increased to 8 mg/day after 1 week, was given to 10 patients with glucose intolerance who had received a renal transplant; ciclosporin and tacrolimus whole blood concentrations were unchanged (139).

In 40 patients with post-transplant diabetes using rosiglitazone 4 mg/day, with increased doses as necessary, there were no significant interactions with tacrolimus or ciclosporin; the patients were followed for 3–12 months (mean 26 weeks) (140).

In 22 patients with recent renal transplants using rosiglitzone 4 and 8 mg/day there were no significant changes in blood ciclosporin and tacrolimus concentrations (141).

Metformin

In 16 healthy men taking metformin 500 mg bd and/or rosiglitazone 2 mg bd for 4 days there were no significant effects on the steady-state pharmacokinetics of either drug (142).

Rifampicin

Rosiglitazone is metabolized by CYP2C8 and to a lesser extent by CYP2C9. No unchanged drug is excreted in the urine. Rifampicin induces hepatic and intestinal CYP isozymes. When 10 healthy Korean men aged 22–26 years were given rifampicin 600 mg/day for 6 days and then rosiglitazone 8 mg on day 7 the plasma AUC was reduced to 65% and the half-life shortened from 3.9 to 1.5 hours compared with placebo (143).

Similar studies have shown increased plasma concentrations of rosiglitazone after the addition of ketoconazole (144) and trimethoprim (145).

Simvastatin

Troglitazone has been reported to reduce the effect of simvastatin, probably by induction of CYP3A4 (146).

Trimethoprim

Rosiglitazone is mainly metabolized by the CYP2C8, and CYP2C9 has a minor role. Trimethoprim is a competitive inhibitor of CYP2C8 and it increases rosiglitazone concentrations, with increased risks of peripheral edema and pulmonary edema. Genotype may influence the ability of trimethoprim to inhibit CYP2C8 (147).

References

1. Schwartz MW, Kahn SE. Insulin resistance and obesity. Nature 1999;402(6764):860–1.
2. Barroso I, Gurnell M, Crowley VE, Agostini M, Schwabe JW, Soos MA, Maslen GL, Williams TD, Lewis H, Schafer AJ, Chatterjee VK, O'Rahilly S. Dominant negative mutations in human PPARgamma associated with severe insulin resistance, diabetes mellitus and hypertension. Nature 1999;402(6764):880–3.
3. Auwerx J. PPARgamma, the ultimate thrifty gene. Diabetologia 1999;42(9):1033–49.
4. Furnsinn C, Waldhausl W. Thiazolidinediones: metabolic actions in vitro. Diabetologia 2002;45(9):1211–23.
5. Willi SM, Kennedy A, Brant BP, Wallace P, Rogers NL, Garvey WT. Effective use of thiazolidinediones for the treatment of glucocorticoid-induced diabetes. Diabetes Res Clin Pract 2002;58(2):87–96.
6. Imano E, Kanda T, Nakatani Y, Nishida T, Arai K, Motomura M, Kajimoto Y, Yamasaki Y, Hori M. Effect of troglitazone on microalbuminuria in patients with incipient diabetic nephropathy. Diabetes Care 1998;21(12):2135–9.
7. Camp HS, Li O, Wise SC, Hong YH, Frankowski CL, Shen X, Vanbogelen R, Leff T. Differential activation of peroxisome proliferator-activated receptor-gamma by troglitazone and rosiglitazone. Diabetes 2000;49(4):539–47.
8. Mori Y, Murakawa Y, Okada K, Horikoshi H, Yokoyama J, Tajima N, Ikeda Y. Effect of troglitazone on body fat distribution in type 2 diabetic patients. Diabetes Care 1999;22(6):908–12.
9. Frias JP, Yu JG, Kruszynska YT, Olefsky JM. Metabolic effects of troglitazone therapy in type 2 diabetic, obese, and lean normal subjects. Diabetes Care 2000;23(1):64–9.
10. Fujibayashi K, Nagasaka S, Itabashi N, Kawakami A, Nakamura T, Kusaka I, Ishikawa S, Saito T. Troglitazone efficacy in a subject with glucocorticoid-induced diabetes. Diabetes Care 1999;22(12):2088–9.
11. Yu JG, Kruszynska YT, Mulford MI, Olefsky JM. A comparison of troglitazone and metformin on insulin requirements in euglycemic intensively insulin-treated type 2 diabetic patients. Diabetes 1999;48(12):2414–21.
12. Day C. Thiazolidinediones: a new class of antidiabetic drugs. Diabet Med 1999;16(3):179–92.
13. Scheen AJ, Lefebvre PJ. Troglitazone: antihyperglycemic activity and potential role in the treatment of type 2 diabetes. Diabetes Care 1999;22(9):1568–77.
14. Saleh YM, Mudaliar SR, Henry RR. Metabolic and vascular effects of the thiazolidinedione troglitazone. Diabetes Rev 1999;7:55–76.
15. Plosker GL, Faulds D. Troglitazone: a review of its use in the management of type 2 diabetes mellitus. Drugs 1999;57(3):409–38.
16. Balfour JA, Plosker GL. Rosiglitazone. Drugs 1999;57(6):921–30.
17. Caspi A. The promise of a new generation: rosiglitazone for the treatment of type 2 diabetes. P&T 1999;24:313–22.
18. Ducobu J, Sternon J. Les glitazones (thiazolidinediones). [Glitazones (thiazolidinediones).] Rev Med Brux 2000;21(5):441–6.
19. Scheen AJ, Charbonnel B. Effets antidiabétiques des thiazolidinediones. Med Ther 2001;7:672–9.
20. Werner AL, Travaglini MT. A review of rosiglitazone in type 2 diabetes mellitus. Pharmacotherapy 2001;21(9):1082–99.
21. Chilcott J, Tappenden P, Jones ML, Wight JP. A systematic review of the clinical effectiveness of pioglitazone in the treatment of type 2 diabetes mellitus. Clin Ther 2001;23(11):1792–823.
22. Wagstaff AJ, Goa KL. Rosiglitazone: a review of its use in the management of type 2 diabetes mellitus. Drugs 2002;62(12):1805–37.
23. Parulkar AA, Fonseca VA. Recent advances in pharmacological treatment of type 2 diabetes mellitus. Compr Ther 1999;25(8–10):418–26.
24. Freed MI, Allen A, Jorkasky DK, DiCicco RA. Systemic exposure to rosiglitazone is unaltered by food. Eur J Clin Pharmacol 1999;55(1):53–6.
25. Gerber P, Lübben G, Heusler S, Dodo A. Effects of pioglitazone on metabolic control and blood pressure: a randomized study in patients with type 2 diabetes mellitus. Curr Med Res Opin 2003;6:532–9.
26. Schöfl C, Lübben G. Postmarketing surveillance study of the efficacy and tolerability of pioglitazone in insulin-resistant patents with type 2 diabetes mellitus in general practice. Clin Drug Invest 2003;23:725–34.
27. Hayashi Y, Miyachi N, Takeuchi T, Takeuchi Y, Kamiya F, Kato T, Imaeda K, Okayama N, Shimizu M, Itoh M. Clinical evaluation of pioglitazone in patients with type 2

diabetes using alpha-glucosidase inhibitor and examination of its efficacy profile. Diabetes Obesity Metab 2003;5:58–65.

28. Seino H, Yamaguchi H, Misaki A, Sakata Y, Kitagawa M, Yarnazaki T, Kikuchi H, Abe R. Clinical effect of combination therapy of pioglitazone and an alpha-glucosidase inhibitor. Curr Med Res Opin 2003;8:676–82.

29. King AB. A comparison in a clinical setting of the efficacy and side effects of three thiazolidinediones. Diabetes Care 2000;23(4):557.

30. St John Sutton M, Rendell M, Dandona P, Dole JF, Murphy K, Patwardhan R, Patel J, Freed M. A comparison of the effects of rosiglitazone and glyburide on cardiovascular function and glycemic control in patients with type 2 diabetes. Diabetes Care 2002;25(11):2058–64.

31. Lebovitz HE, Dole JF, Patwardhan R, Rappaport EB, Freed MIRosiglitazone Clinical Trials Study Group. Rosiglitazone monotherapy is effective in patients with type 2 diabetes. J Clin Endocrinol Metab 2001;86(1):280–8.

32. Nolan JJ, Jones NP, Patwardhan R, Deacon LF. Rosiglitazone taken once daily provides effective glycaemic control in patients with type 2 diabetes mellitus. Diabet Med 2000;17(4):287–94.

33. Wolffenbuttel BH, Gomis R, Squatrito S, Jones NP, Patwardhan RN. Addition of low-dose rosiglitazone to sulphonylurea therapy improves glycaemic control in Type 2 diabetic patients. Diabet Med 2000;17(1):40–7.

34. Phillips LS, Grunberger G, Miller E, Patwardhan R, Rappaport EB, Salzman ARosiglitazone Clinical Trials Study Group. Once- and twice-daily dosing with rosiglitazone improves glycemic control in patients with type 2 diabetes. Diabetes Care 2001;24(2):308–15.

35. Aronoff S, Rosenblatt S, Braithwaite S, Egan JW, Mathisen AL, Schneider RLThe Pioglitazone 001 Study Group. Pioglitazone hydrochloride monotherapy improves glycemic control in the treatment of patients with type 2 diabetes: a 6-month randomized placebo-controlled dose-response study. Diabetes Care 2000;23(11):1605–11.

36. Shimono D, Kuwamura N, Nakamura Y, Koshiyama H. Lack of effect of pioglitazone on postprandial triglyceride levels in type 2 diabetes. Diabetes Care 2001;24(5):971.

37. Kipnes MS, Krosnick A, Rendell MS, Egan JW, Mathisen AL, Schneider RL. Pioglitazone hydrochloride in combination with sulfonylurea therapy improves glycemic control in patients with type 2 diabetes mellitus: a randomized, placebo-controlled study. Am J Med 2001;111(1):10–7.

38. Zhu X-X, Pan C-Y, Li G-W, Shi H-L, Tian H, Yang W-Y, Jiang J, Sun X-C, Davies C, Chow W-H. Addition of rosiglitazone to existing sulfonylurea treatment in Chinese patients with type 2 diabetes and exposure to hepatitis B or C. Diabetes Technol Ther 2003;5:33–42.

39. Inzucchi SE. Oral antihyperglycemic therapy for type 2 diabetes: scientific review. JAMA 2002;287(3):360–72.

40. Holmboe ES. Oral antihyperglycemic therapy for type 2 diabetes: clinical applications. JAMA 2002;287(3):373–6.

41. Van Gaal LF, De Leeuw IH. Rationale and options for combination therapy in the treatment of type 2 diabetes. Diabetologia 2003;46(Suppl 1):M44–50.

42. Fonseca V, Rosenstock J, Patwardhan R, Salzman A. Effect of metformin and rosiglitazone combination therapy in patients with type 2 diabetes mellitus: a randomized controlled trial. JAMA 2000;283(13):1695–702.

43. Gomez-Perez FJ, Fanghanel-Salmon G, Antonio Barbosa J, Montes-Villarreal J, Berry RA, Warsi G, Gould EM. Efficacy and safety of rosiglitazone plus metformin in Mexicans with type 2 diabetes. Diabetes Metab Res Rev 2002;18(2):127–34.

44. Masoudi FA, Wang Y, Inzucchi SE, SetaroJF, Havranek EP, Foody JM, Krumholz HM. Metformin and thiazolidinedione use in Medicare patients with heart failure. J Am Med Assoc 2003;290:81–5.

45. Dailey GE III, Noor MA, Park J-S, Bruce S, Fiedorek FT. Glycemic control with glyburide/metformin tablets in combination with rosiglitazone in patients with type 2 diabetes: a randomised double-blind trial. Am J Med 2004;116:223–9.

46. Rosenstock J, Shen SG, Gatlin MR, Foley JE. Combination therapy with nateglinide and a thiazolidinedione improves glycemic control in type 2 diabetes. Diabetes Care 2002;25(9):1529–33.

47. Raskin P, Jovanovic L, Berger S, Schwartz S, Woo V, Ratner R. Repaglinide/troglitazone combination therapy: improved glycemic control in type 2 diabetes. Diabetes Care 2000;23(7):979–83.

48. Javanovic L, Hassman DR, Gooch B, Jain R, Greco S, Khutoryansky N, Hale PM. Treatment of type 2 diabetes with a combination regimen of repaglinide plus pioglitazone. Diabetes Res Clin Pract 2004;63:127–34.

49. Raskin P, McGill J, Saad MF, Cappleman JM, Kaye W, Khutoryansky N, Hale PM. Combination therapy for type 2 diabetes: repaglinide plus rosiglitazone. Diabetic Med 2004;21:329–35.

50. Buysschaert M, Bobbioni E, Starkie M, Frith LTroglitazone Study Group. Troglitazone in combination with sulphonylurea improves glycaemic control in Type 2 diabetic patients inadequately controlled by sulphonylurea therapy alone. Diabet Med 1999;16(2):147–53.

51. Kerenyi Z, Samer H, James R, Yan Y Stewart M. Combination therapy with rosiglitazone and glibenclamide compared with upward titration of glibenclamide alone in patients with type 2 diabetes mellitus. Diabetes Res Clin Pract 2004;63:213–23.

52. Strowig SM, Aviles-Santa ML, Raskin P. Comparison of insulin monotherapy and combination therapy with insulin and metformin or insulin and troglitazone in type 2 diabetes. Diabetes Care 2002;25(10):1691–8.

53. Raskin P, Rendell M, Riddle MC, Dole JF, Freed MI, Rosenstock JRosiglitazone Clinical Trials Study Group. A randomized trial of rosiglitazone therapy in patients with inadequately controlled insulin-treated type 2 diabetes. Diabetes Care 2001;24(7):1226–32.

54. Huang A, Raskin P. Thiazolidinediones and insulin. Treat Endocrinol 2005;4:205–20.

55. Ng RSH, Darko DA, Hillson RM. Street drug use among young patients with type 1 diabetes in the UK. Diabetic Med 2004;21:295–6.

56. Page II RL, Gozansky WS, Ruscin JM. Possible heart failure exacerbation associated with rosiglitazone: case report and literature review. Pharmacotherapy 2003;23:945–54.

57. Walker AB, Naderali EK, Chattington PD, Buckingham RE, Williams G. Differential vasoactive effects of the insulin sensitizers rosiglitazone (BRL 49653) and troglitazone on human small arteries in vitro. Diabetes 1998;47:810–4.

58. Delea TE, Edelsberg JS, Hagiwara MH, Oster G, Phillips LS. Use of thiazolidinediones and risk of heart failure in people with type 2 diabetes: a retrospective cohort study. Diabetes Care 2003;26:2983–9.

59. Karter AJ, Ahmed AT, Liu J, Moffet HH, Parker MM, Ferrara A, Selby JV. Use of thiazolidinediones and risk of heart failure in people with type 2 diabetes: a retrospective cohort study. Diabetes Care 2004;27:850–1.

60. Delea TE, Edelsberg JS, Hagiwara MH, Oster G, Phillips LS. Use of thiazolidinediones and risk of heart failure in people with type 2 diabetes: a retrospective cohort study. Diabetes Care 2004;27:852.

61. Manley HJ, Allcock NM Thiazolidinedione safety and efficacy in ambulatory patients receiving hemodialysis. Pharmacotherapy 2003;23:861–5.

62. Jun JK, Gong WC, Mathur R. Effects of pioglitazone on diabetes related outcomes in Hispanic patients. Am J Health-Syst Pharm 2003;60:469–73.

63. Igarashi M, Jimbu, Y, Hirato A, Yamaguchi H, Kato T, Tominaga M. Effect of pioglitazone on the plasma concentration of brain natriuretic peptide in patients with type 2 diabetes. Ther Res 2003;24:1873–81.

64. Koshida H, Shibata K, Kametani T. Pleuropulmonary disease in a man with diabetes who was treated with troglitazone. N Engl J Med 1998;339(19):1400–1.

65. Maher TD, Mirza SA. Ataxia and reversible dementia-like syndrome associated with troglitazone. Diabetes 1999;48(Suppl 1):A85.

66. Ledl M, Hohenecker J, Francesconi C, Roots I, Bauer MF, Roden M. Acute myopathy in a type 2 diabetic patient on combination therapy with metformin, fenofibrate and rosiglitazone. Diabetologia 2005;48:1996–8.

67. Colucciello M. Vision loss due to macular edema induced by rosiglitazone treatment of diabetes mellitus. Arch Ophthalmol 2005;123:1273–5.

68. Levin F, Kazim M, Smith TJ, Marcovici E. Rosiglitazone-induced proptosis. Arch Ophthalmol 2005;123:119–21.

69. Valyasevi RW, Harteneck DA, Dutton CM, Bahn RS. Stimulation of adipogenesis, peroxisome proliferator-activated receptor-gamma (PPARγ) and thyrotropin receptor by PPARγ agonists in human orbital preadipocyte fibroblasts. J Clin Endocrinol Metab 2002;87:2352–2358.

70. Starkey K, Heufelder A, Baker G, Joba W, Evans M, Davies S, Ludgate M. Peroxisome proliferator activated receptor-gamma in thyroid eye disease: contraindication for thiazolidinedione use? J Clin Endocrinol Metab 2003;88:55–9.

71. Philips J-C, Petite C, Willi J-P, Buchegger F, Meier CA. Effect of peroxisome proliferator-activated receptor δ agonist rosiglitazone on dedifferentiated thyroid cancers. Nucl Med Comm 2004;25:1183–6.

72. Akazawa S, Sun F, Ito M, Kawasaki E, Eguchi K. Efficacy of troglitazone on body fat distribution in type 2 diabetes. Diabetes Care 2000;23(8):1067–71.

73. Ciaraldi TP, Kong AP, Chu NV, Kim DD, Baxi S, Loviscach M, Plodkowski R, Reitz R, Caulfield M, Mudaliar S, Henry RR. Regulation of glucose transport and insulin signaling by troglitazone or metformin in adipose tissue of type 2 diabetic subjects. Diabetes 2002;51(1):30–6.

74. Katoh S, Hata S, Matsushima M, Ikemoto S, Inoue Y, Yokoyama J, Tajima N. Troglitazone prevents the rise in visceral adiposity and improves fatty liver associated with sulfonylurea therapy—a randomized controlled trial. Metabolism 2001;50(4):414–7.

75. Scheen AJ. Combined thiazolidinedione-insulin therapy should we be concerned about safety? Drug Saf 2004;27:841–56.

76. Promrat K, Lutchman G, Uwaifo GI, Freedman RJ, Soza A, Heller T, Doo E, Ghany M, Premkumar A, Park Y, Liang J, Yanovski JA, Kleiner DE, Hoofnagle JH. A pilot study of pioglitazone treatment for non-alcoholic steatohepatitis. Hepatology 2004;39:188–96.

77. Tan MH, Johns D, Strand J, Hlse J, Madsbad S, Eriksson JW, Clausen J, Konkoy CS, Herz M, for the GLAC Study Group. Sustained effects of pioglitazone vs. glibenclamide on insulin sensitivity, glycaemic control and lipid profiles in patients with type 2 diabetes. Diabetic Med 2004;21:859–66.

78. Smith SR, de Jonge L, Volaufova J, Li Y, Xie H, Bray GA. Effect of pioglitazone on body composition and energy expenditure: a randomized controlled trial. Metab Clin Exp 2005;54:24–32.

79. Iwamoto Y, Kosaka K, Kuzuya T, Akanuma Y, Shigeta Y, Kaneko T. Effects of troglitazone: a new hypoglycemic agent in patients with NIDDM poorly controlled by diet therapy. Diabetes Care 1996;19(2):151–6.

80. Khan MA, St Peter JV, Xue JL. A prospective, randomized comparison of the metabolic effects of pioglitazone or rosiglitazone in patients with type 2 diabetes who were previously treated with troglitazone. Diabetes Care 2002;25(4):708–11.

81. Miyazaki Y, Mahankali A, Matsuda M, Glass L, Mahankali S, Ferrannini E, Cusi K, Mandarino LJ, DeFronzo RA. Improved glycemic control and enhanced insulin sensitivity in type 2 diabetic subjects treated with pioglitazone. Diabetes Care 2001;24(4):710–9.

82. Kiayias JA, Vlachou ED, Theodosopoulou E, Lakka-Papadodima E. Rosiglitazone in combination with glimepiride plus metformin in type 2 diabetic patients. Diabetes Care 2002;25(7):1251–2.

83. Pavo I, Jermendi G, Varkonyi TT, Kerenyi Z, Gymesi A, Shoustov S, Shestakova M, Herz M, Johns D, Schluchter BJ, Festa A, Tan MH. Effect of pioglitazone compared with metformin on glycemic control and indicators of insulin sensitivity in recently diagnosed patients with type 2 diabetes. J Clin Endocrinol Metab 2003;88:1637–45.

84. Calmy A, Hirschel B, Hans D, Karsegard VL, Meier CA. Glitazones in lipodystrophy syndrome induced by highly active antiretroviral therapy. AIDS 2003;17:770–2.

85. Sutinen J, Häkkinen A-M, Westerbacka J, Seppälä-Lindroos A, Vehkavaara S, Halavaara J, Järvinen A, Ristola M, Yki-Järvinen H. Rosiglitazone in the treatment of HAART-associated lipodystrophy—a randomized double-blind placebo-controlled study. Antiviral Ther 2003;8:199–207.

86. Nagai Y, Abe T, Nomura G. Does pioglitazone, like troglitazone, increase serum levels of lipoprotein(a) in diabetic patients? Diabetes Care 2001;24(2):408–9.

87. Sarafidis PA, Lasaridis AN, Nilsson PM, Hitoglou-Makedou AD, Pagkalos EM, Yovos JG, Pliakos CI, Tourkantonis AA. The effect of rosiglitazone on urine albumin excretion in patients with type 2 diabetes mellitus and hypertension. Am J Hypertens 2005;18:227–34.

88. Sarker A, Semple RK, Dinneen SF, O'Rahilly S, Martin SC. Sever hypo-α-lipoproteinemia during treatment with rosiglitazone. Diabetes Care 2004;27:2577–80.

89. Mafong DD, Lee GA, Yu S, Tien P, Mauro T, Grunfeld C. Development of multiple lipomas during treatment with rosiglitazone in a patient with HIV-associated lipoatrophy. AIDS 2004;18:1742–4.

90. Sarafidis PA, Lasaridis AN, Nilsson PM, Hitoglou-Makedou AD, Pagkalos EM, Yovos JG, Pliakos CI, Tourkantonis AA. The effect of rosiglitazone on urine albumin excretion in patients with type 2 diabetes mellitus and hypertension. Am J Hypertens 2005;18:227–34.

91. Thomas ML, Lloyd SJ. Pulmonary edema associated with rosiglitazone and troglitazone. Ann Pharmacother 2001;35(1):123–4.

92. Baba T, Shimada K, Neugebauer S, Yamada D, Hashimoto S, Watanabe T. The oral insulin sensitizer, thiazolidinedione, increases plasma vascular endothelial growth factor in type 2 diabetic patients. Diabetes Care 2001;24(5):953–4.

93. Hanefeld M, Belcher G. Safety profile of pioglitazone. Int J Clin Pract Suppl 2001;(121):27–31.

94. Hussein Z, Wentworth JM, Nankervis AJ, Proietto J, Colman PG. Effectiveness and side effects of thiazolidinediones for type 2 diabetes: real-life experience from a tertiary hospital. Med J Aust 2004;181:536–9.

95. King KA, Levi VE. Prevalence of edema in patients receiving combination therapy with insulin and thiazolidinedione. Am J Health-Syst Pharm 2004;61:390–3.

96. Raskin P, Rendell M, Riddle MC, Dole JF, Freed MI, Rosenstock J; Rosiglitazone Clinical Trials Study Group. A randomised trial of rosiglitazone therapy in patients with inadequately controlled insulin-treated type 2 diabetes. Diabetes Care 2001;24:1226–32.

97. Rosenstock J, Einhorn D, Hershon K, Glazer NB, Yu S; Pioglitazone 014 Study Group. Efficacy and safety of pioglitazone in type 2 diabetes: a randomised placebo controlled study in patients receiving stable insulin therapy. Int J Clin Pract 2002;56:251–7.

98. Singh N. Rosiglitazone and heart failure: long term vigilance. J Cardiovasc Pharmacol Ther 2004;9:21–5.

99. Scheen AJ. Combined thiazolidinedione-insulin therapy should we be concerned about safety? Drug Saf 2004;27:841–56.

100. Marceille JR, Goins JA, Soni R, Biery JC, Lee TA. Chronic heart failure-related interventions after starting rosiglitazone in patients receiving insulin. Pharmacotherapy 2004;24:1317–22.

101. Raskin P, Rappaport EB, Cole ST, Yan Y, Patwardhan R, Freed MI. Rosiglitazone short-term monotherapy lowers fasting and post-prandial glucose in patients with type II diabetes. Diabetologia 2000;43(3):278–84.

102. Kuzuya T, Iwamoto Y, Kosaka K, Takebe K, Yamanouchi T, Kasuga M, Kajinuma H, Akanuma Y, Yoshida S, Shigeta Y, et al. A pilot clinical trial of a new oral hypoglycemic agent, CS-045, in patients with non-insulin dependent diabetes mellitus. Diabetes Res Clin Pract 1991;11(3):147–53.

103. Tolman KG. Thiazolidinedione hepatotoxicity: a class effect? Int J Clin Pract Suppl 2000;(113):29–34.

104. Maeda K. Hepatocellular injury in a patient receiving pioglitazone. Ann Intern Med 2001;135(4):306.

105. May LD, Lefkowitch JH, Kram MT, Rubin DE. Mixed hepatocellular–cholestatic liver injury after pioglitazone therapy. Ann Intern Med 2002;136(6):449–52.

106. Pinto AG, Cummings OW, Chalasani N. Severe but reversible cholestatic liver injury after pioglitazone therapy. Ann Intern Med 2002;137(10):857.

107. Arotcarena R, Bigue J-P, Etcharry F, Pariente A. Hepatite aiguë sévère à la pioglitazone Gastroenterol Clin Biol 2004;28:610–1.

108. Farley-Hills E, Sivasankar R, Martin M. Fatal liver failure associated with pioglitazone. BMJ 2004;329:429.

109. Al-Salman J, Arjomand H, Kemp DG, Mittal M. Hepatocellular injury in a patient receiving rosiglitazone. A case report. Ann Intern Med 2000;132(2):121–4.

110. Forman LM, Simmons DA, Diamond RH. Hepatic failure in a patient taking rosiglitazone. Ann Intern Med 2000;132(2):118–21.

111. Ravinuthala RS, Nori U. Rosiglitazone toxicity. Ann Intern Med 2000;133(8):658.

112. Hachey DM, O'Neil MP, Force RW. Isolated elevation of alkaline phosphatase level associated with rosiglitazone. Ann Intern Med 2000;133(9):752.

113. Dhawan M, Agrawal R, Ravi J, Gulati S, Silverman J, Nathan G, Raab S, Brodmerkel G Jr. Rosiglitazone-induced granulomatous hepatitis. J Clin Gastroenterol 2002;34(5):582–4.

114. Kuschel U, Hesselbarth N, Herrmann A, Hippius M, Hoffmann A. Schwere Elektrolytstorung und Ödeme unter Therapie mit Rosiglitazon. [Severe electrolyte imbalance and edema in therapy with rosiglitazone.] Med Klin (Munich) 2002;97(9):553–5.

115. Nag S, McCulloch A. Liver enzymes and rosiglitazone. Br J Diabetic Vasc Dis 2003;3:62–3.

116. Menees SB, Anderson MA, Chensue SW, Moseley RH. Hepatic injury in a patient taking rosiglitazone. J Clin Gastroenterol 2005;39:638–40.

117. Korytkowski MT. Sulfonylurea treatment of type 2 diabetes mellitus focus on glimepiride. Pharmacotherapy 2004;24:606–20.

118. Berry P. Severe congestive cardiac failure and ischaemic hepatitis associated with rosiglitazone. Pract Diabetes Int 2004;21:199–200.

119. Lebovitz HE, Kreider M, Freed MI. Evaluation of liver function in type 2 diabetic patients during clinical trials: evidence that rosiglitazone does not cause hepatic dysfunction. Diabetes Care 2002;25(5):815–21.

120. Slavin DE, Schlichting CL, Freston JW. Rating the severity of the medical consequences of drug-induced liver injury. Regulatory Toxicol Pharmacol 2005;43:134–40.

121. Yilmaz M, Karakoc A, Töruner FB, Cakir N, Tiras B, Ayvaz G, Arslan M. The effects of rosiglitazone and metformin on menstrual cyclicity and hirsutism in polycystic ovary syndrome. Gynecol Endocrinol 2005;21:154–60.

122. Misbin RI. Troglitazone-associated hepatic failure. Ann Intern Med 1999;130(4 Pt 1):330.

123. Bailey CJ. The rise and fall of troglitazone. Diabet Med 2000;17(6):414–5.

124. Shibuya A, Watanabe M, Fujita Y, Saigenji K, Kuwao S, Takahashi H, Takeuchi H. An autopsy case of troglitazone-induced fulminant hepatitis. Diabetes Care 1998;21(12):2140–3.

125. Iwase M, Yamaguchi M, Yoshinari M, Okamura C, Hirahashi T, Tsuji H, Fujishima M. A Japanese case of liver dysfunction after 19 months of troglitazone treatment. Diabetes Care 1999;22(8):1382–4.

126. Bell DS, Ovalle F. Late-onset troglitazone-induced hepatic dysfunction. Diabetes Care 2000;23(1):128–9.

127. Jick SS, Stender M, Myers MW. Frequency of liver disease in type 2 diabetic patients treated with oral antidiabetic agents. Diabetes Care 1999;22(12):2067–71.

128. Lenhard MJ, Funk WB. Failure to develop hepatic injury from rosiglitazone in a patient with a history of troglitazone-induced hepatitis. Diabetes Care 2001;24(1):168–9.

129. Yokoyama M, Izumiya Y, Yoshizawa M, Usuda R. Acute rhabdomyolysis associated with troglitazone. Diabetes Care 2000;23(3):421–2.

130. Shadid S, Jensen MD. Angioneurotic edema as a side effect of pioglitazone. Diabetes Care 2002;25(2):405.

131. Rajagopalan R, Rerez A, Khan M, Murray FT. Pioglitazone is effective therapy for elderly patients with type 2 diabetes mellitus. Drugs Aging 2004;21:259–71.

132. Budde K, Neumayer H-H, Fritsche L, Sulowicz W, Stompôr T, Eckland D. The pharmacokinetics of pioglitazone in patients with impaired renal function. Br J Clin Pharmacol 2003;55:368–74.

133. Chapelski MC, Thompson-Culkin K, Miller AK, Sack M, Blum R, Freed MI. Pharmacokinetics of rosiglitazone in patients with various degrees of renal insufficiency. J Clin Pharmacol 2003;43:252–9.

134. Agrawal A, Sautter MC, Jones NP. Effects of rosiglitazone maleate when added to a sulfonylurea regimen in patients with type 2 diabetes mellitus and mild to moderate renal impairment: a post hoc analysis. Clin Ther 2003;25:2754–64.

135. Thompson-Culkin K, Zussman B, Miller AK, Freed MI. Pharmacokinetics of rosiglitazone in patients with end-stage renal disease J Int Med Res 2002;30(4): 391–9.

136. Kirchheiner J, Roots I, Goldammer M, Rosenkranz B, Brockmöller J. Effect of genetic polymorphisms in cytochrome P450 (CYP) 2C9 and CYP2C8 on the pharmacokinetics of oral antidiabetic drugs: clinical relevance. Clin Pharmacokinet 2005;44(12):1209–25.

137. Niemi M. Backman JT, Granfors M, Laitila J, Neuvonen M, Neuvonen PJ. Gemfobrizil considerably increases the plasma concentrations of rosiglitazone. Diabetologia 2003;46:1319–23.

138. Jaakkola T, Backman JT, Neuvonen M, Neuvonen P. Effects of gemfibrozil, itraconazole and their combination on the pharmacokinetics of pioglitazone. Clin Pharmacol Ther 2005;77:404–14.

139. Viytovich MH, Simonsen C, Jenssen T, Hjelmesaeth J, Asberg A, Hartsmann A. Short-term treatment with rosiglitazone improves glucose tolerance, insulin sensitivity and endothelial function in renal transplant recipients. Nephrol Dial Transplant 2005;20:413–8.

140. Villanueva G, Baldwin D. Rosiglitazone therapy of post-transplant diabetes mellitus. Transplantation 2005;80:1402–5.

141. Pietruck F, Kribben A, Van TN, Patschan D, Herget-Rosenthal S, Janssen O, Mann K, Philipp T, Witzke O. Rosiglitazone is as safe and effective treatment option of new-onset diabetes mellitus after renal transplantation. Transplant Int 2005;18:483–6.

142. Di Cicco RA, Allen A, Carr A, Fowles S, Jorkasky DK, Freed MI. Rosiglitazone does not alter the pharmacokinetics of metformin. J Clin Pharmacol 2000;40(11):1280–5.

143. Park J-Y, Kim K-A, Kang M-H, Kim S-L, Shin J-G. Pharmacokinetics and drug disposition. Effect of rifampicin on the pharmacokinetics of rosiglitazone in healthy subjects. Clin Pharmacol Ther 2004;75:157–62.

144. Park J-Y, Kim K-A, Shin J-G, Lee KY. Effect of ketoconazole on the pharmacokinetics of rosiglitazone in healthy subjects. Br J Clin Pharmacol 2004;58:397–402.

145. Niemi M, Backman JT, Neuvonen PJ. Effects of trimethoprim and rifampicin on the pharmacokinetics of the cytochrome P450 2C8 substrate rosiglitazone. Clin Pharmacol Ther 2004;76:239–49.

146. Lin JC, Ito MK. A drug interaction between troglitazone and simvastatin. Diabetes Care 1999;22(12):2104–6.

147. Hruska MW, Amico JA, Langaee TY, Ferrell RE, Fitzgerald SM, Frye RF. The effect of trimethoprim on CYP2C8 mediated rosiglitazone metabolism in human liver microsomes and healthy subjects. Br J Clin Pharmacol 2005;59:70–9.

OTHER HORMONES AND RELATED DRUGS

Calcitonin

General Information

Calcitonin inhibits osteoclastic bone resorption, increases the urinary excretion of calcium and phosphate, and reduces serum calcium. It is established in the treatment of disorders of high bone turnover, including Paget's disease and postmenopausal osteoporosis, but is less effective than the bisphosphonates. Calcitonin is less effective than other therapeutic measures in the treatment of acute hypercalcemia. Long-term administration of calcitonin reduces morbidity in cases of osteogenesis imperfecta and algoneurodystrophy (SEDA-13, 1307) (1,2). The role of calcitonin in treating acute pain due to osteoporotic crush fractures has been reviewed, but the mechanism of its analgesic effect is not known (3).

When used continuously in high doses, the therapeutic effect of calcitonin is sustained for only a few months, probably because of down-regulation of osteoclast receptors. The duration of the response to calcitonin can be extended by periodically interrupting treatment. A number of regimens, ranging from cycles of a few days to several months, are effective both as prophylaxis in healthy postmenopausal women and in women with established osteoporosis; however, the risk of fractures is not reduced (4). Calcitonin also has a potent analgesic effect independent of its effect on bone, possibly mediated through endogenous opioids (5). It appears to be more effective when given intranasally than subcutaneously for this indication.

Salmon- and eel-derived calcitonins are more potent than the human and porcine forms. Intranasal calcitonin has a systemic availability of only 3% of the subcutaneous form but is associated with fewer adverse effects, probably because of lower systemic availability. Antibodies against calcitonin are often found after prolonged treatment, more commonly with salmon (30–69%) or eel calcitonin than with human calcitonin. Antibodies do not usually affect the clinical effect of calcitonin and have not been reported to cause any harm to the patient. Antibody-mediated resistance is exceptional.

The adverse effects of calcitonin, although common, are usually mild and are dose-related in the therapeutic range. They include gastrointestinal effects (nausea, cramps, and vomiting), dizziness and flushing, and local reactions either at the injection site (rash, pruritus) or in the nose (rhinitis, dryness, sneezing, and rarely epistaxis). In 40 patients there was nausea and dizziness in 37% of those given rectal salmon calcitonin compared with 6% of those given placebo (6).

Observational studies

The usefulness of intranasally administered salmon calcitonin for 2 years has been evaluated in 44 glucocorticoid-dependent asthmatics (SEDA-19, 378; 7). All were taking calcium supplements (1000 mg/day), but one group also took calcitonin 100 IU every other day. Calcitonin increased spinal bone mass during the first year of treatment, and maintained bone mass in a steady state during the second year. However, the rate of vertebral fractures was similar in the two groups. The addition of salmon calcitonin did not increase the efficacy of calcium plus vitamin D in the prevention of bone loss in 48 newly diagnosed patients taking glucocorticoids for giant cell arteritis and polymyalgia rheumatica in a double-blind, randomized, placebo-controlled trial (SEDA-21, 418) (8).

Placebo-controlled studies

Salmon calcitonin nasal spray prevented bone loss in the lumbar spine of 31 patients treated with prednisone for polymyalgia rheumatica (SEDA-22, 448) (9). They were randomized to salmon calcitonin nasal spray 200 IU/day or matched placebo for 1 year. Both groups were treated with calcium supplements if their dietary intake was below 800 mg/day. With calcitonin the mean bone mineral density in the lumbar spine fell by 1.3% and with placebo by 5% after 1 year. There were no differences in the hip, including the femoral neck and trochanter, or in total body bone density.

Organs and Systems

Cardiovascular

Flushing occurs soon after administration of calcitonin in up to 20% of patients and usually settles within several minutes (10).

Respiratory

When salmon calcitonin 100 IU was given intravenously to 18 patients with atopic asthma in a randomized, double-blind, crossover study, to assess any potential anti-inflammatory effect, it significantly reduced FEV1 and FVC, but the effect lasted less than 1 hour (11). Three subjects had dyspnea that did not require specific treatment.

Ear, nose, throat

In a randomized, placebo-controlled trial 22% of 1255 postmenopausal women taking calcitonin compared with 15% of women taking placebo had rhinitis (nasal congestion, discharge, or sneezing) (12). Almost all cases were of mild to moderate severity.

Mineral balance

Calcitonin can cause abnormalities of calcium balance.

- A 46-year-old woman with low back pain and osteoporosis took salmon calcitonin subcutaneously 100 U/day and calcium carbonate orally 1.5 g/day for 7 days before developing nausea and facial flushing (13). Calcitonin was continued for a further 8 days and then stopped. The next day she developed intermittent generalized convulsions. She was subsequently found to have breast cancer with skeletal metastases and hypercalcemia (3.9 mmol/l) without a reduced parathyroid hormone concentration (115 pg/ml). She was given fluids and the hypercalcemia promptly resolved.

The authors suggested that this was the first report of exogenous calcitonin causing hypercalcemia. There were several unknowns in this case, including the calcium concentration before treatment and the concentration of PTHrp, which would have helped to determine the cause of the hypercalcemia. Calcitonin is usually associated with a reduction in calcium concentration rather than a rise. The authors postulated that calcitonin could alter PTHrp concentrations, with different effects depending on cell type. They also provided evidence of hypercalcemia caused by calcitonin in non-human models (14).

- A 72-year-old woman received calcitonin 100 IU twice a week intramuscularly, calcitriol 0.25 micrograms bd, and daily calcium supplements for 3 years, before presenting with a raised calcium concentration (2.7 mmol/l) and linear calcification in the knee joints. The parathormone concentration was raised (151 pg/ml; reference range 7–53) and a parathyroid adenoma was demonstrated on ultrasound (15).

Primary hyperparathyroidism was the likely explanation in this patient, rather than a direct effect of calcitonin.

Gastrointestinal

Nausea is common with calcitonin, and vomiting or diarrhea occur more rarely. These symptoms usually settle without treatment if the drug is continued and may also be reduced by giving the dose at bedtime.

In 46 patients with Paget's disease given synthetic salmon thyrocalcitonin 80 IU/day for 3 months, there were hot flushes in 35% and nausea in 24%; in only one case was it necessary to stop treatment because of intractable diarrhea (16).

Urinary tract

In postmenopausal osteoporosis treatment with calcitriol plus etidronate or calcitonin produced improvement in spinal bone mineral density, but a high rate of nephrotoxic adverse events (17).

Skin

Rash and pruritus can occur at the site of subcutaneous injections of calcitonin (18).

Immunologic

Calcitonin allergy is very rare.

- A 60-year-old woman tolerated daily intranasal calcitonin for 6 months of the year for 4 years (19). She developed nasal watering, nasal and ocular pruritus, and sweating immediately after the administration of nasal calcitonin when she restarted after a 6-month break. These symptoms recurred 2 years later, with abdominal pain and hypotension, after 10 months of

intramuscular calcitonin, and were again reproduced by a lower dose intramuscularly.

- A 65-year-old woman, who had previously tolerated calcitonin nasal spray, developed eye and nose congestion, an itchy nose, and sneezing minutes after using intranasal salmon calcitonin (20). She was later given intramuscular salmon calcitonin and developed generalized urticaria and nasal itching within minutes. Skin testing was positive with eel and salmon calcitonins but not human calcitonin, and she was treated with human calcitonin without adverse effects.

Drug Administration

Drug formulations

Intranasal calcitonin is associated with fewer adverse effects than parenteral formulations, probably because of low systemic availability. However, a meta-analysis has confirmed that adverse events are poorly reported in clinical trials (21). The pooled relative risk for rhinitis from four trials ($n = 1663$) was 1.72, but this did not reach statistical significance.

The adverse effects of parenteral and intranasal calcitonin have been compared (22). Parenteral salmon calcitonin is commonly associated with flushing of the face, ears, hands, and feet within minutes of the injection. Nausea and vomiting can occur within 30 minutes. The flushing needs to be distinguished from the less common but serious and potentially fatal hypersensitivity reactions that have been reported. The nausea, which is mild, usually abates with continued therapy. Intranasal calcitonin is better tolerated; rhinitis of mild or moderate severity is the most frequent adverse effect.

Drug–Drug Interactions

Lithium

In four women serum lithium concentrations fell significantly within 3 days of starting calcitonin (23) because of increased renal clearance of lithium (23,24). Serum lithium concentrations should therefore be monitored in patients who start to take calcitonin.

Serum lithium concentration should be monitored at the start of calcitonin therapy.

Serum lithium concentrations fell significantly within 3 days of starting calcitonin in four women (23), due to increased renal clearance of lithium (23,24).

After they had received 100 units of salmon calcitonin subcutaneously for 3 days, four patients had a 30% mean reduction in serum lithium concentration, which was attributed to reduced absorption and/or increased renal excretion (23).

References

1. Nishi Y, Hamamoto K, Kajiyama M, Ono H, Kihara M, Jinno K. Effect of long-term calcitonin therapy by injection

and nasal spray on the incidence of fractures in osteogenesis imperfecta. J Pediatr 1992;121(3):477–80.

2. Gobelet C. Place de la calcitonine dans le traitement de l'algoneurodystrophie. [The role of calcitonin in the treatment of algoneurodystrophy.] Schweiz Rundsch Med Prax 1986;75(1–2):7–9.

3. Maksymowych WP. Managing acute osteoporotic vertebral fractures with calcitonin. Can Fam Physician 1998;44:2160–6.

4. Meunier PJ. Evidence-based medicine and osteoporosis: a comparison of fracture risk reduction data from osteoporosis randomised clinical trials. Int J Clin Pract 1999;53(2):122–9.

5. Lyritis GP, Paspati I, Karachalios T, Ioakimidis D, Skarantavos G, Lyritis PG. Pain relief from nasal salmon calcitonin in osteoporotic vertebral crush fractures. A double blind, placebo-controlled clinical study. Acta Orthop Scand Suppl 1997;275:112–4.

6. Lyritis GP, Ioannidis GV, Karachalios T, Roidis N, Kataxaki E, Papaioannou N, Kaloudis J, Galanos A. Analgesic effect of salmon calcitonin suppositories in patients with acute pain due to recent osteoporotic vertebral crush fractures: a prospective double-blind, randomized, placebo-controlled clinical study. Clin J Pain 1999;15(4):284–9.

7. Luengo M, Pons F, Martinez de Osaba MJ, Picado C. Prevention of further bone mass loss by nasal calcitonin in patients on long term glucocorticoid therapy for asthma: a two year follow up study. Thorax 1994;49(11):1099–102.

8. Healey JH, Paget SA, Williams-Russo P, Szatrowski TP, Schneider R, Spiera H, Mitnick H, Ales K, Schwartzberg P. A randomized controlled trial of salmon calcitonin to prevent bone loss in corticosteroid-treated temporal arteritis and polymyalgia rheumatica. Calcif Tissue Int 1996;58(2):73–80.

9. Adachi JD, Bensen WG, Bell MJ, Bianchi FA, Cividino AA, Craig GL, Sturtridge WC, Sebaldt RJ, Steele M, Gordon M, Themeles E, Tugwell P, Roberts R, Gent M. Salmon calcitonin nasal spray in the prevention of corticosteroid-induced osteoporosis. Br J Rheumatol 1997;36(2):255–9.

10. Gennari C, Fischer JA. Cardiovascular action of calcitonin gene-related peptide in humans. Calcif Tissue Int 1985;37(6):581–4.

11. Kawalski H, Polanowicz U, Jonderko G, Kucharz EJ, Krol W, Klimmek K, Gina AR, Pieczyrak R, Slifirski J, Shani J. Immunological parameters and respiratory functions in patients suffering from atopic bronchial asthma after intravenous treatment with salmon calcitonin. Immunol Lett 1999;70(1):15–9.

12. Chesnut CH 3rd, Silverman S, Andriano K, Genant H, Gimona A, Harris S, Kiel D, LeBoff M, Maricic M, Miller P, Moniz C, Peacock M, Richardson P, Watts N, Baylink DPROOF Study Group. A randomized trial of nasal spray salmon calcitonin in postmenopausal women with established osteoporosis: the prevent recurrence of osteoporotic fractures study. Am J Med 2000;109(4):267–76.

13. Chung SY, Chen TH, Lai SL, Huang CH, Chen WH. Hypercalcaemia and status epilepticus relates to salmon calcitonin administration in breast cancer. Breast 2005;14(5):399–402.

14. Fouchereau-Peron M, Arlot-Bonnemains Y, Moukhtar MS, Milhaud G. Calcitonin induces hypocalcaemia in grey mullet and immature freshwater and sea-water adapted rainbow trout. Comp Biochem Physiol A 1987;87:1051–3.

15. Ozcajar L, Akinci A. Linear joint calcifications while treating osteoporosis: in flagrante delicto. Rheumatol Int 2005;25:154–5.

16. Bouvet JP. Traitement de la maladie de Paget par la thyrocalcitonine de saumon. Etude cooperative en double insu. [Treatment of Paget's disease with salmon thyrocalcitonin. Cooperative double-blind study.] Nouv Presse Méd 1976;6(17):1447–50.

17. Gurlek A, Bayraktar M, Gedik O. Comparison of calcitriol treatment with etidronate–calcitriol and calcitonin–calcitriol combinations in Turkish women with postmenopausal osteoporosis: a prospective study. Calcif Tissue Int 1997;61(1):39–43.

18. Siminoski K, Josse RG. Prevention and management of osteoporosis: consensus statements from the Scientific Advisory Board of the Osteoporosis Society of Canada. 9. Calcitonin in the treatment of osteoporosis. CMAJ 1996;155(7):962–5.

19. Porcel SL, Cumplido JA, de la Hoz B, Cuevas M, Losada E. Anaphylaxis to calcitonin. Allergol Immunopathol (Madr) 2000;28(4):243–5.

20. Rodriguez A, Trujillo MJ, Herrero T, Baeza ML, de Barrio M. Allergy to calcitonin. Allergy 2001;56(8):801.

21. Cranney A, Tugwell P, Zytaruk N, Robinson V, Weaver B, Shea B, Wells G, Adachi J, Waldegger L, Guyatt G. Osteoporosis Methodology Group and The Osteoporosis Research Advisory Group. Meta-analyses of therapies for postmenopausal osteoporosis. VI. Meta-analysis of calcitonin for the treatment of postmenopausal osteoporosis. Endocr Rev 2002;23(4):540–51.

22. Munoz-Torres M, Alonso G, Raya PM. Calcitonin therapy in osteoporosis. Treat Endocrinol 2004;3:117–32.

23. Passiu G, Bocchetta A, Martinelli V, Garau P, Del Zompo M, Mathieu A. Calcitonin decreases lithium plasma levels in man. Preliminary report. Int J Clin Pharmacol Res 1998;18(4):179–81.

24. Bachofen M, Bock H, Beglinger C, Fischer JA, Thiel G. Calcitonin, ein proximal tubular wirkendes Diuretikum: Lithium-Clearance-Messungen am Menschen. [Calcitonin, a proximal-tubular-acting diuretic: lithium clearance measurements in humans.] Schweiz Med Wochenschr 1997;127(18):747–52.

Desmopressin

See also Vasopressin and analogues

General Information

Desmopressin (*N*-deamino-8-D-arginine vasopressin, dDAVP) is a longer acting analogue of vasopressin. It has very little vasoactive effect but is antidiuretic by an action on vasopressin V_2 receptors in the renal tubule and is used to treat central diabetes insipidus and nocturnal enuresis.

At higher doses desmopressin also has significant hematological effects and can significantly boost concentrations of factor VIII and von Willebrand factor (VWF) in the blood. Desmopressin is therefore a valuable agent for the treatment of mild and moderate hemophilia A (congenital or acquired) and type 1 von Willebrand disease, in which the VWF protein structure is normal but the plasma concentration is reduced (1). By contrast with conventional coagulation factor concentrates, desmopressin is cheap and is free from the risk of transmission of viral infections, which have proved such a problem in the past. It is also very useful in the treatment of carriers of hemophilia A, many of whom have significant reductions in the baseline concentration of factor VIII. By contrast, desmopressin has no effect on the concentration of factor IX, and is thus of no value in hemophilia B (Christmas disease). It is also of little value in type 2 (abnormal VWF structure) von Willebrand's disease, which accounts for about 15–20% of all cases. The administration of desmopressin to patients with type 2B von Willebrand's disease can be hazardous, as it is likely to cause thrombocytopenia (2). The use of desmopressin in bleeding disorders has been reviewed (3). Tachyphylaxis develops if desmopressin is used for prolonged periods to control bleeding disorders, because desmopressin causes release of stored factor VIII and von Willebrand factor, after which it takes time for them to accumulate again.

Intravenous injection is the most common route although subcutaneous injection may also be used. A concentrated nasal spray formulation has been proved to be efficient for home treatment of patients with bleeding episodes or even minor surgical procedures and has also been used prophylacticly (4). The nasal spray used to treat diabetes insipidus (Desmospray) is too dilute for use in disorders of hemostasis. Similarly, desmopressin in tablet form (Desmotabs) is intended for treatment of nocturnal enuresis in children and is of no use in the treatment of hemostatic disorders.

Desmopressin also shortens the prolonged skin bleeding time in patients with renal insufficiency (5,6), hepatic cirrhosis (7,8), and congenital or acquired defects of platelet function (9–11), including aspirin-induced platelet dysfunction (12).

Desmopressin reduces blood loss in patients without bleeding disorders during surgical procedures, including cardiac surgery (13,14). However, similar benefits have also been observed with other agents, including aprotinin, tranexamic acid, and aminocaproic acid. Meta-analyses have confirmed the efficacy of these agents and have shown that aprotinin is the most effective of these agents in reducing blood loss, while desmopressin was the least effective (15,16).

Children with nocturnal enuresis treated with desmopressin have fewer wet nights per week, but this effect does not persist after therapy is stopped. A meta-analysis showed an overall rate of 7.1 adverse events per 100 children (17). These were almost all local nasal reactions, including nasal irritation and epistaxis.

In an open trial of high-dose desmopressin 1.5 mg intranasally to control bleeding in 278 patients with congenital bleeding disorders, headache occurred in 3.6% and flushing in 3.2% of patients (18). Dizziness and nausea were reported in 1–1.5% and edema in 0.3% of patients.

General adverse effects

The adverse effects of desmopressin include headache, tachycardia, facial flushing, abdominal pain, tremor, and sweating during or shortly after intravenous administration (1). These symptoms are quite common but are usually simply the consequence of rapid intravenous infusion, and symptoms usually quickly subside after slowing, or even temporarily stopping, the infusion. The incidence of these relatively minor adverse effects increases with the dose of desmopressin.

Organs and Systems

Cardiovascular

Facial flushing occurred in two of 25 children with either hemophilia or von Willebrand disease given high-dose intranasal desmopressin (150 micrograms) in a single-dose open study (19).

Marked hypotension with circulatory collapse has occasionally been reported with desmopressin (20,21), although both of these reports related to patients with pre-existing cardiac conditions.

Thrombotic disorders
Desmopressin stimulates the release from endothelial cells of all the multimeric forms of von Willebrand factor found in normal plasma, including large forms that are not normally present (22). These abnormal multimers can aggregate platelets, particularly at the high levels of fluid shear stress that occur at sites of arterial stenosis.

Myocardial thrombosis
There have been several reports of arterial thrombosis associated with the use of desmopressin, including myocardial infarction (23–27). One of these reports concerned a case of fatal myocardial infarction in a blood donor in excellent health, with no risk factors and no signs of vascular disease (25).

- A 59-year-old woman with hemolytic–uremic syndrome and a recent history of atypical chest pain was given prophylactic desmopressin 0.4 micrograms/kg immediately before a renal biopsy (28). Within 30 minutes she developed chest pain and bradycardia due to myocardial infarction.

Three other cases of myocardial infarction in the absence of desmopressin have been reported in patients with hemolytic–uremic syndrome, who already have an increased risk of thrombosis.

People with hemophilia can develop atherosclerosis, but they are usually protected from ischemic coronary events. However, such events can occur when desmopressin is given.

- A 59-year-old man with mild hemophilia A was given a test dose of desmopressin 30 micrograms (0.19 micrograms/kg) in 100 ml of saline by intravenous infusion over 30 minutes (29). Shortly afterwards, having had a cigarette, he developed chest pain. An electrocardiogram showed ST elevation, and a myocardial infarction was confirmed.

Cardiovascular evaluation may be appropriate before using desmopressin.

A meta-analysis of placebo-controlled trials of desmopressin in 702 cardiac surgery patients showed a significantly increased risk of myocardial infarction in treated patients (RR = 2.39, CI = 1.02, 5.60) (30). Overall mortality was not different from placebo. Desmopressin was less efficacious in reducing perioperative blood loss than either aprotinin or lysine analogues.

Cerebral thrombosis

Cerebral infarction has also been reported in association with the use of desmopressin in children (31,32). One of these cases involved a 7-month-old child with congenital nephrotic syndrome who developed a cerebral infarction after surgery (31). One child developed cerebral ischemia after *Varicella* infection and desmopressin for enuresis (32).

Thromboembolism

There are isolated reports of thromboembolic complications in recipients of desmopressin; most occurred in patients with pre-existing vascular disease. However, in nine trials of the hemostatic efficacy of desmopressin in reducing blood and transfusion requirements in 763 patients, there were no significant differences between the frequencies of thromboembolism in subjects treated with desmopressin and controls (33). An analysis of 31 clinical trials of desmopressin in patients undergoing cardiac, vascular, orthopedic, or other major surgery showed that desmopressin did not increase the incidence of thrombosis (34).

Most of the reported thromboembolic complications occurred in elderly patients and desmopressin should not be used in patients with documented arterial disease or even in elderly patients, in whom some degree of latent arterial disease may be assumed to be present (34). Concomitant use of antifibrinolytic agents, such as tranexamic acid, should also be avoided.

Nervous system

In 64 women mean age 53 years enrolled in a randomized, placebo-controlled, crossover study of desmopressin 40 micrograms by nasal spray for the treatment of severe daytime urinary incontinence, there were drug-related adverse events in 25 women taking desmopressin and 24 adverse drug reactions in 15 women taking placebo (35). The most common adverse event with desmopressin was headache (36%). Nausea occurred in 10%.

Ear, nose, throat

Nasal irritation and rhinitis are common adverse effects of nasal desmopressin: treatment does not normally have to be altered as a result (36,37).

Electrolyte balance

Hyponatremia has often been reported with desmopressin although significant hyponatremia is rare, provided that guidelines are adhered to (38,39).

The pharmacokinetics of one dose of desmopressin 400 micrograms have been investigated in 15 men and nine women with nocturia aged over 65 years (40). They then entered a placebo-controlled crossover evaluation period. Peak concentrations occurred at 1–2 hours after administration and gradually fell over 6–7 hours. The women had significantly higher concentrations than the men, even after adjustment for body weight. Four women were withdrawn from the crossover period because of hyponatremia.

An analysis of trials reporting the risk of hyponatremia in older adults using desmopressin for nocturia has suggested that the risk is much higher in this group, estimated at 7.6% (41). However, the analysis was limited by problems with definitions of hyponatremia, varying ages studied, and the lengths of the studies. This is a similar incidence to another report of 5% (42). In this report it was suggested that the highest risk was in those over the age of 65 years, in whom sodium monitoring was recommended.

In 224 women aged 20–89 years, desmopressin 0.1–0.4 mg/day was used for treating nocturia (43). There were five adverse events, four of which were reported in the dose-titration period. Of these four events, two were deaths that were not thought to be due to hyponatremia and two were due to serious hyponatremia. The fifth case occurred during the double–blind period in the placebo group. In 27 patients serum sodium concentrations were below the reference range and in 13 they were less than 130 mmol/l; 11 of the 13 were aged 65 years or older.

- A 55-year-old woman with Von Willebrand's disease was found comatose (44). She had received desmopressin as prophylaxis for bleeding several times before without problems. On this occasion she had also received ibuprofen as a pain killer. She was hyponatremic.

NSAIDs inhibit prostaglandin synthesis. This can potentiate the effect of water reabsorption in the renal tubules of vasopressin.

About 900 000 children with primary nocturnal enuresis are treated with tablets and 400 000 with spray annually. Hyponatremia is rare (42), possibly as low as 1 per 20 000 patients exposed.

- A 3.5-year-old girl with mild hemophilia A received desmopressin 0.3 micrograms/kg intravenously 30 minutes before adenotonsillectomy. She drank 600 ml of fluid within the first 10 hours and then received 300 ml of intravenous 5% dextrose in 0.45% saline. She developed hyponatremia, headache, nausea, and seizures.

This case is a reminder that even one dose can result in problems if fluid intake is inappropriate (45).

- An 11-year-old girl was given desmopressin 10 micrograms by nasal spray per nostril for nocturnal enuresis (46). On the second night she took 3 puffs and at 3 a.m. awoke with a tonic–clonic fit. Her serum sodium concentration was 115 mmol/l.

This case highlights the importance of clear guidance for the use of desmopressin when taken for bedwetting:

- the prescribed dose should never be exceeded;
- if using a nasal spray and uncertain if the spray was successful, never repeat the dose;
- fluid intake should be kept to a minimum from one hour before taking the desmopressin and for the following 8 hours;
- if there is vomiting or diarrhea desmopressin should be withdrawn;
- inform the doctor if starting any other drugs.

Mineral balance

There was a slight but significant increase in calcium excretion in 15 girls and 17 boys, median age 9.8 years, who received desmopressin 30 micrograms by intranasal spray for 4 weeks, withdrawn for 2 weeks, and then continued for at least 3 further weeks (47). This is unlikely to be significant in the short term and whether it would have any significance in the long term is uncertain.

Fluid balance

A potential risk of desmopressin is of water intoxication with resultant hyponatremia (48), and rapid falls in serum sodium concentration can result in seizures. The risk is increased in infants and patients receiving hypotonic intravenous fluids, and such patients need to be carefully monitored.

- A 37-year-old woman with primary enuresis continued her customary daily fluid intake (2 liters) when she started intranasal desmopressin 30 micrograms at night. Within 2 days she became severely hyponatremic, with loss of consciousness, generalized seizures, and cerebral edema.
- An 80-year-old woman with a high baseline fluid intake developed severe hyponatremia, with loss of consciousness and seizures, after a single dose of desmopressin 0.2 mg (49).
- An 89-year-old woman, who had previously been stable on desmopressin, developed severe hyponatremia and became confused and unresponsive after an increase in fluid intake (49).
- A 47-year-old woman with von Willebrand disease, who was given desmopressin and intravenous fluids perioperatively, developed hyponatremia and seizures, which resolved after water restriction (50).

In a double-blind study of desmopressin, 10 of 224 adult men had serum sodium concentrations below 130 mmol/l during a 3-week, open, dose-titration period. Men aged 65 years and over were more likely to develop hyponatremia (51).

In another open study of elderly men and women, one of 30 subjects developed generalized weakness in association with a serum sodium concentration of 125 mmol/l and a serum potassium concentration of 3.1 mmol/l (52).

In a double-blind, crossover study, 20 men aged 52–80 years were given desmopressin for nocturia. Three of them had symptoms due to fluid retention, particularly bloating, headache, and reversible weight gain, and two of these had a significant fall in plasma sodium (53). In a meta-analysis of 14 studies of serum sodium in 529 patients treated with desmopressin there was mild asymptomatic hyponatremia in up to 10% of patients (54).

Fluid balance and plasma electrolytes should be monitored to prevent this complication, particularly if repeated doses are required. Children seem to be particularly vulnerable to this complication (55). In a long-term, open study of 245 Swedish children given intranasal desmopressin 20–40 micrograms at night for enuresis, five had an asymptomatic fall in plasma sodium (36). Mild hyponatremia, which did not cause symptoms, was found in five of 399 children in an open, multicenter trial (56).

Convulsions have been reported after desmopressin administration, some associated with excessive fluid intake.

- In a 12-year-old boy taking desmopressin for nocturnal enuresis, hyponatremia and cerebral edema developed after high fluid intake before a urodynamic procedure (57).
- A 13 kg 3-year-old boy given 40 micrograms of desmopressin intravenously and 1.6 liters of hypotonic fluid over 12 hours had convulsions and a respiratory arrest: his plasma sodium fell to 114 mmol/l (58).

There have been several reports of seizures in association with hyponatremia after intravenous administration of desmopressin to cover surgery in young children with congenital bleeding disorders such as mild hemophilia A or von Willebrand's disease (58–60). Hyponatremia and convulsions have occurred in children without congenital bleeding disorders who received desmopressin for urine concentration tests or to treat nocturnal enuresis (54,61,62).

Pulmonary edema associated with fluid retention occurred in a 27-year-old man after the administration of desmopressin to reduce blood loss during surgery (63).

Excess water intake during desmopressin therapy was implicated in seven cases of cerebral edema in children, which occurred over a 5-year period in the Czech Republic (64). A non-metered dropper was used for the desmopressin, so overdosage may have contributed.

Hematologic

Thrombocytopenia is rarely reported in patients who receive desmopressin, and is probably due to increased platelet aggregation (SEDA-13, 1310; 65).

- In a 50-year-old woman with uremia the platelet count fell from 149×10^9/l to 45×10^9/l after an abdominal hysterectomy with prophylactic desmopressin, and she developed a fatal subdural hemorrhage (65).

- A 38-year-old man with von Willebrand disease type 2B developed severe thrombocytopenia after a single dose of desmopressin (66).

Desmopressin also stimulates fibrinolysis (67), and this may have contributed to the outcome in the first patient.

In four patients with von Willebrand disease, desmopressin caused a significant but transient reduction in platelet count without an increase in plasma glycocalicin concentrations nor enhanced expression of P selectin, suggesting that acute thrombocytopenia after the administration of desmopressin in type 2B von Willebrand disease is not related to platelet activation and consumption (68).

In 224 adult men, mean age 65 (range 37–88) years, thrombocytopenia developed in one man during a 1-week washout period after dose titration to up to 0.4 mg of oral desmopressin daily over the preceding 3 weeks; thrombocytopenia did not recur on rechallenge (51).

Desmopressin induces factor VIII and von Willebrand factor (vWF) activity, resulting in an increase in ultra-large vWF multimers. In thrombotic thrombocytopenic purpura there is a deficiency in the von Willebrand factor-cleaving protease (ADAMTS13), which is responsible for degradation of vWF multimers. These ultra-large vWF multimers accumulate and facilitate platelet adhesion.

- A 42-year-old woman with thrombotic thrombocytopenic purpura received a number of therapies, including desmopressin 20 micrograms in 100 ml of saline over 1 hour. One hour later she developed a fever of 38.4°C, headache, and an expressive aphasia (69).

Pancreas

A scientific registry of transplant recipients has been used to determine the effect of cadaveric organ donor treatment with desmopressin on the incidence of pancreas graft thrombosis in clinical pancreas transplantation (70). Of 2804 cases with sufficient information between 5 April 1994 and 27 September 2002, 1287 (46%) had received desmopressin. The mean follow up was 1.5 years (1 month to 8.4 years). There was pancreatic graft thrombosis in 4.3%, of whom 5.1% had received desmopressin and 3.5% had not; this was just statistically significant. There was no information about dose, timecourse, or duration of desmopressin use. It is not known whether this finding is clinically significant.

Second-Generation Effects

Pregnancy

There is growing evidence that desmopressin can be used safely in pregnant women and no adverse effects have been reported in either mothers with diabetes insipidus or their babies (71), or in women with clotting factor deficiencies (72). However, the manufacturers advise that it should be used with caution in women with bleeding disorders, who require high doses.

One report described adverse reactions in two pregnant women with von Willebrand disease (73). One went into premature labor after a single dose (attributed to the oxytocic effect of desmopressin) and the other had severe hyponatremia associated with seizures after repeated administration of desmopressin to cover a cesarean section.

Lactation

Insignificant quantities of desmopressin pass into breast milk (74), and so breastfeeding is not contraindicated in association with desmopressin administration to a nursing mother.

Susceptibility factors

Age

Participants in a short-term study were invited to continue in an open study of the long-term use of desmopressin for nocturia (75). The study was completed by 95 men aged 24 –88 years and 87 women aged 21 –85 years, who took therapy for 11–13 months. The dosage was the dose (0.1, 0.2, or 0.4 mg orally at bedtime) that was found to be optimal during the short-term study by dose titration. Adverse events were more common in those aged 65 years or older, 27% versus 21% in men and 41% versus 19% in women. Hyponatremia was more common, but it was unclear which other events occurred more commonly. The authors recommended monitoring of sodium concentrations, particularly when starting therapy and when changing dose.

Drug–Drug Interactions

Carbamazepine

Carbamazepine increases the release of endogenous antidiuretic hormone and can therefore potentiate the antidiuretic effect of desmopressin. Of 103 children with cranial diabetes insipidus included in a retrospective analysis, 10% became hyponatremic (76). The risk of hyponatremia was three-fold higher when desmopressin and carbamazepine were given in combination.

Chlorpromazine

Chlorpromazine increases the release of endogenous antidiuretic hormone and can therefore potentiate the antidiuretic effect of desmopressin (77).

Lamotrigine

In 103 children with cranial diabetes insipidus, 3 children who started or had an increase in dose of lamotrigine needed a larger dose of desmopressin, suggesting an effect on the renal tubule or on drug clearance (76). Lamotrigine also increased desmopressin dosage requirements in two other children with cranial diabetes insipidus (78).

Tricyclic antidepressants

Tricyclic antidepressants increase the release of endogenous antidiuretic hormone and can therefore potentiate the antidiuretic effect of desmopressin. A hyponatremic convulsion occurred in a child who was given desmopressin and imipramine (79).

References

1. Mannucci PM. Desmopressin (DDAVP) in the treatment of bleeding disorders: the first 20 years. Blood 1997;90(7):2515–21.
2. Holmberg L, Nilsson IM, Borge L, Gunnarsson M, Sjorin E. Platelet aggregation induced by 1-desamino-8-D-arginine vasopressin (DDAVP) in Type IIB von Willebrand's disease. N Engl J Med 1983;309(14):816–21.
3. Sutor AH. Desmopressin (DDAVP) in bleeding disorders of childhood. Semin Thromb Hemost 1998;24(6):555–66.
4. Lethagen S, Ragnarson Tennvall G. Self-treatment with desmopressin intranasal spray in patients with bleeding disorders: effect on bleeding symptoms and socioeconomic factors. Ann Hematol 1993;66(5):257–60.
5. Mannucci PM, Remuzzi G, Pusineri F, Lombardi R, Valsecchi C, Mecca G, Zimmerman TS. Deamino-8-D-arginine vasopressin shortens the bleeding time in uremia. N Engl J Med 1983;308(1):8–12.
6. Watson AJ, Keogh JA. 1-Deamino-8-D-arginine vasopressin as a therapy for the bleeding diathesis of renal failure. Am J Nephrol 1984;4(1):49–51.
7. Burroughs AK, Matthews K, Qadiri M, Thomas N, Kernoff P, Tuddenham E, McIntyre N. Desmopressin and bleeding time in patients with cirrhosis. BMJ (Clin Res Ed) 1985;291(6506):1377–81.
8. Mannucci PM, Vicente V, Vianello L, Cattaneo M, Alberca I, Coccato MP, Faioni E, Mari D. Controlled trial of desmopressin in liver cirrhosis and other conditions associated with a prolonged bleeding time. Blood 1986;67(4):1148–53.
9. Kobrinsky NL, Israels ED, Gerrard JM, Cheang MS, Watson CM, Bishop AJ, Schroeder ML. Shortening of bleeding time by 1-deamino-8-D-arginine vasopressin in various bleeding disorders. Lancet 1984;1(8387):1145–8.
10. Schulman S, Johnsson H, Egberg N, Blomback M. DDAVP-induced correction of prolonged bleeding time in patients with congenital platelet function defects. Thromb Res 1987;45(2):165–74.
11. DiMichele DM, Hathaway WE. Use of DDAVP in inherited and acquired platelet dysfunction. Am J Hematol 1990;33(1):39–45.
12. Chard RB, Kam CA, Nunn GR, Johnson DC, Meldrum-Hanna W. Use of desmopressin in the management of aspirin-related and intractable haemorrhage after cardiopulmonary bypass. Aust NZ J Surg 1990;60(2):125–8.
13. Salzman EW, Weinstein MJ, Weintraub RM, Ware JA, Thurer RL, Robertson L, Donovan A, Gaffney T, Bertele V, Troll J, et al. Treatment with desmopressin acetate to reduce blood loss after cardiac surgery. A double-blind randomized trial. N Engl J Med 1986;314(22):1402–6.
14. Cattaneo M, Mannucci PM. Desmopressin and blood loss after cardiac surgery. Lancet 1993;342(8874):812.
15. Fremes SE, Wong BI, Lee E, Mai R, Christakis GT, McLean RF, Goldman BS, Naylor CD. Metaanalysis of prophylactic drug treatment in the prevention of postoperative bleeding. Ann Thorac Surg 1994;58(6):1580–8.
16. Laupacis A, Fergusson D. Drugs to minimize perioperative blood loss in cardiac surgery: meta-analyses using perioperative blood transfusion as the outcome. The International Study of Peri-operative Transfusion (ISPOT) Investigators. Anesth Analg 1997;85(6):1258–67.
17. Glazener CM, Evans JH. Desmopressin for nocturnal enuresis in children. Cochrane Database Syst Rev 2000;(2):CD002112.
18. Leissinger C, Becton D, Cornell C Jr, Cox Gill J. High-dose DDAVP intranasal spray (Stimate) for the prevention and treatment of bleeding in patients with mild haemophilia A, mild or moderate type 1 von Willebrand disease and symptomatic carriers of haemophilia A. Haemophilia 2001;7(3):258–66.
19. Gill JC, Ottum M, Schwartz B. Evaluation of high concentration intranasal and intravenous desmopressin in pediatric patients with mild hemophilia A or mild-to-moderate type 1 von Willebrand disease. J Pediatr 2002;140(5):595–9.
20. D'Alauro FS, Johns RA. Hypotension related to desmopressin administration following cardiopulmonary bypass. Anesthesiology 1988;69(6):962–3.
21. Israels SJ, Kobrinsky NL. Serious reaction to desmopressin in a child with cyanotic heart disease. N Engl J Med 1989;320(23):1563–4.
22. Ruggeri ZM, Mannucci PM, Lombardi R, Federici AB, Zimmerman TS. Multimeric composition of factor VIII/von Willebrand factor following administration of DDAVP: implications for pathophysiology and therapy of von Willebrand's disease subtypes. Blood 1982;59(6):1272–8.
23. Bond L, Bevan D. Myocardial infarction in a patient with hemophilia treated with DDAVP. N Engl J Med 1988;318(2):121.
24. van Dantzig JM, Duren DR, Ten Cate JW. Desmopressin and myocardial infarction. Lancet 1989;1(8639):664–5.
25. McLeod BC. Myocardial infarction in a blood donor after administration of desmopressin. Lancet 1990;336(8723):1137–8.
26. Hartmann S, Reinhart W. Fatal complication of desmopressin. Lancet 1995;345(8960):1302–3.
27. Anonymous. Desmopressin and arterial thrombosis. Lancet 1989;1(8644):938–9.
28. Stratton J, Warwicker P, Watkins S, Farrington K. Desmopressin may be hazardous in thrombotic microangiopathy. Nephrol Dial Transplant 2001;16(1):161–2.
29. Virtanen R, Kauppila M, Itala M. Percutaneous coronary intervention with stenting in a patient with haemophilia A and an acute myocardial infarction following a single dose of desmopressin. Thromb Haemost 2004;92:1154–6.
30. Levi M, Cromheecke ME, de Jonge E, Prins MH, de Mol BJ, Briet E, Buller HR. Pharmacological strategies to decrease excessive blood loss in cardiac surgery: a meta-analysis of clinically relevant endpoints. Lancet 1999;354(9194):1940–7.
31. Grunwald Z, Sather SD. Intraoperative cerebral infarction after desmopressin administration in infant with end-stage renal disease. Lancet 1995;345(8961):1364–5.
32. Wieting JM, Dykstra DD, Ruggiero MP, Robbins GB, Galusha K. Central nervous system ischemia after Varicella infection and desmopressin therapy for enuresis. J Am Osteopath Assoc 1997;97(5):293–5.
33. Mannucci PM, Lusher JM. Desmopressin and thrombosis. Lancet 1989;2(8664):675–6.
34. Mannucci PM, Carlsson S, Harris AS. Desmopressin, surgery and thrombosis. Thromb Haemost 1994;71(1):154–5.
35. Robinson D, Cardozo L, Akeson M, Hvistendahl G, Riis A, Norgaard JP. Antidiuresis: a new concept in managing female daytime urinary incontinence. BJU Int 2004;93:996–1000.
36. Tullus K, Bergstrom R, Fosdal I, Winnergard I, Hjalmas K. Efficacy and safety during long-term treatment of primary

monosymptomatic nocturnal enuresis with desmopressin. Swedish Enuresis Trial Group. Acta Paediatr 1999;88(11):1274–8.

37. Chiozza ML, del Gado R, di Toro R, Ferrara P, Fois A, Giorgi P, Giovannini M, Rottoli A, Segni G, Biraghi M. Italian multicentre open trial on DDAVP spray in nocturnal enuresis. Scand J Urol Nephrol 1999;33(1):42–8.

38. Del Gado R, Del Gaizo D, Cennamo M, Auriemma R, Del Gado G, Verni M. Desmopressin is a safe drug for the treatment of enuresis. Scand J Urol Nephrol 2005;39:308–12.

39. Triantafyllidis A, Charalambous S, Papatsoris AG, Papathanasiou A, Kalaitzis C, Rombis V, Touloupidis S. Management of nocturnal enuresis in Greek children. Pediatr Nephrol 2005;20:1343–5.

40. Hvistendahl GM, Riis A, Nørgaard JP, Djurhuus JC. The pharmacokinetics of 400 µg of oral desmopressin in elderly patients with nocturia, and the correlation between the absorption of desmopressin and clinical effect. BJU Int 2005;95:804–9.

41. Weatherall M. The risk of hyponatremia in older adults using desmopressin for nocturia: a systematic review and meta-analysis. Neurourol Urodyn 2004;23:302–5.

42. Norgaard JP. Hyponatremia in desmopressin treated patients—what is evidence based? J Urol Urogynäkol 2004;11:7.

43. Lose G, Lalos O, Freeman RM, Van Kerrebroeck P, the Nocturia study group. Efficacy of desmopressin (Minirin) in the treatment of nocturia: a double-blind placebo-controlled study in women. Am J Obstet Gynecol 2003;189:1106–13.

44. Garcia EBG, Ruitenberg A, Madrestsma GS, Hintzen RQ. Hyponatraemic coma induced by desmopresssin and ibuprofen in a woman with von Willebrand's disease. Haemophilia 2003;9:232–4.

45. Molnár Z, Farkas V, Nemes L, Reusz GS, Szabó AJ. Hyponatraemic seizures resulting from inadequate postoperative intake following a single dose of desmopressin. Nephrol Dial Transplant 2005;20:2265–7.

46. Passi GR, Shad R. Seizures and coma after desmopressin for nocturnal enuresis. Indian Pediatr 2004;41:1276–7.

47. Muller D, Kuehnle K, Eggert P. Increased urinary calcium excretion in enuretic children treated with desmopressin. J Urol 2004;171:2618–20.

48. Odeh M, Oliven A. Coma and seizures due to severe hyponatremia and water intoxication in an adult with intranasal desmopressin therapy for nocturnal enuresis. J Clin Pharmacol 2001;41(5):582–4.

49. Shindel A, Tobin G, Klutke C. Hyponatremia associated with desmopressin for the treatment of nocturnal polyuria. Urology 2002;60(2):344.

50. Pruthi RS, Kang J, Vick R. Desmopressin induced hyponatremia and seizures after laparoscopic radical nephrectomy. J Urol 2002;168(1):187.

51. Mattiasson A, Abrams P, Van Kerrebroeck P, Walter S, Weiss J. Efficacy of desmopressin in the treatment of nocturia: a double-blind placebo-controlled study in men. BJU Int 2002;89(9):855–62.

52. Kuo HC. Efficacy of desmopressin in treatment of refractory nocturia in patients older than 65 years. Urology 2002;59(4):485–9.

53. Cannon A, Carter PG, McConnell AA, Abrams P. Desmopressin in the treatment of nocturnal polyuria in the male. BJU Int 1999;84(1):20–4.

54. Robson WL, Norgaard JP, Leung AK. Hyponatremia in patients with nocturnal enuresis treated with DDAVP. Eur J Pediatr 1996;155(11):959–62.

55. Sutor AH. DDAVP is not a panacea for children with bleeding disorders. Br J Haematol 2000;108(2):217–27.

56. Hjalmas K, Hanson E, Hellstrom AL, Kruse S, Sillen U. Long-term treatment with desmopressin in children with primary monosymptomatic nocturnal enuresis: an open multicentre study. Swedish Enuresis Trial (SWEET) Group. Br J Urol 1998;82(5):704–9.

57. Brodzikowska-Pytel A, Giembicki J. Hyponatremia as a complication of nocturnal enuresis treatment with desmopressin in a child. Pediatr Pol 1999;74:79–83.

58. Francis JD, Leary T, Niblett DJ. Convulsions and respiratory arrest in association with desmopressin administration for the treatment of a bleeding tonsil in a child with borderline haemophilia. Acta Anaesthesiol Scand 1999;43(8):870–3.

59. Shepherd LL, Hutchinson RJ, Worden EK, Koopmann CF, Coran A. Hyponatremia and seizures after intravenous administration of desmopressin acetate for surgical hemostasis. J Pediatr 1989;114(3):470–2.

60. Smith TJ, Gill JC, Ambruso DR, Hathaway WE. Hyponatremia and seizures in young children given DDAVP. Am J Hematol 1989;31(3):199–202.

61. Apakama DC, Bleetman A. Hyponatraemic convulsion secondary to desmopressin treatment for primary enuresis. J Accid Emerg Med 1999;16(3):229–30.

62. Schwab M, Ruder H. Hyponatraemia and cerebral convulsion due to DDAVP administration in patients with enuresis nocturna or urine concentration testing. Eur J Pediatr 1997;156(8):668.

63. Cone A, Riley R. DDAVP and pulmonary oedema. Anaesth Intensive Care 1994;22(4):502–3.

64. Lebl J, Kolska M, Zavacka A, Eliasek J, Gut J, Biolek J. Cerebral oedema in enuretic children during low-dose desmopressin treatment: a preventable complication. Eur J Pediatr 2001;160(3):159–62.

65. Sun HL, Chien CC. Thrombocytopenia and subdural hemorrhage after desmopressin administration. Anesthesiology 1998;88(4):1115–7.

66. Gomez Garcia EB, Brouwers GJ, Kappers-Klunne MC, Leebeek FW, van Vliet HH. Intermitterende trombocytopenie als uiting van de ziekte van von Willebrand. [Intermittent thrombocytopenia as a manifestation of Von Willebrand's disease.] Ned Tijdschr Geneeskd 2002;146(25):1192–5.

67. Burroughs AK, Planas R, Svoboda P. Optimizing emergency care of upper gastrointestinal bleeding in cirrhotic patients. Scand J Gastroenterol Suppl 1998;226:14–24.

68. Casonato A, Steffan A, Pontara E, Zucchetto A, Rossi C, De Marco L, Girolami A. Post-DDAVP thrombocytopenia in type 2B von Willebrand disease is not associated with platelet consumption: failure to demonstrate glycocalicin increase or platelet activation. Thromb Haemost 1999;81(2):224–8.

69. Overman M, Brass E. Worsening of thrombotic thrombocytopenic purpura symptoms associated with desmopressin administration. Thromb Haemost 2004;92:886–7.

70. Marques RG, Rogers J, Chavin KD, Baliga PK, Lin A, Emovon O, Afzal F, Baillie GM, Taber DJ, Ashcraft EE, Rajagopalan PR. Does treatment of cadaveric organ donors with desmopressin increase the likelihood of pancreas graft thrombosis? Results of a preliminary study. Transplant Proc 2004;36:1048–9.

71. Ray JG. DDAVP use during pregnancy: an analysis of its safety for mother and child. Obstet Gynecol Surv 1998;53(7):450–5.

72. Mannucci PM. Use of desmopressin (DDAVP) during early pregnancy in factor VIII-deficient women. Blood 2005;105(8):3382.

73. Chediak JR, Alban GM, Maxey B. von Willebrand's disease and pregnancy: management during delivery and outcome of offspring. Am J Obstet Gynecol 1986;155(3):618–24.
74. Burrow GN, Wassenaar W, Robertson GL, Sehl H. DDAVP treatment of diabetes insipidus during pregnancy and the post-partum period. Acta Endocrinol (Copenh) 1981;97(1):23–5.
75. Lose G, Mattiasson A, Walter S, Lalos O, van Kerrerbroeck P. Abrams P, Freeman R. Clinical experiences with desmopressin for long-term treatment of nocturia. J Urol 2004;172:1021–5.
76. Rizzo V, Albanese A, Stanhope R. Morbidity and mortality associated with vasopressin replacement therapy in children. J Pediatr Endocrinol Metab 2001;14(7):861–7.
77. Wilke RA. Posterior pituitary sigma receptors and drug-induced syndrome of inappropriate antidiuretic hormone release. Ann Intern Med 1999;131(10):799.
78. Mewasingh L, Aylett S, Kirkham F, Stanhope R. Hyponatraemia associated with lamotrigine in cranial diabetes insipidus. Lancet 2000;356(9230):656.
79. Hamed M, Mitchell H, Clow DJ. Hyponatraemic convulsion associated with desmopressin and imipramine treatment. BMJ 1993;306(6886):1169.

Follitropin

General Information

The first gonadotropins available for clinical use were extracted from the urine of postmenopausal women. Human menopausal gonadotropin (hMG) is in limited supply and contains other proteins, which may be allergenic, as well as luteinizing hormone. Purified preparations of follicle-stimulating hormone (FSH; urofollitropin and highly purified urofollitropin) are also extracted from human urine. Recombinant FSH (follitropin-alfa) prepared from a Chinese hamster ovarian cell line is likely to replace other gonadotropins because of its purity and ease of patient self-administration.

Follitropin treatment for infertility has been reviewed in detail (1,2). Multiple pregnancy occurs in 20% of patients, 80% being twin pregnancies. There is no documented increase in congenital abnormalities in children conceived after ovulation induction with follitropin.

Organs and Systems

Nervous system

- A 32-year-old woman who was not obese developed benign intracranial hypertension in association with ovarian hyperstimulation syndrome after ovulation induction using goserelin, follitropin, and human chorionic gonadotropin (hCG) (3). The syndrome did not recur during a second pregnancy in which follitropin and hCG were not used

Reproductive system

Ovarian hyperstimulation syndrome (OHSS) is characterized by massive ovarian enlargement and fluid shift from the intravascular space to the peritoneal, pleural, and pericardial cavities. Rates of up to 20% for all grades and 1–2% for severe OHSS have been documented and do not differ between preparations of follitropin. Women with polycystic ovarian syndrome are at higher risk of this complication. In rare cases women have died of pulmonary embolism, disseminated intravascular coagulation, or adult respiratory distress syndrome. If the patient is pregnant, OHSS is more severe and prolonged (1). Generally, it resolves within 7 days if the patient is not pregnant or in 10–20 days if she is. The underlying cause of this adverse effect is not known.

References

1. Vollenhoven BJ, Healy DL. Short- and long-term effects of ovulation induction. Endocrinol Metab Clin North Am 1998;27(4):903–14.
2. Goa KL, Wagstaff AJ. Follitropin alpha in infertility. Biodrugs 1998;9:235–60.
3. Lesny P, Maguiness SD, Hay DM, Robinson J, Clarke CE, Killick SR. Ovarian hyperstimulation syndrome and benign intracranial hypertension in pregnancy after in-vitro fertilization and embryo transfer: case report. Hum Reprod 1999;14(8):1953–5.

Gonadorelin and analogues

General Information

The effects of gonadorelin depend on the duration of use. Gonadotropin release is stimulated in the short term, but is later suppressed owing to down-regulation of hypophyseal receptors. Its therapeutic indications have been summarized (SEDA-13, 1311) (1). Long-acting and depot formulations have the same adverse effects as shorter-acting analogues. The available gonadorelin analogues include buserelin, goserelin, leprorelin, nafarelin, and triptorelin (all rINNs).

Gonadorelin and its analogues cause an initial surge in follicle-stimulating hormone (FSH), luteinizing hormone (LH), and gonadal steroids. Receptor down-regulation and gonadotropin suppression occur after prolonged administration. Thus, both the clinical and adverse effects depend on the duration of administration. Biological activity and adverse effects also vary between gonadorelin agonists.

Comparative studies

In 67 premenopausal Japanese women randomized to 4-weekly, low-dose buserelin 1.8 mg or leuprorelin 1.88 mg, women given leuprorelin had a more rapid clinical response and a higher rate of hot flushes (2).

Adverse effects and quality of life have been compared in 431 men with prostate cancer treated with a gonadorelin agonist or orchidectomy (3). Of the men who reported normal sexual function before treatment, 51% had reduced libido and 69% became impotent. Of those given gonadorelin, 57% had hot flushes. Breast swelling was more common in those given gonadorelin (25% compared with 10% after orchidectomy).

Of 547 men randomized to leuprorelin plus flutamide for 3 or 8 months, those treated for 8 months had a higher overall rate of adverse events, and 87% had hot flushes, compared with 72% of those who were treated for 3 months (4).

Placebo-controlled studies

In a randomized, placebo-controlled study in women who received leuprolide acetate depot 11.25 mg intramuscularly with tibolone 2.5 mg/day (n = 36), leuprolide acetate depot 11.25 mg with placebo (n = 37), or a placebo injection with placebo tablets (n = 39), irritable bowel syndrome related to the menstrual cycle improved in those who received leuprolide (5). There were hot flushes in those who took leuprolide compared with placebo; no data were given about the frequency of hot flushes, but there were no withdrawals because of this symptom. Amenorrhea also occurred. Both flushing and amenorrhea are expected adverse effects of leuprolide.

Organs and Systems

Cardiovascular

Gonadorelin inhibits nitric oxide-mediated arterial relaxation, which disappears within 3 months after stopping treatment. This effect was abolished with "add-back" hormone replacement in a prospective, randomized study of 50 women treated for 6 months (6).

Respiratory

- A 75-year-old man developed a high fever and cough immediately after an injection of leuprorelin acetate 3.75 mg and 8 days after starting flutamide 375 mg/day (7). He died of respiratory failure after a month, and interstitial pneumonitis was confirmed postmortem.

There have been two other reports of pneumonitis associated with gonadorelin agonists.

Ear, nose, throat

Local irritation or rhinitis occurs uncommonly when gonadorelin agonists are taken intranasally.

- A 34-year-old woman had to stop using nafarelin nasal spray after 14 days because of exacerbation of maxillary sinusitis (8).

Nervous system

Pituitary apoplexy (hemorrhagic infarction presenting with sudden severe headache, often followed by pituitary

hormone deficiency) has been reported after intravenous gonadorelin testing to investigate a pituitary macroadenoma and in several patients with gonadotropin-secreting pituitary macroadenomas who were given gonadorelin to treat prostate cancer (9). It may be advisable to assess gonadotropin status prior to therapy in such patients.

- A 43-year-old woman with a pituitary macroadenoma, who took quinagolide 37.5 micrograms/day for 33 months, developed a severe headache, nausea and vomiting, and photophobia 30 minutes after diagnostic testing with gonadorelin 50 micrograms intravenously (10). Although a CT scan at the time showed no evidence of hemorrhage, an MRI scan 18 months later showed a partial empty sella.
- A 67-year-old man with prostate cancer and an unsuspected pituitary macroadenoma developed a severe frontal headache, nausea and vomiting, and blindness within 12 hours of insertion of a goserelin implant (11).

Two further cases have been reported, in which gonadorelin was administered either alone (12) or with insulin (13). The mechanism of pituitary apoplexy in these cases is unclear. Gonadorelin may have a direct effect on vascular tone or may increase tumor metabolic activity.

There has been one previous report of seizure exacerbation during leuprorelin treatment, in a girl with pre-existing brain damage (14), and a case of de novo seizures has also been reported (15).

- A 13-year-old girl, who had previously had surgery and radiotherapy for a medulloblastoma, developed atypical absence seizures for the first time after 3 months of therapy with leuprorelin. The seizures stopped 1 month after treatment was withdrawn and did not recur until 30 months later. The seizures were not related to estradiol concentrations or the menstrual cycle.

Neuromuscular function

Prolonged administration of gonadorelin is commonly associated with reduced muscle bulk and voluntary muscle function. In a prospective, uncontrolled study of 62 men with prostate cancer, treatment with cyproterone acetate and goserelin caused an increase in fatigue scores and increased muscle fatiguability on objective testing within 6 weeks, in 66% of subjects (16). Fatigue was unrelated to psychological complaints or to self-reported functional ability.

Sensory systems

Blurred vision, sometimes associated with headache and dizziness, is common soon after the commencement of treatment and usually resolves within 2–3 weeks. It has recurred in some patients after rechallenge (17).

Psychological, psychiatric

Depressed mood and emotional lability occur in up to 75% of gonadorelin recipients, and there are rare reports of more severe mood disturbances (18). Defects of verbal memory have been described and may be reversed by "add-back" estrogen treatment (18) and sertraline (19).

- A 32-year-old woman had psychotic symptoms of persecutory delusions, agitation, and auditory hallucinations a few days after her second injection of triptorelin (20). Her symptoms recurred after a pregnancy, suggesting that they were due to the rapid fall in estrogen in both instances.

During a 6-month, randomized trial, men randomized to gonadorelin agonists had reduced attention and memory test scores, compared with men who were not given gonadorelin agonists but were closely monitored, in whom there was no change (21).

Endocrine

Gonadotropin-releasing hormone analogues initially stimulate the pituitary gland, resulting in increased concentrations of luteinizing hormone and testosterone in men. Subsequently, the pituitary receptors down-regulate and testosterone concentrations fall. On withdrawal of the agonist the effects have been thought to be reversible. However, they can be sustained for substantial periods in men receiving prolonged courses for prostate cancer (22). Patients receiving intermittent androgen therapy for prostate cancer were treated with leuprolide acetate 7.5 mg monthly and nilutamide orally for 8 months. Full testosterone recovery during the off treatment period was documented in 61% of cycles. In cycles during which recovery occurred, the median time to recovery was 23 (4–61) weeks (23).

Of 247 men with prostate cancer who received goserelin 3.6 mg subcutaneously every 28 days or 10.8 mg every 84 days, 27% and 18% respectively had a rise in serum testosterone concentration to above the castrate range [24]. Only 1.7% had a testosterone concentration within the age-specific reference range. There were no clinical symptoms of tumor flare reaction.

In Japanese children with precocious puberty treated with leuprolide the time between the last injection and the median onset of menarche was 15 (range 3.6–63) months (25). The age at menarche was higher than that of the healthy population (13 versus 12 years).

For in vitro fertilization the use of triptorelin 0.1 mg/day, with early withdrawal, caused suppressed endogenous luteinizing hormone for 10–14 days after withdrawal (26).

Symptoms of hypoestrogenism, including hot flushes, vaginal dryness, reduced libido, and mood changes, occur in almost all women on long-term gonadorelin. Men also experience hypogonadal symptoms with prolonged gonadorelin administration, including hot flushes and reduced libido, although this is a therapeutic effect rather than an adverse effect. Gynecomastia occasionally occurs in men.

"Add-back" estrogen replacement reduces the frequency and severity of these symptoms without apparently compromising the effectiveness of gonadorelin in women with endometriosis (19,27). In a randomized, multicenter, double-blind comparison of intranasal nafarelin twice daily and depot leuprolide acetate monthly for 6 months in 192 young women with endometriosis, nafarelin caused fewer hypoestrogenic symptoms, although the difference between the two groups was statistically significant only after 3 months of therapy (28).

"Draw-back" therapy, in which the dosage of nafarelin was reduced after 4 weeks, had similar efficacy, but a smaller degree of bone loss and fewer vasomotor adverse effects compared with full-dose therapy, in a randomized study in 15 premenopausal women (29).

- A 47-year-old woman developed symptoms of thyrotoxicosis (palpitation, tremor, tachycardia, and goiter) due to Graves' disease, after using goserelin acetate for 13 months (30).
- A 45-year-old woman developed transient thyroiditis associated with antithyroid antibodies in taking leuprorelin (31).

The second patient had other risk factors for autoimmune thyroid disease, and the association was probably coincidental, but the episode may have been precipitated by low estrogen concentrations, as is hypothesized in postpartum thyroiditis.

Further reports of autoimmune thyroid disease in association with gonadorelin analogues have appeared (32).

- A 49-year-old woman developed Graves' disease after receiving buserelin acetate for 4 months.
- A 41-year-old woman developed painless thyroiditis after receiving leuprolide acetate for 4 months.
- A 29-year-old woman developed Graves' disease 4 months after starting to receive buserelin acetate.

Metabolism

In 20 premenopausal women treated with triptorelin for 8 weeks, the mean LDL concentration rose from 2.7 to 3.9 mmol/l and HDL fell from 1.6 to 1.5 mmol/l (33). Although the change in HDL was not clinically relevant in isolation, the increases in LDL and LDL:HDL ratio were significant, suggesting an increased risk of atherogenesis. "Add-back" conjugated equine estrogen did not reverse these changes over 24 weeks.

- A woman with type 2 diabetes had worse glycemic control while receiving buserelin (34). Her blood glucose returned to its previous concentration after withdrawal.

Two men developed hyperglycemia after using leuprolide acetate (35).

- A 61-year-old Japanese man with prostate cancer had had well controlled diabetes for 6 years (Hb_{A1c} less than 6.4%). He received leuprolide acetate subcutaneously 3.75 mg/month and oral flutamide 250 mg/day. Three weeks after the second injection his fasting glucose was 18 mmol/l and Hb_{A1c} 8.0%.
- An 81-year-old Japanese man not known to have diabetes developed prostate cancer. His Hb_{A1c} concentration was 5.1%. He received three injections of leuprolide acetate 3.75 mg/month subcutaneously then 11.25 mg every 3 months. After 7 months he complained of thirst and his blood glucose had increased to 19 mmol/l and Hb_{A1c} to 9.9%.

There is increasing evidence of a link between low testosterone concentrations and type 2 diabetes mellitus.

Hematologic

The relation between androgens and erythropoiesis is well known. In 42 patients with adenocarcinoma of the prostate, leuprolide acetate and flutamide (an antiandrogen) were used in combination (36). Hemoglobin concentrations fell by more than 25% in six patients who developed symptomatic anemia. Checking the hemoglobin at 3 months was thought to be useful in predicting those who would become symptomatic.

Leuprolide acetate has been reported to cause normochromic normocytic anemia in patients with benign prostatic hyperplasia (37). The anemia is usually transient, and the hemoglobin returns to baseline 6 months after stopping androgen suppression. There is a single case report of more serious red cell aplasia in a patient receiving gonadorelin, with resolution after treatment was withdrawn (38).

A coagulopathy has been attributed to leuprolide (39).

- A 65-year-old man, with metastatic carcinoma of the prostate was treated with flutamide 250 mg/day orally followed after 6 days by 7.5mg leuprolide intramuscularly. Two days later he developed bleeding and hematomas. His hemoglobin fell from 12.4 to 7.8 g/dl and he had a disseminated intravascular coagulopathy.

The timing in this case suggested that testosterone release may have occurred despite androgen blockade by flutamide. As a result, tumor cell growth and coagulopathy may have occurred. In some patients with prostate cancer taking fluoxymesterone (an androgenic hormone) there was activation of clotting (40).

Skin

Injection site reactions are common with gonadorelin receptor agonists. In 119 women randomized to subcutaneous triptorelin a local reaction (redness, pain, or bruising) was present after 1 hour in 24% and persisted for 24 hours in 9.5% (41). In another study in 105 women randomized to leuprorelin acetate, moderate local reactions occurred in 24% and severe reactions in 1% (42).

- A 48-year-old woman developed an itchy skin eruption and spotted dark brown pigmentation 3 weeks after starting nasal buserelin 900 micrograms/day. The lesions resolved when buserelin was withdrawn, and recurred with rechallenge; some persisted for up to 2 years (43).
- A 78-year-old man treated with subcutaneous leuprorelin acetate had repeated local reactions, with erythema, induration, abscesses, and an ulcer on one hip (44).

Altered skin pigmentation has been previously reported in pregnancy and after sex hormone administration, so the initial surge in gonadotropins after gonadorelin treatment was a probable cause for the first patient's presentation.

In the second case the lactic acid/glycolic acid vehicle may have caused the reaction rather than leuprorelin.

Epithelioid granulomata have been attributed to leuprorelin (45).

- A 73-year-old man with prostate cancer received leuprorelin acetate injections and developed a subcutaneous nodule at the injection site. Histology showed epithelioid granulomata with multinuclear giant cells.

These lesions were suggested to have been caused by a type IV allergic response to the co-polymer of lactic and glycolic acids used as a vehicle.

Three further cases of granulomatous reactions at leuprorelin injection sites in Japanese men have led to speculation that they occur more often in Japan because of the use of subcutaneous injection rather than intramuscular injection, which is used in Western countries (46). The exact mechanism of this reaction is unknown, and whether it is due to the co-polymer or leuprorelin itself is debated. Local reactions can cause reduced efficacy (47).

Musculoskeletal

Osteoporosis, trabecular bone being most affected, has been regularly observed in both sexes with chronic gonadorelin agonist treatment (48), and the duration of therapy for prostate cancer is inversely related to bone mineral density (49,50). Intravenous pamidronate may prevent bone loss in these patients (51,52).

- A 44-year-old woman with no previous history of widespread pain, depression, or anxiety developed a diffuse pain syndrome consistent with fibromyalgia after leuprorelin treatment. Her symptoms increased in severity with three successive monthly injections, and persisted for several months (53).

In 47 children treated with depot leuprolide acetate for precocious puberty for 2 years, bone mineral density decreased significantly and markers of bone turnover increased significantly during treatment but were normal for age 2 years after treatment was withdrawn (54).

Of 25 girls with idiopathic precocious puberty, 11 had not been treated and 14 had received leuprolide acetate monthly for at least 1 year; they were compared with 19 healthy controls (55). There was no significant difference between the groups. There was no osteopenia or osteoporosis after therapy.

Since women have a lower initial bone mass than men their fracture risk is higher. Osteoporosis is reversible in premenopausal patients after gonadorelin withdrawal (56). However, the treatment period should be limited to 6 months.

Cross-sectional (57) and longitudinal (58) studies of men with prostate cancer have shown a significant relation between the duration of gonadorelin treatment and bone loss.

Estrogens, etidronate, and parathyroid hormone have been used with partial success to prevent gonadorelin-induced bone loss. In a prospective study of 49 women treated with goserelin and randomized to estradiol plus norethisterone or placebo, bone loss persisted 6 years after stopping therapy, and the hormone replacement therapy had only a minor protective effect (59).

- An 87-year-old man developed progressive proximal limb weakness 1 year after starting leuprolide therapy for prostate cancer (60). Electromyography showed a moderately severe non-inflammatory myopathy without evidence of fiber necrosis or associated biochemical changes. Within 6 months after stopping leuprolide he was able to resume his usual activities.

Three men developed rheumatoid arthritis 1–9 months after starting antiandrogen therapy with either cyproterone acetate or leuprolide acetate (61).

Reproductive system

Ovarian hyperstimulation syndrome (OHSS) affects up to 33% of women undergoing ovulation induction with gonadorelin receptor agonists and gonadotropins given in combination (62), or with gonadotropins alone (63). Gonadotropins are usually withheld if the diagnosis is made before conception (62,64).

OHSS is characterized by cystic ovarian enlargement, increased capillary permeability, and third space fluid accumulation (that is in an extracellular compartment that is not in equilibrium with either the extracellular or intracellular fluid, for example the bowel lumen, subcutaneous tissues, retroperitoneal space, or peritoneal cavity). Risk factors include a previous history of OHSS, age under 30 years (probably because more follicles are available), and polycystic ovary syndrome. Non-pregnant patients usually recover within 14 days with supportive treatment. The severe form (with ascites or pleural effusion and hemoconcentration) occurs in 1–10% of patients (64,65). In critical cases, hypoxemia, renal insufficiency, thromboembolism, and rarely death can occur (66).

- A 29-year-old woman with polycystic ovary syndrome had her first in vitro fertilization cycle of leuprorelin acetate, FSH, and human chorionic gonadotropin (hCG) (67). Within 2 days she complained of abdominal distension, shortness of breath, and abdominal pain. Over the next few days she developed massive ovarian enlargement, ascites, hyponatremia, respiratory failure, and renal insufficiency. This was further complicated by duodenal perforation, probably due to severe physical stress.
- Ovarian hyperstimulation syndrome occurred in a woman with polycystic ovarian syndrome, 3 weeks after an intramuscular injection of leuprorelin acetate for endometriosis (68). She was later given further courses of the drug without this complication.
- A 35-year-old obese woman with a previously undiagnosed pituitary gonadotroph adenoma developed multiple ovarian cysts and abdominal distension after 1 month of leuprolide therapy (69).
- A 32-year-old woman who was not obese developed benign intracranial hypertension in association with ovarian hyperstimulation syndrome after ovulation induction using goserelin, FSH, and hCG (70). The syndrome did not recur during a second pregnancy in which FSH and hCG were not used.

It is unclear which of the hormonal agents used was responsible for this complication in the last case.

Gonadorelin receptor antagonists have been reported to lower the risk of OHSS significantly. A meta-analysis showed that cetrorelix but not ganirelix reduced the incidence of OHSS by 75%, both overall and the severe form (71).

Thromboembolism is a serious complication of OHSS (72–75).

- A previously healthy 34-year-old woman who underwent ovulation induction with leuprorelin acetate and FSH developed abdominal ascites due to OHSS, followed by acute aphasia and right hemiparesis (76). The stroke was caused by a large intracardiac thrombus.

A review identified 54 other reports of thromboembolic disease associated with ovulation induction; 60% were in upper limb veins and two-thirds of the patients had OHSS (77). The mechanism for the increased risk of thrombosis in these patients has not been determined, but hemoconcentration or a hypercoagulable state associated with high estrogen concentrations could be responsible.

One of 66 women randomized to receive goserelin acetate for uterine fibroids withdrew from the study owing to severe pelvic pain (78).

Immunologic

Altered immune function has been reported in several cases associated with gonadorelin agonist therapy. This is possibly related to the initial surge in sex steroids that occurs with these agents, but there is no evidence that this is the mechanism. Cardiac allograft rejection occurred in three men within months of starting gonadorelin therapy for prostate cancer. One died of heart failure, but the other two recovered cardiac function after the gonadorelin agonist was withdrawn (79).

Systemic lupus erythematosus can be exacerbated in the initial gonadotropin-stimulating phase of gonadorelin therapy: in one case this was fatal (80).

Long-Term Effects

Tumorigenicity

Tumor flare occurs in up to 30% of treated patients after the first 4–7 days of gonadorelin therapy, due to an initial surge in gonadotropin concentrations (81). For this reason antiandrogen treatment is often given before gonadorelin in men with prostate cancer. However, despite tumor flare there was no difference in survival in a prospective, multicenter comparison of gonadorelin and surgical oophorectomy in 136 patients (82).

Second-Generation Effects

Pregnancy

Of 34 women who conceived while receiving triptorelin acetate for infertility, five developed gestational diabetes (17%) compared with a background rate of 5% (83). The increased incidence could not be explained by obesity, as only one of these five women had a BMI over 35 kg/m^2; nor could it be explained by polycystic ovary syndrome. Larger studies are required to confirm this finding.

Teratogenicity

Pregnancies have occurred both after low-dose gonadorelin agonist therapy for ovulation induction and after higher-dose therapy for endometriosis or other indications: these have been reviewed in the context of a report of a 36-year-old woman who stopped monthly goserelin injections at 16 weeks of gestation and delivered a healthy girl. Congenital abnormalities have been reported in a few cases, including one child with trisomy 13, one with trisomy 18, and an intrauterine death due to thrombosis; however most pregnancies have had normal outcomes (84).

There was one case of polydactyly with no major defects (3.4%) in the children of 35 women who had conceived while using triptorelin (78). This was probably coincidental.

Drug Administration

Drug formulations

There is no difference in the adverse effects profiles of long-acting or depot formulations compared with shorter-acting analogues used continuously.

Drug dosage regimens

Intermittent courses of gonadotropin analogues for prostate cancer may reduce the frequency of adverse effects. In 95 patients who received 245 cycles of leuprolide acetate and nilutamide for 8 months, testosterone concentrations recovered during the rest periods (61% of cycles) and sexual function improved (47%) (23).

Drug-Drug Interactions

Oral contraceptives

There were mild increases in serum triglyceride and cholesterol concentrations in 13 hirsute women treated with triptorelin and a triphasic oral contraceptive, in a randomized comparison of triptorelin with flutamide + cyproterone acetate (85). Altered lipid profiles have not been described before in patients receiving gonadorelin agonists and oral contraceptives.

Management of adverse drug reactions

The use of gonadorelin analogues is commonly associated with reduced bone mineral density. In 50 premenopausal women with uterine leiomyomas who received leuprolide acetate depot 3.75 mg every 28 days for 18 cycles with raloxifene 60 mg/day, there was a reduction in leiomyoma size with no significant change in bone mineral density or markers of bone metabolism [86].

References

1. Filicori M. Gonadotrophin-releasing hormone agonists. A guide to use and selection. Drugs 1994;48(1):41–58.
2. Takeuchi H, Kobori H, Kikuchi I, Sato Y, Mitsuhashi N. A prospective randomized study comparing endocrinological and clinical effects of two types of GnRH agonists in cases of uterine leiomyomas or endometriosis. J Obstet Gynaecol Res 2000;26(5):325–31.
3. Potosky AL, Knopf K, Clegg LX, Albertsen PC, Stanford JL, Hamilton AS, Gilliland FD, Eley JW, Stephenson RA, Hoffman RM. Quality-of-life outcomes after primary androgen deprivation therapy: results from the Prostate Cancer Outcomes Study. J Clin Oncol 2001;19(17):3750–7.
4. Gleave ME, Goldenberg SL, Chin JL, Warner J, Saad F, Klotz LH, Jewett M, Kassabian V, Chetner M, Dupont C, Van Rensselaer SCanadian Uro-Oncology Group. Randomized comparative study of 3 versus 8-month neoadjuvant hormonal therapy before radical prostatectomy: biochemical and pathological effects. J Urol 2001;166(2):500–6.
5. Palomba S, Orio F, Manguso F, Russo T, Falbo A, Lombardi G, Doldo P, Zullo F. Leuprolide acetate treatment with and without coadministration of tibolone in premenopausal women with menstrual cycle-related irritable bowel syndrome. Fertil Steril 2005;83:1012–20.
6. Yim SF, Lau TK, Sahota DS, Chung TK, Chang AM, Haines CJ. Prospective randomized study of the effect of "add-back" hormone replacement on vascular function during treatment with gonadotropin-releasing hormone agonists. Circulation 1998;98(16):1631–5.
7. Azuma T, Kurimoto S, Mikami K, Oshi M. Interstitial pneumonitis related to leuprorelin acetate and flutamide. J Urol 1999;161(1):221.
8. Heinig J, Coenen-Worch V, Cirkel U. Acute exacerbation of chronic maxillary sinusitis during therapy with nafarelin nasal spray. Eur J Obstet Gynecol Reprod Biol 2001;99(2):266–7.
9. Morsi A, Jamal S, Silverberg JD. Pituitary apoplexy after leuprolide administration for carcinoma of the prostate. Clin Endocrinol (Oxf) 1996;44(1):121–4.
10. Foppiani L, Piredda S, Guido R, Spaziante R, Giusti M. Gonadotropin-releasing hormone-induced partial empty sella clinically mimicking pituitary apoplexy in a woman with a suspected non-secreting macroadenoma. J Endocrinol Invest 2000;23(2):118–21.
11. Eaton HJ, Phillips PJ, Hanieh A, Cooper J, Bolt J, Torpy DJ. Rapid onset of pituitary apoplexy after goserelin implant for prostate cancer: need for heightened awareness. Intern Med J 2001;31(5):313–4.
12. Hiroi N, Ichijo T, Shimojo M, Ueshiba H, Tsuboi K, Miyachi Y. Pituitary apoplexy caused by luteinizing hormone-releasing hormone in prolactin-producing adenoma. Intern Med 2001;40(8):747–50.

13. Matsuura I, Saeki N, Kubota M, Murai H, Yamaura A. Infarction followed by hemorrhage in pituitary adenoma due to endocrine stimulation test. Endocr J 2001;48(4):493–8.

14. Minagawa K, Sueoka H. [Seizure exacerbation by the use of leuprorelin acetate for treatment of central precocious puberty in a female patient with symptomatic localization-related epilepsy.]No To Hattatsu 1999;31(5):466–8.

15. Akaboshi S, Takeshita K. A case of atypical absence seizures induced by leuprolide acetate. Pediatr Neurol 2000;23(3):266–8.

16. Stone P, Hardy J, Huddart R, A'Hern R, Richards M. Fatigue in patients with prostate cancer receiving hormone therapy. Eur J Cancer 2000;36(9):1134–41.

17. Fraunfelder FT, Edwards R. Possible ocular adverse effects associated with leuprolide injections. JAMA 1995;273(10):773–4.

18. Warnock JK, Bundren JC, Morris DW. Depressive symptoms associated with gonadotropin-releasing hormone agonists. Depress Anxiety 1998;7(4):171–7.

19. Moghissi KS, Schlaff WD, Olive DL, Skinner MA, Yin H. Goserelin acetate (Zoladex) with or without hormone replacement therapy for the treatment of endometriosis. Fertil Steril 1998;69(6):1056–62.

20. Mahe V, Nartowski J, Montagnon F, Dumaine A, Gluck N. Psychosis associated with gonadorelin agonist administration. Br J Psychiatry 1999;175:290–1.

21. Green HJ, Pakenham KI, Headley BC, Yaxley J, Nicol DL, Mactaggart PN, Swanson C, Watson RB, Gardiner RA. Altered cognitive function in men treated for prostate cancer with luteinizing hormone-releasing hormone analogues and cyproterone acetate: a randomized controlled trial. BJU Int 2002;90(4):427–32.

22. Heyns CF. Triptorelin in the treatment of prostate cancer. Clinical efficacy and tolerability Am J Cancer 2005;4:169–83.

23. Malone S, Perry G, Segal R, Dahrouge S, Crook J. Long-term side-effects of intermittent androgen suppression therapy in prostate cancer: results of a phase II study. BJU Int 2005;96:514–20.

24. Zinner NR, Bidair M, Ceneno A, Tomera K. Similar frequency of testosterone surge after repeat injections of goserelin (Zoladex) 3.6 mg and 10.8 mg: results of a randomised open-label trial. Urology 2004;64:1177–81.

25. Tanaka T, Niimi H, Matsuo N, Fujieda K, Tachibana K, Ohyama K, Satoh M, Kugu K. Results of long-term follow-up after treatment of central precocious puberty with leuprorelin acetate: evaluation of effectiveness of treatment and recovery of gonadal function. The TAP-144-SR Japanese study group on central precocious puberty. J Clin Endocrinol Metab 2005;90:1371–6.

26. Simons AHM, Roelolofs HJM, Schmoutziguer APE, Roozenburg BJ, van't Hof-van den Brink EP, Schoonderwoerd SA. Early cessation of triptorelin in in vitro fertilization: a double-blind, randomized study. Fertil Steril 2005;83:889–96.

27. Freundl G, Godtke K, Gnoth C, Godehardt E, Kienle E. Steroidal "add-back" therapy in patients treated with GnRH agonists. Gynecol Obstet Invest 1998;(45 Suppl 1):22–30discussion 35.

28. Zhao SZ, Kellerman LA, Francisco CA, Wong JM. Impact of nafarelin and leuprolide for endometriosis on quality of life and subjective clinical measures. J Reprod Med 1999;44(12):1000–6.

29. Tahara M, Matsuoka T, Yokoi T, Tasaka K, Kurachi H, Murata Y. Treatment of endometriosis with a decreasing

30. Morita S, Ueda Y. Graves' disease associated with goserelin acetate. Acta Med Nagasaki 2002;47:79–80.

31. Kasayama S, Miyake S, Samejima Y. Transient thyrotoxicosis and hypothyroidism following administration of the GnRH agonist leuprolide acetate. Endocr J 2000;47(6):783–5.

32. Amino N, Hidaka Y, Takano T, Tatsumi K, Izumi Y, Nakata Y. Possible induction of Graves' disease and painless thyroiditis by gonadotrophin-releasing hormone analogues. Thyroid 2003;8:815–8.

33. Al-Omari WR, Nassir UN, Izzat B. Estrogen "add-back" and lipid profile during GnRH agonist (triptorelin) therapy. Int J Gynaecol Obstet 2001;74(1):61–2.

34. Imai A, Takagi A, Horibe S, Fuseya T, Takagi H, Tamaya T. A gonadotropin-releasing hormone analogue impairs glucose tolerance in a diabetic patient. Eur J Obstet Gynecol Reprod Biol 1998;76(1):121–2.

35. Inaba M, Otani Y, Nishimura K, Takaha N, Okuyama A, Koga M, Azuma J, Kawase I, Kasayama S. Marked hyperglycemia after androgen-deprivation therapy for prostate cancer and usefulness of pioglitazone for its treatment. Metabolism 2005;54(1):55–9.

36. Bogdanos J, Karamanolakis D, Milathianakis C, Repousis P, Tsintavis A, Koutsilieris M. Combined androgen blockade-induced anemia in prostate cancer patients without bone involvement. Anticancer Res 2003;23:1757–62.

37. Strum SB, McDermed JE, Scholz MC, Johnson H, Tisman G. Anaemia associated with androgen deprivation in patients with prostate cancer receiving combined hormone blockade. Br J Urol 1997;79(6):933–41.

38. Maeda H, Arai Y, Aoki Y, Okubo K, Okada T, Ueda Y. Leuprolide causes pure red cell aplasia. J Urol 1998;160(2):501.

39. Bern MM. Coagulopathy, following medical therapy, for carcinoma of the prostate. Haematology 2005;10(1):65–8.

40. Al-Mondhiry H, Manni A, Owen J, Gordon R. Hemostatic effects of hormonal stimulation in patients with metastatic prostate cancer. Am J Hematol 1988;28:141–5.

41. van Hooren HG, Fischl F, Aboulghar MA, Nicollet B, Behre HM, Van der Ven H, Simon A, Kilani Z, Barri PN, Haberle M, Braat DD, Lambalk NEuropean and Middle East Orgalutran Study Group. Comparable clinical outcome using the GnRH antagonist ganirelix or a long protocol of the GnRH agonist triptorelin for the prevention of premature LH surges in women undergoing ovarian stimulation. Hum Reprod 2001;16(4):644–51.

42. Fluker M, Grifo J, Leader A, Levy M, Meldrum D, Muasher SJ, Rinehart J, Rosenwaks Z, Scott RT Jr, Schoolcraft W, Shapiro DBNorth American Ganirelix Study Group. Efficacy and safety of ganirelix acetate versus leuprolide acetate in women undergoing controlled ovarian hyperstimulation. Fertil Steril 2001;75(1):38–45.

43. Kono T, Ishii M, Taniguchi S. Intranasal buserelin acetate-induced pigmented roseola-like eruption. Br J Dermatol 2000;143(3):658–9.

44. Hirashima N, Shinogi T, Sakashita N, Narisawa Y. A case of cutaneous injury induced by the subcutaneous injection of leuprolide acetate. Nishinihon J Dermatol 2001;63:384–6.

45. Yamano Z, Kusuda Y, Hara S, Shimogaki H, Hamani G. Cutaneous epithelioid granulomas caused by subcutaneous infusion of leuprorelin acetate. A case report. Acta Urol Japan 2004;50:199–202.

46. Yasukawa K, Sawamura D, Sugawara H, Kato N. Leuprorelin acetate granulomas: case reports and review of the literature. Br J Dermatol 2005;152:1045–7.

47. Tonini G, Marioni S, Forleo V, Rustico M. Local reactions to luteinizing hormone releasing hormone analog therapy. J Pediatr 1995;126:159–60.

48. Fogelman I. Gonadotropin-releasing hormone agonists and the skeleton. Fertil Steril 1992;57(4):715–24.

49. Stoch SA, Parker RA, Chen L, Bubley G, Ko YJ, Vincelette A, Greenspan SL. Bone loss in men with prostate cancer treated with gonadotropin-releasing hormone agonists. J Clin Endocrinol Metab 2001;86(6):2787–91.

50. Kiratli BJ, Srinivas S, Perkash I, Terris MK. Progressive decrease in bone density over 10 years of androgen deprivation therapy in patients with prostate cancer. Urology 2001;57(1):127–32.

51. Smith MR, McGovern FJ, Zietman AL, Fallon MA, Hayden DL, Schoenfeld DA, Kantoff PW, Finkelstein JS. Pamidronate to prevent bone loss during androgen-deprivation therapy for prostate cancer. N Engl J Med 2001;345(13):948–55.

52. Diamond TH, Winters J, Smith A, De Souza P, Kersley JH, Lynch WJ, Bryant C. The antiosteoporotic efficacy of intravenous pamidronate in men with prostate carcinoma receiving combined androgen blockade: a double blind, randomized, placebo-controlled crossover study. Cancer 2001;92(6):1444–50.

53. Toussirot E, Wendling D. Fibromyalgia developed after administration of gonadotrophin-releasing hormone analogue. Clin Rheumatol 2001;20(2):150–2.

54. van der Sluis IM, Boot AM, Krenning EP, Drop SL, de Muinck Keizer-Schrama SM. Longitudinal follow-up of bone density and body composition in children with precocious or early puberty before, during and after cessation of GnRH agonist therapy. J Clin Endocrinol Metab 2002;87(2):506–12.

55. Unal O, Berberoglu M, Evliyaoglu O, Adiyaman P, Aycan Z, Ocal G. Effects of bone mineral density of gonadotropin releasing hormone analogs used in the treatment of central precocious puberty. J Pediatr Endocrinol Metab 2003;16:407–11.

56. Paoletti AM, Serra GG, Cagnacci A, Vacca AM, Guerriero S, Solla E, Melis GB. Spontaneous reversibility of bone loss induced by gonadotropin-releasing hormone analogue treatment. Fertil Steril 1996;65(4):707–10.

57. Wei JT, Gross M, Jaffe CA, Gravlin K, Lahaie M, Faerber GJ, Cooney KA. Androgen deprivation therapy for prostate cancer results in significant loss of bone density. Urology 1999;54(4):607–11.

58. Daniell HW, Dunn SR, Ferguson DW, Lomas G, Niazi Z, Stratte PT. Progressive osteoporosis during androgen deprivation therapy for prostate cancer. J Urol 2000;163(1):181–6.

59. Pierce SJ, Gazvani MR, Farquharson RG. Long-term use of gonadotropin-releasing hormone analogues and hormone replacement therapy in the management of endometriosis: a randomized trial with a 6-year follow-up. Fertil Steril 2000;74(5):964–8.

60. Van Gerpen JA, McKinley KL. Leuprolide-induced myopathy. J Am Geriatr Soc 2002;50(10):1746.

61. Pope JE, Joneja M, Hong P. Anti-androgen treatment of prostatic carcinoma may be a risk factor for development of rheumatoid arthritis. J Rheumatol 2002;29(11):2459–62.

62. Whelan JG 3rd, Vlahos NF. The ovarian hyperstimulation syndrome. Fertil Steril 2000;73(5):883–96.

63. Mancini A, Milardi D, Di Pietro ML, Giacchi E, Spagnolo AG, Di Donna V, De Marinis L, Jensen L. A case of forearm amputation after ovarian stimulation for in vitro fertilization–embryo transfer. Fertil Steril 2001;76(1):198–200.

64. Beerendonk CC, van Dop PA, Braat DD, Merkus JM. Ovarian hyperstimulation syndrome: facts and fallacies. Obstet Gynecol Surv 1998;53(7):439–49.

65. Chillik C, Young E, Gogorza S, Estofan D, Neuspiller N, Antunes N Jr, Borges E Jr, Vantman D, Fabres C, Montoya JM, Madero JI, Gutierrez-Najar A, Bronfenmajer S, Kovacs A, Kroeze S, Out HJLatin-American Puregon IVF Study Group. A double-blind clinical trial comparing a fixed daily dose of 150 and 250 IU of recombinant follicle-stimulating hormone in women undergoing in vitro fertilization. Fertil Steril 2001;76(5):950–6.

66. Abramov Y, Elchalal U, Schenker JG. Febrile morbidity in severe and critical ovarian hyperstimulation syndrome: a multicentre study. Hum Reprod 1998;13(11):3128–31.

67. Uhler ML, Budinger GR, Gabram SG, Zinaman MJ. Perforated duodenal ulcer associated with ovarian hyperstimulation syndrome: Case Report. Hum Reprod 2001;16(1):174–6.

68. Jirecek S, Nagele F, Huber JC, Wenzl R. Ovarian hyperstimulation syndrome caused by GnRH-analogue treatment without gonadotropin therapy in a patient with polycystic ovarian syndrome. Acta Obstet Gynecol Scand 1998;77(9):940–1.

69. Castelbaum AJ, Bigdeli H, Post KD, Freedman MF, Snyder PJ. Exacerbation of ovarian hyperstimulation by leuprolide reveals a gonadotroph adenoma. Fertil Steril 2002;78(6):1311–3.

70. Lesny P, Maguiness SD, Hay DM, Robinson J, Clarke CE, Killick SR. Ovarian hyperstimulation syndrome and benign intracranial hypertension in pregnancy after in-vitro fertilization and embryo transfer: case report. Hum Reprod 1999;14(8):1953–5.

71. Ludwig M, Katalinic A, Diedrich K. Use of GnRH antagonists in ovarian stimulation for assisted reproductive technologies compared to the long protocol. Meta-analysis. Arch Gynecol Obstet 2001;265(4):175–82.

72. Ludwig M, Tolg R, Richardt G, Katus HA, Diedrich K. Myocardial infarction associated with ovarian hyperstimulation syndrome. JAMA 1999;282(7):632–3.

73. Belaen B, Geerinckx K, Vergauwe P, Thys J. Internal jugular vein thrombosis after ovarian stimulation. Hum Reprod 2001;16(3):510–2.

74. Loret de Mola JR, Kiwi R, Austin C, Goldfarb JM. Subclavian deep vein thrombosis associated with the use of recombinant follicle-stimulating hormone (Gonal-F) complicating mild ovarian hyperstimulation syndrome. Fertil Steril 2000;73(6):1253–6.

75. Yoshii F, Ooki N, Shinohara Y, Uehara K, Mochimaru F. Multiple cerebral infarctions associated with ovarian hyperstimulation syndrome. Neurology 1999;53(1):225–7.

76. Worrell GA, Wijdicks EF, Eggers SD, Phan T, Damario MA, Mullany CJ. Ovarian hyperstimulation syndrome with ischemic stroke due to an intracardiac thrombus. Neurology 2001;57(7):1342–4.

77. Stewart JA, Hamilton PJ, Murdoch AP. Thromboembolic disease associated with ovarian stimulation and assisted conception techniques. Hum Reprod 1997;12(10):2167–73.

78. Donnez J, Vivancos BH, Kudela M, Audebert A, Jadoul P. A randomised placebo-controlled, dose-ranging trial

comparing fulvestrant with goserelin in premenopausal patients with uterine fibroids awaiting hysterectomy. Fertil Steril 2003;79:1380–9.

79. Schofield RS, Hill JA, McGinn CJ, Aranda JM. Hormone therapy in men and risk of cardiac allograft rejection. J Heart Lung Transplant 2002;21(4):493–5.

80. Casoli P, Tumiati B, La Sala G. Fatal exacerbation of systemic lupus erythematosus after induction of ovulation. J Rheumatol 1997;24(8):1639–40.

81. Mahler C. Is disease flare a problem? Cancer 1993;72(Suppl 12):3799–802.

82. Taylor CW, Green S, Dalton WS, Martino S, Rector D, Ingle JN, Robert NJ, Budd GT, Paradelo JC, Natale RB, Bearden JD, Mailliard JA, Osborne CK. Multicenter randomized clinical trial of goserelin versus surgical ovariectomy in premenopausal patients with receptor-positive metastatic breast cancer: an intergroup study. J Clin Oncol 1998;16(3):994–9.

83. Mayer A, Lunenfeld E, Wiznitzer A, Har-vardi I, Bentov Y, Levitas E. Increased prevalence of gestational diabetes mellitus in in vitro fertilization pregnancies inadvertently conceived during treatment with long-acting triptorelin acetate. Fertil Steril 2005;84:789–92.

84. Jimenez-Gordo AM, Espinosa E, Zamora P, Feliu J, Rodriguez-Salas N, Gonzalez-Baron M. Pregnancy in a breast cancer patient treated with a LHRH analogue at ablative doses. Breast 2000;9(2):110–2.

85. Pazos F, Escobar-Morreale HF, Balsa J, Sancho JM, Varela C. Prospective randomized study comparing the long-acting gonadotropin-releasing hormone agonist triptorelin, flutamide, and cyproterone acetate, used in combination with an oral contraceptive, in the treatment of hirsutism. Fertil Steril 1999;71(1):122–8.

86. Palomba S, Orio F Jr, Russo T, Falbo A, Cascella T, Doldo P, Nappi C, Mastrantonio P, Zullo F. Long-term effectiveness and safety of GnRH agonist plus raloxifene administration in women with uterine leiomyomas. Hum Reprod 2004;6:1308–14.

Gonadorelin antagonists

General Information

The gonadorelin antagonists include abarelix, cetrorelix, degarelix, detirelix, ganirelix, iturelix, prazarelix, ramorelix, and teverelix (all rINNs).

Gonadorelin agonists suppress the release of gonadotropin after an initial surge: pituitary suppression takes up to 2 weeks to develop. Competitive antagonists at gonadorelin receptors cause immediate inhibition of gonadotropin secretion without down-regulating the receptor. This class of agents would therefore be preferable to gonadorelin agonists when a rapid clinical effect is desired, for example in controlled ovarian stimulation.

Early gonadorelin antagonists were of low potency and tended to cause histamine release (1). However, ganirelix and cetrorelix are better tolerated (1,2). They do not share the lipophilic and histamine-releasing properties of earlier generation gonadorelin antagonists and neither do they lead to depot formation. There appears to be a narrow therapeutic margin in ovarian stimulation

protocols. Ganirelix concentrations correlate with body weight, and it has been suggested that the dose should be adjusted to weight to maximize pregnancy rates (3). The adverse effects of ganirelix are usually mild and include minor injection site reactions, mild nausea, and malaise (1).

The adverse effects of cetrorelix and ganirelix have been reviewed (4). Those most commonly reported are headache, fatigue, and injection site reactions. In the development of LHRH antagonists one problem was their ability to induce systemic histamine release; however, structural changes solved this problem (5) and no symptoms attributed to systemic histamine release have been reported so far.

Organs and Systems

Endocrine

In a small, controlled study of 10 healthy men, cetrorelix increased concentrations of insulin, leptin, and apolipoprotein A-I compared with placebo (6). The clinical significance of these findings has yet to be determined.

Skin

Local injection reactions are common and probably dose-related. In an open study of cetrorelix in its lowest effective dose of 0.25 mg/day, 3 of 346 women described local reactions (7). In another study of 154 women, 115 of whom were randomized to one 3 mg dose of cetrorelix, 25% had transitory redness or itching at the injection site (2). In a multicenter European study of 463 women randomized to ganirelix and 238 to buserelin, 17% of those given ganirelix had moderate skin redness, bruising, pain, or itching 1 hour after subcutaneous injection; this had mostly disappeared after 4 hours (8).

Five of 168 men with prostate cancer treated with abarelix had urticaria and pruritus, which resolved without treatment (9).

Reproductive system

Ovarian hyperstimulation syndrome is far less common with gonadorelin receptor antagonists than agonists in induction of ovulation (2,7). Hot flushes are rare, in contrast to gonadorelin receptor agonists: in a prospective, uncontrolled study of 346 women given cetrorelix, there was only one case of hot flushes (7).

References

1. Gillies PS, Faulds D, Balfour JA, Perry CM. Ganirelix. Drugs 2000;59(1):107–11.

2. Olivennes F, Belaisch-Allart J, Emperaire JC, Dechaud H, Alvarez S, Moreau L, Nicollet B, Zorn JR, Bouchard P, Frydman R. Prospective, randomized, controlled study of in vitro fertilization-embryo transfer with a single dose of a luteinizing hormone-releasing hormone (LH-RH) antagonist (cetrorelix) or a depot formula of an LH-RH agonist (triptorelin). Fertil Steril 2000;73(2):314–20.

3. Trew GH. Optimizing gonadotrophin-releasing hormone antagonist protocols. Hum Fertil (Camb) 2002;5(1):G13–6.
4. Griesinger G, Felberbaum RE, Schultze-Mosgau A, Diedrich K. Gonadotropin-releasing hormone antagonists for assisted reproductive techniques. Are there clinical differences between agents? Drugs 2004;64:563–75.
5. Reissman T, Schally AV, Bouchard P, Riethmuller H, Engel J. The LHRH antagonist cetrorelix: a review. Hum Reprod Update 2000;6:322–31.
6. Buchter D, Behre HM, Kliesch S, Chirazi A, Nieschlag E, Assmann G, von Eckardstein A. Effects of testosterone suppression in young men by the gonadotropin releasing hormone antagonist cetrorelix on plasma lipids, lipolytic enzymes, lipid transfer proteins, insulin, and leptin. Exp Clin Endocrinol Diabetes 1999;107(8):522–9.
7. Felberbaum RE, Albano C, Ludwig M, Riethmuller-Winzen H, Grigat M, Devroey P, Diedrich K. Ovarian stimulation for assisted reproduction with HMG and concomitant midcycle administration of the GnRH antagonist cetrorelix according to the multiple dose protocol: a prospective uncontrolled phase III study. Hum Reprod 2000;15(5):1015–20.
8. Borm G, Mannaerts BThe European Orgalutran Study Group. Treatment with the gonadotrophin-releasing hormone antagonist ganirelix in women undergoing ovarian stimulation with recombinant follicle stimulating hormone is effective, safe and convenient: results of a controlled, randomized, multicentre trial. Hum Reprod 2000;15(7):1490–8.
9. Trachtenberg J, Gittleman M, Steidle C, Barzell W, Friedel W, Pessis D, Fotheringham N, Campion M, Garnick MBAbarelix Study Group. A phase 3, multicenter, open label, randomized study of abarelix versus leuprolide plus daily antiandrogen in men with prostate cancer. J Urol 2002;167(4):1670–4.

Melatonin

General Information

Melatonin (*N*-acetyl-5-methoxytryptamine) is a neurohormone secreted by the pineal gland from the amino acid precursor L-tryptophan. Its endogenous secretion is photosensitive and has a circadian rhythm—plasma melatonin concentrations are highest at night in both diurnal and nocturnal animals, and fall with age (1). The nocturnal melatonin peak coincides with a drop in body temperature and increased sleepiness in healthy humans. Oral melatonin has a short half-life (30–50 minutes) and extensive first-pass metabolism. Its clearance is reduced in severe liver disease (2).

Uses

Melatonin has been promoted as a treatment for conditions ranging from jet lag to cancer (1,3–5) and is sometimes used for sleep induction (1) and shift work (6). Because melatonin is present in small amounts in some foods, it is licensed as a nutritional supplement in the USA.

General adverse effects

Acute exogenous administration of melatonin causes sedation, fatigue, self-reported vigor, confusion, and a reduction in body temperature in healthy subjects. The effects of chronic treatment have not been studied, and adverse effects have not been systematically reported.

Timing is critical for melatonin to be effective: if it is given at the wrong time for sleep disorders or jet lag, it can cause increased daytime sleepiness (5,7) and worsened mental performance (8). Drowsiness and a small fall in body temperature are commonly reported effects (9), particularly after daytime administration, when endogenous concentrations of melatonin are low.

Organs and Systems

Cardiovascular

There was an increase in blood pressure throughout 24 hours in a double-blind, placebo-controlled, crossover study in 47 hypertensive patients who were also taking nifedipine (10). This finding differs from other studies in which melatonin had a mild hypotensive effect (11) and may indicate an interaction between melatonin and nifedipine. Tachycardia, chest pain, and cardiac dysrhythmias have also been reported, although the relation to melatonin was not clearly established (5).

Nervous system

Four of six children with pre-existing severe neurological disorders had increased seizure activity within 2 weeks of starting oral melatonin 5 mg at bedtime (12). Seizure frequency returned to baseline after treatment was stopped, and increased again after rechallenge with melatonin 1 mg. A convulsion during melatonin treatment, which recurred when medication was continued, has been reported to the WHO database but not published (5). Headache, which recovered after melatonin was withdrawn, has also been reported in a few cases (5).

Dyskinesia and akathisia have been reported after withdrawal of long-term melatonin (13).

- A 22-year-old woman of Ashkenazi origin, with spastic diplegia resulting from cerebral palsy and severe mental retardation, had insomnia for 6 years. She had taken melatonin 5 mg each night at 8 p.m. for the past year, with a good response. However, 1 week after melatonin was stopped, because of repeated vomiting, she gradually developed involuntary lip-smacking movements and tongue protrusion, with extreme restlessness, moaning, and shouting. These symptoms continued for 2 weeks, accompanied by marked worsening of insomnia. She was restless, could not sit still, and was shouting, moaning, and grunting. Melatonin was reintroduced in gradually increasing doses, and 2 days after a dose of 5 mg was reached, the involuntary movements disappeared and her agitated state and insomnia improved. A month later, another episode of abdominal pain and vomiting made her discontinue melatonin again. Within 2 days she developed identical involuntary lip and tongue movements and akathisia. Melatonin 5 mg was re-administered and all her symptoms disappeared by the next day. No antiemetic drugs were given during these episodes.

This case raises an important question regarding the dopamine-blocking effect of melatonin. Like dopamine receptor antagonists, melatonin should be used with care, because of the risk of tardive dyskinesia, which has serious morbidity and a low remission rate. Melatonin should be used with special caution in patients with organic brain damage.

Asperger's disease is a rare neuropsychiatric disorder classified among the spectrum of autistic disorders. Its cause is unknown, but it is thought to be associated with genetic and neurodevelopment factors (14). Sleep disturbances are common in patients with Asperger's disease. Although these sleep problems often persist and can significantly impair the child's daytime well-being, no treatment studies have been reported. In an open trial, the effectiveness of melatonin 3 mg/day for 14 days was studied in 15 children (13 boys) with Asperger's disease aged 6-17 years (15). Sleep patterns improved in all the children, and half of them had excellent responses. However, one child suffered from excessive tiredness, dizziness, and headache. This was surprising, because in another study 100 children with sleep-related problems took melatonin with no adverse effects (16).

Sensory systems

- Loss of visual acuity, reduced color vision, and altered light adaptation developed in a 42-year-old woman 2 weeks after she started to take a high protein diet and melatonin 1 mg/day (17). She had also been taking sertraline for the past 4 years. Her vision improved within 2 months of stopping the melatonin and the high protein diet.

This patient's retinal melatonin concentration may have been boosted by increased serotonin (a melatonin precursor) from the effect of sertraline, the high protein intake, and the exogenous melatonin.

Retinal damage has been briefly reported as an adverse effect of melatonin (9).

Psychological, psychiatric

A severely depressed woman developed a mixed affective state after taking melatonin for 7 days in a clinical trial (18). Confusion, hallucinations, and paranoia temporally related to melatonin have also been described (5).

Endocrine

There was suppression of endogenous melatonin secretion in two of five patients with bipolar disorder after 12 weeks of treatment with high-dose melatonin (10 mg/day) (19).

Gynecomastia has been attributed to melatonin (8,20).

- A 56-year-old man complained of painful asymmetrical breast enlargement, gradually developing over 3 months (20). He had had amyotrophic lateral sclerosis for 3 years and had taken riluzole 50 mg bd for 2 years and melatonin for 1.5 years (1 mg/day during the first year then gradually increasing to 2 mg/day). He had bilateral painful gynecomastia and homogeneously enlarged breasts. There was no galactorrhea. There were no signs or symptoms of other endocrine dysfunction. Withdrawal of melatonin resulted in complete regression of the gynecomastia within a few weeks.

This is a warning against the uncontrolled use of apparently innocuous substances. The absence of adverse effects in healthy people taking melatonin for various reasons does not mean complete safety, particularly in people who are unwell.

Metabolism

Impaired insulin-dependent glucose utilization occurred in a double-blind study of postmenopausal women given melatonin 1 mg in the morning (21). The authors also cited isolated reports of increased blood glucose in healthy individuals and in two men with Parkinson's disease taking melatonin.

Liver

- Autoimmune hepatitis was diagnosed in a previously healthy, 39-year-old woman 4 weeks after she started to take melatonin 3 mg at bedtime (22).

It is unclear whether this was a direct hepatotoxic effect of melatonin (or a contaminant), or if hepatitis was caused indirectly by an immunomodulatory mechanism.

Skin

Vesicular plaques and erosions developed on the penis in two men after they took melatonin for jet lag: one man had two such episodes 4 months apart (23). The lesions resolved within 10 days without any sequelae, and recurred within 8 hours of rechallenge.

Reproductive system

Melatonin affects reproduction in seasonally breeding animals. In humans, findings of increased endogenous melatonin in hypogonadism and low concentrations in precocious puberty imply an interaction between melatonin and gonadotropins; however, data on the effects of exogenous melatonin are limited (1). In a randomized study in 16 women, melatonin enhanced LH and FSH responses to submaximal GnRH stimuli in the follicular but not the luteal phase of the menstrual cycle (24).

A very high dose of melatonin (300 mg) partially inhibited ovulation in healthy young women: norethisterone enhanced the effect (25).

Immunologic

There has been a single report of a subject in a controlled trial of melatonin who had difficulty in swallowing and breathing within 20 minutes of taking melatonin 0.5 mg.

The symptoms resolved without treatment after 45 minutes and recurred in a milder form after rechallenge (26).

Long-Term Effects

Drug withdrawal

There was suppression of endogenous melatonin secretion in two of five patients with bipolar disorder after 12 weeks of treatment with high-dose melatonin (10 mg/day) (19). One woman developed an unentrained sleep–wake cycle after melatonin was withdrawn (not previously a feature of her illness), which persisted for several months.

Involuntary movements of the lip and tongue, restlessness, and insomnia developed twice when chronic melatonin therapy was abruptly withdrawn in a young woman with cerebral palsy: these symptoms resolved when melatonin was restarted, but did not recur with gradual withdrawal over 2 months (13). This again suggests that endogenous melatonin secretion is suppressed after chronic use.

Drug Administration

Drug contamination

The reliability and consistency of commercial melatonin has been questioned (3). One group analysed three commercial melatonin formulations and identified analogues of the contaminant of L-tryptophan compounds implicated in an epidemic of eosinophilia–myalgia syndrome in the 1980s (27). There have been no reports of this condition associated with melatonin consumption, but food supplements are not required to comply with the same manufacturing and monitoring quality control standards as drugs.

Drug overdose

Melatonin overdose has been reported in three patients, all of whom were also taking psychotropic drugs. Drug interactions with antidepressants may have played a part in the resulting symptoms, which were not reported in cancer trials using higher doses of melatonin (1).

- A 73-year-old woman developed an acute psychosis after taking melatonin 30 mg as well as her usual fluoxetine (28).
- A 14-year-old girl became drowsy and dizzy and complained of blurred vision after taking melatonin 24–36 mg as well as her usual trazodone and paroxetine (29).
- A 66-year old man became lethargic, confused, and disoriented after taking melatonin 24 mg with his usual amitriptyline and chlordiazepoxide (30).

All three patients recovered fully within 24 hours without specific treatment.

A 14-year-old girl with major depressive disorder had drowsiness, dizziness, blurred vision, and confusion after taking an overdose of melatonin (24-36 mg) (31).

The Texas Poison Center Network has received reports of 779 cases of exposure to melatonin during 1998–2003 (32). The annual number of cases was 114–146 with no annual trend. Melatonin was the only reported exposure in 644 (83%) of the cases. Of the patients whose ages were known, 59% were under 6 years, 14% were 6–19 years, and 27% were over 19 years. The majority of pre-school age patients were male, while more of the older patients were female. Most of the exposures to melatonin among children under 6 years were unintentional, while most of the exposures among the older age groups were intentional. Exposure was more likely to occur in the patient's home than anywhere else. Of the cases with a known outcome, the proportion with at least minor effects rose with increasing age. There were no deaths. The most common effects among the 394 cases during 2000–2003 in whom melatonin was the only exposure were drowsiness or lethargy, which affected 58 (18%). No other categories of clinical effects were reported in more than four cases. These included chest pain, tachycardia, abdominal pain, nausea, vomiting, hypothermia, agitation/irritability, ataxia, confusion, vertigo/dizziness, headache, slurred speech, and tremors.

Drug–Drug Interactions

Nifedipine

Melatonin has a hypotensive effect in both normotensive and hypertensive subjects. In a double-blind, randomized, crossover study designed to evaluate whether evening ingestion of melatonin potentiates the antihypertensive effect of nifedipine monotherapy in 50 patients with well-controlled mild to moderate hypertension aged 38–65 years (28 men, 22 women), there was a surprising significant increase in blood pressure and heart rate throughout 24 hours (33). The authors suggested that there was competition between melatonin and nifedipine, with impairment of the antihypertensive efficacy of the calcium channel blocker.

SSRIs

Fluvoxamine increases the systemic availability of oral melatonin, probably by reducing its first-pass clearance (34). In a crossover study in seven healthy subjects, serum melatonin concentrations were increased by fluvoxamine but not citalopram (35). In another study fluoxetine, paroxetine, citalopram, imipramine, and desipramine did not affect the biotransformation of melatonin at therapeutic concentrations in vitro (36).

Warfarin

There have been several reports of altered prothrombin time in patients taking warfarin and melatonin. In some cases bleeding or purpura was the presenting symptom, despite a reduced prothrombin time (5).

References

1. Brzezinski A. Melatonin in humans. N Engl J Med 1997;336(3):186–95.
2. Lane EA, Moss HB. Pharmacokinetics of melatonin in man: first pass hepatic metabolism. J Clin Endocrinol Metab 1985;61(6):1214–6.
3. Caley CF. Dehydroepiandrosterone and melatonin: two neurohormones. J Pharm Pract 1999;12:251–65.
4. Avery D, Lenz M, Landis C. Guidelines for prescribing melatonin. Ann Med 1998;30(1):122–30.
5. Herxheimer A, Petrie KJ. Melatonin for preventing and treating jet lag. Cochrane Database Syst Rev 2001;(1):CD001520.
6. Lamberg L. Melatonin potentially useful, but safety, efficacy remain uncertain. JAMA 1996;276:1011–4.
7. Middleton BA, Stone BM, Arendt J. Melatonin and fragmented sleep patterns. Lancet 1996;348(9026):551–2.
8. Rogers NL, Phan O, Kennaway DJ, Dawson D. Effect of daytime oral melatonin administration on neurobehavioral performance in humans. J Pineal Res 1998;25(1):47–53.
9. Lamberg L. Melatonin potentially useful but safety, efficacy remain uncertain. JAMA 1996;276(13):1011–4.
10. Lusardi P, Piazza E, Fogari R. Cardiovascular effects of melatonin in hypertensive patients well controlled by nifedipine: a 24-hour study. Br J Clin Pharmacol 2000;49(5):423–7.
11. Arangino S, Cagnacci A, Angiolucci M, Vacca AM, Longu G, Volpe A, Melis GB. Effects of melatonin on vascular reactivity, catecholamine levels, and blood pressure in healthy men. Am J Cardiol 1999;83(9):1417–9.
12. Sheldon SH. Pro-convulsant effects of oral melatonin in neurologically disabled children. Lancet 1998;351(9111):1254.
13. Giladi N, Shabtai H. Melatonin-induced withdrawal emergent dyskinesia and akathisia. Mov Disord 1999;14(2):381–2.
14. Gilberg C. Disorders of empathy: autism and autism spectrum disorders (including childhood onset schizophrenia). In: Clinical Child Neuropsychiatry. Gillberg C (editor). Cambridge: Cambridge University Press, 1995:54–111.
15. Paavonen EJ, Nieminen-von Wendt T, Vanhala R, Aronen ET, Von Wendt L. Effectiveness of melatonin in the treatment of sleep disturbances in children with Asperger disorder. J Child Adolesc Psychopharmacol 2003;13:83–95.
16. Jan JE, O'Donnell ME. Use of melatonin in the treatment of paediatric sleep disorders. J Pineal Res 1996;21:193–9.
17. Lehman NL, Johnson LN. Toxic optic neuropathy after concomitant use of melatonin, Zoloft, and a high-protein diet. J Neuroophthalmol 1999;19(4):232–4.
18. Dalton EJ, Rotondi D, Levitan RD, Kennedy SH, Brown GM. Use of slow-release melatonin in treatment-resistant depression. J Psychiatry Neurosci 2000;25(1):48–52.
19. Leibenluft E, Feldman-Naim S, Turner EH, Wehr TA, Rosenthal NE. Effects of exogenous melatonin administration and withdrawal in five patients with rapid-cycling bipolar disorder. J Clin Psychiatry 1997;58(9):383–8.
20. De Bleecker JL, Lamont BH, Verstraete AG, Schelfhout VJ. Melatonin and painful gynecomastia. Neurology 1999;53(2):435–6.
21. Cagnacci A, Arangino S, Renzi A, Paoletti AM, Melis GB, Cagnacci P, Volpe A. Influence of melatonin administration on glucose tolerance and insulin sensitivity of postmenopausal women. Clin Endocrinol (Oxf) 2001;54(3):339–46.
22. Hong YG, Riegler JL. Is melatonin associated with the development of autoimmune hepatitis? J Clin Gastroenterol 1997;25(1):376–8.
23. Bardazzi F, Placucci F, Neri I, D'Antuono A, Patrizi A. Fixed drug eruption due to melatonin. Acta Derm Venereol 1998;78(1):69–70.
24. Cagnacci A, Paoletti AM, Soldani R, Orru M, Maschio E, Melis GB. Melatonin enhances the luteinizing hormone and follicle-stimulating hormone responses to gonadotropin-releasing hormone in the follicular, but not in the luteal, menstrual phase. J Clin Endocrinol Metab 1995;80(4):1095–9.
25. Voordouw BC, Euser R, Verdonk RE, Alberda BT, de Jong FH, Drogendijk AC, Fauser BC, Cohen M. Melatonin and melatonin–progestin combinations alter pituitary–ovarian function in women and can inhibit ovulation. J Clin Endocrinol Metab 1992;74(1):108–17.
26. Spitzer RL, Terman M, Williams JB, Terman JS, Malt UF, Singer F, Lewy AJ. Jet lag: clinical features, validation of a new syndrome-specific scale, and lack of response to melatonin in a randomized, double-blind trial. Am J Psychiatry 1999;156(9):1392–6.
27. Williamson BL, Tomlinson AJ, Naylor S, Gleich GJ. Contaminants in commercial preparations of melatonin. Mayo Clin Proc 1997;72(11):1094–5.
28. Force RW, Hansen L, Bedell M. Psychotic episode after melatonin. Ann Pharmacother 1997;31(11):1408.
29. Balentine J, Hagman J. More on melatonin. J Am Acad Child Adolesc Psychiatry 1997;36(8):1013.
30. Holliman BJ, Chyka PA. Problems in assessment of acute melatonin overdose. South Med J 1997;90(4):451–3.
31. Balentine J, Hagman J. More on melatonin. J Am Acad Child Adolesc Psychiatry 1997;36:1013–8.
32. Forrester MB. Melatonin exposures reported to Texas Poison Centers in 1998–2003. Vet Hum Toxicol 2004;46:345–6.
33. Lusardi P, Piazza E, Fogari R. Cardiovascular effects of melatonin in hypertensive patients well controlled by nifedipine: a 24-hour study. Br J Clin Pharmacol 2000;49(5):423–7.
34. Hartter S, Grozinger M, Weigmann H, Roschke J, Hiemke C. Increased bioavailability of oral melatonin after fluvoxamine coadministration. Clin Pharmacol Ther 2000;67(1):1–6.
35. von Bahr C, Ursing C, Yasui N, Tybring G, Bertilsson L, Rojdmark S. Fluvoxamine but not citalopram increases serum melatonin in healthy subjects—an indication that cytochrome P450 CYP1A2 and CYP2C19 hydroxylate melatonin. Eur J Clin Pharmacol 2000;56(2):123–7.
36. Hartter S, Wang X, Weigmann H, Friedberg T, Arand M, Oesch F, Hiemke C. Differential effects of fluvoxamine and other antidepressants on the biotransformation of melatonin. J Clin Psychopharmacol 2001;21(2):167–74.

Oxytocin and analogues

General Information

Oxytocin is a hypothalamic nonapeptide that selectively stimulates the smooth muscle of the uterus and mammary glands. It is used in the induction or augmentation of labor and to prevent postpartum hemorrhage, and is well tolerated and effective in a wide range of infusion rates and concentrations. Contraindications to its use include placenta previa or vasa previa, a previous classical uterine incision, pelvic structural deformities, and an abnormal fetal presentation. Large fetal size and high maternal parity are relative contraindications. Prior non-classical cesarean delivery should not preclude oxytocin therapy.

Uterine contractions and fetal heart rate should be monitored during oxytocin administration (SEDA-13, 1310) (1,2). There is no significant increase in uterine complications or in fetal morbidity or mortality in women with a previous cesarean section, although oxytocin-treated patients had a higher rate of failed trial of labor for reasons that are unclear (3). Oxytocin is structurally similar to vasopressin, and like the latter has water-retaining properties when used in pharmacological doses.

Oxytocin is in common use during induction of labor and in the third stage of labor to prevent uterine atony and postpartum hemorrhage. Carbetocin, a synthetic analogue with a half-life 4–10 times longer than the native hormone, has been studied in trials; both agents cause a small transient fall in blood pressure (less than 4 mmHg) (4). Common mild adverse effects of both drugs include headache, flushing, a feeling of warmth, a metallic taste, and abdominal pain.

Organs and Systems

Cardiovascular

Tachycardia and a fall in blood pressure are common and usually short-lived after oxytocin administration during labor. There has been one reported maternal death after a hypovolemic woman was given a bolus dose of oxytocin 10 units (5).

In 34 women undergoing cesarean section at full term under spinal anesthesia, heart rate and cardiac output increased significantly within 2 minutes of the rapid administration of either 5 or 10 units of oxytocin, with an associated 10 mmHg fall in mean arterial pressure in those who received 10 units (6). There were significant ST segment changes in 11 of 26 women undergoing cesarean section, with raised concentrations of troponin I in two; however, the relationship to oxytocin administration was not clear in this report (7).

- A previously fit 19-year-old woman had severe ST segment depression and increased troponin concentrations after a bolus dose of oxytocin 5 units (8).

Ventricular tachycardia has been reported in two patients with pre-existing prolongation of the QT interval, immediately after oxytocin was begun (9).

Fluid balance

Fluid retention causing severe hyponatremia and convulsions has been observed in neonates after administration of oxytocin and salt-poor fluids to the mother during labor.

Acute water intoxication has produced maternal cerebral edema and convulsions in under 50 reported cases, both with intravenous and intranasal administration (10). The risk is higher in women given high doses of the drug in combination with salt-poor intravenous fluids. In rare cases this has been fatal.

Hematologic

Maternal oxytocin administration increases the rate of neonatal physiological jaundice in a dose-dependent manner (SEDA-13, 1310) (11). This effect may be due to hemodilution and an increased rate of hemolysis.

Immunologic

Anaphylactoid reactions to oxytocin have been described (12).

- A 41-year-old woman treated for shock after a septic abortion received an intravenous infusion of oxytocin 40 mU/minute. Just after the infusion started she developed tachypnea, bronchospasm, and laryngeal stridor. Her symptoms disappeared only when the oxytocin was withdrawn.

Second-Generation Effects

Pregnancy

In a retrospective analysis of 2774 women who had had one prior cesarean delivery, there was a 1% incidence of uterine rupture in women who were given oxytocin, compared with 0.4% in non-augmented controls with spontaneous labor (13). Six women needed emergency hysterectomy. The odds ratio for uterine rupture in the oxytocin-treated women was 4.6 by logistic regression analysis (CI = 1.5,14). The small number of events limited the study: it had only 30% power to detect changes of that magnitude. However, it is reasonable to proceed cautiously, with close clinical observation, given the potentially severe outcome.

- Uterine rupture occurred when oxytocin was started 5 hours after the administration of a second misoprostol tablet for induction of labor, although the usual recommendation is to wait at least 12 hours (14).
- A 36-year-old multiparous woman had a ruptured uterus after labor was induced at 24 weeks with misoprostol 200 µg and augmented with oxytocin (15).

The risk of uterine rupture is increased by previous cesarean section, fetal weight over 4 kg, and the use of oxytocin (SEDA-24, 506) (16,17). In 24 women with uterine rupture after oxytocin, the dose and duration of use of oxytocin were 10% higher than in controls; this difference was not statistically significant, but the power of the study was limited by the small sample size (18).

High-dose and low-dose oxytocin have been compared in augmentation or induction of labor (19). There was large variation in the doses given in the studies reviewed, particularly among the high doses used. In some studies low-dose oxytocin resulted in higher rates of cesarean section but fewer fetal heart rate abnormalities. In one study women given high-dose oxytocin had a higher rate of cesarean sections as result of fetal distress. Studies were often underpowered.

References

1. Owen J, Hauth JC. Oxytocin for the induction or augmentation of labor. Clin Obstet Gynecol 1992;35(3):464–75.
2. ACOG. Technical Bulletin Number 157. Int J Obstet 1991;39:139.
3. Chelmow D, Laros RK Jr. Maternal and neonatal outcomes after oxytocin augmentation in patients undergoing a trial of labor after prior cesarean delivery. Obstet Gynecol 1992;80(6):966–71.
4. Dansereau J, Joshi AK, Helewa ME, Doran TA, Lange IR, Farine D, Schulz ML, Horbay GL, Griffin P, Wassenaar W. Double-blind comparison of carbetocin versus oxytocin in prevention of uterine atony after cesarean section. Am J Obstet Gynecol 1999;180(3 Pt 1):670–6.
5. Why mothers die 1997–1999. The confidential enquiries into maternal deaths in the United KingdomLondon: RCOG Press;. 2001.
6. Pinder AJ, Dresner M, Calow C, Shorten GD, O'Riordan J, Johnson R. Haemodynamic changes caused by oxytocin during caesarean section under spinal anaesthesia. Int J Obstet Anesth 2002;11(3):156–9.
7. Moran C, Ni Bhuinneain M, Geary M, Cunningham S, McKenna P, Gardiner J. Myocardial ischaemia in normal patients undergoing elective Caesarean section: a peripartum assessment. Anaesthesia 2001;56(11):1051–8.
8. Spence A. Oxytocin during Caesarean section. Anaesthesia 2002;57:710–1.
9. Liou SC, Chen C, Wong SY, Wong KM. Ventricular tachycardia after oxytocin injection in patients with prolonged Q-T interval syndrome—report of two cases. Acta Anaesthesiol Sin 1998;36(1):49–52.
10. Mayer-Hubner B. Pseudotumour cerebri from intranasal oxytocin and excessive fluid intake. Lancet 1996;347(9001):623.
11. Sakala EP, Kaye S, Murray RD, Munson LJ. Oxytocin use after previous cesarean: why a higher rate of failed labor trial? Obstet Gynecol 1990;75(3 Pt 1):356–9.
12. Cabestrero D, Perez-Paredes C, Fernandez-Cid R, Arribas MA. Bronchospasm and laryngeal stridor as an adverse effect of oxytocin treatment. Crit Care 2003;7:392.
13. Zelop CM, Shipp TD, Repke JT, Cohen A, Caughey AB, Lieberman E. Uterine rupture during induced or augmented labor in gravid women with one prior cesarean delivery. Am J Obstet Gynecol 1999;181(4):882–6.
14. Fletcher H, McCaw-Binns A. Rupture of the uterus with misoprostol (prostaglandin El) used for induction of labour. J Obstet Gynaecol 1998;18(2):184–5.
15. Al-Hussaini TK. Uterine rupture in second trimester abortion in a grand multiparous woman. A complication of misoprostol and oxytocin. Eur J Obstet Gynecol Reprod Biol 2001;96(2):218–9.
16. Aboyeji AP, Ijaiya MD, Yahaya UR. Ruptured uterus: a study of 100 consecutive cases in Ilorin, Nigeria. J Obstet Gynaecol Res 2001;27(6):341–8.
17. Diaz SD, Jones JE, Seryakov M, Mann WJ. Uterine rupture and dehiscence: ten-year review and case-control study. South Med J 2002;95(4):431–5.
18. Goetzl L, Shipp TD, Cohen A, Zelop CM, Repke JT, Lieberman E. Oxytocin dose and the risk of uterine rupture in trial of labor after cesarean. Obstet Gynecol 2001;97(3):381–4.
19. Patka JH, Lodolce AE, Johnston AK. High-versus low-dose oxytocin for augmentation or induction of labor. Ann Pharmacother 2005;39:95–101.

Parathyroid hormone and analogues

General Information

Both intact parathyroid hormone (e.g. PTH_{1-34}, teriparatide) and smaller N-terminal fragments PTH_{1-84} are used. No adverse reactions have been reported with single infusions of up to 60 mg of synthetic human parathyroid hormone in diagnostic procedures (SEDA-13, 1307; 1,2). Although bone resorption increases if the hormone is given continuously or in high doses, it has an anabolic effect on bone when given intermittently. Synthetic parathyroid hormone fragments have therefore been used in the treatment of slow turnover osteoporosis. However, no improvement in fracture risk has been documented, and the anabolic effect may only be present in the first 12 months (3). The use of parathyroid hormone in the treatment of hypoparathyroidism is also under investigation, with the optimum dosage and target calcium concentrations yet to be determined.

Reviews of parathyroid hormone have suggested that it is generally well tolerated (4,5,6). The adverse effects of parathyroid hormone that have been reported in clinical trials are mild and include transient bone pain, nausea, dizziness and local irritation at the injection site (7). Hypercalcemia, which is common, is usually mild and asymptomatic. Adverse effects, including hypercalcemia, appear to be dose related in the therapeutic range.

Parathyroid hormone has potent anabolic effects on the skeleton if given intermittently; being used in clinical trials. Initial concerns about the development of osteosarcoma in rats after prolonged treatment with high doses of parathyroid hormone have not been confirmed in human trials, but surveillance continues (8). In one study there was a mild increase in creatinine, which was thought not to have clinical significance (9). Mild nausea (10) and arthralgia (10,11) have also been reported.

Nausea was reported in 18% and headache in 13% of 552 women who took parathyroid hormone 40 micrograms, compared with 8% of the 544 women who took placebo (12).

Organs and Systems

Cardiovascular

Parathyroid hormone lowers the blood pressure by a direct effect on vascular smooth muscle, and there are isolated instances of hypotension or tachycardia (13).

Pre-injection blood pressure was normal in 1093 women randomized to parathyroid hormone (PTH_{1-34}), and dizziness was reported infrequently in 541 women taking 20 micrograms/day but not in 552 taking 40 micrograms/day (12).

Metabolism

Most studies of parathormone have involved PTH_{1-34}. In 238 women with post-menopausal osteoporosis randomly assigned to subcutaneous PTH_{1-84} plus placebo, parathormone plus alendronate, or alendronate plus placebo, there was a significant increase in mean serum uric acid concentrations in those taking parathormone (14). Three women had gout, one in the parathormone-only group and two in the combination group

Mineral balance

Mild asymptomatic hypercalcemia is common during treatment with parathyroid hormone (15). The hypercalcemia is persistent, and requires dosage reduction in 3% of patients using 20 micrograms/day and in 11% using 40 micrograms/day (16). Transient mild hypercalciuria and increased serum phosphate are common but do not usually limit therapy.

In a randomized study in premenopausal women also treated with nafarelin, four of 23 women randomized to PTH_{1-34} 500 IU/day had a serum calcium concentration over 2.67 mmol/l 4 hours after the injection; the concentration normalized after the dose of parathyroid hormone was reduced and other treatment was continued (10).

In another study, two of 10 men who were randomized to receive subcutaneous PTH_{1-34} 400 IU/day for 18 months had serum calcium concentrations over 2.6 mmol/l after 1 or 3 months; the concentrations normalized after reduction of the dose of parathyroid hormone (11).

Hypercalcemia was present in 11% of 541 women 4–6 hours after parathyroid hormone 20 micrograms/day and in 28% of 552 women after 40 micrograms/day (12). The dose was halved because of hypercalcemia in 3 and 11% of the women taking 20 and 40 micrograms/day respectively. Nine of the women taking 40 micrograms/day stopped treatment because hypercalcemia persisted after dosage reduction.

Patients randomly assigned to PTH_{1-84} at doses of 50 micrograms/day (n = 50), 75 micrograms/day (n = 52), 100 micrograms/day (n = 51), or to placebo (n = 53) had a dose-related increase in serum total calcium concentrations. This effect was most evident in the first 6 months and appeared to improve at 6–12 months. There was transient hypercalcemia in 24 patients, of whom 11 were taking 100 micrograms/day (17).

There was hypercalcemia in 12% of 119 patients taking PTH_{1-84} 100 micrograms/day with daily calcium and vitamin D and in 14% of 59 taking additional alendronate. After stopping the calcium supplements only two women needed a dosage reduction of parathormone (14,17).

Combining parathyroid hormone with antiresorptive agents may prevent or minimize hypercalcemia. None of

27 women randomized to estrogen plus parathyroid hormone PTH_{1-34} 25 micrograms/day became hypercalcemic during a 3-year study (18).

Skin

Local reactions at sites of subcutaneous injection are common (17) but are usually limited to transitory redness (10,11).

Subcutaneous nodules at the injection site developed in two of 17 women after more than 2 years of administration in a clinical trial (19). Two of 27 women randomized to parathyroid hormone developed nodules at injection sites; however, this could have been due to a contaminant, as both women received parathyroid hormone from the same batch (18).

Immunologic

Dose-dependent antiparathyroid hormone antibodies developed in under 10% of 1093 women in one study; however, there was no reduction in efficacy (12).

Long-Term Effects

Tumorigenicity

The rate of osteosarcoma in animal and human trials of parathyroid hormone has been reviewed (20,6). Rats treated with parathyroid hormone for 2 years had a high dose-dependent rate of osteosarcoma, up to 48% in animals given 75 micrograms/kg; human trials were therefore interrupted (21). However, the anabolic effect of parathyroid hormone is much greater and occurs much earlier in rats than in humans, possibly because of fundamental differences in bone biology: moreover, osteosarcoma has never been associated with primary, secondary, or tertiary hyperparathyroidism in humans (20). There has been no evidence of osteosarcoma in several hundred patients involved in parathyroid hormone clinical trials lasting up to 3 years, after 5 years minimum follow-up (20).

Drug–Drug Interactions

Bisphosphonates

Alendronate significantly reduced the anabolic effect of parathyroid hormone when the two were used in combination, both in postmenopausal women (22) and in men (23). It seems likely that this interaction will also apply to other bisphosphonates, although the mechanism has not been determined.

References

1. Mallette LE. Synthetic human parathyroid hormone 1–34 fragment for diagnostic testing. Ann Intern Med 1988;109(10):800–4.
2. Mallette LE, Kirkland JL, Gagel RF, Law WM Jr, Heath H 3rd. Synthetic human parathyroid hormone-(1–34) for the

study of pseudohypoparathyroidism. J Clin Endocrinol Metab 1988;67(5):964–72.

3. Dempster DW, Cosman F, Parisien M, Shen V, Lindsay R. Anabolic actions of parathyroid hormone on bone. Endocr Rev 1993;14(6):690–709.

4. Olszynski WP, Davison KS, Adachi JD, Brown JP, Cummings SR, Hanley DA, Harris ST, Hodsman AB, Kendler D, McClumg MR, Miller PD, Yuen CK. Osteoporosis in men: epidemiology, diagnosis, prevention and treatment. ClinTher 2004;26:15–28.

5. Keam SJ, Plosker GL. Prevention and treatment of osteoporosis in postmenopausal women. Dis Manage Health Outcomes 2004;12:19–37.

6. McClung M. Parathyroid hormone for the treatment of osteoporosis. Obstet Gynaecol Surv 2004;59:826–32.

7. Winer KK, Yanovski JA, Cutler GB Jr. Synthetic human parathyroid hormone 1-34 vs calcitriol and calcium in the treatment of hypoparathyroidism. JAMA 1996;276(8):631–6.

8. Whitfield J, Morley P, Willick G. The parathyroid hormone, its fragments and analogues—potent bone-builders for treating osteoporosis. Expert Opin Investig Drugs 2000;9(6):1293–315.

9. Hodsman AB, Fraher LJ, Watson PH, Ostbye T, Stitt LW, Adachi JD, Taves DH, Drost D. A randomized controlled trial to compare the efficacy of cyclical parathyroid hormone versus cyclical parathyroid hormone and sequential calcitonin to improve bone mass in postmenopausal women with osteoporosis. J Clin Endocrinol Metab 1997;82(2):620–8.

10. Finkelstein JS, Klibanski A, Arnold AL, Toth TL, Hornstein MD, Neer RM. Prevention of estrogen deficiency-related bone loss with human parathyroid hormone-(1–34): a randomized controlled trial. JAMA 1998;280(12):1067–73.

11. Kurland ES, Cosman F, McMahon DJ, Rosen CJ, Lindsay R, Bilezikian JP. Parathyroid hormone as a therapy for idiopathic osteoporosis in men: effects on bone mineral density and bone markers. J Clin Endocrinol Metab 2000;85(9):3069–76.

12. Neer RM, Arnaud CD, Zanchetta JR, Prince R, Gaich GA, Reginster JY, Hodsman AB, Eriksen EF, Ish-Shalom S, Genant HK, Wang O, Mitlak BH. Effect of parathyroid hormone (1–34) on fractures and bone mineral density in postmenopausal women with osteoporosis. N Engl J Med 2001;344(19):1434–41.

13. Morley P, Whitfield JF, Willick GE. Parathyroid hormone: an anabolic treatment for osteoporosis. Curr Pharm Des 2001;7(8):671–87.

14. Black DM, Greespan SL, Ensrud KE, Palmero L, McGowan JA, Lang TF, Garnero P, Bouxsein ML, Bilezikian JP, Rosen CJ. The effects of parathyroid hormone and alendronate alone or in combination in postmenopausal osteoporosis. New Engl J Med 2003;349:1207–15.

15. Body JJ, Gaich GA, Scheele WH, Kulkarni PM, Miller PD, Peretz A, Dore RK, Correa-Rotter R, Papaioannou A, Cumming DC, Hodsman AB. A randomized double-blind trial to compare the efficacy of teriparatide [recombinant human parathyroid hormone (1–34)] with alendronate in postmenopausal women with osteoporosis. J Clin Endocrinol Metab 2002;87(10):4528–35.

16. Rubin MR, Bilezikian JP. The potential of parathyroid hormone as a therapy for osteoporosis. Int J Fertil Womens Med 2002;47(3):103–15.

17. Hodsman AB, Hanley DA, Ettinger MP, Bolognese MA, Fox J, Metcalfe AJ, Lindsay R. Efficacy and safety of human parathyroid hormone (1–84) in increasing bone mineral density in postmenopausal osteoporosis. J Clin Endocrinol Metab 2003;88:5212–20.

18. Cosman F, Nieves J, Woelfert L, Formica C, Gordon S, Shen V, Lindsay R. Parathyroid hormone added to established hormone therapy: effects on vertebral fracture and maintenance of bone mass after parathyroid hormone withdrawal. J Bone Miner Res 2001;16(5):925–31.

19. Lindsay R, Nieves J, Formica C, Henneman E, Woelfert L, Shen V, Dempster D, Cosman F. Randomised controlled study of effect of parathyroid hormone on vertebral-bone mass and fracture incidence among postmenopausal women on oestrogen with osteoporosis. Lancet 1997;350(9077):550–5.

20. Tashjian AH Jr, Chabner BA. Commentary on clinical safety of recombinant human parathyroid hormone 1–34 in the treatment of osteoporosis in men and postmenopausal women. J Bone Miner Res 2002;17(7):1151–61.

21. Vahle JL, Sato M, Long GG, Young JK, Francis PC, Engelhardt JA, Westmore MS, Linda Y, Nold JB. Skeletal changes in rats given daily subcutaneous injections of recombinant human parathyroid hormone (1–34) for 2 years and relevance to human safety. Toxicol Pathol 2002;30(3):312–21.

22. Black DM, Greenspan SL, Ensrud KE, Palermo L, McGowan JA, Lang TF, Garnero P, Bouxsein ML, Bilezikian JP, Rosen CJPaTH Study Investigators. The effects of parathyroid hormone and alendronate alone or in combination in postmenopausal osteoporosis. N Engl J Med 2003;349(13):1207–15.

23. Finkelstein JS, Hayes A, Hunzelman JL, Wyland JJ, Lee H, Neer RM. The effects of parathyroid hormone, alendronate, or both in men with osteoporosis. N Engl J Med 2003;349(13):1216–26.

Somatostatin and analogues

General Information

Somatostatin was first isolated from the hypothalamus, and was shown to inhibit growth hormone release. It has since been found in neuroendocrine tissues throughout the body. It has multiple effects, via five distinct receptors, and acts as a neurotransmitter, in the regulation of growth hormone and thyrotropin release, as a regulator of gastrointestinal and pancreatic function, and as an immune modulator. Synthetic analogues are selective for receptor subtypes 2 and 5, and have different clinical and adverse effects profiles to the native hormone, as well as having longer half-lives. Analogues of somatostatin include depreotide, edotreotide, ilatreotide, lanreotide, octreotide, pasireotide, pentetreotide, and vapreotide (all rINNs).

Octreotide, an octapeptide somatostatin analogue, is usually given subcutaneously in three divided doses per day. Longer-acting analogues, such as lanreotide, with similar efficacy and adverse effects to octreotide, but which can be given every 14–28 days, have been developed (1,2). The therapeutic indications and adverse effects of octreotide have been reviewed (SEDA-13, 1309; 3).

A review of octreotide LAR has suggested that the most common adverse effects are gastrointestinal effects and injection site reactions (4). Injection site pain is also common and dose related. The cardiovascular, biliary, and glucose metabolism effects were also reviewed.

Organs and Systems

Cardiovascular

Both somatostatin and octreotide cause transient increases in mean arterial pressure and mean pulmonary pressure when given intravenously to patients with cirrhosis, more marked with bolus administration than with continuous infusion (5). This may be either direct or mediated by inhibition of gut vasodilatory peptides (SEDA-24, 505; 6) and is not usually associated with significant clinical effects.

Severe hypertension with associated headache, nausea, and vomiting was reported within 2 weeks of administration of octreotide LAR 20 mg in a 26-year-old diabetic woman with autonomic neuropathy (6). Rechallenge with octreotide 75 µg resulted in a transient hypertensive episode lasting 3 hours.

- Exacerbation of pre-existing hypertension was also reported in a 22-month-old boy during octreotide infusion (7).

There has been one report of acute pulmonary edema during octreotide and intravenous fluid therapy for variceal bleeding (8).

Sinus bradycardia (less than 50/minute) is reported in up to 25% of acromegalic patients taking octreotide, and conduction abnormalities are also commonly reported in these patients. This adverse effect is reported only rarely in other recipients of somatostatin or octreotide, probably reflecting the high rate of cardiac abnormalities due to acromegaly (9).

- A 67-year-old man who was receiving subcutaneous octreotide 100 micrograms bd underwent abdominal laparotomy for metastatic carcinoid tumor (10). He was given an intravenous bolus of octreotide 100 micrograms 10 minutes after induction and immediately after surgical incision. His heart rate fell to 35/minute and his blood pressure to 85/40 mmHg. He was given ephedrine 20 mg intravenously and recovered. He was given a further bolus of octreotide 100 micrograms 30 minutes later. His heart rate immediately fell to 45/minute and he developed complete heart block. He was given ephedrine 20 mg and glycopyrrolate 0.2 mg intravenously and recovered.

The authors suggested that intravenous octreotide should be infused slowly when possible.

The records of 21 children who received infusions of octreotide (1–2 micrograms/kg/hour) for 35 gastrointestinal bleeds have been reviewed (11). There was one case of asymptomatic bradycardia and one case of a sudden unexplained cardiac event in a patient who appeared to be hemodynamically stable just before the event 5 hours after starting octreotide.

Octreotide increases systemic vascular resistance, and bradycardia may be a baroreceptor-induced response. Octreotide also has direct effects on the heart, the main effects being reduced heart rate, reduced myocardial contractility, and slowing of the propagation velocity along the cardiac conduction system.

Respiratory

Octreotide has been used in premature neonates for closure of enterocutaneous fistulae complicating necrotizing enterocolitis. Two cases of oxygen desaturation have been reported (12). The authors suggested that the effect may relate to pre-existing hyaline membrane disease.

Nervous system

Dizziness occurred in 7.4% of 68 patients randomized to somatostatin and 8.2% of 73 randomized to octreotide, both by rapid infusion, to control variceal bleeding, in which the effectiveness of somatostatin and its analogues is probably via a transient reduction in heart rate and cardiac output (13).

Endocrine

Of 7 infants with congenital chylothorax whose cases were reviewed, one had been treated with continuous intravenous somatostatin (60 micrograms/kg/day) at 33 days (14). Therapy was withdrawn after 10 days as the symptoms had improved. Thyroid function had been normal at 13 days but was found to be abnormal at 57 days, during routine screening for congenital hypothyroidism (T_4 26 µg/l, TSH 116 mU/l). The infant had recurrent sepsis and received further somatostatin. Levothyroxine was given and thyroid function was monitored over several months. At 11 months thyroid function was normal, levothyroxine having been withdrawn at 8 months. The other six infants with chylothorax did not receive somatostatin and did not develop hypothyroidism. It was therefore thought that the somatostatin could have been responsible, although the mechanism was unclear. Somatostatin inhibits TSH secretion and is useful for treating TSH-secreting adenomas.

Metabolism

Somatostatin and its analogues inhibit insulin secretion in the short term, before receptor down-regulation. Mild hyperglycemia occurs during octreotide infusion in up to 23% of adults (15,16), and occasionally in children (17). This is not usually clinically significant (3). However, in an open, retrospective comparison of octreotide and lanreotide in 38 patients with acromegaly, one patient in each group stopped therapy because of worsening glycemic control (18).

In a meta-analysis of trials for variceal bleeding, hyperglycemia occurred in 41 of 310 patients who received somatostatin, octreotide, or vapreotide, compared with 26 of 318 patients who received placebo (19).

Reports of the effects of octreotide on glucose metabolism in acromegaly are inconsistent and are complicated by the high prevalence of insulin resistance and overt diabetes in acromegaly. In 10 patients with acromegaly who used modified-release lanreotide for 19 months followed by modified-release octreotide for 21 months after a 3-month washout period, mean fasting glucose, the glucose response to oral glucose tolerance testing, and glycated hemoglobin all increased after octreotide but not lanreotide (20). However, the study was small and the order of the two medications was not randomized.

In 24 patients with acromegaly, glucose homeostasis was assessed before and after 6 months of either 2-weekly lanreotide (n = 14) or monthly octreotide (n = 10) (21). Insulin resistance and triglyceride concentrations improved. Glucose homeostasis, measured by HbA_{1c}, deteriorated. This was probably due to impaired insulin secretion. There were no distinct differences between the analogues, but the numbers were small.

In patients with insulinoma, octreotide can cause clinically important hypoglycemia, because of suppression of counter-regulatory hormone secretion (22).

- A 62-year-old woman with multiple carcinoid hepatic metastases was given octreotide LAR 20 mg and developed severe hypoglycemia 6 hours later. Parenteral dextrose was continued for a month. Prednisolone was needed to discontinue the dextrose.

The authors suggest that in patients at risk of hypoglycemia, short-acting somatostatin may be useful to assess response (23).

Hematologic

Thrombosis of a splenic artery pseudoaneurysm has been reported in a patient receiving octreotide (24).

- A 55-year-old woman with a history of chronic pancreatitis developed epigastric pain and melena and was found to have a splenic artery pseudoaneurysm expanding a pseudocyst. She was given an intravenous bolus of octreotide followed by an infusion of 50 micrograms/ hour. A CT scan subsequently suggested thrombosis of the pseudoaneurysm, with segmental splenic infarction. Nine months later the pseudoaneurysm had recanalized.

The octreotide may have contributed by causing vasoconstriction. A case of thrombosis in a splenic artery pseudoaneurysm in a patient receiving somatostatin has previously been reported (25).

- A 42-year-old woman, treated with octreotide infusion 50 mg/hour for cirrhosis-related gastrointestinal bleeding on two occasions 9 months apart, had an immediate fall in platelet count on both occasions, resolving after octreotide withdrawal (26). The thrombocytopenia was not severe (nadir platelet counts 62 and 55 × 10^9/l) and did not require specific treatment.

The rapid fall in platelet count in this case suggests an immunological mechanism, although this was not directly demonstrated.

Gastrointestinal

Transient gastrointestinal symptoms (nausea, diarrhea, abdominal discomfort, and flatulence) occur in up to 50% of patients during the first few days of treatment, but usually resolve spontaneously after the first 1–2 weeks of treatment (13,27). Nausea and vomiting occur in up to 25% of patients after somatostatin and are also common after octreotide (28). Two of 15 patients in a phase I trial of malignant gastrinoma had to stop using long-acting octreotide because of severe nausea (29).

Radiolabelled isotopes of somatostatin analogues are used in managing patients with neuroendocrine gastroenteropancreatic tumors. The somatostatin analogue (DOTA0,Tyr3)octreotate has been radiolabelled with ^{177}Lu and used in 35 patients (30). Nausea and vomiting within the first 24 hours of administration were common (up to 30%) and abdominal pain occurred in 11%.

Diarrhea is common soon after starting octreotide but usually resolves within 2 weeks without specific treatment. In a randomized, double-blind, placebo-controlled trial in 203 mostly postmenopausal women with locally recurrent or metastatic breast carcinoma, all of whom were also taking tamoxifen, and who had estrogen-receptor positive and/or progesterone-receptor positive tumors, octreotide was added to the basic treatment in 99 cases (31). The adverse events experienced by 10% or more of the patients and attributed to octreotide were gastrointestinal: diarrhea (53%), nausea (16%), and abdominal pain (11%); diarrhea occurred in only 11% of the controls.

Of 24 patients with hepatocellular carcinoma receiving octreotide LAR, 11 had mild diarrhea (32). The effect of octreotide on bowel transit appears to be variable. In some patients, such as those with carcinoid syndrome, it is useful for the management of diarrhea.

In 10 non-acromegalic controls, 11 patients with acromegaly not receiving octreotide, and 11 receiving long-term octreotide subcutaneously, large bowel transit time was increased in acromegaly and prolonged further in those receiving octreotide (33). The total fecal count of anerobic bacteria was higher and bile acid activity was increased in those who received octreotide.

One of 10 patients with rheumatoid arthritis in an open study stopped using long-acting octreotide because of severe diarrhea and weight loss of 3 kg (34). These effects are dose-related and are similar in healthy volunteers, acromegalic patients, and patients with gastrointestinal tumors (3).

Octreotide 100 μg given subcutaneously to five healthy subjects 30 minutes before meals for 7 days increased fecal fat excretion; however, steatorrhea occurred in only two cases; fecal bile acid excretion fell to about 25% (35)

Liver

There have been isolated reports of hepatic dysfunction due to octreotide (36).

- A 41 year old woman with hepatocellular carcinoma was treated with chemotherapy. Octreotide 100 micrograms bd and LAR 20 mg was added to her therapy to control symptoms of diarrhea, but 10 days later she developed severe abdominal pain and 10-fold increases in transaminases, which returned to normal 6 weeks after octreotide was withdrawn.

Biliary tract

Biliary sludge and gallstones are frequent adverse effects of both octreotide (2) and its longer acting analogues, compared with 10–25% of the general population (37). Cholelithiasis develops in up to 20% of patients in the long term, secondary to reduced gall-bladder contractility, but only 1% of patients develop symptoms per year of treatment (38). There is prospective evidence that gallstones develop earlier in patients on higher doses of octreotide (24). Rebound gall-bladder hypermotility can occur on withdrawal of octreotide and can be associated with biliary colic or pancreatitis (SEDA-13, 1309; 39,40).

Patients treated with octreotide have impaired meal-stimulated gall-bladder emptying and altered bile chemical composition, similar to spontaneous cholelithiasis. In 16 patients with acromegaly the serum deoxycholic acid concentration increased in proportion to large bowel transit time (41). In 11 patients gall-bladder emptying was slower in patients given octreotide LAR than lanreotide SR, but was impaired in both groups compared with pretreatment values (42).

Fasting gall-bladder volume increased progressively in seven patients with acromegaly treated with once-monthly long-acting octreotide; gallstones formed de novo in six patients within 8 months and one had symptomatic biliary colic (43). Gallstones have also been reported in children receiving prolonged octreotide therapy (17).

Ursodiol appeared to reverse gall-bladder abnormalities in seven of 10 patients. Data from this study also showed earlier development of sludge in recipients of higher doses of octreotide (37).

Urinary tract

Of 12 patients with ascites due to cirrhosis of the liver, who received subcutaneous octreotide 300 micrograms bd for 11 days, 11 had increased renal plasma flow and 10 had a reduced GFR (44). Creatinine concentrations did not change. The effects of octreotide on the kidneys have been variably reported in previous studies. In patients with cirrhosis the effects are likely to be affected by the activated renin–angiotensin–aldosterone system.

Skin

There have been three cases of lipoatrophy in women taking subcutaneous octreotide for acromegaly (45). One had used octreotide 600 micrograms/day for 6 years, another had used octreotide 300 micrograms /day for 30 months, and the third developed problems 4 years after using octreotide 800 micrograms/day. The patients were given intramuscular octreotide instead; in one the lipoatrophy regressed. The mechanism is not known. Long-term subcutaneous octreotide has been used less often since the development of long-acting somatostatin analogues, but when it is used follow-up for lipoatrophy is

appropriate. No data were given as to whether the lipoatrophy affected the absorption of octreotide.

Hair

Reversible hair loss has been reported in a few patients after both octreotide (46) and lanreotide (47).

- Hair loss in a 36-year-old man began after he had taken octreotide for acromegaly for 1 month (48). Therapy was changed to lanreotide after 6 months and hair loss reversed. This may have been coincidental.

Four patients who developed hair loss whilst receiving octreotide found that the loss stopped after 3–6 months (4).

Immunologic

Antibodies to somatostatin analogues have been reported only rarely. However, in one study octreotide antibodies were demonstrated in 63 (27%) of 231 patients treated with subcutaneous octreotide for more than 3 years, rising to 57% after 5 years and 72% after 8 years (49). The antibodies did not reduce clinical efficacy.

- A 64-year-old woman, who had had monthly intramuscular injections of long-acting octreotide in the buttocks for 6 years, had increased uptake of ^{111}In-pentetreotide in both buttocks, thought to represent granuloma formation at the injection sites (50). Localized granulomas have previously been described in isolated cases after intramuscular somatostatin analogues, and somatostatin receptors are expressed in high density in activated lymphocytes.

Allergic reactions to somatostatin are rare. Of 97 cirrhotic patients randomized to subcutaneous octreotide, one stopped therapy because of erythematous itchy skin, which then resolved (16).

Body temperature

Of 12 patients (7 men, 5 women) with malignant mid-gut carcinoid tumors, median age 50 years, who received intramuscular octreotide pamoate 160 mg every 2 weeks for 2 months and then every month for 12 months, six developed unexplained episodic fever (51). No infection or cause was found.

Second-Generation Effects

Pregnancy

Octreotide is a small peptide that can pass the placental barrier, and it is not recommended for use in pregnant women.

Placental transfer was significant in the first reported pregnancy with long-acting octreotide (52). The dose of octreotide was reduced after an ultrasound suggested intrauterine growth retardation. The female infant had a low birth weight (11th percentile) but caught up to the 50th percentile by 3 months of age. Her development was normal during 18 months of follow-up.

Of seven women who took somatostatin analogues during pregnancy, five stopped taking it when the pregnancy was diagnosed (53). One had a single injection of modified-release lanreotide before pregnancy was diagnosed, with no apparent adverse effects on the infant (54). No fetal malformations or delay in postnatal development have been reported.

Susceptibility Factors

Age

Children are generally not given long-term octreotide because of concerns about its effect on growth. Although growth was reported as normal in a few case series, "catch-up" growth was also described after octreotide was withdrawn (17).

Drug–Drug Interactions

Erythromycin

Pretreatment with octreotide enhanced the gastric prokinetic effects of erythromycin in eight healthy subjects, suggesting that octreotide may be clinically useful in patients with tachyphylaxis to this effect of erythromycin (55).

Midodrine

In a controlled study of octreotide and midodrine (an alpha-adrenoceptor agonist) in patients with orthostatic hypotension, the pressor effect of the two drugs was synergistic (56).

Morphine

Somatostatin and its analogues have been reported to be OP_3 (μ) opioid receptor antagonists (57). Somatostatin infusions significantly reduced the effectiveness of morphine analgesia in a case report of three patients with cancer.

References

1. Caron P, Morange-Ramos I, Cogne M, Jaquet P. Three year follow-up of acromegalic patients treated with intramuscular slow-release lanreotide. J Clin Endocrinol Metab 1997;82(1):18–22.
2. Davies PH, Stewart SE, Lancranjan L, Sheppard MC, Stewart PM. Long-term therapy with long-acting octreotide (Sandostatin-LAR) for the management of acromegaly. Clin Endocrinol (Oxf) 1998;48(3):311–6.
3. Lamberts SW, van der Lely AJ, de Herder WW, Hofland LJ. Octreotide. N Engl J Med 1996;334(4):246–54.
4. McKeage K, Cheer S, Wagstaff AJ. Octreotide long-acting release (LAR) a review of its use in management of acromegaly. Drugs 2003;63:2473–99.
5. Hadengue A. Somatostatin or octreotide in acute variceal bleeding. Digestion 1999;60(Suppl 2):31–41.
6. Pop-Busui R, Chey W, Stevens MJ. Severe hypertension induced by the long-acting somatostatin analogue Sandostatin LAR in a patient with diabetic autonomic neuropathy. J Clin Endocrinol Metab 2000;85(3):943–6.
7. Beckman RA, Siden R, Yanik GA, Levine JE. Continuous octreotide infusion for the treatment of secretory diarrhea caused by acute intestinal graft-versus-host disease in a child. J Pediatr Hematol Oncol 2000;22(4):344–50.
8. Jenkins SA, Shields R, Davies M, Elias E, Turnbull AJ, Bassendine MF, James OF, Iredale JP, Vyas SK, Arthur MJ, Kingsnorth AN, Sutton R. A multicentre randomised trial comparing octreotide and injection sclerotherapy in the management and outcome of acute variceal haemorrhage. Gut 1997;41(4):526–33.
9. Herrington AM, George KW, Moulds CC. Octreotide-induced bradycardia. Pharmacotherapy 1998;18(2):413–6.
10. Dilger JA, Rho EH, Que FG, Sprung J. Octreotide-induced bradycardia and heart block during surgical resection of a carcinoid tumour. Anesth Analg 2004;98:318–20.
11. Eroglu Y, Emerick KM, Whitingon PF, Alonso EM. Octreotide therapy for control of acute gastrointestinal bleeding in children. J Ped Gastroenterol Nutr 2004;38:41–7.
12. Arevalo RP, Bullabh P, Krauss AN, Auld PAM, Spigland N. Octreotide-induced hypoxemia and pulmonary hypertension in premature neonates. J Pediatr Surg 2003;38:251–3.
13. Zhang HB, Wong BC, Zhou XM, Guo XG, Zhao SJ, Wang JH, Wu KC, Ding J, Lam SK, Fan DM. Effects of somatostatin, octreotide and pitressin plus nitroglycerine on systemic and portal haemodynamics in the control of acute variceal bleeding. Int J Clin Pract 2002;56(6):447–51.
14. Maayan-Metzger A, Sack J, Mazkereth R, Vardi A, Kuint J. Somatostatin treatment of congenital chylothorax may induce transient hypothyroidism in newborns. Acta Paediatr 2005;94:785–9.
15. Corley DA, Cello JP, Adkisson W, Ko WF, Kerlikowske K. Octreotide for acute esophageal variceal bleeding: a meta-analysis. Gastroenterology 2001;120(4):946–54.
16. Erstad BL. Octreotide for acute variceal bleeding. Ann Pharmacother 2001;35(5):618–26.
17. Lam JC, Aters S, Tobias JD. Initial experience with octreotide in the pediatric population. Am J Ther 2001;8(6):409–15.
18. Razzore P, Colao A, Baldelli R, Gaia D, Marzullo P, Ferretti E, Ferone D, Jaffrain-Rea ML, Tamburrano G, Lombardi G, Camanni F, Ciccarelli E. Comparison of six months therapy with octreotide versus lanreotide in acromegalic patients: a retrospective study. Clin Endocrinol (Oxf) 1999;51(2):159–64.
19. Banares R, Albillos A, Rincon D, Alonso S, Gonzalez M, Ruiz-del-Arbol L, Salcedo M, Molinero LM. Endoscopic treatment versus endoscopic plus pharmacologic treatment for acute variceal bleeding: a meta-analysis. Hepatology 2002;35(3):609–15.
20. Ronchi C, Epaminonda P, Cappiello V, Beck-Peccoz P, Arosio M. Effects of two different somatostatin analogues on glucose tolerance in acromegaly. J Endocrinol Invest 2002;25(6):502–7.
21. Baldelli R, Battista C, Leonetti F, Ghiggi M-R, Ribaudo M-C, Paoloni A, D'Amico E, Ferretti E, Baratta R, Liuzzi A, Trishitta V, Tamburrano G. Glucose homeostasis in acromegaly: effects of long-acting somatostatin analogues treatment. Clin Endocrinol 2003;59:492–9.
22. Stehouwer CD, Lems WF, Fischer HR, Hackeng WH, Naafs MA. Aggravation of hypoglycemia in insulinoma patients by the long-acting somatostatin analogue

octreotide (Sandostatin). Acta Endocrinol (Copenh) 1989;121(1):34–40.

23. Sari H, Altunbas H, Ozdogan M, Gurer EI, Karayalcin U. Severe and prolonged hypoglycemia triggered by long-acting octreotide in a patient with malignant mesenchymal tumor: case report. J Chemother 2003;15:85–8.

24. Tang LJ, Zipser S, Kang YS. Temporary spontaneous thrombosis of a splenic artery pseudoaneurysm in chronic pancreatitis during intravenous octreotide administration. J Vasc Interv Radiol 2005;16(6):863–6.

25. De Rone T, VanBeers B, de Canniere L, Trigaux JP, Melange M. Thrombosis of splenic artery pseudoaneurysm complicating pancreatitis Gut 1993;34:1271–3.

26. Demirkan K, Fleckenstein JF, Self TH. Thrombocytopenia associated with octreotide. Am J Med Sci 2000;320(4):296–7.

27. Bienvenu B, Timsit J. Sauna-induced diabetic ketoacidosis. Diabetes Care 1999;22(9):1584.

28. Abraldes JG, Bosch J. Somatostatin and analogues in portal hypertension. Hepatology 2002;35(6):1305–12.

29. Shojamanesh H, Gibril F, Louie A, Ojeaburu JV, Bashir S, Abou-Saif A, Jensen RT. Prospective study of the antitumor efficacy of long-term octreotide treatment in patients with progressive metastatic gastrinoma. Cancer 2002;94(2):331–43.

30. Kwekkeboom DJ, Bakker WH, Kam BL, Teunissen JJM, Kooij PPM, Herder WW, Feelders RA, Eijck CHJ, Jong M, Srinivasan A, Erion JL, Krenning EP. Treatment of patients with gastro-entero-pancreatic (GEP) tumours with the novel radiolabelled somatostatin analogue (177Lu-DOTA0, Tyr3)octreotate. Eur J Nucl Med Mol Imaging 2003;30:417–22.

31. Bajetta E, Procopio G, Ferrari L, Martinetti A, Zilembo N, Catena L, Alu M, Della TS, Alberti D, Buzzoni R. A randomized, multicenter prospective trial assessing long-acting release octreotide pamoate plus tamoxifen as a first line therapy for advanced breast carcinoma. Cancer 2002;94(2):299–304.

32. Slijkuis WA, Stadheim L, Hassoun ZM, Nzeako UC, Kremers WK, Talwalkar JA, Gores GJ. Octreotide therapy for advanced hepatocellular carcinoma. J Clin Gastroenterol 2005;39:333–8.

33. Thomas LA, Veysey MJ, Murphy GM, Russell-Jones D, French GL, Wass JAH, Dowling RH. Octreotide induced prolongation of colonic transit increases fecal anaerobic bacteria, bile acid metabolizing enzymes, and serum deoxycholic acid in patients with acromegaly. Gut 2005;54:630–5.

34. Paran D, Elkayam O, Mayo A, Paran H, Amit M, Yaron M, Caspi D. A pilot study of a long acting somatostatin analogue for the treatment of refractory rheumatoid arthritis. Ann Rheum Dis 2001;60(9):888–91.

35. Nakamura T, Kudoh K, Takebe K, Imamura K, Terada A, Kikuchi H, Yamada N, Arai Y, Tando Y, Machida K, et al. Octreotide decreases biliary and pancreatic exocrine function, and induces steatorrhea in healthy subjects. Intern Med 1994;33(10):593–6.

36. Uygur-Bayramicli O, Gemici C. Is liver disease an octreotide side effect? J Clin Gastroenterol 2003;37:86–7.

37. Avila NA, Shawker TH, Roach P, Bradford MH, Skarulis MC, Eastman R. Sonography of gallbladder abnormalities in acromegaly patients following octreotide and ursodiol therapy: incidence and time course. J Clin Ultrasound 1998;26(6):289–94.

38. Hussaini SH, Pereira SP, Veysey MJ, Kennedy C, Jenkins P, Murphy GM, Wass JA, Dowling RH. Roles of gall bladder emptying and intestinal transit in the pathogenesis of octreotide induced gall bladder stones. Gut 1996;38(5):775–83.

39. Rhodes M, James RA, Bird M, Clayton B, Kendall-Taylor P, Lennard TW. Gallbladder function in acromegalic patients taking long-term octreotide: evidence of rebound hypermotility on cessation of treatment. Scand J Gastroenterol 1992;27(2):115–8.

40. Sadoul JL, Benchimol D, Thyss A, Freychet P. Acute pancreatitis following octreotide withdrawal. Am J Med 1991;90(6):763–4.

41. Veysey MJ, Thomas LA, Mallet AI, Jenkins PJ, Besser GM, Wass JA, Murphy GM, Dowling RH. Prolonged large bowel transit increases serum deoxycholic acid: a risk factor for octreotide induced gallstones. Gut 1999;44(5):675–81.

42. Turner HE, Lindsell DR, Vadivale A, Thillainayagam AV, Wass JA. Differing effects on gall-bladder motility of lanreotide SR and octreotide LAR for treatment of acromegaly. Eur J Endocrinol 1999;141(6):590–4.

43. Moschetta A, Stolk MF, Rehfeld JF, Portincasa P, Slee PH, Koppeschaar HP, Van Erpecum KJ, Vanberge-Henegouwen GP. Severe impairment of postprandial cholecystokinin release and gall-bladder emptying and high risk of gallstone formation in acromegalic patients during Sandostatin LAR. Aliment Pharmacol Ther 2001;15(2):181–5.

44. Kalambokis G, Economou M, Fotopoulos A, Bokharhii JA, Pappas C, Katsaraki A, Tsianos EV. The effects of chronic treatment with octreotide versus octreotide plus midodrine on systemic hemodynamics and renal hemodynamics and function in nonazotemic cirrhotic patients with ascites. Am J Gastroenterol 2005;100:879–85.

45. Atmaca A, Erbas, T. Lipoatrophy induced by subcutaneous administration of octreotide in the treatment of acromegaly. Exp Clin Endocrinol Diabetes 2005;113:340–3.

46. Vecht J, Lamers CB, Masclee AA. Long-term results of octreotide-therapy in severe dumping syndrome. Clin Endocrinol (Oxf) 1999;51(5):619–24.

47. Suliman M, Jenkins R, Ross R, Powell T, Battersby R, Cullen DR. Long-term treatment of acromegaly with the somatostatin analogue SR-lanreotide. J Endocrinol Invest 1999;22(6):409–18.

48. Lami M-C, Hadjadj S, Guillet G. Hair loss in three patients with acromegaly treated with octreotide. Br J Dermatol 2003;149:655–6.

49. Kaal A, Orskov H, Nielsen S, Pedroncelli AM, Lancranjan I, Marbach P, Weeke J. Occurrence and effects of octreotide antibodies during nasal, subcutaneous and slow release intramuscular treatment. Eur J Endocrinol 2000;143(3):353–61.

50. Rideout DJ, Graham MM. Buttock granulomas: a consequence of intramuscular injection of Sandostatin detected by In-111 octreoscan. Clin Nucl Med 2001;26(7):650.

51. Welin SV, Janson ET, Sundin A, Stridsberg M, Lavenius E, Granberg D, Skogseid B, Oberg KE, Eriksson BK. High-dose treatment with a long-acting somatostatin analogue in patients with advanced midgut carcinoid tumours. Eur J Endocrinol 2004;151:107–12.

52. Fassnacht M, Capeller B, Arlt W, Steck T, Allolio B. Octreotide LAR treatment throughout pregnancy in an acromegalic woman. Clin Endocrinol (Oxf) 2001;55(3):411–5.

53. Herman-Bonert V, Seliverstov M, Melmed S. Pregnancy in acromegaly: successful therapeutic outcome. J Clin Endocrinol Metab 1998;83(3):727–31.

54. de Menis E, Billeci D, Marton E, Gussoni G. Uneventful pregnancy in an acromegalic patient treated with slow-

release lanreotide: a case report. J Clin Endocrinol Metab 1999;84(4):1489.

55. Athanasakis E, Chrysos E, Zoras OJ, Tsiaoussis J, Karkavitsas N, Xynos E. Octreotide enhances the accelerating effect of erythromycin on gastric emptying in healthy subjects. Aliment Pharmacol Ther 2002;16(8):1563–70.

56. Hoeldtke RD, Horvath GG, Bryner KD, Hobbs GR. Treatment of orthostatic hypotension with midodrine and octreotide. J Clin Endocrinol Metab 1998;83(2):339–43.

57. Ripamonti C, De Conno F, Boffi R, Ascani L, Bianchi M. Can somatostatin be administered in association with morphine in advanced cancer patients with pain? Ann Oncol 1998;9(8):921–3.

Somatropin (growth hormone)

General Information

Established indications for somatropin (growth hormone) include growth hormone deficiency in children, Turner's syndrome, Noonan's syndrome, and renal insufficiency in children. Other well-studied indications include idiopathic short stature, adult growth hormone deficiency, osteoporosis, and catabolic states associated with acute and chronic illness and injury. Body composition, respiratory muscle function, physical strength, and height improved in a 12-month trial of somatropin in 54 children with Prader–Willi syndrome (1).

The adverse effects of somatropin differ between adults and children. In adults, adverse effects are commoner in men, in heavier patients, and in adult-onset growth hormone deficiency. Efficacy is no greater in those who develop adverse effects. The higher rate of adverse effects is due to the higher dose of somatropin when calculated according to body weight, and also to lower sensitivity to somatropin in women than in men (2–4). Rapid dose escalation also increases the rate of adverse effects. To minimize adverse effects, it is recommended that treatment be started at a low dosage, that is 0.4–0.8 U/day, and titrated according to the age-specific concentration of IGF-1 (2,3,5).

Adverse effects are commoner in patients using higher doses. Starting at a low dose, increasing the dose gradually, and titrating individual doses against age-specific IGF-I concentrations may minimize adverse events.

The potential immediate and long-term hazards in athletes who use growth hormone in supraphysiological doses have been reviewed (6). They were:

Acute:

- exacerbation of lipolysis and increasing lactate production during exercise, which could impair an athlete's performance;
- reduced glycogen storage in muscle and liver, which would make exercise recovery more difficult;
- increased fatty acid concentrations, with a possible risk of cardiac dysrhythmias.

Chronic:

- poor exercise tolerance;
- evidence of reduced fat; although muscle appears better defined it can show myopathic features.

Organs and Systems

Cardiovascular

The effect of somatropin on cardiovascular risk is complex, as growth hormone reduces visceral fat and total cholesterol and increases HDL cholesterol concentrations (7–9).

Edema, both generalized and peripheral, is common in adults given somatropin, as is hypertension. Symptoms are usually mild and resolve in many patients despite continuing treatment (10). Increased left ventricular wall thickness has been reported in both adults and children, although in children this is thought to reflect an increase in overall mass and is not thought to be of clinical significance (11,12).

In an open study in five patients with severe dilated cardiomyopathy given high-dose somatropin 4 IU/day (1.3 mg/day) for 3 months, ventricular dysrhythmias worsened in all patients during treatment, from Lown class 2 or 3 to 4A or 4B, and returned to baseline when treatment was stopped (13).

- A 7-year-old boy developed cardiomegaly and edema within a month of starting somatropin, 0.7 IU/kg/week; when the dose was reduced to 0.35 IU/kg/week his heart size returned to normal (14).

This is a reminder that the adverse effects of somatropin are dose-related within the therapeutic range and that dose escalation should be gradual.

In 80 postmenopausal women with osteoporosis aged 50–70 years, two doses of growth hormone, 1.0 U/day (n = 28) or 2.5 U/day (n = 27) for 3 years, were compared with placebo (15). Plasma fibrinogen increased in both growth hormone groups at 4 years only; the significance of this finding is uncertain. Fibrinogen concentrations are raised in acromegaly and since fibrinogen is a risk factor for cardiovascular disease, especially stroke, people with acromegaly have an increased risk of cardiovascular disease.

Of 23 adolescent patients with growth hormone deficiency in childhood who were reassessed when they had reached adult bone age and completed puberty, eight were no longer thought to be growth hormone deficient and therapy was withdrawn (16). The other 15 had a 6-month break from growth hormone therapy and then restarted. Compared with a control group at the time of withdrawal, the eight patients without growth hormone deficiency had increased thickness of the carotid intima media, which fell to normal values by 12 months. These results support the recommendation that children with idiopathic growth hormone deficiency should be retested after completion of growth to assess the need for continued administration of growth hormone.

Respiratory

In 31 elderly frail women, mean age 86 years, who were randomized to receive growth hormone or placebo for 14 days after surgery for hip fracture, there was an excess of thromboembolic events and chest infections; the mechanism was not clear (17).

Nervous system

Somatropin extracted from cadaveric human pituitaries was used to treat growth hormone-deficient patients until several cases of the fatal degenerative neurological disorder Creutzfeldt–Jakob disease were reported in the mid-1980s. Of 267 cases of iatrogenic Creutzfeldt–Jakob disease, 139 were caused by human cadaver-derived somatropin (SEDA-25, 479).

This disease develops when an abnormal prion protein present in the cadaveric material induces a cascade of conformational changes in host protein. Creutzfeldt–Jakob disease in recipients of somatropin differs from the sporadic form, in that it usually presents with cerebellar signs rather than cognitive impairment, and also in the prominence of prion protein amyloid plaques in nervous tissue (18). In a review, 139 cases of Creutzfeldt–Jakob disease were identified worldwide in people treated with cadaveric somatropin before recombinant human growth hormone became available in the mid-1980s (19). The prevalence of this fatal neurodegenerative condition in recipients of somatropin ranges from 0.3% in the USA to 4.4% in France. Creutzfeldt–Jakob disease has been reported to start at 4–30 years after therapy with cadaveric somatropin (18), so that further cases are anticipated and continue to be reported (20).

- A case has been reported in Brazil, 28 years after somatropin therapy (21).
- An 18-year-old man from Qatar presented with a 3-month history of unsteadiness, dysarthria, and left-sided weakness, followed by visual, hearing, and memory loss, 13 years after somatropin therapy (22).

This is the first case from Qatar, but it is possible that other cases there have not been reported.

People exposed to a contaminated batch of somatropin have about a 6% chance of developing Creutzfeldt–Jakob disease (23), although there are no reliable predictors of risk in an individual. The risk varies to some extent with the mode of preparation of the product, but it seems unlikely that it can be entirely eliminated. The natural product was therefore withdrawn from the market in most countries, but was rapidly replaced by biosynthetic somatropin preparations

Carpal tunnel syndrome due to somatropin is probably dose-dependent and was reported in 4.8% of subjects in a double-blind trial (10).

Headache is a common adverse effect of somatropin. It often occurs early in treatment and usually responds to temporary dosage reduction followed by gradual re-escalation (1,24). It can be an early indicator of the rare complication pseudotumor cerebri (idiopathic intracranial hypertension), particularly in high-risk groups, such

as children with renal insufficiency, and may require further investigation. Headache was reported in 13% of 75 prepubertal children treated with a modified-release formulation of somatropin over 12 months (25).

Somatropin can cause idiopathic intracranial hypertension (pseudotumor cerebri), characterized by headache, papilledema, visual disturbance, and sometimes nausea and vomiting (26). Less common features include extraocular palsy, present in up to 48% of affected patients (26), mood changes, and somnolence. There have been 30 cases reported worldwide (27); chronic renal insufficiency, Turner's syndrome, obesity, and biochemical growth hormone deficiency are all associated with an increased risk. About half of the reported cases occurred within the first 8 weeks of treatment, and all responded to dose reduction or withdrawal of human growth hormone. Fundoscopy is recommended before starting somatropin and regularly during the first few months, although the absence of papilledema does not exclude the diagnosis. Up to 48% of children with intracranial hypertension due to somatropin also develop a sixth nerve palsy (27).

The National Cooperative Growth Study Multicentre Observational Surveillance Registry started in 1985. It is a post-marketing surveillance programme in children treated with biosynthetic growth hormone from Genentech. Data collected up to January 2002 have shown that the risk of intracranial hypertension is related to the indication for growth hormone (28). There were 62 cases per 1000 patient years in children with renal insufficiency, 3.7 cases per 1000 patient years in children with Turner's syndrome, 1.6 cases per 1000 patient years in children with growth hormone deficiency, and no cases in children with idiopathic short stature. This suggests that a prior condition may be required for the development of intracranial hypertension. Most cases are reversible after withdrawal of growth hormone.

- A 13-month-old girl with Turner's syndrome developed mild papilledema (29). At the age of 4 years she was considered for growth hormone therapy and investigation showed intracranial hypertension before therapy was started.
- A 6-year-old girl with Turner's syndrome was treated with growth hormone. There was no papilledema before therapy, but intracranial hypertension was diagnosed at the age of 10 years (29).
- A non-obese 6-year-old girl with Ullrich–Turner syndrome developed headache, vomiting, and blurred vision, with papilledema and increased cerebrospinal fluid pressure 5 months after starting somatropin 0.9 IU/kg/week (30). The cerebrospinal fluid pressure normalized after somatropin was withdrawn, and increased again when therapy was restarted. Her visual acuity was reduced to less than 30% in the right eye.

According to the authors there have been 40 cases of pseudotumor cerebri associated with somatropin therapy worldwide, owing to stimulation of cerebrospinal fluid production or reduced drainage.

Sensory systems

Retinal changes, clinically indistinguishable from diabetic retinopathy, were reported in two non-diabetic recipients of somatropin (31).

- An obese 31-year-old man developed non-proliferative retinopathy and macular edema with reduced visual acuity after 14 months' therapy, which improved after somatropin was withdrawn.
- An 11-year-old girl with Turner's syndrome developed unilateral neovascularization after receiving somatropin for 22 months.

These patients improved but did not completely resolve after somatropin was withdrawn.

Somatropin concentrations correlate with retinopathy in patients with diabetes. There are no prospective clinical reports of retinal findings in adult recipients of somatropin, and these are awaited to determine the true frequency of this complication.

Psychological

In 20 women (mean age 67 years) who received intramuscular triptorelin 3.75 mg 6-weekly for endometriosis, nine developed mood disturbance after the second injection and appeared to be cumulative, since the symptoms only started after the second injection and worsened with successive injections (32). One woman withdrew after the third injection because of severe irritability.

Endocrine

Thyroid function tests are often altered by somatropin because of increased conversion of T4 to T3, but this is clinically insignificant at low doses (SEDA-21, 453). One child with Prader–Willi syndrome had a fall in serum thyroxine concentration during somatropin therapy and needed thyroxine replacement (33). Hypothyroidism developed in 11 of 46 growth hormone-deficient children treated with somatropin (34). Prior abnormalities in hypothalamic-pituitary function and alterations in thyroid hormone metabolism, probably both, contributed to the high incidence of hypothyroidism, which was similar to that in previous studies.

Three adolescent boys with chronic renal insufficiency, treated with somatropin during the pubertal growth spurt, developed severe hyperparathyroidism (35). It is unclear whether this was coincidental or whether growth hormone and sex steroid hormones had a synergistic effect.

There have been occasional reports of gynecomastia attributed to somatropin (SEDA-21, 453).

Metabolism

Hyperinsulinemia is common in recipients of somatropin, but the long-term effects are controversial. This issue is becoming increasingly important as more adult patients are treated and the duration of therapy is extended. Growth hormone deficiency is itself associated with insulin resistance (36). Plasma concentrations of glucose and hemoglobin A_{1C} increase, especially in the first 6–12

months, indicating relative insulin resistance (37,38); the increases are often within the reference ranges (4,39).

Plasma glucose is inconsistently described as showing a sustained increase within the reference range, a transient increase, or no change. This reflects both the small non-controlled populations reported and possible selection bias, with exclusion of some patients because of hyperglycemia before the start of a cohort study (39). Hyperglycemia has occasionally been reported in patients receiving very high doses of human growth hormone for catabolic conditions, but has usually not required specific treatment (40). In a 6-month randomized study of 74 men and 57 women aged over 65 years, diabetes or glucose intolerance developed in 18 men treated with somatropin compared with seven controls (41).

Diabetes mellitus was previously not thought to be more common in recipients of somatropin than in the general population (SEDA-13, 1308) (42). However, longer-term observations have shown a three-fold incidence compared with predicted rates of type II diabetes, probably representing a younger age of onset rather than an increase in de novo cases (43).

In 78 children treated with somatropin for 7 years the mean fasting glucose concentration increased significantly compared with baseline after both 1 and 6 years of somatropin treatment, but remained the reference range and was not higher at 6 years than at 1 year (37).

In a 5-year study, 67 children treated with somatropin all had a sustained increase in fasting and oral glucose-stimulated insulin concentrations. This was most significant in children on dialysis and with renal transplants (44). In another study, insulin secretion in response to intravenous glucose was increased in 14 children with renal insufficiency, but returned to baseline after 12 months. However, increased insulin concentrations persisted in nine girls with Turner's syndrome (45). Concomitant glucocorticoid and somatropin treatment in children with juvenile arthritis caused a small but significant rise in blood glucose and glycosylated hemoglobin, which returned to pretreatment concentrations after somatropin was withdrawn (46).

Of 21 children, 15 developed hyperglycemia in a study of high-dose somatropin (0.2 mg/kg/day) for burns (47). In another study of 29 children with renal insufficiency (a group known to have insulin resistance), integrated insulin concentrations increased significantly in the first year of somatropin treatment, with no associated change in plasma glucose or glycated hemoglobin (48).

In a retrospective study, the fasting glucose:insulin ratio, a marker of insulin resistance, fell more in girls with Turner syndrome than in children with idiopathic short stature during somatropin therapy. The lower glucose:insulin ratio was due to increased fasting insulin and correlated with increased body mass index (49).

- Diabetes occurred 2 months after somatropin was begun in a 14 year-old girl, with restoration of normoglycemia after it was withdrawn (50).

In a postmarketing review of over 20 000 patients, type II diabetes was three times more common than expected, probably because at-risk individuals became diabetic at an earlier age than predicted (43). In a postmarketing review of 23 333 children and adolescents (52 375 treatment years), the incidence of type I diabetes was not significantly increased. However, type II diabetes occurred in 46 and 28 per 100 000 treatment years in children aged 10–19 and 6–14 years respectively (six times greater in both age groups than published reference values). There was no difference in incidence between boys and girls. A further 42 children developed abnormal glucose tolerance (51). Diabetes and glucose intolerance did not resolve after somatropin was withdrawn. Children who became diabetic were usually pubertal and had received somatropin for a longer period. Obesity, a risk factor for type II diabetes in the general population, was uncommon in these children.

Experience in adults is more limited, and monitoring is essential (52). Studies of somatropin in adults have consistently shown increased plasma concentrations of glucose, glycated hemoglobin, and insulin (53,54). Glucose intolerance and frank diabetes mellitus have been frequently reported in small series (53,55). Hyperglycemia not requiring specific treatment has been reported more often in adult patients (10) and in patients receiving high-dose somatropin to treat wasting associated with burns or HIV infection (40,56), but the overall incidence has not been compared with that in the general population.

In 25 patients a depot formulation of somatropin was associated with a non-sustained increase in glucose and insulin concentrations, more pronounced in men (57).

In a double-blind, placebo-controlled study of 24 growth hormone-deficient adults treated for 4 months with somatropin 2 IU/day, the treated patients had a significant increase in fasting plasma glucose and insulin concentrations, and increased insulin resistance, determined by insulin AUC during oral and intravenous glucose tolerance testing (9). Similarly, a group of 30 adolescents who were not growth hormone-deficient, and who were treated with somatropin for a mean of 7.9 years, had significantly reduced insulin sensitivity and raised plasma glucose concentrations during treatment, returning to control concentrations after somatropin was withdrawn (58). One of these patients developed glucose intolerance.

In a study of high-dose somatropin (0.1 mg/kg/day) in 20 patients with severe burns (a condition that causes insulin resistance), 60% of the treated patients required insulin therapy for hyperglycemia compared with 25% of the controls (59). This study was limited by the fact that the treated patients had more severe burns than the controls.

In a high-dose study in eight HIV-positive men, oral glucose tolerance worsened in the first month of human growth hormone 3 mg/day, then improved toward baseline. Mild glucose intolerance was still present after 6 months, despite a reduction in visceral fat. One man with pre-existing glucose intolerance developed symptomatic diabetes within 2 weeks of starting somatropin (60).

- Acanthosis nigricans, which is characterized by dark velvety thickening of the skin on the nape of the neck and in the groins and axillae, has been described in a non-obese 10-year-old boy with achondroplasia who received somatropin 3–4 IU/week for 7 years (61).

There has been one previous report of acanthosis nigricans in a woman who received human pituitary extract (62). This condition is usually seen in hyperinsulinemic states, including diabetes mellitus and acromegaly; overstimulation at the IGF-I receptor is probably the final common pathway.

- A 13-year-old boy with Prader–Willi syndrome and steatohepatitis was given growth hormone 0.23 mg/kg/week (63). His Hb_{A1c} concentration before treatment was 5.6%. Four weeks later he developed diabetic ketoacidosis. He was given insulin and the growth hormone was withdrawn. Insulin was then gradually withdrawn and blood glucose concentrations remained normal for the next 6 months.

The KIGS/KIMS (Pharmacia International Growth Database) has reported 233 patients with Prader–Willi syndrome, of whom three developed carbohydrate intolerance.

Premenopausal women who received leuprolide acetate depot 3.75 mg every 28 days for 6 cycles had slightly but statistically significant higher concentrations of total cholesterol, LDL-cholesterol, and HDL-cholesterol, and increased insulin resistance (64). Whether these changes are clinically significant is not known.

Mineral balance

Hypercalcemia, usually mild and not requiring specific treatment, was reported in 43 of 100 patients receiving high-dose somatropin in intensive care (SEDA-13, 1308; 65).

Fluid balance

Edema is three times more frequent with a dose of somatropin of 0.025 mg/kg/day than 0.0125 mg/kg/day (66). In a randomized, controlled study of 33 obese women, three of nine who received somatropin and two of seven who received somatropin plus insulin-like growth factor-1 withdrew from the study, because of intolerable edema, compared with none in the placebo group. Most patients receiving somatropin required diuretic treatment for edema in this study, in which dose was calculated according to body weight (67). In a randomized, placebo-controlled trial of growth hormone replacement in 166 hormone-deficient adults, 48% of the treated group and 30% of the placebo group reported mild to moderate edema, which resolved in 70% of subjects despite continued treatment (10).

Hematologic

Leukemia has been reported in several patients treated with somatropin. However, when other risk factors are accounted for, there is no current evidence that it increases the risk significantly above population levels (SEDA-23, 468; 68).

- Acute myelogenous leukemia was diagnosed in a 25-year-old man with hypopituitarism, 4 months after he started to use somatropin three times a week (69).

The time interval in this case was too short to implicate somatropin as a definite cause.

Gastrointestinal

Nausea, which did not require specific treatment, occurred within 72 hours after an injection of long-acting somatropin in six of 25 patients (57).

Skin

Injection site reactions to somatropin are common and include nodules, pain, and erythema. They usually resolve spontaneously (25,34). In a 2-year study of once- or twice-monthly injections of a modified-release formulation of somatropin in 56 prepubertal children, injection site reactions were common, especially in the first year of treatment. These included skin nodules in 56% of injections, erythema in 49%, and lipoatrophy in 12% (70).

- A 12-year-old boy developed lipohypertrophy at the site of somatropin injection (71). Site rotation gave partial resolution.
- A 51-year-old woman with both panhypopituitarism and liver disease developed localized abdominal lipohypertrophy during somatropin therapy (72).

The authors of the second report speculated that hepatic IGF-1 secretion was compromised and that peripheral somatropin reached supraphysiological concentrations.

Lipoatrophy, a transient loss of subcutaneous fat identifiable as skin dimpling, occurred in 11% of injections in 75 children who were given modified-release somatropin for 12 months (25) and in one of 68 children in another study (34). Site rotation is recommended to prevent lipodystrophy.

Non-neoplastic pigmented nevi may increase in number in patients treated with somatropin (SEDA-21, 453).

Musculoskeletal

Arthralgia and proximal myalgia are common with somatropin, especially with large doses or rapid dose escalation (3,56,66,67).

A slipped capital femoral epiphysis was reported in 26 of 16 500 patients in one study: it is less common in children with idiopathic short stature than those with a known cause of growth failure (73).

- Avascular necrosis of the femoral head and another of slipped capital femoral epiphysis with avascular necrosis have been reported in two children with growth hormone deficiency receiving growth hormone (74).

However, in a North American register of patients with chronic renal insufficiency and end-stage renal disease there was no excess of cases of slipped capital femoral epiphysis or avascular necrosis in those receiving growth hormone (75).

Growth acceleration makes scoliosis more apparent in less than 1% of children treated with somatropin, many of whom also receive spinal irradiation. A causative role for somatropin has not been substantiated (76).

There are conflicting reports on a possible increased risk of fractures in children with osteogenesis imperfecta treated with somatropin, many of whom have a qualitative defect in collagen (77,78).

- A boy with osteogenesis imperfecta, with no previous fractures, who received somatropin from age 5 to 14, had four fractures during his pubertal growth spurt, similar to two previous case reports (79).

Of 21 of 151 patients who were treated with growth hormone for growth hormone deficiency for 2–12 years, some developed acromegalic features: eight had a foot size greater than the 97th centile and four had a jaw length greater than +2 standard deviations (80).

In 85 Japanese children with various skeletal dysplasias there was no gain in height from growth hormone therapy in those with pseudochondroplasia (n = 4) or congenital spondyloepiphyseal dysplasia (n = 4) (81). Patients with spondyloepiphyseal dysplasia in particular found that when growth was promoted weakness in their ligaments resulted in worsening kyphosis and lordosis.

Of 35 children with achondroplasia randomized to either low-dose growth hormone (0.1 IU/kg/day) or high-dose growth hormone (0.2 IU/kg/day), two in the low-dose group developed worsening of bow legs, requiring surgery; one in the high-dose group developed incomplete paraplegia, requiring thoracic laminectomy, and another had surgery for a narrow foramen magnum (82). There was no control group, and although it was thought that all the events had been related to the achondroplasia rather than the growth hormone, it is not known whether problems had been exacerbated.

- A girl with floating harbor syndrome (short stature, delayed bone age, typical facies, and delayed speech development) received growth hormone from the age of 3.5 years for 14 months (83). At 6 years she developed an abnormal gait due to a tethered cord.

A tethered cord is a developmental abnormality that does not usually manifest until mid-childhood. Floating harbor syndrome is associated with severe short stature, and tethered cord is not usually a manifestation. It is possible that altered growth velocity associated with growth hormone may have been implicated.

Reproductive system

A change in prostate size has been reported in patients receiving growth hormone, but no change in the concentration of prostate-specific antigen (84).

Immunologic

Patients treated with recombinant somatropin commonly develop antibodies against growth hormone; the incidence is 22–88% (85). There were low titers of antigrowth hormone antibody, with no reduction in growth response, in 44% of children who used modified-release somatropin once a month and in 68% who used it twice a month (25). Antibodies almost never have clinical significance, but the fourth case of reduced growth due to neutralizing antibodies against growth hormone has been reported in a 9-year-old boy; growth resumed after he was changed to a methionyl-free human formulation of somatropin (85).

Systemic allergic reactions to somatropin are very rare, but can be overcome by desensitization (SEDA-13, 1308; 86). Although early studies suggested a higher rate of renal transplant rejection in recipients of somatropin than in controls (SEDA-21, 452), this was not confirmed in a long-term prospective study (87).

- In a 15-year-old boy with previously quiescent lupus nephritis, laboratory markers of disease activity rose during somatropin treatment and returned to baseline concentrations within 3 months after withdrawal (88).

Death

Nine deaths have been reported in children with Prader–Willi syndrome receiving growth hormone. Pfizer issued a safety warning for growth hormone and Prader–Willi syndrome after reviewing seven deaths in male subjects (89). There was an association with severe obesity and severe respiratory impairment.

- A 4-year-old, severely obese boy with Prader–Willi syndrome received growth hormone 0.3 mg/day for 2 weeks, 0.6 mg/day for 2 further weeks, and then 1 mg/day (0.16 mg/kg/week actual body weight and 0.41 mg/kg/week ideal body weight) (90). He started to have headaches within a few weeks of using the highest dosage, which was reduced. The dosage was then increased without recurrence of symptoms to 1 mg/day, but he was found dead 3 days later, 67 days after starting growth hormone.

Reports of sudden unexplained death in Prader–Willi syndrome in association with growth hormone have generally been in boys. Two deaths in girls have now been reported (91).

- A 4-year-old girl with Prader–Willi syndrome had an adenoidectomy for severe snoring, and growth hormone was started at a dose of 0.24 mg/kg/week. Suddenly, 7 weeks later, she died at home of cardiorespiratory failure.
- A 9-year-old girl with trisomy 21 and Prader–Willi syndrome started growth hormone treatment 0.14 mg/kg/week. She had previously received growth hormone 0.28 mg/kg/week for 12 months at the age of 7 years, but therapy had been stopped at the family's request. Six months later she developed a respiratory infection and died.

In a review of sudden death in patients with Prader–Willi syndrome, those who received growth hormone were compared with those who had not (92). Death between the ages of 3 and 15 years seemed to be more common in those who had received growth hormone than in those who had not. The dose of growth hormone, obesity, and respiratory problems may have been

contributing factors. Six of seven patients who had received growth hormone died within 4 months of starting treatment.

Long-Term Effects

Tumorigenicity

The incidence of malignancy is increased in acromegaly, in which growth hormone is present in excess. Patients treated with growth hormone have therefore been carefully monitored. The cancer risk of growth hormone has been reviewed (93).

The first report of leukemia in Japanese children treated with growth hormone (94) prompted a worldwide survey. There have been reports of 44 new cases of leukemia in growth hormone recipients, of which only 20 were acute lymphoblastic leukemia. This is much less than the expected 80–85% of new childhood leukemia (95).

A review of Japanese patients found that of the 15 patients who had developed hematological malignancies since 1975, 6 had other risk factors for leukemia, such as Fanconi's syndrome or prior chemotherapy or radiotherapy. The incidence of leukemia in this study was 3 per 100 000, similar to that in the general population of the same age (68). The National Cooperative Growth Study (NCGS—a postmarketing database that includes 19 846 patient-years since the time of growth hormone exposure) similarly reported no increase in the incidence of new leukemia when patients with other risk factors were excluded from the analysis (96).

The recurrence rate of intracranial tumors has been addressed in a number of large observational studies. Reports from the NCGS database (which includes 1262 children with brain tumors) and from England have shown no increase in intracranial tumor recurrence in patients treated with growth hormone (97,98). For patients with craniopharyngioma, postoperative irradiation reduced the recurrence rate, but growth hormone therapy did not increase the risk (99).

A higher incidence of intracranial neoplasia has been reported in the Pharmacia (originally Pharmacia & Upjohn) International Metabolic Surveillance (KIMS) study; however, this could be an effect of increased surveillance (100).

Japanese patients with growth hormone deficiency who had taken part in a placebo-controlled study (n = 64) were entered into an open 48-week study of growth hormone; one had a recurrence of craniopharyngioma and required withdrawal from the study (101). Whether growth hormone was contributory is not known.

In the NCGS study extracranial non-leukemia malignancy rates were similarly not increased in patients treated with growth hormone compared with those who were not (102).

Despite theoretical concerns, there is no evidence that either intracranial or extracranial malignancy, new or recurrent, is increased in subjects treated with growth hormone (97,98,99). Despite this, certain precautions are still recommended for children who have previously been treated for cancer. The diagnosis of growth hormone deficiency should be clearly established (95) and it is recommended that treatment be delayed for at least 1 year after tumor therapy has been completed (43).

In a cohort study in 1848 British patients who received human pituitary-derived growth hormone from 1959 to 1985 (30 000 patient-years), there were two cases of colorectal cancer (0.25 expected) and two cases of Hodgkin's disease (0.85 expected); the standardized mortality ratios were 10.8 and 11.4 respectively (103). However, the number of cancers was small and the doses used were higher than typically today, and these results should be interpreted with caution.

In 1848 patients treated with growth hormone during childhood there was an 11-fold increase in the incidence of colorectal cancer after a mean 16 years of follow-up and a 15-fold increase in mortality from colorectal cancer and Hodgkin's disease after 21 years of follow-up. However, there were too few deaths to draw any firm conclusions.

Diamond–Blackfan anemia is rare: only about 400 cases have been reported world wide. Six patients have developed an osteosarcoma, three after receiving growth hormone (104).

- A Caucasian girl with Diamond–Blackfan anemia received growth hormone to treat short stature, and 6 weeks later developed pain in the right thigh; an osteosarcoma was diagnosed.

The short time period in this case makes the tumor less likely to have been induced by growth hormone. It is also unlikely that the growth hormone hastened the growth of a pre-existing tumor; the mean survival of the other five patients was 1.6 years from the time of diagnosis and this patient was alive 1.6 years after the diagnosis.

The safety of growth hormone treatment for idiopathic short stature has been discussed in two reports of studies involving pharmaceutical companies. The doses and durations of therapy varied. Comparison of adverse event rates with those in the background population did not show an increased risk of new malignancies. However, this was a post-marketing surveillance study and it is uncertain that it had sufficient power to detect a small increase in risk (105). In a similar report, adverse events in patients with idiopathic short stature were compared with those in patients with growth hormone deficiency and Turner's syndrome (106). While malignancy was not attributed to the use of growth hormone, long-term safety data are essential to establish whether there is a small increased risk of life-threatening events.

Second-Generation Effects

Teratogenicity

Only a few pregnancies have been reported in women treated with somatropin. Eight women with hypopituitarism were followed prospectively during 12 pregnancies at a mean daily pregestation dose of 0.5 mg/day. The dose of somatropin was gradually reduced during the second trimester and withdrawn at the start of the third trimester. No congenital abnormalities were observed and weight and length at birth were normal (107).

Susceptibility Factors

Age

Most of the information about the long-term safety of somatropin in children has been derived from databases voluntarily maintained by two pharmaceutical companies; thus, there may be under-reporting. Other trials have generally been of short duration, with few participants, and may thus have been subject to type II error. The effectiveness and safety of somatropin in children has been the subject of a systematic review (108).

The use of growth hormone in adults over the age of 60 years without growth hormone deficiency has been reviewed (109). The adverse effects were the same as those found in adults deficient in growth hormone: peripheral edema, paresthesia, carpal tunnel syndrome, glucose intolerance, and gynecomastia in men. The adverse effects were dose-related. There were no long-term data available about safety, in particular the risk of cancer.

Sex

Somatropin is being increasingly prescribed for growth hormone-deficient adults. Men have more adverse effects than women, probably because of a greater IGF-1 response (110). This was also seen in 74 elderly men and 57 elderly women in a controlled trial, and was not influenced by concomitant sex steroid therapy (41).

In 47 men and 37 women aged 18–70 years, who received growth hormone 0.0125 mg/kg/day for 1 month and then 0.025 mg/kg/day in a placebo-controlled trial for 12 months, the dose was adjusted if adverse effects occurred (111). The mean serum IGF-1 concentration in women rose into the reference range. In contrast the mean serum IGF-1 concentration in men exceeded the age-adjusted reference range. Arthralgia was more common in men who received growth hormone than placebo (34% versus 10%) and edema in was more common in women (70% versus 40%). Ring size increased in both men (5.4% versus 0.7%) and women (3.5 versus –1.7%).

Drug Administration

Drug formulations

Human growth hormone with a molecular mass of 20 kDa comprises 6–7% of circulating growth hormone. Rat studies have suggested that 20 kDa growth hormone may have fewer adverse effects than the commonly prescribed 22 kDa variety. In 56 subjects aged 20–64 years with growth hormone deficiency, who received 20 kDa growth hormone, 0.006mg/kg/day (n=19), 0.012 mg/kg/day (n=18), or 0.024 mg/kg/day (n=19) for 16 weeks, adverse effects were similar to those that occur with 22 kDa growth hormone (112). Peripheral edema developed in six patients (31%) who received the lowest dose and in 15 patients (79%) who received the highest dose. Arthralgia, headache, and glucose intolerance also occurred. There were no significant advantages of 20 kDa growth hormone.

The proprietary product hGH-Biosphere is a dry powder containing microspheres of growth hormone, which is reconstituted and injected subcutaneously. In eight patients with growth hormone deficiency who took part in a phase I/II study, there were two peaks of growth hormone concentration: the first was 0.83 μg/l at 7.7 hours and the second was 1.2 μg/l after 7.2 days (113). The concentrations fell to baseline from days 10 to 28. There were no serious adverse events. One patient had fatigue, headache, and cramps, which resolved over 28 hours, one had myalgia, and two had erythema. The long-term suitability of long-acting growth hormone replacement is not known.

Drug dosage regimens

One recommended regimen is to start somatropin in a dosage of 0.15 mg/day and titrate upward (SEDA-14, 1521). Very high dosages (0.1–0.2 mg/kg/day, 10–20 times higher than replacement dosages given to adults with growth hormone deficiency) were given to 532 critically ill patients in intensive care units in two placebo-controlled trials (114). Mortality was significantly higher in the treated group than in the placebo group (42 versus 18%). Morbidity was also increased in somatropin recipients, who needed longer ventilator times.

Early studies using doses of somatropin that have been derived from pediatric experience had a high rate of adverse effects, and doses have been progressively reduced. In a 6-month, multicenter, randomized study, 302 adults were given somatropin 3 micrograms/kg/day, increasing to 6 micrograms/kg/day after 3 months, and 293 were given 6 micrograms/kg/day, increasing to 12 micrograms/kg/day (115). The lower dose was associated with significantly fewer adverse events (in particular, arthralgia in 12 versus 20%). However, 78% of women or patients with childhood-onset growth hormone deficiency had subnormal IGF-1 concentrations, suggesting that treatment should be titrated to IGF-1 concentrations and adverse effects.

Drug–Drug Interactions

Ciclosporin

Growth hormone increases the activity and regulates the gene expression of hepatic CYP3A4 (116). Mean blood concentrations of ciclosporin were lower during somatropin therapy in an open study in 16 prepubertal kidney transplant recipients, despite stable weight-related doses, suggesting that the metabolism of ciclosporin was increased by somatropin. Two patients had acute episodes of rejection during somatropin therapy; one of these may have been related to the fall in ciclosporin concentration (117).

Estradiol

In eight postmenopausal growth hormone-deficient women randomized to estradiol, either orally 2 mg/day or transdermally 100 micrograms/day, together with incremental doses of somatropin in an 8-week, crossover study, oral but not transdermal estrogen reduced IGF-1 concentrations, protein synthesis, and postprandial lipid oxidation rates (118). This confirms the results of a previous report (119). The mechanism is not known, but high portal estrogen concentrations after oral estrogen administration probably alter hepatic growth hormone metabolism.

References

1. Carrel AL, Myers SE, Whitman BY, Allen DB. Growth hormone improves body composition, fat utilization, physical strength and agility, and growth in Prader–Willi syndrome: a controlled study. J Pediatr 1999;134(2):215–21.
2. Blethen S. Dosing, monitoring, and safety in adults with growth hormone deficiency. Endocrinologist 1998;16:994–9.
3. Drake WM, Coyte D, Camacho-Hubner C, Jivanji NM, Kaltsas G, Wood DF, Trainer PJ, Grossman AB, Besser GM, Monson JP. Optimizing growth hormone replacement therapy by dose titration in hypopituitary adults. J Clin Endocrinol Metab 1998;83(11):3913–9.
4. Hayes FJ, Fiad TM, McKenna TJ. Gender difference in the response of growth hormone (GH)-deficient adults to GH therapy. Metabolism 1999;48(3):308–13.
5. Meling TR. Growth hormone deficiency in adults: the role of replacement therapy. Biodrugs 1998;9:351–62.
6. Rennie MJ. Claims for the anabolic effects of growth hormone: a case of the Emperor's new clothes? Br J Sports Med 2003;37:100–5.
7. Weaver JU, Monson JP, Noonan K, John WG, Edwards A, Evans KA, Cunningham J. The effect of low dose recombinant human growth hormone replacement on regional fat distribution, insulin sensitivity, and cardiovascular risk factors in hypopituitary adults. J Clin Endocrinol Metab 1995;80(1):153–9.
8. Attanasio AF, Lamberts SW, Matranga AM, Birkett MA, Bates PC, Valk NK, Hilsted J, Bengtsson BA, Strasburger CJAdult Growth Hormone Deficiency Study Group. Adult growth hormone (GH)-deficient patients demonstrate heterogeneity between childhood onset and adult onset before and during human GH treatment. J Clin Endocrinol Metab 1997;82(1):82–8.
9. Rosenfalck AM, Fisker S, Hilsted J, Dinesen B, Volund A, Jorgensen JO, Christiansen JS, Madsbad S. The effect of the deterioration of insulin sensitivity on beta-cell function in growth-hormone-deficient adults following 4-month growth hormone replacement therapy. Growth Horm IGF Res 1999;9(2):96–105.
10. Cuneo RC, Judd S, Wallace JD, Perry-Keene D, Burger H, Lim-Tio S, Strauss B, Stockigt J, Topliss D, Alford F, Hew L, Bode H, Conway A, Handelsman D, Dunn S, Boyages S, Cheung NW, Hurley D. The Australian Multicenter Trial of Growth Hormone (GH) Treatment in GH-Deficient Adults. J Clin Endocrinol Metab 1998;83(1):107–16.
11. Daubeney PE, McCaughey ES, Chase C, Walker JM, Slavik Z, Betts PR, Webber SA. Cardiac effects of growth

hormone in short normal children: results after four years of treatment. Arch Dis Child 1995;72(4):337–9.

12. Crepaz R, Pitscheider W, Radetti G, Paganini C, Gentili L, Morini G, Braito E, Mengarda G. Cardiovascular effects of high-dose growth hormone treatment in growth hormone-deficient children. Pediatr Cardiol 1995;16(5):223–7.

13. Frustaci A, Gentiloni N, Russo MA. Growth hormone in the treatment of dilated cardiomyopathy. N Engl J Med 1996;335(9):672–3.

14. Oczkowska U. Przejsciowe powiekszenie sylwetki serca jako nietypowe powiklanie leczenia hormonen wzrostu. [Transient cardiac enlargement: an unusual adverse event associated with growth hormone therapy.] Endokrynol Diabetol Chor Przemiany Materii Wieku Rozw 2001;7(1):53–6.

15. Landin-Wilhelmsen K, Nilsson A, Bosaeus I, Bengtsson BA. Growth hormone increases bone mineral content in postmenopausal osteoporosis: a randomised placebo-controlled trial. J Bone Mineral Res 2003;18:393–405.

16. Calao A, Di Somma C, Rota F, Di Maio S, Salerno M, Klain A, Spiezia S, Lombardi G. Common carotid intima-media thickness in growth hormone (GH) deficient adolescents: a prospective study after GH withdrawal and restarting GH replacement. J Clin Endocrinol Metab 2005;90:2659–65.

17. Yeo AL, Levy D, Martin FC, Sonksen P, Sturgess I, Wheeler MM, Young A. Frailty and the biochemical effects of recombinant human growth hormone in women after surgery for hip fracture. Growth Hormone IGF Res 2003;13:361–70.

18. Brown P, Preece MA, Will RG. "Friendly fire" in medicine: hormones, homografts, and Creutzfeldt–Jakob disease. Lancet 1992;340(8810):24–7.

19. Brown P, Preece M, Brandel JP, Sato T, McShane L, Zerr I, Fletcher A, Will RG, Pocchiari M, Cashman NR, d'Aignaux JH, Cervenakova L, Fradkin J, Schonberger LB, Collins SJ. Iatrogenic Creutzfeldt–Jakob disease at the millennium. Neurology 2000;55(8):1075–81.

20. Gibbons RV, Holman RC, Belay ED, Schonberger LB. Creutzfeldt–Jakob disease in the United States: 1979-1998. JAMA 2000;284(18):2322–3.

21. Caboclo LO, Huang N, Lepski GA, Livramento JA, Buchpiguel CA, Porto CS, Nitrini R. Iatrogenic Creutzfeldt–Jakob disease following human growth hormone therapy: case report. Arq Neuropsiquiatr 2002;60(2-B):458–61.

22. Hamad A, Hamad A, Sokrab TE, Momeni S. Iatrogenic Creutzfeldt–Jakob disease at the millennium. Neurology 2001;56(7):987.

23. Huillard d'Aignaux J, Alperovitch A, Maccario J. A statistical model to identify the contaminated lots implicated in iatrogenic transmission of Creutzfeldt–Jakob disease among French human growth hormone recipients. Am J Epidemiol 1998;147(6):597–604.

24. Toogood AA, Shalet SM. Growth hormone replacement therapy in the elderly with hypothalamic–pituitary disease: a dose-finding study. J Clin Endocrinol Metab 1999;84(1):131–6.

25. Reiter EO, Attie KM, Moshang T Jr, Silverman BL, Kemp SF, Neuwirth RB, Ford KM, Saenger PGenentech, Inc.-Alkermes, Inc. Collaborative Study Group. A multicenter study of the efficacy and safety of sustained release GH in the treatment of naive pediatric patients with GH deficiency. J Clin Endocrinol Metab 2001;86(10):4700–6.

26. Malozowski S, Tanner LA, Wysowski DK, Fleming GA, Stadel BV. Benign intracranial hypertension in children with growth hormone deficiency treated with growth hormone. J Pediatr 1995;126(6):996–9.

27. Crock PA, McKenzie JD, Nicoll AM, Howard NJ, Cutfield W, Shield LK, Byrne G. Benign intracranial hypertension and recombinant growth hormone therapy in Australia and New Zealand. Acta Paediatr 1998;87(4):381–6.

28. Wyatt D. Lessons from the National Cooperative Growth Study. Eur J Endocrinol 2004;151:S55–9.

29. Bala P, McKiernan J, Gardiner C, O'Connor G, Murray A. Turner's syndrome and benign intracranial hypertension with or without growth hormone treatment. J Ped Endocrinol Metab 2004;17:1243–4.

30. Bechtold S, Butenandt O, Meidert A, Boergen KP, Schmidt H. Persistent papilledema in Ullrich–Turner syndrome treated with growth hormone. Clin Pediatr (Phila) 2001;40(11):629–31.

31. Koller EA, Green L, Gertner JM, Bost M, Malozowski SN. Retinal changes mimicking diabetic retinopathy in two nondiabetic, growth hormone-treated patients. J Clin Endocrinol Metab 1998;83(7):2380–3.

32. Wong AYK, Tang L. An open and randomised study comparing the efficacy of standard danazol and modified triptorelin regimens for postoperative disease management of moderate to severe endometriosis. Fertil Steril 2004;81:1522–7.

33. Lindgren AC. Side effects of growth hormone treatment in Prader–Willi syndrome. Endocrinologist 2000;10(Suppl 1):S63–4.

34. Bercu BB, Murray FT, Frasier SD, Rudlin C, O'Dea LS, Brentzel J, Hanson B, Landy H. Long-term therapy with recombinant human growth hormone (Saizen) in children with idiopathic and organic growth hormone deficiency. Endocrine 2001;15(1):43–9.

35. Picca S, Cappa M, Rizzoni G. Hyperparathyroidism during growth hormone treatment: a role for puberty? Pediatr Nephrol 2000;14(1):56–8.

36. Johansson JO, Fowelin J, Landin K, Lager I, Bengtsson BA. Growth hormone-deficient adults are insulin-resistant. Metabolism 1995;44(9):1126–9.

37. Sas T, Mulder P, Aanstoot HJ, Houdijk M, Jansen M, Reeser M, Hokken-Koelega A. Carbohydrate metabolism during long-term growth hormone treatment in children with short stature born small for gestational age. Clin Endocrinol (Oxf) 2001;54(2):243–51.

38. Wuhl E, Haffner D, Offner G, Broyer M, van't Hoff W, Mehls OEuropean Study Group on Growth Hormone Treatment in Children with Nephropathic Cystinosis. Long-term treatment with growth hormone in short children with nephropathic cystinosis. J Pediatr 2001;138(6):880–7.

39. Jeffcoate W. Growth hormone therapy and its relationship to insulin resistance, glucose intolerance and diabetes mellitus: a review of recent evidence. Drug Saf 2002;25(3):199–212.

40. Singh KP, Prasad R, Chari PS, Dash RJ. Effect of growth hormone therapy in burn patients on conservative treatment. Burns 1998;24(8):733–8.

41. Blackman MR, Sorkin JD, Munzer T, Bellantoni MF, Busby-Whitehead J, Stevens TE, Jayme J, O'Connor KG, Christmas C, Tobin JD, Stewart KJ, Cottrell E, St Clair C, Pabst KM, Harman SM. Growth hormone and sex steroid administration in healthy aged women and men: a randomized controlled trial. JAMA 2002;288(18):2282–92.

42. Czernichow P, Albertsson-Wikland K, Tuvemo T, Gunnarsson R. Growth hormone treatment and diabetes: survey of the Kabi Pharmacia International Growth Study. Acta Paediatr Scand Suppl 1991;379:104–7.

43. Frisch H. Pharmacovigilance: the use of KIGS (Pharmacia and Upjohn International Growth Database) to monitor the safety of growth hormone treatment in children. Endocrinol Metabol 1997;4(Suppl B):83–6.

44. Haffner D, Nissel R, Wuhl E, Schaefer F, Bettendorf M, Tonshoff B, Mehls O. Metabolic effects of long-term growth hormone treatment in prepubertal children with chronic renal failure and after kidney transplantation. The German Study Group for Growth Hormone Treatment in Chronic Renal Failure. Pediatr Res 1998;43(2):209–15.

45. Filler G, Amendt P, Kohnert KD, Devaux S, Ehrich JH. Glucose tolerance and insulin secretion in children before and during recombinant growth hormone treatment. Horm Res 1998;50(1):32–7.

46. Touati G, Prieur AM, Ruiz JC, Noel M, Czernichow P. Beneficial effects of one-year growth hormone administration to children with juvenile chronic arthritis on chronic steroid therapy. I. Effects on growth velocity and body composition. J Clin Endocrinol Metab 1998;83(2):403–9.

47. Hart DW, Wolf SE, Chinkes DL, Lal SO, Ramzy PI, Herndon DN. Beta-blockade and growth hormone after burn. Ann Surg 2002;236(4):450–6.

48. Hertel NT, Holmberg C, Ronnholm KA, Jacobsen BB, Olgaard K, Meeuwisse GW, Rix M, Pedersen FB. Recombinant human growth hormone treatment, using two dose regimens in children with chronic renal failure—a report on linear growth and adverse effects. J Pediatr Endocrinol Metab 2002;15(5):577–88.

49. Burgert TS, Vuguin PM, DiMartino-Nardi J, Attie KM, Saenger P. Assessing insulin resistance: application of a fasting glucose to insulin ratio in growth hormone-treated children. Horm Res 2002;57(1-2):37–42.

50. Filler G, Franke D, Amendt P, Ehrich JH. Reversible diabetes mellitus during growth hormone therapy in chronic renal failure. Pediatr Nephrol 1998;12(5):405–7.

51. Cutfield WS, Wilton P, Bennmarker H, Albertsson-Wikland K, Chatelain P, Ranke MB, Price DA. Incidence of diabetes mellitus and impaired glucose tolerance in children and adolescents receiving growth-hormone treatment. Lancet 2000;355(9204):610–3.

52. Jeffcoate W. Can growth hormone therapy cause diabetes? Lancet 2000;355(9204):589–90.

53. Florakis D, Hung V, Kaltsas G, Coyte D, Jenkins PJ, Chew SL, Grossman AB, Besser GM, Monson JP. Sustained reduction in circulating cholesterol in adult hypopituitary patients given low dose titrated growth hormone replacement therapy: a two year study. Clin Endocrinol (Oxf) 2000;53(4):453–9.

54. Rosenfalck AM, Maghsoudi S, Fisker S, Jorgensen JO, Christiansen JS, Hilsted J, Volund AA, Madsbad S. The effect of 30 months of low-dose replacement therapy with recombinant human growth hormone (rhGH) on insulin and C-peptide kinetics, insulin secretion, insulin sensitivity, glucose effectiveness, and body composition in GH-deficient adults. J Clin Endocrinol Metab 2000;85(11):4173–81.

55. Fernholm R, Bramnert M, Hagg E, Hilding A, Baylink DJ, Mohan S, Thoren M. Growth hormone replacement therapy improves body composition and increases bone metabolism in elderly patients with pituitary disease. J Clin Endocrinol Metab 2000;85(11):4104–12.

56. Nguyen BY, Clerici M, Venzon DJ, Bauza S, Murphy WJ, Longo DL, Baseler M, Gesundheit N, Broder S, Shearer G, Yarchoan R. Pilot study of the immunologic effects of recombinant human growth hormone and recombinant insulin-like growth factor in HIV-infected patients. AIDS 1998;12(8):895–904.

57. Cook DM, Biller BM, Vance ML, Hoffman AR, Phillips LS, Ford KM, Benziger DP, Illeperuma A, Blethen SL, Attie KM, Dao LN, Reimann JD, Fielder PJ. The pharmacokinetic and pharmacodynamic characteristics of a long-acting growth hormone (GH) preparation (Nutropin Depot) in GH-deficient adults. J Clin Endocrinol Metab 2002;87(10):4508–14.

58. Bareille P, Azcona C, Matthews DR, Conway GS, Stanhope R. Lipid profile, glucose tolerance and insulin sensitivity after more than four years of growth hormone therapy in non-growth hormone deficient adolescents. Clin Endocrinol (Oxf) 1999;51(3):347–53.

59. Demling RH. Comparison of the anabolic effects and complications of human growth hormone and the testosterone analogue, oxandrolone, after severe burn injury. Burns 1999;25(3):215–21.

60. Lo JC, Mulligan K, Noor MA, Schwarz JM, Halvorsen RA, Grunfeld C, Schambelan M. The effects of recombinant human growth hormone on body composition and glucose metabolism in HIV-infected patients with fat accumulation. J Clin Endocrinol Metab 2001;86(8):3480–7.

61. Downs AM, Kennedy CT. Somatotrophin-induced acanthosis nigricans. Br J Dermatol 1999;141(2):390–1.

62. Nordlund JJ, Lerner AB. Cause of acanthosis nigricans. N Engl J Med 1975;293(4):200.

63. Yigit S, Estrada E, Bucci K, Hyams J, Rosengren S. Diabetic ketoacidosis secondary to growth hormone treatment in a boy with Prader–Willi syndrome and steatohepatitis. J Ped Endocrinol Metab 2004;17:361–4.

64. Palomba S, Russo T, Orio F Jr, Sammartino A, Sbano FM, Nappi C, Colao A, Mastantonio P, Lombardi G, Zullo F. Lipid, glucose and homocysteine metabolism in women treated with GnRH agonist with or without raloxifene. Hum Reprod 2004;19:415–21.

65. Knox JB, Demling RH, Wilmore DW, Sarraf P, Santos AA. Hypercalcemia associated with the use of human growth hormone in an adult surgical intensive care unit. Arch Surg 1995;130(4):442–5.

66. Blethen S. Dosing, monitoring, and safety of growth hormone-replacement therapy in adults with growth hormone deficiency. Endocrinologist 1998;8:S36–40.

67. Thompson JL, Butterfield GE, Gylfadottir UK, Yesavage J, Marcus R, Hintz RL, Pearman A, Hoffman AR. Effects of human growth hormone, insulin-like growth factor I, and diet and exercise on body composition of obese postmenopausal women. J Clin Endocrinol Metab 1998;83(5):1477–84.

68. Nishi Y, Tanaka T, Takano K, Fujieda K, Igarashi Y, Hanew K, Hirano T, Yokoya S, Tachibana K, Saito T, Watanabe S. Recent status in the occurrence of leukemia in growth hormone-treated patients in Japan. GH Treatment Study Committee of the Foundation for Growth Science, Japan. J Clin Endocrinol Metab 1999;84(6):1961–5.

69. Aktan M, Tanakol R, Nalcaci M, Dincol G. Leukemia in a patient treated with growth hormone. Endocr J 2000;47(4):471–3.

70. Silverman BL, Blethen SL, Reiter EO, Attie KM, Neuwirth RB, Ford KM. A long-acting human growth

hormone (Nutropin Depot): efficacy and safety following two years of treatment in children with growth hormone deficiency. J Pediatr Endocrinol Metab 2002;15(Suppl 2):715–22.

71. Ruvalcaba RH, Kletter GB. Abdominal lipohypertrophy caused by injections of growth hormone: a case report. Pediatrics 1998;102(2 Pt 1):408–10.

72. Mersebach H, Feldt-Rasmussen UF. Lokaliseret lipohy-pertrophia under behandling med vaeksthormon. [Localized lipohypertrophy during growth hormone ther-apy.] Ugeskr Laeger 2002;164(14):1930–2.

73. Blethen SL, Rundle AC. Slipped capital femoral epiphysis in children treated with growth hormone. A summary of the National Cooperative Growth Study experience. Horm Res 1996;46(3):113–6.

74. Smida M, Nouri H, Kandara H, Jalel C, Ghachem MB. Bone diseases in children receiving growth hormone. Acta Orthopaed Belg 2003;69:458–62.

75. Fine RN, Ho M, Tejani A, Blethen S. Adverse events with rhGH treatment of patients with chronic renal insuffi-ciency and end-stage renal disease. J Pediatr 2003;142:539–45.

76. Allen DB. Safety of human growth hormone therapy: cur-rent topics. J Pediatr 1996;128(5 Pt 2):S8–S13.

77. Antoniazzi F, Bertoldo F, Mottes M, Valli M, Sirpresi S, Zamboni G, Valentini R, Tato L. Growth hormone treat-ment in osteogenesis imperfecta with quantitative defect of type I collagen synthesis. J Pediatr 1996;129(3):432–9.

78. Kodama H, Kubota K, Abe T. Osteogenesis imperfecta: are fractures and growth hormone treatment linked? J Pediatr 1998;132(3 Pt 1):559–60.

79. Noda H, Onishi H, Saitoh K, Nakajima H. Growth hor-mone therapy may increase fracture risk in a pubertal patient with osteogenesis imperfecta. J Pediatr Endocrinol Metab 2002;15(2):217–8.

80. Carvalho LR, Justamante de Faria ME, Osorio MGF, Arnhold IJP, Mendonca BB. Acromegalic features in growth hormone (GH)-deficient patients after long-term GH therapy. Clin Endocrinol 2003;59:788–92.

81. Kanazawa H, Tanaka H, Inoue M, Yamanaka Y, Namba N, Seino Y. Efficacy of growth hormone therapy for patient with skeletal dysplasia. J Bone Mineral Metab 2003;21:307–10.

82. Hertel NT, Eklöf O, Ivarsson S, Aronson S, Westphal O, Sipilä I, Kaitila I, Bland J, Veimo D, Müller J, Mohnike K, Neumeyer L, Ritzen M, Hagenäs L. Growth hormone treatment in 35 prepubertal children with achondroplasia: a five-year dose-response trial. Acta Paediatr 2005;94:1402–10.

83. Wiltshire E, Wickremesekera A, Dixon J. Floating-Harbor syndrome complicated by tethered cord: a new association and potential contribution from growth hormone therapy. Am J Med Genet A 2005;136(1):81–3.

84. Colao A, Di Somma C, Spiezia S, Filippella M, Pivonello R, Lombardi G. Effect of growth hormone (GH) and/or testosterone replacement on the prostate in GH-deficient adult patients. J Clin Endocrinol Metab 2003;88:88–94.

85. Pitukcheewanont P, Schwarzbach L, Kaufman FR. Resumption of growth after methionyl-free human growth hormone therapy in a patient with neutralizing antibodies to methionyl human growth hormone. J Pediatr Endocrinol Metab 2002;15(5):653–7.

86. Walker SB, Weiss ME, Tattoni DS. Systemic reaction to human growth hormone treated with acute desensitization. Pediatrics 1992;90(1 Pt 1):108–9.

87. Guest G, Berard E, Crosnier H, Chevallier T, Rappaport R, Broyer M. Effects of growth hormone in short children after renal transplantation. French Society of Pediatric Nephrology. Pediatr Nephrol 1998;12(6):437–46.

88. Yap HK, Loke KY, Murugasu B, Lee BW. Subclinical activation of lupus nephritis by recombinant human growth hormone. Pediatr Nephrol 1998;12(2):133–5.

89. Allen DB, Carrel AL, Growth hormone therapy for Prader–Willi syndrome: a critical appraisal. J Ped Endocrinol Metab 2004;17:1297–306.

90. Van Vliet G, Deal CL, Crock PA, Robitaille Y, Oligny LL. Sudden death in growth hormone-treated children with Prader–Willi syndrome. J Pediatr 2004;144:129–31.

91. Riedl S, Blümel P, Zwiauer K, Frisch H. Death in two female Prader–Willi syndrome patients during the early phase of growth hormone treatment. Acta Paediatr 2005;94:974–7.

92. Nagai T, Obata K, Tonoki H, Temma S, Murakamai N, Katada Y, Yoshino A, Sakazume S, Takahashi E, Sakuta R, Niikawa N. Cause of sudden, unexpected death of Prader–Willi syndrome patients with or without growth hormone treatment. Am J Med Genet A 2005;136(1):45–8.

93. Murray RD Adult growth hormone replacement: current understanding. Curr Opin Pharmacol 2003;3:642–9.

94. Anonymous. Leukaemia in patients treated with growth hormone. Lancet 1988;1(8595):1159–60.

95. Moshang T Jr. Use of growth hormone in children surviv-ing cancer. Med Pediatr Oncol 1998;31(3):170–2.

96. Allen DB, Rundle AC, Graves DA, Blethen SL. Risk of leukemia in children treated with human growth hormone: review and reanalysis. J Pediatr 1997;131(1 Pt 2):S32–6.

97. Moshang T Jr, Rundle AC, Graves DA, Nickas J, Johanson A, Meadows A. Brain tumor recurrence in chil-dren treated with growth hormone: the National Cooperative Growth Study experience. J Pediatr 1996;128(5 Pt 2):S4–7.

98. Ogilvy-Stuart AL, Ryder WD, Gattamaneni HR, Clayton PE, Shalet SM. Growth hormone and tumour recurrence. BMJ 1992;304(6842):1601–5.

99. Price DA, Wilton P, Jonsson P, Albertsson-Wikland K, Chatelain P, Cutfield W, Ranke MB. Efficacy and safety of growth hormone treatment in children with prior cra-niopharyngioma: an analysis of the Pharmacia and Upjohn International Growth Database (KIGS) from 1988 to 1996. Horm Res 1998;49(2):91–7.

100. Monson JP Long-term experience with GH replacement therapy: efficacy and safety. Eur J Endocrinol 2003;148:S9–14.

101. Chihara K, Koledova E, Shimatsu A, Kato Y, Kohno H, Tanaka T, Teramoto A, Bates PC, Attanasio AF. An individualized GH dose regimen for long-term GH treat-ment in Japanese patients with adult GH deficiency. Eur J Endocrinol 2005;153:57–65.

102. Tuffli GA, Johanson A, Rundle AC, Allen DB. Lack of increased risk for extracranial, nonleukemic neoplasms in recipients of recombinant deoxyribonucleic acid growth hormone. J Clin Endocrinol Metab 1995;80(4):1416–22.

103. Swerdlow AJ, Higgins CD, Adlard P, Preece MA. Risk of cancer in patients treated with human pituitary growth hormone in the UK, 1959–85: a cohort study. Lancet 2002;360(9329):273–7.

104. Lee RS, Higgs D, Haddo O, Pringle J, Briggs TWR. Osteosarcoma associated with Diamond–Blackfan anae-mia: a case of a child receiving growth hormone therapy. Sarcoma 2004;8:47–9.

105. Kemp SF, Kuntze J, Attie KM, Maneatis T, Butler MS, Frane J, Lippe B. Efficacy and safety results of long-term growth hormone treatment of idiopathic short stature. J Clin Endocrinol Metab 2005;90:5247–53.

106. Quigley CA, Gill AM, Crowe BJ, Robling K, Chipman JJ, Rose SR, Ross JL, Cassorla FG, Wolka AM, Wit JM, Rekers-Mombarg LTM, Cutler GB. Safety of growth hormone treatment in pediatric patients with idiopathic short stature. J Clin Endocrinol Metab 2005;90:5188–96.

107. Wiren L, Boguszewski CL, Johannsson G. Growth hormone (GH) replacement therapy in GH-deficient women during pregnancy. Clin Endocrinol (Oxf) 2002;57(2):235–9.

108. Bryant J, Cave C, Mihaylova B, Chase D, McIntyre L, Gerard K, Milne R. Clinical effectiveness and cost-effectiveness of growth hormone in children: a systematic review and economic evaluation. Health Technol Assess 2002;6(18):1–168.

109. Toogood AA. The somatopause. An indication for growth hormone therapy. Treat Endocrinol 2004;3:201–9.

110. Attanasio AF, Bates PC, Ho KK, Webb SM, Ross RJ, Strasburger CJ, Bouillon R, Crowe B, Selander K, Valle D, Lamberts SWHypoptiuitary Control and Complications Study International Advisory Board. Human growth hormone replacement in adult hypopituitary patients: long-term effects on body composition and lipid status—3-year results from the HypoCCS Database. J Clin Endocrinol Metab 2002;87(4):1600–6.

111. Hoffman AR, Kuntze JE, Baptista J, Baum HBA, Baumann GP, Biller BMK, Clark RV, Cook D, Inzucchi SE, Kleinberg D, Klibanski A, Phillips LS, Ridgway EC, Robbins RJ, Schlechte J, Sharma M, Thorner MO, Vance ML. Growth hormone (GH) replacement therapy in adult-onset GH deficiency: effects on body composition in men and women in a double-blind, randomised, placebo-controlled trial. J Clin Endocrinol Metab 2004;89:2048–56.

112. Hayakawa M, Shimazaki Y, Tsushima T, Kato Y, Takano K, Chihara K, Shimatsu A, Irie M. Metabolic effects of 20-kilodalton human growth hormone (20k-hGH) for adults with growth hormone deficiency: results of an exploratory uncontrolled multicenter clinical trial of 20k-hGH. J Clin Endocrinol Metab 2004;89:1562–71.

113. Jostel A, Mukherjee A, Alenfall J, Smethurst L, Shalet S. A new sustained-release preparation of human growth hormone and its pharmacokinetic, pharmacodynamic and safety profile. Clin Endocrinol 2005;62:623–7.

114. Takala J, Ruokonen E, Webster NR, Nielsen MS, Zandstra DF, Vundelinckx G, Hinds CJ. Increased mortality associated with growth hormone treatment in critically ill adults. N Engl J Med 1999;341(11):785–92.

115. Kehely A, Bates PC, Frewer P, Birkett M, Blum WF, Mamessier P, Ezzat S, Ho KK, Lombardi G, Luger A, Marek J, Russell-Jones D, Sonksen P, Attanasio AF. Short-term safety and efficacy of human GH replacement therapy in 595 adults with GH deficiency: a comparison of two dosage algorithms. J Clin Endocrinol Metab 2002;87(5):1974–9.

116. Liddle C, Goodwin BJ, George J, Tapner M, Farrell GC. Separate and interactive regulation of cytochrome P450 3A4 by triiodothyronine, dexamethasone, and growth hormone in cultured hepatocytes. J Clin Endocrinol Metab 1998;83(7):2411–6.

117. Sanchez CP, Salem M, Ettenger RB. Changes in cyclosporine A levels in pediatric renal allograft recipients receiving recombinant human growth hormone therapy. Transplant Proc 2000;32(8):2807–10.

118. Wolthers T, Hoffman DM, Nugent AG, Duncan MW, Umpleby M, Ho KK. Oral estrogen antagonizes the metabolic actions of growth hormone in growth hormone-deficient women. Am J Physiol Endocrinol Metab 2001;281(6):E1191–6.

119. Cook DM, Ludlam WH, Cook MB. Route of estrogen administration helps to determine growth hormone (GH) replacement dose in GH-deficient adults. J Clin Endocrinol Metab 1999;84(11):3956–60.

Somatropin (growth hormone) receptor antagonists

General Information

Pegvisomant is a new genetically engineered growth hormone analogue that acts as a growth hormone receptor antagonist. Its role in managing acromegaly is evolving (1).

Organs and Systems

Nervous system

In 112 patients with active acromegaly who received pegvisomant in a 12 week, randomized, double-blind study of three different daily subcutaneous doses of pegvisomant (10,15, and 20 mg), headache was reported in the placebo group as often as in the active treatment groups (12%) (2). In a longer follow-up study for up to 18 months, 26% of 160 patients had headache, but there was no control group for comparison (3).

Endocrine

Two patients receiving pegvisomant had significant growth of their pituitary tumors after several months, requiring further therapy. There was no control group to show if this was significant, but regular assessment of the pituitary anatomy is recommended (3). Pegvisomant inhibits the action of growth hormone at its receptor, reducing serum IGF-1 concentrations. Growth hormone concentrations increase and appear to plateau by 6 months. Whether a Nelson's syndrome-like effect will occur in patients receiving pegvisomant requires long-term follow up.

Metabolism

Fasting glucose concentrations fell and Hb_{A1c} concentrations improved in people with acromegaly who used pegvisomant (4). This occurred in those with and without diabetes, although there was a larger change in the former. However, this was an uncontrolled study and some change may have occurred because of closer monitoring.

Pegvisomant does not alter insulin concentrations directly but does so through its action in blocking the effects of growth hormone. Monitoring blood glucose concentrations in those with diabetes receiving pegvisomant is advisable, in order to ensure appropriate treatment when necessary.

Gastrointestinal

In a 12-week study there was diarrhea in four of 29 patients taking pegvisomant 20 mg/day compared with one patient taking placebo (2). One patient taking 10 mg/day and none taking 15 mg/day reported diarrhea. In a longer follow-up study (18 months) 14% reported diarrhea.

Liver

Two patients developed significantly abnormal liver function tests after receiving pegvisomant for 12 weeks (2,3). Transaminase activities rose to more than 10-fold the upper limits of the reference ranges and returned to normal after withdrawal. One of the two was treated for autoimmune hepatitis (5). Monitoring of liver enzymes every 4-6 weeks is recommended for 6 months or if symptoms of hepatitis develop.

In a non-randomized, open, 32-week study in 53 people with acromegaly, 48 of whom had previously received pegvisomant, all of whom had used octreotide LAR for at least 3 months, pegvisomant 10 mg/day subcutaneously was given 4 weeks after the last dose of octreotide and the dose was adjusted depending on IGF1 concentrations; 51 completed 12 weeks of the study and 49 completed 32 weeks (4). Three patients developed abnormal liver function tests but continued the study. In one the alanine transaminase activity rose to more than 7 times the upper limit of the reference at week 20, and in another it rose to more than 4.5 times at week 24; a third had fluctuating activity, but never more than 3.5 times the upper limit of the reference range. The dose of pegvisomant was not reduced and liver function returned to normal with continued therapy.

Skin

In a placebo-controlled study, six of 80 patients taking pegvisomant had injection site reactions, which were mild, erythematous, and self-limiting and did not require treatment (2).

Long-Term Effects

Tumorigenicity

In one patient who switched to pegvisomant, a large aggressive pituitary tumor continued to grow (4). A second patient, who had been treated initially with surgery and then with a dopamine receptor agonist and octreotide LAR for 4 years, switched to pegvisomant for 21 months and subsequently octreotide LAR for 18 months and had stable disease with a tumor volume of 1.33 cm³. When

pegvisomant was given again at week 32 the tumor increased in size to 2.24 cm³. When pegvisomant was continued for a further 12 months there was no further growth. Regular long-term follow-up by scanning when using pegvisomant is advisable.

References

1. Rowles S, Paisley A, Trainer PJ. Somastatin analogue versus growth-hormone antagonist treatment for acromegaly: who should get what? Curr Opin Endocrinol Diabetes 2003;10:265–71.
2. Trainer PJ, Drake WM, Katznelson L, Freda PU, Herman-Bonert V, Van der Lely AJ, Dimarki EV, Stewart PM, Friend KE, Vance ML, Besser GM, Scarlett JA, Thorner MO, Parkinson C, Klibanski A, Powell JS, Barkan AL, Sheppard MC, Maldonado M, Rose DR, Clemmons DR, Johannson G, Bengtsson B-A, Stavrou S, Kleinberg DL, Cook DM, Phillips LS, Bidlingmaier M, Strasburger CJ, Hackett S, Zib K, Bennett WF, Davis RJ. Treatment of acromegaly with growth hormone-receptor antagonist pegvisomant. New Engl J Med 2000;342:1171–7.
3. Van der Lely AJ, Hutson RK, Trainer PJ, Besser GM, Barkan AL, Katznelson L, Klibnaski A, Herman-Bonert V, Melmed S, Vance ML, Freda PU, Stewart PM, Friend KE, Clemmons DR, Johannsson G, Stavrou S, Cook DM, Phillips LS, Strasburger CJ, Hacker S, Zib KA, Davis RJ, Scarlett JA, Thorner MO. Long-term treatment of acromegaly with pegvisomant, a growth hormone receptor antagonist. Lancet 2001;358:1754–9.
4. Barkan AL, Burman P, Clemmons DR, Drake WM, Gagel RF, Harris PE, Trainer PJ, van der Lely AJ, Vance ML. Glucose homeostasis and safety in patients with acromegaly converted from long-acting octreotide to pegvisomant. J Clin Endocrinol Metab 2005;90:5684–91.
5. Melmed S, Vance ML, Barkan AL, Bengtsson B-A, Kleinberg D, Klibanski A, Trainer PJ. Current status and future opportunities for controlling acromegaly. Pituitary 2002;5:185–96.

Vasopressin and analogues

See also Desmopressin

General Information

Vasopressin, a hypothalamic octapeptide that is secreted by the neurohypophysis, has both antidiuretic and vasoconstrictor properties. Its short half-life (about 10 minutes) necessitates continuous intravenous infusion or frequent nasal application.

Because its vasoconstrictor effects limit the use of the native hormone, analogues with greater or lesser affinity for vasopressin V_2 receptors and more selective antidiuretic effects have been developed:

- argipressin (8-arginine vasopressin)
- desmopressin (*N*-deamino-8-D-arginine vasopressin, DDAVP); desmopressin is covered in a separate monograph
- felypressin (2-phenylalanine, 8-lysine vasopressin)

- lypressin (8-lysine vasopressin; pig vasopressin)
- ornipressin (8-onithine vasopressin)
- terlipressin (triglycyl-lysine vasopressin).

Vasopressin receptor antagonists, such as relcovaptan (an antagonist at V_{1a} receptors), lixivaptan and tolvaptan (V_2), and conivaptan (mixed V_{1a}/V_2), are also under development (1).

Desmopressin has little vasoconstrictor effect but has potent antidiuretic action, through renal vasopressin V_2 receptors, and at high doses hemostatic properties, by increasing concentrations of factor VIII and von Willebrand factor in the blood.

Ornipressin is a selective agonist at vasopressin V_1 receptors and has weaker antidiuretic activity than the native hormone.

Terlipressin, a long-acting vasopressin analogue, is metabolized to the active drug lysine vasopressin. The use of terlipressin to treat acute variceal bleeding has been reviewed (2,3).

A review has suggested that terlipressin has fewer adverse effects than vasopressin; however, the studies on which this was based were rated as low in quality (4).

The use of vasopressin and terlipressin for the management of septic shock has been reviewed; a maximum dose of 0.04 U/minute is recommended (5). Vasopressin 0.23 U/minute in patients with hepatorenal syndrome did not appear to be associated with the adverse effects that occur at the lower doses that are used to treat other critically ill patients (6).

Although vasopressin and its analogues have been used in the acute management of bleeding esophageal varices, they do not reduce mortality (2,3) and the rate of adverse effects is higher than with octreotide (3).

Uterine and abdominal cramps, nausea, and an urge to defecate have been reported in vasopressin-treated patients.

Organs and Systems

Cardiovascular

Dose-related adverse effects of vasopressin include skin pallor, hypertension, cardiac dysrhythmias, and myocardial ischemia or infarction; treatment has to be stopped in 20–30% of patients because of these effects (3).

Intestinal and peripheral vasoconstriction can follow prolonged infusion, resulting in gangrene of intestinal segments or of skin, fingers, or limbs. This has been fatal in several cases, and vasopressin should be withdrawn if skin necrosis occurs (SEDA-13, 1310; 7).

Of 10 patients with hepatorenal syndrome one had to be withdrawn 2 hours after receiving 12 units of ornipressin (6 IU/hour) because of a ventricular tachydysrhythmia, and an infusion of dopamine 2–3 micrograms/kg/minute was started (8).

Terlipressin has similar, but less pronounced, systemic hemodynamic effects to vasopressin, including increases in mean arterial pressure and reduced heart rate (9). Of 105 patients who had continuous terlipressin infusions for variceal bleeding in a multicenter study, lower limb ischemia developed in two and cardiac ischemia in one (10).

Of 86 cirrhotic patients treated with terlipressin 10 developed a tachycardia, four developed atrial fibrillation, and one developed ventricular tachycardia. Four patients in the same study developed hypertension (11). In another study, tachycardia occurred in 23% of patients randomized to pitressin for acute variceal bleeding and 8% developed transient hypertension (12).

Myocardial ischemia has been associated with terlipressin (13).

- A 61-year-old man with coronary artery stenosis became hypotensive during elective surgery, refractory to ephedrine (cumulative dose of 36 mg over 45 minutes). Immediately after terlipressin 1 mg, he developed hypertension and bradycardia, with evidence of myocardial ischemia.

One of 21 patients with hepatorenal syndrome developed finger ischemia on the fourth day of intermittent intravenous terlipressin and recovered after terlipressin was stopped (14).

Respiratory

An elderly patient (over 70 years old) with cirrhosis and hepatorenal syndrome developed severe bronchospasm and died after intravenous terlipressin administration; the mechanism was not determined (15).

Nervous system

Six unselected patients (four women), mean age 27 years, with acute liver failure and grade IV hepatic encephalopathy received terlipressin 0.005 mg/kg as a single intravenous bolus (16). There was an increase in cerebral blood flow 1 hour after the bolus, which returned to baseline at 5 hours, and an increase in intracranial pressure at 1 hour, which returned to baseline at 2 hours. The authors speculated that terlipressin could have a deleterious effect on cerebral hemodynamics in patients with severe hepatic encephalopathy.

Electrolyte balance

Profound hyponatremia due to reduced free water clearance is a predictable dose-related effect of vasopressin (17). This is a particular risk in patients who are unconscious or who have disturbed thirst sensation (SEDA-22, 487).

Hyponatremia has been attributed to vasopressin in children undergoing cardiac surgery (18).

- A 36-week-old 2.3 kg girl undergoing cardiac surgery received vasopressin 0.0003 units/kg/minute, titrated up to a maximum dose of 0.0012 units/kg/minute. After 82 hours vasopressin was discontinued because of hyponatremia (sodium 117 mmol/l).
- A 3.6 kg boy born at term underwent cardiac surgery and received similar doses of vasopressin, which was discontinued after 60 hours because of a sodium concentration of 119 mmol/l.

The falls in sodium were gradual and resolved on withdrawal of vasopressin. The authors recommended that when vasopressin is used for more than 24 hours sodium concentrations should be monitored.

Of 105 patients who had continuous infusions of terlipressin for variceal bleeding in a multicenter study, four developed hyponatremia, severe in one case (10).

High-dose terlipressin (1 mg intravenously every 4 hours for 5 days) was associated with severe hyponatremia and loss of consciousness in one of 45 cirrhotic patients in a randomized trial (11). Of course, cirrhosis itself is associated with hyponatremia.

Hematologic

Mild lymphangitis was reported in one of 105 patients in a multicenter study of the effects of terlipressin (10).

Gastrointestinal

Tongue ischemia and ischemic colitis have been described after 4–9 days of treatment with ornipressin 6 IU/hour combined with plasma volume expansion (19).

When arginine vasopressin is used in high single doses (4–16 IU), to control upper gastrointestinal tract bleeding, gut ischemia has been reported (20). Continuous infusions at lower doses have shown changes suggestive of splanchnic hypoperfusion.

It has also been suggested that terlipressin has vasoconstrictor activity within the splanchnic vascular territory (21). Hypotension developed under general anesthesia in 32 patients undergoing carotid endarterectomy treated with renin-angiotensin inhibitors (22). They were randomized to received terlipressin 1 mg (n = 16) or noradrenaline infusion. Compared with baseline those who received terlipressin had reduced gastric mucosal perfusion for at least 4 hours. There was also reduced oxygen delivery and oxygen consumption index at 30 minutes and 4 hours in those who received terlipressin.

Skin

Skin necrosis is often reported after vasopressin therapy. In a retrospective study, two of five patients treated with a continuous infusion of terlipressin developed skin necrosis at the infusion site and a third developed scrotal necrosis (15).

In a retrospective analysis of 63 patients treated with arginine vasopressin for catecholamine resistant vasodilatory shock, 30% developed ischemic skin lesions (23). Pre-existing peripheral arterial occlusive disease and septic shock were independent susceptibility factors.

Multiple logistic regression analysis has shown that the presence of septic shock and pre-existing peripheral arterial occlusive disease are significant independent risk factors for the development of ischemic skin lesions during vasopressin infusion (24). The authors of a review have suggested that low-dose vasopressin should not be given peripherally when treating septic shock owing to the risk of severe skin necrosis that can occur after extravasation (25).

- A 46-year-old woman with septic shock had a peripheral venous infusion of vasopressin 0.04 U/minute in addition to dobutamine, via the subclavian vein; extravasation of vasopressin to local soft tissue resulted in ischemic skin necrosis (26).

Purpuric skin necrosis, due to local vasoconstriction, has been reported in 19 patients within a few days of starting vasopressin infusion (27).

Bullous necrosis developed within 48 hours of starting an infusion of terlipressin in a 44-year-old man (28). There have been only four previous reports of skin necrosis.

Musculoskeletal

Rhabdomyolysis has been attributed to terlipressin (29).

- A 36-year-old man with nephrotic syndrome was given an infusion of terlipressin (an intravenous bolus of 2 mg followed by 2 mg over 24 hours) to treat diffuse gastric bleeding, and 12 hours later developed acute pain and livedo reticularis in both legs. High plasma concentrations of myoglobin and creatine kinase confirmed the diagnosis of toxic rhabdomyolysis, thought to be due to the vasoconstrictor action of terlipressin. He made a gradual recovery over the next few weeks after terlipressin was withdrawn.

Pre-existing blood vessel disease due to amyloidosis may have contributed to the outcome in this patient.

Drug Administration

Drug dosage regimens

A review of trials has suggested that vasopressin is more likely to cause adverse effects at doses of 0.04 U/minute or more when it is used to treat septic shock; mesenteric ischemia and cardiac dysfunction and ischemia were particularly associated with high doses (30). The authors suggested that limiting the dosage to 0.03 U/minute may minimize these effects. This suggestion has been supported by a retrospective audit of the effects of continuous vasopressin infusion in septic shock in 102 men and women, mean age 53 years (31). There were adverse events that may have been linked to vasopressin in 18 patients: cardiac arrest (n = 9); ischemic/mottled digits (n = 8); myocardial infarction (n = 1); and hyponatremia (n = 1). Adverse events occurred with doses of vasopressin of 0.04 units/minute and over, except in one patient (dose not stated).

Further data have come from a review of the use of high doses of vasopressin (mean dose 0.47 U/minute) to replace noradrenaline (24). There were reductions in heart rate, cardiac index, and oxygen delivery. The authors recommended that the dose of vasopressin should not exceed 0.04 U/minute and that vasopressin should not be used as a single vasopressor agent in septic shock.

References

1. Serradeil-Le Gal C, Wagnon J, Valette G, Garcia G, Pascal M, Maffrand JP, Le Fur G. Nonpeptide vasopressin receptor antagonists: development of selective and orally active V1a, V2 and V1b receptor ligands. Prog Brain Res 2002;139:197–210.

2. Avgerinos A. Approach to the management of bleeding esophageal varices: role of somatostatin. Digestion 1998;59(Suppl 1):1–22.

3. Burroughs AK, Planas R, Svoboda P. Optimizing emergency care of upper gastrointestinal bleeding in cirrhotic patients. Scand J Gastroenterol Suppl 1998;226:14–24.

4. Ioannou GN, Doust J, Rockey DC. Systematic review: terlipressin in acute oesophageal variceal haemorrhage. Aliment Pharmacol Ther 2003;17:53–64.

5. Delmas A, Leone M, Rousseau S, Albanése J, Martin C. Clinical review: vasopressin and terlipressin in septic shock patients. Crit Care 2005;9:212–22.

6. Kiser TH, Fish DN, Obritsch MD, Jung R, MacLaren R, Parikh CR. Vasopressin, not octreotide, may be beneficial in the treatment of hepatorenal syndrome: a retrospective study. Nephrol Dial Transplant 2005;20:1813–20.

7. Moreno-Sanchez D, Casis B, Martin A, Ortiz P, Castellano G, Munoz MT, Vanaclocha F, Solis-Herruzo JA. Rhabdomyolysis and cutaneous necrosis following intravenous vasopressin infusion. Gastroenterology 1991;101(2):529–32.

8. Gulberg V, Bilzer M, Gerbes AL. Long-term therapy and retreatment of hepatorenal syndrome type 1 with ornipressin and dopamine. Hepatology 1999;30(4):870–5.

9. Romero G, Kravetz D, Argonz J, Bildozola M, Suarez A, Terg R. Terlipressin is more effective in decreasing variceal pressure than portal pressure in cirrhotic patients. J Hepatol 2000;32(3):419–25.

10. Escorsell A, Ruiz del Arbol L, Planas R, Albillos A, Banares R, Cales P, Pateron D, Bernard B, Vinel JP, Bosch J. Multicenter randomized controlled trial of terlipressin versus sclerotherapy in the treatment of acute variceal bleeding: the TEST study. Hepatology 2000;32(3):471–6.

11. Bruha R, Marecek Z, Spicak J, Hulek P, Lata J, Petrtyl J, Urbanek P, Taimr P, Volfova M, Dite P. Double-blind randomized, comparative multicenter study of the effect of terlipressin in the treatment of acute esophageal variceal and/or hypertensive gastropathy bleeding. Hepatogastroenterology 2002;49(46):1161–6.

12. Zhang HB, Wong BC, Zhou XM, Guo XG, Zhao SJ, Wang JH, Wu KC, Ding J, Lam SK, Fan DM. Effects of somatostatin, octreotide and pitressin plus nitroglycerine on systemic and portal haemodynamics in the control of acute variceal bleeding. Int J Clin Pract 2002;56(6):447–51.

13. Medel J, Boccara G, Van de Steen E, Bertrand M, Godet G, Coriat P. Terlipressin for treating intraoperative hypotension: can it unmask myocardial ischemia? Anesth Analg 2001;93(1):53–5.

14. Ortega R, Gines P, Uriz J, Cardenas A, Calahorra B, De Las Heras D, Guevara M, Bataller R, Jimenez W, Arroyo V, Rodes J. Terlipressin therapy with and without albumin for patients with hepatorenal syndrome: results of a prospective, nonrandomized study. Hepatology 2002;36(4 Pt 1):941–8.

15. Halimi C, Bonnard P, Bernard B, Mathurin P, Mofredj A, di Martino V, Demontis R, Henry-Biabaud E, Fievet P, Opolon P, Poynard T, Cadranel JF. Effect of terlipressin (Glypressin) on hepatorenal syndrome in cirrhotic patients: results of a multicentre pilot study. Eur J Gastroenterol Hepatol 2002;14(2):153–8.

16. Shawcross DL, Davies NA, Mookerjee RP, Hayes PC, Williams R, Lee A, Jalan R. Worsening of cerebral hyperemia by the administration of terlipressin in acute liver failure with severe encephalopathy. Hepatology 2004;39:471–5.

17. Robson WL, Norgaard JP, Leung AK. Hyponatremia in patients with nocturnal enuresis treated with DDAVP. Eur J Pediatr 1996;155(11):959–62.

18. Scheurer MA, Bradley SM, Atz AM. Vasopressin to attenuate pulmonary hypertension and improve systemic blood pressure after correction of obstructed total anomalous pulmonary venous return. J Thorac Cardiovasc Surg 2005;129:464–6.

19. Crowther CA, Hiller JE, Haslam RR, Robinson JSACTOBAT Study Group. Australian Collaborative Trial of Antenatal Thyrotropin-Releasing Hormone: adverse effects at 12-month follow-up. Pediatrics 1997;99(3):311–7.

20. Dunser MW, Wenzel V, Mayr AJ, Hasibeder WR. Management of vasodilatory shock defining the role of arginine vasopressin. Drugs 2003;63:237–56.

21. Fellahi JL, Benard P, Daccache G, Mourgeon E, Gerard JL. Vasodilatory septic shock refractory to catecholamines: is there a role for terlipressin? Ann Fr Anesth Reanim 2003;22:631–4.

22. Morelli A, Tritapepe L, Rocco M, Conti G, Orecchioni A, De Gaetano A, Picchini U, Pelaia P, Reale C, Pietropaoli P. Terlipressin versus norepinephrine to counteract anesthesia-induced hypotension in patients treated with renin–angiotensin system inhibitors: effects on systemic and regional hemodynamics. Anesthesiology 2005;102:12–19.

23. Dunser MW, Mayr AJ, Tur A, Pajk W, Barbara F, Knotzer H, Ulmer H, Hasibeder WR. Ischemic skin lesions as a complication of continuous vasopressin infusion in catecholamine-resistant vasodilatory shock: incidence and risk factors. Crit Care Med 2003;31:1394–8.

24. Holmes CL, Walley KR. Vasopressin in the ICU. Curr Opin Crit Care 2004;10:442–8.

25. Kam PCA, Williams S, Yoong FFY. Vasopressin and terlipressin: pharmacology and its clinical relevance. Anaesthesia 2004;59:993–1001.

26. Kahn JM, Kress JP, Hall JB. Skin necrosis after extravasation of low-dose vasopressin administered for septic shock. Crit Care Med 2002;30(8):1899–901.

27. Lemlich G, Di Grandi S, Szaniawski WK. Cutaneous reaction to vasopressin. Cutis 1996;57(5):330–2.

28. Tomassini E, Guiot P, Poussel JF, De Cubber J, Schnitzler B. Bullous disease following intravenous terlipressin infusion. Reanim Urgences 2000;9:313–4.

29. Rolla D, Cannella G, Ravetti JL. Toxic rhabdomyolysis induced by terlipressin infusion in a uraemic patient suffering from AA-type amyloidosis. Nephron 1999;83(2):167–8.

30. Obritsch MD, Bestul DJ, Jung R, Fish DN, MacLaren R. The role of vasopressin in vasodilatory septic shock. Pharmacotherapy 2004;24:1050–63.

31. Obritsch MD, Jung R, Fish DN, MacLaren R. Effects of continuous vasopressin infusion in patients with septic shock. Ann Pharmacother 2004;38:1117–22.

Vasopressin receptor antagonists

General Information

Non-peptide vasopressin receptor antagonists include relcovaptan (an antagonist at V_{1a} receptors), lixivaptan, satavaptan, and tolvaptan (V_2), and conivaptan (mixed $V_{1a/V2}$). They have been used in the treatment of hyponatremia.

Placebo-controlled studies

Conivaptan

In 142 patients with symptomatic heart failure (New York Heart Association classes III and IV) randomized to double-blind, placebo-controlled short-term treatment with a single intravenous dose of conivaptan 10, 20, or 40 mg, conivaptan significantly reduced pulmonary capillary wedge pressure and right atrial pressure and increased urine output (1).

In a 5-day, double-blind, randomized, placebo-controlled study in 74 patients with euvolemic or hypervolemic hyponatremia, oral conivaptan (40 or 80 mg/day) significantly increased serum sodium concentrations (2). The most common adverse events were headache, hypotension, nausea, constipation, and postural hypotension.

In 84 patients with euvolemic or hypervolemic hyponatremia randomized to intravenous placebo or conivaptan 20 mg over 30 minutes followed by a 96-hour infusion of either 40 or 80 mg/day, conivaptan increased serum sodium concentrations (3). Infusion site reactions led to withdrawal of one and four of the patients who were given conivaptan 40 and 80 mg/day respectively.

Satavaptan

In 110 patients with cirrhosis, ascites, and hyponatremia in a multicenter, double-blind, randomized, placebo-controlled study of three fixed doses of satavaptan (5, 12.5, or 25 mg/day) for 14 days plus spironolactone 100 mg/day, satavaptan was associated with improved control of ascites. Thirst was the main adverse effect (4).

Tolvaptan

In a double-blind placebo-controlled study of the effects of three doses of tolvaptan (30, 45, or 60 mg/day) in 254 patients with chronic heart failure taking stable doses of furosemide there were significant reductions in body weight and increased urine volumes; edema improved and serum sodium normalized in those with hyponatremia (5). There were no significant changes in heart rate, blood pressure, serum potassium, or renal function.

In two multicenter, randomized, double-blind, placebo-controlled studies of tolvaptan in 448 patients with euvolemic or hypervolemic hyponatremia, tolvaptan 15–60 mg/day increased serum sodium concentrations significantly compared with placebo (6). The main adverse effects associated with tolvaptan included increased thirst, dry mouth, and increased urination.

In a multicenter randomized, double-blind, placebo-controlled study in 4133 patients with heart failure, tolvaptan 30 mg/day for a minimum of 60 days in addition to standard therapy significantly improved dyspnea, body weight, and edema; in patients with hyponatremia, serum sodium concentrations increased significantly (7). The main adverse effects were increased thirst and a dry mouth.

In two double-blind, randomized, placebo-controlled studies in 17 subjects in all, the main adverse effects of tolvaptan 60–240-mg/day were excess thirst, frequent urination, and a dry mouth (8).

Organs and Systems

Cardiovascular

Intravenous conivaptan had no effects on the electrocardiogram in a randomized, single-blind, placebo- and positive-controlled, parallel-group study, in which an intravenous loading dose of conivaptan of 20 mg was followed by a continuous infusion of 40 or 80 mg/day for 4 days or moxifloxacin 400 mg/day for 4 days (9).

Drug-Drug Interactions

Diuretics

Pharmacokinetic and pharmacodynamic interactions of single doses of tolvaptan 30 mg with furosemide 80 mg or hydrochlorothiazide 100 mg have been determined in a randomized, open, parallel-arm, 3-period, crossover study in 12 healthy men (10). There were no clinically significant changes in the pharmacokinetics of tolvaptan and either furosemide or hydrochlorothiazide during coadministration. Free water clearance, 24-hour urine volume, plasma sodium and argentine vasopressin concentrations, and plasma osmolality were higher, and urine osmolality was lower when tolvaptan was administered either alone or in combination with furosemide or hydrochlorothiazide, compared with furosemide or hydrochlorothiazide alone. At 24 hours after the dose plasma renin activity was increased after furosemide or hydrochlorothiazide administered alone or with tolvaptan, but it was unchanged after tolvaptan alone. Thus, tolvaptan did not significantly affect the natriuretic activity of furosemide or hydrochlorothiazide and neither furosemide nor hydrochlorothiazide significantly affected the aquaretic effect of tolvaptan.

References

1. Udelson JE, Smith WB, Hendrix GH, Painchaud CA, Ghazzi M, Thomas I, Ghali JK, Selaru P, Chanoine F, Pressler ML, Konstam MA. Acute hemodynamic effects of conivaptan, a dual V(1A) and V(2) vasopressin receptor antagonist, in patients with advanced heart failure. Circulation 2001;104(20):2417–23.
2. Ghali JK, Koren MJ, Taylor JR, Brooks-Asplund E, Fan K, Long WA, Smith N. Efficacy and safety of oral conivaptan: a $V_{1A/V2}$ vasopressin receptor antagonist, assessed in a

randomized, placebo-controlled trial in patients with euvolemic or hypervolemic hyponatremia. J Clin Endocrinol Metab 2006;91(6):2145–52.

3. Zeltser D, Rosansky S, van Rensburg H, Verbalis JG, Smith N; Conivaptan Study Group. Assessment of the efficacy and safety of intravenous conivaptan in euvolemic and hypervolemic hyponatremia. Am J Nephrol 2007;27(5):447–57.

4. Ginès P, Wong F, Watson H, Milutinovic S, del Arbol LR, Olteanu D; HypoCAT Study Investigators. Effects of satavaptan, a selective vasopressin V(2) receptor antagonist, on ascites and serum sodium in cirrhosis with hyponatremia: a randomized trial. Hepatology 2008;48(1):204–13.

5. Gheorghiade M, Niazi I, Ouyang J, Czerwiec F, Kambayashi J, Zampino M, Orlandi C; Tolvaptan Investigators. Vasopressin V_2-receptor blockade with tolvaptan in patients with chronic heart failure: results from a double-blind, randomized trial. Circulation 2003;107(21):2690–6.

6. Schrier RW, Gross P, Gheorghiade M, Berl T, Verbalis JG, Czerwiec FS, Orlandi C; SALT Investigators. Tolvaptan, a selective oral vasopressin V_2-receptor antagonist, for hyponatremia. N Engl J Med 2006;355(20):2099–112.

7. Konstam MA, Gheorghiade M, Burnett JC Jr, Grinfeld L, Maggioni AP, Swedberg K, Udelson JE, Zannad F, Cook T, Ouyang J, Zimmer C, Orlandi C; Efficacy of Vasopressin Antagonism in Heart Failure Outcome Study With Tolvaptan (EVEREST) Investigators. Effects of oral tolvaptan in patients hospitalized for worsening heart failure: the EVEREST Outcome Trial. JAMA 2007;297(12):1319–31.

8. Shoaf SE, Wang Z, Bricmont P, Mallikaarjun S. Pharmacokinetics, pharmacodynamics, and safety of tolvaptan, a nonpeptide AVP antagonist, during ascending single-dose studies in healthy subjects. J Clin Pharmacol 2007;47(12):1498–507.

9. Lasseter KC, Dilzer SC, Smith N. Intravenous conivaptan: effects on the QT_c interval and other electrocardiographic parameters in healthy volunteers. Adv Ther 2007;24(2):310–8.

10. Shoaf SE, Bramer SL, Bricmont P, Zimmer CA. Pharmacokinetic and pharmacodynamic interaction between tolvaptan, a non-peptide AVP antagonist, and furosemide or hydrochlorothiazide. J Cardiovasc Pharmacol 2007;50(2):213–22.

LIPID – REGULATING DRUGS

Acipimox

General Information

Acipimox (S-methylpyrazine-2-carboxylic acid 4-oxide) is structurally related to nicotinic acid. There were flushing and gastrointestinal disturbances in 7137 patients, of whom 15% stopped taking the drug because of adverse effects; there were no adverse effects on blood glucose or uric acid (1). Of 32 patients with hypertriglyceridemia, excessive hypertriglyceridemia, and combined hyperlipidemia, acipimox had to be withdrawn in 10 cases, because of adverse effects or absence of clinical response (2). The other 22 completed 6 months of treatment with no adverse effects. The authors claimed that acipimox is much better tolerated than nicotinic acid; it has fewer adverse effects and can therefore be used as a second-line drug.

Organs and Systems

Metabolism

In an open study, blood glucose was on average slightly lowered in 3009 type II diabetics given acipimox for at least 2 months (3).

References

1. Ganzer BM. Langzeitstudie zu acipimox. Pharmazie 1990;135:31.
2. Yeshurun D, Hamood H, Morad N, Naschitz J. [Acipimox (Olbetam) as a secondary hypolipemic agent in combined hypertriglyceridemia and hyperlipidemia.]Harefuah 2000;138(8):650–3710.
3. Lavezzari M, Milanesi G, Oggioni E, Pamparana F. Results of a phase IV study carried out with acipimox in type II diabetic patients with concomitant hyperlipoproteinaemia. J Int Med Res 1989;17(4):373–80.

Atorvastatin

See also HMG Co-A reductase inhibitors

General Information

Atorvastatin is an HMG Co-A reductase inhibitor. Pooled data from 21 completed and 23 continuing trials representing 3000 patient-years have shown that constipation, flatulence, dyspepsia, abdominal pain, headache, and myalgia occur in 1–3% of patients. Under 2% of atorvastatin-treated patients discontinued treatment because of an adverse event (1). Serious events in this review amounted to one patient with pancreatitis and one with cholestatic jaundice (1). There were no differences in adverse effects in 177 patients randomized for 52 weeks to either simvastatin or atorvastatin (2).

Combination with ezetimibe

Ezetimibe plus atorvastatin was also well tolerated in 628 patients, with a safety profile similar to that of atorvastatin alone and to placebo. When co-administered with atorvastatin, ezetimibe provided significant incremental reductions in LDL cholesterol and triglycerides and increased HDL cholesterol (3).

Ezetimibe given with simvastatin and atorvastatin is well tolerated, with a safety profile similar to the statin alone and to placebo (SEDA-28, 534). However, there are concerns about the use of ezetimibe in patients with impaired oxidation of fatty acids, as in familial combined hyperlipidemia. Of more than 300 patients with intolerance of lipid-lowering therapies a subgroup had common features, including raised fasting respiratory exchange ratios while not taking lipid-lowering drugs and hypertriglyceridemia (4). An interaction of ezetimibe with statins was suspected in two men aged 43 and 53 years, both of whom had raised creatine kinase activity and one of whom also had myalgia (5). However, co-administration of ezetimibe and lovastatin in 48 healthy men resulted in no significant changes in laboratory test results, including enzymes indicative of muscle or liver damage (6).

Organs and Systems

Nervous system

A peripheral neuropathy has been reported with atorvastatin.

- A 60-year-old woman had painless horizontal diplopia, vertigo, blurry vision, and paresthesia in both arms after taking atorvastatin 10 mg/day (7). Neurological improvement began 2 days after drug withdrawal. Antiacetylcholine receptor antibodies were 10 times the upper limit of the reference range.

Although some features of this patient's external ophthalmoplegia were similar to myasthenia and there was a reversible rise in antiacetylcholine receptor antibody titer, a negative edrophonium test and a negative repetitive stimulation test on electromyography argued against a myasthenia-like drug reaction.

- A 57-year-old man in good health took atorvastatin 5 mg and aspirin 75 mg/day and had progressive numbness and burning in both feet for 6 months (8). Muscle punch biopsies showed a neuropathic process affecting small-caliber sensory nerve fibers. The symptoms resolved 3 months after withdrawal of atorvastatin.

Peripheral neuropathy has also been reported in a case-control study (9).

Sensory systems

In 696 patients taking atorvastatin and 235 taking lovastatin for 1 year there were no significant differences in the distribution of lenticular opacities or cortical opacities and spokes between the two drugs (10).

Metabolism

Co-enzyme Q10 concentrations were measured in blood from hypercholesterolemic subjects before and after exposure to atorvastatin 80 mg/day for 14 and 30 days in 34 subjects eligible for statin treatment (11). The mean blood concentration of co-enzyme Q10 was 1.26 µg/ml at baseline, and fell to 0.62 after 30 days of atorvastatin therapy. There was a statistically significant fall detectable after 14 days of treatment. The authors concluded that widespread inhibition of co-enzyme Q10 synthesis could explain the exercise intolerance, myalgia, and myoglobinuria that are observed with statin treatment.

Hematologic

Thrombocytopenia occurred in a 46-year-old man coinciding with atorvastatin treatment; he had already tolerated simvastatin (12).

Leukopenia with oral ulceration has been attributed to atorvastatin in a patient with insulin allergy who had received a pancreatic transplant; the symptoms resolved on withdrawal (13).

Liver

Acute hepatitis has been attributed to statins.

- A 65-year-old woman developed fatigue, jaundice, and altered liver function tests while taking atorvastatin (20 mg/day for some weeks) (14). On the basis of clinical, serological, and histological findings, a diagnosis of autoimmune hepatitis was made.

The authors suggested that atorvastatin may have unmasked an underlying autoimmune hepatitis.

Based on the low frequency of raised alanine transaminase activity and the lack of clinical evidence of hepatotoxicity, some clinicians have called for a change in the current practice of monitoring liver function tests. However, a 71-year-old woman taking atorvastatin had raised transaminase activity on two occasions and developed pruritus on rechallenge. Thus, clinicians should be aware of asymptomatic rises in liver function tests in patients taking atorvastatin who do not have known susceptibility factors for liver damage (15).

Pancreas

Pancreatitis has been observed with atorvastatin (16).

Skin

Potentially life-threatening toxic epidermal necrolysis occurred in a 73-year-old moderately obese woman with type 2 diabetes and hypertension after she had taken 40 mg of atorvastatin (17).

- A 59-year-old man developed urticaria while taking atorvastatin for hypercholesterolemia (18). Scratch tests with his medications gave a strong positive reaction only with atorvastatin. Atorvastatin was withdrawn and his urticaria resolved over the next 10 days.

Linear IgA bullous dermatosis (19) and dermographism (20) have been described in patients taking atorvastatin.

Musculoskeletal

In one study of 133 patients there was myalgia in 3% of those taking atorvastatin, but no patient had persistent increases in creatine kinase activity above 10 times the top of the reference range (21).

Immunologic

Hypersensitivity reactions to atorvastatin have been reported.

- Antinuclear and antihistone antibodies developed in a 26-year-old man who was taking atorvastatin (22). He had constitutional symptoms and slight headaches but no definite symptoms of lupus. After some months without medication he became seronegative and asymptomatic.

This case was similar to other previous reports with other statins.

- A patient developed atorvastatin-induced severe autoimmune hepatitis and a lupus-like syndrome. Although the drug was immediately withdrawn, the disease persisted and deteriorated to a fulminant form with acute hepatic failure. There was no response to conventional immunosuppression with glucocorticoids and azathioprine. Only the introduction of intense immunosuppressive therapy, as used in solid organ transplantation, led to a complete and sustained recovery. The patient had the HLA haplotypes DR3 and DR4, which are well-known genetic factors associated with autoimmune diseases.

This case is the first report of drug-induced lupus-like syndrome concomitant with severe autoimmune hepatitis in a genetically predisposed patient (23).

Drug Administration

Drug dosage regimens

In a comparison of atorvastatin 80 mg/day and 10 mg/day in 10 001 patients adverse events related to treatment occurred in 406 of those who took 80 mg/day (n = 4955) compared with 289 of those who took 10 mg/day (n = 5006) (8.1 versus 5.8%) (24). The respective rates of withdrawal because of treatment-related adverse events were 7.2% and 5.3%. Treatment-related myalgia was reported by 241 patients taking 80 mg/day and by 234 patients taking 10 mg/day (4.8% and 4.7% respectively). There were persistent rises in the activities of alanine transaminase, aspartate transaminase, or both in 60 patients taking 80 mg/day compared with nine taking 10 mg/day. There were five cases of rhabdomyolysis, two in those taking 80 mg/day and three in those taking 10 mg/day. At the start of the study 131 patients were excluded because of abnormal liver function tests, but in all the study showed that high-dose atorvastatin is relatively safe. This finding has been supported by the results of another study, in which the proportion of patients who developed rises in liver enzymes with atorvastatin 80 mg/day was low and comparable to the results of other similar studies (25).

Drug–Drug Interactions

Cardiac glycosides

Atorvastatin 80 mg/day increased the AUC and C_{max} of digoxin 0.25 mg/day by 15% and 20% respectively during steady-state therapy, without affecting renal digoxin clearance (26).

Ciclosporin

Rhabdomyolysis occurred when atorvastatin was combined with ciclosporin for 2 months in a woman with systemic lupus erythematosus and a renal transplant (27).

Diltiazem

Rhabdomyolysis and acute hepatitis have been reported in association with the co-administration of diltiazem and atorvastatin (28).

- A 60-year-old African-American man developed abdominal pain, a racing heart, and shortness of breath over 24 hours. He had also noticed increasing fatigue and reduced urine output over the previous 2–3 days. He had been taking several medications, including atorvastatin, for more than 1 year, but diltiazem had been added 3 weeks before for atrial fibrillation. On the basis of laboratory findings and physical examination, a diagnosis of acute hepatitis and rhabdomyolysis with accompanying acute renal insufficiency was made. His renal function gradually normalized and his CK activity reached a maximum of 2092 units/l on day 1 and fell to 623 units/l on discharge. His liver function tests returned to normal by 3 months.

While rhabdomyolysis from statins is rare, the risk is increased when they are used in combination with agents that share similar metabolic pathways. Atorvastatin is metabolized by CYP3A4, which is inhibited by diltiazem.

Erythromycin

When erythromycin was co-administered with atorvastatin, the mean C_{max} and AUC of atorvastatin increased by more than 30% (29,30).

In 12 healthy volunteers, erythromycin increased both the maximal plasma concentration and AUC of co-administered atorvastatin (31).

Esomeprazole

Rhabdomyolysis was associated with third-degree atrioventricular block in a patient taking atorvastatin with esomeprazole and clarithromycin.

- A 51-year-old white woman developed severe weakness, near syncope, shortness of breath, and chest pain. She had complete heart block. The creatine kinase activity was over 7000 U/l. She had taken atorvastatin for more than 1 year, esomeprazole for 6 weeks, and three doses of clarithromycin 500 mg just before the episode. Her symptoms coincided with starting to take esomeprazole.

The pharmacokinetic profiles of these agents suggested that esomeprazole had inhibited P glycoprotein, reducing the normal first-pass clearance of atorvastatin (32).

Itraconazole

Itraconazole increases serum concentrations of atorvastatin by inhibiting CYP3A4. In a randomized, double-blind, crossover study in 10 healthy volunteers, itraconazole 200 mg increased the AUC and half-life of atorvastatin 40 mg about three-fold, with a change in C_{max} (33). The AUC of atorvastatin lactone was increased about 4-fold, and the C_{max} and half-life were increased more than 2-fold. Itraconazole significantly reduced the C_{max} and AUC of 2-hydroxyatorvastatin acid and 2-hydroxyatorvastatin lactone and increased the half-life of 2-hydroxyatorvastatin lactone. The concomitant use of itraconazole and other potent inhibitors of CYP3A4 with atorvastatin should therefore be avoided, or the dose of atorvastatin should be reduced accordingly.

Terfenadine

Atorvastatin, although a substrate for CYP3A4, does not affect blood terfenadine concentrations to a clinically significant extent (34).

Warfarin

In 12 patients chronically maintained on warfarin, atorvastatin 80 mg/day for 2 weeks reduced mean prothrombin times slightly, but only for the first few days of the 2-week treatment period (35). Thus, atorvastatin had no consistent effect on the anticoagulant activity of warfarin and adjustments in warfarin doses should not be necessary.

References

1. Yee HS, Fong NT. Atorvastatin in the treatment of primary hypercholesterolemia and mixed dyslipidemias. Ann Pharmacother 1998;32(10):1030–43.
2. Dart A, Jerums G, Nicholson G, d'Emden M, Hamilton-Craig I, Tallis G, Best J, West M, Sullivan D, Bracs P, Black D. A multicenter, double-blind, one-year study comparing safety and efficacy of atorvastatin versus simvastatin in patients with hypercholesterolemia. Am J Cardiol 1997;80(1):39–44.
3. Ballantyne CM, Houri J, Notarbartolo A, Melani L, Lipka LJ, Suresh R, Sun S, Le Beaut AP, Sager PT, Veltri EP, for the Ezetimibe Study Group . Effect of ezetimibe coadministered with atorvastatin in 628 patients with primary hypercholesterolemia: a prospective, randomized, double-blind trial. Circulation 2003;107:2409–15.
4. Phillips PS. Ezetimibe and statin-associated myopathy. Ann Intern Med 2004;141(8):649.
5. Fux R, Mörike K, Gundel UF, Hartmann R, Gleiter CH. Ezetimibe and statin-associated myopathy. Ann Intern Med 2004;140(8):671–2.

6. Kosoglou T, Statkevich P, Meyer I, Cutler DL, Musiol B, Yang B, Zhu Y, Maxwell SE, Veltri EP. Effects of ezetimibe on the pharmacodynamics and pharmacokinetics of lovastatin. Curr Med Res Opin 2004;20(6):955–65.

7. Negevesky GJ, Kolsky MP, Laureno R, Yau TH. Reversible atorvastatin-associated external ophthalmoplegia, anti-acetylcholine receptor antibodies, and ataxia. Arch Ophthalmol 2000;118(3):427–8.

8. Silverberg C. Atorvastatin-induced polyneuropathy. Ann Int Med 2003;139:792–3.

9. Gaist D, Jeppesen U, Andersen M, Garcia Rodriguez LA, Hallas J, Sindrup SH. Statins and risk of polyneuropathy: a case-control study. Neurology 2002;58:P1333–7.

10. Reid L, Bakker-Arkema R, Black D. The effect of atorvastatin on the human lens after 52 weeks of treatment. J Cardiovasc Pharmacol Ther 1998;3(1):71–6.

11. Rundek T, Naini A, Sacco R, Coates K, DiMauro S. Atorvastatin decreases the coenzyme Q10 level in the blood of patients at risk for cardiovascular disease and stroke. Arch Neurol 2004;61(6):889–92.

12. Gonzalez-Ponte ML, Gonzalez-Ruiz M, Duvos E, Gutierrez-Iniguez MA, Olalla JI, Conde E. Atorvastatin-induced severe thrombocytopenia. Lancet 1998;352(9136):1284.

13. Malaise J, Leonet J, Goffin E, Lefebvre C, Tennstedt D, Vandeleene B, Buysschaert M, Squifflet J. Pancreas transplantation for treatment of generalised allergy to human insulin in type I diabetes. Transplant Proc 2005;37:2839.

14. Pelli N. Autoimmune hepatitis revealed by atorvastatin. Eur J Gastroenterol Hepatol 2003;15:921–4.

15. Gershovich OE, Lyman AE Jr. Liver function test abnormalities and pruritus in a patient treated with atorvastatin: case report and review of the literature. Pharmacotherapy 2004;24:150–4.

16. Belaiche G, Ley G, Slama JL. Pancreatite aiguë associée a la prise d'atorvastatine. [Acute pancreatitis associated with atorvastatine therapy.] Gastroenterol Clin Biol 2000;24(4):471–2.

17. Pfeiffer CM, Kazenoff S, Rothberg HD. Toxic epidermal necrolysis from atorvastatin. JAMA 1998;279(20):1613–4.

18. Anliker MD, Wuthrich B. Chronic urticaria to atorvastatin. Allergy 2002;57(4):366.

19. Konig C, Eickert A, Scharfetter-Kochanek K, Krieg T, Hunzelmann N. Linear IgA bullous dermatosis induced by atorvastatin. J Am Acad Dermatol 2001;44(4):689–92.

20. Adcock BB, Hornsby LB, Jenkins K. Dermographism: an adverse effect of atorvastatin. J Am Board Fam Pract 2001;14(2):148–51.

21. Lea AP, McTavish D. Atorvastatin. A review of its pharmacology and therapeutic potential in the management of hyperlipidaemias. Drugs 1997;53(5):828–47.

22. Jimenez-Alonso J, Jaimez L, Sabio JM, Hidalgo C, Leon L. Atorvastatin-induced reversible positive antinuclear antibodies. Am J Med 2002;112(4):329–30.

23. Graziadei IW. Drug-induced lupus-like syndrome associated with severe autoimmune hepatitis. Lupus 2003;12:409–12.

24. LaRosa JC, Grundy SM, Waters DD, Shear C, Barter P, Fruchart JC, Gotto AM, Greten H, Kastelein JJP, Shepherd J, Wenger NK; for the Treating to Target (TNT) Investigators. Intensive lipid lowering with atorvastatin in patients with stable coronary disease. N Engl J Med 2005;352(14):1425–35.

25. Pedersen TR, Faergeman O, Kastelein JJP, Olsson AG, Tikkanen MJ, Holme I, Larsen ML, Bendiksen FS, Lindahl C, Szarek M, Tsai J; for the Incremental Decrease

in End Points Through Aggressive Lipid Lowering (IDEAL) Study Group. High-dose atorvastatin vs usual-dose simvastatin for secondary prevention after myocardial infarction. The IDEAL Study: a randomized controlled trial. JAMA 2005;294(19):2437–45.

26. Boyd RA, Stern RH, Stewart BH, Wu X, Reyner EL, Zegarac EA, Randinitis EJ, Whitfield L. Atorvastatin coadministration may increase digoxin concentrations by inhibition of intestinal P-glycoprotein-mediated secretion. J Clin Pharmacol 2000;40(1):91–8.

27. Maltz HC, Balog DL, Cheigh JS. Rhabdomyolysis associated with concomitant use of atorvastatin and cyclosporine. Ann Pharmacother 1999;33(11):1176–9.

28. Lewin JJ 3rd, Nappi JM, Taylor MH, Lugo SI, Larouche M. Rhabdomyolysis with concurrent atorvastatin and diltiazem. Ann Pharmacother 2002;36(10):1546–9.

29. Rubinstein E. Comparative safety of the different macrolides. Int J Antimicrob Agents 2001;18(Suppl 1):S71–6.

30. Williams D, Feely J. Pharmacokinetic–pharmacodynamic drug interactions with HMG-CoA reductase inhibitors. Clin Pharmacokinet 2002;41(5):343–70.

31. Siedlik PH, Olson SC, Yang BB, Stern RH. Erythromycin coadministration increases plasma atorvastatin concentrations. J Clin Pharmacol 1999;39(5):501–4.

32. Sipe BE, Jones RJ, Bokhart GH. Rhabdomyolysis causing AV blockade due to possible atorvastatin, esomeprazole, and clarithromycin interaction. Ann Pharmacother 2003;37:808–11.

33. Kantola T, Kivisto KT, Neuvonen PJ. Effect of itraconazole on the pharmacokinetics of atorvastatin. Clin Pharmacol Ther 1998;64(1):58–65.

34. Stern RH, Smithers JA, Olson SC. Atorvastatin does not produce a clinically significant effect on the pharmacokinetics of terfenadine. J Clin Pharmacol 1998;38(8):753–7.

35. Stern R, Abel R, Gibson GL, Besserer J. Atorvastatin does not alter the anticoagulant activity of warfarin. J Clin Pharmacol 1997;37(11):1062–4.

Cerivastatin

See also HMG Co-A reductase inhibitors

General Information

Weight for weight, cerivastatin is the most potent statin. Like other statins, the chance of rhabdomyolysis increases when cerivastatin is taken together with certain other drugs (1). Although cerivastatin is degraded by two different isoforms of P_{450} in the liver, and therefore should be less likely to take part in drug interactions than most of the other statins, clinically important interactions do occur, and reports of drug interactions in 2001 triggered its withdrawal, after 31 people in the USA taking cerivastatin, 12 of whom had also taken gemfibrozil, died of severe rhabdomyolysis (2).

In other respects, the adverse effects of cerivastatin are similar to those of other statins (3), and a pooled analysis of studies of cerivastatin 100–400 micrograms/day taken for at least 8 weeks showed no differences in drug-related adverse events between cerivastatin and placebo (4). There was no association between plasma transaminase or creatine kinase activities and cerivastatin dosages.

Cerivastatin 800 micrograms/day for 4 weeks had only mild transient adverse effects (5).

Organs and Systems

Liver

There were increases in serum transaminase activities to more than three times the top end of the reference range in under 1% of patients taking cerivastatin, which is similar to findings with other statins (6).

Musculoskeletal

There were no cases of myalgia in 94 patients taking cerivastatin 50–300 micrograms/day for 72 weeks, whereas in the same study, two of 59 patients taking simvastatin had myalgia (7). At dosages of 300–400 micrograms/day for 8 weeks in 349 patients there were no rises in creatine kinase activity above 10 times the upper limit of the reference range, and asymptomatic increases (to over three times the upper limit of the reference range) occurred more often with placebo (2.8%) than with cerivastatin (1.4% with 0.4 mg; none with 0.3 mg) (8).

Drug–Drug Interactions

Cardiac glycosides

In 20 healthy men, cerivastatin had no effect on the steady-state pharmacokinetics of digoxin (11). Digoxin had no significant effect on the pharmacokinetics of cerivastatin.

Ciclosporin

Cerivastatin 0.2 mg/day was well tolerated when given together with ciclosporin, although there were 3- to 5-fold increases in the plasma concentrations of cerivastatin and its metabolites when single-dose cerivastatin was given to 12 kidney transplant recipients taking ciclosporin 200 mg bd and to 12 healthy controls (9). Ciclosporin may have affected both the distribution of cerivastatin and its biotransformation in the liver.

Gemfibrozil

Cerivastatin was withdrawn in 2001 after 31 people in the USA taking cerivastatin, 12 of whom had also taken gemfibrozil, died of severe rhabdomyolysis (2).

- Myalgia and a marked increase in creatine kinase was precipitated in a 74-year-old woman with normal renal function who took gemfibrozil 1200 mg/day 3 weeks after she had started to take cerivastatin 300 µg/day (10).

Itraconazole

Cerivastatin uses a secondary CYP2C8-mediated metabolic pathway, which is unaffected by itraconazole (12). The effects of itraconazole on the pharmacokinetics of cerivastatin and its major metabolites have been investigated in a randomized, double-blind, crossover study (13). Inhibition of the CYP3A4-mediated M-1 pathway led to raised serum concentrations of cerivastatin, cerivastatin lactone, and metabolite M-23, resulting in increased concentrations of active HMG-CoA reductase inhibitors. However, the effect was modest.

References

1. Horsmans Y. Differential metabolism of statins: importance in drug–drug interactions. Eur Heart J Suppl 1999;1(Suppl T):T7–T12.
2. Thompson CA. Cerivastatin withdrawn from market. Am J Health Syst Pharm 2001;58(18):1685.
3. McClellan KJ, Wiseman LR, McTavish D. Cerivastatin. Drugs 1998;55(3):415–20.
4. Stein E, Schopen U, Catagay M. A pooled efficacy analysis of cerivastatin in the treatment of primary hyperlipidaemia. Clin Drug Invest 1999;18:433–44.
5. Stein E, Isaacsohn J, Stoltz R, Mazzu A, Liu MC, Lane C, Heller AH. Pharmacodynamics, safety, tolerability, and pharmacokinetics of the 0.8-mg dose of cerivastatin in patients with primary hypercholesterolemia Am J Cardiol 1999;83(10):1433–6.
6. Anonymous. Cerivastatin for hypercholesterolemia. Med Lett Drugs Ther 1998;40(1018):13–4.
7. Leiter LA, Hanna K. Efficacy and safety of cerivastatin in primary hypercholesterolemia: a long term comparative titration study with simvastatin. Can J Cardiol 1999;15(5):545–55.
8. Davignon J, Hanefeld M, Nakaya N, Hunninghake DB, Insull W Jr, Ose L. Clinical efficacy and safety of cerivastatin: summary of pivotal phase IIb/III studies. Am J Cardiol 1998;82(4B):J32–9.
9. Muck W, Mai I, Fritsche L, Ochmann K, Rohde G, Unger S, Johne A, Bauer S, Budde K, Roots I, Neumayer HH, Kuhlmann J. Increase in cerivastatin systemic exposure after single and multiple dosing in cyclosporine-treated kidney transplant recipients. Clin Pharmacol Ther 1999;65(3):251–61.
10. Pogson GW, Kindred LH, Carper BG. Rhabdomyolysis and renal failure associated with cerivastatin–gemfibrozil combination therapy. Am J Cardiol 1999;83(7):1146.
11. Weber P, Lettieri JT, Kaiser L, Mazzu AL. Lack of mutual pharmacokinetic interaction between cerivastatin, a new HMG-CoA reductase inhibitor, and digoxin in healthy normocholesterolemic volunteers. Clin Ther 1999;21(9):1563–75.
12. Gubbins PO, McConnell SA, Penzak SR. Antifungal Agents. In: Piscitelli SC, Rodvold KA, editors. Drug Interactions in Infectious Diseases. Totowa, NJ: Humana Press Inc, 2001:185–217.
13. Kantola T, Kivisto KT, Neuvonen PJ. Effect of itraconazole on cerivastatin pharmacokinetics. Eur J Clin Pharmacol 1999;54(11):851–5.

Ezetimibe

General Information

Ezetimibe is a selective potent inhibitor of the intestinal absorption of dietary and biliary cholesterol. A total of 432 patients were included in a pooled analysis of two phase-II studies, both lasting for 12 weeks; ezetimibe was well tolerated, with an adverse events profile similar to that of placebo (1). In 668 patients who took ezetimibe with simvastatin, the adverse effects were similar to those with simvastatin alone (2).

In 432 patients included in a pooled analysis of two phase 2 studies, both lasting for 12 weeks, ezetimibe was well tolerated, with an adverse events profile similar to that of placebo (3).

Organs and Systems

Liver

In several studies of co-administration of ezetimibe with a statin there have been small numbers of patients with raised serum transaminase activities at or above three times the upper limit of the reference range.

- A 50-year-old woman with previous autoimmune thyroid disease taking atorvastatin developed acute hepatitis when she also was given ezetimibe (4). Further investigations, including liver biopsy, showed a probable drug-induced autoimmune hepatitis.

Ezetimibe was considered to be the most likely causal agent, although atorvastatin could not be ruled out.

Musculoskeletal

Myotoxicity linked to ezetimibe has been described in a 45-year-old overweight man with McArdle disease, which is the most common disorder of muscle carbohydrate metabolism, caused by mutations in the gene that encodes myophosphorylase (5).

Drug-drug interactions

Fibrates

Co-administration of ezetimibe and fenofibrate in 32 healthy subjects with hypercholesterolemia (6) resulted in no significant changes in laboratory test results, including enzymes indicative of muscle or liver injury.

In a randomized, open, three-way crossover, multiple-dose study in 12 healthy adult men there was no clinically significant interaction of ezetimibe with gemfibrozil (7).

HMG Co-A reductase inhibitors

In 668 patients ezetimibe was given with simvastatin and adverse effects were similar to those experienced with simvastatin alone (8).

Ezetimibe plus atorvastatin was also well tolerated in 628 patients, with a safety profile similar to that of atorvastatin alone and to placebo. When co-administered with atorvastatin, ezetimibe provided significant incremental reductions in LDL cholesterol and triglycerides and increased HDL cholesterol (9).

Ezetimibe given with simvastatin and atorvastatin is well tolerated, with a safety profile similar to the statin alone and to placebo (SEDA-28, 534). However, there are concerns about the use of ezetimibe in patients with impaired oxidation of fatty acids, as in familial combined hyperlipidemia. Of more than 300 patients with intolerance of lipid-lowering therapies a subgroup had common features, including raised fasting respiratory exchange ratios while not taking lipid-lowering drugs and hypertriglyceridemia (10). An interaction of ezetimibe with statins was suspected in two men aged 43 and 53 years, both of whom had raised creatine kinase activity and one of whom also had myalgia (11). However, co-administration of ezetimibe and lovastatin in 48 healthy men resulted in no significant changes in laboratory test results, including enzymes indicative of muscle or liver damage (12)

Vitamins

Ezetimibe has no major effect on the absorption of fat-soluble vitamins (13).

References

1. Bays HE, Moore PB, Drehobl MA, Rosenblatt S, Toth PD, Dujovne CA, Knopp RH, Lipka LJ, Lebeaut AP, Yang B, Mellars LE, Cuffie-Jackson C, Veltri EPEzetimibe Study Group. Effectiveness and tolerability of ezetimibe in patients with primary hypercholesterolemia: pooled analysis of two phase II studies. Clin Ther 2001;23(8):1209–30.
2. Davidson MH, McGarry T, Bettis R, Melani L, Lipka LJ, LeBeaut AP, Suresh R, Sun S, Veltri EP. Ezetimibe coadministered with simvastatin in patients with primary hypercholesterolemia. J Am Coll Cardiol 2002;40(12):2125–34.
3. Bays HE, Moore PB, Drehobl MA, Rosenblatt S, Toth PD, Dujovne CA, Knopp RH, Lipka LJ, LeBeaut AP, Yang B, Mellars LE, Cuffie-Jackson C, Veltri EP, for the Ezetimibe Study Group. Effectiveness and tolerability of ezetimibe in patients with primary hypercholesterolemia: pooled analysis of two phase II studies. Clin Ther 2001;23:1209–30.
4. Heyningen CV. Drug-induced acute autoimmune hepatitis during combination therapy with atorvastatin and ezetimibe. Ann Clin Biochem 2005;42:402–4.
5. Perez-Calvo J, Civeira-Murillo F, Cabello A. Worsening myopathy associated with ezetimibe in a patient with McArdle disease. Q J Med 2005;98(6):461–2.
6. Kosoglou T, Statkevich P, Fruchart JC, Pember LJ, Reyderman L, Cutler DL, Guillaume M, Maxwell SE, Veltri EP. Pharmacodynamic and pharmacokinetic interaction between fenofibrate and ezetimibe. Curr Med Res Opin 2004;20(8):1197–207.
7. Reyderman L, Kosoglou T, Statkevich P, Pember L, Boutros T, Maxwell SE, Affrime M, Batra V. Assessment of a multiple-dose drug interaction between ezetimibe, a novel selective cholesterol absorption inhibitor and gemfibrozil. International J Clin Pharmacol Ther 2004;42(9):512–8.
8. Davidson MH, McGarry T, Bettis R, Melani L, Lipka LJ, LeBeaut AP, Suresh R, Sun S, Veltri EP. Ezetimibe

coadministered with simvastatin in patients with primary hypercholesterolemia. J Am Coll Cardiol 2002;40:2125–34.

9. Ballantyne CM, Houri J, Notarbartolo A, Melani L, Lipka LJ, Suresh R, Sun S, Le Beaut AP, Sager PT, Veltri EP, for the Ezetimibe Study Group . Effect of ezetimibe coadministered with atorvastatin in 628 patients with primary hypercholesterolemia: a prospective, randomized, double-blind trial. Circulation 2003;107:2409–15.

10. Phillips PS. Ezetimibe and statin-associated myopathy. Ann Intern Med 2004;141(8):649.

11. Fux R, Mörike K, Gundel UF, Hartmann R, Gleiter CH. Ezetimibe and statin-associated myopathy. Ann Intern Med 2004;140(8):671–2.

12. Kosoglou T, Statkevich P, Meyer I, Cutler DL, Musiol B, Yang B, Zhu Y, Maxwell SE, Veltri EP. Effects of ezetimibe on the pharmacodynamics and pharmacokinetics of lovastatin. Curr Med Res Opin 2004;20(6):955–65.

13. Murdoch D, Scott LJ. Ezetimibe/simvastatin: a review of its use in the management of hypercholesterolemia. Am J Cardiovasc Drugs 2004;4(6):405–22.

Fibrates

General Information

Fibrates reduce plasma triglycerides by inhibiting their hepatic synthesis and increasing their catabolism. They reduce the synthesis of triglyceride–very low density lipoprotein (VLDL) by increasing the beta-oxidation of fatty acids in the liver. They increase triglyceride catabolism by inducing lipoprotein lipase gene transcription and reducing apoC-III gene transcription. Fibrates increase high-density lipoprotein (HDL) cholesterol by increasing apoA-I and apoA-II gene transcription. These effects are due to activation of peroxisome proliferator-activated receptors (PPAR) alpha and induction of the over-expression of genes containing a peroxisome proliferator response element (PPRE) in their promoter (1).

The fibrates include beclobrate, bezafibrate, biclofibrate, binifibrate, ciprofibrate, clinofibrate, clofibrate, dulofibrate, etofibrate, fenirofibrate, fenofibrate, gemfibrozil, lifibrate, nicofibrate, picafibrate, pirifibrate, ponfibrate, ronifibrate, salafibrate, serfibrate, simfibrate, sitofibrate, tiafibrate, timofibrate, tocofibrate, urefibrate, and xantifibrate (all rINNs).

The adverse events of the fibrates are essentially the same with all members of the class and are generally mild or absent during short-term treatment. The observed frequency of adverse effects with a micronized formulation of fenofibrate is comparable to that associated with the usual formulation (SEDA-22, 490).

Organs and Systems

Nervous system

Nervous system adverse effects are rare, constituting 0.5% of all adverse effects (2). Gemfibrozil-induced headache has been reported (3) and occurred in one patient who had taken bezafibrate for 24 hours (4). Peripheral neuropathy has been observed with bezafibrate (SEDA-13, 1324; 5).

Metabolism

Of 70 patients with cutaneous T cell lymphomas, three who were taking gemfibrozil had to have it withdrawn because of increases in serum triglycerides (6).

- A 76-year-old woman with type 2 diabetes taking gemfibrozil for pronounced hypertriglyceridemia had recurrent episodes of hypoglycemia; her insulin requirements fell by 65% and her HbA_{1c} concentration fell from 9 to 6.5% over 5 months (7).

In patients taking fenofibrate and atorvastatin, increased concentrations of plasma homocysteine were attributed to an action of the fibrates themselves and not indirectly via their lipid-lowering effect (8). Concomitant administration of folic acid, at least in part, offset this adverse effect (9). The degree of rise in homocysteine differs among the various fibrates. It has been reported with fenofibrate and bezafibrate, and a study of fenofibrate and gemfibrozil substantiated a difference between the drugs (10). Because the concentration of plasma homocysteine depends on renal function, increased plasma homocysteine concentrations could result from renal function impairment caused by fenofibrate. In contrast, gemfibrozil does not affect renal function. This was tested in a crossover study in 22 patients who had hypertriglyceridemia, by giving them gemfibrozil 900 mg/day or fenofibrate 200 mg/day for 6 weeks (11). Lipids were altered similarly, but homocysteine, creatinine, and cystatin C were raised by fenofibrate but not by gemfibrozil. In another report, there was a 57% increase in homocysteine in 26 individuals who took ciprofibrate and a 17% reduction in homocysteine in 12 patients who took bezafibrate.

Fibrates

Fenofibrate and bezafibrate can cause hyperhomocysteinemia, which is a risk factor for coronary heart disease. The authors of a review suggested using gemfibrozil instead or adding vitamin B_{12} and folic acid (12).

Fluid balance

Clofibrate has a mild antidiuretic effect (13), and animal studies suggest that this is due to release of antidiuretic hormone (ADH) (14). This effect has been used in the treatment of cranial diabetes insipidus (15).

Hematologic

Leukopenia has been reported with bezafibrate (16), clofibrate (17), and fenofibrate (18).

Gastrointestinal

Abdominal discomfort occurs in 5–10% of all patients taking fibrates. Epigastric fullness, nausea, meteorism, and mild diarrhea have been repeatedly described, and stomatitis has been incidentally mentioned. There are wide discrepancies in the figures given for such complications, ranging as they do from 2 (2) to 20%; the truth appears to be that during the first few days and weeks of treatment, mild discomfort of one sort or another is quite common, although some of it is due to a placebo effect; serious symptoms are most unusual. Bezafibrate is better tolerated than gemfibrozil (19). In a double-blind trial with fenofibrate, the incidence of gastrointestinal adverse effects was not different from that seen with placebo (20). Five of 1213 individuals taking beclobrate complained of diarrhea (21).

Liver

Assurance of good renal and hepatic function is mandatory before beginning treatment with the fibrates (22). Serum transaminase changes are regularly seen and hepatitis occurs (23). Several cases of hepatitis due to fenofibrate have been reviewed (24) and it has also been observed with etofibrate (25). One case of liver failure, probably due to beclobrate, has been reported (SEDA-13, 1324; 26). Liver biopsies showed a lymphoplasmacytic infiltrate in all of five cases of chronic hepatitis associated with fibrates (27).

Cirrhosis has been attributed to fenofibrate (28).

- A 62-year-old Indian man developed abnormal liver function tests after taking fenofibrate for 11 months. Liver biopsy confirmed the presence of cirrhosis; there was no steatosis or cholestasis.

Possible mechanisms of fenofibrate-induced liver injury include activation of peroxisome proliferation-activator receptors, a hypersensitivity reaction, and immune-mediated injury from cross-reactivity of the drug with autoantigens. The authors referred to six reported cases of hepatic fibrosis attributed to fenofibrate. Raised transaminase activities occur commonly with fenofibrate but are generally transient, reverse on withdrawal, and do not result in long-term injury. Fenofibrate should be withdrawn if higher than normal enzyme activities persist, and a liver biopsy should be considered if liver enzymes do not normalize after withdrawal.

Biliary tract

Fibrates produce bile that is supersaturated with cholesterol. Although gallstones are common with clofibrate, no excess frequency has been observed with fenofibrate (23). In the WHO study, 59 patients taking clofibrate had to be operated on for gallstones, compared with 24 and 25 respectively in the two placebo groups (29).

Pancreas

Pancreatitis has been attributed to bezafibrate.

- A 75-year-old white woman had fever and raised amylase on three consecutive occasions after taking a tablet of bezafibrate (30). After stopping taking the drug, she remained free of symptoms.

Urinary tract

Unexpected acute renal insufficiency occurred in four patients after uncomplicated cardiac surgery; each was taking a fibrate (31). Renal insufficiency occurred rapidly within 3 days of surgery and was associated with increased concentrations of skeletal muscle-derived creatine kinase. One patient developed myoglobinuria. Presumably, patients taking lipid-lowering drugs are at higher risk of acute renal insufficiency after cardiac surgery, because of rhabdomyolysis. This suggests that patients taking either statins or fibrates should discontinue them before cardiac surgery.

Fenofibrate was the probable cause of rises in serum creatinine concentrations in six patients in one clinic (32). The authors therefore recommended routine serum creatinine monitoring at baseline and at 1 month after starting fenofibrate.

Severe reversible renal insufficiency has been reported with fibrates (33).

Reversible acute renal allograft dysfunction occurred in three patients taking fenofibrate (34). Serum concentrations of immunosuppressant agents remained within the target ranges throughout. On withdrawal of fenofibrate the renal dysfunction resolved. The pathological changes in the proximal tubules in all three biopsy specimens were in keeping with a toxic rather than an ischemic etiology. Although the control of hyperlipidemia is crucial in patients with transplants, the authors suggested that caution should be exercised and serum creatinine concentrations be closely monitored in patients who start to take fibrates.

Skin

Non-specific rashes have been reported in patients taking fibrates. With fenofibrate, rashes are reported significantly more often than with placebo (35), and occur in some 0.6% of patients (23). In a double-blind trial, the incidence of cutaneous adverse effects was 11% with fenofibrate and less than 1% with placebo; they included hives and urticaria (20). In another study, the difference was 6% (36).

- Chronic radiodermatitis after cardiac catheterization has been observed in a 62-year-old woman taking ciprofibrate. A second catheterization performed when she had stopped taking it did not provoke new lesions (37).

Photosensitivity due to fenofibrate (38) was confirmed by systemic photochallenge (39). Photodermatitis has been associated with cross-reactivity between ketoprofen and fenofibrate; this was thought to be due to chemical similarities between these two drugs (40).

Psoriasis was exacerbated by gemfibrozil in one case (41).

Stevens–Johnson syndrome has been associated with bezafibrate (42) and clofibrate (43).

Musculoskeletal

Rhabdomyolysis is a problem with several lipid-lowering drugs (SEDA-13, 1325; SEDA-13, 1328; SEDA-13, 1330;

SEDA-19, 409; 44–46), especially when they are used in combination (47). In individuals with pre-existing renal insufficiency, this can lead to an earlier need for chronic dialysis (48). Also, interactions between various hypolipidemic drugs and other drugs sometimes cause rhabdomyolysis (SEDA-18, 426).

Creatine kinase activity increased in five out of 1213 patients taking beclobrate (21). Myopathy during treatment has been reported with gemfibrozil (49) and ciprofibrate (50,51).

- A 30-year-old white man with hypertension, type 1 diabetes mellitus, and hyperlipidemia developed myalgias, nausea, and vomiting, which began 4 days after he started working as a jackhammer operator (52). His medications were lisinopril, aspirin, insulin, and gemfibrozil. Creatine kinase and creatinine, which had previously been respectively mildly raised and normal, were markedly raised, consistent with rhabdomyolysis with acute renal insufficiency.

Fibrate monotherapy of hyperlipidemia may predispose to rhabdomyolysis with acute renal insufficiency. Patients using fibrates should be cautioned regarding strenuous exertion, dehydration, and the need for prompt evaluation of myalgia.

Hypothyroidism predisposes to rhabdomyolysis (53,54) and screening of thyroid function has been advocated before starting hypolipidemic drugs (SEDA-21, 458). This notion has been supported by observations in a 69-year-old man taking fenofibrate 200 mg daily (55). The muscular syndrome appears to be a special risk in patients with nephrotic syndrome (SEDA-13, 1325; 56).

- Two women, 55 and 57 years old, with renal insufficiency, had rhabdomyolysis after taking micronized fenofibrate in dosages a little higher than recommended (57). Both had mild hypothyroidism.

Reduced renal function in the elderly appears to be a risk factor for myopathy (SEDA-23, 472).

- A 73-year-old woman had an increase in serum creatinine concentration while she was taking long-acting bezafibrate and again when she was re-challenged by self-medication (58).
- Low-dose bezafibrate was associated with myositis in a patient with mild chronic renal insufficiency (serum creatinine 210 µmol/l) (59). She was a 58-year-old obese diabetic with isolated hypertriglyceridemia.

Sexual function

Erectile dysfunction has been reported in 12% of 339 men treated with fibrate derivatives or statins, compared with 5.6% of similar patients not taking these drugs (60). The mechanism is unknown and should be confirmed in randomized studies.

Gemfibrozil was suspected to have reduced libido in two cases (61,62), an effect that is well-known with clofibrate, and four cases of loss of libido and impotence involving gemfibrozil have previously been reported (SEDA-13, 1325; 63,64).

Immunologic

Vasculitis, Raynaud's phenomenon, and polyarthritis have been reported with gemfibrozil (65).

Allergic reactions have been reported with some fibrates.

- A 61-year-old woman with penicillin allergy suffered generalized urticaria, chest tightness, wheezing, nausea, vomiting, hypotension, and loss of consciousness (66). Two hours earlier, she had taken Eulitop Retard after lunch. She had intense positive responses to intradermal Eulitop Retard and its active component, bezafibrate; skin tests in control subjects were negative. Specific IgE tests (RAST) to Eulitop Retard were negative. The positive skin tests suggested that an IgE mechanism was responsible for this adverse reaction.
- A 69-year-old woman developed a major allergic reaction after taking fenofibrate 300 mg/day for 10 days (67). The clinical features included weakness, hyperthermia, and slight muscular pain. Biological abnormalities were mildly raised muscle enzymes and pancytopenia, which developed rapidly.

Long-Term Effects

Tumorigenicity

It has been suspected that low concentrations of serum cholesterol might be associated with an increased risk of cancer or overall mortality. All fibrates and statins cause cancer in rodents, but the relevance of this finding to man has been questioned (68). In an epidemiological study these risks were almost non-existent after adjusting for confounding factors.

Second-Generation Effects

Fetotoxicity

In pregnant mice given etofylline clofibrate and fenofibrate in doses of 12, 117, and 586 mg/kg orally from day 7 to day 16 of gestation, terminal maternal body weight was significantly reduced by all doses of etofylline clofibrate (69). The low and middle doses of etofylline clofibrate and fenofibrate had no adverse effects on embryofetal development, but the highest dose of etofylline clofibrate significantly reduced fetal weight at term. Postimplantation loss was significantly higher after the highest dose of fenofibrate. There were no teratogenic effects. The significance of these results to human pregnancy is unknown.

Drug–Drug Interactions

Bexarotene

Of 70 patients with cutaneous T cell lymphomas, three who were taking gemfibrozil had to have it withdrawn because of increases in serum concentrations of triglycerides and bexarotene, an RXR-selective retinoid "rexinoid", which is used for all stages of cutaneous T cell lymphoma (6).

Colchicine

Rhabdomyolysis due to the combination of colchicine with gemfibrozil has been reported in a 40-year-old man with amyloidosis and chronic liver disease (70).

HMG coenzyme-A reductase inhibitors

The increased risk of myopathy observed during concomitant treatment with statins and fibrates may be partly pharmacokinetic in origin. In interactions between fibrates and statins there may be differences between the various fibrates (71). Eleven healthy volunteers took bezafibrate 400 mg/day, gemfibrozil 1200 mg/day, or placebo for 3 days. On day 3, each took a single dose of lovastatin 40 mg. Plasma concentrations of lovastatin, lovastatin acid, gemfibrozil, and bezafibrate were measured for up to 24 hours. Gemfibrozil markedly increased plasma concentrations of lovastatin acid, but bezafibrate did not. The risk of myopathy during concomitant therapy with lovastatin and a fibrate may be smaller with bezafibrate than with gemfibrozil.

In 80 patients with primary mixed hyperlipidemia, gemfibrozil used together with lovastatin resulted in 3% discontinuation because of myositis, but none attributable to rhabdomyolysis or myoglobinuria (72).

In a retrospective series, 4 (5%) out of 80 subjects taking lovastatin and gemfibrozil developed a myopathy. Based on this and on reports to US Food and Drug Administration the combined use of the two drugs is discouraged, especially in patients with compromised renal and/or hepatic function. Elderly women may be at special risk (73,74).

Some investigators have concluded that rare drug-induced reversible hepatotoxicity calls for close monitoring of liver enzymes in long-term treatment with statin-fibrate combinations (75).

Combination therapy with fluvastatin and bezafibrate 400 mg/day in 71 patients with persistent hypertriglyceridemia resulted in no significant increase in creatine kinase activity or in the frequency of myalgia (76).

- In contrast, although in vitro studies have not shown any evidence of pharmacokinetic interactions between cerivastatin and gemfibrozil (77), there was myalgia and a marked increase in creatine kinase in a 74-year-old woman with normal renal function who took gemfibrozil 1200 mg/day 3 weeks after she started to take cerivastatin 0.3 mg/day (78).

Since then several other cases have been described:

- a 64-year-old woman (79)
- a 63-year-old man with diabetes mellitus (80)
- a 75-year-old man (81)
- a 68-year-old man (82).

The last patient fared well on a combination of gemfibrozil and cerivastatin until he received influenza vaccination. Rhabdomyolysis has been reported with various viruses, including influenza A and B and inactivation of the virus does not totally prevent this.

Gemfibrozil also increased plasma concentrations of simvastatin and its active form, simvastatin acid, in a randomized, double-blind, crossover study in 10 healthy volunteers given gemfibrozil or placebo orally for 3 days before a single dose of simvastatin (83). This suggests that the increased risk of myopathy in combination treatment is at least partly pharmacokinetic in origin. Because gemfibrozil does not inhibit CYP3A4 in vitro, the mechanism of the pharmacokinetic interaction is probably inhibition of non-CYP3A4-mediated metabolism of simvastatin acid.

Ibuprofen

Acute renal insufficiency occurred in one patient taking ciprofibrate 100 mg/day and ibuprofen 400 mg/day (84). Both drugs are highly protein-bound and contain propionic acid groups. Thus, ibuprofen may displace ciprofibrate.

Repaglinide

Possible interactions of gemfibrozil, itraconazole, and their combination with repaglinide have been investigated in a randomized crossover study in 12 healthy volunteers who took gemfibrozil 600 mg bd, itraconazole 100 mg/day (first dose 200 mg), both gemfibrozil and itraconazole, or placebo, each for 3 days (85). On day 3 they took a single dose of repaglinide 0.25 mg. Plasma drug and blood glucose concentrations were followed for 7 hours and serum insulin and C peptide concentrations for 3 hours after the dose. Gemfibrozil increased the AUC of repaglinide 8 (range 5.5–15) times and prolonged its half-life from 1.3 to 3.7 hours. Although itraconazole alone increased the AUC of repaglinide only 1.4 (1.1–1.9) times, the combination of gemfibrozil + itraconazole increased it 19 (13–25) times and prolonged the half-life of repaglinide to 6.1 hours. The plasma repaglinide concentration at 7 hours was increased 29 times by gemfibrozil and 70 times by the combination of gemfibrozil + itraconazole. Gemfibrozil alone and in combination with itraconazole considerably enhanced and prolonged the blood glucose-lowering effect of repaglinide. Concomitant use of gemfibrozil and repaglinide is best avoided.

Rosiglitazone

Gemfibrozil increases plasma concentrations of rosiglitazone, probably by inhibiting the metabolism of rosiglitazone by CYP2C8. Co-administration of gemfibrozil, or another potent inhibitor of CYP2C8, and rosiglitazone could increase the efficacy of rosiglitazone, but could also increase the risk of adverse effects (86).

Sulfonylureas

Fibrates are highly bound to albumin and displace other similarly bound drugs. This can affect treatment with sulfonylureas. Hypoglycemia occurred in a diabetic patient taking glibenclamide plus gemfibrozil (87).

In 10 healthy volunteers, gemfibrozil 600 mg bd increased the mean total AUC of a single dose of glimepiride 0.5 mg by 23% (range 6–56%) (88). The mean half-life of glimepiride was prolonged from 2.1 to 2.3 hours. This effect may have been caused by inhibition of CYP2C9. However, there were no statistically significant effects on serum insulin or blood glucose variables.

Warfarin

Several interactions between warfarin and hypolipidemic drugs have been described (SEDA-21, 459), including clinically important potentiation of warfarin by bezafibrate (89) and gemfibrozil (90). Two patients developed a significantly increased anticoagulant effect of warfarin while taking fenofibrate (91). A 20% reduction in warfarin dosage, followed by close INR monitoring, has been suggested (92).

References

1. Duriez P. Mécanismes d'action des statines et des fibrates. [Mechanisms of actions of statins and fibrates.] Therapie 2003;58(1):5–14.
2. Adkins JC, Faulds D. Micronised fenofibrate: a review of its pharmacodynamic properties and clinical efficacy in the management of dyslipidaemia. Drugs 1997;54(4):615–33.
3. Alvarez-Sabin J, Codina A, Rodriguez C, Laporte JR. Gemfibrozil-induced headache. Lancet 1988;2(8622):1246.
4. Hodgetts TJ, Tunnicliffe C. Bezafibrate-induced headache. Lancet 1989;1(8630):163.
5. Ellis CJ, Wallis WE, Caruana M. Peripheral neuropathy with bezafibrate. BMJ 1994;309(6959):929.
6. Talpur R, Ward S, Apisarnthanarax N, Breuer-Mcham J, Duvic M. Optimizing bexarotene therapy for cutaneous T cell lymphoma. J Am Acad Dermatol 2002;47(5):672–84.
7. Klein J, Ott V, Schutt M, Klein HH. Recurrent hypoglycaemic episodes in a patient with Type 2 diabetes under fibrate therapy. J Diabetes Complications 2002;16(3):246–8.
8. Giral P, Bruckert E, Jacob N, Chapman MJ, Foglietti MJ, Turpin G. Homocysteine and lipid lowering agents. A comparison between atorvastatin and fenofibrate in patients with mixed hyperlipidemia. Atherosclerosis 2001;154(2):421–7.
9. Stulc T, Melenovsky V, Grauova B, Kozich V, Ceska R. Folate supplementation prevents plasma homocysteine increase after fenofibrate therapy. Nutrition 2001;17(9):721–3.
10. Westphal S, Dierkes J, Luley C. Effects of fenofibrate and gemfibrozil on plasma homocysteine. Lancet 2001;358(9275):39–40.
11. Harats D, Yodfat O, Doolman R, Gavendo S, Marko D, Shaish A, Sela BA. Homocysteine elevation with fibrates: is it a class effect? Isr Med Assoc J 2001;3(4):243–6.
12. Dierkes J, Westphal S, Luley C. Fenofibrate-induced hyperhomocysteinemia: clinical implications and management. Drug Saf 2003;26:81–91.
13. Rado JP. Evidence for permanent enhancement of residual ADH induced by antidiuretic agents (chlorpropamide, carbamazepine, clofibrate) in patients with pituitary diabetes insipidus. Endokrinologie 1975;64(2):217–22.
14. Czako L, Nagy E, Szilagyi I, Laszlo FA. Study of the antidiuretic effect of clofibrate in rat. Endokrinologie 1976;68(2):235–8.
15. Perlemuter L, Hazard J, Kazatchkine M, Guilhaume B, Bernheim R. Action comparée de la carbamazepine et du clofibrate dans le diabète insipide. Etude de 7 cas. [Comparative action of carbamazepine and clofibrate in diabetes insipidus. Study of 7 cases.] Nouv Presse Méd 1975;4(32):2307–10.
16. Ariad S, Hechtlinger V. Bezafibrate-induced neutropenia. Eur J Haematol 1993;50(3):179.
17. Janke EM. Reaction to clofibrate. Can Med Assoc J 1974;111(8):752.
18. Roberts WC. Safety of fenofibrate–US and worldwide experience. Cardiology 1989;76(3):169–79.
19. Kremer P, Marowski C, Jones C, Acacia E. Therapeutic effects of bezafibrate and gemfibrozil in hyperlipoproteinaemia type IIa and IIb. Curr Med Res Opin 1989;11(5):293–303.
20. Brown WV. Treatment of hypercholesterolaemia with fenofibrate: a review. Curr Med Res Opin 1989;11(5):321–30.
21. Capurso A. Drugs affecting triglycerides. Cardiology 1991;78(3):218–25.
22. Brown WV. Fibric acid derivatives. J Drug Dev 1990;3:211–6.
23. Roberts WC. Safety of fenofibrate—US and worldwide experience. Cardiology 1989;76(3):169–79.
24. Rigal J, Furet Y, Autret E, Breteau M. Hépatite mixte sévère au fénofibrate? Revue de la littérature à propos d'un cas. [Severe mixed hepatitis caused by fenofibrate? A review of the literature apropos of a case.] Rev Med Interne 1989;10(1):65–7.
25. Macedo G, Ribeiro T. Etofibrate induced acute hepatitis mimicking biliary tract disease. Arch Med 1996;10:185–6.
26. Vartiainen E, Puska P, Pekkanen J, Tuomilehto J, Lonnqvist J, Ehnholm C. Serum cholesterol concentration and mortality from accidents, suicide, and other violent causes. BMJ 1994;309(6952):445–7.
27. Ganne-Carrie N, de Leusse A, Guettier C, Castera L, Levecq H, Bertrand HJ, Plumet Y, Trinchet JC, Beaugrand M. Hépatites d'allure auto-immune induites par les fibrates. [Autoimmune hepatitis induced by fibrates.] Gastroenterol Clin Biol 1998;22(5):525–9.
28. Ahmed F, Petrovic L, Rosen E, Gonzalez R, Jacobson IM. Fenofibrate-induced cirrhosis. Dig Dis Sci 2005;50(2):312–3.
29. Anonymous. Trial of clofibrate in the treatment of ischaemic heart disease. Five-year study by a group of physicians of the Newcastle upon Tyne region. BMJ 1971;4(5790):767–75.
30. Gang N, Langevitz P, Livneh A. Relapsing acute pancreatitis induced by re-exposure to the cholestrol lowering agent bezafibrate. Am J Gastroenterol 1999;94(12):3626–8.
31. Sharobeem KM, Madden BP, Millner R, Rolfe LM, Seymour CA, Parker J. Acute renal failure after cardiopulmonary bypass: a possible association with drugs of the fibrate group. J Cardiovasc Pharmacol Ther 2000;5(1):33–9.
32. Ritter JL, Nabulsi S. Fenofibrate-induced elevation in serum creatinine. Pharmacotherapy 2001;21(9):1145–9.
33. Lipkin GW, Tomson CR. Severe reversible renal failure with bezafibrate. Lancet 1993;341(8841):371.
34. Angeles C, Lane BP, Miller F, Nord EP. Fenofibrate-associated reversible acute allograft dysfunction in 3 renal transplant recipients: biopsy evidence of tubular toxicity. Am J Kidney Dis 2004;44(3):543–50.

35. Zimetbaum P, Frishman WH, Kahn S. Effects of gemfibrozil and other fibric acid derivatives on blood lipids and lipoproteins. J Clin Pharmacol 1991;31(1):25–37.

36. Knopp RH. Review of the effects of fenofibrate on lipoproteins, apoproteins, and bile saturation: US studies. Cardiology 1989;76(Suppl 1):14–22.

37. Gironet N, Jan V, Machet MC, Machet L, Lorette G, Vaillant L. Radiodermite chronique post cathétérisme cardiaque: role favorisant du ciprofibrate (Lipanor)?. [Chronic radiodermatitis after heart catheterization: the contributing role of ciprofibrate (Lipanor)?.] Ann Dermatol Venereol 1998;125(9):598–600.

38. Leroy D, Dompmartin A, Lorier E, Leport Y, Audebert C. Photosensitivity induced by fenofibrate. Photodermatol Photoimmunol Photomed 1990;7(3):136–7.

39. Leenutaphong V, Manuskiatti W. Fenofibrate-induced photosensitivity. J Am Acad Dermatol 1996;35(5 Pt 1):775–7.

40. Leroy D, Dompmartin A, Szczurko C, Michel M, Louvet S. Photodermatitis from ketoprofen with cross-reactivity to fenofibrate and benzophenones. Photodermatol Photoimmunol Photomed 1997;13(3):93–7.

41. Fisher DA, Elias PM, LeBoit PL. Exacerbation of psoriasis by the hypolipidemic agent, gemfibrozil. Arch Dermatol 1988;124(6):854–5.

42. Sawamura D, Umeki K. Stevens–Johnson syndrome associated with bezafibrate. Acta Dermatol Venereol 2000;80(6):457.

43. Wong SS. Stevens–Johnson syndrome induced by clofibrate. Acta Dermatol Venereol 1994;74(6):475.

44. Ory JP, Cleau D, Jobard JM, Bourscheid D. Interaction miconazole–cipofibrate responsable d'une rhabdomyolyse. A propos d'un cas. Ann Med Nancy Est 1993;32:305.

45. Mantell G, Burke MT, Staggers J. Extended clinical safety profile of lovastatin. Am J Cardiol 1990;66(8):B11–5.

46. Reaven P, Witztum JL. Lovastatin, nicotinic acid, and rhabdomyolysis. Ann Intern Med 1988;109(7):597–8.

47. van Puijenbroek EP, Du Buf-Vereijken PW, Spooren PF, van Doormaal JJ. Possible increased risk of rhabdomyolysis during concomitant use of simvastatin and gemfibrozil. J Intern Med 1996;240(6):403–4.

48. Biesenbach G, Janko O, Stuby U, Zazgornik J. Terminales myoglobinurisches Nierenversagen unter Lovastatintherapie bei präexistenter chronischer Nierenfunktionsstorung. [Terminal myoglobinuric renal failure in lovastatin therapy with pre-existing chronic renal insufficiency.] Wien Klin Wochenschr 1996;108(11):334–7.

49. Magarian GJ, Lucas LM, Colley C. Gemfibrozil-induced myopathy. Arch Intern Med 1991;151(9):1873–4.

50. Harvengt C. Drugs recently released in Belgium. Mefloquine—ciprofibrate. Acta Clin Belg 1991;46(2):117–9.

51. Buck N, Devlin HB, Lunn JN. The Report of A Confidential Enquiry into Perioperative DeathsLondon: Buttfield Provincial Hospitals Trust and King's Fund;. 1987.

52. Layne RD, Sehbai AS, Stark LJ. Rhabdomyolysis and renal failure associated with gemfibrozil monotherapy. Ann Pharmacother 2004;38(2):232–4.

53. Tregouet B. L'hypothyroïdie favorise-t-elle la toxicité musculaire des fibrates?. [Does hypothyroidism predispose muscular toxicity of fibrates?.] Rev Med Interne 1991;12(2):159.

54. Hattori N, Shimatsu A, Murabe H, Nishimura M, Nakamura H, Imura H. Clofibrate-induced myopathy in a patient with primary hypothyroidism. Jpn J Med 1990;29(5):545–7.

55. Neuvonen PJ, Jalava KM. Itraconazole drastically increases plasma concentrations of lovastatin and lovastatin acid. Clin Pharmacol Ther 1996;60(1):54–61.

56. Bridgman JF, Rosen SM, Thorp JM. Complications during clofibrate treatment of nephrotic-syndrome hyperlipoproteinaemia. Lancet 1972;2(7776):506–9.

57. Clouatre Y, Leblanc M, Ouimet D, Pichette V. Fenofibrate-induced rhabdomyolysis in two dialysis patients with hypothyroidism. Nephrol Dial Transplant 1999;14(4):1047–8.

58. Terrovitou CT, Milionis HJ, Elisaf MS. Acute rhabdomyolysis after bezafibrate re-exposure. Nephron 1998;78(3):336–7.

59. Gotsman I, Haviv YS, Nir-Paz R. Low-dose bezafibrate-associated myositis in a patient with chronic renal failure. Clin Drug Invest 1999;18:481–3.

60. Bruckert E, Giral P, Heshmati HM, Turpin G. Men treated with hypolipidaemic drugs complain more frequently of erectile dysfunction. J Clin Pharm Ther 1996;21(2):89–94.

61. Bain SC, Lemon M, Jones AF. Gemfibrozil-induced impotence. Lancet 1990;336(8727):1389.

62. Pizarro S, Bargay J, D'Agosto P. Gemfibrozil-induced impotence. Lancet 1990;336(8723):1135.

63. Figueras A, Castel JM, LaPorte JR, Capella D. Gemfibrozil-induced impotence. Ann Pharmacother 1993;27(7–8):982.

64. Alcala Pedrajas JN, Prada Pardal JL. Impotencia por gemfibrozil. [Gemfibrozil induced impotence.] An Med Interna 1998;15(3):175–6.

65. Smith GW, Hurst NP. Vasculitis, Raynaud's phenomenon and polyarthritis associated with gemfibrozil therapy. Br J Rheumatol 1993;32(1):84–5.

66. de Barrio M, Matheu V, Baeza ML, Tornero P, Rubio M, Zubeldia JM. Bezafibrate-induced anaphylactic shock: unusual clinical presentation. J Investig Allergol Clin Immunol 2001;11(1):53–5.

67. Rabasa-Lhoret R, Rasamisoa M, Avignon A, Monnier L. Rare side-effects of fenofibrate. Diabetes Metab 2001;27(1):66–8.

68. Cattley RC. Carcinogenicity of lipid-lowering drugs. JAMA 1996;275(19):1479.

69. Ujhazy E, Onderova E, Horakova M, Bencova E, Durisova M, Nosal R, Balonova T, Zeljenkova D. Teratological study of the hypolipidaemic drugs etofylline clofibrate (VULM) and fenofibrate in Swiss mice. Pharmacol Toxicol 1989;64(3):286–90.

70. Atmaca H, Sayarlioglu H, Kulah E, Demircan N, Akpolat T. Rhabdomyolysis associated with gemfibrozil–colchicine therapy. Ann Pharmacother 2002;36(11):1719–21.

71. Kyrklund C, Backman JT, Kivisto KT, Neuvonen M, Laitila J, Neuvonen PJ. Plasma concentrations of active lovastatin acid are markedly increased by gemfibrozil but not by bezafibrate. Clin Pharmacol Ther 2001;69(5):340–5.

72. Jacobson RH, Wang P, Glueck CJ. Myositis and rhabdomyolysis associated with concurrent use of simvastatin and nefazodone. JAMA 1997;277(4):296–7.

73. Goldstein MR. Myopathy and rhabdomyolysis with lovastatin taken with gemfibrozil. JAMA 1990;264(23):2991–2.

74. Kogan AD, Orenstein S. Lovastatin-induced acute rhabdomyolysis. Postgrad Med J 1990;66(774):294–6.

75. Athyros VG, Papageorgiou AA, Hatzikonstandinou HA, Didangelos TP, Carina MV, Kranitsas DF, Kontopoulos AG. Safety and efficacy of long-term statin–fibrate combinations in patients with refractory familial combined hyperlipidemia. Am J Cardiol 1997;80(5):608–13.

76. Spieker LE, Noll G, Hannak M, Luscher TF. Efficacy and tolerability of fluvastatin and bezafibrate in patients with hyperlipidemia and persistently high triglyceride levels. J Cardiovasc Pharmacol 2000;35(3):361–5.

77. Plosker GL, Dunn CI, Figgitt DP. Cerivastatin: a review of its pharmacological properties and therapeutic efficacy in the management of hypercholesterolaemia. Drugs 2000;60(5):1179–206.

78. Pogson GW, Kindred LH, Carper BG. Rhabdomyolysis and renal failure associated with cerivastatin–gemfibrozil combination therapy. Am J Cardiol 1999;83(7):1146.

79. Bermingham RP, Whitsitt TB, Smart ML, Nowak DP, Scalley RD. Rhabdomyolysis in a patient receiving the combination of cerivastatin and gemfibrozil. Am J Health Syst Pharm 2000;57(5):461–4.

80. Ozdemir O, Boran M, Gokce V, Uzun Y, Kocak B, Korkmaz S. A case with severe rhabdomyolysis and renal failure associated with cerivastatin–gemfibrozil combination therapy—a case report. Angiology 2000;51(8):695–7.

81. Alexandridis G, Pappas GA, Elisaf MS. Rhabdomyolysis due to combination therapy with cerivastatin and gemfibrozil. Am J Med 2000;109(3):261–2.

82. Plotkin E, Bernheim J, Ben-Chetrit S, Mor A, Korzets Z. Influenza vaccine—a possible trigger of rhabdomyolysis induced acute renal failure due to the combined use of cerivastatin and bezafibrate. Nephrol Dial Transplant 2000;15(5):740–1.

83. Backman JT, Kyrklund C, Kivisto KT, Wang JS, Neuvonen PJ. Plasma concentrations of active simvastatin acid are increased by gemfibrozil. Clin Pharmacol Ther 2000;68(2):122–9.

84. Ramachandran S, Giles PD, Hartland A. Acute renal failure due to rhabdomyolysis in presence of concurrent ciprofibrate and ibuprofen treatment. BMJ 1997;314(7094):1593.

85. Niemi M, Backman JT, Neuvonen M, Neuvonen PJ. Effects of gemfibrozil, itraconazole, and their combination on the pharmacokinetics and pharmacodynamics of repaglinide: potentially hazardous interaction between gemfibrozil and repaglinide. Diabetologia 2003;46:347–51.

86. Niemi M. Gemfibrozil considerably increases the plasma concentrations of rosiglitazone. Diabetologia 2003;46:1319–23.

87. Ahmad S. Gemfibrozil: interaction with glyburide. South Med J 1991;84(1):102.

88. Niemi M, Neuvonen PJ, Kivisto KT. Effect of gemfibrozil on the pharmacokinetics and pharmacodynamics of glimepiride. Clin Pharmacol Ther 2001;70(5):439–45.

89. Beringer TR. Warfarin potentiation with bezafibrate. Postgrad Med J 1997;73(864):657–8.

90. Rindone JP, Keng HC. Gemfibrozil–warfarin drug interaction resulting in profound hypoprothrombinemia. Chest 1998;114(2):641–2.

91. Ascah KJ, Rock GA, Wells PS. Interaction between fenofibrate and warfarin. Ann Pharmacother 1998;32(7–8):765–8.

92. Kim KY, Mancano MA. Fenofibrate potentiates warfarin effects. Ann Pharmacother 2003;37:212–5.

Fish oils

General Information

Omega-3 fatty acids are long-chain polyunsaturated fatty acids. The parent fatty acid of this group is alpha-linolenic acid, an essential fatty acid that the body is unable to synthesize; alpha-linolenic acid can be converted in the body to eicosapentaenoic acid (EPA) and docosahexaenoic acid (DHA). In animals and man, these acids reduce the production of several compounds that are involved in inflammation and thrombosis, such as eicosanoids (prostaglandins, thromboxanes, prostacyclin, and leukotrienes) and cytokines (interleukin II-1) (1). The extent of the conversion of alpha-linolenic acid to EPA and DHA is unclear. The conversion process appears to be inhibited by a high intake of linoleic acid, another essential fatty acid (2). In addition, alpha-linolenic acid is found in dark green vegetables and the oils of certain nuts and seeds, especially rape seeds and soya beans.

Oily fish and extracted fish oils contain high concentrations of EPA and DHA. Fish oils also contain vitamins A and D. Oil derived from cod, halibut, or shark liver, or from fish body, typically contains about 200 mg/ml of long-chain omega-3 fatty acids. In addition, cod liver oil provides 50 μg/ml of vitamin A and 2 μg/ml of vitamin D. Many fish oil supplements are artificially enriched with omega-3 fatty acids.

The safety of drugs containing EPA and DHA has been reviewed; the reported adverse effects were similar to those in control groups (3). Even 3–7 g/day for several months did not change liver enzyme activities, and there were no bleeding problems. Consumption of fish oils reduces the resistance of LDL to oxidative modification, and this is partly opposed by the addition of vitamin E (4). Belching or eructation with a fishy taste or smell, vomiting, flatulence, diarrhea, and constipation are relatively common.

Organs and Systems

Cardiovascular

Some of the beneficial effects of fish oils after acute myocardial infarction have been attributed to an antidysrhythmic effect on the heart (5). However, the results of a randomized trial in 200 patients with implantable cardioverter defibrillators are at variance with this: the rate of cardioversion was higher in those taking fish oils 1.8 g/day than in a control group who took olive oil (6). The lack of benefit and the suggestion that fish oil supplementation may increase the risk of ventricular tachycardia or ventricular fibrillation in some patients with implantable cardioverter defibrillators can reasonably be interpreted as evidence that the routine use of fish oil supplementation in patients with implantable cardioverter defibrillators and recurrent ventricular dysrhythmias should be avoided.

Respiratory

Fish oils can cause exacerbation of asthma in aspirin-sensitive patients (7).

Cod liver oil supplements can cause lipoid pneumonia (8).

Metabolism

In high doses, fish oils can cause a rise in blood glucose concentration in patients with non-insulin-dependent diabetes mellitus (9).

Hematologic

Bleeding times can increase in patients taking fish oils (10), leading to more prolonged and frequent nose-bleeds (11). Fish oil supplements should be used with care in patients with hemophilia and anyone taking high doses of anticoagulants or aspirin.

Gastrointestinal

Of 39 patients with Crohn's disease, treated with an enteric-coated fish oil formulation, 4 were withdrawn because of diarrhea, the only reported adverse effect in this investigation (12).

In 814 patients randomly allocated to fish oils for 18 weeks for the reduction of re-stenosis after percutaneous transluminal coronary angioplasty, gastrointestinal adverse effects, most commonly bloating and burping, were reported in 37% of patients taking fish oils, versus 31% of those taking placebo (13).

Liver

Two individuals with serum triglyceride concentrations over 11.3 mmol/l (1000 mg/dl) were referred to a pharmacist-managed lipid clinic by their primary-care provider because of either treatment failure or intolerance of conventional therapies (14). Fish oils were used in one case in lieu of and in the other in addition to conventional treatments. Although fish oil has not been reported to cause hepatotoxicity, both of these patients had increased transaminases while taking fish oil. Whether fish oil truly causes hepatic injury remains to be elucidated.

Second-Generation Effects

Pregnancy

During early pregnancy, high doses of vitamin A (as found in halibut and shark liver oils) can lead to birth defects (15). Fish oil supplements rich in vitamin A should therefore be avoided by women in the first trimester and those who might become pregnant.

Drug–Drug Interactions

Acetylsalicylic acid

In eight healthy men who took a total of 485 mg of aspirin over 3 days before beginning 2 weeks of fish oil supplementation (4.5 g of n-3 fatty acids/day), aspirin alone prolonged the bleeding time by 34% and fish oil alone prolonged it by only 9%; however, aspirin + fish oil prolonged the bleeding time by 78% (16). Although fish oil alone did not significantly raise aggregation thresholds for collagen, arachidonic acid, or platelet activating factor, it did reduce the extent of aggregation with collagen. When challenged by single or dual agonists, the combination of fish oil and aspirin did not make platelets less sensitive than aspirin alone.

However, in 18 healthy men randomly allocated to N-3 polyunsaturated fatty acids 10 g/day or placebo for 14 days, the addition of a single intravenous dose of acetylsalicylic acid 100 mg did not alter the small effect of polyunsaturated fatty acids on platelet aggregation (17).

In four subjects given a single oral dose of aspirin 37.5 mg before and after a natural stable fish oil daily for 1 week, serum thromboxane A_2 fell by 40% after aspirin alone, but by 62% after fish oil + aspirin, and leukotriene B_4 rose by 19% after aspirin and fell by 69% after fish oil + aspirin; serum prostacyclin fell equally in both cases (18).

In healthy subjects who took either fish oil or olive oil (control) daily for 3 weeks before exposure to aspirin or no aspirin, fish oil had no significant effect on mucosal prostaglandin E_2 or $F_{2\alpha}$ content or on the damaging effect of aspirin on the stomach, despite the fact that fish oil reduced serum triglyceride concentrations significantly (19).

Warfarin

In a placebo-controlled, randomized, double-blind study of the effect of fish oil supplements 3–6 g/day for 4 weeks on the International Normalized Ratio (INR) in 16 patients taking chronic warfarin therapy there was no statistically significant effect on anticoagulation (20).

However, fish oils can affect hemostasis, and there has been an anecdotal report of a possible interaction.

- A 67-year-old white woman who had been taking warfarin for 18 months doubled her dose of fish oil from 1000 to 2000 mg/day. The INR increased from 2.8 to 4.3 within 1 month and fell to 1.6 within 1 week of reduction of the dose of fish oil (21).

References

1. Sanders TA. Marine oils: metabolic effects and role in human nutrition. Proc Nutr Soc 1993;52(3):457–72.
2. Sanders TA, Roshanai F. The influence of different types of omega 3 polyunsaturated fatty acids on blood lipids and platelet function in healthy volunteers. Clin Sci (Lond) 1983;64(1):91–9.
3. Harris WS. Dietary fish oil and blood lipids. Curr Opin Lipidol 1996;7(1):3–7.
4. Wander RC, Du SH, Ketchum SO, Rowe KE. Effects of interaction of RRR-alpha-tocopheryl acetate and fish oil on low-density-lipoprotein oxidation in postmenopausal women with and without hormone-replacement therapy. Am J Clin Nutr 1996;63(2):184–93.
5. Marchioli R, Barzi F, Bomba E, Chieffo C, Di Gregorio D, Di Mascio R, Franzosi MG, Geraci E, Levantesi G, Maggioni AP, Mantini L, Marfisi RM, Mastrogiuseppe G, Mininni N, Nicolosi GL, Santini M, Schweiger C, Tavazzi L, Tognoni G, Tucci C, Valagussa F, on behalf of the GISSI-Prevenzione Investigators. Early protection against sudden death by n-3 polyunsaturated fatty acids after myocardial infarction: time-course analysis of the results of the Gruppo Italiano per lo Studio della Sopravvivenza nell'Infarto

Miocardico (GISSI)-Prevenzione. Circulation 2002;105(23):1897–903.

6. Raitt MH, Connor WE, Morris C, Kron J, Halperin B, Chugh SS, McClelland J, Cook J, MacMurdy K, Swenson R, Connor SL, Gerhard G, Kraemer DF, Oseran D, Marchant C, Calhoun D, Shnider R, McAnulty J. Fish oil supplementation and risk of ventricular tachycardia and ventricular fibrillation in patients with implantable defibrillators: a randomized controlled trial. JAMA 2005;293(23):2884–91.

7. Ritter JM, Taylor GW. Fish oil in asthma. Thorax 1988;43(2):81–3.

8. Dawson JK, Abernethy VE, Graham DR, Lynch MP. A woman who took cod-liver oil and smoked. Lancet 1996;347(9018):1804.

9. Vessby B, Boberg M. Dietary supplementation with n-3 fatty acids may impair glucose homeostasis in patients with non-insulin-dependent diabetes mellitus. J Intern Med 1990;228(2):165–71.

10. Tracy RP. Diet and hemostatic factors. Curr Atheroscler Rep 1999;1(3):243–8.

11. Clarke JT, Cullen-Dean G, Regelink E, Chan L, Rose V. Increased incidence of epistaxis in adolescents with familial hypercholesterolemia treated with fish oil. J Pediatr 1990;116(1):139–41.

12. Belluzzi A, Brignola C, Campieri M, Pera A, Boschi S, Miglioli M. Effect of an enteric-coated fish-oil preparation on relapses in Crohn's disease. N Engl J Med 1996;334(24):1557–60.

13. Cairns JA, Gill J, Morton B, Roberts R, Gent M, Hirsh J, Holder D, Finnie K, Marquis JF, Naqvi S, Cohen E. Fish oils and low-molecular-weight heparin for the reduction of restenosis after percutaneous transluminal coronary angioplasty. The EMPAR Study. Circulation 1996;94(7):1553–60.

14. Caron MF, Nguyen IT, Folstad JE. Treatment of very high triglycerides with fish oils: a review of 2 cases. J Pharm Technol 2003;19:14–18.

15. Rothman KJ, Moore LL, Singer MR, Nguyen US, Mannino S, Milunsky A. Teratogenicity of high vitamin A intake. N Engl J Med 1995;333(21):1369–73.

16. Harris WS, Silveira S, Dujovne CA. The combined effects of N-3 fatty acids and aspirin on hemostatic parameters in man. Thromb Res 1990;57(4):517–26.

17. Svaneborg N, Kristensen SD, Hansen LM, Bullow I, Husted SE, Schmidt EB. The acute and short-time effect of supplementation with the combination of N-3 fatty acids and acetylsalicylic acid on platelet function and plasma lipids. Thromb Res 2002;105(4):311–6.

18. Engstrom K, Wallin R, Saldeen T. Effect of low-dose aspirin in combination with stable fish oil on whole blood production of eicosanoids. Prostaglandins Leukot Essent Fatty Acids 2001;64(6):291–7.

19. Faust TW, Redfern JS, Podolsky I, Lee E, Grundy SM, Feldman M. Effects of aspirin on gastric mucosal prostaglandin E2 and F2 alpha content and on gastric mucosal injury in humans receiving fish oil or olive oil. Gastroenterology 1990;98(3):586–91.

20. Bender NK, Kraynak MA, Chiquette E, Linn WD, Clark GM, Bussey HI. Effects of marine fish oils on the anticoagulation status of patients receiving chronic warfarin therapy. J Thromb Thrombolysis 1998;5(3):257–61.

21. Buckley MS, Goff AD, Knapp WE. Fish oil interaction with warfarin. Ann Pharmacother 2004;38(1):50–2.

Fluvastatin

See also HMG Co-A reductase inhibitors

General Information

It has been suggested that the pharmacokinetics of fluvastatin, including extensive biliary excretion and absence of circulating active metabolites, might be associated with a low incidence of systemic adverse effects compared with other statins. In over 1800 patients treated for an average of 61 weeks, fluvastatin was safe and tolerable (SEDA-19, 408). Pooled data from clinical trials have shown that gastrointestinal symptoms occurred in 14% of fluvastatin recipients compared with 9% taking placebo; other complaints occurred 0.5–5% more often with fluvastatin, including insomnia, sinusitis, hypesthesia, tooth disorders, and urinary tract infections. Fluvastatin was withdrawn because of adverse events in 3.5% of 2585 patients taking monotherapy and in 3.2% of 842 patients taking placebo (1).

Organs and Systems

Liver

Hepatotoxicity has been reported with fluvastatin.

- Cholestatic hepatitis developed in a 71-year-old man with nephrotic syndrome (2). Hepatic function was normal after several months of fluvastatin 20 mg/day. Some weeks after the dose was increased to 40 mg/day, his gamma-glutamyl transpeptidase activity rose from normal to 1818 IU/l, with negative serology for viruses. After normalization, re-introduction of fluvastatin 20 mg/day was not tolerated, but he did tolerate simvastatin 20 mg/day.
- A 61-year-old woman developed symptoms of acute hepatitis 6 weeks after she began to take fluvastatin sodium 20 mg/day for hypercholesterolemia (3). Ultrasonography and liver biopsy confirmed the diagnosis of non-obstructive intrahepatic jaundice. Studies of viral markers and autoimmune factors excluded viral hepatitis and autoimmune hepatitis. There was a high serum concentration of a metabolite of fluvastatin, suggesting a possible anomaly of drug metabolism. All liver function tests normalized 8 weeks after the withdrawal of fluvastatin.

Pancreas

Acute pancreatitis has been attributed to fluvastatin (4).

- A 36-year-old man took fluvastatin 40 mg/day for 3 months and developed mild acute pancreatitis, which settled with medical treatment. Other causes were ruled out. Some months later, he started taking fluvastatin again and had a recurrence of pancreatitis within a few days.

According to the authors, statin-induced acute pancreatitis can occur on the first day of therapy or after several months. It is generally mild and runs a benign course; no deaths have been reported. Its frequency is unknown but it is probably rare.

Musculoskeletal

In a pooled analysis of a large population of patients with hypercholesterolemia taking fluvastatin 20 mg/day, 40 mg/day, and fluvastatin modified-release 80 mg/day, the frequency of significant rises in creatine kinase activity was low and not different from placebo (5). This applied to men and women both above and below the age of 65 years. There were no increases in the frequency of rises in creatine kinase activity with higher doses of fluvastatin.

Immunologic

- A 67-year-old woman had a fatal reaction 1 week after she started to take fluvastatin 20 mg/day. When the drug was withdrawn 10 weeks later, she had arthralgia, myalgia, an erythematous maculopapular rash, and breathlessness due to a widespread alveolitis (6).

Drug Administration

Drug formulations

Once-daily administration of modified-release formulation of fluvastatin 80–320 mg/day was generally safe and well tolerated in 40 patients with primary hypercholesterolemia over 13 days (7). However, fluvastatin 640 mg in this formulation was not well tolerated: six of seven patients had adverse events, including diarrhea, headache, and rises in serum transaminases. In addition, the pharmacokinetics of fluvastatin were non-linear at this dose, possibly because of saturation of first-pass metabolism, causing higher than expected serum drug concentrations.

Drug–Drug Interactions

Bezafibrate

Concomitant administration of fluvastatin and bezafibrate resulted in a 50% increase in the AUC of fluvastatin (SEDA-21, 460).

Cardiac glycosides

A single dose of fluvastatin increased the steady-state C_{max} of digoxin 0.125–0.5 mg/day by 11% and renal clearance by 15%, without changing AUC or t_{max} (8).

Ion-exchange resins

The systemic availability of fluvastatin is reduced by bile acid sequestrants (1).

Itraconazole

The effects of itraconazole 100 mg on the pharmacokinetics of fluvastatin 40 mg have been studied in a randomized, placebo-controlled, crossover study in 10 healthy volunteers (9). Itraconazole had no significant effect on the C_{max} or total AUC of fluvastatin, but slightly prolonged its half-life.

Rifampicin

The systemic availability of fluvastatin is reduced by the hepatic enzyme inducer rifampicin (1).

References

1. Plosker GL, Wagstaff AJ. Fluvastatin: a review of its pharmacology and use in the management of hypercholesterolaemia. Drugs 1996;51(3):433–59.
2. Gascon A, Zabala S, Iglesias E. Acute cholestasis during long-term treatment with fluvastatin in a nephrotic patient. Nephrol Dial Transplant 1999;14(4):1038.
3. Wachi K, Ishii K, Ikehara T, Shinohara M, Kawafune T, Sumino Y, Nonaka H. A case of acute cholestatic hepatitis associated with fluvastatin sodium. J Med Soc Toho 2001;48:153–8.
4. Tysk C, Al-Eryani AY, Shawabkeh AA. Acute pancreatitis induced by fluvastatin therapy. J Clin Gastroenterol 2002;35(5):406–8.
5. Benghozi R, Bortolini M, Jia Y, Isaacsohn JL, Troendle AJ, Gonasun L. Frequency of creatine kinase elevation during treatment with fluvastatin. Am J Cardiol 2002;89(2):231–3.
6. Sridhar MK, Abdulla A. Fatal lupus-like syndrome and ARDS induced by fluvastatin. Lancet 1998;352(9122):114.
7. Sabia H, Prasad P, Smith HT, Stoltz RR, Rothenberg P. Safety, tolerability, and pharmacokinetics of an extended-release formulation of fluvastatin administered once daily to patients with primary hypercholesterolemia. J Cardiovasc Pharmacol 2001;37(5):502–11.
8. Garnett WR, Venitz J, Wilkens RC, Dimenna G. Pharmacokinetic effects of fluvastatin in patients chronically receiving digoxin. Am J Med 1994;96(6A):S84–6.
9. Kivisto KT, Kantola T, Neuvonen PJ. Different effects of itraconazole on the pharmacokinetics of fluvastatin and lovastatin. Br J Clin Pharmacol 1998;46(1):49–53.

HMG coenzyme-A reductase inhibitors

General Information

Statins inhibit HMG-CoA reductase and reduce cellular cholesterol synthesis (1). Lower intracellular cholesterol concentrations cause over-expression of the LDL receptor in the plasma membrane of hepatocytes. This over-expression increases the clearance of circulating LDL, reducing plasma concentrations of LDL cholesterol.

The statins include atorvastatin, bervastatin, cerivastatin, crilvastatin, dalvastatin, fluvastatin, glenvastatin, lovastatin, mevastatin, pitavastatin, pravastatin, rosuvastatin, simvastatin, and tenivastatin (all rINNs). Atorvastatin, cerivastatin, fluvastatin, lovastatin, pravastatin, and simvastatin are covered in separate monographs.

The adverse effects of the statins are mostly limited to slight increases in liver and muscle enzymes in the blood. Hypersensitivity reactions are very rare. There is no evidence of tumor-inducing effects. Second-generation effects are suspected, and statins should not be used during pregnancy.

The adverse effects of statins have been reviewed in the light of the ever increasing dosages that are being used to lower LDL cholesterol to a minimum (2). In another review high doses of atorvastatin and simvastatin were specially emphasized (3).

Observational studies

In a multicenter, open, phase III study in 104 Korean patients there were eight adverse drug reactions in six patients taking pitavastatin and 19 adverse drug reactions in 12 patients taking simvastatin (4). However, there were no reports of serious reactions in either group.

Organs and Systems

Cardiovascular

In 14 asymptomatic patients statin therapy worsened left ventricular diastolic function; co-enzyme Q10 supplementation produced improvement. There were several limitations of this study, including a small sample size and the lack of a control arm, but the patients did serve as contemporary controls for themselves. Because baseline concentrations of co-enzyme Q10 do not predict dysfunction, routine concomitant co-enzyme Q10 administration, especially in patients at risk, may be prudent (5).

Nervous system

Statins interfere with the production of isoprene which is somehow connected with sleep, but there have been neither changes in sleep EEG measures relevant to insomnia nor changes in the quality of sleep (SEDA-13, 1327) (6). However, there has been a report of sleep disturbances (7).

- Three months after starting to take metoprolol 100 mg bd and simvastatin 10 mg/day, a 55-year-old man reported restless nights and nightmares, which he had not previously experienced. The dose of metoprolol was reduced to 50 mg bd, with no observable benefit. Simvastatin was withdrawn 2 weeks later and pravastatin 20 mg/day was prescribed, with substantial improvement in the quality of sleep; however, some unpleasant nightmares still occurred. Four weeks later, metoprolol was also withdrawn and atenolol 100 mg/day was prescribed. Thereafter, the quality of sleep was significantly improved, and 6 months later the patient did not report any nightmares. Sleep disturbances recurred after a later attempt to reintroduce simvastatin in place of pravastatin. The same effect

occurred when, during treatment with pravastatin, substitution of atenolol with metoprolol was attempted.

In this case, the statins may have interacted with metoprolol, and it may have been relevant that metoprolol is more lipid-soluble than atenolol.

Peripheral neuropathy occurs with statins, and perhaps with all cholesterol-lowering drugs, and may be related to reduced production of ubiquinone, as suggested in a review (8). The possible link between statins and peripheral neuropathy, has been evaluated (9). Based on epidemiologic studies and case reports risk appears to be minimal. These findings should alert prescribers to a potential risk of peripheral neuropathy in patients taking any statin; that is, statins should be considered the cause of peripheral neuropathy when other causes have been excluded. It appears that once a statin produces a neuropathy, rechallenge with any other statin is likely to cause a recurrence. This is reported to occur 1–3 weeks after rechallenge, whereas the resolution takes 4–6 weeks after withdrawal (8).

In a series of seven cases of neuropathy, all were axonal peripheral neuropathies and both thick and thin nerve fibers were affected (10). No cause of peripheral neuropathy other than statin treatment could be identified. In this series at least four of the cases were irreversible, probably due to long exposure to statins (4–7 years versus 1–2 years in previous reports). Besides an effect on ubiquinone, interference with cholesterol synthesis may alter nerve membrane function, since cholesterol is a ubiquitous component of human cell membranes. Neuropathy has not been observed in extensive long-term trials of lipid-lowering drugs. It could be due to patient selection, a low frequency of the adverse effect, or lack of attention to symptoms of peripheral neuropathy. The observed association may also not be causal.

In a case-control study of 166 cases of idiopathic polyneuropathy, of which 35 had a definite diagnosis, the odds ratio for neuropathy was 14 for statin users compared with non-users (11).

- A 58-year-old man developed a disorder resembling Guillain–Barré syndrome at the start of simvastatin therapy (12). He had had a similar but milder episode after taking pravastatin 6 months before.

This case suggests that acute polyradiculoneuropathy may represent a rare but serious adverse effect of statin treatment. The pathophysiology of acute neuropathy on statin exposure is unknown; a hypersensitivity reaction resulting in an immune-mediated process has been suggested. It is possible that this patient had relapsing Guillain–Barré syndrome unrelated to the use of statins.

With the current level of information, it is prudent to consider withdrawal of statins in patients with symptoms compatible with polyneuropathy.

Sensory systems

One should be alert to the possibility of color blindness due to statins (13), although the risk is uncertain.

Owing to the high cholesterol content of the human lens, ocular changes have been looked for during trials with statins. It has been concluded that cataract does not occur. Although the degree of lens opacities increases during treatment, the incidence does not differ from that seen in an untreated control population (14). With fenofibrate serving as control, lovastatin or simvastatin did not reduce visual acuity during treatment for 2 years (SEDA-13, 1328) (15). According to a review, there is no danger during long-term treatment and there should be no requirement for regular ophthalmological examination (16).

Psychological

Animal and cross-sectional studies have suggested that serum lipid concentrations can cause altered cognitive function, mood, and behavior (16).

When the MedWatch drug surveillance system of the Food and Drug Administration (FDA) from November 1997 to February 2002 was searched for reports of statin-associated memory loss, 60 patients were identified; 36 had taken simvastatin, 23 atorvastatin, and one pravastatin (17). About a half of the patients noted cognitive adverse effects within 2 months of therapy and 14 of 25 patients noted improvement when the statin was withdrawn. Memory loss recurred in four patients who were rechallenged. The current literature is conflicting with regard to the effects of statins on memory loss. Experimental studies support links between cholesterol intake and amyloid synthesis; however, observational studies suggest that patients taking statins have a reduced risk of dementia. However, available prospective studies show no cognitive or antiamyloid benefits of any statin.

Psychiatric

Emerging data associate statins with a reduced risk of Alzheimer's disease; however, two women had significant cognitive impairment temporally related to statin therapy (18). One took atorvastatin, and the other first took atorvastatin then simvastatin. Cognitive impairment and dementia as potential adverse effects associated with statins has been reviewed (17).

In 308 hypercholesterolemic adults aged 35–70 years, daily treatment with placebo, simvastatin 10 mg, or simvastatin 40 mg for 6 months was associated with decremental effects of simvastatin on tests previously observed to be sensitive to statins and on tests not previously administered, but not on tests previously observed to be insensitive to statins (19). For the three tests specifically affected by simvastatin, effects on cognitive performance were small, manifesting only as a failure to improve during the 6 months of treatment, and were confounded by baseline differences on one test. This study provides partial support for minor decrements in cognitive functioning with statins. Whether such effects have any long-term sequelae or occur with other cholesterol-lowering interventions is not known.

Ratings on a depression scale rose in four out of six men given cholesterol-lowering drugs, in two of them to a degree that met the criteria for mild clinical depression (20).

Some studies have shown increased risks of violent death and depression in subjects with reduced serum cholesterol concentrations. Serum and membrane cholesterol concentrations, the microviscosity of erythrocyte membranes, and platelet serotonin uptake have been determined in 17 patients with hypercholesterolemia (21). There was a significant increase in serotonin transporter activity only during the first month of simvastatin therapy. This suggests that within this period some patients could be vulnerable to depression, violence, or suicide. This is an important paper, in that it explains why mood disorders are not regularly seen in clinical trials with statins, as has been summarized in a recent review (3).

Metabolism

Although the statins seem to be similar in their ability to lower LDL, there are also dissimilarities. For instance, simvastatin increases HDL cholesterol with increasing doses, whereas atorvastatin does not (22). The clinical significance of this is unknown.

Hematologic

Hematological adverse effects can occur during treatment with both simvastatin and atorvastatin, according to a brief review (23). They include thrombotic thrombocytopenic purpura and severe thrombocytopenic purpura.

Liver

HMG CoA reductase inhibitors can be associated with small rises in alanine transaminase activity, but have not been definitely associated with severe morbidity involving altered hepatic function. The results of randomized trials do not suggest that statins in standard doses are hepatotoxic. In none of the large randomized studies in which standard doses were assessed (atorvastatin 10 mg/day, fluvastatin 40–80 mg/day, pravastatin 40 mg/day, simvastatin 20–40 mg/day) was there any clear excess risk of hepatitis or any other serious liver-related adverse events. Long-term large randomized trials have confirmed an excess of persistent rises in transaminases with atorvastatin 80 mg/day compared with lower doses or placebo, and similarly some excess with simvastatin 80 mg/day, but hepatitis and liver failure were not reported (4).

All cases of acute liver failure related to the use of lovastatin have been reviewed, and probably the frequency is similar to the background rate. This suggests that periodic monitoring of alanine transaminase in these patients would be burdensome and expensive (24).

The term "transaminitis" has been coined to describe a rise in the activities of serum transaminases without clinical symptoms. One author has suggested that in such cases one should switch from one statin to another, thereby preventing unnecessary withdrawal of statin treatment in dyslipidemic patients at high cardiovascular risk (25).

A return to normal or only slightly increased values of transaminases is often seen after a short period. The overall probability of having an increase in transaminase activity more than three times the top of the reference range is 0.7% (26). The probability may be increased in patients with pre-existing minor hepatic changes, as has been seen in one patient with systemic lupus erythematosus (27). There seems to be no difference between the various drugs in this respect (16), but when simvastatin and atorvastatin, each at a dose of 80 mg/day, were compared in 826 hypercholesterolemic patients there were fewer drug-related gastrointestinal symptoms and clinically significant transaminase rises with simvastatin (28). Frank hepatitis is rare. A cholestatic picture has also been reported (29). The mechanisms of these reactions are not known.

In one series, the frequency of liver toxicity was similar in patients taking pravastatin or simvastatin (30), while in another study there was a difference 6 months after the start of the study when the simvastatin group showed increases in liver enzymes (SEDA-13, 1327; 31).

In a comparison of atorvastatin with pravastatin, of 224 patients taking atorvastatin, two had clinically significant increases in alanine transaminase activity (32). They recovered during the next 4 months, one after withdrawal of atorvastatin and the other after a dosage reduction. Withdrawals due to adverse effects were similar in the two groups. One patient developed hepatitis while taking atorvastatin, but was able to tolerate simvastatin (33). The authors concluded that this adverse effect was not a class effect. Eosinophils in a liver-biopsy specimen pointed to an immunological mechanism.

Pancreas

Pancreatitis has been observed during treatment with simvastatin (q.v.).

- A 77-year-old woman taking rosuvastatin developed acute pancreatitis, which resolved on withdrawal (34). No other cause for the pancreatitis was found. She had had a similar episode 1 year before precipitated by atorvastatin, which resolved on withdrawal.

The authors suggested that pancreatitis may be a class effect of the statins.

Skin

Adverse effects of statins on the skin are rare, although statins can affect cutaneous lipid content. A series of skin reactions have been described in patients using statins (35).

A 59-year-old woman developed a lichenoid eruption while taking a statin (36).

Musculoskeletal

Myopathy and rhabdomyolysis

DoTS classification (BMJ 2003; 327: 1222-5):
Dose-relation: Collateral
Time-course: Intermediate
Susceptibility factors: Drug-drug interactions (for example, with fibrates)

Rhabdomyolysis is a problem with several lipid-lowering drugs (SEDA-13, 1325; SEDA-13, 1328; SEDA-13, 1330; SEDA-19, 409), especially when they are used in combination (37). In individuals with pre-existing renal insufficiency this can lead to an earlier need for chronic dialysis (38). All statins can cause myopathy and rhabdomyolysis, but not all statins are alike. For example, the evidence to date, based on almost 2 decades of experience, points to an extremely low risk of myopathy and rhabdomyolysis with lovastatin, and lovastatin 20 mg tablets are being considered for non-prescription availability in several countries (39). Furthermore, muscle adverse effects do not necessarily occur after a change from one statin to another (40). Interactions between various hypolipidemic drugs and other drugs also sometimes cause rhabdomyolysis (SEDA-18, 426). For instance, itraconazole markedly increases plasma concentrations of lovastatin, and in one subject plasma creatine kinase was increased 10-fold within 24 hours of administration of this combination (41).

- A 59-year-old woman taking pravastatin 20 mg/day tolerated immunosuppression with ciclosporin, prednisone, and mycophenolate mofetil for 4 years after heart transplantation. After switching from pravastatin to simvastatin she developed severe muscle weakness and laboratory evidence of muscle breakdown. The biochemical markers of rhabdomyolysis did not normalize until after repeat hemodialysis. Clinical improvement did not occur until after 5 months.

For all types of statin the risk is higher with higher doses in the therapeutic range. The risk is not clearly related to LDL-lowering efficacy; for example, cerivastatin was not particularly effective but was much more likely than other statins to cause rhabdomyolysis. Despite the fact that they can cause a myopathy, there is no clear evidence from randomized trials that statins cause myalgia, and reports of muscle cramp do not seem to be increased (2). However, these assertions, which are based on results from randomized clinical trials, are difficult to reconcile with observations made in the Primo study (42). This was an observational study in an unselected population in France taking high doses of various statins. Muscle symptoms were reported by 832 of 7924 patients (11%), with a median time of onset of 1 month after the start of statin therapy. Muscle pain prevented even moderate exertion during everyday activities in 315 patients (38%), while 31 (4%) were confined to bed or unable to work. Among individual statins fluvastatin was associated with the lowest rate of muscular symptoms (5.1%). Creatine kinase activity was not measured.

The incidence of rhabdomyolysis in patients taking different statins and fibrates, alone and in combination, has been estimated using data from 11 managed health care plans across the USA (43). The incidences of rhabdomyolysis were 0.44 per 10 000 person-years of treatment with atorvastatin, pravastatin, or simvastatin, 5.34 with cerivastatin, and 2.82 with fibrates. The incidence increased to 5.98 when atorvastatin, pravastatin, or simvastatin was with a fibrate, and to 1035 when cerivastatin was combined with a fibrate.

The clinical course and muscle biopsy findings have been described in eight patients with hyperlipoproteinemia taking lipid-lowering drugs who developed myalgias or proximal muscle weakness (44). All became asymptomatic after withdrawal of the drug, although creatine kinase activity remained high. Muscle biopsy in six cases from 3 months to 2 years after withdrawal of the drug showed variation in fiber diameters in all cases, with necrosis of fibers in five cases, inflammatory infiltration in one, vacuolated fibers in one, and ragged-red fibers in three. Although the muscle biopsy findings were not specific, the authors concluded that prolonged use of statins or fibrates might cause a chronic myopathy, even in the absence of symptoms.

In four patients with muscle symptoms while taking statins, creatine kinase activity was normal, but they were subsequently able to distinguish from their symptoms whether they were taking drug or placebo; muscle biopsies showed evidence of mitochondrial dysfunction (45).

Hypothyroidism predisposes to rhabdomyolysis and screening thyroid function has been advocated before starting hypolipidemic drugs (SEDA-21, 458).

Myopathic symptoms, predominantly stiffness and tenderness of proximal limb muscles and difficulty in rising from a low chair, can develop within a month of starting therapy and most cases develop within 3 months. Most patients recover after withdrawal. Sometimes a glucocorticoid is needed to reverse the myopathy. In one patient, histological investigation of muscle biopsies suggested that the myopathy was due, at least in part, to an inflammatory reaction (46). The serum coenzyme Q concentration is reduced by about 30% during statin treatment, because the enzyme is carried by LDL particles, although the concentrations during long-term treatment are equal to those in healthy controls (SEDA-13, 1328; 47,48). Ubiquinone (coenzyme-Q) is part of the oxidative respiratory pathway generating ATP, and deficiency could impede the function of myocytes, leading to an increase in serum creatine kinase and even cell destruction, with release of myoglobin, which in its turn can block kidney tubules and thereby produce anuria.

- Simvastatin 5 mg/day caused rhabdomyolysis in a 61-year-old man who was not taking concomitant interacting drugs (49).
- An elderly lady with chronic renal insufficiency developed rhabdomyolysis during simvastatin therapy (50). Her symptoms of muscle pain, fatigue, myoglobulinuria, oliguria, and pulmonary edema occurred 48 hours after the first dose of simvastatin. Simvastatin was immediately withdrawn, and she was dialysed for 1 week.

Myopathy, defined as muscle symptoms with a rise in creatine kinase greater than 10 times the upper limit of the reference range, was found in one study in only one patient who was taking 40 mg od and in four patients taking 80 mg/day, out of a total of 8245 patients. The number of patients with rhabdomyolysis was, according to postmarketing reporting from the first million

individuals taking lovastatin, 24 in all. Seventeen of those had taken other medications that are known to increase the risk (51). There is some evidence that patients with other concomitant illnesses may be at greater risk of myopathy than would be anticipated from experience in controlled trials.

Diplopia may be an early sign of generalized drug-induced muscle dysfunction. Altogether, 71 cases of diplopia, possibly related to various HMG-CoA inhibitors, have been collected from adverse drug reactions-reporting databases. The information was mostly too scanty to judge a causal relation, but improvement occurred in 33 on withdrawal, and two patients had positive rechallenge data (52).

- A 67-year-old woman had ocular myasthenia while taking various statins and also bezafibrate (53). Atorvastatin had the smallest effect.

The authors suggested that this was a variant of a generalized myopathy and was due to a low co-enzyme Q10 concentration.

Exercise-induced muscle pain, without myopathy and a rise in creatine kinase activity, can probably be caused by statins. This has been described in seven patients with heterozygous familial hypercholesterolemia and consisted of pain during exercise and cramps in the following hours (54).

Symptomatic rises in creatine kinase activity to over 10 times the upper end of the reference range occurred in 0, 1, and 0.9% of patients taking placebo, cerivastatin 0.4 mg, or cerivastatin 0.8 mg respectively (55), and rhabdomyolysis has been described in patients taking cerivastatin (56,57). However, in a review of the pharmacological properties and therapeutic efficacy of cerivastatin in hypercholesterolemia, it was stated that cerivastatin only infrequently causes rhabdomyolysis when given alone (58).

Chinese red rice products include natural HMG CoA reductase inhibitors (primarily lovastatin) and are used as cholesterol-lowering agents.

- A 50-year-old man presented with joint pain and muscle weakness in his upper right arm (59). His history was unremarkable, except for the fact that he had started taking a Chinese red rice preparation 3 months earlier, 1 month before the onset of symptoms. He was instructed to stop taking this medicine, and 3 weeks later his symptoms had completely resolved.

Other effects

Four cases of tendinopathy have been reported in three men and one woman taking statins (60). The diagnoses were extensor tenosynovitis in the hands, tenosynovitis of the tibialis anterior tendon, and Achilles tendinopathy. Two patients were taking simvastatin and two atorvastatin. The tendinopathy developed 1–2 months after the start of treatment. The outcome was consistently favorable within 1–2 months after drug withdrawal.

A few cases of dermatomyositis and polymyositis due to cholesterol-lowering drugs have previously been reported. Symptoms in four men and one woman, median age 68 years, were compatible with a diagnosis of polymyositis. Antinuclear antibodies were positive in four cases and muscle biopsies showed polymyositic infiltrates in four cases. Treatment (four statins and one fibrates) was withdrawn, with partial clinical improvement in three cases. Clinical remission was obtained with glucocorticoids. Antinuclear antibody screening, especially in cases of proximal muscular weakness and increased muscle enzyme activity, is warranted (61).

Sexual function

Erectile dysfunction has been reported in 12% of 339 men treated with fibrate derivatives or statins, compared with 5.6% of similar patients not taking these drugs (62). The mechanism is unknown and should be confirmed in randomized studies. A class effect has been suggested by the case of a 57-year-old man who had impotence after taking lovastatin for 2 weeks and also when he later tried pravastatin (63).

Immunologic

Lupus-like symptoms have been reported in patients taking statins (64).

- A 59-year-old patient (sex not specified) developed anti-dsDNA antibodies in the serum while taking a statin (65).

Statin-induced lupus-like syndrome is characterized by a long delay between the start of therapy and the skin eruption. Antinuclear antibodies can persist for many months after drug withdrawal. The causal relation may be therefore difficult to establish, and probably many cases are unrecognized. Early diagnosis may avoid unnecessary immunosuppressive therapy.

Long-Term Effects

Tumorigenicity

It has been suspected that low concentrations of serum cholesterol might be associated with an increased risk of cancer or overall mortality. All fibrates and statins cause cancer in rodents, but the relevance of this finding to man has been questioned (66). In an epidemiological study these risks were almost non-existent after adjusting for confounding factors. However, in the CARE study, breast cancer occurred in one patient in the control group and 12 in the pravastatin group (67). The incidence of cancers, both during clinical studies and up to 9 years after, has been reassuring (68).

Drug–Drug Interactions

General

Many statins are metabolized by CYP3A4, and this and other mechanisms of drug interactions involving statins have been reviewed (69). Other drugs metabolized by CYP3A4 can greatly increase statin concentrations in the body and precipitate rhabdomyolysis. Although the statins are similar in their ability to lower cholesterol

concentrations, there are dissimilarities in their interactions with other drugs.

With the exception of fluvastatin and pravastatin, the statins are metabolized by CYP3A4. Selective inhibition of CYP3A4 or of P-glycoprotein (69) in the small intestine probably increases the systemic availability of CYP3A4 substrates. Some drugs that are metabolized by this enzyme, such as the macrolide antibiotics and the antidepressant nefazodone, can greatly enhance the concentrations of statins in the body and thereby precipitate rhabdomyolysis. However, other drugs that are metabolized by CYP3A4, such as cimetidine, have not been reported to have this effect.

Antifungal azoles

The antifungal azoles inhibit CYP isozymes and can therefore interact with some statins.

Fluconazole

In a randomized, double-blind, crossover study in 12 healthy volunteers, fluconazole increased the plasma concentrations of fluvastatin and prolonged its elimination; the mechanism was probably inhibition of the CYP2C9-mediated metabolism of fluvastatin (70). Care should be taken if fluconazole or other potent inhibitors of CYP2C9 are given to patients using fluvastatin.

- A 76-year-old man taking antimicrobial drug treatment including fluconazole switched from pravastatin to atorvastatin 40 mg/day (71). After 1 week he began to feel tired and became oliguric, and on day 2 the serum myoglobin concentration was 16 120 µg/l. After 8 days in intensive care he died in multiorgan failure.

Itraconazole

The effects of itraconazole, a potent inhibitor of CYP3A4, on the pharmacokinetics of atorvastatin, cerivastatin, and pravastatin have been evaluated in an open, randomized, crossover study in 18 healthy subjects who took single doses of atorvastatin 20 mg, cerivastatin 0.8 mg, or pravastatin 40 mg, with and without itraconazole 200 mg (72). Itraconazole markedly raised atorvastatin plasma concentrations (2.5-fold) and produced modest rises in the plasma concentrations of cerivastatin (1.3-fold) and pravastatin (1.5-fold). These results suggest that in patients taking itraconazole, cerivastatin or pravastatin may be preferable to atorvastatin.

Physicians should check for lipid-lowering drugs before treating elderly individuals with itraconazole (73). Susceptibility to this interaction varies from statin to statin, in that simvastatin is more affected than pravastatin (74). Concomitant use of simvastatin with itraconazole should be avoided, and the same holds true for atorvastatin (75). In another study, the blood concentration of fluvastatin was not significantly increased, whereas that of lovastatin was (76).

Ketoconazole

Ketoconazole can also cause rhabdomyolysis when taken with both lovastatin and simvastatin (77).

Carbamazepine

In twelve Caucasian men concomitant use of carbamazepine reduced the serum concentration of simvastatin and simvastatin acid by 83%, through induction of CYP3A4 (78).

Chlorzoxazone

- A 73-year-old woman had rhabdomyolysis, cholestatic hepatitis, and mild renal insufficiency 14 days after she started to take the centrally acting muscle relaxant chlorzoxazone while also taking simvastatin (79). Withdrawal of the causal medication and conservative therapy with volume substitution and forced diuresis was followed by almost complete resolution of the symptoms.

The authors believed that either the two drugs had interacted by metabolism through the same hepatic enzyme, or that chlorzoxazone had caused cholestasis which then increased the blood concentration of simvastatin.

Ciclosporin

Most drug interactions associated with rhabdomyolysis occur when ciclosporin is combined with simvastatin or lovastatin. It has been suggested that if a statin is to be combined with ciclosporin, pravastatin or fluvastatin should be chosen instead (80).

Clopidogrel

Clopidogrel is a prodrug that is converted to its active form by CYP3A4. The active drug irreversibly blocks one specific platelet adenosine 5'-diphosphate (ADP) receptor (P2Y12). As certain lipophilic statins (atorvastatin, lovastatin, simvastatin) are substrates of CYP3A4, drug interactions are possible. It has therefore been suggested that the use of a statin that is not metabolized by CYP3A4 and platelet function testing are warranted in patients taking clopidogrel (81). However, this predicted interaction was not observed in a post hoc analysis of a placebo-controlled study (82). The comments of others show that this question is not yet settled (83).

In 45 patients with acute coronary syndrome randomized to receive either atorvastatin 10 mg/day or pravastatin 40 mg/day neither atorvastatin nor pravastatin significantly affected clopidogrel-induced inhibition of platelet activation; nor did clopidogrel affect the therapeutic efficacy of atorvastatin (84).

Platelet biomarkers were studied 4 and 24 hours after clopidogrel in 75 patients taking statins or placebo before coronary stenting (85). There were no significant differences in measured platelet characteristics among the study groups, with the exception of a lower collagen-induced aggregation at 24 hours and a constantly reduced expression of G-protein-coupled protease-activated thrombin receptor in patients treated with statins. Thus statins do not affect the ability of clopidogrel to inhibit platelet function in patients undergoing coronary stenting.

The inhibitory potency of clopidogrel on ADP-induced platelet activation was not attenuated when it was co-administered with atorvastatin (20 mg/day) for 5 weeks in 51 patients with acute coronary syndromes (86). Atorvastatin had no effect on either clopidogrel-induced inhibition of platelet aggregation initiated by ADP 5 or 10 µmol/l or clopidogrel-induced reduction of the membrane expression of P-selectin and CD40L induced by ADP.

Colchicine

Interactions of statins with colchicine have been reported.

- A 70-year-old man with hyperlipidemia and gout had been taking fluvastatin 80 mg/day for 2 years (87). After taking colchicine 1.5 mg/day for acute gouty arthritis for 3 days he developed stomach ache and nausea followed by severe pains and weakness in his arms and legs. After 10 days he developed rhabdomyolysis and non-oliguric myoglobinuric acute renal insufficiency.

- A 65-year-old woman who had been taking pravastatin 20 mg/day for 6 years developed acute gout (88). Her blood urea nitrogen and serum creatinine concentrations were 48 mg/dl and 1.3 mg/dl respectively. She was given colchicine 1.5 mg/day but 20 days later developed symmetrical proximal muscle weakness in the legs. Examination, laboratory findings, and electromyelography suggested myopathy. The weakness improved 7 days after withdrawal of colchicine and pravastatin and the enzyme activities returned to normal. Colchicine 1 mg/day was restarted 5 days later and the myopathy did not recur.

Colchicine is cleared by a different CYP450 isozyme than fluvastatin and pravastatin are, but another possible mechanism is synergistic myotoxicity, since colchicine causes myopathy by disrupting tubular function with subsequent vacuolization. Patients taking colchicine should be informed about possible muscular and gastrointestinal adverse effects and advised to stop.

Coumarin anticoagulants

Interactions of statins with warfarin, resulting in an increased bleeding tendency, have been reported (51), including interactions of anticoagulants with both lovastatin (51) and fluvastatin (89).

Three patients taking fluvastatin 20 mg/day had raised international normalized ratios (INRs), with a risk of bleeding (90).

- A 67-year-old man receiving a stable maintenance dosage of warfarin experienced an increased INR without bleeding when his atorvastatin therapy was switched to fluvastatin. His warfarin dosage was reduced and his INR stabilized. The fluvastatin was switched back to atorvastatin, and the warfarin dosage was increased to maintain the patient's goal INR (91).

In 46 adults taking warfarin, a change from pravastatin to simvastatin caused a significant increase in INR from 2.42 to 2.74 without an overall change in the dose of warfarin; there were no unusual episodes of bleeding (92).

In three patients taking stable warfarin dosages with INRs in the target range, the INRs increased when fluvastatin was added (89). Although none had a bleeding episode, they did require a reduction in their weekly warfarin dosage to achieve an appropriate degree of anticoagulation.

In contrast, in 12 patients chronically maintained on warfarin, atorvastatin 80 mg/day for 2 weeks had no important effect on mean prothrombin time (92).

In 21 healthy men, cerivastatin 300 micrograms did not alter the pharmacokinetics of R- and S-warfarin, or the pharmacodynamics of a single oral dose of warfarin 25 mg (93).

In a patient given the anticoagulant acenocoumarol, the INR increased from the target range (2–3.5) to 9.0, 3 weeks after starting simvastatin 20 mg/day. It is conceivable either that the two drugs competed for hepatic metabolism or that the oral anticoagulant was displaced from plasma albumin by simvastatin (94). The former mechanism is supported by the observation that pravastatin, which is only bound 50% to albumin, interacted with the anticoagulant fluindione and raised the INR (95).

Diltiazem

Diltiazem interacts with lovastatin but not with pravastatin (96). In 10 healthy volunteers given lovastatin orally with or without intravenous diltiazem in a randomized, two-way, crossover design, the interaction of diltiazem with lovastatin was primarily a first-pass effect, due to inhibition of CYP3A4 (97). Thus, drug interactions with diltiazem may become evident when a patient is switched from intravenous to oral dosing.

Fibrates

In a retrospective series, 4 (5%) out of 80 subjects taking lovastatin and gemfibrozil developed a myopathy. Based on this and on reports to US Food and Drug Administration the combined use of the two drugs is discouraged, especially in patients with compromised renal and/or hepatic function. Elderly women may be at special risk (98,99).

Some investigators have concluded that rare drug-induced reversible hepatotoxicity calls for close monitoring of liver enzymes in long-term treatment with statin-fibrate combinations (100).

In a randomized crossover study gemfibrozil increased the AUC of atorvastatin and its metabolites (101). Low doses of atorvastatin should be used if gemfibrozil is co-administered.

Combination therapy with fluvastatin and bezafibrate 400 mg/day in 71 patients with persistent hypertriglyceridemia resulted in no significant increase in creatine kinase activity or in the frequency of myalgia (102).

- In contrast, although in vitro studies have not shown any evidence of pharmacokinetic interactions between cerivastatin and gemfibrozil (58), there was myalgia and a marked increase in creatine kinase in a 74-year-old woman with normal renal function who took gemfibrozil 1200 mg/day 3 weeks after she started to take cerivastatin 0.3 mg/day (57).

Since then several other cases have been described:

- a 64-year-old woman (103)
- a 63-year-old man with diabetes mellitus (104)
- a 75-year-old man (105)
- a 68-year-old man (106).

The last patient fared well on a combination of gemfibrozil and cerivastatin until he received influenza vaccination. Rhabdomyolysis has been reported with various viruses, including influenza A and B and inactivation of the virus does not totally prevent this.

Gemfibrozil also increased plasma concentrations of simvastatin and its active form, simvastatin acid, in a randomized, double-blind, crossover study in 10 healthy volunteers given gemfibrozil or placebo orally for 3 days before a single dose of simvastatin (107). This suggests that the increased risk of myopathy in combination treatment is at least partly pharmacokinetic in origin. Because gemfibrozil does not inhibit CYP3A4 in vitro, the mechanism of the pharmacokinetic interaction is probably inhibition of non-CYP3A4-mediated metabolism of simvastatin acid.

Fusidic acid

Rhabdomyolysis has been attributed to the combination of fusidic acid with statins.

- A 71-year-old man developed nausea, abdominal discomfort, and myalgia after taking fusidic acid for 4 weeks. The next day he had myoglobinuria. Simvastatin, which he had taken for 8 years, was withdrawn. Prompt clinical improvement followed (108).

Grapefruit juice

Grapefruit juice inhibits CYP3A4, and serum concentrations of atorvastatin, but not of pravastatin, increased after administration of double-strength grapefruit juice 200 ml tds for 2 days (109).

When 10 healthy volunteers took simvastatin 24 hours after a large amount of grapefruit juice in a non-randomized, crossover study, the effect on the AUC of simvastatin was only about 10% of the effect observed when grapefruit juice and simvastatin were taken together (110). The interaction potential of even large amounts of grapefruit juice with CYP3A4 substrates dissipates within 3–7 days after ingestion of the last dose.

HIV protease inhibitors

Healthy volunteers were given protease inhibitors and statins, and the authors concluded that simvastatin should be avoided and that atorvastatin could be used with caution in people taking ritonavir and saquinavir (111). Dosage adjustment of pravastatin may be necessary with co-administration of ritonavir and saquinavir. Pravastatin does not alter the pharmacokinetics of nelfinavir, and thus appears to be safe for co-administration.

Macrolides

The macrolide antibiotic erythromycin together with statins enhances the risk of rhabdomyolysis (SED-13, 1328) (112), as do clarithromycin and azithromycin (113).

Severe myopathy has been attributed to the combination of simvastatin with clarithromycin and amiodarone (114).

- A 56-year-old man taking simvastatin was given clarithromycin and amiodarone for pneumonia and a supraventricular tachycardia. He found it difficult to move and complained of general weakness and muscle pain. The blood creatine kinase activity was over 20 000 IU/l. Simvastatin was withdrawn on day 19 and during days 22–31 he steadily improved.

Nefazodone

The antidepressant nefazodone increases the risk of rhabdomyolysis from statins (115).

Red yeast rice

Rhabdomyolysis in a stable renal transplant recipient was attributed to the presence of red yeast rice (*Monascus purpureus*) in a herbal mixture (116). The condition resolved when he stopped taking the product. Rice fermented with red yeast contains several types of mevinic acids, including monacolin-K, which is identical to lovastatin. The authors postulated that the interaction of ciclosporin with these compounds through cytochrome P450 had resulted in the adverse effect. Transplant recipients must be cautioned against using herbal products to lower their lipid concentrations, in order to prevent such complications.

Rifampicin

In a randomized crossover study rifampicin reduced the total AUC of atorvastatin and increased the C_{max} of 2-hydroxyatorvastatin acid by 68% (101). It is advisable to increase the dosage of atorvastatin and preferable to administer it in the evening to guarantee adequate concentrations during the period of rapid cholesterol synthesis that occurs at night when rifampicin or other potent inducers of CYP3A4 are co-administered.

St John's wort (*Hypericum perforatum*)

St John's wort induces CYP3A4 and reduces blood concentrations of CYP3A4 substrates. In one study, St John's wort reduced plasma concentrations of simvastatin but not pravastatin (117).

Troglitazone

When troglitazone was added in four men with diabetes using insulin and taking atorvastatin, serum LDL cholesterol and triglycerides increased by 23 and 21% respectively (118). This suggests a drug interaction, but further studies are warranted to substantiate this.

References

1. Duriez P. Mécanismes d'action des statines et des fibrates. [Mechanisms of actions of statins and fibrates.] Thérapie 2003;58(1):5–14.
2. Armitage J. The safety of statins in clinical practice. Lancet 2007;370(9601):1781–90.
3. Waters DD. Safety of high-dose atorvastatin therapy. Am J Cardiol 2005;96(5A Suppl):69F-75F.
4. Park S, Kang HJ, Rim SJ, Ha JW, Oh BH, Chung N, Cho SY. A randomized, open-label study to evaluate the efficacy and safety of pitavastatin compared with simvastatin in Korean patients with hypercholesterolemia. Clin Ther 2005;27(7):1074–82.
5. Silver MA, Langsjoen PH, Szabo S, Patil H, Zelinger A. Effect of atorvastatin on left ventricular diastolic function and ability of coenzyme Q10 to reverse that dysfunction. Am J Cardiol 2004;94(10):1306–10.
6. Eckernas SA, Roos BE, Kvidal P, Eriksson LO, Block GA, Neafus RP, Haigh JR. The effects of simvastatin and pravastatin on objective and subjective measures of nocturnal sleep: a comparison of two structurally different HMG CoA reductase inhibitors in patients with primary moderate hypercholesterolaemia. Br J Clin Pharmacol 1993;35(3):284–9.
7. Boriani G, Biffi M, Strocchi E, Branzi A. Nightmares and sleep disturbances with simvastatin and metoprolol. Ann Pharmacother 2001;35(10):1292.
8. Ziajka PE, Wehmeier T. Peripheral neuropathy and lipid-lowering therapy. South Med J 1998;91(7):667–8.
9. Chong PH, Boskovich A, Stevkovic N, Bartt RE. Statin-associated peripheral neuropathy: review of the literature. Pharmacotherapy 2004;24(9):1194–203.
10. Jeppesen U, Gaist D, Smith T, Sindrup SH. Statins and peripheral neuropathy. Eur J Clin Pharmacol 1999;54(11):835–8.
11. Gaist D, Jeppesen U, Andersen M, Garcia Rodriguez LA, Hallas J, Sindrup SH. Statins and risk of polyneuropathy: a case-control study. Neurology 2002;58(9):1333–7.
12. Rajabally YA, Varakantam V, Abbott RJ. Disorder resembling Guillain–Barré syndrome on initiation of statin therapy. Muscle Nerve 2004;30(5):663–6.
13. Lintott CJ, Scott RS, Nye ER, Robertson MC, Sutherland WH. Simvastatin (MK 733): an effective treatment for hypercholesterolemia. Aust NZ J Med 1989;19(4):317–20.
14. Laties AM, Shear CL, Lippa EA, Gould AL, Taylor HR, Hurley DP, Stephenson WP, Keates EU, Tupy-Visich MA, Chremos AN. Expanded clinical evaluation of lovastatin (EXCEL) study results. II. Assessment of the human lens after 48 weeks of treatment with lovastatin. Am J Cardiol 1991;67(6):447–53.
15. Schmidt J, Schmitt C, Hockwin O, Paulus U, von Bergmann K. Ocular drug safety and HMG-CoA-reductase inhibitors. Ophthalmic Res 1994;26(6):352–60.
16. Farmer JA, Torre-Amione G. Comparative tolerability of the HMG-CoA reductase inhibitors. Drug Saf 2000;23(3):197–213.
17. Wagstaff LR, Mitton MW, Arvik BM, Doraiswamy PM. Statin-associated memory loss: analysis of 60 case reports and review of the literature. Pharmacotherapy 1920;23:871–80.
18. King DS. Cognitive impairment associated with atorvastatin and simvastatin. Pharmacotherapy 2003;23:1663–7.

19. Muldoon MF, Ryan CM, Sereika SM, Flory JD, Manuck SB. Randomized trial of the effects of simvastatin on cognitive functioning in hypercholesterolemic adults. Am J Med 2004;117(11):823–9.

20. Davidson KW, Reddy S, McGrath P, Zitner D, MacKeen W. Increases in depression after cholesterol-lowering drug treatment. Behav Med 1996;22(2):82–4.

21. Vevera J, Fisar Z, Kvasnicka T, Zdenek H, Starkova L, Ceska R, Papezova H. Cholesterol-lowering therapy evokes time-limited changes in serotonergic transmission. Psychiatry Res 2005;133(2-3):197–203.

22. Mikhailidis DP, Wierzbicki AS. HDL-cholesterol and the treatment of coronary heart disease: contrasting effects of atorvastatin and simvastatin. Curr Med Res Opin 2000;16(2):139–46.

23. Groneberg DA, Barkhuizen A, Jeha T. Simvastatin-induced thrombocytopenia. Am J Hematol 2001;67(4):277.

24. Tolman KG. The liver and lovastatin. Am J Cardiol 2002;89(12):1374–80.

25. Dujovne CA. Side effects of statins: hepatitis versus "transaminitis"-myositis versus "CPKitis". Am J Cardiol 2002;89(12):1411–3.

26. Black DM, Bakker-Arkema RG, Nawrocki JW. An overview of the clinical safety profile of atorvastatin (Lipitor), a new HMG-CoA reductase inhibitor. Arch Intern Med 1998;158(6):577–84.

27. Jimenez-Alonso J, Osorio JM, Gutierrez-Cabello F, Lopez de la Osa A, Leon L, Mediavilla Garcia JD. Atorvastatin-induced cholestatic hepatitis in a young woman with systemic lupus erythematosus. Grupo Lupus Virgen de las Nieves. Arch Intern Med 1999;159(15):1811–2.

28. Illingworth DR, Crouse JR 3rd, Hunninghake DB, Davidson MH, Escobar ID, Stalenhoef AF, Paragh G, Ma PT, Liu M, Melino MR, O'Grady L, Mercuri M, Mitchel YBSimvastatin Atorvastatin HDL Study Group. A comparison of simvastatin and atorvastatin up to maximal recommended doses in a large multicenter randomized clinical trial. Curr Med Res Opin 2001;17(1):43–50.

29. Spreckelsen U, Kirchhoff R, Haacke H. Cholestatischer Iikterus Wahrend Lovastatin-Einnahme. [Cholestatic jaundice during lovastatin medication.] Dtsch Med Wochenschr 1991;116(19):739–40.

30. Ballare M, Campanini M, Catania E, Bordin G, Zaccala G, Monteverde A. Acute cholestatic hepatitis during simvastatin administration. Recenti Prog Med 1991;82(4):233–5.

31. Muggeo M, Travia D, Querena M, Zenti MG, Bagnani M, Branzi P, et al. Long term treatment with pravastatin, simvastatin and gemfibrozil in patients with primary hypercholesterolaemia, a controlled study. Drug Invest 1992;4:376–85.

32. Assmann G, Huwel D, Schussman KM, Smilde JG, Kosling M, Withagen AJ, Wunderlich J, Stoel I, Van Dormaal JJ, Neuss J, et al. Efficacy and safety of atorvastatin and pravastatin in patients with hypercholesterolemia. Eur J Intern Med 1999;10:33–9.

33. Nakad A, Bataille L, Hamoir V, Sempoux C, Horsmans Y. Atorvastatin-induced acute hepatitis with absence of cross-toxicity with simvastatin. Lancet 1999;353(9166):1763–4.

34. Singh S, Nautiyal A, Dolan JG. Recurrent acute pancreatitis possibly induced by atorvastatin and rosuvastatin. Is statin induced pancreatitis a class effect? JOP 2004;5(6):502–4.

35. Adcock BB, Hornsby LB, Jenkins K. Dermographism: an adverse effect of atorvastatin. J Am Board Fam Pract 2001;14(2):148–51.

36. Sebök B, Toth M, Anga B, Harangi F, Schneider I. Lichenoid drug eruption with HMG-CoA reductase inhibitors (fluvastatin and lovastatin). Acta Derm Venereol 2004;84(3):229–30.

37. van Puijenbroek EP, Du Buf-Vereijken PW, Spooren PF, van Doormaal JJ. Possible increased risk of rhabdomyolysis during concomitant use of simvastatin and gemfibrozil. J Intern Med 1996;240(6):403–4.

38. Biesenbach G, Janko O, Stuby U, Zazgornik J. Terminales myoglobinurisches Niereneversagen unter Lovastatintherapie bei praexistenter chronischer Nierenfunktionsstorungo. [Terminal myoglobinuric renal failure in lovastatin therapy with pre-existing chronic renal insufficiency.] Wien Klin Wochenschr 1996;108(11):334–7.

39. Wortmann RL, Tipping RW, Levine JG, Melin JM. Frequency of myopathy in patients receiving lovastatin. Am J Cardiol 2005;95(8):983–5.

40. Sochman J, Podzimkova M. Not all statins are alike: induced rhabdomyolysis on changing from one statin to another one. Int J Cardiol 2005;99(1):145–6.

41. Neuvonen PJ, Jalava KM. Itraconazole drastically increases plasma concentrations of lovastatin and lovastatin acid. Clin Pharmacol Ther 1996;60(1):54–61.

42. Bruckert E, Hayem G, Dejager S, Yau C, Begaud B. Mild to moderate muscular symptoms with high-dosage statin therapy in hyperlipidemic patients—the PRIMO Study. Cardiovasc Drugs Ther 2005;19(6):403–14.

43. Graham DJ, Staffa JA, Shatin D, Andrade SE, Schech SD, Grenade LL, Gurwitz JH, Chan KA, Goodman MJ, Platt R. Incidence of hospitalized rhabdomyolysis in patients treated with lipid-lowering drugs. JAMA 2004;292(21):2585–90.

44. Carvalho AA, Lima UW, Valiente RA. Statin and fibrate associated myopathy: study of eight patients. Arq Neuro-Psiquiatria 2004;62(2A):257–61.

45. Phillips PS, Haas RH, Bannykh S, Hathaway S, Gray NL, Kimura BJ, Vladutiu GD, England JDScripps Mercy Clinical Research Center. Statin-associated myopathy with normal creatine kinase levels. Ann Intern Med 2002;137(7):581–5.

46. Giordano N, Senesi M, Mattii G, Battisti E, Villanova M, Gennari C. Polymyositis associated with simvastatin. Lancet 1997;349(9065):1600–1.

47. Laaksonen R, Ojala JP, Tikkanen MJ, Himberg JJ. Serum ubiquinone concentrations after short- and long-term treatment with HMG-CoA reductase inhibitors. Eur J Clin Pharmacol 1994;46(4):313–7.

48. Laaksonen R, Jokelainen K, Sahi T, Tikkanen MJ, Himberg JJ. Decreases in serum ubiquinone concentrations do not result in reduced levels in muscle tissue during short-term simvastatin treatment in humans. Clin Pharmacol Ther 1995;57(1):62–6.

49. Pershad A, Cardello FP. Simvastatin and rhabdomyolysis—a case report and brief review. J Pharm Technol 1999;15:88–9.

50. Al Shohaib S. Simvastatin-induced rhabdomyolysis in a patient with chronic renal failure. Am J Nephrol 2000;20(3):212–3.

51. Mantell G, Burke MT, Staggers J. Extended clinical safety profile of lovastatin. Am J Cardiol 1990;66(8):B11–5.

52. Fraunfelder FW, Fraunfelder FT, Edwards R. Diplopia and HMG-CoA reductase inhibitors. J Toxicol Cutaneous Ocul Toxicol 1999;18:287–9.

53. Parmar B, Francis PJ, Ragge NK. Statins, fibrates, and ocular myasthenia. Lancet 2002;360(9334):717.

54. Sinzinger H, Schmid P, O'Grady J. Two different types of exercise-induced muscle pain without myopathy and CK-elevation during HMG-Co-enzyme-A-reductase inhibitor treatment. Atherosclerosis 1999;143(2):459–60.

55. Insull W Jr, Isaacsohn J, Kwiterovich P, Ra P, Brazg R, Dujovne C, Shan M, Shugrue-Crowley E, Ripa S, Tota RCerivastatin Study Group. Efficacy and safety of cerivastatin 0.8 mg in patients with hypercholesterolaemia: the pivotal placebo-controlled clinical trial J Int Med Res 2000;28(2):47–68.

56. Rodriguez ML, Mora C, Navarro JF. Cerivastatin-induced rhabdomyolysis. Ann Intern Med 2000;132(7):598.

57. Pogson GW, Kindred LH, Carper BG. Rhabdomyolysis and renal failure associated with cerivastatin–gemfibrozil combination therapy. Am J Cardiol 1999;83(7):1146.

58. Plosker GL, Dunn CI, Figgitt DP. Cerivastatin: a review of its pharmacological properties and therapeutic efficacy in the management of hypercholesterolaemia. Drugs 2000;60(5):1179–206.

59. Smith DJ, Olive EO. Chinese red rice-induced myopathy. South Med J 2003;96:1265–7.

60. Chazerain P, Hayem G, Hamza S, Best C, Ziza JM. Four cases of tendinopathy in patients on statin therapy. Joint Bone Spine 2001;68(5):430–3.

61. Fauchais AL, Iba Ba J, Maurage P, Kyndt X, Bataille D, Hachulla E, Parent D, Queyrel V, Lambert M, Michon Pasturel U, Hatron PY, Vanhille P, Devulder B. Polymyosites induites ou associées aux traitements hypolipémiants? A propos de cinq cas. Rev Med Interne 2004;25(4):294–8.

62. Bruckert E, Giral P, Heshmati HM, Turpin G. Men treated with hypolipidaemic drugs complain more frequently of erectile dysfunction. J Clin Pharm Ther 1996;21(2):89–94.

63. Halkin A, Lossos IS, Mevorach D. HMG-CoA reductase inhibitor-induced impotence. Ann Pharmacother 1996;30(2):192.

64. Antonov D, Kazandjieva J, Etugov D, Gospodinov D, Tsankov N. Drug-induced lupus erythematosus. Clin Dermatol 2004;22(2):157–66.

65. Noel B, Panizzon RG. Lupus-like syndrome associated with statin therapy. Dermatology 2004;208(3):276–7.

66. Cattley RC. Carcinogenicity of lipid-lowering drugs. JAMA 1996;275(19):1479.

67. Sacks FM, Pfeffer MA, Moye LA, Rouleau JL, Rutherford JD, Cole TG, Brown L, Warnica JW, Arnold JM, Wun CC, Davis BR, Braunwald E. The effect of pravastatin on coronary events after myocardial infarction in patients with average cholesterol levels. Cholesterol and Recurrent Events Trial investigators. N Engl J Med 1996;335(14):1001–9.

68. Dalen JE, Dalton WS. Does lowering cholesterol cause cancer? JAMA 1996;275(1):67–9.

69. Horsmans Y. Differential metabolism of statins: importance in drug–drug interactions. Eur Heart J Suppl 1999;1(Suppl T):T7–T12.

70. Kantola T, Backman JT, Niemi M, Kivisto KT, Neuvonen PJ. Effect of fluconazole on plasma fluvastatin and pravastatin concentrations. Eur J Clin Pharmacol 2000;56(3):225–9.

71. Kahri J, Valkonen M, Bäcklund T, Vuoristo M, Kivistö KT. Rhabdomyolysis in a patient receiving atorvastatin and fluconazole. Eur J Clin Pharmacol 2005;60(12):905–7.

72. Mazzu AL, Lasseter KC, Shamblen EC, Agarwal V, Lettieri J, Sundaresen P. Itraconazole alters the pharmacokinetics of atorvastatin to a greater extent than either cerivastatin or pravastatin. Clin Pharmacol Ther 2000;68(4):391–400.

73. Horn M. Coadministration of itraconazole with hypolipidemic agents may induce rhabdomyolysis in healthy individuals. Arch Dermatol 1996;132(10):1254.

74. Neuvonen PJ, Kantola T, Kivisto KT. Simvastatin but not pravastatin is very susceptible to interaction with the CYP3A4 inhibitor itraconazole. Clin Pharmacol Ther 1998;63(3):332–41.

75. Kantola T, Kivisto KT, Neuvonen PJ. Effect of itraconazole on the pharmacokinetics of atorvastatin. Clin Pharmacol Ther 1998;64(1):58–65.

76. Kivisto KT, Kantola T, Neuvonen PJ. Different effects of itraconazole on the pharmacokinetics of fluvastatin and lovastatin. Br J Clin Pharmacol 1998;46(1):49–53.

77. Gilad R, Lampl Y. Rhabdomyolysis induced by simvastatin and ketoconazole treatment. Clin Neuropharmacol 1999;22(5):295–7.

78. Ucar M, Neuvonen M, Luurila H, Dahlqvist R, Neuvonen PJ, Mjorndal T. Carbamazepine markedly reduces serum concentrations of simvastatin and simvastatin acid. Eur J Clin Pharmacol 2004;59(12):879–82.

79. Bielecki JW, Schraner C, Briner V, Kuhn M. Rhabdomyolyse und cholestatische Hepatitis unter der Behandlung mit Simvastatin und Chlorzoxazon. [Rhabdomyolysis and cholestatic hepatitis under treatment with simvastatin and chlorzoxazone.] Schweiz Med Wochenschr 1999;129(13):514–8.

80. Stirling CM, Isles CG. Rhabdomyolysis due to simvastatin in a transplant patient: Are some statins safer than others? Nephrol Dial Transplant 2001;16(4):873–4.

81. Lau WC. Atorvastatin reduces the ability of clopidogrel to inhibit platelet aggregation: a new drug-drug interaction. Circulation 2003;107:32–7.

82. Saw J. Lack of adverse clopidogrel-atorvastatin clinical interaction from secondary analysis of a randomized, placebo-controlled clopidogrel trial. Circulation 2003;108:921–4.

83. Serebruany VL. Are antiplatelet effects of clopidogrel inhibited by atorvastatin? A research question formulated but not yet adequately tested. Circulation 2003;107:1568–9.

84. Mitsios JV, Papathanasiou AI, Rodis FI, Elisaf M, Goudevenos JA, Tselepis AD. Atorvastatin does not affect the antiplatelet potency of clopidogrel when it is administered concomitantly for 5 weeks in patients with acute coronary syndromes. Circulation 2004;109(11):1335–8.

85. Serebruany VL, Midei MG, Malinin AI, Oshrine BR, Lowry DR, Sane DC, Tanguay JF, Steinhubl SR, Berger PB, O'Connor CM, Hennekens CH. Absence of interaction between atorvastatin or other statins and clopidogrel: results from the interaction study. Arch Intern Med 2004;164(18):2051–7.

86. Mitsios JV, Papathanasiou AI, Elisaf M, Goudevenos JA, Tselepis AD. The inhibitory potency of clopidogrel on ADP-induced platelet activation is not attenuated when it is co-administered with atorvastatin (20 mg/day) for 5 weeks in patients with acute coronary syndromes. Platelets 2005;16(5):287–92.

87. Atasoyu EM, Evrenkaya TR, Solmazgul E. Possible colchicine rhabdomyolysis in a fluvastatin-treated patient. Ann Pharmacother 2005;39(7-8):1368–9.

88. Alayli G, Cengiz K, Canturk F, Durmus D, Akyol Y, Menekse EB. Acute myopathy in a patient with concomitant use of pravastatin and colchicine. Ann Pharmacother 2005;39(7):1358–61.

89. Trilli LE, Kelley CL, Aspinall SL, Kroner BA. Potential interaction between warfarin and fluvastatin. Ann Pharmacother 1996;30(12):1399–402.

90. Kline SS, Harrell CC. Potential warfarin–fluvastatin interaction. Ann Pharmacother 1997;31(6):790.

91. Andrus MR. Oral anticoagulant drug interactions with statins: case report of fluvastatin and review of the literature. Pharmacotherapy 2004;24(2):285–90.

92. Stern R, Abel R, Gibson GL, Besserer J. Atorvastatin does not alter the anticoagulant activity of warfarin. J Clin Pharmacol 1997;37(11):1062–4.

93. Schall R, Muller FO, Hundt HK, Ritter W, Duursema L, Groenewoud G, Middle MV. No pharmacokinetic or pharmacodynamic interaction between rivastatin and warfarin. J Clin Pharmacol 1995;35(3):306–13.

94. Grau E, Perella M, Pastor E. Simvastatin–oral anticoagulant interaction. Lancet 1996;347(8998):405–6.

95. Trenque T, Choisy H, Germain ML. Pravastatin: interaction with oral anticoagulant? BMJ 1996;312(7035):886.

96. Azie NE, Brater DC, Becker PA, Jones DR, Hall SD. The interaction of diltiazem with lovastatin and pravastatin. Clin Pharmacol Ther 1998;64(4):369–77.

97. Masica AL, Azie NE, Brater DC, Hall SD, Jones DR. Intravenous diltiazem and CYP3A-mediated metabolism. Br J Clin Pharmacol 2000;50(3):273–6.

98. Goldstein MR. Myopathy and rhabdomyolysis with lovastatin taken with gemfibrozil. JAMA 1990;264(23):2991–2.

99. Kogan AD, Orenstein S. Lovastatin-induced acute rhabdomyolysis. Postgrad Med J 1990;66(774):294–6.

100. Athyros VG, Papageorgiou AA, Hatzikonstandinou HA, Didangelos TP, Carina MV, Kranitsas DF, Kontopoulos AG. Safety and efficacy of long-term statin–fibrate combinations in patients with refractory familial combined hyperlipidemia. Am J Cardiol 1997;80(5):608–13.

101. Backman JT, Luurila H, Neuvonen M, Neuvonen PJ. Rifampin markedly decreases and gemfibrozil increases the plasma concentrations of atorvastatin and its metabolites. Clin Pharmacol Ther 2005;78(2):154–67.

102. Spieker LE, Noll G, Hannak M, Luscher TF. Efficacy and tolerability of fluvastatin and bezafibrate in patients with hyperlipidemia and persistently high triglyceride levels. J Cardiovasc Pharmacol 2000;35(3):361–5.

103. Bermingham RP, Whitsitt TB, Smart ML, Nowak DP, Scalley RD. Rhabdomyolysis in a patient receiving the combination of cerivastatin and gemfibrozil. Am J Health Syst Pharm 2000;57(5):461–4.

104. Ozdemir O, Boran M, Gokce V, Uzun Y, Kocak B, Korkmaz S. A case with severe rhabdomyolysis and renal failure associated with cerivastatin–gemfibrozil combination therapy—a case report. Angiology 2000;51(8):695–7.

105. Alexandridis G, Pappas GA, Elisaf MS. Rhabdomyolysis due to combination therapy with cerivastatin and gemfibrozil. Am J Med 2000;109(3):261–2.

106. Plotkin E, Bernheim J, Ben-Chetrit S, Mor A, Korzets Z. Influenza vaccine—a possible trigger of rhabdomyolysis induced acute renal failure due to the combined use of cerivastatin and bezafibrate. Nephrol Dial Transplant 2000;15(5):740–1.

107. Backman JT, Kyrklund C, Kivisto KT, Wang JS, Neuvonen PJ. Plasma concentrations of active simvastatin acid are increased by gemfibrozil. Clin Pharmacol Ther 2000;68(2):122–9.

108. Yuen SL, McGarity B. Rhabdomyolysis secondary to interaction of fusidic acid and simvastatin. Med J Aust 2003;179:172.

109. Lilja JJ, Kivisto KT, Neuvonen PJ. Grapefruit juice increases serum concentrations of atorvastatin and has no effect on pravastatin. Clin Pharmacol Ther 1999;66(2):118–27.

110. Lilja JJ, Kivisto KT, Neuvonen PJ. Duration of effect of grapefruit juice on the pharmacokinetics of the CYP3A4 substrate simvastatin. Clin Pharmacol Ther 2000;68(4):384–90.

111. Fichtenbaum CJ, Gerber JG, Rosenkranz SL, Segal Y, Aberg JA, Blaschke T, Alston B, Fang F, Kosel B, Aweeka FNIAID AIDS Clinical Trials Group. Pharmacokinetic interactions between protease inhibitors and statins in HIV seronegative volunteers: ACTG Study A5047. AIDS 2002;16(4):569–77.

112. Spach DH, Bauwens JE, Clark CD, Burke WG. Rhabdomyolysis associated with lovastatin and erythromycin use. West J Med 1991;154(2):213–5.

113. Grunden JW, Fisher KA. Lovastatin-induced rhabdomyolysis possibly associated with clarithromycin and azithromycin. Ann Pharmacother 1997;31(7–8):859–63.

114. Chouhan UM, Chakrabarti S, Millward LJ. Simvastatin interaction with clarithromycin and amiodarone causing myositis. Ann Pharmacother 2005;39(10):1760–1.

115. Jacobson RH, Wang P, Glueck CJ. Myositis and rhabdomyolysis associated with concurrent use of simvastatin and nefazodone. JAMA 1997;277(4):296–7.

116. Prasad GV, Wong T, Meliton G, Bhaloo S. Rhabdomyolysis due to red yeast rice (Monascus purpureus) in a renal transplant recipient. Transplantation 2002;74(8):1200–1.

117. Sugimoto K, Ohmori M, Tsuruoka S, Nishiki K, Kawaguchi A, Harada K, Arakawa M, Sakamoto K, Masada M, Miyamori I, Fujimura A. Different effects of St John's wort on the pharmacokinetics of simvastatin and pravastatin. Clin Pharmacol Ther 2001;70(6):518–24.

118. DiTusa L, Luzier AB. Potential interaction between troglitazone and atorvastatin. J Clin Pharm Ther 2000;25(4):279–82.

Ion exchange resins

General Information

The ion exchange resins colestyramine (rINN) and colestipol (rINN) are not absorbed, and their main adverse effects are therefore on the gastrointestinal tract. They can also interfere with the absorption of other drugs or fat-soluble vitamins.

Organs and Systems

Metabolism

The ion exchange resins tend to increase serum triglyceride concentrations, especially in patients with hypertriglyceridemia (1).

Nutrition

Serum total carotenoid and vitamin A concentrations fell by 30% in patients taking colestipol 30 g/day (2).

Acid–base balance

Colestyramine has been reported to have caused a hyperchloremic metabolic acidosis.

- A 70-year-old woman with a 2-year history of primary biliary cirrhosis confirmed by histological and immunological criteria took colestyramine sachets twice daily for 2 months and developed lethargy, confusion, and drowsiness (3). She had signs of chronic liver disease, portal hypertension, and hepatic encephalopathy. Laboratory investigations confirmed a metabolic acidosis (pH 7.15) and hyperchloremia. Multiple cultures failed to reveal sepsis, and a urinary pH of 4.85 together with tests of renal acidification excluded renal tubular acidosis. No other cause was found and she responded to 600 mmol of sodium bicarbonate intravenously over 36 hours.

Hematologic

Inhibition of vitamin K absorption can cause vitamin K deficiency, leading to hypoprothrombinemia and hence to bleeding (4).

Gastrointestinal

Patients taking colestyramine often have constipation, abdominal discomfort, and heartburn, but dietary fiber, such as psyllium, can reduce the symptoms (5,6). Other effects are flatulence, nausea, and fecal impaction; a mild laxative may be needed, particularly in the elderly. Many other patients complain of anorexia and occasionally there is diarrhea. Doses of colestyramine higher than the 10–16 g normally used can cause steatorrhea (7).

A small child died when impacted resin obstructed the colon (SEDA-8, 935; 8).

The most common adverse effect of colestipol is constipation (30%). In the first months of therapy nausea and bloating can also occur. There is disappointingly poor adherence to therapy in young patients (9). The encapsulated form of the drug is better tolerated (10).

Liver

- A 65-year-old man with type IIa dyslipidemia who took flavored colestipol granules 2 scoops/day for 3 months developed asymptomatic hepatotoxicity (11). Several of his liver enzymes were raised to 10 times the upper limit of the reference range. One week after withdrawal of colestipol, his serum transaminases fell dramatically and 3 weeks later all his liver function tests were normal.

Rechallenge was not attempted, but other potential causes of hepatocellular injury were ruled out.

Musculoskeletal

A degree of osteoporosis or osteomalacia can occur because of reduced vitamin D absorption (12).

Drug–Drug Interactions

General

Ion-exchange resins do not have systemic adverse effects, but they can affect the absorption of other drugs from the gut, particularly if they undergo enterohepatic or enteroenteric recirculation, since they will adsorb them in the gut and prevent their reabsorption.

There is reason to anticipate problems if the resin is given along with acidic drugs and some other drugs that have a narrow safety margin, such as oral anticoagulants (coumarins), cardiac glycosides, and thyroid hormones (thyroxine, triiodothyronine). Interference with the absorption of other acidic drugs, including the barbiturates, naproxen, phenylbutazone and its congeners, and the thiazide diuretics, can almost certainly occur, but is of little or no clinical importance, since the doses of these drugs can easily be adjusted as time goes by, to allow for any reduction in absorption, or alternative drugs can be used. Interference with anticoagulants and cardiac glycosides presents the most serious problems, because they have a low therapeutic index. It has often been said that problems can be avoided provided the drugs are not given simultaneously; however, this is not true when the drug in question undergoes enterohepatic circulation, as is the case with digitoxin and phenprocoumon, as a result of which these substances are present in the gastrointestinal tract for a long time and can be exposed to an ion exchange resin at any time. The interval principle for other drugs is useful, but the interval should be at least 1 hour and in the case of thyroxine 4–5 hours, in which case the drug should be given before the resin.

Cardiac glycosides

Colestyramine and colestipol bind digoxin and digitoxin and can affect their absorption. When the ion exchange resins and digoxin are co-administered the absorption of digoxin is reduced (13). However, even when they are not administered together, the resins can bind cardiac glycosides that have re-entered the gut after absorption by virtue of enterohepatic recycling and enteral secretion, increasing their rate of elimination. This action has been used to treat digoxin toxicity (14–16), digitoxin toxicity (17), and toxicity from derivatives of digoxin (18).

Coumarin anticoagulants

The interaction of colestyramine with coumarins is due to the enterohepatic recirculation of coumarins, which is interrupted by colestyramine.

Phenprocoumon undergoes enterohepatic recycling, and its elimination can be enhanced by ion exchange resins, sometimes with fatal consequences (19).

Warfarin also undergoes enterohepatic recycling, and its elimination can be enhanced by ion exchange resins (20); this has been used to treat warfarin toxicity (21).

Fluvastatin

The systemic availability of fluvastatin is reduced by bile acid sequestrants (22).

Folic acid

Malabsorption of folic acid has been reported in patients taking colestyramine (SEDA-13, 1326) (23).

In children taking colestipol supplementary folic acid may need to be provided (24).

Valproic acid

The systemic availability of valproic acid is reduced by colestyramine unless they are given 3 hours apart (25).

References

1. Ryan JR, Jain A. The effect of colestipol or cholestyramine on serum cholesterol and triglycerides in a long-term controlled study. J Clin Pharmacol New Drugs 1972;12(7):268–73.
2. Probstfield JL, Lin TL, Peters J, Hunninghake DB. Carotenoids and vitamin A: the effect of hypocholesterolemic agents on serum levels. Metabolism 1985;34(1):88–91.
3. Eaves ER, Korman MG. Cholestyramine induced hyperchloremic metabolic acidosis. Aust NZ J Med 1984;14(5):670–2.
4. Vroonhof K, van Rijn HJ, van Hattum J. Vitamin K deficiency and bleeding after long-term use of cholestyramine. Neth J Med 2003;61(1):19–21.
5. Maciejko JJ, Brazg R, Shah A, Patil S, Rubenfire M. Psyllium for the reduction of cholestyramine-associated gastrointestinal symptoms in the treatment of primary hypercholesterolemia. Arch Fam Med 1994;3(11):955–60.
6. Spence JD, Huff MW, Heidenheim P, Viswanatha A, Munoz C, Lindsay R, Wolfe B, Mills D. Combination therapy with colestipol and psyllium mucilloid in patients with hyperlipidemia. Ann Intern Med 1995;123(7):493–9.
7. Zurier RB, Hashim SA, Van Itallie TB. Effect of medium chain triglyceride on cholestyramine-induced steatorrhea in man. Gastroenterology 1965;49(5):490–5.
8. Cohen MI, Winslow PR, Boley SJ. Intestinal obstruction associated with cholestyramine therapy. N Engl J Med 1969;280(23):1285–6.
9. Kruse W, Kohlmeier M, Nikolaus T, Vogel G, Schlierf G. Langzeitbehandlung mit colestipol. Munch Med Wochenschr 1989;131:407–9.
10. Linet OI, Grzegorczyk CR, Demke DM. The effect of encapsulated, low-dose colestipol in patients with hyperlipidemia. J Clin Pharmacol 1988;28(9):804–6.
11. Sirmans SM, Beck JK, Banh HL, Freeman DA. Colestipol-induced hepatotoxicity. Pharmacotherapy 2001;21(4):513–6.
12. Heaton KW, Lever JV, Barnard D. Osteomalacia associated with cholestyramine therapy for postileectomy diarrhea. Gastroenterology 1972;62(4):642–6.
13. Brown DD, Schmid J, Long RA, Hull JH. A steady-state evaluation of the effects of propantheline bromide and cholestyramine on the bioavailability of digoxin when administered as tablets or capsules. J Clin Pharmacol 1985;25(5):360–4.
14. Roberge RJ, Sorensen T. Congestive heart failure and toxic digoxin levels: role of cholestyramine. Vet Hum Toxicol 2000;42(3):172–3.
15. Krivoy N, Eisenman A. [Cholestyramine for digoxin intoxication.]Harefuah 1995;128(3):145–7199.
16. Payne VW, Secter RA, Noback RK. Use of colestipol in a patient with digoxin intoxication. Drug Intell Clin Pharm 1981;15(11):902–3.
17. Hantson P, Vandenplas O, Mahieu P, Wallemacq P, Hassoun A. Repeated doses of activated charcoal and cholestyramine for digitoxin overdose: pharmacokinetic data and urinary elimination. J Toxicol Clin Exp 1991;11(7–8):401–5.
18. Kuhlmann J. Use of cholestyramine in three patients with beta-acetyldigoxin, beta-methyldigoxin and digitoxin intoxication. Int J Clin Pharmacol Ther Toxicol 1984;22(10):543–8.
19. Balmelli N, Domine F, Pfisterer M, Krahenbuhl S, Marsch S. Fatal drug interaction between cholestyramine and phenprocoumon. Eur J Intern Med 2002;13(3):210–1.
20. Jahnchen E, Meinertz T, Gilfrich HJ, Kersting F, Groth U. Enhanced elimination of warfarin during treatment with cholestyramine. Br J Clin Pharmacol 1978;5(5):437–40.
21. Roberge RJ, Rao P, Miske GR, Riley TJ. Diarrhea-associated over-anticoagulation in a patient taking warfarin: therapeutic role of cholestyramine. Vet Hum Toxicol 2000;42(6):351–3.
22. Plosker GL, Wagstaff AJ. Fluvastatin: a review of its pharmacology and use in the management of hypercholesterolaemia. Drugs 1996;51(3):433–59.
23. Kane JP, Malloy MJ. Treatment of hypercholesterolemia. Med Clin North Am 1982;66(2):537–50.
24. Glueck CJ. Colestipol and probucol: treatment of primary and familial hypercholesterolemia and amelioration of atherosclerosis. Ann Intern Med 1982;96(4):452–82.
25. Malloy MJ, Ravis WR, Pennell AT, Diskin CJ. Effect of cholestyramine resin on single dose valproate pharmacokinetics. Int J Clin Pharmacol Ther 1996;34(5):208–11.

Lorenzo's oil

General Information

Lorenzo's oil is a 4:1 mixture of glyceryl trioleate and glyceryl trierucate. It is used in patients with adrenoleukodystrophy. The dyslipidemia in patients with adrenoleukodystrophy consists of increased blood concentrations of very-long-chain saturated fatty acids, particularly hexacosaenoic acid (C26:0). Treatment with Lorenzo's oil has tended to normalize the abnormality in the blood while the patient deteriorates. Neurological changes are unrelated to the fatty acid changes in the blood, and, moreover, erucic acid does not seem to enter the brain. It is not known whether it works.

Registration of adverse effects with Lorenzo's oil has been hampered by the absence of controlled trials. In 22 patients treated for at least 12 months, although Lorenzo's oil did not seem to be beneficial, there were possible adverse effects, such as mild increases in liver enzymes (55%), thrombocytopenia (55%), gastrointestinal complaints (14%), and gingivitis (14%). Furthermore, there were falls in hemoglobin concentration and leukocyte count, and an increase in the plasma alkaline phosphatase concentration; the reduction in platelet count did not result in hemorrhage (1). Whether some of the adverse effects of Lorenzo's oil are due to low concentrations of essential fatty acids or caused by reduced dietary fat intake is not known.

Organs and Systems

Hematologic

Lorenzo's oil affected blood platelet counts in 39 patients followed for 1 year (2). Blood platelet aggregation studies in those patients were normal and there were no platelet-associated immunoglobulins. It has been suggested that the thrombocytopenia might be due to platelet activation, resulting from an increase in the concentration of erucic acid in the platelet membrane (1).

References

1. van Geel BM, Assies J, Haverkort EB, Koelman JH, Verbeeten B Jr, Wanders RJ, Barth PG. Progression of abnormalities in adrenomyeloneuropathy and neurologically asymptomatic X-linked adrenoleukodystrophy despite treatment with "Lorenzo's oil". J Neurol Neurosurg Psychiatry 1999;67(3):290–9.
2. Kickler TS, Zinkham WH, Moser A, Shankroff J, Borel J, Moser H. Effect of erucic acid on platelets in patients with adrenoleukodystrophy. Biochem Mol Med 1996;57(2):125–33.

Lovastatin

General Information

The adverse events profile of lovastatin in 8245 patients with moderate hypercholesterolemia has been evaluated in a double-blind, diet- and placebo-controlled trial (1). The difference between lovastatin and placebo in the incidence of adverse events that required discontinuation was small, ranging from 1.2% at 20 mg bd to 1.9% at 80 mg/day. Among a variety of symptoms, only constipation differed significantly between drug and placebo, with a slightly higher frequency in the treated group. The treated patients also gained on average 0.4 kg more weight than controls. Deaths were few. Lovastatin-induced rhabdomyolysis can occur (2), even in the absence of other drug therapy (SEDA-12, 1101) (3).

Organs and Systems

Psychological, psychiatric

In a double-blind study, 209 healthy adults were randomized to placebo or lovastatin 20 mg/day for 6 months (4). Placebo-treated subjects improved between baseline and post-treatment periods on neuropsychological tests in all performance domains (neuropsychological performance, depression, hostility, and quality of life), consistent with the effects of practice on test performance, whereas those treated with lovastatin improved only on tests of memory recall. Comparisons of the changes in performance between placebo and lovastatin showed small but significant differences for tests of attention

and psychomotor speed, and were consistent with greater improvement with placebo. Psychological well-being was not affected by lovastatin. The authors concluded that treatment of hypercholesterolemia with lovastatin did not cause psychological distress or substantially alter cognitive function. However, treatment did result in slight impairment of performance in neuropsychological tests of attention and psychomotor speed, the clinical importance of which is uncertain.

Skin

Ichthyosiform eruptions on the abdomen and back occurred in a Korean patient after 3 months of lovastatin therapy; they disappeared on withdrawal (5). Similar lesions occurred in a 54-year-old Chinese man (6).

Reproductive system

Hypospermia has been reported in a patient taking lovastatin (7).

Immunologic

There were 25 serious hypersensitivity reactions (such as arthralgia and thrombocytopenia) among the first million patients taking lovastatin; at least some of these were considered to be due to the drug (8).

Body temperature

Severe hyperthermia has been attributed to lovastatin (9).

Drug–Drug Interactions

Diltiazem

The effects of co-administration of oral diltiazem, a potent inhibitor of CYP3A, on the pharmacokinetics of lovastatin have been evaluated in a randomized study in 10 healthy volunteers (10). Lovastatin is oxidized by CYP3A to active metabolites. Diltiazem significantly increased the oral AUC and maximum serum concentration of lovastatin, but did not alter its half-life. The magnitude of the increase of plasma concentration of lovastatin suggested that caution is necessary when co-administering diltiazem and lovastatin.

In another study by the same investigators, 10 healthy volunteers were randomized in a two-way, crossover study either to oral lovastatin or to intravenous diltiazem followed by oral lovastatin. Intravenous diltiazem did not significantly affect the pharmacokinetics of lovastatin (oral AUC, C_{max}, t_{max}, or half-life), suggesting that the interaction does not occur systemically and is primarily a first-pass effect (11). Drug interactions with diltiazem may therefore become evident when a patient is changed from intravenous to oral dosing.

Diuretics

Potassium-depleting diuretics, except indapamide, can attenuate the effect of lovastatin on blood lipid concentrations (12).

Erythromycin

Rhabdomyolysis due to a short course of erythromycin in a 73-year-old man who had taken lovastatin for 7 years was accompanied by signs of multiple organ toxicity so severe as to mimic sepsis (13).

Rhabdomyolysis with or without renal impairment has been reported in patients taking both erythromycin and lovastatin (14). The exact mechanism is unknown, but lovastatin is extensively metabolized by CYP3A4 and its metabolism may therefore be inhibited by erythromycin. The manufacturers have advised that careful monitoring is required when these two drugs are given together.

Gemfibrozil

Lovastatin in combination with gemfibrozil caused a rise in creatine kinase activity 234 000 U/l, with complete remission after both drugs had been withdrawn (15).

Itraconazole

The effects of itraconazole 100 mg on the pharmacokinetics of lovastatin 40 mg have been studied in a randomized, placebo-controlled, crossover study in 10 healthy volunteers (16). Itraconazole, even in this low dosage, greatly increased plasma concentrations of lovastatin and its active metabolite, lovastatin acid, and increased the C_{max} of lovastatin about 15-fold and the total AUC by more than 15-fold; similarly, the C_{max} and total AUC of lovastatin acid were increased about 12-fold and 15-fold respectively.

Macrolide antibiotics

Based on case reports or small studies, the potential for drug interactions between macrolides and lovastatin should be considered (17).

- Rhabdomyolysis, acute renal insufficiency, pancreatitis, ileus, livedo reticularis, and raised transaminase activities developed in a patient who had taken lovastatin for 7 years and took erythromycin before a dental procedure.
- Rhabdomyolysis requiring short-term dialysis occurred in a 57-year-old man with chronic renal insufficiency treated with lovastatin 40 mg/day, gemfibrozil 600 mg bd, and clarithromycin 500 mg tds (18).

In a review of the literature, three other reported instances of erythromycin and lovastatin interaction presenting with rhabdomyolysis, raised transaminase activities, and acute renal insufficiency were identified (19).

Quetiapine

Lovastatin caused prolongation of the QT interval in a patient taking quetiapine.

- A 46-year-old African-American woman with schizophrenia, taking quetiapine 800 mg/day and sertraline 100 mg/day, was given lovastatin 10 mg/day for dyslipidemia (20). Although 2 months later her lipid concentrations had improved, a routine electrocardiogram

showed prolongation of the QT_c interval to 569 milliseconds; it had been 416 milliseconds 6 months before. There were no electrolyte abnormalities and no history of cardiac conduction abnormalities. The dose of lovastatin was reduced to 5 mg/day and an electrocardiogram the next day showed a normal QT_c interval (424 milliseconds). Later she switched from lovastatin to niacin and subsequent electrocardiograms were all normal.

Probably lovastatin caused an increase in plasma quetiapine concentrations through competitive inhibition of CYP3A4.

References

1. Bradford RH, Shear CL, Chremos AN, Dujovne C, Downton M, Franklin FA, Gould AL, Hesney M, Higgins J, Hurley DP, et al. Expanded Clinical Evaluation of Lovastatin (EXCEL) study results. I. Efficacy in modifying plasma lipoproteins and adverse event profile in 8245 patients with moderate hypercholesterolemia. Arch Intern Med 1991;151(1):43–9.
2. Jacobson RH, Wang P, Glueck CJ. Myositis and rhabdomyolysis associated with concurrent use of simvastatin and nefazodone. JAMA 1997;277(4):296–7.
3. Mantell G, Burke MT, Staggers J. Extended clinical safety profile of lovastatin. Am J Cardiol 1990;66(8):B11–5.
4. Muldoon MF, Barger SD, Ryan CM, Flory JD, Lehoczky JP, Matthews KA, Manuck SB. Effects of lovastatin on cognitive function and psychological well-being. Am J Med 2000;108(7):538–46.
5. Seong JJ, Wong TK. A case of acquired ichthyosis developed during cholesterol-lowering treatment. Korean J Dermatol 1997;35:546–50.
6. Park JH, Oh KS, Lee HJ, Whang KU. Ichthysiform skin eruptions possibly due to lovastatin (Mevacor). Korean J Dermatol 1999;37:535–7.
7. Hildebrand RD, Hepperlen TW. Lovastatin and hypospermia. Ann Intern Med 1990;112(7):549–50.
8. Tobert JA, Shear CL, Chremos AN, Mantell GE. Clinical experience with lovastatin. Am J Cardiol 1990;65(12):F23–6.
9. von Pohle WR. Recurrent hyperthermia due to lovastatin. West J Med 1994;161(4):427–8.
10. Azie NE, Brater DC, Becker PA, Jones DR, Hall SD. The interaction of diltiazem with lovastatin and pravastatin. Clin Pharmacol Ther 1998;64(4):369–77.
11. Masica AL, Azie NE, Brater DC, Hall SD, Jones DR. Intravenous diltiazem and CYP3A-mediated metabolism. Br J Clin Pharmacol 2000;50(3):273–6.
12. Aruna AS, Akula SK, Sarpong DF. Interaction between potassium-depleting diuretics and lovastatin in hypercholesterolemic ambulatory care patients. J Pharm Technol 1997;13:21–6.
13. Wong PW, Dillard TA, Kroenke K. Multiple organ toxicity from addition of erythromycin to long-term lovastatin therapy. South Med J 1998;91(2):202–5.
14. Garnett WR. Interactions with hydroxymethylglutaryl-coenzyme: a reductase inhibitors. Am J Health Syst Pharm 1995;52(15):1639–45.
15. Deltoro MG, Rocati G, Cavanilles CR, Cervellera AG, Catala JC, Belda JE, De Lelis FP, Rodena JV, Gonzalez EO, Ballester AH. Rhabdomyolysis and renal

failure due to lovastatin–gemfibrozil. A case report. Endocrinologia 1998;45:35–7.

16. Kivisto KT, Kantola T, Neuvonen PJ. Different effects of itraconazole on the pharmacokinetics of fluvastatin and lovastatin. Br J Clin Pharmacol 1998;46(1):49–53.

17. Ayanian JZ, Fuchs CS, Stone RM. Lovastatin and rhabdomyolysis. Ann Intern Med 1988;109(8):682–3.

18. Landesman KA, Stozek M, Freeman NJ. Rhabdomyolysis associated with the combined use of hydroxymethylglutaryl-coenzyme A reductase inhibitors with gemfibrozil and macrolide antibiotics. Conn Med 1999;63(8):455–7.

19. Wong PW, Dillard TA, Kroenke K. Multiple organ toxicity from addition of erythromycin to long-term lovastatin therapy. South Med J 1998;91(2):202–5.

20. Furst BA, Champion KM, Pierre JM, Wirshing DA, Wirshing WC. Possible association of QTc interval prolongation with co-administration of quetiapine and lovastatin. Biol Psychiatry 2002;51(3):264–5.

Nicotinic acid and derivatives

General Information

Nicotinic acid is an antilipidemic agent that effectively reduces serum concentrations of total cholesterol, low-density lipoprotein (LDL) cholesterol, very low density lipoprotein (VLDL) cholesterol, and triglycerides, and increases concentrations of high-density lipoprotein (HDL) cholesterol. It has been suggested that the marked lowering of serum cholesterol seen during treatment of dyslipidemia with nicotinic acid results from hepatotoxicity (1).

Nicotinic acid is also a potent vasodilator, probably by a direct action on smooth muscle cells. It produces cutaneous vasodilatation, itching of the skin, facial flushing, a sensation of feeling hot, pounding in the head, gastric irritation, diarrhea, raised transaminases, hyperglycemia, and hyperuricemia. These unpleasant adverse effects limit its acceptability for many patients. Nicotinic acid as such is not used in the treatment of vascular disorders, but some of its derivatives are, albeit with poor evidence of clinical efficacy.

Modified-release formulations of nicotinic acid do not appear to be better tolerated than regular formulations, flushing and itching being the most common adverse effects (SEDA-19, 206). There have also been several reports of hepatotoxicity with this form of the drug (SEDA-16, 438). Other adverse effects are hepatotoxicity (apparently a dose-related direct toxic effect), hyperglycemia, and hyperuricemia. It has been questioned whether the modified-release formulation, which is available over the counter in some countries, ought to continue to be available for self-medication in view of its serious adverse effects (2,3).

Given its many adverse reactions, the safety of using nicotinic acid continues to be discussed. Some are of the opinion that it should only be given to patients with marked dyslipidemia and under close monitoring, and that the initial expectations of fewer adverse reactions

with the modified-release form of the drug do not seem to have been borne out in practice (4,5). Others recommend its continued use (6,7). A general warning against indiscriminate use of nicotinic acid as a vitamin supplement has been given (8).

In two studies of accelerated radiotherapy with carbogen and nicotinamide in patients with cancer the adverse effects of nicotinamide have been documented (9,10). In the first study, 62 patients with stage III-IV laryngeal carcinoma were treated with accelerated radiotherapy (total radiation 64 Gy) combined with carbogen breathing in 11 patients and with both carbogen and nicotinamide (Arcon) in 51 patients. Adverse effects attributed to nicotinamide in the 51 patients were nausea in 35 patients, vomiting in 20, flushing, dizziness, epigastric pain, and headache in two patients each, and gastrointestinal bleeding, sweating, fatigue, and emotional disturbances in one patient each.

In the second study nicotinamide (Nicobion) 6 g was given in tablet form to 15 patients with advanced head and neck and non-small cell lung carcinomas 90 minutes before radiotherapy. Toxicity (nausea and vomiting) did not correlate with any of the pharmacokinetic parameters, such as t_{max}, C_{max}, half-life, or AUC. Gastrointestinal toxicity reached grade 1 (nausea not requiring antiemetics) in four patients, grade 2 (nausea and/or vomiting requiring antiemetics) in four patients, and grade 3 (nausea and/or vomiting requiring nasogastric intubation or parenteral support) in two patients.

It has been hypothesized that long-term survival after recovery from myocardial infarction could be improved with only 1 g of nicotinic acid daily (11).

The beneficial and adverse effects of nicotinic acid (niacin) have been reviewed (12). Standard nicotinic acid from an immediate-release formulation is metabolized primarily by conjugation, which results in a high frequency of flushing. Long-acting nicotinic acid is metabolized through the nicotinamide pathway, which results in less flushing but increases the risk of hepatotoxicity. Modified-release nicotinic acid, on the other hand, has a more balanced metabolism and causes fewer of both types of adverse effects.

Nicotinic acid derivatives

Nicotinic acid derivatives include acipimox, aluminium nicotinate, nicotinyl alcohol, and xanthinol nicotinate. The adverse effects of these compounds appear to be identical to those of nicotinic acid.

Acipimox (S-methylpyrazine-2-carboxylic acid 4-oxide) is structurally related to nicotinic acid. Flushing and gastrointestinal disturbances, but there were no effects on blood glucose or uric acid in 7137 patients, of whom 15% stopped taking the drug because of adverse effects (13). In another open study blood glucose was on average slightly lowered in 3009 patients with type 2 diabetes given acipimox for at least 2 months (14).

Acipimox had to be withdrawn in 10 of 32 patients with hypertriglyceridemia, excessive hypertriglyceridemia, and combined hyperlipidemia because of adverse effects or absence of clinical response (15). The other 22 completed

6 months of treatment with no adverse effects. The authors claimed that acipimox is much better tolerated than nicotinic acid, that it has fewer adverse effects, and can therefore be used as a second-line drug.

Aluminium nicotinate perhaps causes slightly less gastrointestinal distress than nicotinic acid, but the same can be achieved by buffering the acid, and neither approach in fact solves the problem, which is probably not primarily one of acidity.

Severe toxicoderma has been reported with xanthinol nicotinate and confirmed by a provocation test (SEDA-1, 333). Flushing is claimed to be less frequent with xanthinol nicotinate than with nicotinic acid, but has nevertheless been repeatedly observed, and its other adverse effects are likely to be the same as those of nicotinic acid.

Organs and Systems

Cardiovascular

Symptoms observed after high doses of nicotinic acid (such as giddiness, faintness, and vasovagal attacks) result from dilatation of the small arteries and arterioles, resulting in reduced peripheral resistance and blood pressure (6). Flushing occurs transiently in all patients and persists in 10-15% of cases. When starting with a high dose, hypotension can occur (16). The flushing of the skin with pruritus is transitory.

Coronary steal with worsening of myocardial ischemia related to vasodilatation has been reported in a patient taking nicotinic acid (17), which should therefore perhaps be withheld in patients with unstable angina.

Nervous system

Electroencephalographic abnormalities associated with vitamin B therapy have been reported (SEDA-15, 412; 18). Tingling of the fingertips, faintness, and dizziness have been observed. Peripheral neuropathy has been reported (19). Tingling in the orofacial region has been attributed to a neuropathic effect, but this could have been due to vasodilatation.

Sensory systems

Ocular adverse effects of nicotinic acid include sicca syndrome, blurred vision, and eyelid edema.

A few cases of advanced cystoid macular edema have been reported in the older literature; these took months to resolve once nicotinic acid was withdrawn (SEDA-14, 331; SEDA-20, 191; 15,20). Four new cases have been added in patients who took nicotinic acid 2-4.5 g/day (21,22). The first symptoms of blurred vision appeared 1-18 months after the start of therapy. Withdrawal of nicotinic acid resulted in improvement of visual acuity and resolution of the cystoid macular edema within 1-2 months. A particular feature that distinguishes this form of maculopathy is the absence of leakage on fluorescein angiography. Retinal edema, when it occurs, will abate on withdrawal of nicotinic acid (15).

Three cases of impaired vision occurred after the administration of high-dose nicotinic acid (23).

- A 51-year old man increased his dose of nicotinic acid from 1 to 4.5 g/day. Within 4 weeks, he noted blurred vision in both eyes. Nicotinic acid was discontinued and his vision improved within a month.
- A 53-year old man increased his dose of nicotinic acid from 1 to 3 g/day over a year. After he had been taking 3 g/day for 6 months, he noticed a gradual darkening of vision. His symptoms improved within 3 days of withdrawal.
- A 51-year old man took nicotinic acid 2 g bd. After 18 months he noted visual symptoms, which resolved within two months of withdrawal.

Endocrine

Prolonged administration of nicotinic acid can have a diabetogenic effect and decompensation of previously stable diabetes can occur. Severe hyperglycemia has been precipitated by nicotinic acid treatment of hyperlipidemia (24).

Metabolism

During long-term treatment with nicotinic acid, uric acid concentrations tend to rise slightly, but the change is clinically insignificant (25) .

Nicotinic acid has a hyperglycemic action (SED-13, 1330), and is therefore not recommended as a first-line hypolipidemic drug in patients with type 2 diabetes mellitus (26).

Lactic acidosis has been observed in patients taking nicotinic acid (SED-13, 1330).

Hematologic

- A 55-year-old man with localized prostate cancer was given pravastatin (10 mg/day) and aspirin (325 mg/day) (27). He also took food supplements containing about 30 different ingredients, most notably nicotinic acid 2250 g/day. During preparation for prostate surgery it was discovered that his prothrombin time was slightly prolonged (17 seconds, normal 11.4-14.4 seconds). All prescribed medications were withheld, but his prothrombin time continued to be abnormal (24 seconds).

The authors thought that the high dose of nicotinic acid had caused this abnormality.

Intravenous administration of nicotinic acid or nicotinyl alcohol tartrate can cause short-lived fibrinolytic activity (28).

Teeth

Two patients complained of dental and gingival pain, not previously reported adverse effects of nicotinic acid (29). The pain abated on withdrawal and in one case recurred on rechallenge.

Gastrointestinal

General gastrointestinal symptoms include heartburn, vomiting, persistent nausea (30), abdominal pain, and hunger pains.

In patients with squamous cell carcinomas of the head and neck accelerated radiotherapy with carbogen and nicotinamide 6 g/day (ARCON) was carried out to determine the feasibility and the adverse effects of this therapeutic approach (31). Accelerated fractionation was combined with carbogen (n = 11), daily nicotinamide (n = 10), or both (n = 17). There were no significant differences in local adverse effects in the three groups. Systemic adverse effects took the form of nausea or vomiting. The authors concluded that in future ARCON trials a lower dose of nicotinamide will be needed to reduce severe upper gastrointestinal toxicity.

Of 61 patients with ischemic heart disease and dyslipidemia treated with nicotinic acid 1.5 and 3.0 g/day, 32 patients were withdrawn, 18 because of adverse effects and 14 for reasons not related to nicotinic acid (32). Of the 29 patients who finished the study, adverse effects included dryness of the skin (14%), acanthosis nigricans (10%), fatigue (6.9%), nausea (6.9%), abdominal pain (3.4%), diarrhea (3.4%), and anorexia (3.4%); the figures in parentheses were the incidences at 33 weeks. Flushing occurred more often at 18 weeks than at 33 weeks (24 versus 6.9%), as did pruritus (35 versus 28%), suggesting tolerance to these effects.

Liver

Nicotinic acid is hepatotoxic, and it is suspected that the modified-release formulation increases the risk (SED-13, 1330; 33).

Late adverse effects include hepatic dysfunction, with altered liver function tests and hyperbilirubinemia. After prolonged use of nicotinic acid and nicotinyl alcohol, histological changes, for example parenchymal cell injury, portal fibrosis, cholangitis, cholestasis, biliary casts, and lymphocytic infiltrations around the bile ducts, have occasionally been seen.

Rechallenge with crystalline formulations in people in whom liver damage has occurred with the modified-release formulation has been tolerated (34). However, three cases of hepatic dysfunction in patients taking crystalline nicotinic acid 1.5-3.0 g/day have been reported (1). They were all associated with a reduced ratio of esterified cholesterol to free cholesterol in LDL, a reduction in lecithin cholesteryl acyl transferase activity (LCAT), and other evidence of liver dysfunction, including prolonged prothrombin time. Transaminases were in the reference ranges. On reduction of the dosage or withdrawal of nicotinic acid all the abnormalities resolved within 4 weeks. Others have pointed out that some observations suggest that lipid-lowering with nicotinic acid always is part of a generalized hepatotoxic effect (1).

A "starry sky liver" has been reported in a patient with nicotinic acid-induced hepatitis (35).

- A 50-year-old man developed recurrent sharp lower abdominal pain and nausea, having taken modified-release nicotinic acid 500-2000 mg/day for 8 weeks for hypercholesterolemia. He had a low-grade fever, tachycardia, and hypotension. Abdominal ultrasonography showed a markedly hypoechoic liver of normal size,

with relatively echogenic conspicuous portal triads. Aspartate transaminase activity and prothrombin time were raised. Nicotinic acid was withdrawn and the signs and symptoms resolved within several days.

Nicotinic acid can cause hepatic steatosis and clinical hepatic abnormalities that together can simulate the presentation of hepatobiliary neoplasia (36).

- A 52-year-old man with long-standing tetraplegia, who had been taking oral nicotinic acid 2 g/day for several months, developed nausea, vomiting, and fever, raised liver enzymes and total and indirect bilirubin. Ultrasonography showed several hyperechoic intrahepatic lesions and CT scan showed several hypoattenuating lesions, some of which were associated with interrupted vessels and had convex borders, suggestive of a tumor. Other lesions had CT features typical of fatty infiltration of the liver. Niacin was withdrawn. The liver function tests normalized within 4 days and the nausea and vomiting abated. The hepatic lesions on CT scan improved within 1 month and resolved after 9 months.

Skin

Nicotinic acid disturbs the normal cornification of the skin, occasionally leading to reversible ichthyosis and acanthosis nigricans (SEDA-19, 206). Two mechanisms are advanced to explain this effect: insulin resistance induced by nicotinic acid, with compensatory hyperinsulinemia (which in turn leads to increased insulin binding to insulin-like growth factor receptors and stimulation of keratinocytes), or a disturbance of epidermal lipid homeostasis.

Skin problems can be persistent in a proportion of patients, variously estimated at 10-59%, and this can severely limit adherence to therapy. The skin reaction can be ameliorated by concomitant use of non-steroidal anti-inflammatory drugs such as aspirin and indometacin (SEDA-15, 412). Transient exanthems, pruritus, and sometimes wheals are seen, as well a uniform dryness and scaling of the epidermis, brown pigmentation, and even on occasion an acanthosis nigricans-like dermatosis (15). Persistent rashes can also occur. Doses in excess of 5 g/day are routinely associated with skin manifestations and can on occasion cause liver damage, gout and ulcer formation. These reactions can be associated with nicotinic acid rather than nicotinamide, which is sometimes recommended as an alternative (37). Increased hair loss has been described.

Musculoskeletal

Nicotinic acid has been associated with the development of myopathy with nocturnal leg aching and cramps, symptoms that can be exacerbated by simultaneous use of other lipid lowering drugs associated with similar adverse effects, or alcohol, which also has myopathic effects (SEDA-15, 413; 38).

Immunologic

Anaphylactic shock can occur with nicotinic acid (6).

A pseudoallergic reaction has been reported in a patient who took several nicotinic acid-containing formulations (39).

- A previously healthy 40-year-old woman developed a generalized macular erythematous rash associated with palpitation and light-headedness, recurring every few days. The rash started behind the neck and arms, with a sensation of tingling, progressing to a general feeling of heat. She felt ill and had to lie down until the episode subsided after 45-90 minutes, with residual fatigue for several hours. Laboratory findings were all in the reference ranges. She was taking two multivitamin tablets a day, each containing nicotinic acid 20 mg, one B complex tablet containing nicotinic acid 50 mg, and 1-3 tablets of an antiemetic containing nicotinic acid 50 mg. Thus, she had unknowingly taken nicotinic acid up to 240 mg/day. Graded oral challenge with nicotinic acid 20-200 mg reproduced her symptoms.

Drug Administration

Drug formulations

Since nicotinic acid can cause unpleasant flushing and other symptoms of vasodilatation, attempts have been made to develop modified-release formulations. Modified-released nicotinic acid formulations may be better tolerated than the immediate-release formulation, because they reduce the vasodilatory effects of the drug. However, the low frequency of flushing produced by modified-release formulations may be offset by an increased risk of hepatotoxicity. Some reports have suggested a higher frequency of hepatic dysfunction with traditional modified-release nicotinic acid formulations compared with immediate-release products (2, 40).

In a double-blind, placebo-controlled study of a modified-release formulation in 128 patients pruritus was reported in 10 patients taking nicotinic acid (11%) and rash in 9 patients (10%); there were no similar effects in those taking placebo (41).

In 517 patients taking a modified-release formulation the most commonly reported adverse events were headache in 92 patients (13%), pain in any part of the body except the abdomen in 46 (6%), abdominal pain in 54 (8%), diarrhea in 97 (13%), dyspepsia in 46 (6%), nausea in 72 (10%), vomiting in 38 (5%), rhinitis in 30 (4%), pruritus in 56 (8%), and rash in 51 (7%) (24).

In a study of the efficacy and tolerability of a modified-release formulation in 269 adults and 230 additional adults for whom short-term safety data were available, 13 of 269 patients (4.8%) withdrew because of flushing (42). During the first 4 weeks about half had flushing. The mean intensity was about 4.0 on a visual analogue scale (representing "none" to "intolerable"). Patients were encouraged to use aspirin prophylactically to minimize flushing. Other nicotinic acid-related adverse effects leading to withdrawal included nausea (3.3%) sometimes with vomiting, other gastrointestinal symptoms (1.5%), and pruritus (2.6%). Once case each of gout, acanthosis nigricans, headache, palpitation, raised glucose concentrations, and shoulder pain led to patient withdrawal. Certain adverse events thought to be associated with nicotinic acid were uncommon in the study group. There was one case of peptic ulcer, amblyopia occurred in three patients, and leg aches and myalgias in one patient taking nicotinic acid with simvastatin, with a normal creatine kinase activity.

The efficacy and adverse effects of a modified-release formulation have been studied in 32 patients with type 2 diabetes (43). Of 22 patients who completed 6 months of therapy, 17 took 1000 mg/day, three 1500 mg/day, and two 2000 mg/day. Seven of 32 patients discontinued therapy. Of these, three withdrew after 2, 5, and 6 months because of flushing and itching. Three other patients withdrew within 2 months because of nausea, diarrhea, and dyspepsia. One patient withdrew after 7 days because of increased blood glucose concentrations. There were no significant increases in mean transaminase activities, which remained within the reference ranges in all patients.

The safety and efficacy of escalating doses of modified-release tablets of nicotinic acid (Niaspan) have been evaluated in a multicenter, placebo-controlled study in 131 patients with primary hyperlipidemia (44). The dose of nicotinic acid was initially 375 mg/day, then 500 mg/day, and then increasing in 500 mg increments at 4-week intervals to a maximum of 3000 mg/day. Changes in biochemical measurements in patients taking nicotinic acid were significant only for uric acid and phosphorus. Fasting blood glucose, bilirubin, transaminases, alkaline phosphatase, lactate dehydrogenase, and amylase were not altered. Of the 131 patients, 80 completed the study. Of the patients who withdrew, 31 did so for medical reasons (3% taking nicotinic acid and 11% placebo). Eight of the 26 patients who stopped taking nicotinic acid withdrew because of flushing (all before the 2000 mg/day dose) and five because of a rash. These reasons accounted for half of the drop-outs with nicotinic acid. The number of patients who had episodes of flushing fell with each dose increment of nicotinic acid, suggesting tolerance. Of other adverse events, only nausea (18% and 9%), vomiting (10% and 2%), pruritus (11% and 0%), and rash (10% and 0%) were more common with nicotinic acid.

Drug-Drug Interactions

Ethanol

An apparent interaction between nicotinic acid and alcohol caused toxic delirium and lactic acidosis (45).

HMG co-A reductase inhibitors

Nicotinic acid increased the risk of rhabdomyolysis associated with HMG-CoA reductase inhibitors (SEDA-19, 206; 46).

Nicotine

An interaction between nicotinic acid and nicotine transdermal patches has also been observed, causing flushing and dizziness (47).

References

1. Effects of crystalline nicotinic acid-induced hepatic dysfunction on serum low-density lipoprotein cholesterol and lecithin cholesteryl acyl transferase. Am J Cardiol 1998;81(6):805–7.

2. McKenney JM, Proctor JD, Harris S, Chinchili VM. A comparison of the efficacy and toxic effects of sustained-vs immediate-release niacin in hypercholesterolemic patients. JAMA 1994;271(9):672–7.

3. Lasagna L. Over-the-counter niacin. JAMA 1994;271(9):709–10.

4. Gibbons LW, Gonzalez V, Gordon N, Grundy S. The prevalence of side effects with regular and sustained-release nicotinic acid. Am J Med 1995;99(4):378–85.

5. Crouse JR 3rd. New developments in the use of niacin for treatment of hyperlipidemia: new considerations in the use of an old drug. Coron Artery Dis 1996;7(4):321–6.

6. ASHP Therapeutic Position Statement on the safe use of niacin in the management of dyslipidemias. American Society of Health-System Pharmacists. Am J Health Syst Pharm 1997;54(24):2815–9.

7. Knopp RH. Clinical profiles of plain versus sustained-release niacin (Niaspan) and the physiologic rationale for nighttime dosing. Am J Cardiol 1998;82(12A):24U-28U; discussion 39U-41U.

8. Miller SM. Potential perils of niacin therapy. Clin Lab Sci 1991;4:156–8.

9. Kaanders JHAM, Pop LAM, Marres HAM, Liefers J, Van Den Hoogen FJA, Van Daal WAJ, Van Der Kogel AJ. Accelerated radiotherapy with carbogen and nicotinamide (ARCON) for laryngeal cancer. Radiother Oncol 1998; 48: 115–22.

10. Bernier J, Stratford MRL, Denekamp J, Dennis MF, Bieri S, Hagen F., Kocagöncü O, Bolla M, Rojas A. Pharmacokinetics of nicotinamide in cancer patients treated with accelerated radiotherapy: the experience of the co-operative group of radiotherapy of the European Organization for Research and Treatment of Cancer. Radiother Oncol 1998; 48: 123–33.

11. Luria MH. Atherosclerosis: the importance of HDL cholesterol and prostacyclin: a role for niacin therapy. Med Hypotheses 1990;32(1):21–8.

12. McKenney J. Niacin for dyslipidemia: considerations in product selection. Am J Health-Syst Pharm 2003;60:995–1005.

13. Ganzer BM. Langzeitstudie zu acipimox. Pharmazie 1990;135:31.

14. Lavezzari M, Milanesi G, Oggioni E, Pamparana F. Results of a phase IV study carried out with acipimox in type II diabetic patients with concomitant hyperlipoproteinaemia. J Int Med Res 1989;17(4):373–80.

15. Yeshurun D, Hamood H, Morad N, Naschitz J. Acipimox as a secondary hypolipidemia in combined hypertriglyceridemia and hyperlipidemia. Harefuah 2000; 138: 650–3.

16. Carlson LA. Nicotinic acid: the broad-spectrum lipid drug. J Drug Dev Suppl 1990;3:223–6.

17. Pasternak RC, Kolman BS. Unstable myocardial ischemia after the initiation of niacin therapy. Am J Cardiol 1991;67(9):904–6.

18. Santanelli P, Gobbi G, Albani F, Gastaut H. Apparition d'anomalies EEG chez deux patients en traitement chronique par des vitamines B. [Appearance of EEG abnormalities in two patients during long-term treatment with B vitamins.] Neurophysiol Clin 1988;18(6):549–53.

19. Ziajka PE, Wehmeier T. Peripheral neuropathy and lipid-lowering therapy. South Med J 1998;91(7):667–8.

20. Fraunfelder FW, Fraunfelder FT, Illingworth DR. Adverse ocular effects associated with niacin therapy. Br J Ophthalmol 1995;79(1):54–6.

21. Callanan D, Blodi BA, Martin DF. J Macular edema with nicotinic acid (niacin). J Am Med Assoc 1998; 279: 1702.

22. Devaney DM. Maculopathy induced by nicotinic acid. Clin Eye Vis Care 1998; 10: 67–71.

23. Anonymous. Nicotinic acid—visual loss. WHO Newsletter 1998; 11/12: 6.

24. Schwartz ML. Severe reversible hyperglycemia as a consequence of niacin therapy. Arch Intern Med 1993;153(17):2050–2.

25. Capuzzi DM, Guyton JR, Morgan JM, Goldberg AC, Kreisberg RA, Brusco OA, Brody J. Efficacy and safety of an extended-release niacin (Niaspan): a long-term study. Am J Cardiol 1998;82(12A):74U-81U; discussion 85U-86U.

26. Garg A, Grundy SM. Nicotinic acid as therapy for dyslipidemia in non-insulin-dependent diabetes mellitus. JAMA 1990;264(6):723–6.

27. D'Amico AV, Toupless G, Lopes L, Valentine KJ, Cormack RA, Tempany CM, Kumar S, Marks PJ. Self-administration of untested medical therapy for treatment of prostate cancer can lead to clinically significant adverse events. Int J Radiation Oncol Biol Phys 2002; 54: 1311–13.

28. Robertson BR. Effect of nicotinic acid on fibrinolytic activity in health, in thrombotic disease and in liver cirrhosis. Acta Chir Scand 1971;137(7):643–8.

29. Leighton RF, Gordon NF, Small GS, Davis WJ, Ward ES Jr. Dental and gingival pain as side effects of niacin therapy. Chest 1998; 114: 1472–4.

30. Kaanders JH, Pop LA, Marres HA, van der Maazen RW, van der Kogel AJ, van Daal WA. Radiotherapy with carbogen breathing and nicotinamide in head and neck cancer: feasibility and toxicity. Radiother Oncol 1995;37(3):190–8.

31. Bernier J, Denekamp J, Rojas A, Minatel E, Horiot J-C, Hamers H, Antognoni P, Dahl O, Richaud P, Van Glabbeke M, Pierart M. ARCON: Accelerated Radiotherapy with Carbogen and Nicotinamide in head and neck squamous cell carcinomas. The experience of the Co-operative Group of Radiotherapy of the European Organization for Research and Treatment of Cancer (EORTC). Radiother Oncol 2000; 55: 111–19.

32. Morato Hernandez MDL, Del Sagrario Ichazo Cerro M, Alvarado Vega AG, Zamora Gonzalez J, Cardoso Saldana GC, Posadas Romero C. Immediate release niacin in the treatment of ischemic heart disease. Arch Inst Cardiol Mex 2000; 70: 367–76.

33. Gibaldi M. Adverse drug effects. Perspect Clin Pharm 1991;9:3–8.

34. Henkin Y, Johnson KC, Segrest JP. Rechallenge with crystalline niacin after drug-induced hepatitis from sustained-release niacin. JAMA 1990;264(2):241–3.

35. Scheer MS, Perlmutter S, Ross W, Katz DS. Ultrasonographic findings in niacin-induced hepatitis. J Ultrasound Med 1999; 18: 321–3.

36. Kristensen T, Olcott EW. Effects of niacin therapy that simulate neoplasia: Hepatic steatosis with concurrent hepatic dysfunction. J Comput Assisted Tomogr 1999; 23: 314–7.

37. Warady B, Kriley M, Alon U, Hellerstein S. Nicotinic acid-induced flush. Perit Dial Int 1989;9(1):81–2.
38. Litin SC, Anderson CF. Nicotinic acid-associated myopathy: a report of three cases. Am J Med 1989;86(4):481–3.
39. Grouhi M, Sussman G. Pseudoallergic toxic reaction. Ann Allergy Asthma Immunol 2000; 85: 269–71.
40. Keenan JM, Fontaine PL, Wenz JB, Myers S, Huang ZQ, Ripsin CM. Niacin revisited. A randomized, controlled trial of wax-matrix sustained-release niacin in hypercholesterolemia. Arch Intern Med 1991;151(7):1424–32.
41. Goldberg AC. Clinical trial experience with extended-release niacin (Niaspan): dose-escalation study. Am J Cardiol 1998;82:35U-38U.
42. Guyton JR, Goldberg AC, Kreisberg RA, Sprecher DL, Superko HR, O'Connor CM. Effectiveness of once-nightly dosing of extended-release niacin alone and in combination for hypercholesterolemia. Am J Cardiol 1998;82:737–43.
43. Kane MP, Hamilton RA, Addesse E, Busch RS, Bakst G. Cholesterol and glycemic effects of Niaspan in patients with type 2 diabetes. Pharmacotherapy 2001; 21: 1473–8.
44. Goldberg A, Alagona DP Jr, Capuzzi DM, Guyton J, Morgan JM, Rodgers J, Sachson R, Samuel P. Multiple-dose efficacy and safety of an extended-release form of niacin in the management of hyperlipidemia. Am J Cardiol 2000;85:1100–5.
45. Schwab RA, Bachhuber BH. Delirium and lactic acidosis caused by ethanol and niacin coingestion. Am J Emerg Med 1991;9(4):363–5.
46. Reaven P, Witztum JL. Lovastatin, nicotinic acid, and rhabdomyolysis. Ann Intern Med 1988;109(7):597–8.
47. Rockwell KA Jr. Potential interaction between niacin and transdermal nicotine. Ann Pharmacother 1993;27(10):1283– 8.

Pravastatin

See also HMG Co-A reductase inhibitors

General Information

In a placebo-controlled study of 1142 hypercholesterolemic patients treated with pravastatin for 8–16 weeks, the numbers of "adverse drug experiences" were similar in the treated and untreated individuals (1). Rash was the only adverse clinical event that was different (4.0 versus 1.1%). However, in the same patients withdrawal of therapy during follow-up was thought to be necessary in 3.2% of those given pravastatin alone. Myopathy was observed in one instance only, and increases in creatine kinase activity in those taking pravastatin did not differ significantly from controls. There were marked persistent increases in transaminases in 1.1%, with no cases of symptomatic hepatitis. Pravastatin is believed to have a particularly low potential for nervous system-related adverse effects, as it has not been shown to enter the cerebrospinal fluid, and clinical experience suggests that muscle toxicity occurs less often with pravastatin than with lovastatin (2).

Organs and Systems

Respiratory

- A 41-year-old man, who had been taking pravastatin for 2 years, developed a hypersensitivity pneumonitis with eosinophilia; the symptoms gradually resolved after withdrawal of pravastatin (3).

Metabolism

- After short-term treatment with pravastatin, a 77-year-old woman transiently developed symptoms diagnosed as porphyria cutanea tarda (4).

Liver

Acute cholestatic hepatitis occurred after 7 weeks of pravastatin 20 mg/day. There was no evidence of allergy (5). It is possible that pravastatin enhances the toxicity of simultaneously administered drugs, for instance, metoprolol in the present case.

- A 64-year-old woman who was twice treated with pravastatin had cholestasis on both occasions with minimal hepatocellular injury (6).

Musculoskeletal

Although myopathy is rarely seen with pravastatin in clinical trials, it does occur.

- Rhabdomyolysis was suspected in a 67-year-old obese man with an acute myocardial infarction (7).
- A 37-year-old man with sarcoidosis developed marked myotonia during several years while he was taking pravastatin 20 mg/day (8). On drug withdrawal his symptoms improved after 2 months.

This association does not prove a causal relation. The authors of the second report pointed to previous observations of myotonia both in sarcoidosis and during the administration of various drugs.

Reproductive system

- A man taking pravastatin 20 mg/day for 3 months reported gynecomastia, which regressed after withdrawal of the drug; he was also taking allopurinol (9).

Drug–Drug Interactions

Diltiazem

The effects of co-administration of diltiazem, a potent inhibitor of CYP3A, on the pharmacokinetics of pravastatin have been evaluated in a randomized study in 10 healthy volunteers (10). Pravastatin is active alone and is not metabolized by CYP3A. Diltiazem did not alter the oral AUC, maximum serum concentration, or half-life of pravastatin.

Fibrate

Rhabdomyolysis can occur when pravastatin is combined with a fibrate (SEDA-21, 460; 11).

Itraconazole

The effects of itraconazole 200 mg on the pharmacokinetics of pravastatin have been studied in a randomized, double-blind, crossover study in 10 healthy volunteers (12). Itraconazole slightly increased the AUC and C_{max} of pravastatin, but the changes were not statistically significant; the half-life was not altered.

Warfarin

With concurrent administration of warfarin and pravastatin there was no evidence of an interaction as assessed by prothrombin time (13).

References

1. Newman TJ, Kassler-Taub KB, Gelarden RT, et al. Safety of pravastatin in long-term clinical trials conducted in the united states. J Drug Dev 1990;3:275–80.
2. Jungnickel PW, Cantral KA, Maloley PA. Pravastatin: a new drug for the treatment of hypercholesterolemia. Clin Pharm 1992;11(8):677–89.
3. Liscoet-Loheac N, Andre N, Couturaud F, Chenu E, Quiot JJ, Leroyer C. Une pneumopathie iatrogénique rapportée a la prise de pravastatine. [Hypersensitivity pneumonitis in a patient taking pravastatin.] Rev Mal Respir 2001;18(4 Pt 1):426–8.
4. Schindl A, Trautinger F, Pernerstorfer-Schon H, Konnaris C, Honigsmann H. Porphyria cutanea tarda induced by the use of pravastatin. Arch Dermatol 1998;134(10):1305–6.
5. Hartleb M, Rymarczyk G, Januszewski K. Acute cholestatic hepatitis associated with pravastatin. Am J Gastroenterol 1999;94(5):1388–90.
6. Batey RG, Harvey M. Cholestasis associated with the use of pravastatin sodium. Med J Aust 2002;176(11):561.
7. Offman EM, Sabawi N, Melendez LJ. Suspected pravastatin-induced rhabdomyolysis in a patient experiencing a myocardial infarction. Can. J Hosp Pharm 1998;51:233–5.
8. Riggs JE, Schochet SS Jr. Myotonia associated with sarcoidosis: marked exacerbation with pravastatin. Clin Neuropharmacol 1999;22(3):180–1.
9. Aerts J, Karmochkine M, Raguin G. Gynécomastie attributable à la pravastatine. [Gynecomastia due to pravastatin.] Presse Med 1999;28(15):787.
10. Azie NE, Brater DC, Becker PA, Jones DR, Hall SD. The interaction of diltiazem and pravastatin. Clin Pharmacol Ther 1998;64(4):369–77.
11. Colombo P, Olivetto L, Andreoni P. Rabdiomiolisi acuta in corso di trattamento combinato con pravastatina e bezafibrato. Considerationi su un caso clinico. G Gerontol 1996;44:399–402.
12. Neuvonen PJ, Kantola T, Kivisto KT. Simvastatin but not pravastatin is very susceptible to interaction with the CYP3A4 inhibitor itraconazole. Clin Pharmacol Ther 1998;63(3):332–41.
13. Catalano P. Pravastatin safety: an overview. Round Table Ser 1990;16:26–31.

Probucol

General Information

The adverse effects of probucol have been reviewed (1). As the Probucol Quantitative Regression Swedish Trial (PQRST) showed no improvement in lumen volume of the femoral artery in patients given probucol plus colestyramine, as compared with those given colestyramine alone, doubt has been raised about its efficacy (2).

Organs and Systems

Cardiovascular

Prolongation of the QT interval has been seen and 16 cases of tachydysrhythmias, especially torsade de pointes, have been reported in association with probucol, 15 cases in women (SEDA-13, 1331; 3,4).

Gastrointestinal

According to long-term studies covering 7–9 years, probucol seems to be well tolerated with a reasonably low incidence of adverse effects. All the documented adverse effects were concentrated in the gastrointestinal tract. The incidence of diarrhea fell from 19% in the first year to 5% in the next. Only in some 3% of cases do symptoms such as diarrhea or abdominal pain lead to withdrawal of treatment. Diarrhea and flatulence, which resolve after a few months, are common.

References

1. Zimetbaum P, Eder H, Frishman W. Probucol: pharmacology and clinical application. J Clin Pharmacol 1990;30(1):3–9.
2. Sasich LD, Sukkari SR. Probucol—lack of efficacy and market withdrawals. Saudi Pharm J 1997;5:72–3.
3. Gohn DC, Simmons TW. Polymorphic ventricular tachycardia (torsade de pointes) associated with the use of probucol. N Engl J Med 1992;326(21):1435–6.
4. Matsuhashi H, Onodera S, Kawamura Y, Hasebe N, Kohmura C, Yamashita H, Tobise K. Probucol-induced QT prolongation and torsades de pointes. Jpn J Med 1989;28(5):612–5.

Simvastatin

See also HMG Co-A reductase inhibitors

General Information

Simvastatin is an HMG Co-A reductase inhibitor. Its most serious adverse effect is rhabdomyolysis, which is enhanced by other drugs that inhibit CYP3A4 (1).

Organs and Systems

Cardiovascular

Transient hypotension attributable to simvastatin may have been related to reduced production of corticosteroids (2).

Respiratory

Hypersensitivity reactions can occur with statins (SEDA-13, 1328; 3), and an otherwise unexplained case of interstitial lung disease and pleural effusion developed during treatment with simvastatin for 6 months; the number of eosinophils in the bronchoalveolar lavage fluid normalized a few days after withdrawal (4).

Psychological, psychiatric

In the 4S study there were five suicides in the simvastatin group and four in controls (5).

Endocrine

In 521 patients taking simvastatin 40–80 mg/day, serum cortisol concentrations were on average reduced by 3–7% (6). In the men there was a 10% fall in serum testosterone. However, there were no reports of sexual dysfunction.

Simvastatin up to 40 mg/day was given to 98 boys and 75 girls, aged 10–17 years, for 48 weeks without any adverse effects beyond a small fall in dehydroepiandrosterone (7). Of special note was the observation that simvastatin had no adverse effects on growth or pubertal development.

Metabolism

- A 53-year-old man taking simvastatin 40 mg/day developed rhabdomyolysis and hepatitis and had a raised serum lactate concentration (8.3 mmol/l; reference range 0.5–2.2) (8). Everything resolved 7 days after drug withdrawal.

Lactic acidosis in this patient supports the view that interference with the mitochondrial respiratory chain may play a role in the toxicity of the statins.

Hematologic

Thrombocytopenia is a rare adverse effect of simvastatin (9).

- Severe thrombocytopenia occurred in a 75-year-old woman taking simvastatin 5 mg/day and was resistant to therapy until she developed pneumonia. Recovery from the thrombocytopenia coincided with an increased interleukin concentration in the blood (10).
- There was a close temporal association with thrombotic thrombocytopenic purpura in a 43-year-old man after his second dose of simvastatin (11).

Other cases have been reported (12–15).

Liver

Cholestatic hepatitis occurred in a man with cirrhosis of the liver given simvastatin 20 mg/day (16).

Pancreas

Pancreatitis has been reported with simvastatin (17–22).

Urinary tract

It has been claimed that physicians should bear in mind the nephrotoxic potential of this drug (23), but there is no definite evidence that simvastatin is associated with the development of proteinuria (24).

Skin

Generalized exanthematous pustulosis was believed to have been due to simvastatin 20 mg/day for 2 weeks, in that oral rechallenge produced pustular lesions within 3 hours in a 57-year-old man (25).

- A 63-year-old man took simvastatin for hypercholesterolemia for 2 months and 1 month later developed a pruriginous and bullous lichenoid eruption (26). Histological and direct immunofluorescent features were consistent with the diagnosis of lichen planus pemphigoides. Western blot analysis showed antibodies against a 180 kDa antigen. All the lesions disappeared gradually after simvastatin was withdrawn.
- A 66-year-old man had persistent photosensitivity after using simvastatin intermittently (27). The clinical, histopathological, and photobiological features met the criteria for chronic actinic dermatitis.

Musculoskeletal

Rhabdomyolysis has been reported in patients taking simvastatin (28,29). Of 66 patients who took simvastatin for 1 year, two had myalgia and weakness with creatine kinase activity above 3000 (normally less than 100) (30).

- Simvastatin 5 mg/day caused rhabdomyolysis in a 61-year-old man not taking interacting drugs (31).

In a meta-analysis of megatrials with simvastatin, the overall incidence of myopathy was 0.025% (32). The authors suggested that potent inhibitors of CYP3A4 greatly increase the risk, but that weak inhibitors do not. Episodes of gout occurred in three of nine patients with chronic renal insufficiency who took simvastatin (33).

Immunologic

Lupus-like syndrome has been associated with simvastatin, with antibodies to double-stranded DNA in the serum (34).

- Simvastatin-induced lupus erythematosus was suspected in a 79-year-old white man after 3 months (35). He had signs of pleuropericarditis that resolved within 2 weeks of withdrawal.

Second-Generation Effects

Teratogenicity

Of 169 women exposed to simvastatin during pregnancy, three delivered babies with malformations and there were two fetal deaths (36). These results are comparable to what would be expected in the general population. However, based on a general consideration of risk, statins should not be used during pregnancy and only in exceptional circumstances should they be given to any woman of childbearing age.

Drug–Drug Interactions

Amiodarone

An interaction of simvastatin with amiodarone has been described.

- A 63-year-old white man with insulin-dependent diabetes and recent coronary artery bypass surgery developed diffuse muscle pain with generalized muscular weakness after taking amiodarone 1 g/day for 10 days then 200 mg/day plus simvastatin 40 mg/day (37). He had a significant increase in creatine kinase activity, peaking at 40 392 U/l.

Amiodarone may be another drug that necessitates special caution if used with statins metabolized by CYP3A4.

Bosentan

Concomitant treatment with simvastatin and bosentan (the first orally active endothelin receptor antagonist) reduces exposure to simvastatin by about 40%, suggesting that in vivo bosentan is a mild inducer of CYP3A4 (38).

Calcium channel blockers

In a meta-analysis of megatrials of simvastatin, the overall incidence of myopathy was 0.025%; the same proportion of those with myositis had used calcium channel blockers as the proportion overall, suggesting that there is no important interaction between these two groups of drugs (32).

However, diltiazem interacts with lovastatin although not with pravastatin (SEDA-24, 511).

The interaction of diltiazem with simvastatin has been investigated in 135 patients attending a hypertension clinic (39). Cholesterol reduction in the 19 patients taking diltiazem was 33% compared with 25% in the other 116 patients (median difference 8.6%; 95% CI = 1.1, 12). Multivariate analysis showed that concurrent diltiazem therapy, age, and the starting dose of simvastatin were independent predictors of percentage cholesterol response. The authors concluded that patients who take both diltiazem and simvastatin may need lower doses of simvastatin to achieve the recommended reduction in cholesterol.

Results from two clinical studies of the interaction of diltiazem with simvastatin showed that diltiazem increased the C_{max} of simvastatin (40) and enhanced its cholesterol-reducing effect (39).

In 10 healthy volunteers taking oral simvastatin 20 mg/day, diltiazem 120 mg bd for 2 weeks significantly increased the simvastatin C_{max} 3.6-fold, the AUC 5-fold,

and the half-life 2.3-fold (40). There were no changes in the t_{max} of simvastatin or simvastatin acid.

Of 135 patients attending a hypertension clinic who were taking simvastatin for primary or secondary prevention of coronary heart disease, 19 were also taking diltiazem (39). The cholesterol reduction in the 19 patients taking diltiazem was significantly higher than in the other 116 (33 versus 25%), with less interindividual variability. Concurrent diltiazem therapy, age, and the starting dose of simvastatin were significant independent predictors of the percentage cholesterol response.

Rhabdomyolysis due to an interaction of simvastatin with diltiazem has been reported (41).

- A 75-year-old-man taking simvastatin 80 mg/day and diltiazem 240 mg/day developed extreme weakness and diffuse muscle pain. All drugs were withdrawn and he underwent hemodialysis. Within 3 weeks his muscle pain disappeared and he regained function in his legs. The activities of creatine kinase and transaminases gradually returned to normal, but he continued to need hemodialysis.

Ciclosporin

In a patient with glucocorticoid-resistant nephrotic syndrome taking simvastatin and ciclosporin, there was an increase in lactic dehydrogenase activity, suggesting tissue injury, in the absence of an increase in creatine kinase (42).

Danazol

A potential drug interaction between simvastatin and danazol, causing rhabdomyolysis and acute renal insufficiency, has been reported (43). Rhabdomyolysis can occur with all statins when they are used alone and particularly when they are combined with other drugs that are themselves myotoxic or that increase the concentration of the statin. Statins are particularly susceptible to the latter effect because of their metabolism by the CYP450 system and their low oral systemic availability.

Gemfibrozil

- Severe rhabdomyolysis occurred in a 52-year-old woman taking a combination of gemfibrozil and simvastatin (44).

Grapefruit juice

Simvastatin should be avoided in patients using grapefruit juice (45).

In a randomized, two-phase, controlled, crossover study in 10 healthy volunteers one glass of grapefruit juice, taken daily for 3 days considerably increased the plasma concentrations of simvastatin and simvastatin acid (46).

Itraconazole

Itraconazole probably inhibits simvastatin metabolism (SEDA 21, 459).

The effects of itraconazole 200 mg on the pharmacokinetics of simvastatin have been studied in a randomized, double-blind, crossover study in 10 healthy volunteers (47). Itraconazole increased the C_{max} and AUC of simvastatin and simvastatin acid at least 10-fold. The C_{max} and AUC of total simvastatin acid (naive simvastatin acid plus that derived by hydrolysis of the lactone) were increased 17-fold and 19-fold respectively, and the half-life was increased by 25%.

In two cases, rhabdomyolysis was caused by itraconazole in heart transplant recipients taking long-term ciclosporin and simvastatin (48,49). To avoid severe myopathy, ciclosporin concentrations should be monitored frequently and statins should be withdrawn or the dosage should be reduced, as long as azoles need to be prescribed in transplant recipients. Patients need to be educated about signs and symptoms that require immediate physician intervention.

Macrolide antibiotics

Erythromycin interacts with simvastatin, probably by inhibiting its metabolism by CYP3A4. In a randomized, double-blind crossover study in 12 healthy volunteers, erythromycin significantly increased mean peak serum concentration and AUC for both unchanged simvastatin and its active metabolite simvastatin acid. However, there was extensive interindividual variability in the extent of this interaction (50).

Lovastatin has been reported to interact with clarithromycin (SEDA-14, 1531) (51), and a similar reaction has been observed with simvastatin (52).

- A 64-year-old African-American man developed worsening renal insufficiency, raised creatine kinase activity, diffuse muscle pain, and severe muscle weakness. He had been taking simvastatin for about 6 months and clarithromycin for sinusitis for about 3 weeks. He was treated aggressively with intravenous hydration, sodium bicarbonate, and hemodialysis. A muscle biopsy showed necrotizing myopathy secondary to a toxin. He continued to receive intermittent hemodialysis until he died from infectious complications 3 months after admission.

A case-control analysis of 7405 cases and 28 327 controls suggested that concomitant use of simvastatin and erythromycin is associated with an increased risk of cataract (53). Studies in dogs have shown that some statins are associated with cataract when given in excessive doses (54).

A 49-year-old man developed rhabdomyolysis after taking simvastatin 80 mg/day combined with clarithromycin 500 mg bd for 6 weeks (55). This effect was probably causal according to the Naranjo algorithm.

Meglitinides

Concomitant treatment with the CYP3A4 substrate simvastatin altered the mean AUC and mean C_{max} of repaglinide by 2 and 27% respectively (56).

Rifamycins

Rifampicin greatly reduced the plasma concentrations of simvastatin and simvastatin acid in 10 healthy volunteers in a randomized, crossover study (57). Because the half-life of simvastatin was not affected by rifampicin, induction of CYP3A4-mediated first-pass metabolism of simvastatin in the intestine and liver probably explains this interaction.

Thiazolidinediones

Troglitazone has been reported to reduce the effect of simvastatin, probably by induction of CYP3A4 (58).

Warfarin

An interaction with warfarin with resulting acute rhabdomyolysis has been observed in a patient taking simvastatin (59). This has not been observed with other statins.

References

1. Kivisto KT, Kantola T, Neuvonen PJ. Different effects of itraconazole on the pharmacokinetics of fluvastatin and lovastatin. Br J Clin Pharmacol 1998;46(1):49–53.
2. French J, White H. Transient symptomatic hypotension in patients on simvastatin. Lancet 1989;2(8666):807–8.
3. Tobert JA, Shear CL, Chremos AN, Mantell GE. Clinical experience with lovastatin. Am J Cardiol 1990;65(12):F23–6.
4. De Groot RE, Willems LN, Dijkman JH. Interstitial lung disease with pleural effusion caused by simvastatin. J Intern Med 1996;239(4):361–3.
5. Pedersen TR, Tobert JA. Benefits and risks of HMG-CoA reductase inhibitors in the prevention of coronary heart disease: a reappraisal. Drug Saf 1996;14(1):11–24.
6. Stein EA, Davidson MH, Dobs AS, Schrott H, Dujovne CA, Bays H, Weiss SR, Melino MR, Stepanavage ME, Mitchel YB. Efficacy and safety of simvastatin 80 mg/day in hypercholesterolemic patients. The Expanded Dose Simvastatin U.S. Study Group Am J Cardiol 1998;82(3):311–6.
7. de Jongh S, Ose L, Szamosi T, Gagne C, Lambert M, Scott R, Perron P, Dobbelaere D, Saborio M, Tuohy MB, Stepanavage M, Sapre A, Gumbiner B, Mercuri M, van Trotsenburg AS, Bakker HD, Kastelein JJSimvastatin in Children Study Group. Efficacy and safety of statin therapy in children with familial hypercholesterolemia: a randomized, double-blind, placebo-controlled trial with simvastatin. Circulation 2002;106(17):2231–7.
8. Goli AK, Goli SA, Byrd RP Jr, Roy TM. Simvastatin-induced lactic acidosis: a rare adverse reaction? Clin Pharmacol Ther 2002;72(4):461–4.
9. McCarthy LJ, Dlott JS, Orazi A, Waxman D, Miraglia CC, Danielson CF. Thrombotic thrombocytopenic purpura: yesterday, today, tomorrow. Ther Apher Dial 2004;8(2):80–6.
10. Yamada T, Shinohara K, Katsuki K. Severe thrombocytopenia caused by simvastatin in which thrombocyte recovery was initiated after severe bacterial infection. Clin Drug Invest 1998;16:172–4.
11. McCarthy LJ, Porcu P, Fausel CA, Sweeney CJ, Danielson CF. Thrombotic thrombocytopenic purpura and simvastatin. Lancet 1998;352(9136):1284–5.
12. Possamai G, Bovo P, Santonastaso M. Thrombocytopenic purpura during therapy with simvastatin. Haematologica 1992;77(4):357–8.
13. Koduri PR. Simvastatin and thrombotic thrombocytopenic purpura. Lancet 1998;352(9145):2020.
14. Groneberg DA, Barkhuizen A, Jeha T. Simvastatin-induced thrombocytopenia. Am J Hematol 2001;67(4):277.
15. Sundram F, Roberts P, Kennedy B, Pavord S. Thrombotic thrombocytopenic purpura associated with statin treatment. Postgrad Med J 2004;80(947):551–2.
16. Horiuchi Y, Maruoka H. Petechial eruptions due to simvastatin in a patient with diabetes mellitus and liver cirrhosis. J Dermatol 1997;24(8):549–51.
17. Ramdani M, Schmitt AM, Liautard J, Duhamel O, Legroux P, Gislon J, Pariente EA, Agay D, Faure D. Pancreatite aiguë à

la simvastatine: deux cas. [Simvastatin-induced acute pancreatitis: two cases.] Gastroenterol Clin Biol 1991;15(12):986.

18. Couderc M, Blanc P, Rouillon JM, Bauret P, Larrey D, Michel H. Un nouveau cas de pancréatite aiguë après la prise de simvastatine. [A new case of simvastatin-induced acute pancreatitis.] Gastroenterol Clin Biol 1991;15(12):986–7.

19. Andersen V, Sonne J, Andersen M. Spontaneous reports on drug-induced pancreatitis in Denmark from 1968 to 1999. Eur J Clin Pharmacol 2001;57(6–7):517–21.

20. McDonald KB, Garber BG, Perreault MM. Pancreatitis associated with simvastatin plus fenofibrate. Ann Pharmacother 2002;36(2):275–9.

21. Pezzilli R, Ceciliato R, Corinaldesi R, Barakat B. Acute pancreatitis due to simvastatin therapy: increased severity after rechallenge. Dig Liver Dis 2004;36(9):639–40.

22. Lons T, Chousterman M. La simvastatine: une nouvelle molécule responsable de pancréatite aiguë?. [Simvastatin: a new drug responsible for acute pancreatitis?.] Gastroenterol Clin Biol 1991;15(1):93–4.

23. Gorrie MJ, MacGregor MS, Rodger RS. Acute on chronic renal failure induced by simvastatin. Nephrol Dial Transplant 1996;11(11):2328–9.

24. La Belle P, Mantel G. Simvastatin and proteinuria. Lancet 1991;337(8745):864.

25. Oskay T. Acute generalized exanthematous pustulosis induced by simvastatin. Clin Exp Dermatol 2003;28:558–9.

26. Stoebner P. Lichen plan pemphigoide induit par la simvastatine. Ann Dermatol Venereol 2003;130:187–90.

27. Granados MT, de la Torre C, Cruces MJ, Pineiro G. Chronic actinic dermatitis due to simvastatin. Contact Dermatitis 1998;38(5):294–5.

28. Berland Y, Vacher Coponat H, Durand C, Baz M, Laugier R, Musso JL. Rhabdomyolysis with simvastatin use. Nephron 1991;57(3):365–6.

29. Deslypere JP, Vermeulen A. Rhabdomyolysis and simvastatin. Ann Intern Med 1991;114(4):342.

30. Emmerich J, Aubert I, Bauduceau B, Dachet C, Chanu B, Erlich D, Gautier D, Jacotot B, Rouffy J. Efficacy and safety of simvastatin (alone or in association with cholestyramine). A 1-year study in 66 patients with type II hyperlipoproteinaemia. Eur Heart J 1990;11(2):149–55.

31. Pershad A, Cardello FP. Simvastatin and rhabdomyolysis—a case report and brief review. J Pharm Technol 1999;15:88–9.

32. Gruer PJ, Vega JM, Mercuri MF, Dobrinska MR, Tobert JA. Concomitant use of cytochrome P450 3A4 inhibitors and simvastatin. Am J Cardiol 1999;84(7):811–5.

33. Harris DC, Simons LA, Mitchell P, Stewart JH. Management of non-nephrotic hyperlipidaemia of chronic renal failure with simvastatin. Med J Aust 1991;155(8):573.

34. Noel B, Panizzon RG. Lupus-like syndrome associated with statin therapy. Dermatology 2004;208(3):276–7.

35. Khosla R, Butman AN, Hammer DF. Simvastatin-induced lupus erythematosus. South Med J 1998;91(9):873–4.

36. Freyssinges C, Ducrocq MB. Simvastatine et grossesse. [Simvastatin and pregnancy.] Therapie 1996;51(5):537–42.

37. Roten L, Schoenenberger RA, Krahenbuhl S, Schlienger RG. Rhabdomyolysis in association with simvastatin and amiodarone. Ann Pharmacother 2004;38(6):978–81.

38. Dingemanse J. Investigation of the mutual pharmacokinetic interactions between bosentan, a dual endothelin receptor antagonist, and simvastatin. Clin Pharmacokinet 2003;42:293–301.

39. Yeo KR, Yeo WW, Wallis EJ, Ramsay LE. Enhanced cholesterol reduction by simvastatin in diltiazem-treated patients. Br J Clin Pharmacol 1999;48(4):610–5.

40. Mousa O, Brater DC, Sunblad KJ, Hall SD. The interaction of diltiazem with simvastatin. Clin Pharmacol Ther 2000;67(3):267–74.

41. Peces R, Pobes A. Rhabdomyolysis associated with concurrent use of simvastatin and diltiazem. Nephron 2001;89(1):117–8.

42. Ogawa D, Maruyama K, Miyatake N, Kashihara N, Makino H. Concomitant use of simvastatin and cyclosporin A increases LDH in nephrotic syndrome. Nephron 1998;80(3):351–2.

43. Andreou ER. Potential drug interaction between simvastatin and danazol causing rhabdomyolysis. Can J Clin Pharmacol 2003;10:172-4.

44. Tal A, Rajeshawari M, Isley W. Rhabdomyolysis associated with simvastatin–gemfibrozil therapy. South Med J 1997;90(5):546–7.

45. Lilja JJ, Kivisto KT, Neuvonen PJ. Grapefruit juice–simvastatin interaction: effect on serum concentrations of simvastatin, simvastatin acid, and HMG-CoA reductase inhibitors. Clin Pharmacol Ther 1998;64(5):477–83.

46. Lilja JJ, Neuvonen M, Neuvonen PJ. Effects of regular consumption of grapefruit juice on the pharmacokinetics of simvastatin. Br J Clin Pharmacol 2004;58(1):56–60.

47. Neuvonen PJ, Kantola T, Kivisto KT. Simvastatin but not pravastatin is very susceptible to interaction with the CYP3A4 inhibitor itraconazole. Clin Pharmacol Ther 1998;63(3):332–41.

48. Vlahakos DV, Manginas A, Chilidou D, Zamanika C, Alivizatos PA. Itraconazole-induced rhabdomyolysis and acute renal failure in a heart transplant recipient treated with simvastatin and cyclosporine. Transplantation 2002;73(12):1962–4.

49. Maxa JL, Melton LB, Ogu CC, Sills MN, Limanni A. Rhabdomyolysis after concomitant use of cyclosporine, simvastatin, gemfibrozil, and itraconazole. Ann Pharmacother 2002;36(5):820–3.

50. Kantola T, Kivisto KT, Neuvonen PJ. Erythromycin and verapamil considerably increase serum simvastatin and simvastatin acid concentrations. Clin Pharmacol Ther 1998;64(2):177–82.

51. Grunden JW, Fisher KA. Lovastatin-induced rhabdomyolysis possibly associated with clarithromycin and azithromycin. Ann Pharmacother 1997;31(7–8):859–63.

52. Lee AJ, Maddix DS. Rhabdomyolysis secondary to a drug interaction between simvastatin and clarithromycin. Ann Pharmacother 2001;35(1):26–31.

53. Schlienger RG, Haefeli WE, Jick H, Meier CR. Risk of cataract in patients treated with statins. Arch Intern Med 2001;161(16):2021–6.

54. Bernini F, Poli A, Paoletti R. Safety of HMG-CoA reductase inhibitors: focus on atorvastatin. Cardiovasc Drugs Ther 2001;15(3):211–8.

55. Kahri AJ, Valkonen MM, Vuoristo MK, Pentikainen PJ. Rhabdomyolysis associated with concomitant use of simvastatin and clarithromycin. Ann Pharmacother 2004;38(4):719.

56. Hatorp V, Hansen KT, Thomsen MS. Influence of drugs interacting with CYP3A4 on the pharmacokinetics, pharmacodynamics, and safety of the prandial glucose regulator repaglinide. J Clin Pharmacol 2003;43(6):649–60.

57. Kyrklund C, Backman JT, Kivisto KT, Neuvonen M, Laitila J, Neuvonen PJ. Rifampin greatly reduces plasma simvastatin and simvastatin acid concentrations. Clin Pharmacol Ther 2000;68(6):592–7.

58. Lin JC, Ito MK. A drug interaction between troglitazone and simvastatin. Diabetes Care 1999;22(12):2104–6.

59. Mogyorosi A, Bradley B, Showalter A, Schubert ML. Rhabdomyolysis and acute renal failure due to combination therapy with simvastatin and warfarin. J Intern Med 1999;246(6):599–602.

ENDOCRINE AND METABOLIC ADVERSE EFFECTS OF NON-HORMONAL AND NON-METABOLIC DRUGS

Abacavir

While abacavir has been associated with hyperglycemia in individual cases (1), there were no significant effects on blood glucose concentration in clinical trials.

- A 47-year-old man, with normoglycemia and no family history of diabetes mellitus, who was taking highly active antiretroviral therapy, was given abacavir for treatment intensification. He became lethargic and hyperglycemic. Despite metformin and glibenclamide, the hyperglycemia continued. Abacavir was withdrawn, and within 2 weeks his blood glucose concentration returned to baseline and the hypoglycemic drugs were withdrawn.

This patient was also taking hydrochlorothiazide, but the time-course of onset and resolution were consistent with abacavir-induced hyperglycemia.

Acetylsalicylic acid

Aspirin lowers plasma glucose concentrations in C-peptide-positive diabetic subjects and in normoglycemic persons (2). This is of no clinical significance.

Adrenaline

Lactic acidosis has been observed, persisting for some hours after deliberate intravenous misuse of 20 mg adrenaline by an addict (SED-12, 308). Six of 19 patients who were given adrenaline for hypotension after undergoing cardiopulmonary bypass developed lactic acidosis, though the ultimate outcome was favorable (SEDA-22, 154).

Patients with hyperthyroidism are unduly sensitive to the effects of adrenaline (SEDA-14, 179).

Albumin

Acute normovolemic hemodilution to a hematocrit of 22% was performed in a prospective randomized study in 20 patients undergoing gynecological surgery (3). In one group 35% of the blood volume was replaced by 5% albumin while the other group received 6% hydroxyethyl starch solutions containing chloride concentrations of 150 and 15 mmol/l. Neither solution contained bicarbonate or citrate. After acute normovolemic hemodilution the blood volume remained constant in both groups. The plasma albumin concentration fell after hemodilution with hydroxyethyl starch and increased after hemodilution with albumin. There was a slight metabolic acidosis with hyperchloremia and a concomitant fall in anion gap in both groups. The acidosis, which was attributed to hyperchloremia and dilution of bicarbonate in the extracellular volume, was considered to be of no clinical relevance. The authors proposed that acidosis during acute normovolemic hemodilution can be avoided when the composition of electrolytes in colloid solutions is more physiological, as in lactate-buffered solutions.

Aldesleukin

Various hormonal and metabolic effects of aldesleukin are temporally related to hypotension. Transient serum rises in ACTH, cortisol, beta-endorphin, adrenaline and noradrenaline have been found, whereas there were no significant changes in the plasma concentrations of several other hormones (4).

An acute episode of adrenal insufficiency secondary to adrenal hemorrhage occurred in one patient receiving aldesleukin (5).

Thyroid

Since the first reports of hypothyroidism, a number of studies have reported the occurrence of thyroid dysfunction in patients receiving aldesleukin alone or in combination with LAK cells, interferon alfa, interferon gamma, or tumor necrosis factor alfa (SED-13, 1104; 6). Symptoms were usually observed after 2–4 months of treatment (7–9), and mostly consisted of moderate hypothyroidism, which resolved after immunotherapy withdrawal or thyroxine treatment (9,10). Patients treated with aldesleukin plus interferon alfa more commonly developed biphasic thyroiditis with subsequent hypothyroidism or hyperthyroidism (10–13).

The possibility of a positive correlation between the development of thyroid dysfunction and the probability of a favorable tumor response has been debated (7,9,14). The incidence of thyroid dysfunction did not correlate with the dose or the underlying disease, but increased with treatment duration (6). In a large survey of 281 cancer patients receiving low-dose (72 000 IU/kg) or high-dose (720 000 IU/kg) aldesleukin, up to 41% of previously euthyroid cancer patients developed thyroid dysfunction (15). Combined immunotherapy was also associated with more frequent thyroid disorders. Aldesleukin plus interferon alfa produced thyroid dysfunction in 20–91% of patients (6), and the incidence of laboratory thyroid dysfunction reached 100% in patients given five or six cycles of both cytokines (11). Aldesleukin plus interferon alfa also tended to be a risk factor for the development of biphasic thyroiditis (9).

Female sex and the presence of antithyroid antibodies correlated significantly with the development of thyroid disease (9,16). This, together with the findings of strong expression of HLA-DR antigens on thyrocytes or the presence of mononuclear cell infiltrates on histological examination of the thyroid, makes an autoimmune phenomenon likely (9,12). However, a possible direct effect of immunotherapy on thyroid hormonal function has also been suggested in patients who had no detectable thyroid antibodies. There was a significant decrease in TSH concentration, while thyroid autoantibodies were not significantly raised (17).

Reversible insulin-dependent diabetes mellitus has been described in a predisposed patient (SEDA-20, 334).

Aldesleukin can cause lipid disorders. Recurrent and marked hypocholesterolemia with reduced high- and low-density lipoproteins, and slight increases in plasma triglycerides have been observed after high-dose aldesleukin (SEDA-21, 375) (4).

Alemtuzumab

Nine of 27 patients with multiple sclerosis developed antibodics against the thyrotropin receptor and carbimazole-responsive autoimmune hyperthyroidism after a 5-day pulse of alemtuzumab, a finding that was not reported in patients treated for other disorders (18).

Alprazolam

Alprazolam can alter dehydroepiandrosterone and cortisol concentrations. Of 38 healthy volunteers who received a single intravenous dose of alprazolam 2 mg over 2 minutes (phase I), 15 of 25 young men (aged 22–35 years) and all 13 elderly men (aged 65–75 years) responded to alprazolam and agreed to participate in a crossover study of placebo and alprazolam infusion to plateau for 9 hours (19). Plasma samples at 0, 1, 4, and 7 hours were assayed for steroid concentrations. Alprazolam produced:

(a) significant increases in dehydroepiandrosterone concentrations at 7 hours in both the young and elderly men;
(b) significant reductions in cortisol concentrations;
(c) no change in dehydroepiandrosterone-S concentrations.

The results suggest that alprazolam modulates peripheral concentrations of dehydroepiandrosterone and that dehydroepiandrosterone and/or dehydroepiandrosterone-S may have an in vivo role in modulating GABA receptor-mediated responses.

In a double-blind, crossover, placebo-controlled study of the effects of alprazolam 5 mg and dehydroepiandrosterone (DHEA) 100 mg/day, alone and in combination, on hypothalamic–pituitary–adrenal axis activity in 15 men (aged 20–45 years; body mass index 20–25 kg/m^2), alprazolam significantly increased basal growth hormone and blunted the responses to exercise of plasma cortisol, ACTH, AVP, and DHEA (20). DHEA and alprazolam in combination significantly increased the growth hormone response to exercise. The authors concluded that DHEA and alprazolam up-regulate growth hormone during exercise, perhaps by blunting a suppressive (HPA axis) system and potentiating an excitatory (glutamate receptor) system.

In a parallel, double-blind, placebo-controlled study in 13 elderly women and 12 elderly men, alprazolam 0.5 mg bd for 3 weeks caused significant rises in inter-dose morning plasma cortisol concentrations in the women but not in the men (21). In addition, higher morning plasma cortisol concentrations were significantly associated with better cognitive performance. The authors concluded that elderly women had greater inter-dose activation of the hypothalamic–pituitary–adrenal axis during treatment with therapeutic doses of alprazolam than men, but they stated that this could have been related to drug withdrawal.

Aminoglycoside antibiotics

Aminoglycosides can stimulate the formation of reactive oxygen species (free radicals) both in biological and cell-free systems (22,23).

Amiodarone

Testes

Amiodarone can cause endocrine testicular dysfunction, as judged by increases in serum concentrations of FSH and LH and hyper-responsiveness to GnRH (24).

Syndrome of inappropriate ADH secretion

Amiodarone-induced hyponatremia, due to the syndrome of inappropriate secretion of antidiuretic hormone, is rare (SEDA-21, 199; 25). The mechanism is unknown. Unlike other adverse effects of amiodarone, it seems to occur rapidly and to resolve rapidly after withdrawal.

- A 63-year-old man reduced his dietary sodium intake to combat fluid retention and was taking furosemide 40 mg/day, spironolactone 50 mg/day, and enalapril 2.5 mg/day (26). He then took amiodarone 800 mg/day for 7 days and his serum sodium concentration fell to 119 mmol/l; his plasma vasopressin concentration was raised at 2.6 pmol/l. The dose of amiodarone was reduced to 100 mg/day, with fluid restriction; his sodium rose to 130 mmol/l and his vasopressin fell to 1.4 pmol/l.

- An 87-year-old man reduced his dietary sodium intake to combat fluid retention and was taking furosemide 40 mg/day and spironolactone 25 mg/day (26). He then took amiodarone 200 mg/day for 7 days and 100 mg/day for 8 days and his serum sodium concentration fell to 121 mmol/l; his plasma vasopressin concentration was raised at 11 pmol/l. Amiodarone was continued, with fluid restriction; his sodium rose to 133 mmol/l and his vasopressin fell to 2.4 pmol/l.

- A 67-year-old man, who had taken amiodarone 200 mg/day for 3 months, developed hyponatremia (serum sodium concentration 117 mmol/l) (27). He was also taking furosemide 20 mg/day, spironolactone 25 mg/day, and lisinopril 40 mg/day. His urine osmolality was 740 mosmol/kg with a normal serum osmolality. Fluid restriction was ineffective, but when amiodarone was withdrawn the sodium rose to 136 mmol/l.

- A 62-year-old woman with paroxysmal atrial fibrillation who had taken amiodarone 300 mg/day had a serum sodium concentration of 120 mmol/l with a normal serum potassium and a reduced serum osmolality (240 mmol/kg); the urinary sodium concentration was 141 mmol/l and the urine osmolality 422 mmol/kg (25). There was no evident cause of inappropriate secretion of ADH and within 5 days of withdrawal of amiodarone the serum sodium concentration had risen to 133 mmol/l and rose further to 143 mmol/l 14 days later. There was no rechallenge and no recurrence of hyponatremia during the next 6 months. Another case has been reported (28).

In some of these cases other factors may have contributed to the hyponatremia that amiodarone seems to have caused.

Thyroid gland

The effects of amiodarone on thyroid function tests and in causing thyroid disease, both hyperthyroidism and hypothyroidism, have been reviewed in the context of the use of perchlorate, which acts by inhibiting iodine uptake by the thyroid gland (29), and there have been several other reviews (30–34).

Effects on thyroid function tests

Amiodarone causes altered thyroid function tests, with rises in serum concentrations of T4 and reverse T3 and a fall in serum T3 concentration. This is due to inhibition of the peripheral conversion of T4 to T3, causing preferential conversion to reverse T3. These changes can occur in the absence of symptomatic abnormalities of thyroid function.

Hyperthyroidism

DoTS classification
Dose-relation: collateral effect
Time-course: delayed
Susceptibility factors: genetic (unoperated or palliated cyanotic congenital heart disease; beta-thalassemia major); sex (conflicting results); altered physiology (iodine intake, conflicting results)

Frequency

Apart from its effects on thyroid function tests, amiodarone is also associated with both functional hyperthyroidism and hypothyroidism, in up to 6% of patients. The frequency of thyroid disease in patients taking amiodarone has been retrospectively studied in 90 patients taking amiodarone 200 mg/day for a mean duration of 33 months (35). Hypothyroidism occurred in five patients and hyperthyroidism in 11. Hyperthyroidism became more frequent with time and was associated with recurrent supraventricular dysrhythmias in four of the 11 patients.

In a nested case-control analysis of 5522 patients with a first prescription for an antidysrhythmic drug and no previous use of thyroid drugs, cases were defined as all patients who had started a thyroid-mimetic or antithyroid drug no sooner than 3 months after the start of an antidysrhythmic drug and controls were patients with a comparable follow-up period who had not taken any thyroid drugs during the observation period (36). There were 123 patients who had started antithyroid drugs and 96 who had started a thyroid-mimetic drug. In users of amiodarone there was an adjusted odds ratios of 6.3 (95% CI = 3.9, 10) for hyperthyroidism compared with users of other antidysrhythmic drugs. Patients who were exposed to a cumulative dose of amiodarone over 144 g had an adjusted odds ratio of 13 (6, 27) for hyperthyroidism.

Mechanisms

Amiodarone causes two different varieties of hyperthyroidism (SEDA-23, 199), one by the effects of excess iodine in those with latent disease (so-called type 1 hyperthyroidism), the other through a destructive thyroiditis in a previously normal gland (so-called type 2 hyperthyroidism). The two varieties can be distinguished by differences in radio-iodine uptake by the gland: in type 1 hyperthyroidism radio-iodine uptake is normal or increased, whereas in type 2 it is reduced. In type 1 hyperthyroidism, thyroid ultrasound shows a nodular, hypoechoic gland of increased volume, whereas in type 2 the gland is normal. Type 1 typically responds to thionamides and perchlorate while type 2 responds to high-dose glucocorticoids.

Color-flow Doppler sonography can be of use in distinguishing the two types, because type 1 is associated with increased vascularity and type 2 is not. In a retrospective study of 24 patients with amiodarone-induced hyperthyroidism in an iodine-replete environment, 13 had little or no vascularity, of whom seven were prednisolone-responsive; of 11 patients with increased vascularity, four responded to antithyroid drugs alone and only one of seven responded to prednisolone (37). Euthyroidism was achieved twice as rapidly in patients with low vascularity than in those with increased vascularity. Thus, responsiveness to prednisolone was not consistently predicted by lack of vascularity, but the presence of flow appeared to correlate with non-responsiveness to prednisolone.

Iodine intake may be important in determining the type of amiodarone-induced thyroid disease. In 229 patients taking long-term amiodarone hyperthyroidism was more common (9.6 versus 2%) in West Tuscany, where dietary iodine intake is low, and hypothyroidism more common (22 versus 5%) in Massachusetts, where iodine intake is adequate (SEDA-10, 148; 38). However, other factors may play a part. In a retrospective inter-regional study in France there was a greater incidence of amiodarone-induced hyperthyroidism in the maritime areas Aquitaine and Languedoc–Roussillon, and a greater incidence of amiodarone-induced hypothyroidism in Midi–Pyrenees, a non-maritime area, in which iodine intake is lower than in Languedoc–Roussillon (39).

There have also been reports of painful thyroiditis associated with amiodarone (SEDA-15, 170).

Thyroid hormone-producing thyroid carcinoma is an uncommon cause of thyrotoxicosis. Precipitation of thyrotoxicosis by iodine-containing compounds in patients with thyroid carcinoma is rare, but has been attributed to amiodarone in a 77-year-old man with extensive hepatic metastases from a well-differentiated thyroid carcinoma (40).

Susceptibility factors

There has been a retrospective study of the frequency of amiodarone-associated thyroid dysfunction in adults with congenital heart disease (41). Of 92 patients who had taken amiodarone for at least 6 months (mean age 35, range 18–60 years), 36% developed thyroid dysfunction—19 became hyperthyroid and 14 hypothyroid. The mean dosage was 194 (100–300) mg/day, and the median duration of therapy was 3 (0.5–15) years. Female sex (OR = 3) and unoperated or palliated cyanotic congenital heart disease (OR = 7) were significant susceptibility factors for thyroid dysfunction. The risk was also dose-related. Although the authors conceded that they may have over-estimated the risk of thyroid dysfunction, because of the selected nature of the population they studied, the risks were markedly higher than in previous studies of older patients with acquired heart disease, despite a lower maintenance dosage of amiodarone.

In contrast, it has been suggested that men are more susceptible to hyperthyroidism due to amiodarone (42). Of 122 600 patients in 12 practices in the West Midlands in the UK, 142 men and 74 women were taking amiodarone and 27 (12.5%) had thyroid disease. Of those, 11 men (7.7%) and 4 women (5.4%) had hypothyroidism, a nonsignificant difference; however, 12 men (8.5%) had hyperthyroidism compared with no women. This difference is particularly striking because hyperthyroidism is usually more common in women.

Patients with beta-thalassemia major have an increased risk of primary hypothyroidism. In 23 patients with beta-thalassemia amiodarone was associated with a high risk of overt hypothyroidism (33 versus 3% in controls) (43). This occurred at up to 3 months after starting amiodarone. The risk of subclinical hypothyroidism was similar in the two groups. In one case overt hypothyroidism resolved spontaneously after withdrawal, but the other patients were given thyroxine. After 21–47 months of treatment three patients developed thyrotoxicosis, with remission after withdrawal. There were no cases of hyperthyroidism in the controls. The authors proposed that patients with beta-thalassemia may be more susceptible to iodine-induced hypothyroidism, related to an underlying defect in iodine in the thyroid, perhaps associated with an effect of iron overload.

Presentation

Many examples of hyperthyroidism due to amiodarone have been published.

- A 72-year-old woman with dilated cardiomyopathy was given amiodarone for fast atrial flutter and 6 months later developed abnormal thyroid function tests, with a suppressed TSH and a raised serum thyroxine. The autoantibody profile was negative and a thyroid uptake scan showed reduced uptake (44).

Despite the fact that she was clinically euthyroid, the authors suggested that this patient had amiodarone-induced hyperthyroidism. However, amiodarone inhibits the peripheral conversion of thyroxine to triiodothyronine; it can therefore increase the serum thyroxine and suppress the serum TSH, as in this case. On the other hand, the reduced uptake by the thyroid gland is consistent with type 2 amiodarone-induced hyperthyroidism. The authors did not report the serum concentrations of free thyroxine and triiodothyronine.

- A 67-year-old man took amiodarone 200 mg/day for 20 months, after which it was withdrawn; 8 months later his serum TSH was suppressed and the free thyroxine and free triiodothyronine were both raised; there were no thyroid antibodies and an ultrasound scan showed a diffuse goiter with a nodule in the right lobe and reduced iodine uptake (45). Histological examination of the nodule showed a papillary cancer.

The authors attributed these changes to an effect of amiodarone, but it is not clear that amiodarone-induced changes would have taken so long to become manifest after withdrawal. However, the diagnosis of type 2 amiodarone-induced hyperthyroidism was supported by a poor response to prednisone, potassium perchlorate, and methimazole. Lithium produced temporary benefit, but thyroidectomy was required.

- In five patients who presented in Tasmania during 1 year, all of whom were taking amiodarone 200 mg/day, serum TSH was undetectable and the free thyroxine and triiodothyronine concentrations were raised (46). In one case there was a low titer of TSH receptor antibodies and in another a high titer of antithyroid peroxidase antibodies. In all cases the hyperthyroidism was severe and occurred after at least 2 years of treatment with amiodarone. In one of two patients in whom it was measured the serum concentration of interleukin-6 was raised, as has been previously shown (SEDA-19, 193). In two cases the hyperthyroidism was refractory to treatment with propylthiouracil, lithium, and dexamethasone; in these cases thyroidectomy was required. Two patients responded to propylthiouracil, lithium, and dexamethasone, and one responded to carbimazole.

Amiodarone-induced hyperthyroidism can occasionally be fatal (47).

- A 62-year-old man took amiodarone for 2 years and developed hyperthyroidism; carbimazole 40 mg/day, prednisolone, lithium, and colestyramine were ineffective and he died with hepatic encephalopathy and multiorgan failure.
- A 55-year-old man took amiodarone for 4 years and developed hyperthyroidism; carbimazole 60 mg/day, prednisolone, and lithium were ineffective and he died with septicemia and multiorgan failure.

In three other cases reported in the same paper, severe hyperthyroidism responded severally to treatment with carbimazole, carbimazole plus lithium, or propylthiouracil. In one case amiodarone therapy was restarted after prophylactic subtotal thyroidectomy.

Diagnosis

The diagnosis of amiodarone-induced thyroid disorders can be difficult, because amiodarone often alters thyroid function tests without disturbing clinical thyroid function. Although radio-iodine uptake by the thyroid gland is not helpful in making a diagnosis, the discharge of iodine from the thyroid gland in response to perchlorate is reduced in patients with hypothyroidism (48). The test is not abnormal in patients with hyperthyroidism and it is not clear how helpful it is in hypothyroidism.

Since the measurement of serum T3 and T4 concentrations may not be helpful, an alternative would be to measure metabolic status. Measurement of the serum concentration of co-enzyme Q10 may distinguish patients with clinical thyroid dysfunction from those who simply have abnormalities of thyroid function tests (49), but the value of this test remains to be established.

Color-flow Doppler sonography of the thyroid and measurement of serum interleukin-6 (IL-6) have been studied as diagnostic tools in a retrospective case-note study of patients with amiodarone-associated hyperthyroidism (50). There were 37 patients with amiodarone-associated hyperthyroidism (mean age 65, range 20–86 years), and 25 underwent color-flow Doppler sonography. Of those, 10 were classified as type 1 (based on increased vascularity) and 10 as type 2 (based on patchy or reduced vascularity); 5 were indeterminate. In those with type 1 hyperthyroidism, free serum thyroxine tended to be lower (52 versus 75 pmol/l), free serum triiodothyronine was lower (8.8 versus 16 pmol/l), the cumulative amiodarone dose was lower (66 versus 186 g), and less prednisolone was used (because the diagnosis of type 1 disease encouraged steroid withdrawal); however, carbimazole doses were not different and the time to euthyroidism was the same in the two groups (81 versus 88 days). IL-6 was raised in two patients with type 1 and in one patient with type 2 hyperthyroidism. The authors proposed that color-flow Doppler sonography could be used to distinguish the two subtypes, confirming an earlier report (51), but that IL-6 measurement was unhelpful.

Management
The treatment of amiodarone-induced hyperthyroidism is difficult. It often does not respond to conventional therapy with carbimazole, methimazole, or radio-iodine. However, corticosteroids and the combination of methimazole with potassium perchlorate have been reported to be effective (52), even if amiodarone is continued (53). Other regimens that have been used include combinations of corticosteroids with carbimazole (54), corticosteroids and benzylthiouracil (55), or propylthiouracil (SEDA-15, 170). Potassium perchlorate has also been used (SEDA-21, 199). Other forms of treatment that have been successful have been plasma exchange and in very severe cases subtotal thyroidectomy (56) or total thyroidectomy (SEDA-15, 170; SEDA-17, 220; 57).

It has been suggested that potassium perchlorate should be used in the treatment of type 1 hyperthyroidism and glucocorticoids in the treatment of type 2 (SEDA-21, 199). Since hypothyroidism due to amiodarone tends to occur in areas in which there is sufficient iodine in the diet, it has been hypothesized that an iodinated organic inhibitor of hormone synthesis is formed and that the formation of this inhibitor is inhibited by perchlorate to a greater extent than thyroid hormone iodination is inhibited, since the iodinated lipids that are thought to be inhibitors require about 10 times more iodide than the hormone. However, there is a high risk of recurrence after treatment with potassium perchlorate, and it can cause serious adverse effects (SED-13, 1281).

When five patients with type 2 amiodarone-induced hyperthyroidism were treated with a combination of an oral cholecystographic agent (sodium ipodate or sodium iopanoate, which are rich in iodine and potent inhibitors of 5′-deiodinase) plus a thionamide (propylthiouracil or methimazole) after amiodarone withdrawal, all improved substantially within a few days and became euthyroid or

hypothyroid in 15–31 weeks (58). Four of the five became hypothyroid and required long-term treatment with levothyroxine.

In another study, three patients with type 1 disease, two of whom had not responded to methimazole plus perchlorate, were successfully treated with a short course of iopanoic acid 1 g/day, resulting in a marked reduction in the peripheral conversion of T4 to T3 (59). Euthyroidism was restored in 7–12 days, allowing uneventful thyroidectomy. The patients were then treated with levothyroxine for hypothyroidism and amiodarone was safely restarted. The authors suggested that iopanoic acid is the drug of choice for rapid restoration of normal thyroid function before thyroidectomy in patients with drug-resistant type 1 amiodarone-induced hyperthyroidism.

The management of hyperthyroidism due to amiodarone has been reviewed in the light of the practices of 101 European endocrinologists (60). Most (82%) treat type I amiodarone-induced hyperthyroidism with thionamides, either alone (51%) or in combination with potassium perchlorate (31%); the preferred treatment for type II hyperthyroidism is a glucocorticoid (46%). Some initially treat all cases, before the type has been established, with a combination of thionamides and glucocorticoids. After restoration of normal thyroid function, 34% recommend ablative therapy in type I hyperthyroidism and only 8% in type II. If amiodarone therapy needs to be restarted, 65% recommend prophylactic thyroid ablation in type I hyperthyroidism and 70% recommend a wait-and-see strategy in type II.

Thyroid function tests were measured before and after treatment of amiodarone-induced hyperthyroidism (n = 12) and the response to combined antithyroid and glucocorticoid treatment (n = 11) was recorded (61). One patient had type 1 hyperthyroidism, nine had type 2, and two probably had a mixed form. Six patients had diffuse hypoechoic goiters. The median time to euthyroidism (defined as a normal free T3 concentration) with a thionamide + prednisolone (starting dose 20–75 mg/day) was 2 (interquartile range 1.0–2.7) months. Thionamide treatment was stopped after a median duration of 5.7 (4.2–8.7) months and glucocorticoids were completely withdrawn after 6.7 (5.5–8.7) months.

- A 40 year-old patient with severe amiodarone-induced hyperthyroidism after heart transplantation did not respond to high doses of antithyroid drugs combined with glucocorticoids (62). A low dose of lithium carbonate resulted in normalization of thyroid function.

Plasmapheresis, to remove iodine and thyroid hormones, was reportedly successful in treating amiodarone-induced hyperthyroidism in two of three patients, and was followed by thyroidectomy (63). It has been suggested that this would be ineffective in type II hyperthyroidism (64).

Prevention of recurrence of amiodarone-induced hyperthyroidism has been successfully attempted with ^{131}I in 18 patients, in 16 of whom amiodarone was reintroduced (65); the same authors reported the first 15 of these patients in two separate papers (66,67). The problem of whether to restart amiodarone therapy after hyperthyroidism has resolved has been discussed in the light of a case (68).

Some have suggested that the differentiation of amiodarone-induced hyperthyroidism into two types is not helpful in determining suitable therapy (69). Of 28 consecutive patients there was spontaneous resolution of hyperthyroidism in 5 and 23 received carbimazole alone as first-line therapy. Long-term euthyroidism was achieved in 11, 5 became hypothyroid and required long-term thyroxine, and 5 relapsed after withdrawal of carbimazole and became euthyroid with either long-term carbimazole ($n = 3$) or radioiodine ($n = 2$). Four were intolerant of carbimazole and received propylthiouracil, with good effect in three. One was resistant to thionamides and responded to corticosteroids. There was no difference in presentation or outcome between those in whom amiodarone was continued or stopped or between possible type 1 or type 2 disease (defined clinically and by serum IL-6 measurement). The authors concluded that continuing amiodarone has no adverse effect on the response to treatment of hyperthyroidism and that first-line therapy with a thionamide alone, whatever the type of disease, is appropriate in iodine-replete areas, thus avoiding potential complications of other drugs. However, it is not clear how good their differentiation of types 1 and 2 disease was. A previous prospective study in 24 patients showed that differentiation predicted response to treatment (70).

Two patients with cardiomyopathy and resistant dysrhythmias developed thyrotoxicosis while taking amiodarone (71). Despite medical therapy, they failed to improve. Both underwent total thyroidectomy without difficulty or complications. Most reported cases of amiodarone-induced thyrotoxicosis that have been treated surgically have been of type II, i.e. with no underlying thyroid disease.

It is generally recommended that amiodarone should be withdrawn. (72,73) worsening of thyrotoxic symptoms and heart function has been reported after withdrawal of amiodarone. When withdrawal of amiodarone is not an option, near-total thyroidectomy may be preferred. If surgery is not possible plasmapheresis can be helpful.

The use of local anesthesia for total thyroidectomy in patients with amiodarone-induced hyperthyroidism and cardiac impairment has been reviewed in the context of six patients (74).

Hypothyroidism

Amiodarone-induced hypothyroidism has been reviewed in the light of a case of 74-year-old woman (54).

In a nested case-control analysis of 5522 patients with a first prescription for an antidysrhythmic drug and no previous use of thyroid drugs, cases were defined as all patients who had started a thyroid-mimetic or antithyroid drug no sooner than 3 months after the start of an antidysrhythmic drug and controls were patients with a comparable follow-up period who had not taken any thyroid drugs during the observation period (36). There were 123 patients who had started antithyroid drugs and 96 who had started a thyroid-mimetic drug. In users of amiodarone there was an adjusted odds ratios of 6.6 (3.9, 11) for

hypothyroidism compared with users of other antidysrhythmic drugs.

The clinical, biochemical, and therapeutic aspects of amiodarone-induced hypothyroidism have been reviewed in the light of 18 elderly patients (75). Free thyroxine (T_4) concentrations were reduced only in those with severe hypothyroidism and free triiodothyronine (T_3) concentrations were always normal. Withdrawal of amiodarone in five patients led to improvement in four and worsening in one.

The risk of amiodarone-induced hypothyroidism may be greater in patients who have pre-existing thyroid autoimmune disease (76). There is some evidence that the risk of hypothyroidism due to amiodarone is increased in elderly patients (77), but the data are not conclusive.

In amiodarone-induced hypothyroidism the simplest method of treatment is to continue with amiodarone and to add thyroxine as required.

Amiodarone can cause altered serum lipid concentrations (78). Serum cholesterol rises, as can blood glucose and serum triglyceride concentrations. The mechanisms of these effects are not known; nor is it known to what extent they are due to changes in thyroid function.

The major adverse effect on the fetus is altered thyroid function (SEDA-13, 141; SEDA-14, 149; SEDA-19, 194; SEDA-20, 176). There have been individual reports of neonatal hyperthyroxinemia (79), goiter (80), and hypothyroidism (81). In the patient with goiter there was associated hypotonia, bradycardia, large fontanelles, and macroglossia (80).

Of 26 fetuses with hydrops fetalis and supraventricular tachycardias, 25 received transplacental drug therapy; prenatal conversion occurred in 15 (82). Nine fetuses were converted to sinus rhythm using either flecainide ($n = 7$) or amiodarone ($n = 2$) as first-line therapy, while digoxin either alone or in association with sotalol failed to restore sinus rhythm in all cases. After first-line therapy, supraventricular tachycardia persisted in 10 fetuses, nine of whom received amiodarone alone or in association with digoxin as second-line therapy, and five of whom converted to sinus rhythm. Of 11 neonates who received amiodarone in utero, two developed raised thyroid stimulating hormone concentrations on postnatal days 3-4; they received thyroid hormone and had normal outcomes.

Two neonates who had been given intravenous amiodarone as fetuses at 26 and 29 weeks and whose mothers had also taken it orally developed hypothyroidism (83). The authors suggested that low dietary iodine intake by the mothers may have contributed, by enhancing the Wolff–Chaikoff effect.

Amisulpride

Five women with psychoses treated with amisulpride developed hyperprolactinemia and were treated with bromocriptine 10–40 mg/day (84). Prolactin concentrations were markedly reduced in only three of the five; menses recurred in one of four patients with amenorrhea; lactation decreased in one of three patients with galactorrhea, and in two patients with reduced prolactin concentrations the psychotic symptoms exacerbated but fully remitted after withdrawal of bromocriptine. A 40-year-old woman also developed amenorrhea while taking a very low dose of amisulpride for 3 months (100 mg/day) (85).

A prolactinoma has been attributed to amisulpride.

- A 38-year-old woman with a borderline personality disorder developed a prolactinoma, with hyperprolactinemia, amenorrhea, and galactorrhea, probably induced by amisulpride 300 mg/day, which she had taken for 4 months following a bout of delirium with impaired attention, cognitive alteration, anxiety, and agitation (86). She had a microadenoma (5 mm) on the right side of the pituitary gland. Amisulpride was withdrawn and replaced by quetiapine 100 mg/day. The symptoms of hyperprolactinemia resolved.

Amoxapine

A further reminder of the structural resemblance of amoxapine to the neuroleptic drugs has been provided by an adverse effect reported with both amoxapine and its close congener, loxapine (87).

- A 49-year-old woman with no history of diabetes was admitted in unexplained hyperglycemic coma (blood glucose 26 mmol/l) while taking lithium 1500 mg/day and loxapine 150 mg/day. She responded to insulin, but insulin responses on testing were not delayed and suggested an iatrogenic rather than a diabetic cause. The fasting glucose fell to 4.2 mmol/l after withdrawal of loxapine but continuing lithium. Two weeks later amoxapine 150 mg/day was started and she became acutely confused, with a serum glucose of 5.7 mmol/l. Two weeks after stopping amoxapine the serum glucose returned to normal.

The authors speculated that a common metabolite of both drugs, 7-hydroxyamoxapine, was responsible for the hyperglycemia, owing to its antidopaminergic properties.

Amphetamines

Amphetamines can cause retardation of growth (height and weight) in hyperactive children (SED-9, 9).

Angiotensin-converting enzyme inhibitors

Gynecomastia has been reported in a patient taking captopril 75 mg/day; it resolved when captopril was withdrawn but recurred when the patient was given enalapril (88). This suggests that gynecomastia may not be simply attributable to the sulfhydryl group of captopril.

ACE inhibition has been associated with increased insulin sensitivity in diabetic patients, and it has therefore been hypothesized that ACE inhibitors can precipitate hypoglycemia in such patients. A Dutch case-control study suggested that among users of insulin or oral hypoglycemic drugs, the use of ACE inhibitors was significantly associated with an increased risk of hospital admission for hypoglycemia (89). However, a French case/non-case study from the pharmacovigilance database did not confirm this finding (90).

In a matched case-control study of 404 cases of hospitalization for hypoglycemia in diabetic patients and 1375 controls, the risk of hypoglycemia was greater in those who used insulin versus a sulfonylurea and was not influenced by the use of ACE inhibitors (91). However, the use of enalapril was associated with an increased risk of hypoglycemia (OR = 2.4; CI = 1.1, 5.3) in sulfonylurea users. Although the authors emphasized the fact that previous reports of ACE inhibitor-related hypoglycemia were more frequent with enalapril, it is unclear why only enalapril, and not ACE inhibitors as a class, was associated with a significantly increased risk of hypoglycemia, and why this occurred only in sulfonylurea users.

Conversely, it has been suggested that the protective effect of ACE inhibitors against severe hypoglycemia should be tested in high-risk patients with high ACE activity. About 10–20% of patients with type 1 diabetes mellitus have a risk of severe hypoglycemia. In 307 unselected consecutive diabetic outpatients, those with the ACE DD genotype had a relative risk of severe hypoglycemia of 3.2 (95% CI = 1.4, 7.4) compared with those with the genotype II (92). There was a significant relation between serum ACE activity and the risk of severe hypoglycemia.

Antacids

Some antacids contain enough sugar to affect diabetic control (93). Since the sugar is not an active component, it will not be declared on the packaging in many countries.

Antiepileptic drugs

See also individuals agents

Although most anticonvulsants interfere with endocrine function, epilepsy may do so itself, and it is difficult to differentiate the effects of drugs from those of the disease. In any case, symptoms of endocrine dysfunction are less common than biochemical abnormalities.

Growth hormone

Normal growth hormone concentrations are found in carbamazepine-treated patients (94). Growth hormone secretion in response to levodopa stimulation was not affected by carbamazepine or phenobarbital, whereas phenytoin and anticonvulsant polytherapy caused an increase in growth hormone concentration, and valproate a fall at varying times after the administration of levodopa (95). Pubertal growth arrest has been described in a 12-year-old girl who had taken valproate for 18 months (SED-13, 152).

Adrenal–pituitary axis

Neither phenytoin, valproate, carbamazepine, nor phenobarbital altered the circadian ACTH/cortisol rhythm in epileptic patients (95). In some studies, phenytoin and carbamazepine were associated with increased serum concentrations of unbound cortisol (96), but cortisol concentrations were unaffected in other studies (94) and Cushing's syndrome has not been described with these drugs. Valproate can depress ACTH concentrations by inhibiting corticotrophin-releasing factor, and it has been used to treat Nelson's syndrome (97). Serum concentrations of progesterone and cortisol and the excretion of 17-hydroxycorticosteroids have been reported to be lower in untreated patients with epilepsy and to be further reduced by phenytoin (98).

Sex hormones

Carbamazepine, phenobarbital, phenytoin, and anticonvulsant polytherapy increased both basal and stimulated concentrations of prolactin, whereas valproate did not (95). However, in other studies, prolactin was unchanged (94). In boys, phenobarbital lowered baseline LH and FSH concentrations and their response to releasing hormone; baseline prolactin concentration was raised in comparison with healthy children, and the response of prolactin concentrations to stimulation was impaired (99).

Serum concentrations of bound testosterone are increased by phenytoin, carbamazepine, phenobarbital, and primidone owing to increased synthesis of the specific transport protein, sex hormone-binding globulin (SHBG), but concentrations of unbound testosterone, dehydroepiandrosterone sulfate, and 17-α-hydroxyprogesterone and the free androgen index may be reduced (94,100–102). Increased FSH in 31% of carbamazepine-treated men may reflect impairment of spermatogenesis, whereas lower concentrations of inhibin B (in 12% of men) and testosterone/LH ratio (in 50%) indicate impaired function of Sertoli cells and Leydig cells respectively (94). Sexual activity was reduced, while mean plasma concentrations of LH, FSH, PRL, and SHBG were raised in 27 epileptic patients taking phenytoin, primidone, phenobarbital, or combinations of these (103). The often-reported reduction in sexual activity and occasional reports of impotence may be related to the reduction in unbound testosterone caused by enzyme induction. Valproate has been recommended for patients with dysfunctional libido or impotence, because it apparently does not reduce unbound hormone concentrations (104).

In an assessment of the effects of antiepileptic drugs on male sexual function, men taking carbamazepine had higher plasma concentrations of SHBG and lower concentrations of dehydroepiandrosterone compared with controls (105). Patients taking phenytoin had higher total testosterone concentrations and lower dehydroepiandrosterone concentrations. Patients taking carbamazepine and phenytoin also had a lower free androgen index, but free (unbound) testosterone, a more reliable index of active androgen concentrations, did not differ from that of controls. Patients taking valproate showed no differences in hormone concentrations compared with controls. Sexual experience scales showed that treated men embraced a stricter sexual morality than untreated controls, and expressed greater satisfaction with their

marriages. Most of the hormonal changes could be explained by enzyme induction, and there was no evidence of hyposexuality in this population.

Reproductive endocrine disorders and sexual dysfunction have often been attributed to epilepsy itself, but antiepileptic drugs can cause various alterations in endocrine functions. Reproductive endocrine function was prospectively evaluated in 90 men taking valproate ($n = 21$), carbamazepine ($n = 40$), or oxcarbazepine ($n = 29$) as monotherapy for epilepsy, and in 25 healthy controls (106). There were increased serum androgen concentrations in 60% of those who took valproate. Carbamazepine had an opposite effect: men had mean low serum concentrations of dehydroepiandrosterone and a high SHBG concentration. Moreover, 18% of men taking carbamazepine for epilepsy reported reduced libido, impaired potency, or both. Low daily doses of oxcarbazepine (under 900 mg/day) did not have any effects on serum concentrations of reproductive hormones, but men taking high doses of oxcarbazepine (over 900 mg/day) had increased serum testosterone, gonadotropin, and SHBG concentrations. Serum insulin concentrations were high in all patients. Thus, the three antiepileptic drugs affected the serum concentrations of reproductive endocrine hormones in men with epilepsy, but in different ways. Valproate directly affects steroid synthesis or metabolism. Oxcarbazepine and carbamazepine differ in their effects, despite their close structural homology: oxcarbazepine does not reduce the activity of androgens, whereas carbamazepine does. The relevance of these hormonal changes to reproductive or sexual function remains to be demonstrated.

In another study changes in reproductive hormones associated with valproate or carbamazepine were prospectively analysed in 17 women and 22 men with recently diagnosed epilepsy (107). There were no clinical signs of hormonal disorders or weight gain during follow-up at 1 and 3 months. Valproate and carbamazepine caused alterations in reproductive hormonal function during the first month of treatment, and these changes were stable or progressive during the next 2 months. Serum testosterone concentrations increased in half of the women taking valproate; mean serum concentrations of gonadotropins and SHBG also increased, but the concentrations of serum dehydroepiandrosterone sulfate fell. On the other hand, in men after 3 months of valproate treatment, serum FSH concentrations were low and serum progesterone and dehydroepiandrosterone sulfate concentrations were high. Carbamazepine increased serum concentrations of SHBG and dehydroepiandrosterone sulfate, while the free androgen index fell. Thus, valproate was associated with increased serum androgen concentrations, but the profiles of hormonal changes were different in men and women. On the other hand, carbamazepine was associated with reduced sex steroid function in both sexes. Although these results are of interest, the study was not randomized and a large number of statistical comparisons were performed, so that no firm conclusions can be drawn.

Thyroid hormones

Total and free (unbound) thyroxine can be reduced by phenytoin and carbamazepine, but free triiodothyronine is normal or only slightly reduced. Thyroid-stimulating hormone is normal or only slightly altered and patients remain clinically euthyroid (94,108). Reductions in the concentrations of some thyroid hormones are probably related to enzyme induction; the concentrations return to normal after substituting carbamazepine with oxcarbazepine, a less potent enzyme inducer (109). Hypothyroidism has been rarely described in patients taking phenytoin or carbamazepine (110). In contrast to earlier reports, there were no changes in thyroid hormones during treatment with valproate in a later study (111).

Serum thyroid hormones have been compared in 148 healthy children and 141 children with epilepsy who had been taking carbamazepine ($n = 61$), valproate ($n = 51$), or phenobarbital ($n = 29$) for at least 1 year (112). In all the groups mean thyroxine and free thyroxine concentrations were lower than in controls, and those taking carbamazepine and valproate also had lower concentrations of triiodothyronine and thyroid-binding globulin and increased mean TSH concentrations. There was subclinical hypothyroidism, defined as a TSH concentration greater than two standard deviations above the control mean, in 26% of the children taking valproate, 8.2% of those taking carbamazepine, 7.1% of those taking phenobarbital, and 3.6% of controls. However, the magnitude of the TSH increase was usually small and the children were clinically euthyroid.

The effects of antiepileptic drugs on thyroid function have also been studied in an open prospective study in 90 men with epilepsy (40 taking carbamazepine, 29 taking oxcarbazepine, and 21 taking valproate monotherapy) and 25 control subjects (113). Serum thyroxine and/or free thyroxine concentrations were below the reference ranges in 45% of men taking carbamazepine and 24% of men taking oxcarbazepine. Thyroid peroxidase and/or thyroglobulin concentrations were increased in 13% of those taking carbamazepine, 17% of those taking oxcarbazepine, and 6% of controls, but these changes were not associated with altered serum thyroid hormone concentrations. Serum triiodothyronine and thyrotropin (TRH) concentrations in those taking carbamazepine or oxcarbazepine were normal. In men taking valproate, the concentrations of thyroid hormones, thyrotropin, and antithyroid antibodies were normal. Thus, low serum thyroid hormone concentrations appear to be frequent in men taking carbamazepine or oxcarbazepine and are probably not due to liver enzyme induction or activation of immunological mechanisms. The clinical significance of these changes is uncertain: serum TSH was not affected and all the patients were clinically euthyroid. Similar results have been obtained in a retrospective study in 37 children taking valproate or carbamazepine (114).

Phenytoin rarely causes hyperglycemia, and the blood glucose concentration can increase in phenytoin intoxication (SED-13, 139) (115). A reduction in the insulin response to glucose has been noted with therapeutic doses of phenytoin, but glucose intolerance does not arise, probably owing to increased sensitivity to insulin.

Changes in body weight associated with anticonvulsants have been reviewed (116), including the effects of the antiepileptic drugs that have been most commonly associated with this adverse effect (valproic acid, carbamazepine, vigabatrin, and gabapentin) (117). Unlike most anticonvulsants, topiramate, felbamate, and zonisamide can cause weight loss.

Preliminary evidence suggests that certain idiosyncratic reactions to anticonvulsants are mediated by reduced free radical scavenging activity, as indicated by lower selenium concentrations and a higher lipid peroxide index in affected patients (SEDA-19, 62).

Serum lipids

Phenytoin increases high-density lipoprotein (HDL) cholesterol (118), and may also increase total cholesterol and serum triglyceride concentrations (SED-13, 143) (119). In a 5-year prospective study with carbamazepine, there was a persistent rise in total cholesterol and HDL cholesterol, whereas triglycerides and low-density lipoprotein (LDL) cholesterol increased only transiently (120). In a more recent study, total cholesterol fell when 12 patients were switched from carbamazepine to oxcarbazepine, but HDL cholesterol and triglycerides were unchanged (121). In a comparison of 101 epileptic patients with matched controls, valproate was associated with lower total and LDL cholesterol, whereas carbamazepine was associated with higher HDL cholesterol and apolipoprotein A concentrations and phenobarbital with higher concentrations of total and HDL cholesterol and apolipoproteins A and B. The ratio of total to HDL cholesterol was reduced with valproate and carbamazepine but not with phenobarbital (122).

The clinical relevance of these findings is uncertain. The increased HDL cholesterol seen with some drugs might confer some protection against atherosclerosis and coronary heart disease (SEDA-18, 63).

Porphyrin metabolism

Enzyme inducers, such as phenytoin, carbamazepine, and barbiturates, can precipitate attacks in patients with acute intermittent porphyria.

- A patient with uncontrolled posttraumatic epilepsy and acute intermittent porphyria was given phenytoin, carbamazepine, and clonazepam on successive occasions (123). Phenytoin and carbamazepine caused significant increases in porphobilinogen excretion and acute attacks of porphyria. In contrast, clonazepam caused no increase in porphobilinogen excretion.

Valproate (SED-12, 134) (124,125), ethosuximide (126), and some benzodiazepines (127) have also been implicated in the precipitation of acute attacks of porphyria, although valproate is considered safe for patients with porphyria cutanea tarda (SED-13, 150) (128).

Neither vigabatrin nor gabapentin caused porphyrin accumulation in chicken embryo cultured liver cells, whereas felbamate, lamotrigine, and tiagabine were porphyrinogenic in this model (129). For gabapentin, safety in porphyrias has been confirmed in preliminary clinical observations (SEDA-19, 70) (SEDA-20, 62).

Amino acids

Compared with healthy controls, 51 patients with epilepsy taking a variety of antiepileptic drugs (mostly carbamazepine) had higher mean plasma concentrations of homocysteine (130). This effect, which could be related to reductions in the concentrations of folate and vitamin B6, was likely to be drug-induced, but a causative role of the underlying disease could not be excluded. Although homocysteine is an experimental convulsant and a risk factor for atherosclerosis, the clinical relevance of these findings is uncertain.

Phenytoin can reduce blood and CSF thiamine concentrations (131).

Hyperammonemia and carnitine deficiency are adverse effects of valproate, although carnitine deficiency can also be caused by other anticonvulsants (132).

Concentrations of lipoprotein(a) were measured in 51 patients taking long-term carbamazepine, phenobarbital, phenytoin, or valproate and 51 age- and sex-matched controls (133). Lipoprotein(a) concentrations were above 450 µg/ml in 11 patients compared with only 4 controls, and the mean serum lipoprotein(a) concentrations were 330 and 169 µg/ml respectively. The epileptic patients also had a thicker intima media of the common carotid artery. These results suggest that patients taking antiepileptic drugs may be at a higher risk of atherosclerosis.

Weight

The effect of antiepileptic drugs on body weight has been reviewed (134). Valproic acid, carbamazepine, gabapentin, and vigabatrin are associated with weight gain. The mechanisms have not been identified. Increased secretion of insulin and proinsulin, increased appetite for carbohydrates, reduced energy expenditure, reduced leptin concentrations, and reduced beta-oxidation of fatty acids because of carnitine deficiency are proposed mechanisms for valproic acid. Carbamazepine-induced weight gain can arise from edema secondary to increased antidiuretic hormone secretion or from increased appetite and food consumption. Weight gain associated with vigabatrin and gabapentin could be related to GABAergic properties, which can increase carbohydrate consumption and reduce energy expenditure.

Topiramate, felbamate, and zonisamide are associated with weight loss. In animals topiramate reduced food intake, but also reduced energy disposition in the absence of reduced intake. In addition, topiramate increased lipoprotein lipase activity in adipose tissue, possibly reflecting enhanced regulatory thermogenesis. In humans and animals topiramate reduces leptin concentrations. With felbamate weight loss is almost always associated with

anorexia. There is little information on the mechanism of weight loss with zonisamide.

Antihistamines

Appetite stimulation and resulting weight gain is a well-known feature of cyproheptadine, but astemizole also causes weight gain in approximately 3% of patients within weeks of treatment (135,136). Cetirizine also has been reported to cause weight gain (about 2.8%) when it is used for a prolonged time (SEDA-17, 200). Increased body weight occurred in three participants in a trial of azelastine (SEDA-21, 172).

In a double-blind, randomized, placebo-controlled study of the effect of cetirizine, clemastine, and loratadine for 7 days on blood glucose concentration in patients with allergic rhinitis, cetirizine produced a significant increase in postprandial blood glucose and a small rise in fasting blood glucose; clemastine caused a small fall in fasting and a small rise in postprandial blood glucose (137). The mechanisms of these effects are not known.

Antiretroviral drugs

See also individual groups and agents

Metabolic disturbances

Presentation
Dyslipidemia is a common accompaniment of the lipodystrophy syndrome observed in HIV-infected patients. This syndrome presents as a combination of peripheral lipoatrophy and the metabolic syndrome (central adiposity, insulin resistance, and dyslipidemia). The term lipodystrophy syndrome was first used in two case reports to describe a clinical picture of subcutaneous fat wasting in the face and limbs of HIV infected patients treated with indinavir, reminiscent of the rare congenital lipodystrophy syndromes (138,139). In addition, benign symmetric lipomatoses on the trunk and neck were described. A systematic study of this syndrome in the Australian HIV cohort showed co-existence of peripheral lipoatrophy with abdominal visceral obesity, dyslipidemia, and insulin resistance in HIV-infected patients with or without treatment with protease inhibitors (140).

In general, most of the morphological and metabolic changes appear to aggregate in the same population and resemble the so-called "metabolic syndrome", also called "syndrome X". The WHO describes this syndrome as an accumulation of three or more of the following clinical features:

• abdominal obesity;
• raised triglycerides;
• low HDL cholesterol;
• raised blood pressure;
• raised fasting glucose.

More specifically, the ATP III guidelines, from the third report of the National Cholesterol Education Program's expert Adult Treatment Panel on Detection, Evaluation, and Treatment of High Blood Cholesterol in Adults (141), define the metabolic syndrome as involving three or more of the following:

- central/abdominal obesity as measured by waist circumference (men: greater than 102 cm (40 inches); women: greater than 88 cm (35 inches));
- fasting triglycerides greater than or equal to 1.7 mmol/l (150 mg/dl);
- HDL cholesterol (men: less than 1 mmol/l (40 mg/dl); women: less than 1.3 mmol/l (50 mg/ dl));
- blood pressure greater than or equal to 130/85 mmHg;
- fasting glucose greater than or equal to 6.1 mmol/l (110 mg/dl).

In the HIV infected population, further evidence suggested that visceral fat accumulation, dyslipidemia, and insulin resistance are closely linked and associated with antiretroviral treatment, most pronounced with the use of protease inhibitors. In contrast, subcutaneous fat wasting is primarily determined by the choice of nucleoside reverse transcriptase inhibitor (NRTI). Switching studies have supported this notion, since substitution of stavudine has been associated with improvement in fat wasting, while switching a protease inhibitor had no beneficial effect in more than 30 clinical trials (142).

Mechanisms

Several pathophysiological mechanisms have been proposed, including adverse effects of protease inhibitors on hepatocyte and fat cell function (143), mitochondrial toxicity from nucleoside analogues (144), excess of reactive oxygen species (145), and cytokine-mediated events (146). In vitro data and studies in healthy volunteers suggest a role for protease inhibitors in insulin resistance (147) and dyslipidemia (148).

Nucleoside-reverse transcriptase inhibitors (NRTI) have a number of adverse effects on mitochondria. Mitochondrial dysfunction can result in several adverse effects, depending on the affected organ system, as demonstrated by an illustrative case (149).

- A patient taking HAART including didanosine and zidovudine developed a syndrome that evolved over 4 months, starting with weight loss (25%), vomiting, polyuria, bone fracture due to osteoporosis, profound proximal weakness, and a stocking sensory neuropathy. He had a Fanconi-type proximal renal tubular dysfunction, lactic acidosis, myopathy, and pancreatic dysfunction. All signs and symptoms improved markedly after withdrawal of the antiretroviral drugs.

This case demonstrates almost the full clinical spectrum of mitochondrial toxicity.

Depletion of mitochondrial DNA and morphological changes in adipocytes have been assessed in a small study of fat biopsies from HIV-negative patients ($n = 6$), HIV-positive but drug naïve patients ($n = 11$), and patients taking NRTIs, either zidovudine ($n = 9$) or stavudine ($n = 12$) (150). Drug-naïve HIV-infected patients had similar contents of mitochondrial DNA in adipocytes, while patients taking NRTIs had significantly reduced mean mitochondrial DNA content per cell. Compared with HIV-infected controls, mitochondrial DNA depletion was 45% or 87% in those taking zidovudine and stavudine respectively. These results support in vitro findings that stavudine causes more pronounced mitochondrial toxicity than zidovudine (151).

There was significant improvement in signs of mitochondrial toxicity in 49 patients who switched from stavudine to abacavir compared with 63 patients who continued to take stavudine in a non-randomized study for 12 months (152). Only patients who remained on their assigned treatment were included in the analysis. Lactate concentrations were assessed at baseline, week 24, and week 48, and electrical bioimpedance was performed in 22 cases and 12 controls at baseline and week 48. There were significant falls in serum lactate concentrations at weeks 24 and 48 in cases compared with controls. Patients who switched had a trend towards fat gain, while controls had significant reductions in total body fat and percentage of body fat.

Lactic acidosis

Lactic acidosis is a consequence of long-term mitochondrial toxicity of NRTIs. In a systematic review of published cases of lactic acidosis, NRTI use and female sex were identified as significant risk factors (153). Among patients taking a triple drug regimen, all were taking stavudine as one of their NRTIs (52% in combination with didanosine). The most frequent clinical manifestations were gastrointestinal (nausea, vomiting, abdominal pain) in 50%, and 41% had dyspnea and tachypnea. The median lactate concentration in symptomatic patients was 11 mmol/l and liver enzymes were abnormal in 65%. Almost half of the patients died within a median period of 7 days.

Lipids and lipodystrophy

The effects of the protease inhibitor indinavir and the NNRTI efavirenz on lipid concentrations have been compared in a large comparative randomized study (154). Each of the two comparison drugs were used in one arm (with a zidovudine + lamivudine backbone) and the combination of the two drugs in a third arm. Zidovudine and lamivudine did not play a role in the lipid changes. However, both of the comparison drugs significantly increased cholesterol concentrations.

In a prospective, non-randomized analysis of 212 patients treated with a regimen containing a protease inhibitor, the overall incidences of hypertriglyceridemia and hypercholesterolemia at 12 months of treatment were 38% and 25% respectively (155). Increased concentrations of triglycerides and LDL cholesterol were more pronounced in patients taking ritonavir or lopinavir/ritonavir compared with other protease inhibitors.

In a small randomized, open, comparative study patients who switched to abacavir from either stavudine or stavudine plus a protease inhibitor or NNRTI, or a protease inhibitor + NNRTI had improved total and LDL cholesterol (156). Total arm and leg fat mass, measured by DEXA scan, rose significantly in those who switched from stavudine to abacavir, suggesting an important role of stavudine in the pathogenesis of lipodystrophy.

Support for the hypothesis of a casual relation between stavudine and lipodystrophy comes from another randomized study in which stavudine-containing HAART regimens were switched to a combination of zidovudine, lamivudine, and abacavir (157). Eight patients were randomized to continue stavudine and 14 patients switched to the triple combination. Imbalance in the treatment arms resulted from exclusion of patients who maintained treatment for a minimum of 6 months of follow up. Over 48 weeks after randomization, the average leg and arm fat mass fell in the continuation arm but increased in the switch arm. One patient in the switch arm, who had previously taken zidovudine and lamivudine, had a therapeutic failure.

In a retrospective analysis of 36 patients who switched from stavudine to tenofovir while HIV RNA was below 20 copies/ ml for more than 6 months, two switched because of peripheral neuropathy and 34 because of lipoatrophy; the median duration of observation was 36 weeks (158). There was a significant fall in cholesterol concentrations from 5.5 mmol/l to 5.0 mmol/l at week 4, and 4.7 mmol/l at week 36. There was also a non-significant trend toward a fall in triglyceride concentrations.

In patients who had taken their first antiretroviral regimen for more than 6 months, using either stavudine (n = 75) or zidovudine (n = 75) plus lamivudine and indinavir total fat was significantly lower in patients taking stavudine but the lean body mass was similar in the two groups (159). Fat redistribution was common: 20 patients were classified as having lipoatrophy, 33 lipodystrophy, and 41 a mixed syndrome. However, there were no statistically significant differences between the two groups. Lack of physical activity was the only independent predictor of isolated or mixed lipoatrophy. Whether physical activity in fact improves lipodystrophy is not known.

Lipid abnormalities are a major adverse effect of HIV protease inhibitors (160). In a 48-week comparison with nelfinavir, atazanavir did not significantly increase total cholesterol, fasting LDL cholesterol or triglyceride concentrations (+6.8%, −7.1%, +1.5% respectively), while the respective concentrations rose by 28%, 31%, and 42% in those who took nelfinavir. The incidence of grade 1−4 lipodystrophy was infrequent in both groups, but this endpoint was poorly defined in this study.

The effect of the combination of lopinavir + ritonavir on the atherogenic lipid profile has been evaluated in 24 HIV infected patients (161). At baseline, there was an abnormally small LDL density. After 1 month lopinavir + ritonavir increased triglyceride and apolipoprotein CIII concentrations, and LDL size fell further.

Insulin resistance

The independent effect of protease inhibitors on insulin resistance has been investigated. A single dose of indinavir was sufficient to produce a significant reduction in insulin sensitivity, assessed by euglycemic

hyperinsulinemic clamp testing, in both HIV-infected and HIV-negative individuals (162).

Diabetes mellitus

A retrospective analysis of the development of diabetes in 1011 patients has been summarized (163). All were non-diabetic when antiretroviral treatment was started. Over 10 months, diabetes was diagnosed in 16 patients (2.06 per 100 person-years). Older age (HR = 1.1, 1.06-1.16) was associated with a higher risk. In multivariate analysis adjusted for age and sex, the onset of diabetes was not related to CD4 cell count, viral load, or type of antiviral therapy (with or without protease inhibitors). However, patients taking stavudine or indinavir were at significantly higher risks (stavudine HR = 16, 95% CI = 3, 84; indinavir HR = 4.0, 95% CI = 1.3, 13). The strong association of stavudine with diabetes is surprising and needs further confirmation.

In a cohort study (164) in 1785 women, 69 incident cases of diabetes mellitus were diagnosed, with an average incidence of 1.5 cases per 100 patient-years. In patients taking protease inhibitors, incidence rates were about twice as high (2.8 cases per 100 patient-years) as among users of NNRTIs or untreated patients (1.2%) and uninfected controls (1.4%). In a multivariate model use of protease inhibitors (HR = 2.9; 1.5, 5.6), age, and BMI were independent risk factors for diabetes.

Conclusions

Metabolic disturbances are frequent in patients with HIV infection and represent a multifactorial condition related both to the underlying disease and to the antiviral treatment. HIV infection itself appears to cause hyperlipidemia and insulin resistance in some patients. Protease inhibitor therapy is a major contributor to fat accumulation, hyperlipidemia, and insulin resistance. NNRTIs contribute mainly through augmentation of lipid concentrations and NRTIs to the development of lipid-associated toxicity. NRTIs can cause mitochondrial dysfunction.

Apiaceae

Adrenal insufficiency has been attributed to *Cannabis sativum* (165).

- A 28-year-old woman took an extract of *C. sativum* for 7 days to augment lactation while breastfeeding. She developed severe stomach pain and diarrhea and 15 days later resented with dark skin, depression, dehydration, and amenorrhea. A diagnosis of adrenal dysfunction was made, the herbal remedy was withdrawn, and she was treated with dexamethasone, prednisolone, and an oral contraceptive. Her symptoms resolved within 10 days.

Aripiprazole

Galactorrhea has been attributed to aripiprazole after only 2 days of administration (166).

A 29-year-old woman with a schizoaffective disorder took haloperidol 5 mg/day and then 9 mg/day because of acute psychotic episodes. She had no adverse effects such as amenorrhea or galactorrhea. Haloperidol was then replaced by aripiprazole 15 mg/day and on the evening of the second day she developed breast tenderness and marked galactorrhea. The serum prolactin concentration was 32 ng/ml (reference range 5–25 ng/ml). Aripiprazole was withdrawn and haloperidol restarted. The galactorrhea resolved in 1 week.

Artesunate

According to a randomized, open comparison in 113 adults with severe falciparum malaria in Thailand, hypoglycemia seems to occur less often in patients with malaria treated with artesunate (2.4 mg/kg intravenously followed by 1.2 mg/kg 12 hours later and then by 1.2 mg/kg/day intravenously or 12 mg/kg orally for 7 days) compared with those treated with quinine (20 mg/kg intravenously over 4 hours followed by 10 mg intravenously over 2 hours or orally tds for 7 days) (167). Artesunate and quinine had comparable efficacy, but hypoglycemia was only observed in 10% of the patients treated with artesunate whereas it occurred in 28% of those treated with quinine.

Articaine

Articaine has been implicated in an episode of weakness of the limb muscles, fatigue, and anorexia in a patient with a rare respiratory chain disorder due to a genetic defect in mitochondrial DNA (Kearn–Sayre Syndrome).

- A 28 year-old woman with Kearns-Sayre Syndrome, previously exposed multiple times to lidocaine, underwent planned tooth extraction after injection of articaine 1.5 ml (60 mg) with adrenaline (0.009 mg) (168). Within 5 minutes she complained of a feeling of heat, fatigue, weakness, and a desire to sleep. She was unable to walk or stand and had frequent urination. At 20 hours after the injection she had diffuse weakness, reduced tendon and absent patellar reflexes, and subclonic Achilles tendon reflexes. She recovered fully 48 hours after the injection.

The authors assumed a direct mitochondrial toxic effect of articaine, although this was disputed by others in correspondence (169).

Ascorbic acid (vitamin C)

Dehydroascorbic acid appears to have a diabetogenic effect and ascorbic acid causes increased excretion of glucose. High ascorbic acid concentrations can delay the insulin response to a glucose challenge and prolong postprandial hyperglycemia (170).

An increase in serum cholesterol has been reported in patients with atherosclerosis taking high doses of ascorbic acid (171).

Asparaginase

Asparaginase can reduce insulin production (172) and precipitate diabetic ketoacidosis (173,174).

Azathioprine

Hyperprolactinemia has been attributed to azathioprine (175).

- A 24-year-old woman, with a 3-year history of psoriasis, in the last trimester of her first pregnancy developed autoimmune thrombocytic purpura, which resolved after delivery. After 1 year, her liver function tests rose to 10 times normal values, associated with fatigue, weakness, and splenomegaly. Fine-needle liver aspiration showed autoimmune hepatitis. Her transaminases normalized with a glucocorticoid. She was then given azathioprine 50 mg/day instead of the glucocorticoid. After 1 month, her liver function tests rose about seven-fold and her prolactin concentrations by three-fold. She was again given a glucocorticoid and the azathioprine was continued. Six weeks later she was in remission, but her prolactin concentration was still high. There was no galactorrhea or amenorrhea, and the hyperprolactinemia was thought to have been be caused by azathioprine.

Benazepril

Hypoaldosteronism with metabolic acidosis has been reported in a child taking benazepril (176).

- A 4-year-old boy with minimal-change nephrotic syndrome since the age of 11 months had been treated with cyclophosphamide and glucocorticoids. After several relapses and the development of mild hypertension and proteinuria, he was given benazepril 0.3 mg/kg/day. He was admitted 4 months later with a metabolic acidosis (pH 7.28, base excess –15) and mild hyperchloremia (chloride 110 mmol/l). He had mild proteinuria and a normal creatinine clearance. The diagnosis was metabolic acidosis due to gastroenteritis and he was treated with intravenous saline and bicarbonate and discharged, but was re-admitted with anorexia and nausea and the same findings as before. A 24-hour urine sample showed high sodium and a low potassium and chloride excretion. The serum aldosterone concentration was below the limit of detection. The dose of benazepril was reduced to 0.2 mg/kg/day for 1 week and then withdrawn. Ten days later the aldosterone concentration was normal (29 pg/ml). After 9 months of follow-up, he still had mild proteinuria, but there had been no further episodes of metabolic acidosis.

The authors pointed out that there is evidence of ACE inhibitor-induced hypoaldosteronism in adults. This condition should be considered in children and adults taking ACE inhibitors who present with metabolic acidosis.

Benzodiazepines

See also individual agents

Benzodiazepines reduce hypothalamic–pituitary–adrenal axis activity acutely in healthy humans. The acute and chronic effects (3 weeks) of alprazolam and lorazepam on plasma cortisol have been examined in 68 subjects (aged 60–83 years), who took oral alprazolam 0.25 or 0.50 mg bd, or lorazepam 0.50 or 1.0 mg bd, or placebo according to a randomized, double-blind, placebo-controlled, parallel design (177). Plasma cortisol concentrations were significantly affected compared with placebo, but only by the 0.5 mg dose of alprazolam. During the first and last days of treatment, there was a significant fall in cortisol at 2.5 hours after alprazolam compared with placebo. The predose cortisol concentrations increased significantly during chronic alprazolam treatment, and there were correlations between the cortisol changes and changes in depression, anxiety, and memory scores. These findings suggest that even a short period of chronic treatment with alprazolam, but not lorazepam, may result in interdose activation of the hypothalamic–pituitary–adrenal axis in the elderly, consistent with drug withdrawal. If confirmed, this effect may contribute to an increased risk for drug escalation and dependence during chronic alprazolam treatment.

Beta$_2$-adrenoceptor agonists

In obstetrics, the classic effects of beta$_2$-adrenoceptor agonists on glucose metabolism can be absent or harmless in the non-diabetic, but dangerous in women with diabetes, in whom they can cause metabolic acidosis (178); the hyperglycemic effect can be aggravated if glucocorticoids are given (as they may be to prevent hyaline membrane disease in prematurity).

Beta-adrenoceptor antagonists

See also individuals agents

Prolactin

- Reversible hyperprolactinemia with galactorrhea occurred in a 38-year-old woman taking atenolol for hypertension (179).

Thyroid

Propranolol inhibits the conversion of thyroxine (T4) to tri-iodothyronine (T3) by peripheral tissues (180), resulting in increased formation of inactive reverse T3. There have been several reports of hyperthyroxinemia in clinically euthyroid patients taking propranolol for non-thyroid reasons in high dosages (320–480 mg/day) (181,182). The incidence was considered to be higher than could be accounted for by the development of spontaneous hyperthyroidism, but the mechanism is unknown.

The effect of beta-adrenoceptor antagonists on thyroid hormone metabolism is unlikely to play a significant role in their use in hyperthyroidism. Since D-propranolol has similar effects on thyroxine metabolism to those seen with the racemic mixture, membrane-stabilizing activity may be involved (183).

In one case, beta-adrenoceptor blockade masked an unexpected thyroid crisis, resulting in severe cerebral dysfunction before the diagnosis was made (184).

Blood glucose control

In a randomized controlled comparison of the effects of beta-adrenoceptor antagonists with different pharmacological profiles, namely metoprolol and carvedilol, on glycemic and metabolic control in 1235 hypertensive patients with type 2 diabetes already taking a blocker of the renin–angiotensin–aldosterone system, blood pressure reduction was similar in the two groups but the mean glycosylated hemoglobin increased significantly from baseline to the end of the study with metoprolol (0.15%;1 95%CI = 0.08, 0.22) but not carvedilol (0.02%) (185). Insulin sensitivity improved with carvedilol (–9.1%) but not metoprolol (–2.0%). The between-group difefrence was –7.2%. Progression to microalbuminuria was more common with metoprol than with carvedilol. Even if both agents were effective in reducing blood pressure and well tolerated, the use of carvedilol in addition to blockers of the renin–angiotensin–aldosterone system seems to be associated with a better metabolic profile in diabetic patients.

Hypoglycemia

Hypoglycemia, producing loss of consciousness in some cases, can occur in non-diabetic individuals who are taking beta-adrenoceptor antagonists, particularly those who undergo prolonged fasting (186) or severe exercise (187,188). Patients on maintenance dialysis are also at risk (189). It has been suggested that non-selective drugs are most likely to produce hypoglycemia and that cardioselective drugs are to be preferred in at-risk patients (190), but the same effect has been reported with atenolol under similar circumstances (188).

Two children in whom propranolol was used to treat attention deficit disorders and anxiety became unarousable, with low heart rates and respiratory rates, due to hypoglycemia (191). Hypoglycemia can be caused by reduced glucose intake (fasting), increased utilization (hyperinsulinemia), or reduced production (enzymatic defects). One or more of these mechanisms can be responsible for hypoglycemia secondary to drugs. Children treated with propranolol may be at increased risk of hypoglycemia, particularly if they are fasting. Concomitant treatment with methylphenidate can increase the risk of this metabolic disorder.

However, contrary to popular belief, beta-adrenoceptor antagonists do not by themselves increase the risk of hypoglycemic episodes in insulin-treated diabetics, in whom their use was concluded to be generally safe (192). Indeed, in 20 such patients treated with diet or diet plus oral hypoglycemic agents, both propranolol and metoprolol produced small but significant increases in blood glucose concentrations after 4 weeks (193). The rise was considered clinically important in only a few patients.

However, in insulin-treated diabetics who become hypoglycemic, non-selective beta-adrenoceptor antagonists can mask the adrenaline-mediated symptoms, such as palpitation, tachycardia, and tremor; they can cause a rise in mean and diastolic blood pressures, due to unopposed alpha-adrenoceptor stimulation from catecholamines, because the beta$_2$-adrenoceptor-mediated vasodilator response is blocked (194); they can also impair the rate of rise of blood glucose toward normal (195). In contrast, cardioselective drugs mask hypoglycemic symptoms less (196); because of vascular sparing, they are less likely to be associated with a diastolic pressor response in the presence of catecholamines, although this has been reported with metoprolol (197); and delay in recovery from hypoglycemia is either less marked or undetectable with cardioselective drugs, such as atenolol or metoprolol. Thus, if insulin-requiring diabetics need to be treated with a beta-adrenoceptor antagonist, a cardioselective agent should always be chosen for reasons of safety, while allowing that this type of beta-blocker is associated with insulin resistance and can impair insulin sensitivity by 15–30% (SEDA-17, 235), and hence increase insulin requirements.

People with diabetes have a much worse outcome after acute myocardial infarction, with a mortality rate at least twice that in non-diabetics. However, tight control of blood glucose, with immediate intensive insulin treatment during the peri-infarct period followed by intensive subcutaneous insulin treatment, was associated with a 30% reduction in mortality at 1 year, as reported in the DIGAMI study. In addition, the use of beta-blockers in this group of patients had an independent secondary preventive effect (198). The use of beta-blockers in diabetics with ischemic heart disease should be encouraged (199).

In 686 hypertensive men treated for 15 years, beta-blockers were associated with a higher incidence of diabetes than thiazide diuretics (200). This was an uncontrolled study, but the observation deserves further study.

Blood lipids

There is increasing evidence that beta-adrenoceptor antagonists increase total triglyceride concentrations in blood and reduce high-density lipoprotein (HDL) cholesterol. Comparisons of non-selective and cardioselective drugs have shown that lipid changes are less marked but still present with beta$_1$-selective agents (201). Current information suggests that beta$_1$-selective drugs may be preferable in patients with hypertriglyceridemia (202). Topical beta-blockers can cause rises in serum triglyceride concentrations and falls in serum high-density lipoprotein concentrations; this makes them less suitable in patients with coronary heart disease (203,204).

The importance of these effects for the long-term management of patients with hypertension or ischemic heart disease is unknown, but it is recognized that a high serum total cholesterol and a low HDL cholesterol are associated with an increased risk of ischemic heart disease. However, a significant reduction in HDL cholesterol after

treatment for 1 year with timolol was of no prognostic significance and did not attenuate the protective effect of the drug (205). In a 4-year randomized, placebo-controlled study of six antihypertensive monotherapies, acebutolol produced only a small and probably clinically irrelevant (0.17 mmol/l) reduction in total cholesterol (206), which was not statistically different from four of the other antihypertensive drugs.

Obesity

It has been suggested that beta-blockers may predispose to obesity by reducing basal metabolic rate via beta-adrenoceptor blockade (207). Thermogenesis in response to heat and cold, meals, stress, and anxiety is also reduced by beta-adrenoceptor blockade, promoting weight gain (SEDA-16, 193). Beta$_3$-adrenoceptors have been implicated in this mechanism (208,209). Since propranolol blocks beta$_3$-receptors in vivo (210), it would be wise on theoretical grounds to avoid propranolol in obese patients; nadolol is another non-selective beta-blocker that does not act on beta$_3$-adrenoceptors.

A systematic review of eight prospective, randomized trials in 7048 patients with hypertension (3205 of whom were taking beta-blockers) confirmed that body weight was higher in those taking beta-blockers than in controls at the end of the studies (211). The median difference in body weight was 1.2 kg (range –0.4–3.5 kg). There was no relation between demographic characteristics and changes in body weight. The weight gain was observed in the first few months of treatment and thereafter there was no further weight gain compared with controls. This observation suggests that first-line use of beta-blockers in obese patients with hypertension should be considered with caution.

Ophthalmic beta-blockers can cause hypoglycemia in insulin-dependent diabetes (212). Conversely, in diabetic patients taking oral hypoglycemic drugs, hyperglycemia can develop because of impaired insulin secretion (SEDA-21, 487).

Beta-lactam antibiotics

Pivaloyl-containing compounds (baccefuconam, cefetamet pivoxil, cefteram pivoxil, pivampicillin, pivmecillinam) can significantly increase urinary carnitine excretion (213,214). These compounds are esterified prodrugs, which become effective only after the release of pivalic acid, which in turn is esterified with carnitine. Carnitine loss induced by pivaloyl-containing beta-lactams was first described in children and can produce symptoms similar to other types of carnitine deficiency, for example secondary to organic acidurias (213). Carnitine is essential for the transport of fatty acids through the mitochondrial membrane for beta-oxidation. Consequences of its deficiency include skeletal damage, cardiomyopathy, hypoglycemia and reduced ketogenesis, encephalopathy, hepatomegaly, and Reye-like syndromes (215).

The administration of pivaloyl-conjugated beta-lactam antibiotics to healthy volunteers for 54 days reduced mean serum carnitine 10-fold and muscle carnitine, as measured per non-collagen protein, more than 2-fold (215). Long-term treatment of children for 12–37 months to prevent urinary tract infection resulted in serum carnitine concentrations of 0.9–3.6 µmol/l (reference range 23–60 µmol/l). In four cases, muscle carnitine was 0.6–1.4 µmol/g non-collagen protein (reference range 7.1–19) (216).

Although oral carnitine aided the elimination of the pivaloyl moiety, its simultaneous use did not fully compensate for the adverse metabolic effects of pivaloyl-containing beta-lactams (217,218). The consequences of pivaloyl-induced carnitine loss seem to be generally reversible. But as long as the risk of pivaloyl-induced urinary loss of carnitine and particular risk factors are not better defined, it is prudent to use pivaloyl-containing prodrugs only in short-term treatment.

Bile acids

In a randomized controlled study in 86 patients with primary biliary cirrhosis given ursodeoxycholic acid 13–15 mg/kg/day there was significant weight gain (average 3.6 kg) in the first 12 months of treatment, maintained for 4 years, and not related to baseline body mass index (219). In this study patients were. Of 73 patients who took placebo, 43 had an average weight gain of 0.6 kg. The authors postulated that the weight gain may have been due to a sense of improved well-being in patients taking ursodeoxycholic acid, resulting in increased enjoyment and intake of food. They suggested that ursodeoxycholic acid may affect cytokine concentrations, which may influence body mass; alternatively, ursodeoxycholic acid may improve malabsorption and thus increase body mass.

Bisoprolol

Bisoprolol can increase serum triglycerides and reduce HDL cholesterol (220).

Bisphosphonates

A patient who was receiving disodium pamidronate developed gynecomastia, and of another 13 patients, two more men had gynecomastia and one woman had tender swollen breasts (221).

Bromocriptine

Inappropriate secretion of ADH has been described in a single patient (222).

Bumetanide

It has been suggested that bumetanide has a smaller effect on blood glucose than furosemide does, but that is not at all clear.

Caffeine

The major metabolic effects of caffeine are increase in free fatty acids and blood glucose concentration (223,224).

Calcipotriol

Calcipotriol, a biologically active form of vitamin D3, is usually well-tolerated, although it can cause local irritation in up to 30% of patients. Topical calcipotriol in recommended dosages has rarely been associated with hypercalcemia.

- An 85-year-old woman presented with anorexia, oliguria, and acute renal insufficiency 19 days after starting to take calcipotriol (32). She also had raised calcium and sodium concentrations.

Calcium channel blockers

In six hypertensive patients given nitrendipine 20 mg/day for 30 days, there was inhibition of aldosterone response but no significant change in ACTH secretion in response to corticotrophin-releasing hormone (225).

The calcium-dependent pathway of aldosterone synthesis in the zona glomerulosa is blocked by calcium channel blockers, producing a negative feedback increase in the pituitary secretion of ACTH, which in turn causes hyperplasia of the zona glomerulosa. This leads to increased production of androgenic steroid intermediate products and subsequently testosterone, which acts on gingival cells and matrix, giving rise to gingival hyperplasia (see the section on Mouth and teeth).

Calcium transport is essential for insulin secretion, which is therefore inhibited by calcium channel blockers (226). Despite this, calcium channel blockers generally have minimal effects on glucose tolerance in both healthy and diabetic subjects. Oral glucose tolerance is not affected by verapamil, and basal blood glucose concentrations were not altered during long-term verapamil administration (227). Similarly, neither nifedipine nor nicardipine produced significant hyperglycemic effects in either diabetic or non-diabetic patients (228–230). In 117 hypertensive patients nifedipine caused a significant rise in mean random blood glucose of only 0.3 mmol/l (231), an effect that was clearly of no clinical relevance. In the Treatment of Mild Hypertension Study, 4 years of monotherapy with amlodipine maleate caused no change compared with placebo in the serum glucose of 114 hypertensive patients (232). In a review (233) it was concluded that in usual dosages calcium channel blockers do not alter glucose handling. However, in a few patients diabetes appeared de novo or worsened considerably on starting nifedipine (231,234), so there may be a small risk in some individuals.

Cannabinoids

In animals (particularly monkeys), cannabis depresses ovarian and testicular function. In man, chronic use has been associated with reduced serum FSH and LH concentrations in a few people, often accompanied by reduced serum testosterone, oligospermia, reduced sperm motility, and gynecomastia (235). There is no evidence of impairment of male fertility; no studies have been carried out on female fertility. There is evidence of slightly shortened gestation periods in chronic users (236). There are variable non-specific effects on serum prolactin and growth hormone and a rise in plasma cortisol concentrations has been recorded in one study.

Carbamazepine

Carbamazepine therapy in eight women was associated with increased serum concentrations of sex hormone binding globulin (SHBG) and a reduced serum ratio of 17-α-estradiol and estradiol to SHBG. Of 56 women who had been taking carbamazepine for over 5 years, 14 had menstrual disturbances, which tended to be associated with raised SHBG and reduced serum concentrations of 17-α-estradiol (237). Carbamazepine may also reduce serum LH, progesterone, dehydroepiandrosterone, and the free androgen index (238,239), and some of these changes may be associated with anovulatory cycles and menstrual irregularities.

Men taking carbamazepine had mean low serum concentrations of dehydroepiandrosterone and a high SHBG concentration. Moreover, 18% of men taking carbamazepine for epilepsy reported reduced libido, impaired potency, or both.

Changes in body weight have been evaluated in 349 patients taking carbamazepine, phenytoin, or tiagabine. Carbamazepine add-on therapy caused significant mean weight gain of 1.5% (240). Tiagabide add-on therapy caused no significant weight change when added to either phenytoin or carbamazepine.

Some antiepileptic drugs have been associated with low serum and erythrocyte folate concentrations and high total plasma homocysteine concentrations in some patients. The concentrations of folate and homocysteine have been measured in 42 patients taking carbamazepine and 42 matched healthy controls (241). Patients taking carbamazepine had significantly lower serum and erythrocyte folate concentrations. There was hyperhomocystinemia (over 15 μmol/l) in 24% of the patients and 5% of the controls.

Carbenoxolone

- Hyperprolactinemia occurred in a woman with secondary amenorrhea and hypertension who was taking large amounts of liquorice; all the abnormalities reversed on withdrawal (242).

This effect could have reflected involvement of prolactin in adrenal steroidogenesis or salt and water homeostasis.

Carbonic anhydrase inhibitors

Acetazolamide can produce severe lactic acidosis, with an increased lactate:pyruvate ratio, ketosis with a low beta-hydroxybutyrate:acetoacetate ratio, and a urinary organic acid profile consistent with pyruvate carboxylase deficiency. The acquired enzymatic injury that results from inhibition of mitochondrial carbonic anhydrase V, which provides bicarbonate to pyruvate carboxylase, can damage the tricarboxylic acid cycle.

Four preterm neonates with posthemorrhagic ventricular dilatation developed severe metabolic acidosis after being given acetazolamide (33). The acidosis suddenly disappeared after a transfusion of packed erythrocytes, which was attributed to the citrate contained in the blood.

Acetazolamide can cause a metabolic acidosis in 50% of elderly patients (SEDA-11, 199); occasionally (particularly if salicylates are being given or renal function is poor) the acidosis can be severe. It does this by inhibiting renal bicarbonate reabsorption. This effect is of particular use in treating patients with chronic respiratory acidosis with superimposed metabolic alkalosis. Life-threatening metabolic acidosis is rarely observed in the absence of renal insufficiency and/or diabetes mellitus. In three patients with central nervous system pathology alone conventional doses of acetazolamide resulted in severe metabolic acidosis (34). After withdrawal it took up to 48 hours for the metabolic acidosis and accompanying hyperventilation to resolve.

Metabolic acidosis has also been described with the topical carbonic anhydrase inhibitor dorzolamide.

- A 5-day-old boy, weighing 2.3 kg, developed a metabolic acidosis after receiving topical dorzolamide for 1 week for bilateral Peter's anomaly (a congenital corneal disorder characterized by a central leukoma and adhesions at the periphery of the corneal opacity) (35). The maximum base deficit was 20.2 mmol/l. On withdrawal of topical dorzolamide his acidosis resolved within 1 day.

Factors that may have contributed to this metabolic acidosis included low birth weight, renal tubular immaturity, and impaired renal function, which may have resulted in systemic accumulation with repetitive dosing. This case stresses the fact that topical medications can cause systemic effects if a sufficient amount of drug is absorbed in a susceptible subject.

Children with heart disease often require high-dose diuretic therapy, which can lead to hypochloremic metabolic alkalosis. There are limited data on the safety of acetazolamide in the treatment of hypochloremic metabolic alkalosis in children. In 28 patients, median age 2 (range 0.3–20) months who took acetazolamide 5 mg/kg for 3 days, there were no adverse events (36). There was no significant difference in any electrolyte concentration, except for serum HCO_3, which fell from 36 to 31 mmol/l, and serum chloride, which rose from 91 to 95 mmol/l. There was no change in urine output. Acetazolamide appears to be safe in very young patients when given for 3 consecutive days.

Metabolic acidosis due to acetazolamide causes increased minute ventilation, which can cause increased intracranial pressure and result in neurological complications (38).

- A 19-year-old woman with postoperative bilateral raised intracranial pressure was given intravenous acetazolamide 500 mg followed by 250 mg every 6 hours. After 3 days she developed a metabolic acidosis (serum HCO_3 18 mmol/l), which was attributed to acetazolamide. The metabolic acidosis progressed over the next 3 days (HCO_3 15 mmol/l) with appropriate hypocapnia (P_aCO_2 3.2–3.6 kPa). After 6 days she became agitated, and a propofol infusion was begun, but her mechanical respiratory rate was not increased to maintain her prior hypocapnia. After 5 hours her P_aCO_2 was 4.7 kPa and her arterial pH was 7.26. She developed extreme hypertension and a tachycardia. A CT scan of the brain showed cerebral edema, brain stem herniation, and bilateral watershed infarcts. At post mortem there were multiple fat emboli in the brain and lungs.

The use of acetazolamide in the presence of unrecognized cerebral edema due to fat embolism, with sudden normalization of brain CO_2, as occurred in this patient when her previous state of hypocapnia was no longer sustained by ventilatory effort, resulted in cerebral acidosis, vasodilatation, and a further increase in intracranial pressure. This proved catastrophic and led to brainstem herniation and brain death. Acetazolamide should be avoided if at all possible in patients with bony and traumatic brain injuries, particularly during weaning from mechanical ventilation, since it can precipitate coning in patients with raised intracranial pressure.

Thyrotoxic periodic paralysis occurs only occasionally in Caucasians, but for unknown reasons it can be worsened by acetazolamide (SEDA-15, 219).

Topical brinzolamide can be systemically absorbed and could cause systemic adverse effects. In one case it was reported to have caused a metabolic acidosis (39).

- A 66-year-old man with glaucoma was given brinzolamide twice daily to only one eye in addition to topical latanoprost. After 3 months he reported having stopped using brinzolamide because of lethargy and a bad taste in the mouth. He also reported that a silver chain worn around his neck had turned black within 2 days of starting brinzolamide and again soon after it had been cleaned. Electrolyte and acid-base status were not assessed.

Although a metabolic acidosis could occur with topical brinzolamide if sufficient drug were systemically absorbed, a change in the color of a silver chain worn around the neck is hardly an adequate basis for a diagnosis of a metabolic acidosis.

Cardiac glycosides

Digitalis has effects on sex hormones. It causes increased serum concentrations of follicle-stimulating hormone (FSH) and estrogen and reduced concentrations of

luteinizing hormone (LH) and testosterone (243–246). These effects are probably not related to any direct estrogen-like structure of digitalis (despite structural similarities), but rather to an effect involving the synthesis or release of sex hormones. There are three possible clinical outcomes of these effects.

Gynecomastia in men and breast enlargement in women

Effects of cardiac glycosides in the breasts can be associated with demonstrable histological changes (247,248).

Stratification of the vaginal squamous epithelium in postmenopausal women

This can cause difficulty in the pathological interpretation of vaginal smears for cancer diagnosis (249).

A possible modifying effect on breast cancer

Digitalis can reduce the heterogeneity of breast cancer cell populations and reduce the rate of distant metastases (250). There is also evidence that the 5-year recurrence rate after mastectomy is lower in women who have been treated with digitalis (251). Early studies suggested that when breast tumors occurred in women with congestive heart failure taking cardiac glycosides, tumor size was significantly smaller and the tumor cells more homogeneous (SEDA-7, 194). It was originally thought that this action was due to an estrogen-like effect of cardiac glycosides, but more recent evidence suggests that it occurs because inhibition of the Na/K pump is involved in inhibiting proliferation and inducing apoptosis in various cell lines (252–255). Cardiac glycosides have different potencies in their effects on cell lines such as those of ovarian carcinoma and breast carcinoma (order of potency: proscillaridin A > digitoxin > digoxin > ouabain > lanatoside C) (256).

In three patients with diabetes mellitus, withdrawal of digoxin improved blood glucose control, implying that digoxin had impaired glucose tolerance (257). The authors conceded that the effect might have occurred coincidentally, but in one case glucose tolerance deteriorated again after rechallenge. Insulin increases the cellular uptake of glucose and stimulates the sodium/potassium pump, and it may be that inhibition of the sodium/potassium pump by digoxin has the opposite effect.

In 14 patients with morbid obesity, who were being given digoxin in the hope that reduced production of cerebrospinal fluid, with the consequent reduction in pressure, might be associated with weight reduction, the dosage of digoxin (Lanacrist 0.13 mg, equivalent to 0.065 mg of digoxin) was titrated to produce a minimum serum digoxin concentration of 1.0 nmol/l (258). One patient was already diabetic, and five developed fasting blood glucose concentrations greater than 5.0 mmol/l on three consecutive occasions, with accompanying glycosuria. Another had fasting blood glucose concentrations of 6.0–8.5 mmol/l. There was a significant relation between the dose of digoxin and the risk of impaired glucose tolerance. However, the diabetes mellitus did not abate after digoxin withdrawal, and since all these patients were obese, the occurrence of diabetes was probably coincidental.

Carvedilol

Severe diabetes mellitus has been described in a patient with heart failure treated with carvedilol and furosemide (41).

- A 37-year old man with a dilated cardiomyopathy was given furosemide, spironolactone, and candesartan. After 1 year carvedilol was introduced in a maintenance dose of 10 mg/day. HbA_{1c} was 5.1% at the beginning of carvedilol treatment. After 9 months of treatment, he started to feel extremely thirsty and lost 10 kg in 3 months. No viral infections or pancreatitis were detected. The HbA_{1c} concentration increased to 17%, the blood glucose concentration was 31 mmol/l (557 mg/dl). Furosemide was withdrawn and the blood glucose concentration fell within a week to 8.9 mmol/l (160 mg/dl). Carvedilol was then replaced by metoprolol and after 2 further weeks the fasting blood glucose concentration fell to 5.9 mmol/l (106 mg/dl). The patient was stable thereafter.

The mechanisms of carvedilol-induced hyperglycemia are not known, although alpha-blockade in the pancreas could impair insulin secretion. In this case furosemide could have increased insulin resistance.

Ceftriaxone

Although possible interference with the metabolism of carnitine by pivaloylmethyl-esterified beta-lactams is a matter of concern (SEDA-21, 260), new similar prodrug derivatives of cephalosporins continue to be marketed, as do reports that they can be given to healthy volunteers without concern (42).

However, taking a closer look at the data, it is evident that healthy volunteers lost around 10% of their body stores of carnitine within 2 weeks of being given antibiotics containing pivalic acid (43). The authors emphasized that prolonged used of such drugs might result in profound carnitine depletion and that this depletion might be associated with clinical sequelae.

Valproate also causes urinary loss of carnitine (SEDA-12, 209), most probably by a different mechanism than pivalic acid (44). However, the combination can rapidly cause serious adverse effects (45).

- A 72-year-old woman taking valproate as monotherapy for her epilepsy developed a urinary tract infection and was given pivmecillinam 600 mg/day. During the next few days she became stuporose; her serum ammonia concentration was high (113 mmol/l) but liver function was normal. Pivmecillinam and valproate were withdrawn and she recovered rapidly.

The authors recommended caution when treating patients taking valproate with pivmecillinam because of the risk of hyperammonemic encephalopathy. It seems reasonable to assume that this caution should include all beta-lactams that incorporate pivalic acid.

However, there may be another mechanism by which cephalosporins can interfere with carnitine metabolism. Cephalosporins with a quaternary nitrogen (cefepime, cefluprenam, cefoselide, and cefaloridine) compete with carnitine for renal reabsorption due to OCNT2, a major member of the family of organic cationic transporters (46). Mutations in the OCNT2gene are responsible for the genetic disorder primary systemic carnitine deficiency (47,48). Since carnitine and the cephalosporins mentioned above compete for the same substrate-binding site on OCTN2, it is likely that such mutations will interfere with the pharmacokinetics of these drugs. Consequently these cephalosporins should not be given to patients with such mutations.

Celastraceae

Chronic khat chewing increased plasma glucose and C-peptide concentrations in people with type 2 diabetes mellitus (259).

Chlordiazepoxide

A San Francisco woman with a history of diabetes and high blood pressure was hospitalized in January 2001 with a life-threatening low blood sugar concentration after she consumed Anso Comfort capsules (260). The authors conjectured that hospitalization may have been necessitated by a drug interaction of chlordiazepoxide with medications that she was taking for other medical conditions.

Chloroquine and hydroxychloroquine

Hypoglycemia has often been reported in chloroquine-treated patients with malaria, but it is not clear whether the chloroquine or the malaria itself caused the hypoglycemia (SED-14, 952).

- A 16-year old girl was treated empirically with chloroquine (total 450 mg of chloroquine base) for fever, had no malarial parasites in the peripheral blood smear, but had severe hypoglycemia of 1.5 mmol/l (27 mg/dl) (49).

This suggests that therapeutic doses of chloroquine can cause hypoglycemia even in the absence of malaria.

Hypoglycemia was reported in a fatal chloroquine intoxication in a 32-year-old black Zambian male (SEDA-13, 240). Hypoglycemia has also been seen in patients, especially children, with cerebral malaria (SEDA-13, 240). Further studies have shown that the hypoglycemia in these African children was usually present before the antimalarial drugs had been started; in a study in Gambia hypoglycemia occurred after treatment with the drug had been started, although it was not necessarily connected with the treatment (SEDA-13, 240). Convulsions were more common in hypoglycemic children. This commonly unrecognized complication contributes to morbidity and mortality in cerebral *Plasmodium falciparum* malaria. Hypoglycemia is amenable to treatment with intravenous dextrose or glucose, which may help to prevent brain damage (SEDA-13, 804).

Although hydroxychloroquine has been used to treat porphyria cutanea tarda (261), there are reports that it can also worsen porphyria (262,263).

Cibenzoline

Several cases of hypoglycemia have been attributed to cibenzoline (SEDA-18, 204; 264–266). In a case-control study of 14 156 outpatients, 91 had hypoglycemia, and each was matched with five controls (267). Eight of those with hypoglycemia were taking cibenzoline and three were taking disopyramide. In contrast, only seven of the controls were taking cibenzoline, a significant difference. However, 20 of the controls were taking disopyramide, which was not significant from the patients with hypoglycemia, although disopyramide is known to cause hypoglycemia. Insulin was also associated with hypoglycemia, but sulfonylureas were not. Furthermore, there was a positive association with what were termed "thyroid agents." All of these features cast some doubt on the validity of these results in relation to cibenzoline.

- A 65-year-old woman developed hypoglycemia while taking cibenzoline and alacepril (268).

It is possible that hypoglycemia due to cibenzoline can be enhanced by ACE inhibitors, which can increase insulin sensitivity (SED-14, 640).

Ciclosporin

Thyroid

Life-threatening hypothyroidism associated with ciclosporin was reported in a patient treated with reduced-intensity hemopoietic stem cell transplantation for metastatic renal-cell carcinoma (50).

- A 26 year old woman with metastatic renal cell carcinoma underwent reduced-intensity hemopoietic stem cell transplantation after having had a right nephrectomy, pelvic radiotherapy, interferon, and conditioning with busulfan, fludarabine, and antithymocyte globulin. Ciclosporin 3 mg/kg was added and graft-versus-host disease occurred on day 54 after ciclosporin was tapered. Ciclosporin 2 mg/kg was restarted intravenously and she developed malaise and hepatorenal dysfunction. The symptoms resolved after withdrawal of ciclosporin on day 62. One week later, ciclosporin 2 mg/kg was given orally and she developed fatigue, lethargy, and paralytic ileus. Thyroid-stimulating hormone, free triiodothyronine, and free thyroxine were undetectable; thyroid function had previously been normal. A thyrotropin-releasing hormone test showed secondary hypothalamic dysfunction.

The authors suggested that ciclosporin had suppressed the hypothalamic-pituitary axis.

Glucose metabolism and diabetes mellitus

The effect of long-term ciclosporin on glucose metabolism was analysed in heart transplant recipients who developed post-transplant hyperglycemia, 102 with impaired glycemic control and 20 with clinical diabetes (51). There was a significant negative correlation between ciclosporin concentration and insulin in both groups, a significant negative correlation between ciclosporin concentration and proinsulin, C-peptide blood concentration in those with impaired glycemic control and a significant positive correlation between ciclosporin and glucose blood concentration in both groups.

Diabetes mellitus after transplantation is recognized as an important adverse effect of immunosuppressants, and has been extensively reviewed (269). However, the use of ciclosporin in immunosuppressive regimens is not associated with diabetes mellitus after transplantation (10–20%) (270).

Hyperlipidemia

Ciclosporin is potentially more toxic in patients with altered LDL concentrations or a low total serum cholesterol (271). Ciclosporin therapy itself significantly raises plasma lipoprotein concentrations by increasing the total serum cholesterol; this is due to an increase in LDL cholesterol, demonstrated in a prospective, double-blind, randomized, placebo-controlled trial in 36 men with amyotrophic lateral sclerosis (272). In 22 patients there were significant increases in mean serum triglycerides and cholesterol 2 weeks after they started to take low-dose ciclosporin (273). Hypertriglyceridemia developed in seven patients taking ciclosporin 2.0–7.5 mg/kg/day for psoriasis during the first month of therapy; the values were greater than the upper limit in age- and sex-matched controls (274).

The pathology of hyperlipidemia after transplantation is multifactorial, but it is clearly dose-dependently related to immunosuppressive therapy (275). This results in cardiovascular disease, which is one of the most common causes of morbidity and mortality in long-term survivors of organ transplantation (276). Hyperlipidemia can also cause renal atheroma, resulting in graft rejection. The possible impact of ciclosporin on lipids includes an increase in total cholesterol, LDL cholesterol, and apolipoprotein B concentrations, and a reduction in HDL cholesterol (SED-13, 1124). The influence of ciclosporin on lipoprotein(a) concentrations has been debated (SEDA-21, 383; 277). Post-transplant hyperlipidemia is multifactorial and can be affected by impaired renal function, diuretics and beta-blockers, increased age, and female sex. A combination of lipid-lowering drugs and optimization of immunosuppressive regimens compatible with long-term allograft survival is probably required to reduce post-transplantation hyperlipidemia.

Whereas azathioprine is considered to play no role, glucocorticoid use correlates positively with increased serum cholesterol concentrations. It is uncertain whether these lipid changes reflect primarily an effect of ciclosporin alone or an additive/synergistic effect of the drug plus glucocorticoids. Ciclosporin has been considered as a possible independent susceptibility factor by several investigators, but others were unable to find an association between hyperlipidemia and ciclosporin (SEDA-20, 344). There was indirect evidence for a causal role of ciclosporin in several studies; hyperlipidemia developed in non-transplant patients taking ciclosporin alone; there was a transient reduction in hyperlipidemia after ciclosporin withdrawal; there was a significant correlation between ciclosporin blood concentrations and lipid abnormalities; and there was a higher incidence of lipid abnormalities in patients taking ciclosporin alone compared with patients taking azathioprine and prednisolone (SED-8, 1131; SEDA-17, 524; SEDA-21, 383; 275,278). Other studies have provided striking evidence that hyperlipidemia is more frequent in patients taking ciclosporin than in those taking tacrolimus, with more patients classified as having high cholesterol concentrations in the ciclosporin group or a significant fall in total cholesterol or LDL cholesterol in patients switched from ciclosporin to tacrolimus (279,280). Although the glucocorticoid-sparing effect of tacrolimus may account for these differences, the concept that the glucocorticoid dose is a confounding factor has been disputed (SEDA-22, 412). Whether these differences translate to a higher risk of cardiovascular complications in patients taking ciclosporin has not been carefully assessed. The treatment of hyperlipidemia in transplant patients may represent a major dilemma, because of several drug interactions, with an increased risk of myopathy and rhabdomyolysis after the combined use of ciclosporin and several lipid-lowering drugs.

Tacrolimus + sirolimus, tacrolimus + mycophenolate mofetil, and ciclosporin + sirolimus have been compared in recipients of their first kidney transplant (52). One-year patient and graft survival did not differ. Ciclosporin + sirolimus was associated with increased serum creatinine concentrations, reduced creatinine clearance, more frequent protocol discontinuation, more antihyperlipidemic drug therapy, and a higher incidence of post-transplant diabetes mellitus.

Hyperuricemia

Significant hyperuricemia has been observed in as many as 80% of patients taking ciclosporin (281). In one series, hyperuricemia occurred in 72% of male and 82% of female patients taking ciclosporin after cardiac transplantation; there was also an increased incidence of gouty arthritis in these patients (282). Episodes of gout developed mostly in men taking diuretics, but the incidence was lower than in the hyperuricemic population. In renal transplant patients, the incidence of gout was 5–24% and tophi sometimes developed rapidly after the onset of gout (283). The potential mechanisms of hyperuricemia include reduced renal function and impaired tubular secretion of acid uric, with hypertension and diuretics as confounding factors (SEDA-21, 383).

Cimetidine

In the earlier years of cimetidine use there were scattered (although well-documented) reports of the drug having destabilized severe diabetes, resulting in impaired control (284); however, most people with diabetes are unlikely to be affected.

Modest increases in serum high-density lipoproteins have occasionally been noted in patients taking cimetidine (SED-12, 942; 285).

Citric acid and citrates

Although there is a long list of causes of metabolic acidosis with an increased anion gap (286,287), clinical clues can help diagnosis. A case report has illustrated the acute metabolic and hemodynamic effects of ingestion of a massive load of oral citric acid. The principal findings included a metabolic acidosis accompanied by an increase in the plasma anion gap, not due to lactic acidosis, hyperkalemia, and the abrupt onset of hypotension (288).

- A 42-year-old previously healthy male prisoner drank a large volume of a commercial solution of unknown composition. His medical history was non-contributory, except for severe epigastric pain. Within an hour, his condition deteriorated; he was ashen, his blood pressure was 80/40 mmHg, and his pulse rate was 102/minute. His neck vessels were flat and his breath sounds were equal bilaterally, with occasional expiratory wheezes at both bases. There were no cardiac murmurs. The abdomen was soft and the bowel sounds were active. His extremities were warm with no cyanosis or edema. There were no neurological abnormalities. Fortuitously, because of therapy to avoid cardiac complications of hyperkalemia, he was given 1 g of calcium chloride, 50 mmol of sodium bicarbonate, 25 g of glucose, and 10 units of regular insulin intravenously. His blood pressure immediately increased to 116/76 mmHg and his pulse rate fell to 90/minute. By the next morning his plasma acid–base balance was normal, as was his ionized calcium concentration (1.1 mmol/l).

Because of the short duration and severity of the metabolic acidosis, together with a near-normal lactate concentration, acid ingestion was the most likely cause for his acid–base disorder. This diagnosis was confirmed once the composition of the ingested fluid was known.

Clomipramine

Clomipramine has also aroused interest because of an action on prolactin release, which occurs with major tranquillizers but not with other tricyclic antidepressants (289). This action of clomipramine is related to its chemical structure and reflects a greater effect on dopamine metabolism and serotonin uptake compared with other antidepressants.

Clonazepam

In a randomized, double-blind, placebo-controlled, cross-over study in 15 men (mean age 22 years), diazepam 10 mg and clonazepam 1 mg infused over 30 minutes both reduced insulin sensitivity and increased plasma glucose, but the effect of clonazepam was significantly greater (53).

Clonidine and apraclonidine

Clonidine stimulates the release of growth hormone and has been used as a provocation test of growth hormone reserve (290).

Clonidine reduces plasma renin activity and urinary aldosterone and catecholamine concentrations (291).

Clozapine

Diabetes mellitus

Hyperglycemia has been observed in patients taking clozapine (SEDA-26, 59). The effect of clozapine on glucose control and insulin sensitivity has been studied prospectively in 9 women and 11 men with schizophrenia (mean age 31 years) (54). Insulin resistance at baseline was unaffected by clozapine, but 11 of the patients developed abnormal glucose control (mean age 30 years; five women). Mean fasting and 2-hour glucose concentrations increased significantly by 0.55 mmol/l. There was no correlation between change in body mass index and change in fasting glucose concentrations.

Several cases of de novo diabetes mellitus or exacerbation of existing diabetes in patients taking neuroleptic drugs have been reported, including patients taking clozapine (292–295). There was no significant relation to weight gain.

- A 49-year-old man taking olanzapine developed diabetes mellitus and recovered after withdrawal (296).
- Diabetic ketoacidosis occurred in a 31-year-old man who had taken clozapine 200 mg/day for 3 months for refractory schizophrenia (297). Clozapine was withdrawn and he remained metabolically stable. Two months later, clozapine was restarted, and only 72 hours after drug re-exposure he had increased fasting glycemia and insulinemia, suggesting insulin resistance as the underlying mechanism. Apart from slight obesity, he had no predisposing factors.

Hyperglycemia occurs at 2 weeks to 3 months after the start of clozapine treatment and occurs without predisposing factors. Clozapine-induced hyperglycemia can be serious, leading to coma, but it is reversible if clozapine is withdrawn. In some cases, continuation of clozapine is possible by controlling blood glucose concentrations with hypoglycemic drugs. This approach can be useful in refractory schizophrenia responsive to clozapine. All patients should be advised to report altered consciousness, polyuria, or increased thirst.

Glucose metabolism has been studied in 17 patients taking clozapine (298). Six had impaired glucose tolerance and eight had a glycemic peak delay.

Diabetes was also more common in 63 patients taking clozapine than in 67 receiving typical depot neuroleptic drugs (299). The percentages of type 2 diabetes mellitus were 12% and 6% respectively. Nevertheless, the mechanism is not known. In six patients with schizophrenia, clozapine increased mean concentrations of blood glucose, insulin, and C peptide (300). The authors concluded that the glucose intolerance was due to increased insulin resistance.

However, opposite data have been found in a case-control study in 7227 patients with new diabetes and 6780 controls, all with psychiatric disorders (301). Clozapine was not significantly associated with diabetes (adjusted OR = 0.98; 95% CI = 0.74, 1.31) and there was no suggestion of relations between larger dosages or longer durations of clozapine use and an increased risk of diabetes. Among individual non-clozapine neuroleptic drugs, there were significantly increased risks for two phenothiazines: chlorpromazine (OR = 1.31; 95% CI = 1.09, 1.56) and perphenazine (OR = 1.34; 95% CI = 1.11, 1.62). The authors suggested that, in contrast to earlier reports, these results provided some reassurance that clozapine does not increase the risk of diabetes. However, cases of diabetes were identified by the new use of antidiabetic drugs, and it is therefore possible that clozapine was associated with less pronounced glucose intolerance that did not require drug therapy.

Hyperlipidemia

Hyperlipidemia associated with antipsychotic drugs has been reviewed (SEDA-29, 64). Haloperidol and the atypical antipsychotic drugs ziprasidone, risperidone, and aripiprazole would be associated with lower risks of hyperlipidemia, whereas chlorpromazine, thioridazine, and the atypical drugs quetiapine, olanzapine, and clozapine would be associated with higher risks. However, severe clozapine-induced hypercholesterolemia and hypertriglyceridemia has been reported in a patient taking clozapine (55).

- A 42-year-old man with a schizoaffective disorder had new-onset hyperlipidemia while taking clozapine (after failing therapy with traditional antipsychotic drugs). Before taking clozapine his total cholesterol measurements were 2.9–5.5 mmol/l and there were no triglyceride measurements. Despite treatment with various antihyperlipidemic agents, his total cholesterol concentration reached 12 mmol/l and his triglyceride concentration reached 54 mmol/l. His antipsychotic drug therapy was switched to aripiprazole and his lipid concentrations improved dramatically, to the point that antihyperlipidemic treatment was withdrawn. When he was given clozapine again his lipid concentrations again worsened.

Weight gain

Weight gain is often associated with clozapine (SEDA-21, 54). In 42 patients who took clozapine for at least 1 year, men and women gained both weight and body mass, which is more directly related to cardiovascular morbidity (302). Over 10 weeks, leptin concentrations, which correlate with body mass index, increased significantly from baseline in 12 patients taking clozapine (303).

The association between clozapine-related weight gain and increased mean arterial blood pressure has been examined in 61 patients who were randomly assigned to either clozapine or haloperidol in a 10-week parallel-group, double-blind study, and in 55 patients who chose to continue to take clozapine in a subsequent 1-year open study (304). Clozapine was associated with significant weight gain in both the double-blind trial (mean 4.2 kg) and the open trial (mean 5.8 kg). There was no significant correlation between change in weight and change in mean arterial blood pressure.

- The 22-year-old son of healthy parents, with a life-long history of galactosemia, developed weight gain while taking an effective dose of clozapine (56).

Because patients with galactosemia need to avoid weight loss as a result of restrictive dietary measures, the authors suggested that this is an interesting example of weight gain as a positive side effect of clozapine, not necessarily associated with increased appetite and higher caloric intake.

There were no significant associations between cycle length and weight change during clozapine treatment in 13 premenopausal women with psychoses (305).

Sleep apnea associated with clozapine-induced obesity has been reported (306).

- A 45-year-old woman with schizophrenia who took clozapine 300 mg/day for 16 months gained 18 kg and had hypertriglyceridemia and glucose intolerance. She had daytime sedation, difficulty in sleeping at night, loud snoring, and periods of apnea during sleep.

Nasal continuous positive airway pressure produced improvement.

Weight gain with clozapine compared with other neuroleptic drugs has been studied in in-patients who were randomly assigned to switch to open treatment with clozapine (n = 138) or to continue receiving conventional neuroleptic drugs (n = 89) (57). Patients gained weight at the end of 2 years whether they switched to clozapine (5.9 kg, 7%) or continued to take first-generation neuroleptic drugs (2.3 kg, 4%), but weight gain was significantly greater (1 body mass index unit) in those taking clozapine, particularly women.

The relation between genetic variants of the β_3 adrenoceptor and the G-protein β_3 subunit and clozapine-induced body weight change has been investigated in 87 treatment-resistant patients with schizophrenia (58). They gained an average of 2.6 kg. There was no statistically significant relation between weight gain and either the β_3 adrenoceptor Trp6Arg or the G-protein β_3 subunit C8257 polymorphisms.

Substantial interindividual and inter-racial differences suggest that genetic factors may be important in weight gain associated with clozapine. For example, the relation between genetic variants of the β_3 adrenoceptor and the G-protein β_3 subunit and clozapine-induced body weight change has been studied (SEDA-29, 67). Now, in a long-term follow-up study (14 months) of 93 patients with schizophrenia the possible relation between clozapine-induced weight gain and a genetic polymorphism in the adrenoceptor alpha 2a receptor, -1291 C>G, has been examined (59). The GG genotype was associated with a significantly higher mean body weight gain (8.4 kg) than the CC genotype (2.8 kg).

The effect of clozapine on serum ghrelin concentrations has been investigated in 12 patients over 10 weeks after the start of treatment (69). In contrast to increased body mass indices and serum leptin concentrations, there were no significant changes in serum ghrelin concentrations. The authors claimed that these results do not support a causal involvement of ghrelin in clozapine-related weight gain.

Phenylpropanolamine 75 mg/day did not promote weight loss in a randomized, placebo-controlled study in 16 patients with schizophrenia who had gained at least 10% of their body weight while taking clozapine (307).

- A 29-year-old man taking clozapine 800 mg/day gained 46 kg in weight after 25 months, and had myoclonic jerks in the hands, arms, and shoulders on both sides (308). He was treated with topiramate (which causes weight loss). The myoclonic jerks disappeared completely. He lost 21 kg over 5 months, with no significant change in eating habits or food consumption, and felt more energetic, more active, and more motivated to exercise.

Clusiaceae

In a retrospective case-control study, 37 patients with raised TSH concentrations were compared with 37 individuals with normal TSH concentrations (309). Exposure to St. John's wort during the previous 3–6 months increased the odds of a raised TSH concentration by a factor of 2.12 (95% CI = 0.36, 12). The authors concluded that an association between St. John's wort and raised TSH concentrations is probable.

Cocaine

Hypothalamic–pituitary–adrenal axis

The association of cocaine withdrawal with hypothalamic–pituitary–adrenal axis dysregulation has previously been reported and may be important in understanding vulnerability to stress response and relapse (70). The hypothesis that withdrawn cocaine-dependent patients would have higher cerebrospinal fluid concentrations of corticotropin-releasing hormone than healthy controls has been tested in 29 cocaine-dependent men (mean age 40 years) who were abstinent for a minimum of 8 days (mean 29 days) and 66 healthy controls. The subjects were 21 African Americans, two Hispanics, and six Caucasians. There were no significant differences in cerebrospinal fluid concentrations of corticotropin-releasing hormone between the subjects and the controls. There was no correlation between the number of days of cocaine withdrawal and the corticotropin-releasing hormone concentrations. This negative study reflected the fact that the hypothalamic–pituitary–adrenal axis in cocaine abstinence is no longer dysregulated.

Cocaine and nicotine share many similarities, including a strong potential for addiction. In a comparison of the acute effects of cocaine and cigarette smoking on luteinizing hormone, testosterone, and prolactin, 24 men who met criteria for cocaine abuse or nicotine dependence were given intravenous cocaine (0.4 mg/kg) or placebo cocaine, or smoked a low-nicotine or high-nicotine cigarette (72). Placebo-cocaine and low-nicotine cigarette smoking did not change luteinizing hormone, testosterone, or prolactin. Luteinizing hormone increased significantly after both intravenous cocaine and high-nicotine cigarette smoking and correlated significantly with increases in cocaine and nicotine plasma concentrations. However, high-nicotine cigarette smoking stimulated significantly greater increases in luteinizing hormone release than intravenous cocaine. On the other hand, testosterone concentrations did not change significantly after either cocaine or high-nicotine cigarette smoking. Prolactin concentrations fell significantly and remained below baseline after intravenous cocaine. However, after high-nicotine cigarette smoking, prolactin increased to hyperprolactinemic concentrations within 6 minutes and remained significantly above baseline for 42 minutes. The increases in luteinizing hormone were temporally related to behavioral and physiological measures of sexual arousal. The authors commented that the rapid increases in luteinizing hormone and reports of subjective high after both intravenous cocaine and high-nicotine cigarette smoking illustrate the similarities between these drugs and they suggested a possible contribution of luteinizing hormone to their abuse-related effects.

In a prospective study, endocrine responses to hyperthermic stress were assessed in 10 male cocaine users after 4 weeks of abstinence and again after 1 year of abstinence (310). They sat in a sauna for 30 minutes at a temperature of 90°F and a relative humidity of 10%. At the end of the sauna, they rested for another 30 minutes at room temperature. Sublingual temperature, pulse rate, and blood pressure were recorded just before and immediately after the sauna and 30 minutes after the period at room temperature. Venous β-erythropoietin, ACTH, metenkephalin, prolactin, and cortisol were also measured. There were no significant differences between the two groups in heart rate and blood pressure. At baseline and after 1 year of abstinence, plasma prolactin concentrations were higher in the cocaine users than in the controls. Moreover, the hormonal responses in the cocaine users were different from those in controls. Concentrations of all the hormones, except for metenkephalin, were significantly lower in the cocaine users than in the controls at the end of the sauna; the cocaine users did not have significant hormonal changes to hyperthermia after either 4 weeks or 1 year of abstinence. The authors concluded that cocaine abuse produces alterations in the hypothalamic-pituitary axis, which persist during abstinence.

Blood glucose

Blood glucose concentrations can become labile in people with diabetes mellitus who use cocaine, not only because their diet changes, but also because adrenaline concentrations affect the mobilization of glucose (311).

Colchicine

Transient diabetes and hyperlipidemia have been reported. Metabolic acidosis is probably a consequence of heavy, cholera-like diarrhea. Progressive reduction of libido was attributed to colchicine in patients with familial Mediterranean fever (312).

Commiphora mukul (Burseraceae)

Guggulipid is a standardized extract from *Commiphora mukul*, often used in traditional Indian medicine for circulatory problems. The results of several studies have suggested that it lowers cholesterol concentrations. However, a placebo-controlled study showed that it increased LDL cholesterol by 4% (300 mg/day of guggulipid) and 5% (600 mg/day of guggulipid) (73).

Complementary and alternative medicine

Galactorrhea has been associated with acupuncture.

- A 41-year-old woman with breast cancer was treated with acupuncture for pain control (313). She had an episode of galactorrhea 6 days after the first treatment and also during the second acupuncture treatment. No reason for this unusual phenomenon other than acupuncture could be found.

The authors pointed out that in Chinese medicine acupuncture at the points used in this patient promotes lactation.

Coumarin anticoagulants

An antithyroid effect of bishydroxycoumarin has been suspected (314).

Dicoumarol has been reported to have a uricosuric effect (315).

Cucurbitaceae

Momordica charantia can cause hypoglycemic coma and convulsions in children (316).

Cyclophosphamide

Even low-dose intravenous cyclophosphamide can cause a syndrome that resembles inappropriate secretion of antidiuretic hormone, with severe hyponatremia and symptoms of water intoxication (SEDA-19, 347; SEDA-21, 386). A direct effect on the renal tubules is likely, but no other nephrotoxic effects have been documented.

Cytostatic and immunosuppressant drugs

See also individual agents

A rise in body mass index has been reported in young patients with teratomas treated with chemotherapy, still apparent 14 years after the end of treatment (317).

Combined cytostatic drug therapy for Hodgkin's disease in childhood often results in abnormal endocrine function, particularly increases in follicle-stimulating hormone, prolactin, and thyroid-stimulating hormone (318).

Hyperglycemia was reported in 21 of 56 patients who received weekly paclitaxel with oral estramustine and carboplatin (4-weekly); under 10% required pharmacological intervention (319). There was mild hyperphosphatemia in 24.

There was fasting hypoglycemia in 19 of 35 children with acute lymphoblastic leukemia receiving maintenance therapy of daily oral mercaptopurine and weekly oral methotrexate; all the children improved on withdrawal of chemotherapy and 10 of 15 normalized (320).

Tumor lysis syndrome together with increased cytokine release can occur with drugs such as clofarabine; therefore, besides intensified hydration, allopurinol should be given if hyperuricemia is expected (321).

There have been cases of acute tumor lysis syndrome in patients with melanoma (322) and light-chain amyloidosis (323). The authors reviewed the incidence of acute tumor lysis syndrome in these diseases, which are less typically associated with it.

Dexamfetamine

Hyperinsulinemia secondary to chronic administration of dexamfetamine, with a fall in fasting blood sugar after a few weeks of use, has been described (SED-9, 10).

Dextromethorphan

During a double-blind, placebo-controlled study of the effect of high doses of dextromethorphan in children with bacterial meningitis, two of four patients developed type 1 diabetes mellitus; they had received dextromethorphan and the other two placebo (324).

- A 10-year-old boy received dextromethorphan 36 mg/kg/day by nasogastric tube. He developed hyperglycemia with ketoacidosis after 5 days and required insulin. The dose of dextromethorphan was reduced over the next 4 days and withdrawn. Insulin was withdrawn 4 days later.
- A 14-year-old girl received dextromethorphan 26 mg/kg/day by nasogastric tube. She developed hyperglycemia after 2 days and needed insulin for 6 days. A later glucose tolerance test was normal.

Pancreatic beta cells in rats express NMDA receptors, stimulation of which leads to insulin secretion (325). The authors postulated that dextromethorphan inhibits insulin secretion by blocking NMDA receptors and thus impairs glucose tolerance. Both patients had reduced insulin concentrations, implying that peripheral insulin resistance was unlikely to have been the cause of diabetes.

Dextropropoxyphene

Severe hypoglycemia has been reported in the elderly (SEDA-17, 80).

Diamorphine

The syndrome of inappropriate secretion of antidiuretic hormone (SIADH) has been attributed to heroin (326).

- A 23-year-old pregnant woman developed antepartum bleeding at 35 weeks and a tonic-clonic convulsion and hypothermia at 39 weeks, having used heroin 4 hours before. She had further tonic-clonic seizures, became obtunded, and required intubation. She had occasional runs of ventricular bigeminy. A cesarean section was performed. The neonate had poor respiratory effort and required ventilation. Blood chemistry suggested inappropriate secretion of antidiuretic hormone, acute renal insufficiency, and acute pancreatitis. She and the baby recovered after 2 weeks.

Diazepam

Acute diazepam administration causes a reduction in plasma cortisol concentrations, consistent with reduced activity of the hypothalamic–pituitary–adrenal axis, especially in individuals experiencing stress. However, the effects of chronic diazepam treatment on cortisol have been less well studied, and the relation to age, anxiety, duration of treatment, and dose are poorly understood. In a double-blind, placebo-controlled, crossover study, young (19–35 years, n = 52) and elderly (60–79 years, n = 31) individuals with and without generalized anxiety disorder took diazepam 2.5 or 10 mg for 3 weeks (327). The elderly had significant reductions in plasma cortisol concentrations compared with placebo, both after the first dose and during chronic treatment, but the younger subjects did not. A final challenge with the same dose did not produce any significant cortisol effects in either group and the cortisol response in the elderly was significantly reduced compared with the initial challenge. These results are consistent with the development of tolerance to the cortisol-reducing effects of diazepam. The effect was more apparent in the elderly, was not modulated by generalized anxiety disorder or dosage, and was not related to drug effects on performance and on self-ratings of sedation and tension.

Gynecomastia, with raised estradiol, has been reported in men taking diazepam (328).

Diazoxide

Diazoxide can cause hyperglycemia and diabetes mellitus and has been used to treat hyperinsulinism in infancy, although its use may be hazardous (329,330).

Disopyramide

Disopyramide can cause hypoglycemia (SEDA-6, 180; SEDA-17, 222) (331), perhaps due to increased secretion of insulin, and can also potentiate the effects of conventional hypoglycemic drugs (332). This effect may be due to its chief metabolite mono-*N*-dealkyldisopyramide, since many of the reported cases of hypoglycemia have been in patients with renal impairment, in which the metabolite accumulates. In six subjects who were being considered for treatment with disopyramide, serum glucose concentrations were measured at 13, 15, 17, and 19 hours after supper, with no further food, with and without the added administration of two modified-released tablets of disopyramide 150 mg with supper and 12 hours later (333). Disopyramide significantly reduced the serum glucose concentration at all measurement times by an average of 0.54 mmol/l. The fall in serum glucose concentration was not related to the serum concentration of disopyramide or the serum creatinine concentration; it was greater in older patients and in underweight patients.

- Hypoglycemia has also been reported in a 70-year-old woman with type 2 diabetes mellitus taking disopyramide (334).

Diuretics

See also individual agents

Despite their safety record, speculation persists that the metabolic effects of long-term diuretic treatment predispose to myocardial infarction or sudden death, and that diuretic treatment may therefore be hazardous. It is worth noting that much of this speculation is found outside the columns of the legitimate medical press (SEDA-10, 185). The supposed risks of diuretics are broadcast in countless symposium proceedings, monographs, and such like, sponsored by pharmaceutical companies with a vested interest in diverting prescriptions from diuretics to other drugs. Needless to say, these publications do not present a balanced view. Studies of dubious quality are published repeatedly without ever appearing in refereed journals, and eventually come to be cited in independent reviews and articles. There can be no doubt that these publications have a large impact on prescribing practices.

It is relatively easy to foster these concerns, particularly since antihypertensive therapy would be expected to prevent myocardial infarction and sudden death, but in selected studies does not appear to do so. To explain this, it is suggested that the beneficial effects of lowering blood pressure are offset in part by adverse effects related to thiazide-induced biochemical disturbances. Hypokalemia and hypomagnesemia might, for example, be dysrhythmogenic and cause sudden death; or hyperlipidemia and impaired glucose tolerance might be atherogenic and promote myocardial infarction. Some authors have suggested that thiazides should certainly be avoided in left ventricular hypertrophy and coronary heart disease, because of an increased risk of ventricular extra beats (335,336), and that diuretics are not appropriate

options in those who already have hyperglycemia, hyperuricemia, or hyperlipidemia (337). The argument has been taken ad absurdum by a suggestion that the use of diuretics as first-line treatment of hypertension is illogical (338). Others have argued effectively that we should not be impressed by such speculations and that treatment should be based on long-term experience (339), a conclusion similar to that reached in volumes of SEDA, from SEDA-9 to SEDA-19.

Impaired glucose tolerance and insulin resistance

There is little doubt that high dosages of diuretics carry an appreciable risk of impairing diabetic control in patients with established diabetes mellitus. However, their role in causing de novo glucose intolerance is not clear (340). Long-acting diuretics are more likely to alter glucose metabolism. Impaired glucose tolerance is a relatively rare complication with loop diuretics, although isolated cases of non-ketotic hyperglycemia in diabetics have been described (SED-9, 350).

The effects of thiazide-type diuretics on carbohydrate tolerance cannot be ignored (341). There is a definite relation between diuretic treatment, impaired glucose tolerance, and biochemical diabetes, and a possible relation with insulin resistance (342). It is well established that the effect of thiazides on blood glucose is dose-related, probably linearly, while the antihypertensive effect has little relation to dose (343–345). There is relatively little information on the time-course; numerous short-term studies have shown that the blood glucose concentration increases in 4–8 weeks (346). The evidence that current low dosages impair glucose tolerance in the long term is not entirely consistent, perhaps because of differences between studies in dosages, diuretics used, durations of treatment, and types of patient (346,347). In SHEP, low-dosage chlortalidone in elderly patients for 3 years resulted in a non-significant excess of diabetes (8.6 versus 7.5%) compared with placebo (348). The apparent differences between diuretics may be due to comparisons of dosages that are not equivalent (349). Important differences between individual diuretics will be established only when their complete dose–response relations for metabolic variables and blood pressure have been defined (346).

In contrast to the wealth of evidence on impaired glucose tolerance in diabetics, sound clinical trials of the effect on insulin resistance are difficult to find, considering the amount of comment and speculation on the topic (SEDA-15, 216). It is not known whether insulin resistance is completely or even partly responsible for the changes in glucose tolerance that occur during long-term thiazide treatment; impaired insulin secretion may also have a role (350). Hypokalemia or potassium depletion may contribute to impaired glucose tolerance, by inhibiting insulin secretion rather than by causing insulin resistance, but is not the only or even the main cause of impaired glucose tolerance during long-term diuretic treatment (346,347). The routine use of potassium-sparing diuretics with relatively low dosages of thiazides does not prevent impaired glucose tolerance.

Diuretics worsen metabolic control in established diabetes, but it is not known whether this adversely affects prognosis (346). Disturbances of carbohydrate homeostasis have been detected by detailed biochemical testing, but their clinical importance is uncertain (342). The major clinical trials have not shown a major risk of diabetes mellitus. The incidence of diabetes mellitus in diuretic-treated subjects is only about 1%, even when large dosages are used (351). In ALLHAT, among patients classified as non-diabetic at baseline, the incidence of diabetes after more than 4 years was 12% with chlortalidone compared with 9.8% (amlodipine) and 8.1% (lisinopril). Despite these trends, there was no excess of cardiovascular events or mortality from chlortalidone in the entire population or among patients with diabetes. Although these data are reassuring, observational data suggest that diuretic-induced new-onset diabetes carries an increased risk of cardiovascular morbidity and mortality, but that this may take 10–15 years to become fully apparent (352).

Since changes in glucose balance after diuretics tend to be reversible on withdrawal, measures of carbohydrate homeostasis should be assessed after several months of thiazide treatment to detect those few patients who experience significant glucose intolerance (353). With this approach, the small risk of diabetes mellitus secondary to diuretic therapy can be minimized.

Hyperuricemia

Most diuretics cause hyperuricemia. Increased reabsorption of uric acid (along with other solutes) in the proximal tubule as a consequence of volume depletion is one reason; however, diuretics also compete with uric acid for excretory transport mechanisms. There is a small increased risk of acute gout in susceptible subjects (351). In the large outcome trials, about 3–5% of subjects treated with diuretics for hypertension developed clinical gout (354). In those with acute gout during diuretic treatment, attacks were more strongly related to loop diuretics than to thiazides (355). Gout was significantly associated with obesity and a high alcohol intake in the subgroup taking only a thiazide diuretic. About 40% of cases of acute gout may have been prevented by avoiding thiazides in those 20% of men who weighed over 90 kg and/or who consumed more than 56 units of alcohol per week.

Well-conducted studies have shown that diuretic-induced changes in serum uric acid are dose-related (344,356). In low-dosage regimens, as currently recommended, alterations are minor, and other than the risk of gout the long-term consequences of an increased serum uric acid are unknown.

The issues of whether hyperuricemia is an independent risk factor for cardiovascular disease and the clinical relevance of the rise in serum uric acid caused by diuretic treatment are controversial (SED-14, 660; 351). In the Systolic Hypertension in the Elderly Program (SHEP), diuretic-based treatment in 4327 men and women, aged 60 years or more, with isolated systolic hypertension was associated with significant reduction in cardiovascular events (SED-14, 657). Serum uric acid independently predicted cardiovascular events in these patients (357). The benefit of active treatment was not affected by baseline serum uric acid. After randomization, however, an increase in serum uric acid of less than 0.06 mmol/l (median change) in the active treatment group was associated with a hazard ratio (HR) of 0.58 (CI = 0.37, 0.92) for coronary heart disease compared with those whose serum uric acid rose by 0.6 mmol/l or more. This was despite a slight but significantly greater reduction in both systolic and diastolic blood pressures in the latter. Those with serum uric acid increases of 0.6 mmol/l or more in the active group had a similar risk of coronary events as those in the placebo group.

This analysis of the SHEP database confirms the findings of a systematic worksite hypertension program (358). In 7978 treated patients with mild to moderate hypertension, cardiovascular disease was significantly associated with serum uric acid (HR = 1.22; CI = 1.11, 1.35), controlling for known cardiovascular risk factors. The cardioprotective effect of diuretics increased from 31% to 38% after adjustment for serum uric acid.

These observations suggest that persistent elevation of serum uric acid during diuretic-based antihypertensive therapy may detract from the benefit of blood pressure reduction. However, the relation between serum uric acid and cardiovascular disease was independent of the effects of diuretics. Furthermore, low-dose thiazide regimens have a smaller impact on serum uric acid (SED-14, 660).

Lipid metabolism

Reviews of the influence of diuretics on serum lipids (359–362) are in broad agreement as regards short-term effects. Thiazide and loop diuretics increase low-density lipoprotein (LDL) cholesterol, very-low-density lipoprotein (VLDL) cholesterol, total cholesterol, and triglycerides. The effect on high-density lipoprotein (HDL) cholesterol has been variable. The ratio of LDL/HDL or total cholesterol/HDL is generally increased, but not in all studies. Spironolactone 50 mg bd caused modest falls in HDL cholesterol and triglycerides (363). The effects of other potassium-sparing drugs on lipid metabolism have not been well documented. The possible mechanisms of these various short-term effects have been discussed (362).

Diuretic-induced effects on lipid metabolism are dose-related (344,345): at low dosages of thiazides, changes are very slight while antihypertensive efficacy is well maintained. Diuretic-induced lipid changes have not been prominent in studies lasting one year or longer (364,365,359,362,366). An association between thiazide use or antihypertensive treatment and changes in serum lipids has been shown in some population surveys (367,368) but not in others (369).

Most studies of the effects of diuretics on serum lipids have lacked a placebo control to allow identification of time-dependent or environmental changes, or have been confounded intentionally or unknowingly by life-style interventions, including weight loss, diet, and exercise (347). The argument that the effects of diuretics on lipids may limit the beneficial effect of blood pressure reduction is difficult to sustain (341). The effect of thiazides is largely transient, and in the long term total cholesterol and LDL cholesterol are raised only slightly and HDL cholesterol is unchanged. It is not known whether diuretic-induced changes in cholesterol carry the same prognostic significance as naturally occurring hyperlipidemia (365,370). Attempts to calculate a potential impact of diuretic-induced increases in total cholesterol and LDL cholesterol on coronary prognosis are premature. Observations have so far been limited largely to serum concentrations. However, binding of lipids to vascular cells, rather than in the bloodstream, is decisive for atherogenesis, and the effect at the cellular level remains to be investigated.

It has been suggested that even small changes in lipids might be clinically significant (371). However, the study was underpowered to show statistical significance of minor effects. Since under 50% of the patients in each group were followed for 1 year, selection bias may also have been introduced. It should be remembered that lipid changes are subsidiary to mortality. In this respect, diuretics are the best established of the antihypertensive drug classes.

There is little or no evidence that thiazides should be avoided in patients with hyperlipidemia (353), although some physicians continue to make this recommendation. Serum lipids should be checked within 3–6 months of starting thiazides to detect the very few patients who have an increase in total cholesterol or LDL cholesterol. This should not add to the cost of care, since serum chemistry need only be obtained once or twice a year and is no reason to avoid the use of these drugs as initial monotherapy.

Donepezil

In healthy men aged 61–70 years, donepezil 5 mg/day (n = 12) or placebo (n = 12) for 4 weeks, followed by donepezil 10 mg/day for another 4 weeks reversed age-related down-regulation of the growth hormone/insulin-like growth factor-1 (IGF-1) axis (372). In view of this, it would be important to investigate whether donepezil or other cholinesterase inhibitors, such as rivastigmine or galantamine, can restore the senile decline of growth hormone secretion in the long term, and to evaluate the benefit to harm balance as an intervention for the somatopause.

Doxycycline

Doxycycline can cause hypoglycemia.

- A 70-year-old man with type 2 diabetes mellitus presented with sudden confusion, which rapidly progressed to loss of consciousness (373). The only drug he had taken during the previous 2 months was doxycycline (100 mg/day), which he had taken for 5 days for an upper respiratory tract infection. Urine tests for sulfonylureas were negative. Routine hematological and biochemical tests and an electrocardiogram were normal. He improved with intravenous glucose and withdrawal

of doxycycline and had no further episodes of hypoglycemia over the next 3 months.

Plasma insulin was not measured in this case, so the mechanism of hypoglycemia was unclear.

Hypoglycemia has also been attributed to doxycycline in a non-diabetic patient (374).

Efavirenz

In a randomized, double blind study of 327 patients, cholesterol and triglycerides were raised in patients taking efavirenz, although this did not reach statistical significance (375).

In a cross-sectional evaluation of 1018 HIV-infected patients treated with HAART during the previous 12 months in an Italian clinic, isolated hypertriglyceridemia was more common in 183 naive patients taking efavirenz compared with nevirapine, and both hypertriglyceridemia and hypercholesterolemia appeared earlier (376). In the 295 antiretroviral-experienced patients, in whom an NNRTI was introduced for the first time, the frequency of raised triglyceride concentrations was higher and occurred earlier with efavirenz. In the 145 subjects taking salvage HAART, including an NNRTI plus a protease inhibitor-containing regimen, the rates of hypertriglyceridemia, hypercholesterolemia, and hyperglycemia were greater among patients taking efavirenz compared with nevirapine, and the time to peak metabolic alterations in hypercholesterolemia and hyperglycemia, but not hypertriglyceridemia, were more rapid in the whole efavirenz group. Comparing all of the 324 patients who took efavirenz with the 299 subjects who took nevirapine, the frequencies of raised triglyceride, cholesterol, and glucose concentrations were much higher in those taking efavirenz. There was some grade of lipodystrophy in 207 pretreated patients, but there was appreciable improvement after an NNRTI was introduced in patients taking efavirenz compared with those taking nevirapine.

Enalapril

The syndrome of inappropriate secretion of antidiuretic hormone has been reported with enalapril (377, 378).

Encainide

Encainide can cause hyperglycemia (379), perhaps due to insulin resistance.

Enflurane

The endocrine effects of enflurane anesthesia are minimal and clinically insignificant (380).

The effect of enflurane on heme metabolism has been tested in mice (381); the authors suggested that enflurane be added to the list of drugs that can precipitate acute attacks of porphyria.

Ephedra, ephedrine, and pseudoephedrine

One patient with Graves' disease who used pseudoephedrine developed a thyroid storm, suggesting that hyperthyroidism is a susceptibility factor (382).

Erythropoietin, epoetin alfa, epoetin beta, epoetin gamma, and darbepoetin

In two patients with non-insulin-dependent diabetes and uremia, glucose control deteriorated after the introduction of epoetin, requiring insulin therapy (383).

Etacrynic acid

Like other diuretics etacrynic acid can impair glucose tolerance in patients with type 2 diabetes mellitus (384). Non-ketotic hyperglycemia has also been reported (385). However, hypoglycemia has also been reported in two patients with uremia (386).

There has been an anecdotal report of hyperuricemia and acute gout in a patient taking etacrynic acid (387).

Etanercept

- Transient hyperthyroidism occurred after 6 months of etanercept treatment in a 37-year-old woman with rheumatoid arthritis (388).

However, a direct causal relation with etanercept was debatable, because there was complete resolution with propranolol and despite continuation of etanercept.

Type 1 diabetes mellitus occurred after 5 months treatment with etanercept for juvenile rheumatoid arthritis in a 7-year-old girl (389). Antiglutamic acid decarboxylase antibodies were positive both before and during treatment, suggesting that etanercept may have prematurely triggered an underlying disease.

Ethambutol

Blood urate concentrations can be increased because of reduced excretion of uric acid in patients taking ethambutol (390). This is probably enhanced by combined treatment with isoniazid and pyridoxine. Special attention should be paid when tuberculostatic drug combinations include pyrazinamide. However, severe untoward clinical effects are rare, except in patients with gout or renal insufficiency (391,392).

Ethionamide and protionamide

Goitrous hypothyroidism has rarely been described in patients taking ethionamide (393), with recovery after withdrawal (394). Ethionamide inhibits both the uptake of iodine and its incorporation into trichloroacetic acid-precipitable protein (395).

Thionamides lower the blood glucose concentration and also suppress appetite, which influences carbohydrate intake (396).

Etomidate

Etomidate inhibits adrenal function resulting in reduced steroidogenesis after administration of both single boluses and maintenance infusions (397). In a prospective cohort study of 62 critically ill patients who were mechanically ventilated for more than 24 hours, about half developed adrenal insufficiency on the day after intubation. Administration of a single intravenous dose of etomidate 0.2–0.4 mg/kg for intubation led to a 12-fold increased risk of adrenal insufficiency (398). Etomidate should therefore be avoided as an induction agent in critical illness, in particular in patients with septic shock, among whom the incidence of adrenal insufficiency is high (399,400,401).

Adrenocortical function has been assessed in a randomized trial after intravenous etomidate in 30 patients who required rapid-sequence induction and tracheal intubation (402). The controls received midazolam. Etomidate caused adrenocortical dysfunction, which resolved after 12 hours.

Cortisol and aldosterone concentrations were reduced by etomidate in adults (403,404), but the clinical relevance was minimal after a single bolus (405). A reduction in cortisol was reported 2 hours after delivery in 40 infants whose mothers received etomidate for cesarean section. There were also nine cases of severe to moderate hypoglycemia in this study, but the changes in blood glucose concentration were not significantly different from those in controls (406).

Everolimus

Impairment of bile salt synthesis was implicated in everolimus-induced hypercholesterolemia (407).

Fenfluramine

Fenfluramine tends to improve glucose tolerance and to cause small but significant reductions in fasting blood cholesterol and beta-lipoprotein concentrations. Although it has been suggested that metabolic effects may play a role in weight reduction, and that fenfluramine might even be used to reduce blood lipids, the metabolic effects observed are slight and of dubious clinical importance.

Fentanyl

Hypothalamic–pituitary–adrenal (HPA) axis suppression has been attributed to chronic administration of opioids (408).

- A 64-year-old man with chronic sciatic pain had been taking transdermal fentanyl 200 micrograms/hour for 2 years. He developed back pain, miosis, somnolence, and a blood pressure of 70/40 mmHg. Adrenocortical insufficiency was diagnosed, but the cause was unclear, and he was given hydrocortisone 25 mg/day. After poor compliance with hydrocortisone he again presented in adrenal crisis. On re-stabilization, opiate-induced suppression of the HPA axis was suspected. On gradual reduction of the dose of fentanyl, HPA axis function improved markedly.

Fluconazole

Preliminary studies concerning a possible effect on testosterone concentrations and the adrenal response to adrenocorticotropic hormone did not show any changes. However, determinations were performed after only 14 days of fluconazole administration.

- Two critically ill patients, a 77-year-old man with esophageal cancer and a 66-year-old woman with multiple organ failure, developed reversible adrenal insufficiency temporally related to the use of high-dose fluconazole (800 mg loading dose followed by 400 mg/day), as assessed by short stimulation tests with cosyntropin (ACTH) (409). Although anecdotal, these data suggest that the possibility that high-dose fluconazole can cause adrenal insufficiency in already compromised critically ill patients needs to be investigated further.
- A 63-year-old man received high-dose cyclophosphamide for peripheral blood stem-cell harvesting, having been taking fluconazole 200 mg/day (410). On day 3 he developed atrial fibrillation and his blood pressure fell to 78 mmHg. A rapid ACTH stimulation test showed a blunted adrenal response. He was suspected of having adrenal failure, and fluconazole was withdrawn. A rapid ACTH test was normal on day 14. To clarify the association between adrenal failure and fluconazole, he was rechallenged with fluconazole 400 mg/day from day 16 and a rapid ACTH test was performed on day 21; it showed a blunted adrenal response.

In a retrospective analysis of the effects of fluconazole 400 mg/day in 154 critically ill surgical patients the median plasma cortisol concentration was 158 µg/l in 79 patients randomized to fluconazole and 167 µg/l in 75 patients randomized to placebo (411). Patients randomized to fluconazole did not have significantly increased odds of adrenal dysfunction compared with patients randomized to placebo (OR = 0.98; 95%CI = 0.48, 2.01). Randomization to fluconazole was not associated with a significant difference in cortisol concentrations over time. Mortality was not different between patients with and without adrenal dysfunction, nor between patients with adrenal dysfunction who were randomized to fluconazole and those randomized to placebo.

Flumazenil

The effects of flumazenil and midazolam on adrenocorticotrophic hormone and cortisol responses to a corticotrophin-releasing hormone challenge have been assessed in eight healthy men (412). Flumazenil significantly reduced adrenocorticotrophic responses compared with midazolam or placebo, but had no effects on cortisol secretion. The authors suggested that this agonist effect of flumazenil on the pituitary–adrenal axis might account for the anxiolytic activity of flumazenil, which has been observed during simulated stress.

Fluoroquinolones

See also individual agents

There was a higher rate of hyperglycemia with gatifloxacin or levofloxacin compared with ceftriaxone in a retrospective chart review of 17 000 patients (413). Sulfonylurea therapy was identified as an independent risk factor for hypoglycemia.

Fluorouracil

Patients with poorly controlled diabetes are at risk of greater or more severe fluorouracil toxicity, causing hyperglycemia, which has been fatal. This effect seems to be independent of previous diabetic control and or fluorouracil dosage schedules (414)

There have been attempts to unravel the mechanism of fluorouracil-induced hyperammonemia, lactic acidosis, and encephalopathy, a rare adverse effect associated with high-dose therapy. The cause is not known, although Krebs cycle metabolism is almost certainly involved (415,416).

Fluoxetine

Fluoxetine causes weight loss, in contrast to tricyclic antidepressants (417). In one study there was a mean fall in weight of 3.88 pounds over 6 weeks compared with a gain of 4.6 pounds with amitriptyline (418).

Serotonin pathways are involved in the regulation of prolactin secretion. Amenorrhea, galactorrhea, and hyperprolactinemia have been reported in a patient taking SSRIs.

- A 71-year-old woman who had taken fluoxetine (dose unspecified) for a number of weeks noted unilateral galactorrhea and had a raised prolactin of 37 ng/ml (reference range 1.2–24 ng/ml) (419). She was also taking estrogen hormonal replacement therapy, benazapril, and occasional alprazolam. Withdrawal of the fluoxetine led to normalization of the prolactin concentration and resolution of the galactorrhea.

Estrogens also facilitate prolactin release, and so hormone replacement therapy may have played a part in this case.

Flutamide

Flutamide has been implicated in cases of pseudoporphyria (420,421).

- A 75-year-old man with prostatic carcinoma took flutamide for 18 months and developed blisters on the back of the hands and fingers after exposure to the sun (422). The bullae were associated with skin fragility and atrophic scarring. Histopathology and direct immuno-fluorescence showed ultrastructural features similar to those described in porphyria cutanea tarda. However, porphyrin concentrations in the urine and blood were normal. Flutamide was withdrawn and the lesions healed, without relapse after 11 months.

Fluvoxamine

Fluvoxamine causes increased plasma melatonin concentrations. In an in vitro preparation, melatonin was metabolized to 6-hydroxymelatonin by CYP1A2, which was inhibited by fluvoxamine at concentrations similar to those found in the plasma during therapy (423). This effect was not shared by other SSRIs or by tricyclic antidepressants, which do not have prominent effects on melatonin secretion. Whether increased concentrations of melatonin and loss of its normal circadian rhythm might cause symptoms is unclear. However, melatonin is believed to play a role in the regulation of circadian rhythms, including entrainment of the sleep–wake cycle. There have been 10 cases of circadian rhythm sleep disorder associated with fluvoxamine (424). All the patients had delayed sleep-phase syndrome, which is characterized by delayed-sleep onset and late awakening. The delay in falling asleep and waking up in the morning was 2.5–4 hours. In nine of the cases withdrawal of fluvoxamine or a reduced dosage led to resolution of the sleep disorder. When the patients were given alternative serotonin potentiating agents, such as clomipramine or fluoxetine, the sleep disorder did not recur.

Serotonin pathways are involved in the regulation of prolactin secretion. Amenorrhea, galactorrhea, and hyperprolactinemia have been reported in a patient who was already taking an antipsychotic drug after starting treatment with fluvoxamine (SEDA-17, 20).

Three cases of fluvoxamine-induced polydipsia, attributed to the syndrome of inappropriate ADH secretion (SIADH), have been reported (SEDA-18, 20).

Fructose and sorbitol

Infusions of fructose or sorbitol can cause lactic acidosis (425,426), particularly in combination with ethanol.

- In one patient, blood lactate concentration was monitored frequently over 5 days during intravenous feeding with a sorbitol-ethanol-amino acid mixture. During the first five infusions, blood lactate rose only moderately, but with the final infusion, lactate rose to 11 mmol/l and the patient had a severe metabolic acidosis. In retrospect the patient had had worsening renal and hepatic function tests during the preceding 24 hours. On ending the infusions, the blood lactate concentration fell rapidly.

The problems that can result from the administration in total parenteral fluid infusions of D-fructose or sorbitol have been reviewed (427). Either of these can cause life-threatening hypoglycemia, unless glucose is administered concurrently, in patients who have underlying hereditary fructose intolerance. Unless there is a clear clinical history of the condition, it may not be readily identified. In some countries, fructose and D-glucitol (sorbitol) have been eliminated from the pharmacopoeia for this reason.

Furosemide

Furosemide rarely causes the syndrome of inappropriate antidiuretic hormone secretion (SIADH) (although it has been found useful in treating some patients with SIADH who cannot tolerate water restriction (428)). In furosemide-induced cases (SEDA-7, 246), serum ADH concentrations were raised, total body sodium was normal, total body potassium greatly reduced, and intracellular water raised at the expense of extracellular fluid volume. However, such cases are rare, and no new cases have been published since this complication was reported in SEDA-7.

Gabapentin

A 28-year-old woman with bipolar depression developed clinical and biochemical evidence of hyperthyroidism, ascribed to thyroiditis, while taking gabapentin (4800 mg/day) in a clinical trial (429). The condition cleared after withdrawal, and subsequent exposure to a lower dose of gabapentin (1500 mg/day) was uneventful.

Whether gabapentin was responsible for the thyroiditis is doubtful.

Weight gain occurs in up to about one-third of patients and may be more frequent at high dosages (SEDA-20, 61; SEDA-22, 87). Of 44 patients given mean dosages of 3520 mg/day for at least 12 months, 10 gained more than 10% and 15 gained between 5 and 10% of their initial weight (430). The weight gain started after 2–3 months and tended to stabilize after 6–9 months.

Ganciclovir

Six infants with cholestasis (aged 3–16 weeks) and signs of CMV infection were given intravenous ganciclovir for 3–7 weeks (431). One patient with septo-optic dysplasia and hypothyroidism had episodes of symptomatic hypoglycemia during treatment, which was withdrawn.

Gatifloxacin

Gatifloxacin was well tolerated in patients with non-insulin-dependent diabetes mellitus maintained with diet and exercise (432). It had no significant effect on glucose homeostasis, beta cell function, or long-term fasting serum glucose concentrations, but it caused a brief increase in serum insulin concentrations.

However, hyperglycemia was reported in three patients taking gatifloxacin (200 mg/day) and hypoglycemia in one patient (433,434,435). The mechanism of hypoglycemia, shown in vitro, is increased insulin secretion by inhibition of pancreatic beta-cell K_{ATP} channels (436).

In an observational study of spontaneous adverse events reports gatifloxacin was associated with much higher rates of hypoglycemia and hyperglycemia (477 reports per 10^7 retail prescriptions) compared with ciprofloxacin (4 reports), levofloxacin (11 reports), and moxifloxacin (36 reports) (437).

In four pivotal studies in 867 children, low concentrations of fasting and non-fasting glucose occurred more often in children taking gatifloxacin (5.8%) than in those taking co-amoxiclav (2.5%) (438).

Gatifloxacin 600 mg intravenously has been associated with a serious episode of hypoglycemia after cardiopulmonary bypass (439).

Severe hyperglycemia occurred in a non-diabetic patient with progressive renal dysfunction who took gatifloxacin 200 mg/day for 9 days (440). Gatifloxacin was withdrawn and blood glucose concentrations returned to normal within several days after intensive treatment with insulin.

General anesthetics

The effects of anesthesia for more than 10 hours with either isoflurane or sevoflurane on hormone secretion have been studied in 20 patients (441). Adrenaline and noradrenaline concentrations increased continuously during and after surgery in the isoflurane group whereas they increased only after surgery in the sevoflurane group; both concentrations were higher in the isoflurane group during anesthesia. Cortisol increased continuously but adrenocorticotropic hormone increased only during surgery. Antidiuretic hormone increased during surgery and the isoflurane group had significantly higher values than the sevoflurane group. Glucose increased both during and after surgery but insulin increased only after surgery; glucagon fell during surgery in both groups.

he effects of anesthesia with sevoflurane (0.5, 1.0, and 1.5 MAC) and isoflurane (0.5, 1.0, and 1.5 MAC) on glucose tolerance have been studied in a randomized study in 30 patients (442). The insulinogenic index (change in concentration of immunoreactive insulin/change in glucose concentration), the acute insulin response, and the rates of glucose disappearance were significantly lower in all anesthesia groups than in the control group. However, there were no differences among the six anesthesia groups.

Glycerol

Reversible hypothyroidism has been reported in nursing-home residents without a history of thyroid disease, who had been taking iodinated glycerol as an expectorant (443). Hypothyroidism has been reported after long-term treatment with iodinated glycerol (444).

Glycerol can increase plasma insulin concentrations and thereby worsen diabetes; it can particularly cause hyperosmolar non-ketotic hyperglycemia in patients with type 2 diabetes (445,446).

Glycyrrhiza species (Fabaceae)

Of 34 Japanese patients with diabetes and chronic hepatitis, 18 were given glycyrrhizin 240-525 mg for over 1 year (447). This resulted in a significant lowering of total testosterone concentrations and increased arteriosclerotic plaque formation. The authors suggested that glycyrrhizin treatment was an independent risk factor for arteriosclerosis. The testosterone lowering effect of liquorice has been confirmed in another trial (448).

Glycols

Lactic acidosis and convulsions have been associated with the use of propylene glycol (SEDA-15, 537) and polyethylene glycol, the latter after the administration of a high dose of lorazepam (449).

Gold and gold salts

In one case, diabetes was destabilized after 3 weeks of auranofin treatment (450).

Granulocyte colony-stimulating factor (G-CSF)

Several studies have suggested that single or short-term administration of G-CSF did not produce significant changes in the serum concentrations of cortisol, growth hormone, prolactin, follicle-stimulating hormone, luteinizing hormone, or thyrotropin (SEDA-20, 337; SEDA-21, 378).

Thyroid function and thyroid antibodies were not modified in 20 breast cancer patients (451), and only one case of hypothyroidism with increased thyroid antibodies has been reported (SEDA-20, 337). G-CSF had no effect on thyroid function in 33 patients with cancer, even in patients with pre-existing antibodies (452). Subclinical and spontaneously reversible hyperthyroidism occurred in eight patients without thyroid antibodies and with normal thyroid function before treatment, but this was felt to be related to stressful procedures.

Reductions in serum cholesterol concentrations have been sometimes noted in patients receiving G-CSF (453).

Granulocyte–macrophage colony-stimulating factor (GM-CSF)

Three patients with positive thyroid antibodies before GM-CSF treatment developed hypothyroidism or biphasic thyroiditis (454,455), whereas no similar thyroid dysfunction has been observed in patients without pre-existing thyroid antibodies (454). Based on these reports,

GM-CSF has been thought to exacerbate underlying autoimmune thyroiditis.

Serum cholesterol concentrations have reportedly fallen in patients given GM-CSF (456).

Griseofulvin

An estrogen-type effect has been reported in children, affecting the genitals and the breasts (SED-11, 567)(457).

Griseofulvin interferes with porphyrin metabolism. In man, transient increases in erythrocyte protoporphyrin concentrations have been demonstrated, and the production and excretion of porphyrins is increased. Acute intermittent porphyria is an absolute contraindication to griseofulvin. In patients with other forms of porphyria it should also be avoided, in view of the many alternatives (458–463).

Haemophilus influenzae type b (Hib) vaccine

The incidence of diabetes mellitus has been studied in Finnish children born between October 1983 and September 1985 compared with children born between October 1985 and 1987 (464). Of the children born in 1985–87, 50% received Hib vaccine (diphtheria conjugated PRP-D-Hib vaccine) at 3, 4, and 6 months as a primary course and a booster dose at 14–18 months; the other 50% received one dose of the same vaccine at the age of 24 months. Taking into account the documented increase in diabetes in Finnish children, the small difference between the incidence rate of diabetes in children born during the period 1985–87 and immunized at 18 months and the incidence rate of children born in 1983–85 and not immunized against Hib disease was expected, with a slightly higher non-significant incidence in immunized children. In children over 4 years of age primed during the first year of life the incidence rate of diabetes was also slightly but non-significantly higher than in children immunized at 18 months of age. The authors concluded that early PRP-D-Hib immunization does not increase the risk of diabetes during the first 10 years of life.

This study has been criticized on the grounds that the authors did not present data comparing the incidence rates of children born in 1985–87 and primed during the first year of life with children born in 1983–85 and not immunized (465). The critics presented significant differences in the incidence rate of diabetes between the two groups of children and concluded that immunization had increased the risk of diabetes. However, the relative risk of diabetes during the first 10 years of life in the immunized children born in 1985–87 was 1.19 compared with the non-immunized children born in 1983–85.

In another Finnish study, about 116 000 children born in Finland between 1 October 1985 and 31 August 1987 were randomized to receive four doses of Hib vaccine (PPR-D, Connaught) starting at 3 months of life or one dose starting after 24 months of life (466). A control cohort included all 128 500 children born in Finland in the 24 months before the study. The difference in cumulative incidence between those who received four doses of the vaccine and those who received none was 54 cases of diabetes per 100 000 at 7 years (relative risk = 1.26). Most of the extra cases of diabetes occurred in statistically significant clusters starting about 38 months after immunization and lasting about 6–8 months. The authors concluded that exposure to Hib immunization is associated with an increased risk of type 1 diabetes mellitus.

In 1997, US researchers suggested that immunization at 28 days after birth can cause type 1 diabetes mellitus in susceptible individuals. In May 1998, several institutions, including the National Institute of Allergy and Infectious Diseases, the Centers for Disease Control, the World Health Organization, and the UK's Department of Health, sponsored a workshop to assess the evidence of a possible link. Immunologists, diabetologists, epidemiologists, policymakers, and observers debated the available evidence and concluded that a causal link between immunization and type 1 diabetes is not supported. The results of a large, randomized, controlled trial of immunization against Hib carried out in Finland in 1985–87 (467) were also reanalysed and showed no association between the incidence of diabetes mellitus and the addition of another antigen to the schedule, irrespective of timing. Data reanalysis was made possible by prospective linking of individual information on exposure (in this case infant immunization or the administration of placebo) with the Finnish diabetes register (468).

Halogenated quinolines

Diiodohydroxyquinoline can slightly enlarge the thyroid gland (469).

Haloperidol

The relation of prolactin concentrations and certain adverse events has been explored in large randomized, double-blind studies. In 813 women and 1912 men, haloperidol produced dose-related increases in plasma prolactin concentrations in men and women, but they were not correlated with adverse events such as amenorrhea, galactorrhea, or reduced libido in women or with erectile dysfunction, ejaculatory dysfunction, gynecomastia, or reduced libido in men (470).

No further rise in plasma prolactin concentration was observed with dosages of haloperidol over 100 mg/day, which was explained as being related to saturation of the pituitary dopamine receptors by a modest amount of haloperidol (471).

The prevalence of hyperprolactinemia in patients with chronic schizophrenia taking long-term haloperidol has been studied in 60 patients in Korea (28 women; illness mean duration, 15.5 years) (472). There was hyperprolactinemia, defined as a serum prolactin concentration over 20 ng/ml in men and 24 ng/ml in women, in 40; the prevalence of hyperprolactinemia in women (93%) was significantly higher than in men (47%). There was also a significant correlation between haloperidol dose and serum prolactin concentration in women, but not in men.

The time-course of the prolactin increase has been examined in 17 subjects whose prolactin concentrations rose during the first 6–9 days of treatment with haloperidol (473). The increase was followed by a plateau that persisted, with minor fluctuations, throughout the 18 days of observation. Patients whose prolactin concentrations increased above 77 ng/ml ($n = 2$) had hypothyroidism, and it is known that TRH (thyrotropin) stimulates the release of prolactin (474).

The effects of haloperidol and quetiapine on serum prolactin concentrations have been compared in 35 patients with schizophrenia during a drug-free period for at least 2 weeks in a randomized study (475). There was no significant difference in prolactin concentration between the groups at the start of the study; control prolactin concentrations were significantly lower with quetiapine than with haloperidol. Two patients taking haloperidol had galactorrhea related to hyperprolactinemia.

Glucose metabolism has been studied in 10 patients taking haloperidol; none had impaired glucose tolerance and only one had a glycemic peak delay (476).

Heparins

Heparin-induced hypoaldosteronism is well documented, both in patients treated with standard heparin, even at low doses, and in patients treated with low molecular weight heparin (477,478). The most important mechanism of aldosterone inhibition appears to be a reduction in both the number and affinity of angiotensin II receptors in the zona glomerulosa (477). A direct effect of heparin on aldosterone synthesis, with inhibition of conversion of corticosterone to 18-hydroxycorticosterone, has also been suggested. This effect is believed to be responsible for the hyperkalemia that can occur in heparin-treated patients with impaired renal function and particularly in patients on chronic hemodialysis (479), or with diabetes mellitus, or who are taking other potentially hyperkalemic drugs.

Heparin has a strong clearing action on postprandial lipidemia by activating lipoprotein lipase. This has been thought to be associated with an increase in free fatty acid-induced dysrhythmias and death in patients with myocardial infarction.

- Substantial hypertriglyceridemia occurred in a pregnant woman who received long-term subcutaneous heparin treatment (480).

However, the risk of hyperlipidemia seems to have been exaggerated, since the extent of lipolysis is usually small (481).

Hydralazine

Salt and water retention mediated by secondary hyperaldosteronism can complicate hydralazine treatment, leading to weight gain and peripheral edema, loss of blood pressure control, and rarely cardiac failure (SED-8, 474).

Ibuprofen

An increase in serum concentrations of uric acid has been described with ibuprofen (482).

Imipenem

Cilastatin prevents the metabolism of imipenem by renal tubular dipeptidase, which also hydrolyses the glutathione metabolite cysteinylglycine. In patients taking imipenem + cilastatin, plasma concentrations of cysteinylglycine were significantly increased, while cysteine concentrations fell and homocysteine concentrations were unchanged (483). The clinical significance of this is not clear.

Immunoglobulins

Blood glucose should be monitored in patients with diabetes mellitus who receive glucose-containing intravenous immunoglobulin (484).

Indapamide

The metabolic effects of indapamide appear to be as common as those of thiazides (SEDA-14, 185; SEDA-15, 216). The metabolic effects of hydrochlorothiazide 25 mg/day and indapamide 2.5 mg/day for 6 months have been compared in a randomized, double-blind study in 44 patients with mild to moderate hypertension (485). There was little difference between the effects of the drugs on a wide range of lipid parameters, glucose, and potassium. The purported metabolic differences with indapamide are unlikely to be of sufficient magnitude to warrant its preferential use in hyperlipidemia.

Indinavir

Protease inhibitors are associated with hyperglycemia and possible diabetes mellitus. In a prospective study in 12 patients indinavir caused hyperglycemia and reduced insulin sensitivity (486).

Indinavir causes insulin resistance over 4–8 weeks of treatment. Tissue plasminogen activator and plasminogen activator inhibitor antigen are both markedly increased in patients with impaired glucose tolerance. Both markers have been linked to impaired thrombolysis, which is associated with an increased cardiovascular risk. In 11 patients taking indinavir and 14 taking fosamprenavir for 8 weeks indinavir was associated with a statistically significant increase in fasting plasma glucose concentration and with a 30% reduction in insulin sensitivity; there were no significant changes in lipid profiles (487). Amprenavir had no significant effect on glucose concentrations or insulin sensitivity but increased total cholesterol, triglycerides, and free fatty acids. Surprisingly, both drugs reduced tissue plasminogen activator, possibly reflecting a reduction in HIV-related inflammation as implied by a reduction in TNF-α.

Indometacin

Indometacin reduces the area under the corticotropin (ACTH) plasma concentration–time curve after insulin in normal men, possibly because of the role of prostaglandins in the control of ACTH secretion (488).

One report has described low plasma ascorbic acid concentrations during indometacin treatment, and a case of hyperglycemia has been reported (489).

Infliximab

Body composition was assessed in patients with Crohn's disease before and after treatment with infliximab at 1 and 4 weeks (490). There were significant increases in body weight at 4 weeks and serum leptin concentrations at 1 and 4 weeks. The increase in serum leptin occurred at 1 week, when there were no significant changes in weight and fat mass, and was associated with down-regulation of TNF alfa-regulated mediators, solubleTNF receptor type II, and soluble intercellular antiadhesion molecule-1. Moreover, infliximab significantly increased cholesterol concentrations at 1 week compared with the control patients, who received methylprednisolone.

Interferon alfa

Pituitary

Interferon alfa can stimulate the hypothalamic–pituitary–adrenal axis, with a marked increase in cortisol and adrenocorticotrophic hormone secretion after acute administration (SED-13, 1093). No further stimulation was observed after several weeks of treatment, pointing to possible down-regulation of the ACTH secretory system. As a result, long-term treatment with interferon alfa is not thought to influence pituitary hormones significantly, and the concentration of several hormones, for example calcitonin, LH, FSH, prolactin, growth hormone, ACTH, cortisol, testosterone, and estradiol, were not modified by prolonged interferon alfa treatment (491,492). No clinical endocrinopathies attributable to such disorders in the regulation of these hormones have yet been reported.

Although the rate of growth was significantly lower than predicted in 35% of children receiving long-term treatment for recurrent respiratory papillomatosis (493), only one case of growth retardation has been reported in other settings (SEDA-19, 335). A significant reduction in weight and nutritional status was observed during treatment with interferon alfa for 6 months for chronic viral hepatitis in children aged 4–16 years, but this was transient and not associated with growth impairment (494).

Reversible hypopituitarism with antibodies to pituitary GH3 cells and exacerbation of Sheehan's syndrome have been reported (SED-13, 1093; SEDA-21, 371). However, hypopituitarism can occur without antibodies.

- A 44-year-old woman developed severe weakness after 2 months of interferon alfa 9 MU/week (495). Interferon was withdrawn and subsequent treatment with 4.5 MU/week produced similar symptoms within 3 months. Serum cortisol concentrations were dramatically reduced and plasma ACTH was undetectable. Other hormonal concentrations were within the reference ranges and adrenal cortex antibodies were negative. Biological anomalies normalized after interferon alfa withdrawal and 6-month substitutive hydrocortisone treatment.
- A 39-year-old man received interferon alfa-2b 9 MU/week and ribavirin 400 mg/day for 1 year, and amantadine 200 mg/day for 9 months (496). He had major weight gain (23 kg), reduced libido, and neuropsychiatric disturbances during treatment, and there was only partially improvement 1 year after the completion of treatment. There was testosterone, gonadotrophin, and growth hormone deficiency, but antipituitary antibodies were not detected. Although his symptoms markedly improved with recombinant human growth hormone, permanent pituitary impairment was suspected.

The authors suggested that in the second case pituitary dysfunction might have caused persistent symptoms after interferon alfa treatment. Although involvement of the immune system was suggested in both cases, autoantibodies were not detected.

A syndrome resembling inappropriate antidiuretic hormone secretion has been described in a few patients receiving high-dose interferon alfa (SED-13, 1093) (497).

Thyroid

Since the original 1988 report of hypothyroidism in patients with breast cancer receiving leukocyte-derived interferon alfa (498), numerous investigators have provided clear clinical and biological data on thyroid disorders induced by different forms of interferon in patients with various diseases (499,500–503). Two of these reports also mentioned associated adverse effects that developed concomitantly, namely myelosuppression and severe proximal myopathy (Hoffmann's syndrome).

Presentation and outcomes

The spectrum of interferon alfa-induced thyroid disorders ranges from asymptomatic appearance or increase in antithyroid autoantibody titers to moderate or severe clinical features of hypothyroidism, hyperthyroidism, and acute biphasic thyroiditis. Antithyroid hormone antibodies have also been found in one patient, and this could have been the cause of erroneously raised thyroid hormone concentrations (504).

The clinical, biochemical, and thyroid imaging characteristics of thyrotoxicosis resulting from interferon alfa treatment have been retrospectively analysed from data on 10 of 321 patients with chronic hepatitis (75 with chronic hepatitis B and 246 with chronic hepatitis C) who developed biochemical thyrotoxicosis (505). Seven patients had symptomatic disorders, but none had ocular symptoms or a palpable goiter. Six had features of Graves' disease that required interferon alfa withdrawal in four and prolonged treatment with antithyroid drugs in all six. Three presented with transient thyrotoxicosis that subsequently progressed to hypothyroidism and required interferon withdrawal in one and thyroxine treatment in all three.

Although much work on thyroid autoimmunity associated with interferon alfa has accumulated, little is known about the very long-term outcome of this disorder. In 114 patients with chronic hepatitis C and no previous thyroid disease who were treated with interferon alfa-2a for 12 months, data on thyroid status were retrospectively obtained at the end of treatment, 6 months after withdrawal, and after a median of 6.2 years (506). Among 36 patients who had thyroid autoantibodies at the end of treatment, the authors identified three groups according to the long-term outcome: 16 had persistent thyroiditis, 10 had remitting/relapsing thyroiditis (that is antibodies became negative after 6 months of therapy and were again positive thereafter), and 10 had transient thyroiditis. Therefore, 72% of these patients had chronic thyroid autoimmunity at the end of follow-up and 12 developed subclinical hypothyroidism. In contrast, only one of 78 patients negative for thyroid autoantibodies developed thyroid autoantibodies. Although none of the patients had clinical thyroid dysfunction, this study suggests that long-term surveillance of thyroid disorders is useful in patients who have high autoantibody titers at the end of treatment with interferon alfa.

Although thyroid disorders in patients treated with interferon alfa generally follows a benign course after interferon alfa withdrawal or specific treatment, severe long-lasting ophthalmopathy resulting from Graves' disease has been described in a 49-year-old woman (507).

Time-course

Clinical symptoms usually occur after 2–6 months of treatment and occasionally after interferon alfa withdrawal.

- A middle-aged woman developed subacute thyroiditis by the sixth month of treatment with interferon alfa (508). She also had the classic symptoms of hyperthyroidism, although it is clear that these could easily have been mistaken for adverse effects of interferon alfa itself, for example weakness, weight loss, and palpitation.

After 6 months of treatment, 12% of patients with chronic hepatitis C had thyroid disorders, compared with 3% of patients with chronic hepatitis B. This study also suggested a possible relation between low free triiodothyronine serum concentrations before treatment and the subsequent occurrence of thyroid dysfunction. After a follow-up of 6 months after the end of interferon alfa treatment, 60% of affected patients with chronic hepatitis C still had persistent thyroid dysfunction; all had been positive for thyroid peroxidase antibodies before treatment. Long-term surveillance is therefore needed in these patients.

Frequency

In a prospective study, the overall incidence of biochemical thyroid disorders was 12% in 254 patients with chronic hepatitis C randomized to receive ribavirin plus high-dose interferon alfa (6 MU/day for 4 weeks then 9 MU/week for 22 weeks) or conventional treatment (9 MU/week for 26 weeks) (509). There was no difference in the incidence or the time to occurrence of thyroid disorders between the groups. Of the 30 affected patients, 11 (37%) had positive thyroid peroxidase autoantibodies (compared with 1% of patients without thyroid dysfunction), nine developed symptomatic thyroid dysfunction, and only three had to discontinue treatment. There was no correlation between the viral response and the occurrence of thyroid disorders, and only female sex and Asian origin were independent predictors of thyroid disorders.

Data on the incidence of thyroid disorders in interferon alfa-treated patients vary, largely because the follow-up duration, the nature of the study (prospective or retrospective), biological monitoring, diagnostic criteria, and the underlying disease differ from study to study (500). The incidence of clinical or subclinical thyroid abnormalities is generally 5–12% in large prospective studies in patients with chronic hepatitis C treated for 6–12 months, but it reached 34% in one study (499,510). The incidence was far lower in patients with chronic hepatitis B, at 1–3%. A wider range in incidence was found in patients with cancer, with no clinical thyroid disorders in 54 patients treated during a mean of 16 months for hematological malignancies (511), whereas in many other studies there was a 10–45% incidence (500). Even more impressive was the escalating incidence of thyroid disorders in patients with cancer receiving both interferon alfa and interleukin-2 (qv).

Data on interferon alfa-associated thyroid disease have been comprehensively reviewed (512,513). There was a mean prevalence of 6% for incident thyroid dysfunction, and treatment for malignancies was associated with the highest prevalence (11%).

Hypothyroidism occurs more often than hyperthyroidism, and spontaneous resolution is expected in almost 60% of patients with or without interferon alfa withdrawal. Finally, female sex and the presence of baseline thyroid autoimmunity were confirmed to be the most significant risk factors. The mechanisms of interferon alfa-induced thyroid dysfunction are not yet fully clarified. Although an autoimmune reaction or immune dysregulation are the most likely mechanisms, a direct inhibitory effect of interferon alfa on thyrocytes should be considered in patients without thyroid antibodies.

Mechanisms

Possible mechanisms need to be clarified. Since thyroid autoantibodies are detected in most patients who develop thyroid disorders, the induction or exacerbation of pre-existing latent thyroid autoimmunity is the most attractive hypothesis. This is in accordance with the relatively frequent occurrence of other autoantibodies or clinical autoimmune disorders in patients who develop thyroid disorders (514). However, 20–30% of patients who develop thyroid diseases have no thyroid antibodies, and it is thus not yet proven that autoimmunity is the universal or primary mechanism. In fact, there were subtle and reversible defects in the intrathyroidal organification of iodine in 22% of antithyroid antibody-negative patients treated with interferon alfa (515). In addition, the acute systemic administration of interferon alfa in volunteers or chronic hepatitis patients reduces TSH concentrations (SED-13, 1093) (516), and in vitro studies have suggested that interferon alfa directly inhibits thyrocyte function (SED-13, 1093) (517). Finally, the thyroid autoantibody pattern in patients who developed thyroid dysfunction during cytokine treatment was not different from that of patients without thyroid dysfunction, but differed significantly from that of patients suffering from various forms of spontaneous autoimmune thyroid disease (518).

Susceptibility factors

In addition to the underlying disease, there are many potential susceptibility factors (499,519). There is as yet no definitive evidence that age, sex, dose, and duration of treatment play an important role in the development of thyroid disorders. However, patients with previous thyroid abnormalities are predisposed to develop more severe thyroid disease (SEDA-20, 328). The incidence of thyroid disease was not different between natural and recombinant interferon alfa. Although this should be taken into account, a previous familial or personal history of thyroid disease was generally not considered a major risk factor. Finally, only pre-treatment positivity or the development of thyroid antibodies during treatment seem to be strongly associated with the occurrence of thyroid dysfunction.

In 175 patients with hepatitis B or C virus infections, women with chronic hepatitis C and patients with previously high titers of antithyroid autoantibodies were more likely to develop thyroid disorders (520).

The immunological predisposition to thyroid disorders has been studied in 17 of 439 Japanese patients who had symptomatic autoimmune thyroid disorders during interferon alfa treatment (521). There was a significantly higher incidence of the human leukocyte antigen (HLA)-A2 haplotype compared with the general Japanese population (88 versus 41%), suggesting that HLA-A2 is a possible additional risk factor for the development of interferon alfa-induced autoimmune thyroid disease.

Among other potential predisposing factors, treatment with iodine for 2 months in 21 patients with chronic hepatitis C receiving interferon alfa did not increase the likelihood of thyroid abnormalities compared with eight patients who received iodine alone, but abnormal thyroid tests were more frequent compared with 27 patients who received interferon alfa alone (522). This suggests that excess iodine had no synergistic effects on the occurrence of thyroid dysfunction induced by interferon alfa.

The occurrence of thyroid dysfunction in 72 patients treated with interferon alfa plus ribavirin (1.0–1.2 g/day) has been compared with that of 75 age- and sex-matched patients treated with interferon alfa alone for chronic hepatitis C (523). Of the former, 42 patients, and of the latter, 40 patients had received previous treatment with interferon alfa alone. There was no difference in the rate of thyroid autoimmunity (antithyroglobulin, antithyroid peroxidase, and thyroid-stimulating hormone receptor

antibodies) between the two groups, but the patients who received interferon alfa plus ribavirin developed subclinical or overt hypothyroidism more often (15 versus 4%). Similarly, the incidence of hypothyroidism increased to 19% in patients who underwent a second treatment with interferon alfa plus ribavirin compared with 4.8% after the first treatment with interferon alfa alone, while the incidence remained essentially the same in patients who had two consecutive treatments with interferon alfa alone (4.7 and 7.1% respectively). Furthermore, there was no higher incidence of thyroid autoimmunity or clinical disorders after a second course of interferon alfa whether alone or combined with ribavirin in patients who had no thyroid autoantibodies at the end of a first course of interferon alfa alone, suggesting that these patients are relatively protected against the development of thyroid autoimmunity.

Management

The management of clinical thyroid dysfunction depends on the expected benefit of interferon alfa. Assay of thyroid antibodies before treatment, and regular assessment of TSH concentrations in treated patients, even after interferon alfa withdrawal, are useful as a means of predicting and detecting the risk of thyroid disorders. Complete recovery of normal thyroid function is usually observed after thyroxine replacement but sometimes requires interferon alfa withdrawal. Sustained hypothyroidism requiring long-term substitution treatment has occasionally been observed (SED-13, 1092) (524), and is more likely in patients with initially severe hypothyroidism and raised thyroid antibody titers (525). By contrast, hyperthyroidism generally requires the prompt withdrawal of interferon alfa, and severe forms may require radical radioiodine therapy. Although not enough data are available on the long-term consequences of interferon alfa-induced thyroid dysfunction, the recurrence of thyroid abnormalities after the administration of pharmacological doses of iodine should be borne in mind (526).

Parathyroid

Exacerbation of secondary hyperparathyroidism occurred in a 20-year-old renal transplant patient who also developed psoriasis during interferon alfa treatment (527). Both disorders resolved after withdrawal.

Adrenal

Of 62 initially autoantibody-negative patients treated with interferon alfa for chronic hepatitis C for a mean of 8 months, three developed antibodies to 21b-hydroxylase, a sensitive assay of adrenocortical autoimmunity (528). However, there were no cases of Addison's disease or subclinical adrenal insufficiency. This study suggested that the adrenal cortex is another potential target organ of autoimmune effects of interferon alfa, along with thyroid and pancreatic islet cells.

Diabetes mellitus

The development or worsening of insulin-dependent diabetes mellitus is limited to isolated case reports in patients treated with interferon alfa or interferon alfa plus inter-leukin-2 (SEDA-20, 328; SEDA-21, 371). In chronic hepatitis, diabetes mellitus was noted in only 10 of 11 241 treated patients (529). Although a relation between chronic hepatitis C and the occurrence of glucose meta-bolism disorders is possible (530), reports of diabetes mellitus in patients treated with interferon alfa were prob-ably more than coincidental. Indeed, there have been reports of prompt amelioration or complete recovery after interferon alfa withdrawal (SED-13, 1092; 531–533) and of successive episodes of diabetes after each course of interferon alfa (SEDA-21, 371).

- In three middle-aged patients, diabetes was diagnosed after 3–7 months of treatment with interferon alfa-2b and ribavirin, and two presented with severe ketoaci-dosis (534,535). There was a family history of diabetes in one patient and two had high titers of glutamic acid decarboxylase antibodies before treatment. One patient never had diabetes-related serum autoantibo-dies before or after interferon alfa therapy. All three required permanent insulin treatment despite withdra-wal of interferon alfa.
- Insulin-dependent diabetes mellitus has been reported after 2 weeks to 6 months of treatment with interferon alfa in four patients with chronic hepatitis C (536). All discontinued interferon alfa, and one woman who restarted treatment had a subsequent increase in insulin requirements.

A 75 g oral glucose tolerance test was performed before and after 3 months of interferon alfa treatment in 32 patients with chronic hepatitis C, of whom 15 also had an intravenous glucose test (537). Baseline evaluation showed that five patients had mild diabetes mellitus, three had impaired glucose tolerance, and 24 were normal. After 3 months of treatment, two patients with diabetes mellitus shifted to impaired glucose tolerance, and all patients with impaired glucose tolerance had normal glucose tolerance. Only three initially normal patients developed impaired glucose tolerance and none had newly diagnosed diabetes mellitus. From these results, and in contrast to previous reports (SED-14, 1250), it appears that interferon alfa did not have any adverse effects on insulin sensitivity and glucose tolerance after 3 months of treatment.

Interferon alfa may produce more severe changes than interferon beta (538).

- A 39-year-old man with diabetes, stabilized with insulin 22 U/day for 13 years, received interferon beta (6 MU/day) for chronic hepatitis C. His diabetes progressively worsened, necessitating insulin 50 U/day. After 4 weeks, interferon beta was replaced by interferon alfa (10 MU/day). Shortly afterwards he developed severe diabetic ketoacidosis and shock, which reversed after hemody-namic support and continuous hemodiafiltration.

Mechanisms

Autoimmunity was suggested as a likely mechanism, with HLA-DR4 haplotype and/or islet cell antibody (ICA) positivity at the time of diagnosis in several patients. Because the induction of ICA antibodies in patients treated with interferon alfa has never been otherwise demonstrated (499), the triggering, rather than the induc-tion, of a latent autoimmune phenomenon in patients with a genetic susceptibility is probable (539).

More direct interference with glucose metabolism can-not be excluded. Interferon alfa can reduce the sensitivity of peripheral tissues or liver to insulin and accelerate the destruction of stimulated pancreatic beta-cells (540,541); this could be a possible mechanism in patients not exhi-biting islet cell antibodies. This is also in keeping with rare instances of induction or exacerbation of type II non-insulin dependent diabetes mellitus (SEDA-19, 335).

Insulin antibodies were also found in six of 58 patients treated for chronic viral hepatitis (542) and that was associated with signs of insulin allergy in one patient (SEDA-19, 335).

In a randomized trial in 74 patients with chronic hepa-titis C treated with interferon alfa-2b and ribavirin, plus placebo or amantadine, two developed glutamic acid dec-arboxylase (GAD) autoantibodies, but none developed IA-2 or insulin autoantibodies (543). One had an increased titer of GAD autoantibodies during a first sequence of interferon alfa monotherapy, then a further rise during subsequent combination therapy, and finally developed diabetes mellitus after 5 months of treatment. The authors suggested that repetitive treatment with interferon alfa could increase the risk of type 1 diabetes in patients previously positive for islet antibodies.

In patients with chronic hepatic B or C the respective prevalences of pancreatic autoantibodies increased from 2% and 3% at baseline to 5% and 7% after interferon (544). In all, 31 published cases of type 1 diabetes mellitus attributed to interferon alfa treatment were detailed, mostly in patients with hepatitis C. Irreversible diabetes required permanent insulin treatment in all but eight cases. At least one marker of pancreatic autoimmunity was positive in nine of 18 patients before treatment, and in 23 of 30 patients at the onset of diabetes. In accordance with these results and the likelihood of a genetic predis-position, the authors recommended screening for islet cell and glutamic acid decarboxylase autoantibodies before and during interferon alfa treatment. However, owing to the low number of reported cases and the paucity of studies that have examined the relation between pancrea-tic autoimmunity and the occurrence of diabetes, further research on the predictive potential of such a systematic investigation is warranted.

- Autoimmune polyglandular syndrome with progressive thyroid autoimmunity, type 1 diabetes mellitus, ame-norrhea, and adrenal insufficiency has been reported in a 51-year-old woman treated with interferon alfa for chronic hepatitis C (545). Pancreas and pituitary gland autoantibodies, which were undetectable before inter-feron alfa treatment, were present at the time of diag-nosis. After withdrawal, she recovered normal thyroid function, but was still insulin dependent with amenor-rhea and adrenal insufficiency.
- A 39-year-old man who had received peginterferon alfa-2b and ribavirin for 9 months developed diabetes mellitus 3 months after interferon withdrawal (546).

He required oral hypoglycemic drugs and insulin, but fasting plasma glucose and glycosylated hemoglobin concentrations later normalized despite withdrawal of antidiabetic treatment.

Susceptibility factors

Patients with obesity and a family or previous history of glucose intolerance should be considered more predisposed to interferon alfa-induced diabetes, but the association is not consistently found (SEDA-20, 328).

Dyslipidemia

Interferon alfa often affects lipid metabolism and produces a reversible reduction in cholesterol and, more consistently, increases in triglyceride concentrations (SEDA-20, 328; SEDA-21, 371). Meticulous blood lipid investigation showed a significant rise in serum triglyceride and lipoprotein(a) concentrations and reductions in total cholesterol, HDL cholesterol, LDL cholesterol, and apoprotein A1.

Marked hypertriglyceridemia (10–20 μg/ml), which abates when treatment is withdrawn, has sometimes been observed (SED-13, 1093) (547,548). Inhibitory effects of interferon alfa on lipoprotein lipase and triglyceride lipase or increased hepatic lipogenesis have been suggested (549,550). Diet and lipid-lowering drugs have been proposed as means of maintaining acceptable triglyceride concentrations during long-term interferon alfa therapy. Although the possibility of pancreatic or cardiovascular complications should be borne in mind, no secondary clinical consequences of interferon alfa-induced blood lipid disorders have been so far reported.

In a prospective study of lipid changes in 36 patients with chronic hepatitis C treated with interferon alfa for 6 months, the most prominent findings included increases in triglycerides, VLDL cholesterol, and apolipoprotein B, and falls in HLD cholesterol and apolipoprotein A1 (551). Three patients also developed chylomicronemia and two of those had severe hypertriglyceridemia. All three patients had triglycerides over 2 μg/ml before treatment, suggesting that patients with abnormal serum triglyceride concentrations at baseline are more likely to develop marked hypertriglyceridemia.

Severe hypertriglyceridemia (7.5–19 mmol/l; 653–1644 mg/dl) has been reported in three patients receiving adjuvant high-dose interferon alfa for malignant melanoma (552). The authors reviewed the available literature and proposed a detailed surveillance and management plan for this metabolic disorder in patients with melanoma treated with interferon.

Porphyria

- A severe acute flare of porphyria cutanea tarda has been reported in a 61-year-old man after 4 months of treatment with interferon alfa-2b plus ribavirin for chronic hepatitis C (553). No further relapse was observed after chloroquine treatment, despite continuation of the antiviral drugs.

This patient had previously had episodes of small blisters that spontaneously resolved, and hereditary porphyria cutanea tarda was demonstrated by chromatographic and mutation analysis.

Interferon beta

While no evidence of thyroid dysfunction or antithyroid antibodies was found in 20 patients receiving interferon beta during 24 weeks for hematological malignancies (554), antithyroid antibodies were detected in 29% of patients with multiple sclerosis after a prospective follow-up performed at 6, 12, and 18 months of treatment (555). Biological thyroid abnormalities without antithyroid antibodies have also been found (SEDA-20, 332). Overall, thyroid disorders with antithyroid antibodies were reported in only three patients on long-term interferon beta treatment for multiple sclerosis (555,556).

Thyroid disorders before and during the first 9 months of interferon beta-1b treatment have been systematically investigated in eight patients with relapsing–remitting multiple sclerosis (557). Before treatment, one patient had positive thyroperoxidase antibodies and one was taking thyroxine for multinodular goiter. After 3 months three other patients developed sustained positive titers of thyroperoxidase antibodies, of whom one developed hypothyroidism after 9 months. These results are in accordance with a previous similar study and isolated case reports (SEDA-21, 374; SEDA-22, 405), and suggest that interferon beta, like interferon alfa, can cause thyroid autoimmunity.

As suggested in a more comprehensive long-term follow-up study, interferon beta-induced thyroid dysfunction is often transient or has limited clinical consequences (558). Of 31 patients with multiple sclerosis regularly assessed for 30–42 months for thyroid function, 13 developed thyroid disorders during treatment with interferon beta-1b. None withdrew because of thyroid disorders. Of the eight patients with no previous thyroid disorders, one had a persistent but isolated increase in antithyroglobulin titer, six developed transient signs of hypothyroidism or hyperthyroidism during the first year of therapy, and only one had overt hypothyroidism after 12 months of treatment and required thyroxine replacement. Of the five patients with baseline signs of Hashimoto's thyroiditis, one had a transiently positive antithyroglobulin titer, one developed transient hyperthyroidism, and the three patients who had previously had or who newly developed subclinical hypothyroidism remained stable throughout the study. Overall, thyroid disorders occurred only during the first 12 months of treatment and no additional cases were detected after the first year of therapy. In the authors' opinion, pre-existing or new thyroiditis is not a contraindication to continuing interferon beta-1b treatment. Two patients took thyroxine replacement and continued to receive interferon beta-1b (559).

Among 700 patients with multiple sclerosis treated with interferon beta-1a (n = 467) or beta-1b (n = 233), overt hyperthyroidism occurred in five patients treated with interferon-beta-1b, three of whom required withdrawal and long-term carbimazole, while there were two cases of hypothyroidism and one of goiter without thyroid dysfunction in patients treated with interferon beta-1a (560). Clinical abnormalities occurred after a mean of 14 months and there were thyroid antibodies in four of the eight patients. The frequency of clinical thyroid dysfunction was higher, but not statistically different for interferon-beta-1b compared with interferon beta-1a (2.15% versus 0.64%). A severe form of hypothyroidism with signs of Hashimoto's encephalopathy has also been attributed to interferon beta-1a treatment in a 54-year-old woman (561).

In 106 patients (76 women) with multiple sclerosis who received interferon beta-1a or beta-1b for up to 84 (median 42) months, there was baseline thyroid autoimmunity in 8.5% and hypothyroidism in 2.8% (562). Thyroid dysfunction (80% hypothyroidism, 92% subclinical, 56% transient) developed in 24% (68% with autoimmunity) and autoimmunity in 23% (46% with dysfunction), without a significant difference between the two cytokines; 68% of the cases of dysfunction occurred within the first year. Thyroid dysfunction was generally subclinical and was transient in over half of cases. Autoimmunity was the only predictive factor for the development of dysfunction (relative risk = 8.9), but sustained disease was also significantly associated with male sex.

Severe hypertriglyceridemia, a well-known adverse effect of interferon beta, has been reported and fully investigated in a 39-year-old man receiving interferon beta for chronic hepatitis C (563).

Interferon gamma

Interferon gamma can increase serum cortisol concentrations (564).

Reversible dose-dependent hypertriglyceridemia has been attributed to interferon gamma (565).

Hyperglycemia, reversible on interferon gamma withdrawal and a short course of insulin, has been reported in one patient (SEDA-22, 406).

Interleukin-1

Various endocrinological effects have been observed, but without clinically apparent endocrinopathies (SEDA-20, 333).

Interleukin-1-beta has been associated with transient hypoglycemia (566).

Interleukin-4

Permanent hypothyroidism associated with vitiligo was reported in a woman treated with interleukin-4 for metastatic malignant melanoma (SEDA-20, 336).

Interleukin-6

Interleukin-6 reduced serum thyrotropin and thyroid hormone concentrations and increased LH concentrations (SEDA-20, 336).

Iodinated contrast media

Contrast agents contain very large amounts of iodine, though it is in a bound form. Liberation of iodine (567) from these agents can produce some inhibition of thyroid function in healthy subjects for up to 3 months, but can also increase hormonal synthesis in a thyroid adenoma, and cases of frank thyrotoxicosis have been attributed to these agents, the effect starting within a few days (568). Hypothyroidism has also been reported, particularly in neonates. Contrast medium-induced hyperthyroidism is rare and usually occurs in patients with autonomous thyroid function. Treatment is exclusively symptomatic. Prophylaxis with sodium perchlorate should be considered in cardiac patients with a goiter and a subnormal concentration of thyroid stimulating hormone (TSH) (SEDA-21, 478) (569). In premature babies and neonates thyroid complications can develop after intravascular administration of iodinated contrast media and great caution should be exercised during radiological examinations in infants (SEDA-20, 420).

Thyroid metabolism has been prospectively investigated in 102 patients undergoing diagnostic coronary angiography (570). Thyroid function tests (T3, rT3, T4, free T4, and TSH) and urinary iodine excretion were measured before and 3 weeks after diagnostic intra-arterial administration of iodinated contrast agents. Only euthyroid patients were included, in order to determine whether the administration of non-ionic iodine-containing contrast agents causes significant thyroid function changes in euthyroid patients and whether thyroid morphology is a prognostic factor for the risk of hyperthyroidism. Serum concentrations of thyroid autoantibodies (TPO-Ab, Tg-Ab, TSH-receptor-Ab) were measured. Thyroid ultrasound showed that 37 patients had normal thyroid glands. The gland was of normal size but nodular in 16 patients, there was a diffuse goiter in 15 patients, and a nodular goiter in 34 patients. In 25 patients Tg-Ab was positive and in 13 patients TPO-Ab was positive; TSH-receptor-Ab was not detected in any patient. T3 concentrations did not change significantly after the administration of iodine. T4 and free T4 concentrations underwent significantly different changes in the four groups. The amount of iodine given did not affect the changes in the serum concentrations of TSH, T3, T4, free T4, or rT3. Raised concentrations of urinary iodine correlated with the amount of contrast medium given. There were no cases of hyperthyroidism. The study showed that thyroid function was significantly altered after coronary angiography, independent of antibody status and the amount of contrast agent given, but dependent on thyroid morphology.

The effects of iopromide on thyroid function have been investigated in 20 pre-term infants with very low birth weights and 26 matched premature infants who did not receive contrast medium (571). The dose of iopromide (iodine 300 mg/ml) was 0.3–1.0 ml. Iopromide did not affect the concentrations of free thyroxine and thyroid stimulating hormone. This was attributed to the small amount of free iodide that iopromide contains

(0.6 microgram/ml) compared with other contrast media, in which the free iodide concentration ranges from 1.8 micrograms/ml (iohexol) to 4 micrograms/ml (ioxaglate). Furthermore, hypothyroidism has previously been described after the injection of less than 1 ml of ioxaglate 320 in 13 premature infants of less than 34 weeks gestational age and in other children after the injection of iopamidol. The authors concluded that iopromide may be superior to other contrast media in protecting infants of very low birth weight from thyroid dysfunction. It is advisable to monitor thyroid function when contrast media are given to such infants.

- A 54-year-old man developed Graves' disease and hypoadrenalism secondary to adrenocorticotropin deficiency soon after a cranial CT scan with an iodine-containing contrast agent (572).

It was presumed that the iodine load (about 30 g) had precipitated thyrotoxicosis in this patient, who had antibodies to the thyrotropin receptor, which in turn precipitated collapse due to adrenal insufficiency.

In three women (aged 63, 72, and 75 years) with subclinical goiters, hyperthyroidism developed after the intravenous administration of iodinated contrast medium (573). There was a marked rise in the concentration of free T4. The hyperthyroidism improved spontaneously in all three.

The possibility of inducing thyrotoxic crisis after the intravascular use of iodinated contrast media in patients with thyroid carcinoma and thyrotoxicosis has been re-emphasized (574).

Thyrotoxic crisis has been reported after intravascular administration of iodinated contrast media in patients with Graves' disease (575).

- A 41-year-old man had CT pulmonary angiography and developed a tachycardia of 209/minute and hypertension of 220/100 mmHg, which resolved after sublingual and intravenous glyceryl trinitrate and intravenous metoprolol. On further assessment he was found to have thyromegaly with bruit, a fine tremor, and brisk reflexes. He also had a 1-year history of intermittent anxiety, bouts of palpitation, and weight loss. The free thyroxine concentration was 53 ng/l and TSH was less than 0.5 µU/ml. The diagnosis was Graves' disease and thyrotoxicosis triggered by the administration of iodinated contrast medium.

The Contrast Media Safety Committee of the European Society of Urogenital Radiology (ESUR) has produced guidelines on the effects of iodinated contrast media on thyroid function in adults (Table 1) (576).

In 51 sick neonates given two different non-ionic, iodine-containing contrast agents, metrizamide and iohexol, urinary iodine excretion was increased on day 5 after iodine exposure (577). In 17 term neonates given Amipaque, the median TSH concentration was normal after 5 days and 2 weeks, and there was only one case of transient hypothyrotropinemia; median concentrations of T3 and T4 were in the lower reference ranges. However, in 15 neonates given Omnipaque the median TSH was

Table 1 Simple guidelines on iodinated contrast media and thyroid function in adults (http://www.esur.org)

Absolute contraindication	• Iodinated contrast media should not be given to patients with manifest hyperthyroidism

Development of thyrotoxicosis after iodinated contrast media

No risk	• Patients with normal thyroid function
At risk	• Patients with Graves' disease
	• Patients with multinodular goiter and thyroid autonomy, especially if they are elderly and/or live in areas of dietary iodine deficiency
Recommendations	• Prophylaxis is generally not necessary
	• Patients at risk should be closely monitored by endocrinologists after iodinated contrast medium injection
	• In selected high-risk patients prophylactic treatment may be given by an endocrinologist; this is more relevant in areas of dietary iodine deficiency
	• Intravenous cholangiographic contrast media should not be given to patients at risk

Radioactive iodine treatment

Recommendation	• Patients undergoing therapy with radioactive iodine should not have received iodinated contrast media for at least 2 months before treatment

Isotope imaging of the thyroid

Recommendation	• Isotope imaging of the thyroid should be avoided for 2 months after iodinated contrast medium injection.

raised and T3 and T4 concentrations were very low. There was hypothyroidism in six of the eight preterm and one of the seven term neonates.

- Mild hypothyroidism with a goiter developed in a 15-year-old boy 6 weeks after lymphangiography with Lipiodol ultrafluid; the goiter disappeared after 3 months treatment with levothyroxine (SEDA-7, 454).

Iopanoic acid is as potent a uricosuric agent as probenecid and this effect might explain some renal complications; aspirin reduces the uricosuric effect but can also impair X-ray visualization because of competition at plasma protein-binding sites. Fluctuations of serum urate after oral cholecystography can interfere with diagnostic tests and even precipitate an attack of gout (578).

Iron salts

In erythropoietic protoporphyria, iron can cause a relapse of symptoms (579). An involvement of iron overload in the pathogenesis of some cases of porphyria cutanea tarda has been suggested (580).

Isoniazid

Cushing's syndrome, gynecomastia, amenorrhea, and precocious puberty have been regarded as reflecting the enzyme-inhibitory activity of isoniazid, with resulting derangement of hormone metabolism in the liver.

Isoniazid can cause transient hyperglycemia in overdose (581).

In five volunteers taking isoniazid 15 mg/kg/day over a period of 6 weeks, serum cholesterol concentrations were reduced (SEDA-9, 268).

Ketamine

In a double-blind, randomized, placebo-controlled crossover comparison of the effects of ketamine and memantine in 15 male volunteers, ketamine increased serum prolactin and cortisol concentrations, whereas memantine and placebo did not (582).

Ketoconazole

Gynecomastia was occasionally observed in men when ketoconazole first became available. Ketoconazole has a marked effect on steroid concentrations, including a change in the testosterone/estradiol ratio, and this is most likely to be the basis of the gynecomastia. A lowering of testosterone serum concentrations and a reduced response of testosterone concentrations to human gonadotropin have been shown (SED-11, 573) (583). Various studies have shown suppression of testosterone, androstenedione, and dehydroepiandrosterone, with reciprocal increases in gonadotrophins.

Reductions in serum and urinary cortisol concentrations have been reported in patients taking ketoconazole and signs of hypoadrenalism have been seen during high-dose treatment. However, it is not clear whether the asthenia syndrome described in the past (severe muscle weakness, most pronounced in the legs, fatigue, apathy, and anorexia) is related to hypoadrenalism. In some cases, hypoadrenalism has been described shortly after the start of low-dose treatment. Substitution therapy may be required, since simple withdrawal of ketoconazole may not redress hormonal balance quickly enough.

Various studies have shown that ketoconazole interferes with 17- and 20-hydroxylases and inhibits mitochondrial 11-α-hydroxylase and cytochrome P450-dependent steroid hydroxylase enzymes (SED-12, 677; SEDA-12, 228; SEDA-14, 234) (584).

Because of its effects on the pituitary/adrenal system, ketoconazole has been used in the long-term control of hypercortisolism of either pituitary or adrenal origin (SED-12, 677). In seven patients with Cushing's disease and one with an adrenal adenoma, ketoconazole 600–800 mg/day for 3–13 months produced rapid persistent clinical improvement (585). Plasma dehydroepiandrosterone sulfate concentrations and urinary 17-ketosteroid and cortisol excretion fell soon after the start of treatment, and remained normal or nearly so throughout treatment. Urinary tetrahydro-11-deoxycortisol excretion rose

significantly. Plasma cortisol concentrations fell. Plasma ACTH concentrations did not change and individual plasma ACTH and cortisol increments in response to CRH were comparable before and during treatment. The cortisol response to insulin-induced hypoglycemia improved in one patient and was restored to normal in another. The patients recovered normal adrenal suppressibility in response to a low dose of dexamethasone during ketoconazole treatment.

The effect of ketoconazole appears to be mediated by inhibition of adrenal 11-β-hydroxylase and 17,20-lyase, and in some unknown way it prevents the expected rise in ACTH secretion in patients with Cushing's disease (SEDA-12, 228) (SEDA-17, 323). It may, however, cause such a rapid reduction in serum cortisol concentrations that a crisis is precipitated, and patients' adrenal function should be carefully monitored. While ketoconazole (400–800 mg/day) may be a good alternative to other adrenal steroid inhibitors, patients should be observed for signs of hepatotoxicity. Acute adrenal crisis occasionally occurs (586).

Because ketoconazole has antiandrogenic properties, it is particularly suitable for women, in whom it has few effects on menstruation and does not cause hirsutism. In men, however, long-term inhibition of androgen production can be disruptive, especially if it leads to gynecomastia and hypogonadism. Combination with aminoglutethimide and metyrapone has been advocated in order to avoid these effects (SEDA-17, 323).

Ketoconazole (400 mg/day) has been used for the treatment of hirsutism and acne in women, but adverse effects, such as headache, nausea, loss of scalp hair, hepatitis, and biochemical changes, were impressive (587–589).

Lamotrigine

In two children with cranial diabetes insipidus, desmopressin requirements fell while they were taking lamotrigine (590). Lamotrigine may act at voltage-sensitive sodium channels and reduce calcium conductance. Both of these mechanisms of action are shared by carbamazepine, which can cause hyponatremia secondary to inappropriate secretion of antidiuretic hormone.

In a prospective evaluation of the effect of lamotrigine 3.5–14.2 mg/kg on growth in 103 children and adolescents aged 1.6–16 years with epilepsy treated with lamotrigine monotherapy for 6–71 months, the children had normal growth, although the study had several methodological shortcomings (591).

Leflunomide

Life-threatening hypertriglyceridemia has been described during treatment with leflunomide (592).

Levodopa and dopa decarboxylase inhibitors

Occasional increases in protein-bound iodine have occurred (593).

Levodopa usually increases plasma growth hormone concentrations (594).

Disruption of diurnal cortisol rhythm has been detected and could explain some of the sleep disturbances and psychic adverse effects that levodopa can have (SEDA-8, 143).

Levodopa can stimulate glucagon secretion (595).

Carbohydrate tolerance is slightly impaired by levodopa.

There has been interest in the possible effect of anti-Parkinsonian drug therapy to increase plasma homocysteine concentrations and ultimately the risk of vascular disease (although this is currently controversial, given the lack of success of recent interventional trials), and possibly also of progressive cognitive impairment. The effects of catechol-O-methyl transferase (COMT) inhibitors on plasma concentrations of homocysteine and of folic acid and vitamin B_{12}, co-factors in homocysteine metabolism, have been studied in 26 patients with Parkinson's disease taking levodopa, 20 taking levodopa plus a COMT inhibitor, and 32 age-matched controls not suffering from Parkinson's disease (596). Homocysteine concentrations were raised in both groups of Parkinsonian patients, but the effect was less marked in patients taking COMT inhibitors as well as levodopa (18 versus 14 µmol/l; 10 µmol/l in the controls). Plasma folate concentrations were lowest in the patients who took levodopa only but were actually highest in those also taking COMT inhibitors (5.8 versus 8.8 µmol/l; 7.5 µmol/l in the controls). Vitamin B_{12} concentrations were similar in the three groups. The difference in homocysteine concentrations was attributable to the presence of the COMT inhibitor rather than to individual folate concentrations. This is the first time this effect has been described and the authors speculated that it may be due to enzyme inhibition, leading to a reduced supply of S-adenosylhomocysteine, which is then converted to homocysteine. The practical implications are uncertain and designing clinical studies to follow up on this observation may prove quite difficult.

Levofloxacin

Hypoglycemia has uncommonly been reported with levofloxacin and appears to occur most often in elderly patients with type 2 diabetes mellitus who are taking oral hypoglycemics. A new case has been reported (597).

Lidocaine

High systemic doses of lidocaine can cause transient hypoglycemia (SED-12, 255) (598).

Linezolid

Hyperlactatemia and metabolic acidosis are adverse effects of linezolid that could be related to impaired mitochondrial function. Linezolid-induced lactic acidosis occurred in a 70-year-old man during the first 7 days of treatment with linezolid (599). Mitochondria were studied from three patients, in whom weakness and hyperlactatemia developed during therapy with linezolid (600). The results suggested that linezolid interferes with mitochondrial protein synthesis, probably because of similarities between bacterial and mitochondrial ribosomes.

Lisinopril

The syndrome of inappropriate antidiuretic hormone secretion (SIADH) has been attributed to lisinopril (601).

- A 76-year-old woman taking lisinopril 20 mg/day and metoprolol for hypertension developed headaches, nausea, and a tingling sensation in her arms. Her serum sodium was 109 mmol/l, with a serum osmolality of 225 mosm/kg, urine osmolality of 414 mosm/kg, and urine sodium of 122 mmol/l. She had taken diclofenac 75 mg/day for arthritic pain for 6 years and naproxen for about 1 month. Propoxyphene napsylate and paracetamol had then been substituted and zolpidem had been started. A diagnosis of SIADH was postulated and thyroid and adrenal causes were excluded. Lisinopril was withdrawn and fluid was restricted to 100 ml/day. The serum sodium gradually corrected to 143 mmol/l.

The authors referred to three other similar cases, in two of which the diagnosis may have been confused by the concomitant use of diuretics in patients with heart failure. However, the present and one other case had occurred without co-existing risk factors for hyponatremia. They discussed a synergistic effect of zolpidem and/or diclofenac, and suggested a potential mechanism involving non-inhibition of brain ACE, which leaves brain angiotensin II receptors exposed to high circulating concentrations of angiotensin which would strongly stimulate thirst and the release of antidiuretic hormone.

Lithium

Lithium blocks the release of iodine and thyroid hormones from the thyroid and has been used to treat hyperthyroidism, as an adjunct to radioiodine therapy (602–605) and in metastatic thyroid carcinoma (606). However, it can also cause hyperthyroidism. Lithium enhanced the efficacy of radioiodine in 23 patients (607), but was ineffective in a larger comparison of lithium ($n = 175$) or radioiodine alone ($n = 175$) (608). In 24 patients with Graves' disease, lithium attenuated or prevented increases in thyroid hormone concentration after methimazole withdrawal and radioiodine treatment (602,609).

Lithium has been used, with several other drugs, to treat four patients with amiodarone-associated thyrotoxicosis, but the drugs were ineffective in two patients, who required thyroidectomy (610). One hopes that the authors actually used milligram amounts of lithium carbonate rather than the microgram amounts listed in the article.

Lithium therapy in a 17-year-old man with Kleine–Levin syndrome led to remission of the characteristic manifestations, including hyperphagia (611).

Corticotropin (ACTH)

Calcium infusion in lithium patients ($n = 7$) and controls ($n = 7$) caused similar increases in ACTH concentrations across a physiological range of calcium (612).

Prolactin

Serum prolactin concentrations in patients taking long-term ($n = 15$) or short-term ($n = 15$) lithium did not differ from controls (613). In another study, when compared with 17 healthy controls, 20 euthymic bipolar patients who had taken lithium for more than 6 months had significantly lower serum prolactin concentrations (9.72 ng/ml versus 15.56 ng/ml), but prolactin concentrations in short-term lithium users ($n = 15$) did not differ from controls (614). Antipsychotic drugs were not involved.

Diabetes insipidus

Two of ten patients taking long-term lithium therapy were thought to have hypothalamic diabetes insipidus, because of a positive response to desmopressin (615).

- A 63-year-old man taking long-term lithium for a schizoaffective disorder developed a dural sinus thrombosis and severe hypernatremia and died (616).

The authors suggested that the sequence of events was lithium-induced nephrogenic diabetes insipidus resulting in hypernatremia followed by the dural sinus thrombosis.

Hypothalamic–pituitary–adrenal axis

Hypothalamic–pituitary–adrenal axis function in bipolar disorder has been reviewed, but lithium was mentioned only in passing (617). Two studies ($n = 25$, $n = 24$), possibly reporting many of the same patients, showed that lithium augmentation of antidepressant-resistant unipolar depression increased hypothalamic–pituitary–adrenal axis activity, measured by the dexamethasone suppression test, either alone or combined with the corticotropin releasing hormone test (618,619). However, the tests did not distinguish between lithium responders and nonresponders.

Thyroid

The many effects of lithium on thyroid physiology and on the hypothalamic–pituitary axis and their clinical impact (goiter, hypothyroidism, and hyperthyroidism) have been reviewed (620). Lithium has a variety of effects on the hypothalamic–pituitary–thyroid axis, but it predominantly inhibits the release of thyroid hormone. It can also block the action of thyroid stimulating hormone (TSH) and enhance the peripheral degradation of thyroxine (620). Most patients have enough thyroid reserve to remain euthyroid during treatment, although some initially have modest rises in serum TSH that normalize over time.

Both goiter and hypothyroidism continue to be reported as complications of lithium therapy (621,622,623).

In a cross-sectional study of 121 patients taking lithium, there was no difference in thyroid function tests among those taking treatment for 0.7–6 months, 7–10 months, or 61–240 months. However, when compared with healthy volunteers ($n = 24$) and prelithium controls ($n = 11$), there was a significant increase in radioiodine uptake in all lithium groups. Serum TSH concentrations were higher in prelithium patients than controls and highest in those taking lithium. Being from an iodine-deficient area appeared to predispose lithium patients to abnormally high TSH values and clinical hypothyroidism (624).

In 1989, in 150 patients at different stages of lithium therapy, thyroid function was assessed and subsequently 118 were reassessed at least once and 54 completed a 10-year follow-up (625). The annual rates of new cases of thyroid dysfunction were subclinical hypothyroidism 1.7%, goiter 2.1%, and autoimmunity 1.4%. While these figures were little different from those found in the general population, the authors acknowledged that lithium was a potential cause of thyroid dysfunction.

Of 42 bipolar patients who had taken lithium for 4–156 months, three had subclinical hypothyroidism, three had subclinical hyperthyroidism, and one was overtly hyperthyroid (623). Ultrasonography showed that goiter was present in 38% and mild thyroid dysfunction was suggested in 48% because of an apparent increased conversion of free T4 to free T3. There was no correlation between the duration of lithium therapy and thyroid abnormalities.

The antithyroid effect of lithium has occasionally been used to benefit patients. In a case of amiodarone-induced thyrotoxicosis that did not respond to antithyroid drugs and glucocorticoids, low-dose lithium normalized thyroid function (62).

Hypothyroidism

Lithium-induced hypothyroidism has been briefly reviewed (626). Some patients develop more persistent subclinical hypothyroidism (TSH over 5 mU/l, free thyroxine normal) and others overt hypothyroidism (higher risk in women, in those with pre-existing thyroid dysfunction, and those with a family history of hypothyroidism). Since subclinical hypothyroidism is not necessarily asymptomatic, treatment with thyroxine may be necessary in this group (627), as well as in those with more obvious hypothyroidism (628).

In 1705 patients, aged 65 years or over, who had recently started to take lithium, identified from the 1.3 million adults in Ontario receiving universal health care coverage, the rate of treatment with thyroxine was 5.65 per 100 person-years, significantly higher that the rate of 2.70/100 person-years found in 2406 new users of valproate (629). Of 46 adults taking lithium in a psychiatric clinic, 17% developed overt hypothyroidism while 35% had subclinical hypothyroidism (raised concentrations of thyroid stimulating hormone, TSH) (630).

In a controlled, cross-sectional comparison of 100 patients with mood disturbance who had taken lithium for at least 6 months and 100 psychiatrically normal controls, lithium did not increase the prevalence of thyroid autoimmunity; a minimally larger number of control subjects had antithyroid peroxidase antibodies (11 controls versus 7 patients with mood disorders) and anti-thyroglobulin antibodies (15 versus 8) (631).

The prevalence of thyroperoxidase antibodies was higher in 226 bipolar patients (28%) than in population- and psychiatric-control groups (3–18%). While there was no association with lithium exposure, the presence of antibodies increased the risk of lithium-induced hypothyroidism (632).

Thyroid function tests in 101 lithium maintenance patients were compared with their baseline values and with results in 82 controls without psychiatric or endocrine diagnoses. With hypothyroidism defined as a serum TSH above the reference range, 8 patients were hypothyroid at baseline, and another 40 became so during treatment. Women over 60 years of age were at slightly higher risk and had higher TSH values. Patients with a positive family history of hypothyroidism had raised TSH concentrations sooner after starting lithium (3.7 versus 8.7 years). Whether any patients became clinically hypothyroid was not noted (it was stated that those with grade II hypothyroidism were almost free of symptoms) (633).

Serum TSH concentrations were raised (10 mU/l or more) in 13 of 61 children aged 5–17 years taking lithium and valproate for up to 20 weeks (634).

In a review of lithium-induced subclinical hypothyroidism (TSH over 5 mU/l, free thyroxine normal), a prevalence of up to 23% in lithium patients was contrasted with up to 10% in the general population. It was stressed that subclinical hypothyroidism from any cause can be associated with subtle neuropsychiatric symptoms, such as depression, impaired memory and concentration, and mental slowing and lethargy, as well as with other somatic symptoms. Management guidelines were discussed (628).

An abstract reported that 23% of 61 children and adolescents taking lithium and divalproex sodium for up to 20 weeks had a TSH concentration over 10 mU/l (reference range 0.2–6.0); however, no clinical information was provided (635). Another abstract reported that the prevalence of thyroperoxidase antibodies was higher in bipolar outpatients (28% of 226) than in psychiatric inpatients with any diagnosis (10% of 2782) or healthy controls (14% of 225), but this was not related to lithium exposure; on the other hand, hypothyroidism was associated with lithium exposure, especially in the presence of antithyroid antibodies (636).

When 22 men and 38 women who had taken lithium for at least a year (mean 6.9 years) for bipolar disorder were evaluated for adverse effects, hypothyroidism requiring thyroid supplementation was found in 16 (14 women and 2 men); 9 had a goiter (637). The area from which some of the patients came was known to have a high background incidence of thyroid dysfunction.

The observation that Canada, with ample nutritional iodine, has a relatively high rate of lithium-related hypothyroidism compared with relatively low rates in iodine-deficient countries such as Italy, Spain,

and Germany led to the suggestion that ambient iodine may play a role in the genesis of this condition (638). This is reminiscent of the association of amiodarone with hypothyroidism or hyperthyroidism in iodine-replete and iodine-deficient areas respectively (SEDA-10, 148).

Case reports of adverse thyroid effects of lithium have included the following:

- A 56-year-old man taking lithium whose TSH concentration was abnormally high (50 mU/l) (639).
- A 44-year-old woman who had taken lithium for 10 years and who developed swelling of the right lobe of the thyroid and hypothyroidism (640).
- A 63-year-old woman taking long-term lithium who developed subclinical hypothyroidism and primary hyperparathyroidism (641).

Despite the predominantly antithyroid effects of lithium, thyrotoxicosis continues to be described during treatment and after withdrawal (642–644). In a retrospective review of 201 patients taking lithium (mean duration 6.4 years), hypothyroidism requiring supplemental thyroxine developed in 10% (3.4% of men, 15% of women) after a mean duration of 56 months. Women over 50 years of age tended to have an earlier onset. Two patients developed goiter requiring surgery and two others developed thyrotoxicosis (631).

Reports of hyperthyroidism associated with lithium include one in a woman who was also hypercalcemic with a normal parathyroid hormone (PTH) concentration (645) and two discovered while treating lithium toxicity (646).

- A 27-year-old man developed thyrotoxicosis while taking lithium (644).
- A 52-year-old woman became thyrotoxic 2 months after stopping long-term lithium therapy; the authors briefly reviewed 10 previous reports (647).
- A woman with lithium-associated hyperthyroidism lost 2 kg over 3 months, suggesting that lithium may have indirectly caused the weight loss (648).

Thyroiditis

A retrospective record review of 300 patients with Graves' disease and 100 with silent thyroiditis who had undergone thyroid scans showed that the likelihood of lithium exposure was 4.7 times higher in the latter, suggesting a link between lithium and thyrotoxicosis caused by silent thyroiditis (649).

- A 30-year-old man, who had taken lithium for 16 years for bipolar disorder and long-term ciclosporin and prednisolone after a bone-marrow transplant, developed subacute thyroiditis associated with a diffusely enlarged gland that showed heterogeneous echogenicity, but without a clear relation to lithium (650).

Goiter

Euthyroid or hypothyroid goiter can also complicate lithium therapy, although the goiter is seldom of clinical importance and tends to resolve on withdrawal or with thyroxine treatment. In one ultrasound study, there was a

44% incidence of goiter in patients who had taken lithium for 1–5 years compared with 16% in a control group; cigarette smoking was associated with a greater size and frequency of goiter in both groups (651).

Hyperthyroidism has also been associated with lithium use and withdrawal, although a cause-and-effect relation has been more difficult to establish. In fact, lithium has been used with some success to treat hyperthyroidism, particularly in conjunction with propylthiouracil (652) and ^{131}I (603).

Parathyroid and calcium

Mild rises in serum calcium and PTH concentrations have been associated with long-term use of lithium, and, in a review, 27 reports of parathyroid adenoma and 11 of hyperplasia were mentioned (653). The hypercalcemia and raised PTH concentrations are often reversible on withdrawal, but surgical intervention may be necessary. So far, long-term lithium therapy has not emerged as a risk factor for reduced bone mineral density or osteoporosis (654). In one study, there was a greater frequency of electrocardiographic conduction defects in hypercalcemic patients taking lithium than in normocalcemic patients taking lithium (655).

Of 537 patients who had parathyroid glands excised for hyperparathyroidism, 12 (2.2%) had been taking lithium and 11 (2.0%) had been taking it long-term (mean 15.3 years, range 2–30). Manifestations included fatigue, bone pain and fracture, and abdominal pain and constipation. Six had a single adenoma and five had multigland hyperplasia. All resumed lithium, but one had a recurrence after 3 years and one had increased PTH concentrations, but a normal serum calcium. A literature review detected 27 prior reports of parathyroid adenoma and 11 of hyperplasia associated with lithium (653).

When 15 euthymic bipolar patients who had taken lithium for a mean of 49 months were compared with 10 nonlithium euthymic bipolar controls, the former had significantly higher total serum calcium concentrations and intact PTH (iPTH) concentrations (656). The authors advised baseline and periodic serum calcium and iPTH concentrations and bone density measurements in all lithium patients, although whether the benefit outweighs cost is open to question.

Ten patients who had taken lithium for less than 1 year and 13 who had taken it for more than 3 years were assessed for alterations in bone metabolism and parathyroid function (654). There were no differences in bone mineral density, serum calcium concentration, or PTH concentration, but both groups had increased bone turnover and the long-term group had nonsignificantly higher calcium and PTH concentrations (including one hyperparathyroid patient who had an adenoma excised). The authors' conclusion that lithium therapy is not a risk factor for osteoporosis needs to be tempered by the small sample size, the case of adenoma, and the blood concentration trends.

Total serum calcium and iPTH concentrations were measured in 15 patients taking long-term lithium and 10 lithium-naïve patients; both were significantly higher in the lithium group (657). While the number of lithium patients with abnormally high concentrations was not stated, mean iPTH concentrations were almost twice the upper limit of the reference range (102 versus 55 pg/ml).

Of 15 patients who had taken long-term lithium and who had also had surgery for primary hyperparathyroidism, one had recurrent hyperparathyroidism 2 years after the first operation (658). The authors noted that in their experience hyperparathyroidism during lithium treatment was associated with a high incidence of parathyroid adenomas rather than parathyroid gland hyperplasia, and they suggested that lithium might selectively stimulate the growth of parathyroid adenomas in individuals who are susceptible to developing parathyroid adenomas. Furthermore, such adenomas were best treated by excision rather than subtotal parathyroidectomy.

Parathyroid tumors from nine patients with lithium-associated hyperparathyroidism (six multiglandular, three uniglandular) were compared with 13 nonlithium-associated sporadic parathyroid tumors with regard to gross genomic alterations (659). Gross chromosomal alterations were absent in most of the lithium group and were more common in the sporadic group.

In 53 patients studied prospectively at 1, 6, 12, and 24 months, lithium increased serum PTH concentrations (apparent by 6 months) and increased renal reabsorption of calcium in the absence of a significant change in serum calcium (660). A prospective study of 101 lithium maintenance patients and 82 healthy controls showed higher serum calcium concentrations during lithium treatment than at baseline or in the controls, and higher calcium serum concentrations in those lithium patients over 60 years of age (633).

When compared with 12 healthy matched controls, 13 women who had taken lithium for a mean of 8 (range 3–16) years had higher mean ionized and total calcium concentrations, but mean plasma parathormone concentrations did not differ. In eight of the women taking lithium, the calcium concentration was above the upper end of the reference range, and in one the parathormone concentration was abnormally high (661).

Of 15 patients taking long-term lithium who had surgery for primary hyperparathyroidism, 14 had adenomas (11 single, 3 double) and one had four-gland hyperplasia. All restarted lithium successfully after surgery, except one who again developed hyperparathyroidism, resulting in removal of another adenoma (662).

Hyperparathyroidism was considered a possible cause of treatment-resistant manic psychosis in a patient taking lithium (663).

- Hypercalcemia and raised PTH concentrations improved in a woman who had taken lithium for over 20 years after she was switched to divalproex (664).
- A 64-year-old woman who had taken lithium for over 10 years was admitted with altered consciousness, agitation, and disorientation. The serum calcium was 3.35 mmol/l (reference range 2.1–2.6 mmol/l) and the PTH concentration was raised. With hydration and conversion from lithium to valproate, the serum calcium concentration normalized, but 2 years later disorientation and hypercalcemia recurred and a 150 mg parathyroid adenoma was removed surgically (665).

- A 53-year-old woman who had taken lithium for 9 years and carbamazepine for 3 years and had a 3-month history of lethargy was found to be hypercalcemic with a raised concentration of iPTH. She was saved from parathyroid surgery when withdrawal of lithium resolved the hypercalcemia (666).
- A 51-year-old man who had taken lithium for over 10 years presented with nausea, vomiting, anorexia, hypercalcemia (3.1 mmol/l), and increased PTH concentration (iPTH 110 ng/l). Abnormalities resolved after an oxyphilic parathyroid adenoma was excised (667).

Other reports of hyperparathyroidism in patients taking lithium have included the following:

- Three cases among 26 cases of chronic lithium poisoning (668).
- A 78-year-old man who had taken lithium for 30 years who presented with dehydration, azotemia, hypernatremia, hypercalcemia, and increased PTH concentrations (669).
- A 63-year-old woman taking long-term lithium therapy (641).
- A woman who had taken lithium for 15 years who became hypercalcemic and stopped taking lithium, but 2 years later had two parathyroid adenomas removed surgically (670).
- A 42-year-old man who had taken lithium for 17 years and who had raised serum calcium and PTH concentrations which normalized after removal of a parathyroid adenoma (671).
- A 59-year-old man with hypercalcemia and increased PTH concentrations 3 months after starting lithium, which normalized after lithium was withdrawn (672).
- Three cases from Denmark (673) and one from Spain (674);
- A 78-year-old woman who had taken lithium for 25 years (675).
- A 74-year-old man who had an adenoma resected (621).
- Two 77-year-old women who developed hyperparathyroidism which was managed medically (621).
- A 39-year-old (sex unspecified) whose adenoma was resected after taking lithium for 10 years (662).
- A 59-year-old woman with hyperparathyroidism (676).
- A 54-year old man, who had taken lithium for 15 years without problems, suddenly developed food and water aversion, hypercalcemia (2.75 mmol/l), and lithium toxicity, with a serum lithium concentration of 4.3 mmol/l (677). He was confused, delirious, and irritable. Hemodialysis produced a marked improvement in laboratory tests, which became normal after 9 days.

In the last case the authors concluded that the hypercalcemia was due to long-term lithium treatment and cited studies showing that hyperparathyroidism occurs in 5–40% of patients taking long-term lithium, compared with a population frequency of less than 4%. The patient's chief complaint included nausea when he was exposed to food and water, and he therefore refused food and water for 2-3 days before admission. He also had acute renal insufficiency, which was thought to be due to

the hypercalcemia, water aversion, and perhaps "idiosyncratic reasons". The renal insufficiency and water aversion resulted in lithium toxicity.

A lithium chloride solution caused changes in gravicurvature, statocyte ultrastructure, and calcium balance in pea root, believed to be due to effects of lithium on the phosphoinositide second messenger system (678). The implications with regard to human parathyroid function are obscure.

Of 12 patients who underwent parathyroid gland resection while maintaining their intake of lithium, only eight remained normocalcemic (679). Nevertheless, the authors recommended that surgery should be considered if there is hyperparathyroidism.

Diabetes mellitus

It has been reported that diabetes mellitus is three times more common in bipolar patients than in the general population (680). However, lithium does not appear to increase the risk of diabetes mellitus, and its use in patients with pre-existing diabetes is generally safe, assuming that the diabetes is well controlled.

When lithium toxicity has been reported in patients with diabetes mellitus, it has been attributed to impaired glucose intolerance (681).

- An increased lithium dosage requirement in a hyperglycemic 40-year-old woman was attributed to the osmotic diuretic effect of glycosuria, increasing lithium excretion (682).
- Two patients with diabetes mellitus developed lithium toxicity (serum concentrations 3.3 and 3.0 mmol/l) in association with impaired consciousness, and hyperglycemia that resolved after intravenous insulin and fluids (683).

While the authors of the second report concluded that impaired glucose tolerance had predisposed to lithium intoxication, the opposite is also possible.

When a 45-year-old man with severe lithium-induced diabetes insipidus developed hyperosmolar, nonketotic hyperglycemia, it was suggested that poorly controlled diabetes mellitus may have contributed to the polyuria (684). Prior contact with a female patient who had developed hyperosmolar coma secondary to lithium-induced diabetes insipidus (685) allowed physicians 4 years later to treat her safely after a drug overdose and a surgical procedure, by avoiding intravenous replacement fluids with a high dextrose content (despite stopping lithium several years earlier, the patient continued to put out 10 liters of urine daily) (686).

Difficulty in attaining a therapeutic serum concentration of lithium despite increased doses was attributed to increased renal clearance due to the osmotic effect of glycosuria in a 44-year-old man with poorly controlled diabetes mellitus (682).

Weight gain

Weight gain, a well-recognized adverse effect of lithium, occurs in one-third to two-thirds of patients (687). It is more common in those with prior weight problems and at higher dosages of lithium. Possible mechanisms include complex effects on carbohydrate and lipid metabolism, mood stabilization itself, lithium-induced hypothyroidism, the use of high-calorie beverages to treat lithium-induced polydipsia, and the concomitant use of other weight-gaining drugs (for example valproate, olanzapine, mirtazapine). Recognizing and managing weight gain early in the course of treatment can do much to ensure continued adherence to lithium regimens. Two reviews of weight gain with psychotropic drugs mentioned lithium (688,689).

Risk and magnitude

In a review of psychotropic drug-induced weight gain, the prevalence and magnitude of the problem with lithium was discussed together with risk factors, mechanisms, and management (687). Adolescent inpatients treated with risperidone ($n = 18$) or conventional antipsychotic drugs ($n = 19$) over 6 months gained more weight than a control group but concomitant treatment with lithium was not a contributing factor (690).

A review of psychotropic drugs and weight gain included a brief summary of lithium-related weight gain (691). A retrospective evaluation of 176 patients taking long-term lithium showed that weight gain was an adverse effect in 18%. While 34% of the total did not adhere to treatment because of somatic adverse effects, no specific adverse effect (including weight gain) was associated with nonadherence (692).

The prevalence of overweight (BMI 25–29) and obesity (BMI 30 or more) was determined in 89 euthyroid bipolar patients and 445 reference subjects. The rate of obesity in patients taking only lithium was 1.5 times greater than in the reference population (a nonsignificant difference), compared with a statistically significant 2.5 times greater rate associated with antipsychotic drugs (693).

The prevalence of overweight (BMI 20 or more) and obesity (BMI 30 or more) has been evaluated in 89 euthymic bipolar patients and 445 age- and sex-matched controls (693). The bipolar women were more overweight and more obese than the controls and the bipolar men were more obese but not more overweight. Obesity was clearly related to antipsychotic drug use and less so to lithium and anticonvulsants (but patients taking lithium alone had an obesity rate 1.5 times that of the general population).

A review of the effects of mood stabilizers on weight included a section on lithium in which the authors concluded that lithium-related weight gain occurs in one-third to two-thirds of patients, with a mean increase of 4–7 kg; possible mechanisms were discussed (694).

An open chart review of 74 hospitalized patients showed a mean weight gain of 6.3 kg and an increase in BMI of 2.1 kg/m^2 after they had taken lithium for a mean of 89 days (695). Of 47 lithium-treated patients, 14 gained at least 5% of their baseline BMI, 6 gained over 10%, and 2 gained over 15% during an acute treatment phase of unspecified duration, while during the 1-year maintenance phase 11 gained over 5% and 2 gained over 10% (696).

Comparative studies

In a 1-year, placebo-controlled study of bipolar I prophylaxis ($n = 372$), weight gain with divalproex, but not with lithium, was significantly more common than with placebo (697). A patient who gained 18 kg over 18 months while taking lithium and perphenazine lost 16 kg when the latter was changed to loxapine (she also participated in a weight loss program) (698). Whether lithium played a role in the weight gain was unclear.

In a 12-month maintenance study, weight gain was an adverse event in 21% of patients taking divalproex, 13% of those taking lithium, and 7% of those taking placebo (697). The divalproex/placebo difference was statistically significant, but the lithium/placebo difference was not.

Mechanism

In 15 consecutive patients, serum leptin concentrations were measured at baseline and after 8 weeks of lithium treatment. There was a significant mean increase of 3.5 ng/ml and serum leptin correlated positively with weight gain (5.9 kg), increased BMI (24–27), and clinical efficacy (699). The authors suggested that leptin might play a role in lithium-induced weight gain.

Management

The Expert Consensus Guideline Series, Medication Treatment of Bipolar Disorder 2000, has recommended to "continue present medication, focus on diet and exercise" as the preferred first-line treatment for managing weight gain in patients taking lithium or divalproex. The next approach was to continue medication and add topiramate. Second-line treatments included switching from divalproex to lithium or vice versa, reducing the dosage, and switching to another drug. The addition of an appetite suppressant was a lower second-line recommendation (700).

Local anesthetics

Local anesthetics generally have only slight endocrine and metabolic adverse effects, without clinical repercussions.

A small reduction in glucose concentrations, rarely leading to hypoglycemic coma, can occur (SEDA-16, 130). This effect is in keeping with the finding that the catabolic stress response to surgery may be suppressed by epidural analgesia (SED-12, 254) (701). However, in one study, thoracic epidural administration produced a degree of hyperglycemia (SED-12, 252) (702).

- Symptomatic hypoglycemia occurred in a healthy 30-year-old primigravida after a second 5 ml bolus of 0.25% bupivacaine administered epidurally during labor (703). She developed an altered mental state, which responded rapidly to 50 ml of 50% dextrose administered intravenously.

Lopinavir + ritonavir

In 19 patients taking lopinavir + ropinavir, either 533/133 mg bd (in patients co-treated with NNRTIs) or 400/100 mg bd, there were increases in triglyceride and total cholesterol concentrations after 4 weeks; seven patients developed grade 2 or worse rises in lipids and three patients developing grade 3 hyperlipidemia. HDL cholesterol increased over the course of 48 weeks, but LDL did not change significantly (704). At baseline nine patients had lipodystrophy but that did not worsen over the next 48 weeks. However, CT-based standardized analysis showed an increase in total abdominal fat (+14%) and a loss of limb fat (−8%) in the 16 patients who completed the study. There was a significant correlation between lopinavir trough concentrations and changes in limb fat, but no association between lopinavir concentration and changes in total abdominal fat, visceral fat, or subcutaneous abdominal fat. The authors cautioned against interpreting these data as showing a causative relation between lopinavir and lipodystrophy, as the study population was rather small and confounding elements could not be ruled out. However, they advised the use of plasma concentration measurement in order to avoid unnecessarily high lopinavir concentrations, which may be associated with lipodystrophy.

In contrast, in 55 patients taking lopinavir + ropinavir, even though there was a significant increase in triglyceride concentrations over 12 weeks, this did not correlate with higher plasma lopinavir concentrations (705). The authors cautioned against premature dosage adjustments pending larger studies to elucidate this phenomenon.

Lorazepam

Metabolic acidosis and hyperlactatemia have been attributed to lorazepam (706).

- A 34-year-old woman with a history of renal insufficiency induced by long-term use of cocaine developed respiratory failure and was intubated and sedated with intravenous lorazepam (65 mg, 313 mg, and 305 mg on 3 consecutive days). After 2 days she had a metabolic acidosis, with hyperlactatemia and hyperosmolality. Propylene glycol, a component of the lorazepam intravenous formulation, was considered as a potential source of the acidosis, as she had received more than 40 times the recommended amount over 72 hours. Withdrawal of lorazepam produced major improvements in lactic acid and serum osmolality.

Lorcainide

Lorcainide has been reported to cause hyponatremia, attributed to inappropriate secretion of ADH (707).

Manganese

In a series of workers exposed to manganese dust for more than 14 years in a ferroalloy-producing plant, the correlation between prolactin and manganese in blood and in urine was studied (708). In the manganese-exposed workers there was an increase in serum prolactin, which correlated with manganese in both the blood and urine, suggesting impairment of tonic inhibition by tubero-infundibular dopaminergic neurons.

Maprotiline

Galactorrhea occurred in a 23-year-old woman 2 weeks after she started to take maprotiline 50 mg/day (increased to 75 mg after 10 days) and resolved after withdrawal (709).

An often troublesome adverse effect of antidepressant medication is weight gain. Two cases of this adverse effect have been reported in patients taking low doses of maprotiline (710).

Measles, mumps, and rubella vaccines

A total of 20 cases of type I diabetes mellitus suspected to be induced by MMR immunization have been reported to Behringwerke, Marburg, Germany, probably due to the mumps component (711). The earliest case occurred 3 days after receiving the vaccine and the latest 7 months after immunization. Twelve cases were diagnosed within 30 days of immunization. The investigators considered the cases of diabetes mellitus to have a temporal relation to the immunization. For every 5 million children immunized against mumps 50 spontaneous cases of diabetes mellitus are to be expected by random coincidence within a period of 30 days after immunization. In fact, only 12 cases were reported within 30 days after immunization. Mainly based on this analysis the Deutsche Vereinigung zur Bekämpfung der Viruskrankheiten (DVV) could not confirm the relation between mumps immunization and diabetes mellitus (712).

Mefloquine

- A 30-year-old woman took mefloquine, 250 mg/week, and developed abdominal pain, palpitation, and tremor; thyroid function tests were abnormal; 1 month after withdrawal the tests had returned to normal (SEDA-18, 289).

Methadone

Prolonged therapy with methadone causes increases in serum thyroid hormone-binding globulin, triiodothyronine, and thyroxine, as well as albumin, globulin, and prolactin, and these must be monitored (SEDA-15, 71; SEDA-17, 81).

Methyldopa

Acutely methyldopa promotes the release of growth hormone and prolactin, but the long-term significance of this is unclear. However, there have been reports of hyperprolactinemia, leading to amenorrhea and galactor-rhea (713).

Methylphenidate

Methylphenidate has been reported to cause stunting of growth by impairing growth hormone secretion (714).

- A 10-year-old boy with ADHD and chronic asthma, who was using inhaled corticosteroids, developed almost complete growth arrest during methylphenidate treatment. Growth hormone stimulation tests and measurement of growth hormone-dependent growth factors suggested that methylphenidate had altered growth hormone secretion and had impaired growth. Determination of growth velocity was a sensitive marker for the evaluation of growth.

The association between childhood treatment with methylphenidate and adult height and weight has been investigated in 97 boys, aged 4–12 years, who were referred to a child psychiatry out-patients clinic and took methylphenidate for an average of 36 months (715). They were re-evaluated between ages 21 and 23 years. Hierarchical analysis predicted adult height and weight from sets of both nonmedication-related and medication-related variables. Medicated individuals who had attained their final stature did not differ in average height or weight from family, community, or nonmedicated controls. In some individuals, nausea and vomiting and the use of higher doses of methylphenidate were associated with growth impairment. It should be emphasized that the correlations in this study do not demonstrate cause and effect relations between medication and ultimate stature.

Metoclopramide

Hyperprolactinemia and galactorrhea, sometimes with gynecomastia, are classic complications of metoclopramide that can equally well occur in adults, children, or neonates (SEDA-22, 390; 716).

Vasopressin release has been claimed to be enhanced by metoclopramide, while aldosterone release is impaired (SED-12, 940).

Metronidazole

Since anecdotal observations suggested a hypolipidemic effect of metronidazole, the effect of metronidazole 250 mg tds on serum lipids has been evaluated in 30 volunteers who twice took metronidazole for 14 days (717). On both occasions total serum cholesterol fell by 16% and LDL cholesterol by 21%.

Miconazole

Hyperlipidemia has been described in many patients given miconazole; this may be caused by the solvent (SED-12, 679) (718).

Minocycline

A distinctive but rare adverse effect of minocycline is black pigmentation of the thyroid gland, of which about 30 cases have been described (719). It is generally harmless, but can occasionally cause harm (720). Based upon two cases, the authors reviewed 28 previous reports, of which 11 (39%) had been found to harbour papillary carcinoma, strongly suggesting an increased incidence of *thyroid cancer* in these pigmented glands. They referred to an old theory that the pigment is formed by oxidation of minocycline by the enzyme thyroid peroxidase (721). Minocycline is stable in the presence of thyroid peroxidase unless an iodide substrate is added, which accelerates both the oxidation of minocycline and the production of a reactive intermediate benzoquinone iminium ionized product. This process in turn produces competitive inhibition of the coupling of tyrosyl residues with thyroglobulin, a necessary step in the production of thyroid hormone.

Whatever the mechanism may be, the high incidence of associated papillary thyroid cancer mandates at a minimum that one ask about the use of minocycline in any patient who has an enlarged thyroid. The authors recommended that if a patient has taken minocycline in the past, biopsy and possibly removal of the thyroid gland is advisable.

Minoxidil

Pseudoacromegaly has been reported in a patient who had taken large oral doses of minoxidil for about 10 years (722). There have been no reports of pseudoacromegaly associated with topical minoxidil.

Mitotane

Because it inhibits glucocorticoid synthesis, mitotane can cause acute hypoadrenalism (723).

Mitotane 1–5 g daily for 4 weeks was associated with the development of hypercholesterolemia in three cases; the effect had not reverted to normal 3 months later (724).

Mizoribine

There has been a single case report of inappropriate secretion of antidiuretic hormone (SIADH) attributed to mizoribine (725).

A 74-year-old man with rheumatoid arthritis developed nausea and headache 1.5 months after starting to take mizoribine. His serum sodium concentration fell to 118 mmol/l, but his urinary sodium excretion was normal and there was no hypotension or hemoconcentration. His serum antidiuretic hormone concentration was raised at 0.59 pg/ml in spite of a reduced serum osmolality to 254 mosm/kg. He had no organic disease likely to cause SIADH. Despite infusion of hypertonic saline, his serum sodium concentration did not return to normal. Shortly after mizoribine withdrawal, his serum sodium increased from 128 to 139 mmol/l and his plasma osmolality from 265 to 287 mosm/kg.

Additional predisposing factors in this case were the patient's age and difficulty in micturition because of benign prostatic hyperplasia.

In a double-blind, placebo-controlled, multicenter study of mizoribine in 197 children aged 2–19 years with frequently relapsing nephrotic syndrome, transient hyperuricemia was the most common adverse event, occurring in 16% (726).

Moclobemide

A number of antidepressant drugs, particularly SSRIs, can increase plasma prolactin concentrations, although galactorrhea is uncommon. In a prescription event monitoring survey of about 65 000 patients, compared with SSRIs, moclobemide was associated with a relative risk of galactorrhea of 6.7 (95% CI = 2.7, 15) (727). However, this was substantially less than the risk associated with the dopamine receptor antagonist risperidone (relative risk compared with SSRIs 32; 95% CI = 14, 70). Nevertheless, the data suggest that moclobemide may be more likely to cause galactorrhea than other antidepressant drugs.

Monoamine oxidase inhibitors

The syndrome of inappropriate secretion of antidiuretic hormone (SIADH) (728) may be the mechanism of action underlying cases of peripheral edema that have been described (SEDA-2, 12; SEDA-6, 28). Diuretics are not helpful, but dosage reduction produces relief (729).

A number of antidepressant drugs, particularly selective serotonin re-uptake inhibitors (SSRIs), can increase plasma prolactin concentrations, although galactorrhea is uncommon. In a prescription-event monitoring survey of about 65 000 patients, compared with SSRIs, moclobemide was associated with a relative risk of galactorrhea of 6.7 (95% CI = 2.7, 15) (730). However, this was substantially less than the risk associated with the dopamine receptor antagonist risperidone (relative risk compared with SSRIs 32; 95% CI = 14, 70). Nevertheless, the data suggest that moclobemide may be more likely to cause galactorrhea than other antidepressant drugs.

Morphine

Morphine can cause prolactin release (731); this effect is not antagonized by naloxone.

Moxifloxacin

In a pooled analysis of 30 (26 controlled, 4 uncontrolled) prospective, phase II/III studies of oral or intravenous moxifloxacin in 8474 subjects no drug-related hypoglycemic events were reported (732).

Nalidixic acid

Hyperglycemia associated with convulsions has been observed after the use of high single doses of nalidixic acid (733,734).

Nalidixic acid can cause metabolic acidosis in infants (735). This has also been seen in older children and adults with renal insufficiency and can result from disturbed lactate metabolism. Extreme overdosage can cause metabolic acidosis in subjects with normal renal function (734,736).

Naloxone

Marked changes in physiological functions can occur if naloxone is given when the endorphin system has been modified by opioids. Following the use of naloxone, a reduced plasma prolactin concentration was noted (737).

Nabumetone

Nabumetone-induced pseudoporphyria has been described (SEDA-16, 11; SEDA 22, 117), and a further five cases in four adults and a child have been reported (738–740).

Nefazodone

Hypoglycemia occurred in a 54-year-old woman with diabetes mellitus after she started to take nefazodone (741). She also reported weight loss of 5 pounds.

Nelfinavir

The effect of replacing nelfinavir with atazanavir on lipid concentrations has been studied. Atazanavir in combination with stavudine and lamivudine was given to 139 and 144 patients previously treated with atazanavir 400 mg/day or 600 mg/day for 48 weeks who continued their regimen and in 63 patients who had taken nelfinavir 1250 mg bd for 48 weeks and were allowed to switch to atazanavir 400mg/day in an open rollover/switch study (742). Those who took atazanavir during the entire study had no significant changes in lipid profiles compared to baseline. The patients who had previously taken nelfinavir had reductions in total cholesterol, fasting LDL, and triglyceride concentrations and an increase in HDL concentrations at weeks12 and 24.

In an analysis of a randomized comparison of atazanavir and nelfinavir in 467 patients cardiovascular risk modelling was used to estimate the impact of dyslipidemia (743). Concentrations of total cholesterol and low-density lipoprotein cholesterol increased significantly more among patients who used nelfinavir (24% and 28%) than among those who used atazanavir (4% and 1%). Overall, the relative risk of coronary disease, adjusted for risk status, age, and sex, was increased by 50% for nelfinavir versus atazanavir over the next 10 years in men or women, regardless of the presence or absence of other coronary risk factors.

Neuroleptic drugs

See also individual agent

The effects of neuroleptic drugs on menstrual status and the relation between menstrual status and neuroleptic drug efficacy and adverse effects have been explored (744). In contrast to prior reports (SEDA-18, 50), there was not a high prevalence of menstrual irregularities or amenorrhea in 27 premenopausal women with chronic schizophrenia treated with typical neuroleptic drugs.

Treatment of the metabolic disturbances caused by neuroleptic drugs has also been reviewed (745).

Prolactin

Neuroendocrine effects of neuroleptic drugs include a rise in growth hormone, inappropriate ADH and prolactin secretion, and disturbances of sex hormones (SEDA-7, 67). Galactorrhea (SEDA-20, 43) and gynecomastia can follow the rise in prolactin.

A correlation between serum concentrations of neuroleptic drugs and prolactin has been claimed (746,747). In 55 patients who had been taking neuroleptic drugs for more than 10 years, higher doses of medication were associated with increased rates of both hyperprolactinemia and bone mineral density loss, as shown by dual X-ray absorptiometry of their lumbar and hip bones (748).

However, no further rise in plasma prolactin concentration was observed with higher dosages of haloperidol (over 100 mg/day), which was explained as being related to saturation of the pituitary dopamine receptors by a modest amount of haloperidol (747). A low prolactin concentration during maintenance neuroleptic drug treatment predicted relapse after withdrawal, and it was suggested that serum prolactin concentration may be helpful in monitoring treatment (749). Hirsutism, amenorrhea, and a false-positive pregnancy test associated with neuroleptic treatment have also been reported (SED-11, 111) (744,750).

The effects of haloperidol and quetiapine on serum prolactin concentrations have been compared in 35 patients with schizophrenia after a 2-week washout period in a randomized study (751). There was no significant difference in prolactin concentration between the groups at the start of the study, although prolactin concentrations were significantly lower with quetiapine than haloperidol. After 6 weeks, the mean prolactin concentration was significantly increased in those taking haloperidol but not in those taking quetiapine. Two patients taking haloperidol had galactorrhea related to hyperprolactinemia.

There is concern that neuroleptic drugs may increase the risk of breast cancer because of raised prolactin concentrations. For a long time, findings did not confirm this association (752), but a Danish cohort study of 6152 patients showed a slight increase in the risk of breast cancer among schizophrenic women (753).

In eight patients receiving neuroleptic drugs, serum prolactin concentrations were grossly raised (754). The time-course of the prolactin increase was examined in 17 subjects whose prolactin concentrations rose during the first 6–9 days of treatment with haloperidol (755). The increase was followed by a plateau that persisted, with minor fluctuations, throughout the 18 days of observation. Patients whose prolactin concentrations increased above 77 ng/ml ($n = 2$) had hypothyroidism, and it is known that TRH (thyrotropin) stimulates the release of prolactin (756). It was concluded that all patients should have had TSH determinations at the start of therapy with neuroleptic drugs.

Sex differences in hormone concentrations have been investigated in 47 patients (21 men and 26 women) with schizophrenia or related psychoses who were using different neuroleptic drugs (757). The median daily dose and the median body weight-adjusted daily dose were twice as high in men as in women. However, neuroleptic drug-induced hyperprolactinemia was more frequent and occurred at a lower daily dose in women. The growth hormone concentration was normal in all patients.

Some patients who take clozapine take another neuroleptic drug, and the consequences of this practice in terms of prolactin have been studied in five patients (758). After the addition of haloperidol (4 mg/day) to clozapine the mean prolactin concentration increased from 9.7 ng/ml to 16 ng/ml at week 4 and 19 ng/ml at week 6. Each subject had an increase in the percentage of D_2 receptor occupancy, and the group mean increased from 55% at baseline to 79% at week 4; the increased prolactin concentrations correlated with receptor occupancy.

The effects of haloperidol and quetiapine on serum prolactin concentrations have been compared in 35 schizophrenic patients after a 2-week washout period in a randomized study (751). There was no significant difference in prolactin concentration between the groups at the start of the study, although prolactin concentrations were significantly lower with quetiapine than haloperidol. After 6 weeks, the mean prolactin concentration was significantly increased in those taking haloperidol but not in those taking quetiapine. Two patients taking haloperidol had galactorrhea related to hyperprolactinemia.

Hyperprolactinemia with osteopenia has been attributed to neuroleptic drugs (759).

- A 58-year-old schizophrenic woman who had taken haloperidol decanoate 125 mg every 2 weeks had a mildly raised prolactin concentration (505 mIU/l; upper limit of the reference range 450 mIU/liter). Dual X-ray absorptiometry showed osteopenia in her spine and hips. She began taking alendronic acid 5 mg/day and absorptiometry at 1 year showed that her spine and hip had improved by 7% and 9%, although her prolactin concentrations remained mildly raised.

- Three women, aged 61, 53, and 21 years, developed delusions of pregnancy while taking risperidone; their blood prolactin concentrations were 49, 78, and 52 ng/ml, respectively (reference range 2–26) (760).

The relation between prolactin concentrations and osteoporosis has been studied by measuring prolactin concentrations and lumbar spine and hip bone mineral densities in women with schizophrenia taking so-called "prolactin-raising antipsychotic drugs" (n = 26; mean treatment duration, 8.4 years) or olanzapine (n = 12; mean treatment duration, 6.3 years) (761). Prolactin concentrations were 1692 IU/l and 446 IU/l respectively (reference range 50–350 IU/l). Hyperprolactinemia was associated with low bone mineral density: 95% of women with either osteopenia or osteoporosis had hyperprolactinemia, whereas only 11% of those with normal prolactin concentrations had abnormal bone mineral density.

The relation between antipsychotic drug-induced hyperprolactinemia and hypoestrogenism has been studied in 75 women with schizophrenia (762). Serum estradiol concentrations were generally reduced during the entire menstrual cycle compared with reference values. There was hypoestrogenism, defined as serum estradiol concentrations below 30 pg/ml in the follicular phase and below 100 pg/ml in the periovulatory phase, in about 60%.

Inappropriate ADH secretion

Polyuria and polydipsia have long been associated with schizophrenia, and neuroleptic drugs appear to aggravate these symptoms, sometimes with an accompanying syndrome of inappropriate ADH secretion. However, water retention and edema occur very rarely during treatment with neuroleptic drugs. Water intoxication has been reported during treatment with thioridazine and may be due to its pronounced anticholinergic properties and/or direct stimulation of the hypothalamic thirst center (763).

The charts of 94 long-term inpatients have been reviewed retrospectively to examine the changes in weight, fasting glucose, and fasting lipids in those taking either risperidone (*n* = 47) or olanzapine (*n* = 47) (764). The patients had increased weight, triglycerides, and cholesterol, and the changes were significantly higher with olanzapine; olanzapine but not risperidone considerably increased glucose concentrations. One case of new-onset diabetes mellitus occurred in a patient taking olanzapine.

Lipid concentrations

In a cross-sectional study in 44 men, olanzapine had a worse metabolic risk profile than risperidone (765). The men (mean age 29 years) took olanzapine (*n* = 22; mean duration 18 months; mean dose 13 mg/day) or risperidone (*n* = 22; mean duration 17 months; mean dose 2.8 mg/day). Those who took olanzapine had significantly higher plasma triglyceride concentrations, significantly higher very low density lipoprotein cholesterol concentrations, a trend to a lower HDL cholesterol concentration, and a trend to a higher cholesterol/HDL cholesterol ratio. Despite similar mean body weights (olanzapine 84 kg versus risperidone 81 kg), 32% of those who took olanzapine were characterized by the atherogenic metabolic triad (hyperinsulinemia and raised apolipoprotein B and small-density LDL concentrations) compared with only 5% of those who took risperidone.

The effects of neuroleptic drugs on serum lipids in adults have been reviewed (766). Haloperidol and the atypical neuroleptic drugs ziprasidone, risperidone, and aripiprazole, are associated with lower risks of hyperlipidemia, whereas chlorpromazine, thioridazine, and the atypical drugs quetiapine, olanzapine, and clozapine are associated with higher risks.

Diabetes mellitus

DoTS classification (BMJ 2003; 327: 1222-5):
Dose-relation: collateral reaction
Time-course: intermediate
Susceptibility factors: male sex, African–American origin

Several cases of de novo onset or exacerbation of existing diabetes mellitus in patients treated with neuroleptic drugs have been reported and were not significantly related to weight gain. These included eight patients treated with clozapine (767,768) and two patients treated with olanzapine (768).

New-onset diabetes mellitus in such patients is of particular concern, owing to the associated cardiovascular morbidity and the difficulty in managing diabetes in psychiatric patients. Soon after the first neuroleptic drugs were used, associations with weight gain and diabetes were reported (769,770). Nevertheless, even before antipsychotic drugs appeared, diabetes was observed to be more common in patients with schizophrenia (771). The rate of diabetes in patients with schizophrenia has been estimated at 6.2–8.7% (772) and at 0.8% in the general population in the USA (773).

In 48 patients with schizophrenia taking clozapine, olanzapine, risperidone, or typical neuroleptic drugs, and 31 untreated healthy control subjects newer neuroleptic drugs, such as clozapine and olanzapine, compared with typical agents, were associated with adverse effects on blood glucose regulation (774).

The Food and Drug Administration (FDA) has asked all manufacturers of atypical antipsychotic drugs to add the following warning statement describing the increased risk of hyperglycemia and diabetes in patients taking these medications (775): "Hyperglycemia, in some cases extreme and associated with ketoacidosis or hyperosmolar coma or death, has been reported in patients treated with atypical antipsychotic drugs including... (a long list). Assessment of the relationship between atypical antipsychotic use and glucose abnormalities is complicated by the possibility of an increased background risk of diabetes mellitus in patients with schizophrenia and the increasing incidence of diabetes mellitus in the general population. Given these confounders, the relationship between atypical antipsychotic use and hyperglycemia-related adverse events is not completely understood. However, epidemiological studies suggest an increased risk of treatment-emergent hyperglycemia-related adverse events in patients treated with atypical antipsychotic drugs. Precise risk estimates for hyperglycemia-related adverse events in patients treated with atypical antipsychotic drugs are not available.

Patients with an established diagnosis of diabetes mellitus who are started on atypical antipsychotic drugs should be monitored regularly for worsening of glucose control. Patients with risk factors for diabetes mellitus (e.g. obesity, family history of diabetes) who are starting treatment with atypical antipsychotic drugs should undergo fasting blood glucose testing at the beginning of treatment and periodically during treatment. Any patient treated with atypical antipsychotic drugs should be monitored for symptoms of hyperglycemia including polydipsia, polyuria, polyphagia, and weakness. Patients who develop symptoms of hyperglycemia during treatment with atypical antipsychotic drugs should undergo fasting blood glucose testing. In some cases, hyperglycemia has resolved when the atypical antipsychotic was discontinued; however, some patients required continuation of anti-diabetic treatment despite discontinuation of the suspect drug".

Whether diabetes is associated, and to what extent, with a particular antipsychotic drug or a particular type of antipsychotic drug is a matter of debate; since the two most commonly used atypical antipsychotic drugs are risperidone and olanzapine, comparison of these two drugs has been a recent focus of attention. There are more case reports for clozapine and olanzapine, but the studies discussed below have reached conflicting results; further information from clinical trials is needed.

Observational studies

Claims data for the period January 1996 to December 1997 were analysed for patients with mood disorders in two large US health plans (776). In all, 849 patients had been exposed to risperidone, 656 to olanzapine, 785 to high-potency conventional antipsychotic drugs, and 302 to low-potency conventional drugs; 2644 were untreated. Adjusted odds ratios of newly reported type 2 diabetes in patients who took risperidone or high-potency conventional antipsychotic drugs were not significantly different from those in untreated patients at 12 months; on the contrary, patients who took olanzapine or low-potency conventional antipsychotic drugs had a significantly higher risk of type 2 diabetes compared with untreated patients; the 12-month adjusted odds ratios compared with untreated patients were 4.3 (95%CI = 2.1, 8.8) in those who took olanzapine and 4.9 (95%CI = 1.9, 13) in those who took low-potency conventional antipsychotic drugs.

Olanzapine had significantly positive diabetic effects, based on both duration of treatment and dosage. All patients had been exposed to antipsychotic drugs for more than 60 days; because there was less awareness of the diabetic effects of atypical antipsychotic drugs during that period, the use of these data reduced the possibility of selection bias.

Additionally, three other epidemiological studies have identified a higher risk of diabetes associated with olanzapine (Sernyak 777,778). The first of these studies included out-patients with schizophrenia treated over 4 months in 1999 (Sernyak 561). When patients who had taken atypical drugs (n = 22 648) were compared with those who had taken typical antipsychotic drugs (n = 15 984), the adjusted odds ratio of new diagnoses of diabetes was 1.09 (CI = 1.03, 1.15); and was even higher in patients under 40 years of age (OR = 1.63; CI − 1.23, 2.16; n = 3076 and n = 1105). The odds ratios for individual atypical drugs were:

- quetiapine 1.31 (1.11, 1.55; n = 955);
- clozapine 1.25 (1.07, 1.46; n = 1207);
- olanzapine 1.11 (1.04, 1.18; n = 10 970);
- risperidone 1.05 (0.98, 1.12; n = 9903).

In a nested case-control study using information from the UK General Practice Research Database 451 patients with diabetes out of 19 637 patients treated for schizophrenia were matched with 2696 controls (Koro 243). There was a significantly increased risk of diabetes in patients taking olanzapine compared with non-users of antipsychotic drugs (adjusted OR = 5.8; 95% CI = 2, 17) and compared with those taking conventional antipsychotic drugs (adjusted OR = 4.2, 95% CI = 1.5, 12); there was a non-significantly increased risk in those taking risperidone compared with non-users of antipsychotic drugs (adjusted OR = 2.2, 95% CI = 0.9, 5.2) and compared with those taking conventional antipsychotic drugs (adjusted OR = 1.6; 95% CI = 0.7, 3.8).

In a comparison of olanzapine and risperidone, 319 patients out of 19 153 who were given a prescription for olanzapine between 1January 1997 and 31 December 1999 developed diabetes, compared with 217 who were given a prescription for risperidone (n = 14 793) (779). Proportional hazards analysis showed a 20% increased risk of diabetes with olanzapine relative to risperidone (RR = 1.20; CI = 1.00, 1.43).

Finally, a retrospective cohort study carried out with a database that included information from different care plans (Buse 164) showed that the incidence of diabetes mellitus in patients taking any conventional antipsychotic drug was 84 per 1000 patient-years (crude incidence 307 in 19 782) compared with 67 per 1000 patient-years (crude incidence 641 in 38 969) in patients taking any atypical antipsychotic drugs; the estimated incidence in the reference general population was 15.7 per 1000 patients-years (crude incidence 45 513 in 5 816 473). Cox proportional hazards regression, adjusted for age, sex, and duration of antipsychotic drug exposure, showed that the risk of diabetes mellitus was significantly higher for whatever antipsychotic drug than in the general population but not different between the conventional and atypical antipsychotic drugs (HR = 0.97; 95% CI = 0.84, 1.11). The hazard ratios for individual atypical antipsychotic drugs compared with haloperidol were:

- clozapine 1.31 (95% CI, 0.60, 2.86);
- risperidone 1.23 (95% CI, 1.01, 1.50);
- olanzapine 1.09 (95% CI, 0.86, 1.37);
- quetiapine 0.67 (95% CI, 0.46, 0.97).

The data cut-off point for this study was 31 August 2000. Only incident cases of diabetes mellitus that resulted in intervention with antidiabetic drugs were selected and only patients taking antipsychotic drug monotherapy were included; the average duration of antipsychotic drug treatment was not long (68–137 days). One of the main flaws of this study was the possibility of selection bias, since certain patient attributes that influence treatment selection might also affect the likelihood of diabetes mellitus.

Weight gain due to atypical antipsychotic drugs has been addressed in a cross-sectional study of the weight at the time of a single visit compared with that recorded in the clinical chart (780). The proportion of patients with clinically relevant weight gain ($\geq$ 7% increase versus initial weight) was higher with olanzapine (46%; n = 228) than with risperidone (31%; n = 232) or haloperidol (22%; n = 130); no patient had clinically relevant weight gain while taking quetiapine (n = 43). The risk of weight gain was higher in women (OR = 4.4), overweight patients (OR = 3.0) and patients with at least 1 year of treatment (OR = 6.3) in the olanzapine group; these risk factors are not entirely coincidental with other findings (SEDA-26, 56).

In an open non-randomized study of the frequency of undiagnosed impaired fasting glucose and diabetes mellitus in 168 patients taking clozapine, 47 patients were discarded because a fasting plasma glucose was not successfully obtained (n = 20) or because they were identified as diabetic before the fasting plasma glucose screening (n = 27) (781). Of 121 patients not previously diagnosed as diabetic, 93 had normal fasting blood sugar concentrations (below 6 mmol/l or 110 mg/dl), and 2) had a raised plasma glucose concentration (fasting plasma glucose over 6 mmol/l), including seven with type 2 diabetes. Patients with hyperglycemia were significantly older and more commonly had concurrent bipolar affective disorder.

Randomized studies

In a randomized double-blind study, in-patients with schizophrenia were assessed for fasting glucose, cholesterol, and weight gain after 14 weeks of treatment with clozapine (n = 28), haloperidol (n = 25), olanzapine (n = 26), or risperidone (n = 22) (782). There was a statistically significant increase in mean blood glucose concentrations only in the olanzapine group; 14 out of 101 patients (14%) developed raised blood glucose concentrations (over 7 mmol/l or 125 mg/dl) at some time during the study: six while taking clozapine, one haloperidol, four olanzapine, and three risperidone. Similarly, there was a significant increase in cholesterol concentration in the olanzapine group. The largest weight gain was also observed with olanzapine (mean change 7.3 kg), followed by clozapine (4.8 kg) and risperidone (2.4 kg); there was minimal weight gain with haloperidol (0.9 kg). ANCOVA showed no main effect or treatment interaction for the relation between change in blood glucose and weight gain at end-point; however, there was a significant main effect for the association between change in cholesterol and weight gain in the four groups. The rate of hyperglycemia (14%) in this study was about twice the rate of diabetes reported in a large survey of the US population (6–8%) (783) and somewhat higher than the current prevalence

rate of 10% found in extensive samples of patients with schizophrenia (784).

Susceptibility factors and clinical features

Most of the patients who develop diabetes while taking antipsychotic drugs do so in under 6 months; men are at greater risk, and African–Americans are more susceptible than other ethnic groups (785). Weight gain can be present or not; in a retrospective series of 76 patients who developed diabetes while taking olanzapine or risperidone, the increase in fasting blood glucose concentration in patients taking olanzapine did not correlate with changes in weight (786).

Diabetic ketoacidosis is a common presentation of diabetes in patients taking atypical antipsychotic drugs. In 126 patients taking atypical antipsychotic drugs, new-onset, acute, marked glucose intolerance developed in 11 (8.7%) after treatment with clozapine, olanzapine, or quetiapine (787). Of these, six patients required insulin (four only transiently) and five developed diabetic ketoacidosis. The mean and median times to the onset of diabetic ketoacidosis after the start of treatment with an atypical antipsychotic drug were 81 and 33 days respectively. In 45 patients, 19 who presented with ketoacidosis were significantly younger, more often women, and less overweight at baseline than 26 patients who developed diabetes without ketoacidosis (788).

Death due to olanzapine-induced hyperglycemia has been reported (SEDA-27, 61).

Mechanisms

There has been some discussion about whether antipsychotic drug-induced hyperglycemia and diabetes are associated with weight gain (SEDA-25, 65; SEDA-26, 62; SEDA-27, 61). Clozapine and olanzapine have a high propensity to cause both weight gain and diabetes (SEDA-26, 56); however, there have been cases in which diabetes appeared or worsened in the absence of weight gain or even with weight loss (789,790). Both weight gain and diabetes seem to be effects that occur simultaneously, rather than diabetes being an indirect effect of weight gain. Other mechanisms have therefore been suggested (SEDA-21, 67).

Ten patients with schizophrenia taking olanzapine 7.5–20 mg/day were compared with 10 healthy volunteers with regard to body weight, fat mass, and insulin resistance over 8 weeks (791). Fasting serum glucose and insulin increased significantly in the olanzapine group, as did weight gain. The index for insulin resistance increased only in the olanzapine group, whereas beta-cell function did not change significantly. Consistent with this, it has been observed that some antipsychotic drugs inhibit glucose transport into PC12 cells in culture and increase cellular concentrations of glucose, which would in turn cause a homeostatic increase in insulin release.

Insulin resistance is a major but not necessary risk factor for type 2 diabetes. Glucose metabolism in 36 out-patients with schizophrenia aged 18–65 years taking clozapine (n = 12), olanzapine (n = 12), or risperidone (n = 12) has been examined in a cross-sectional study

(792). There was no significant difference in fasting baseline plasma glucose concentrations. Those taking clozapine or olanzapine had significant insulin resistance compared with those taking risperidone. There were no significant differences in total cholesterol, high-density lipoprotein cholesterol, low-density lipoprotein cholesterol, or serum triglyceride concentrations; however, controlling for sex, there was a significant difference (clozapine > olanzapine > risperidone). However, consistent with other results, the small sample size, the cross-sectional design, and the exclusion of obese subjects may limit the generalizability of these findings.

The hormone leptin is synthesized by adipocytes and is important in controlling body weight; plasma leptin concentrations correlate with fat mass and insulin resistance. Leptin could be a link between obesity, insulin resistance syndrome, and treatment with some neuroleptic drugs. Plasma leptin concentrations are raised, regardless of weight, in patients taking clozapine (793).

Management

The relation between the metabolic syndrome and antipsychotic drug therapy has been reviewed (794,795,796). In most patients, diabetes improves or resolves after withdrawing antipsychotic drugs or switching to less diabetogenic drugs. Simple interventions, such as changes in diet and exercise, are recommended for patients with schizophrenia or bipolar disease taking antipsychotic drugs. Patients who develop conditions such as hyperlipidemia or diabetes mellitus often respond to routine treatment. However, managing diabetes in patients with schizophrenia is complicated by their lack of insight, loss of initiative, and cognitive deficits, which are central features of the illness. For patients with type 2 diabetes, the major risk is accelerated coronary heart disease and stroke, greatly aggravated by smoking, which is common in patients with schizophrenia.

In addition to considerations of the diabetogenic potential of each agent, the presence of susceptibility factors, such as obesity, sedentary lifestyle, and a family history of type 2 diabetes, should be taken into account in the selection of a suitable regimen. It is sensible to monitor fasting plasma glucose concentrations, glycosylated hemoglobin, and fasting cholesterol and triglycerides in order to anticipate hyperglycemia and hyperlipidemia. Given the serious implications for morbidity and mortality attributable to diabetes and raised cholesterol, clinicians need to be aware of these risk factors when treating patients with chronic schizophrenia.

Weight gain

Shortly after the typical neuroleptic drugs were introduced in the 1950s, marked increases in body weight were observed, and excessive weight gain has been reported in up to 50% of patients receiving long-term neuroleptic drug treatment (797–803).

Weight gain related to the use of atypical neuroleptic drugs in children and adolescents, in whom this adverse effect is of particular concern, has been reviewed (804). The published data suggest that clozapine and olanzapine are associated with considerable weight gain, risperidone and quetiapine have a moderate risk, and ziprasidone and aripiprazole a low risk. Moreover, obese children have an increased propensity for orthopedic, neurological, pulmonary, and gastroenterological complications.

However, changes in weight during psychosis are also related to the condition; Kraepelin wrote, "The taking of food fluctuates from complete refusal to the greatest voracity · · · Sometimes, in quite short periods, very considerable differences in the body weight are noticed · · ·" (805). It was observed early on that food intake and weight often fell as psychosis worsened, but eating and weight returned to normal or increased when an acute psychotic episode abated. However, since the start of the neuroleptic drug era in the 1950s, a new pattern of sustained increased weight has commonly been detected. The question of whether weight gain is associated with efficacy is important; in one study there was no obvious relation between the magnitude of weight gain and therapeutic efficacy (806).

The association between clozapine-related weight gain and increased mean arterial blood pressure has been examined in 61 patients who were randomly assigned to either clozapine or haloperidol in a 10-week parallel group, double-blind study, and in 55 patients who chose to continue to take clozapine in a subsequent 1-year, open, prospective study (807). Clozapine was associated with significant weight gain in both the double-blind trial (mean 4.2 kg) and the open trial (mean 5.8 kg), but haloperidol was not associated with significant weight gain (mean 0.4 kg). There were no significant correlations between change in weight and change in mean arterial blood pressure for clozapine or haloperidol.

Serum leptin, a peripheral hormone secreted by fat, correlates inversely with body weight; in 22 patients taking clozapine who gained weight, those who had the most pronounced 2-week increase in leptin had the least gain in body weight after 6 and 8 months (808).

Epidemiology

Several reviews have addressed the issue of weight gain (809–813). Comparison of different studies of weight gain during treatment with atypical neuroleptic drugs is hampered by problems with study design, recruitment procedures, patient characteristics, measurement of body weight, co-medications, and duration of therapy. These problems have to be considered when assessing this type of information, particularly figures collected in accordance with the last-observation-carried-forward technique, which is one of the most common approaches taken; this type of analysis can produce marked underestimates of the magnitude of weight gain.

There has been one comprehensive meta-analysis including over 80 studies and over 30 000 patients (814). A meta-analysis of trials of neuroleptic drugs showed the following mean weight gains in kg after 10 weeks of treatment: clozapine, 4.5; olanzapine, 4.2; thioridazine, 3.2; sertindole, 2.9; chlorpromazine, 2.6; risperidone, 2.1; haloperidol, 1.1; fluphenazine, 0.43; ziprasidone 0.04; molindone, −0.39; placebo, −0.74

(815,816). In one study, excessive appetite was a more frequent adverse event in patients treated with olanzapine versus haloperidol (24 versus 12%) (817). Loss of weight has been observed after withdrawal of neuroleptic drugs (818).

The percentages of patients who gain more than 7% of their baseline body weight are highest for olanzapine (29%) and lowest for ziprasidone (9.8%). Although these figures are useful for comparing different drugs, they do not illustrate how weight increases over time, nor the total gain. Body weight tends to increase at first but reaches a plateau by about 1 year; with olanzapine 12.5–17.5 mg/day, patients gained, on average, 12 kg (819).

Risperidone and olanzapine, the two most commonly used atypical drugs, have been compared in trials; patients who took olanzapine gained almost twice as much weight (4.1 kg) as those who took risperidone (2.3 kg) (820). In two groups of inpatients, who took either risperidone ($n = 50$) or olanzapine ($n = 50$) for schizophrenia the mean body weight at baseline was 83 kg in the risperidone group and 85 kg in the olanzapine group; after 4 months of treatment, the mean body weights were 83 and 87 kg respectively (821). The increase in body weight with olanzapine was statistically significant.

In a retrospective chart review of 91 patients with schizophrenia (120 treatment episodes; mean age 38 years), there was weight gain with zotepine (4.3 kg), clozapine (3.1 kg), sulpiride (1.9 kg), and risperidone (1.5 kg), but not in patients treated with typical neuroleptic drugs (mean gain 0.0–0.5 kg) (822). The mean duration of treatment was 28–34 days, the maximum weight gain being in the first 3–5 weeks. The mean increases in weight were 4.3% in the patients with normal weight, 3.0% in those with mild obesity, and 1.9% in those with severe obesity (BMI over 30).

In another retrospective study, 65 patients with schizophrenia who gained weight while taking clozapine for 6 months were followed (823). After that they were switched to a combination of clozapine with quetiapine for 10 months: clozapine was tapered to 25% of the current dose and quetiapine was added proportionately. During clozapine monotherapy the mean weight gain was 6.5 kg and 13 patients developed diabetes. At the end of the combination period, the mean weight loss was 9.4 kg; patients who developed diabetes showed significant improvement, resulting in a rapid fall in insulin requirements and/or withdrawal of insulin and replacement with an oral hypoglycemic agent. The mechanism of clozapine-associated weight gain is uncertain.

A thorough search for studies that addressed obesity in children and adolescents in relation to the new antipsychotic drugs showed that risperidone is associated with less weight gain than olanzapine (824).

Mechanism

The mechanisms of weight gain are not known. Olanzapine, for example, affects at least 19 different receptor sites, may have reuptake inhibition properties, and may affect hormones such as prolactin. Animal models do not help to elucidate mechanisms, since they have not shown clear results: some studies have shown weight gain with neuroleptic drugs in rats and others have not.

However, a serotonergic mechanism has been proposed (825). Most of the atypical drugs, which most commonly cause weight gain, interact with 5-HT$_{2C}$ receptors; however, ziprasidone also binds to 5-HT$_{2C}$ receptors with high affinity and does not cause weight gain or does so to a lesser extent. In 152 patients treated with clozapine, Cys23Ser polymorphism of the 5-HT$_{2C}$ receptor did not explain the weight gain that occurred (826), nor was there an association between specific alleles of the dopamine D$_4$ receptor gene (827). In contrast, in 19-year-old monozygotic twins who gained around 40 kg after taking mainly clozapine, weight gain was related to an unspecified genotype (828). An association between weight gain and a 5-HT$_{2C}$ receptor gene polymorphism has been identified in 123 Chinese Han patients with schizophrenia taking chlorpromazine ($n = 69$), risperidone ($n = 46$), clozapine ($n = 4$), fluphenazine ($n = 3$), or sulpiride ($n = 1$) (829). Weight gain was substantially greater in the patients with the wild-type genotype than in those with a variant genotype (–759C/T), at both 6 and 10 weeks; this effect was seen in men and women.

Susceptibility factors

In general, people with schizophrenia have a greater tendency to be overweight and obese than those who do not have schizophrenia (830). The evidence suggests that weight gain will progress most rapidly during the first 3–20 weeks of treatment with second-generation neuroleptic drugs; there is little evidence that dose affects weight gain. There are no sex differences, but there is a positive correlation between weight gain and age. Smokers treated with neuroleptic drugs may gain less weight than non-smokers (822,831). Patients in hospital are more likely to gain weight than those in the community, perhaps because they have an unrestricted diet and limited physical activity; there is some evidence that those with a lower baseline BMI are likely to gain more weight (810).

However, in the USA, data from a large health and nutrition survey ($n = 17\ 689$) and from patients with schizophrenia to be enrolled in a clinical trial ($n = 420$) showed no differences; the mean BMIs were high and a substantial proportion of the population was obese (830).

The genetic basis of some reactions associated with neuroleptic drugs is of particular interest. An important association between weight gain and a 5-HT$_{2C}$ receptor gene polymorphism has now been identified in 123 Chinese Han schizophrenic patients taking chlorpromazine ($n = 69$), risperidone ($n = 46$), clozapine ($n = 4$), fluphenazine ($n = 3$), or sulpiride ($n = 1$) (829). Weight gain was substantially greater in the patients with the wild-type genotype than in those with a variant genotype (–759C/T), at both 6 and 10 weeks; this effect was seen in men and women. In addition, a homozygous non-functional genotype, CYP2D6*4, was found in a 17-year-old schizophrenic patient who developed severe akathisia, parkinsonism, and drowsiness after taking risperidone 6 mg/day for 3 months; he had a high plasma concentration of risperidone and an active metabolite (832).

Clinical features
Obesity is associated with increased risks of dyslipidemia, hypertension, type 2 diabetes mellitus, cardiovascular disease, osteoarthritis, sleep apnea, and numerous other disorders; all these conditions have been associated with increased mortality. In the EUFAMI (European Federation of Associations of Families of Mentally Ill People) Patient Survey undertaken in 2001 across four countries and involving 441 patients, treatment-induced adverse effects were a fundamental problem; of the 91% of patients who had adverse effects, 60% had weight gain, and of these more than half (54%) rated weight gain as the most difficult problem to cope with (833). Furthermore, weight gain can adversely affect patients' adherence to medication, undermining the success of drug treatment for schizophrenia.

A report has illustrated how extreme the problem of weight gain associated with neuroleptic drugs can be (834).

• A 32-year-old man with schizophrenia taking neuroleptic drugs was switched to olanzapine 20 mg/day for better control. He weighed 101 kg and his BMI was 31 kg/m^2. After 6 months he had gained 4.5 kg and after 1 year 17 kg. Because of poor control, risperidone 4 mg/day was added and 16 months later he had had a 34.6 kg increase from baseline and had a BMI of 42 kg/m^2 (that is in the range of severe obesity). He had both increased appetite and impaired satiety. His serum triglycerides were 4.0 mmol/l, and his fasting blood glucose was 6.7 mmol/l. He and his physician agreed on a goal of losing 12 kg over 12 months and he was referred to a dietician. Over the next 5 weeks, he lost 2.7 kg and after 2 years his BMI was 38 kg/m^2 and 1 year later 39 kg/m^2. He was given nizatidine 300 mg bd and 1 year later his weight was 95 kg (BMI 29 kg/m^2). His triglycerides and fasting blood glucose concentrations were within the reference ranges.

Comparative studies
The charts of 94 long-term inpatients have been reviewed retrospectively to examine the changes in weight, fasting glucose, and fasting lipids in those taking either risperidone ($n = 47$) or olanzapine ($n = 47$) (764). The patients had increased weight, triglycerides, and cholesterol, and the changes were significantly higher with olanzapine; olanzapine but not risperidone considerably increased glucose concentrations. One case of new-onset diabetes mellitus occurred in a patient taking olanzapine. Weight should be monitored in patients taking maintenance atypical neuroleptic drugs, especially dibenzodiazepines.

Management
Behavioral treatment of obesity has given good results in patients taking neuroleptic drugs (835). More dubious is the use of antiobesity drugs, as some of them can cause psychotic reactions.

Good results have been reported with amantadine, which increases dopamine release (836). In 12 patients with a mean weight gain of 7.3 kg during olanzapine treatment, amantadine 100–300 mg/day over 3–6 months produced an average weight loss of 3.5 kg without adverse effects. In contrast, calorie restriction did not lead to weight loss in 39 patients with mental retardation who were taking risperidone, 37 of whom gained weight, the mean gain being 8.3 kg over 26 months (837).

Nevirapine

Lipodystrophy, well recognized with stavudine, has also been reported in nine of 56 patients taking combined HAART therapy including nevirapine, although there must be some doubt as to which drug or combination was responsible (838).

Nicorandil

Nicorandil suppresses the release of insulin from isolated animal pancreatic cells (839). However, this effect is four times weaker than that of diazoxide, and its effect in man is not known.

Nicotinic acid and derivatives

Prolonged administration of nicotinic acid can have a diabetogenic effect and decompensation of previously stable diabetes can occur. Severe hyperglycemia has been precipitated by nicotinic acid treatment of hyperlipidemia (840).

During long-term treatment with nicotinic acid, uric acid concentrations tend to rise slightly, but the change is clinically insignificant (841).

Nicotinic acid has a hyperglycemic action (SED-13, 1330), and is therefore not recommended as a first-line hypolipidemic drug in patients with type 2 diabetes mellitus (842).

Lactic acidosis has been observed in patients taking nicotinic acid (SED-13, 1330).

Nitrofurantoin

One case of hyperlactatemic metabolic acidosis together with hemolytic anemia due to glucose-6-phosphate dehydrogenase deficiency has been reported (843).

Nucleoside analogue reverse transcriptase inhibitors (NRTIs)

See also individual agents

Lipodystrophy

The prevalence of lipodystrophy has been studied during follow-up for 30 months of previously untreated patients who had been randomized to receive different nucleoside analogue combinations for 6 months in the ALBI–ANRS 070 trial (844). After 30 months 37 of 120 patients who had used nucleoside analogues with or without other antiretroviral drugs had at least one morphological change, and 21 of those had isolated peripheral lipoatrophy; the corresponding values for the patients who used only nucleoside analogues during follow-up were 20 of 66 and 14 of 21 respectively. The factors associated with lipodystrophy were initial assignment to stavudine plus didanosine compared with zidovudine plus lamivudine (OR = 6.7), age below 10 years (OR = 3.6), and HIV RNA concentration at month 30 (OR = 0.4). There were no differences in cholesterol and glucose concentrations. Thus, exposure to stavudine and didanosine was associated with lipodystrophy (predominantly lipoatrophy).

In a well-controlled French comparison of changes in body composition, body fat distribution, and insulin secretion, patients taking stavudine (n = 27) or zidovudine (n = 16) were compared with controls (n = 15) (845). The zidovudine group and the control group had similar body composition and regional fat distribution. Stavudine was associated with a significantly lower percentage of body fat than zidovudine (13 versus 15%), a markedly lower ratio of subcutaneous to visceral fat, and a higher mean intake of fat and cholesterol. Triglyceride concentrations were significantly higher with stavudine than in the controls, but did not differ between stavudine and zidovudine or between zidovudine and controls. Free fatty acids tended to be higher with stavudine. Lipodystrophy was observed in 17 patients taking stavudine, and in three taking zidovudine after a median time of 14 months. The relative risk of fat wasting with stavudine compared with zidovudine was 1.95. Five of twelve patients had a major or mild improvement in their lipodystrophy after stavudine was withdrawn. The authors concluded that lipodystrophy may be related to long-term NRTI therapy, particularly if it includes stavudine.

Lactic acidosis

Lactic acidosis is a severe and potentially fatal form of mitochondrial toxicity. Metabolic stress or vitamin deficiencies (riboflavin, carnitine) might provoke it. There is suggestive evidence of clinical benefit with riboflavin therapy (846).

Antiretroviral nucleoside analogues have been associated with hepatic steatosis and lactic acidosis. These compounds require phosphorylation to active triphosphate derivatives by cellular phosphokinases. The triphosphate nucleotide inhibits the growing proviral DNA chain, but it also inhibits host DNA polymerases, and this can result in compensatory glycolysis and lactic acidosis. Abnormal mitochondrial oxidation of free fatty acids causes the accumulation of neutral fat in liver cells, and this manifests as hepatomegaly with macrovesicular steatosis. Hepatic steatosis and lactic acidosis have been reported previously with zidovudine, didanosine, zalcitabine, Combivir (zidovudine plus lamivudine), and lamivudine. Of 349 Australian patients studied for 18 months (516 patient-years) taking NRTIs only two had severe lactic acidosis (847).

Three cases of steatosis/lactic acidosis syndrome associated with stavudine plus lamivudine have been reported (848).

- A 37-year-old HIV-infected woman receiving stavudine, lamivudine, and indinavir developed epigastric pain, anorexia, and vomiting. She had lactic acidosis (serum lactate 4.9 mmol/l), raised liver enzymes, and an increased prothrombin time. She had hepatomegaly and tachypnea and required mechanical ventilation. Her progress was complicated by pancreatitis and acute respiratory distress syndrome. Antiviral medication was stopped and she was treated with co-enzyme Q, carnitine, and vitamin C. The serum lactic acid and transaminases returned to normal over 4 weeks and she was weaned off the ventilator after 4 months.
- A 40-year-old HIV-infected woman receiving stavudine, lamivudine, nelfinavir, and co-trimoxazole developed dyspnea, dysphagia, and vomiting with lactic acidosis (serum lactate 9.4 mmol/l) and hepatomegaly. Despite ventilation for respiratory failure she died after 5 days. Autopsy showed massive hepatomegaly with steatosis.
- A 36-year-old HIV-infected woman who had been receiving stavudine, saquinavir, ritonavir, and didanosine developed lactic acidosis (serum lactate 11.4 mmol/l) and hepatomegaly. She had acute pancreatitis and, despite ventilatory support for respiratory failure, died after 8 weeks.

There have been similar reports related to didanosine plus stavudine (849) and stavudine alone (850).

Routine monitoring of lactate is not recommended, since lactate concentrations do not correlate with symptoms and patients may have asymptomatic lactatemia. Furthermore, technical difficulties in blood collection and processing, and the lack of a standardized definition of lactic acidosis for patients taking NRTIs, prevent any routine monitoring recommendations in the absence of symptoms. In addition, it is possible that NRTIs also cause other forms of mitochondrial dysfunction.

Ofloxacin

Ofloxacin 200 mg bd caused diabetes insipidus in a 25-year-old man (851).

Olanzapine

Prolactin

Olanzapine can cause increased serum prolactin concentrations and galactorrhea, but probably to a lesser extent than haloperidol (SEDA-22, 65).

- A depressed 27-year-old woman taking mirtazapine developed hyperprolactinemia and galactorrhea after taking olanzapine 10 mg/day for 5 weeks (582).
- A 19-year-old woman with mild mental retardation and a history of birth anoxia who took olanzapine 15 mg/day for 3 weeks developed euprolactinemic galactorrhea (853). Laboratory tests were all normal, including

a normal thyroid-stimulating hormone concentration and a prolactin concentration of 13 ng/ml (reference range 3–30 ng/ml). She had mild to moderate akathisia. Both the galactorrhea and the akathisia abated after substitution by quetiapine.

The authors stated that the reason why galactorrhea occurred is unclear but suggested that it may have been due to structural damage and greater sensitivity to prolactin resulting from the patient's anoxia at birth.

- A 35-year-old woman developed hyperprolactinemia, amenorrhea, and galactorrhea after taking risperidone for 2 months; the effects persisted after she switched to olanzapine, mean dose 2.5 mg/day (854).

However, paradoxical cases of improvement in galactorrhea have also been observed (SEDA-23, 67).

Two women with neuroleptic-drug induced hyperprolactinemia, menstrual dysfunction, and galactorrhea had improvement in these adverse effects during treatment with olanzapine (855).

- A 34-year-old woman, who developed amenorrhea while taking risperidone, regained her normal menstrual pattern along with a marked fall in serum prolactin concentration 8 weeks after being switched to olanzapine, whereas amantadine had failed to normalize the menses and had apparently reactivated the psychotic symptoms (856).

The authors suggested that olanzapine may offer advantages for selected patients in whom hyperprolactinemia occurs during treatment with other antipsychotic drugs.

Improvement in galactorrhea has also been observed in a case of trichotillomania refractory to a selective serotonin reuptake inhibitor (857). The patient only had a positive response with risperidone in combination with fluoxetine, but developed hyperprolactinemia and an intolerable galactorrhea. Olanzapine in combination with fluoxetine was started, with significant clinical improvement and without symptoms of galactorrhea; however, the patient had undesired weight gain of 3.6 kg after 22 weeks.

Diabetes mellitus

Hyperglycemia associated with olanzapine has a frequency of 1/100 to 1/1000. Hyperglycemia and diabetes have been associated with olanzapine, and published cases have suggested that these adverse effects may be caused by a mechanism related to weight gain (SEDA-23, 67; SEDA-24, 69; SEDA-25, 65). However, several cases of de novo onset or exacerbation of existing diabetes mellitus in patients treated with neuroleptic drugs have been reported and were not significantly related to weight gain. These included patients taking clozapine (858,859) or olanzapine (859,860).

Diabetes mellitus has been reported in patients taking olanzapine (from 10 mg for 2 months to 25 mg for 22 months) (861). All were switched to quetiapine. Five of the six had known risk factors for diabetes mellitus (positive family history, obesity, race, and hyperlipidemia);

only one gained significant body weight with olanzapine. There was a close temporal relation between the onset of therapy and the appearance of diabetes in three patients. The authors made recommendations about the detection and management of this effect in patients taking neuroleptic drugs; they suggested that consideration should be given to testing for diabetes mellitus 3–7 months after starting neuroleptic drug treatment and that screening is ideally carried out by measuring the fasting plasma glucose concentration. The case of a 39-year-old woman who developed hyperglycemia after the dose of olanzapine was increased from 10 to 15 mg/day has also prompted the recommendation that blood glucose should be monitored in patients taking olanzapine (862).

- A 51-year-old woman with an 18-year history of type II diabetes mellitus developed glucose dysregulation with persistent hyperglycemia within 3 weeks of starting treatment with olanzapine, in the absence of weight gain (863).

The author suggested that olanzapine can cause glucose dysregulation by a mechanism other than weight gain.

- A 32-year-old African-American man with no prior history of diabetes mellitus or glucose intolerance had a raised blood glucose concentration after 6 weeks of olanzapine therapy, and required insulin (864). Olanzapine was withdrawn and blood glucose concentrations returned to normal about 2 weeks later. At rechallenge hyperglycemia occurred again.
- A 50-year-old man developed acute ketoacidosis with de novo diabetes mellitus after 8 months of adjunctive olanzapine (865). His dosage was then gradually titrated to 30 mg/day over 6 months, and after withdrawal of olanzapine his diabetes mellitus disappeared completely.
- A 31-year-old man taking olanzapine 10 mg/day, who had no family history of diabetes and had never had any laboratory evidence of diabetes or glucose intolerance, developed diabetic ketoacidosis; obesity was the only predisposing factor, his BMI being 40 kg/m^2 (866).
- A 45-year-old man with a 4-year history of diet-controlled diabetes had hyperglycemia with polyuria, polydipsia, and blurred vision associated with the use of olanzapine 10 mg/day. Within 1 week after olanzapine was withdrawn his blood glucose returned to normal and insulin was discontinued.
- A 54-year-old woman developed severe glucose dysregulation with exacerbation of type 2 diabetes 12 days after starting to take olanzapine 10 mg/day; she also gained 13 kg (867).

The effects of olanzapine on glucose–insulin homeostasis have been studied in 14 patients in an attempt to elucidate the possible mechanisms of olanzapine-associated weight gain (868). Olanzapine caused weight gain of 1–10 kg in 12 patients and raised concentrations of insulin, leptin, and blood lipids, as well as insulin resistance; three patients developed diabetes mellitus. The authors concluded that both increased insulin secretion and hyperleptinemia may be mechanisms behind olanzapine-induced weight gain. They also suggested that the metabolite

N-desmethylolanzapine has a normalizing effect on the metabolic abnormalities.

In an open study in seven men and four women taking olanzapine (mean daily dose 12 mg and mean treatment duration 23 months), although the mean fasting triglyceride concentrations and mean fasting plasma glucose concentrations were similar to those found in the previous study, the mean fasting insulin concentrations were lower (143 pmol/l versus 228 pmol/l), and four of the subjects had hyperinsulinemia, compared with ten in the other study (869). However, the small sample sizes precluded any clear conclusions.

Susceptibility factors, such as family history, obesity, and concomitant medications can predispose an individual taking olanzapine to diabetes mellitus. New-onset diabetes mellitus developed after olanzapine was given to a 31-year-old man and a 44-year-old man (870). In both cases, the family history included diabetes mellitus, type unknown. The patients were taking various psychotropic drugs. In the first case body weight increased by about 12 kg (BMI 32 kg/m^2) 6 weeks after starting olanzapine, when his diabetes mellitus started; in the second case (BMI 26 kg/m^2, weight 81 kg) the previous weight was unknown.

Olanzapine-induced non-ketotic hyperglycemia has also been reported in the absence of obesity (871).

- A non-obese 51-year-old man without a history of diabetes mellitus had a serum glucose concentration of 89 mmol/l and was non-ketotic. Treatment with olanzapine had been started less than 6 months before; about 2 months before the event, his blood glucose concentration was 6.0 mmol/l, and 8 days after withdrawal the glucose concentration returned to normal; he no longer required insulin nor any other hypoglycemic drug.

The authors suggested that olanzapine can cause hyperglycemia by a mechanism other than weight gain.

Glucose concentrations have been studied in 47 patients with non-responsive schizophrenia taking olanzapine (872). Three of them, who had taken olanzapine for 3–6 months, had persistently high blood glucose concentrations. However, this is similar to what would be expected on the basis of the prevalence of diabetes mellitus in US adults.

Death from olanzapine-induced hyperglycemia has been reported (873).

- A 31-year-old man took olanzapine 10 mg/day for 1 week, and his fasting blood glucose rose to 11 mmol/l (200 mg/dl). For more aggressive treatment of his psychosis, the dosage of olanzapine was increased to 20 mg/day, and his fasting blood glucose rose to 16 mmol/l (280 mg/dl). He became progressively weaker and developed polydipsia and polyuria and died 3 weeks after starting to take olanzapine. He had no personal or family history of diabetes mellitus and was taking no other drugs at the time of his death. Death was attributed to hyperosmolar non-ketotic hyperglycemia.

The authors recommended including vitreous glucose and gammahydroxybutyrate analysis as part of postmortem toxicology work-up when the drug screen reveals either olanzapine or clozapine.

On the other hand, seven cases of asymptomatic lowered blood glucose concentrations have also been reported in patients with Tourette's syndrome who were taking olanzapine (mean dose 12 mg/day) during an 8-week, open-label trial (874). The mean serum glucose concentration was 4.8 mmol/l at baseline and 4.1 mmol/l during the study; the average weight gain was 4.5 kg. The authors suggested that increased insulin release may have been responsible for the changes observed; however, non-insulin mechanisms, such as a low carbohydrate intake, may also have played a role.

Weight gain

Significant weight gain occurs more often with olanzapine than with haloperidol or risperidone (SEDA-24, 69; SEDA-25, 65; SEDA-26, 57; SEDA-27, 61).

Weight gain of 38.5 kg occurred in a 15-year-old adolescent who had taken olanzapine 5–10 mg/day for 14 months (875).

The medical records of ten patients with a DSM-IV diagnosis of cluster B personality disorder (narcissistic personality disorder) who had taken olanzapine 2.5–20 mg/day for 8 weeks have been reviewed (876). The mean Social Dysfunction and Aggression Scale score was 29 for the 8 weeks before olanzapine therapy and improved to 14 after 8 weeks of treatment. Five of the ten patients developed severe weight gain.

In 15 patients with excessive weight gain associated with olanzapine the mean weight gain was 11 (range 3.6–25) kg and the mean duration of treatment was 7 (range 2–11) months (877).

In a retrospective study of 16 patients (7 men, 9 women) taking olanzapine (mean dose 14 mg/day, range 10–30) there was weight gain of over 7% in 15 of them; no change in diet, access to food, or change in exercise pattern had occurred (878).

Weight gain was observed in nine patients (seven men, two women, mean age 41 years) treated with olanzapine (mean dose 19, range 10–30, mg/day) (879). The patients had a mean weight gain of 9.9 kg and triglyceride concentrations (reference range 0.3–2.3 mmol/l) increased from a mean of 1.9 mmol/l (range 0.8–4.3) to a mean of 2.7 mmol/l (range 1.5–4.2).

Average weight gain was 8 kg in patients with refractory schizophrenia (*n* = 8) who were taking olanzapine in high doses (20–40 mg over an average of 40 weeks) (880).

In a retrospective chart review, 20 consecutive patients, who requested a switch from their previous neuroleptic drug therapy to olanzapine, were monitored over 12 months to note changes in weight. After 12 months of olanzapine treatment, 13 had a mean weight gain of 7.3 kg and three had no significant change in weight (881). Paradoxically, four patients lost weight when taking olanzapine, and the authors claimed that this is the first report of patients who had weight loss with olanzapine, although in these cases it is difficult to determine which factors contributed to the weight loss.

There was significant weight gain in 12 drug-naive patients with a first-episode of psychosis who took olanzapine for 3–4 months (mean dose 10.7 mg/day) compared with a control group of four healthy volunteers (8.8 kg versus 1.2 kg) (882).

Long-term olanzapine has been assessed in 27 outpatients with schizophrenia or schizoaffective disorders (mean age 40 years; 13 men) (883). At entry to the study the mean dose of olanzapine was 8.52 mg/day and the mean body mass index (BMI) 25 (range 19–35). At the end (mean treatment duration 22 months, range, 6–42) the mean dose of olanzapine was 8.70 mg/day and the mean BMI was 29 (range 20–40). Weight gain was more pronounced in the first year than in the second (7.7 versus 1.7 kg), especially during the first 3 months. Weight gain per month was significantly higher in patients with lower BMIs, but the greatest weight gain was in the most obese patient (BMI 35, weight gain 29 kg).

Weight gain has also been reported in 26 patients with bipolar affective disorder who were followed for 1 year while taking the combination of topiramate + olanzapine (mean modal doses 271 and 9.9 mg/day respectively). Although most of them gained weight during the first month of combined therapy (mean weight gain 0.7 kg), there was slight weight loss after 12 months (0.5 kg); weight loss was more pronounced in the obese patients ($n = 5$), and no patient with a low BMI ($n = 3$) lost weight (884). Patients who were switched to quetiapine from olanzapine lost weight after 10 weeks (mean weight loss 2.02 kg; n = 16 (885); although most of the patients lost weight, four gained about 2.6 kg.

In a randomized double-blind study there was weight gain in nine of 29 patients with alcohol dependence treated with olanzapine versus four of 31 taking placebo (886).

There was a mean weight gain of 7.9 kg (range 0–25 kg) between baseline and end-point weights in eight adolescents with psychoses (age range 12–18 years) who took olanzapine for 17.5 (range 4–26) weeks (887).

In contrast, in a study sponsored by Eli Lilly, there was improvement in 21 hospitalized elderly patients with schizophrenia or schizoaffective disorder who were taking olanzapine, mean final dose 13 mg/day. There was no significant weight gain (mean baseline weight 73.6 kg, mean final weight, 72.8 kg; mean treatment duration around 10 months) (888). However, the propensity for studies that are sponsored by pharmaceutical companies to be more favorable to their drug is well known (889).

In a study supported by the market authorization holder risperidone data from two double-blind trials in 552 adult and elderly patients with schizophrenia or schizoaffective disorders, weight gain after 8 weeks was higher with olanzapine than risperidone (mean doses not stated) in the adult and elderly patients and in smokers and non-smokers (890). For example, among the elderly patients, weight gain with olanzapine was 1.18 kg on average in smokers (n = 27) and 1.30 kg in non-smokers (n = 35); with risperidone weight gain was 0.08 kg in smokers (n = 20) and 1.06 kg in non-smokers (n = 31).

In 55 subjects randomized to olanzapine10 mg/day, risperidone 4 mg/day, or placebo for 2 weeks, there were significant increases in weight with olanzapine (2.25 kg) and risperidone (1.05 kg) (891).

Taking advantage of this effect on weight, olanzapine 10 mg has been used in an open trial in 20 patients with anorexia nervosa (892). Of the 14 patients who completed the 10-week study, 10 gained an average of 3.9 kg and three of these attained their ideal body weight. The other four patients who completed the study lost a mean of 1.0 kg. The most common adverse effects were sedation ($n = 13$), headache ($n = 5$), fatigue ($n = 4$), and hypoglycemia ($n = 4$).

The genetic basis of some reactions associated with neuroleptic drugs is of particular interest. Different polymorphisms have been studied in connection with atypical neuroleptic drug-induced weight gain (SEDA-26, 57). The relation between the CYP2D6 genotype and weight gain in patients taking atypical neuroleptic drugs has been addressed in a study in 11 Caucasian patients taking a fixed dose of olanzapine 7.5–20 mg/day for up to 47 weeks (893). They had their DNA analysed for the CYP2D6*1, CYP2D6*3, and CYP2D6*4 alleles; six had two *1 alleles and the other five had either *1/*3 or *1/*4. Subjects with a heterozygous genotype (*1/*3 or *1/*4) had a statistically significantly larger percentage change in body mass index than those who were homozygous for the *1 allele.

Histamine H_2 receptor antagonists, like nizatidine, can control appetite in overweight patients (894).

- A 23-year-old man, who had had repeated episodes of weight gain during olanzapine treatment, had good control and subsequent weight reduction after 4–5 weeks of therapy with nizatidine.

In a double-blind trial, the efficacy of nizatidine in limiting weight gain has been evaluated in 175 patients with schizophrenia and related disorders who took olanzapine 5-20 mg, nizatidine 150 mg or 300 mg, or placebo for up to 16 weeks (895). There was significantly less weight gain on average at weeks 3 and 4 with olanzapine plus nizatidine 300 mg compared with olanzapine plus placebo, but the difference was not statistically significant at 16 weeks.

On the other hand, famotidine did not prevent or attenuate weight gain in 14 patients taking olanzapine who were randomly assigned to either famotidine 40 mg/day (n = 7) or placebo (n = 7) in addition to olanzapine 10 mg/day for 6 weeks (mean weight gain 4.8 kg versus 4.9 kg respectively) (896).

Omeprazole

In patients with Zollinger–Ellison syndrome, omeprazole causes significant weight gain, perhaps because of shifts in hormonal balance (SEDA-17, 419; 897,898).

Opioid analgesics

Morphine reduces the response of the hypothalamus to afferent stimulation (899). In many species, opioids alter the equilibrium point of the hypothalamic heat-regulatory mechanisms.

In patients undergoing surgery, opioids inhibit the stress-induced release of ACTH (900).

Secretion of luteinizing hormone (LH) and thyrotropin is suppressed by opioids, whereas the release of prolactin and, in some cases, growth hormone is enhanced (901).

Oxaprozin

Drug-induced pseudoporphyria has been ascribed to oxaprozin (SEDA-21, 106).

Pancreatic enzymes

The effects of pancreatic exocrine supplements (four capsules with meals, two with snacks; each capsule containing lipase 10 000 units, protease 37 500 units, amylase 33 200 units) on glucose metabolism have been studied in a 2-week parallel, randomized, placebo-controlled trial in 29 patients with chronic pancreatitis who had stool fat excretion of over 10 g/day, 18 of whom were diabetic and 15 of whom were malnourished (902). There were major problems with blood glucose control in 28 of the 29 patients.

Pantothenic acid derivatives

As a pantothenic acid analogue, hopantenate can affect lactate generation, glucose metabolism, and ammonia disposal, and there have been two fatal cases in elderly people who developed disturbances of consciousness with lactic acidosis, hypoglycemia, and hyperammonemia (903).

Paracetamol

Hypoglycemia has been recorded with paracetamol, particularly in children (904).

Parenteral nutrition

Ammonium

Hyperammonemia has occurred during parenteral nutrition as a component of therapy for renal insufficiency (905). The hyperammonemia presented as a change in mental status, developing about 3 weeks after initiation of parenteral nutrition therapy; in most cases the episodes are of increasing duration and paroxysmal. In three of the patients, serum amino acid analysis in the acute phase showed reduced concentrations of ornithine and citrulline (the respective substrate and product of condensation with carbamyl phosphate at its entry into the urea cycle). Concentrations of arginine, the precursor to ornithine, were raised.

Carbohydrates

The effects of parenteral nutrition on endocrine and exocrine functions of the pancreas have been investigated in experimental rats (906). The conclusion was that after parenteral nutrition treatment the insulin secretory response to glucose is impaired, the exocrine pancreas is hypoplastic, and the storage pattern of pancreatic exocrine enzymes is altered.

Lipids have an adverse effect on carbohydrate metabolism under basal conditions. The infusion of 20% triglyceride emulsion with heparin during basal insulin and glucose turnover conditions resulted in a rise of plasma free fatty acids from 0.4 to 0.8 mmol/l at a low rate of infusion (0.5 ml/minute for 2 hours) to between 1.6 and 2.1 mmol/l at a high rate (1.5 ml/minute for 2 hours). There were similar increases in plasma concentrations of glycerol, acetoacetate, and hydroxybutyrate. The infusions resulted in significant increases in C-peptide concentrations, but had no effects on any of the other indices of carbohydrate metabolism that were examined (plasma glucose, lactate, and pyruvate concentrations), or on carbohydrate oxidation rates. By blocking the compensatory release of insulin by the intravenous administration of somatostatin and by simultaneous replacement of basal insulin and glucagon concentrations, these workers found that there was a significant increase in plasma glucose and in hepatic glucose output, and reduced glucose clearance. It was concluded that exogenous lipids may have adverse effects on carbohydrate metabolism under basal conditions, and that healthy individuals normally compensate for this by additional secretion of insulin (907).

Preoperative parenteral nutrition can be a major cause of hyperglycemia, which has been associated with an increased risk of postoperative infection. The frequency of hyperglycemia and infectious complications has been studied in a prospective, randomized, controlled, non-blind trial in 40 patients who required parenteral nutrition for at least 5 days (908). They were given either a hypocaloric regimen (1 liter containing nitrogen 70 g and dextrose 1000 kcal) or a standard weight-based regimen begun with similar amounts initially but with gradual increases in calorie and nitrogen contents to 25 kcal and 1.5 g nitrogen/kg, up to one-third of the calories being given as fat. There were no significant differences between the two groups with regard to hyperglycemia or infections. The higher calorie regimen provided significant nutritional benefit in terms of nitrogen balance compared with the hypocaloric regimen.

Some children receiving parenteral nutrition have abnormal glucose tolerance. When this was studied in 12 patients, aged 5.7–19 years, receiving cyclic nocturnal parenteral nutrition, patients with normal glucose tolerance had an insulin response to intravenous glucose tolerance testing similar to that of normal people of the same age (909). Two patients with abnormal glucose tolerance had a reduced capacity to release insulin, whereas insulin sensitivity was unchanged in one of them. Patients with a limited capacity to release insulin, either constitutional or acquired, may not be able to produce enough insulin in these conditions and they may develop glucose intolerance during parenteral nutrition. Insulin sensitivity was not a key factor in the alteration of glucose tolerance in this study.

In five patients with multiple trauma given sodium lactate as part of parenteral nutrition there was a 20%

fall in glycemia, a 43% fall in insulinemia, a 34% reduction in net carbohydrate oxidation (assessed by indirect calorimetry), and a 54% fall in plasma glucose oxidation (assessed using $^{13}CO_2$). Respiratory oxygen exchange was increased by 3.7% owing to a 20% thermic effect of lactate, but respiratory CO_2 exchange was not altered. PaO_2 fell by 11.3 mmHg, suggesting that the increased oxygen consumption was matched by an appropriate increase in spontaneous ventilation. Arterial pH increased from 7.41 to 7.46. It appears that sodium lactate given in parenteral nutrition during short intravenous nutrition in critically ill patients as a metabolic substrate limits hyperglycemia but contributes to metabolic alkalosis and does not spare ventilatory demand (910).

Lipids

The fat overload syndrome, characterized by a sudden rise in serum triglycerides, hepatosplenomegaly, intravascular coagulopathy, and end-organ dysfunction, is today an uncommon complication of intravenous administration of fat emulsion. Its higher incidence in the past may have been due to the greater phospholipid content of intravenous solutions in use at the time. The syndrome is a consequence of fat sludging within the microvasculature in organs such as the spleen, liver, kidney, lungs, brain, and retina. Necrosis in these organs suggests that emboli are responsible for the clinical symptoms and functional impairment that results. Plasma exchange has been successfully used in a patient with this syndrome who had not responded adequately to conventional medical therapy (911).

Critically ill patients are at greatest risk of fat overload syndrome when they are given lipid emulsions intravenously. Some of these patients already have impaired lipid metabolism and they are at risk of developing fat intolerance. These are the very patients who are likely to be given parenteral nutrition, including fat emulsions. Patients with increased serum triglyceride concentrations (for example, in hypothyroidism, with inborn errors of lipid metabolism, renal insufficiency, and severe sepsis, especially gram-negative sepsis) are at greatest risk. There is impaired metabolism of fats in advanced liver disease. Continuous heparin infusion may also lead to a decreased elimination capacity (912).

Fatty acids

Patients undergoing home parenteral nutrition for severe malabsorption or reduced oral intake can exhaust their stores of essential fatty acids, causing clinical effects, mainly dermatitis. In a comparative study of fatty acid profiles in 37 healthy control subjects and 56 patients receiving home parenteral nutrition, reduced small bowel length was associated with aggravated biochemical signs of essential fatty acid deficiency (913). This applied to total *n*-6 fatty acids and not to *n*-3 fatty acids. There were skin problems in 25 of the 56 patients receiving home parenteral nutrition. Patients receiving home parenteral nutrition had biochemical signs of essential fatty acid deficiency. Parenteral fluids did not increase the concentration of essential fatty acids to values

comparable with those of control subjects. However, 500 ml of 20% fat emulsion (Intralipid) once a week was sufficient to prevent an increase in the Holman index (an indicator that reflects optimum proportions of polyunsaturated fatty acids).

Linoleic acid and alpha-linoleic acid are essential fatty acids that are provided in any long-term parenteral nutrition by administering fat emulsions at least twice a week. Fatty acid deficiency is a common complication of severe end-stage liver disease. The ability of short-term intravenous lipid supplementation to reverse fatty acid deficiencies has been studied in patients with chronic liver disease and low plasma concentrations of fatty acids (914). Short-term supplementation failed to normalize triglycerides.

Phospholipids

Although choline is not regarded as an essential nutrient for humans, it has been described as being "conditionally essential" in patients receiving parenteral nutrition. Choline is a methyl-group donor, a component of phospholipids, and a precursor of acetylcholine and lecithin. In animal models and healthy human beings, choline deficiency impairs liver function. Studies in patients receiving long-term parenteral nutrition have shown that low levels of plasma choline are common and are associated with hepatic steatosis.

- Choline deficiency developed in a 41-year-old woman with advanced cervical cancer who underwent prolonged parenteral nutrition (915). Her liver function tests became abnormal and she became jaundiced and complained of nausea and vomiting. The serum choline concentration was 5.77 mmol/l and there was histological evidence of hepatic steatosis. There was steady improvement with oral choline supplementation, 3 g/day, and with oral glutamine 15 g/day. There was a 45% improvement in serum choline concentration over baseline.

Intravenous fat emulsions contain choline, but not in sufficient amounts to prevent choline deficiency (915,916).

Uric acid

Hypouricemia commonly occurs after several days of parenteral nutrition, although occasional reports of gout have been reported. In one case polyarticular gout developed on two occasions after a sudden fall in serum uric acid after the start of purine-free parenteral nutrition (917).

- A 61 year old man with a Stage I adenocarcinoma and a history of polymyalgia rheumatica, hypertension, atrial fibrillation, and cardiomyopathy, who was taking quinapril, warfarin, atorvastatin, digoxin, and atenolol, had a radical esophagogastrectomy. Three days after successful surgery and starting parenteral nutrition he developed generalized stiffness and joint swelling. He had flexion contractures of both knees and effusions in both ankles and the left wrist. There were no tophi or other joint deformities. Hazy yellow fluid was aspirated from one knee. Culture was negative but the fluid contained a moderate number of white blood cells and numerous intracellular negatively birefringent crystals. He was treated with intravenous methylprednisolone 40 mg 12 hourly, with marked functional improvement and resolution of joint effusions after 24-48 hours. The serum uric acid concentration was 270 μmol/l (4.6 mg/dl). He was readmitted 2.5 months later with vomiting, dehydration, and failure to gain weight. Parenteral nutrition was begun again, and after 4 days he developed a painful left shoulder and swelling of the right knee. He was again successfully treated with glucocorticoids. The serum uric acid was 460 μmol/l (7.7 mg/dl) before admission and fell to 200 μmol/l (3.5 mg/dl) by the fifth day of parenteral nutrition.

The causes of parenteral nutrition-related hypouricemia are not known, although it is postulated that the high glycine content of some parenteral nutrition regimens may be one relevant factor. This case illustrates that gout can be precipitated in susceptible patients; parenteral nutrition in such patients requires careful management. The authors suggested that routine daily monitoring of uric acid concentrations may be helpful in alerting clinicians to falling serum concentrations and potential subsequent exacerbation in patients with a history of gout.

Paroxetine

Serotonin pathways are involved in the regulation of prolactin secretion. Galactorrhea has been associated with paroxetine (918).

Serotonin pathways are involved in the regulation of prolactin secretion. Amenorrhea, galactorrhea, and hyperprolactinemia have been reported in a patient taking SSRIs.

- A 32-year-old woman taking paroxetine 40 mg/day had a raised prolactin concentration (46 ng/ml) and galactorrhea, both of which resolved a few days after paroxetine withdrawal (919).

Increases in cholesterol are most commonly reported in association with atypical antipsychotic drugs, such as olanzapine; however, similar reactions have been reported with some antidepressants, including mirtazapine and doxepin (SEDA-29, 19), which cause significant weight gain, probably through histamine H_1 receptor blockade. Serum cholesterol concentrations have been measured in 38 patients (23 men and 15 women) suffering from panic disorder before and after 3 months of treatment with paroxetine (20–40 mg/day) (920). At baseline the mean total cholesterol concentrations of the patients did not differ from those of controls (4.06 versus 4.29 mmol/l; 156 versus 165 mg/dl). However, after paroxetine the cholesterol concentrations rose significantly to 4.55 mmol/l (175 mg/dl).

Of the SSRIs, paroxetine is the agent most likely to cause weight gain; however, in this study the authors reported no change in body mass index during the 3 months of treatment, suggesting a more direct effect of paroxetine on metabolism. Further work will be needed to see if similar metabolic effects are associated with other SSRIs and in patients with other treatment indications.

Penicillamine

A few patients are on record with suspected penicillamine-induced thyroiditis, one case being associated with a myasthenic reaction (921,922).

Penicillamine had a small effect on urinary glucaric acid excretion in patients with rheumatoid arthritis (923). This effect was thought to be the result of an indirect effect on hepatic metabolism and not to be related to disease activity.

Anti-insulin antibodies and hypoglycemia

One of the remarkable autoimmune phenomena that penicillamine can cause is the induction of anti-insulin antibodies, with resultant hypoglycemia (autoimmune hypoglycemia) (924,925). In these patients, there are high concentrations of immunoreactive insulin, despite undetectable free insulin. When penicillamine is withdrawn antibody titers fall sharply. The occurrence of hypoglycemia rather than hyperglycemia is not fully understood (926).

In two previously well-controlled diabetic patients taking penicillamine who developed hypoglycaemia, no reference was made to anti-insulin antibodies (927).

In a study using a competitive radiobinding assay, as many as 43% of patients with rheumatoid arthritis using penicillamine had autoantibodies against insulin (928). These antibodies did not appear to affect pancreatic beta-cells, as the response to intravenous glucose was normal and there were no episodes of hypoglycemia. Other sulfhydryl compounds that have occasionally been reported to cause autoimmune hypoglycemia are tiopronin, pyritinol, and thiamazole (methimazole) (929).

Enzyme inhibition

In in vitro studies penicillamine inhibited angiotensin-converting enzyme (ACE) and carboxypeptidase (930). Penicillamine interferes with the functions of the copper-containing enzyme ceruloplasmin, and some of the penicillamine- and copper-containing complexes formed in vivo have a superoxide dismutase effect (931). In patients with scleroderma, penicillamine normalized collagen metabolism, by inhibiting beta-galactosidase activity (932).

Penicillins

Lipoatrophy can occur after the injection of some drugs, including penicillin (933).

- A 2-year-old boy developed a non-tender, hypopigmented, atrophic patch measuring about 2 × 6 cm on his right buttock. He had been well until 5 months before, when he had received an injection of penicillin into the right buttock.

The incidence of this adverse effect is unknown, as is the mechanism.

In six healthy subjects, ampicillin caused an increase in urinary uric acid excretion; this effect was attributed to competition for active renal tubular reabsorption of urate (SEDA-13, 212).

Pentamidine

Hypoglycemia can be a serious and life-threatening effect of pentamidine and is seen in 10–30% of cases, mainly with parenteral use, although it can also occur with inhalation. In one 21-day study it was equally common with either form of therapy. Higher doses and longer durations of treatment increase the likelihood, as does prior treatment with pentamidine (SEDA-16, 314); uremia also increases the risk. In one study there was nephrotoxicity in all cases with hypoglycemia. The hypoglycemia is the result of a direct toxic effect on the pancreatic beta cells, resulting in insulin release and transient hypoglycemia, which is followed by beta cell destruction and insulin deficiency, which in turn can eventually lead to an irreversible state of diabetes mellitus (SEDA-13, 825; SEDA-16, 315; SEDA-17, 331) (934).

Phenylbutazone

Because of interference with iodine uptake, hypothyroidism and goiter can result (935). The condition is reversible, but an obstructive syndrome due to thyroid enlargement has been observed (935).

Phenytoin and fosphenytoin

Phenytoin can cause a rise in growth hormone concentration (936).

Phenytoin can cause acromegaly-like facial features, possibly related to its osteogenic actions (SEDA-20, 65).

Phosphates

A 39-year-old woman with oncogenic osteomalacia caused by an osteosarcoma of the right scapula developed tertiary hyperparathyroidism after taking oral phosphate and vitamin D (937). The uniqueness of this case was the co-existence of hyperparathyroidism and oncogenic osteomalacia. All patients previously reported as having developed tertiary hyperparathyroidism with phosphate supplements had taken them for 10–14 years before diagnosis, but this patient had taken it for only 2 years. The proposed mechanism is that exogenous phosphate stimulates parathyroid activity through sequestration of calcium.

X-linked hypophosphatemic rickets is characterized by defective proximal renal tubular phosphate transport and impaired renal production of 1,25-dihydroxycolecalciferol. These abnormalities lead to renal phosphate wasting, hypophosphatemia with normocalcemia, low plasma 1,25-dihydroxycolecalciferol concentrations, and defective bone mineralization. The clinical features include rickets, skeletal deformities, growth retardation, and dental abscesses (938).

Anecdotal observations suggest that excessive use of oral phosphates may be a risk factor for the development of tertiary hyperparathyroidism in patients with X-linked hypophosphatemic rickets. Of 13 patients with X-linked hypophosphatemic rickets two developed tertiary hyperparathyroidism and 11 secondary hyperparathyroidism during treatment (939). Patients with tertiary hyperparathyroidism had on average earlier and longer treatment and higher doses of phosphates (over 100mg/kg/day) than the 11 patients with secondary hyperparathyroidism. Those who later developed tertiary hyperparathyroidism had very high serum parathormone concentrations (over 42 pmol/l).

Photochemotherapy (PUVA)

Severe hyperlipidemia possibly related to PUVA has been observed once (SEDA-19, 155).

Pizotifen

In 47 patients with severe migraine unresponsive to clonidine, pizotifen 1.5 mg for 6 months more than halved the incidence of attacks in 30 patients and 12 became headache-free. Weight gain was a problem in some subjects (940). In an open, multicenter study of the use of pizotifen 1.5 mg at night to prevent migraine in 834 patients, the most frequent adverse effects were drowsiness, although in one-third of the affected patients this was transient, and weight gain, with an average increase of 0.7 kg over 2 months (941).

Platinum-containing cytostatic drugs

The endocrine effects of cisplatin-based chemotherapy were studied in 22 men 9–24 or more months after completion of treatment for germ cell tumors (942). Mean basal FSH and stimulated LH and FSH concentrations were increased but serum testosterone concentrations were similar to untreated controls. Younger patients (under 25 years old) appeared more resistant to these effects of chemotherapy, and the hormonal abnormalities recovered with time.

The long-term effects on Leydig cell function of chemotherapy in 244 patients with germ cell tumors have been studied by measuring concentrations of sex hormone-binding globulin, luteinizing hormone, and follicle-stimulating hormone at least 74 months after chemotherapy (943). The population was divided into groups by cumulative cisplatin exposure (above and below 400 mg/m^2). Low-dose cisplatin exposure had no effect on Leydig cell function, but cumulative high-dose chemotherapy caused persistent impairment.

- Hyperosmolar non-ketotic hyperglycemia occurred in a 61-year-old patient 6 days after a first cycle of cisplatin therapy (944). The patient recovered with conventional conservative management.

Prazosin

Prazosin and other quinazolines are associated with small but significant changes in plasma lipid profiles. Generally these are potentially beneficial changes, with reductions in LDL cholesterol, total cholesterol, and triglycerides, and increases in HDL cholesterol.

Propafenone

Propafenone can cause hyponatremia due to inappropriate secretion of ADH (945).

Propofol

Hyperlipidemia

Five cases of hyperlipidemia have been reported in 12 patients who received propofol infusions 3–8 mg/kg/hour for 10–187 hours for sedation in an intensive care unit (946). Propofol was their only source of lipids.

Propofol 2% has been compared with midazolam for sedation in 63 ventilated patients in intensive care (947). They were randomly assigned to either propofol 1.5–6.0 mg/kg/hour or midazolam 0.10–0.35 mg/kg/hour. Sedation was considered a failure if greater rates were required or if triglyceride concentrations were over 5.7 mmol/l (500 mg/dl) on one occasion or greater than 4.0 mmol/l (350 mg/dl) on two occasions. Hemodynamic, respiratory, and neurological variables were similar. Sedation failure occurred in 15 patients given propofol, three with increased triglyceride concentrations and 12 with poor sedation. In comparison, sedation failed in only one of the patients given midazolam. Average serum triglyceride concentrations were higher in the propofol group. In a separate retrospective comparison, triglyceride concentrations were lower than in similar patients treated with 1% propofol, and the sedation failure rate was lower using 2% propofol (9 versus 36%). The authors concluded that 2% propofol is safe but may be less efficient than midazolam. It should be noted that the dose ranges that they used may not have been comparable, leading to an artificially high rate of failure to provide adequate sedation in the propofol group.

The frequency and severity of hypertriglyceridemia and pancreatitis have been studied in 159 adults in intensive care who were given propofol for 24 hours or longer (948). There was hypertriglyceridemia in 29 (18%), of whom six had a serum triglyceride concentration of 11 mmol/l or more; the median maximum serum triglyceride concentration was 8.0 (range 4.6–20) mmol/l. At the time when hypertriglyceridemia was detected, the median infusion rate of propofol was 50 (range 5–110) micrograms/kg/minute. The median time from the start of propofol therapy to identification of hypertriglyceridemia was 54

(range 14–319) hours. Pancreatitis developed in three of the 29 patients with hypertriglyceridemia.

Propofol infusion syndrome

Propofol infusion syndrome is a syndrome of cardiac failure (bradycardia, hypotension, low cardiac output), metabolic acidosis, and rhabdomyolysis, first described in children receiving high-dose propofol infusions for more than 48 hours.

- Severe lactic acidosis occurred in a 7-year-old child with osteogenesis imperfecta during short-term (150 minutes) propofol infusion anesthesia (mean infusion rate 13.5 mg/kg/hour) (949). The peak arterial lactate concentration occurred 160 minutes after withdrawal of propofol (lactate 9.2 mmol/l, bicarbonate 16 mmol/l, base deficit 8.3 mmol/l). The hyperlactatemia settled within 18 hours.

The authors suggested that the combination of a prolonged preoperative fast and a high dose of propofol had contributed to the lactic acidosis. Osteogenesis imperfecta is also associated with malignant hyperthermia, but the temperature was not raised in this case.

Although it was initially recognized in children, the propofol infusion syndrome is now known to occur in both children (950,951) and adults (952).

Three fatal cases of propofol infusion syndrome in adults have been reported (953):a 27-year-old woman who developed a metabolic acidosis, hypotension, and bradycardia;

- a 64-year-old man who developed a metabolic acidosis, hypotension, and rhabdomyolysis;
- a 24-year-old woman who developed hypotension, metabolic acidosis, and bradydysrhythmias.

Propofol infusion syndrome can present with one component only, such as lactic acidosis (954) or rhabdomyolysis (955) (see below). It has been suggested that patients who are susceptible to metabolic acidosis or rhabdomyolysis after propofol administration may have subclinical forms of mitochondrial diseases that affect either the respiratory chain complex or fatty acid oxidation (956). In order to minimize the development of propofol infusion syndrome as a potentially lethal complication, a maximum dose of 3 mg/kg/hour has been recommended for sedation in intensive care patients.

Initially, the syndrome was thought to result from cumulative toxicity, with reports after high-dose infusion as well as after prolonged administration of lower doses. However, recent reports suggest that it can occur even after short-term use and low-dose administration (957). Two cases of isolated severe lactic acidosis in adults during short-term (6–7 hours) propofol infusion sedation and anesthesia (infusion rates 1.5–7.5 mg/kg/hour) have been reported (958,959). Lactic acidosis resolved on withdrawal of propofol. These two reports were accompanied by an editorial, in which anesthesiologists were advised to check arterial blood gases and lactate concentrations in the event of unexpected tachycardia during propofol anesthesia (960). The authors concluded that in adults propofol can occasionally produce cytopathic hypoxia by impairing the electron transport chain or fatty acid oxidation.

It has been proposed that the mechanism of propofol toxicity might be attributed to impaired fatty acid oxidation, causing increased concentrations of malonyl-carnitine and C5-carnitine. Disturbed fatty acid oxidation might be caused by impaired entry of long-chain acylcarnitine ester into mitochondria. This, in turn, may be due to effects of propofol on mitochondrial electron transport, which has been shown in animals (particularly in cardiac myocytes). Support for this theory has been obtained in an investigation of the stored serum of a 5-month-old child who developed life-threatening propofol infusion syndrome after a mean infusion rate of 11.7 mg/kg/hour for 62 hours (961). The baby recovered after withdrawal of propofol, charcoal hemoperfusion, and continuous venovenous hemofiltration. Serum samples taken while the baby was critically ill showed increased concentrations of acetyl and hydroxybutyryl species, with generalized increases in fatty acylcarnitine intermediates, especially medium-chain unsaturated and dicarboxylic species. A follow-up sample taken when the child had recovered was entirely normal.

Propofol infusion syndrome might be precipitated by a combination of prolonged propofol infusion and carbohydrate intake insufficient to suppress fat metabolism. Support for this hypothesis has come from a case report of a child with catastrophic epilepsy who developed fatal propofol infusion syndrome after a ketogenic diet was introduced in an attempt to control severe intractable epilepsy (962).

- A 10-year-old child had status epilepticus controlled with a combination of valproate, oxcarbazepine, and 48 hours of propofol infusion in a dose of 5.5 mg/kg/hour. After weaning from propofol, a classic ketogenic diet was instituted in an attempt to provide long-term control of the seizures. A day later status epilepticus recurred and propofol was restarted at a rate of 6–9 mg/kg/hour to suppress seizure activity (the diet, valproate, and oxcarbazepine were also continued). Shortly thereafter, he developed the classical constellation of malignant ventricular arrhythmias, hyperlipidemia, rhabdomyolysis, lactic acidosis, and biventricular cardiac failure. He did not survive.

The use of extracorporeal cardiac support in the successful management of the cardiac failure associated with propofol infusion syndrome has been described (963).

- A 13-year-old boy underwent a 17-hour craniotomy in an attempt to resect an arteriovenous malformation with propofol-based anesthesia. He developed frank propofol infusion syndrome after 74 hours of postoperative propofol sedation in the neurosurgical ICU (used to manage intracranial hypertension). Echocardiography showed severe biventricular dysfunction despite extraordinary pharmacological support. Extracorporeal circulation with membrane oxygenation (ECMO) was instituted at the bedside via cannulation of the left femoral vessels. Hemofiltration

was added to the circuit. ECMO was discontinued 60 hours later, as there was normal ventricular function on echocardiography. He made a full recovery and returned to school.

Several case reports have ascribed survival to the early use of hemofiltration, but this case shows that very aggressive invasive cardiovascular support can also be useful.

There have been several reports of lactic acidosis with and without rhabdomyolysis after propofol infusion, and two fatal cases have been reported (964).

- Two men, aged 7 and 17 years, presented with refractory status epilepticus. Both were treated with high-dose propofol infusions to achieve burst suppression on the electroencephalogram. During the second day of propofol infusion there was progressive severe lactic acidosis, hypoxia, pyrexia, and rhabdomyolysis, followed by hypotension, bradydysrhythmias, and renal dysfunction, leading to death. The total doses of propofol were 1275 mg/kg over 2.7 days and 482 mg/kg over 2 days.

Lactic acidosis and rhabdomyolysis have been reported in a child receiving an infusion of propofol for sedation in an intensive care unit (965).

- A previously healthy 10-month-old boy with an esophageal foreign body was given endotracheal intubation to protect his airway. Midazolam and morphine did not produce satisfactory sedation and he was given propofol by infusion, increased from 3.5 to 7 mg/kg/hour over 2 hours to a total dose of about 500 mg/kg over the next 2 days. Other drugs given included cefotaxime, flucloxacillin, and ranitidine. He developed green urine, triglyceridemia of 907 mg/dl (10 mmol/l), and lactic acidosis, with a peak lactate concentration of 18 mmol/l. He also developed hypotension, with first-degree atrioventricular block and right bundle branch block, unresponsive to atropine, external cardiac pacing, or isoprenaline. Continuous venovenous hemofiltration was instituted. He slowly improved over the next 2 days, but developed a raised creatine kinase activity (over 30 000 U/l) and myoglobinuria. A liver biopsy showed 10% necrosis of zone 3, with fatty infiltration characteristic of a toxic effect. A muscle biopsy showed large areas of muscle necrosis. Extensive investigations showed no underlying infectious or metabolic causes. He slowly recovered over 10 days and appeared to have completely recovered at 3 months.

Lactic acidosis without rhabdomyolysis has been reported in another case (966).

- A 61-year-old woman undergoing mitral valve surgery received fentanyl, midazolam, nitrous oxide, and propofol infusion 3 mg/kg/hour during a 5-hour anesthetic. She developed lactic acidosis soon after the completion of surgery and required reintubation and ventilation. The peak lactate concentration, which occurred 1 day later, was 14.3 mmol/l. There was also mild disturbance of liver function. She eventually recovered.

These cases are important because, unlike previous reports of metabolic acidosis after propofol infusion, the patients had no documented infections and, in at least one case, extensive investigation showed no other causes of the acidosis. The role of propofol in causing the metabolic problems appears to have been more likely in these than in previous reports. In the first three cases the doses of propofol used, both per hour and in all, were extremely high compared with normal therapeutic practice. The subject has also been reviewed, and it was pointed out that, although suggestive, the association of fatal metabolic acidosis with propofol infusion in sick patients is as yet unproven and to date hinges on 11 case reports of patients who had multiple problems (967).

Porphyria

An acute attack of porphyria has been reported in association with propofol (968).

- A 23-year-old man, with a past history of Fallot's tetralogy repaired at age 2, had catheter ablation of an aberrant conduction pathway causing right ventricular tachycardia, a procedure that took 16 hours. He was sedated with propofol at an average rate of 100 micrograms/kg/minute, and required intubation for respiratory insufficiency half way through the procedure. He also received caffeine and isoprenaline during the procedure to induce ventricular tachycardia. After the procedure he could not be roused or extubated for a further 10 hours and remained drowsy for a further day. He had weakness of an arm and a leg and had lancinating abdominal and shoulder pains. Urinary concentrations of porphyrins, aminolevulinic acid, porphobilinogen, and coproporphyrin III were markedly raised. He made a good recovery after administration of dextrose.

Propofol is regarded as being safe in patients with different types of porphyria. This is the first reported case in which propofol had a possible role in causing raised porphyrin concentrations perioperatively. However, severe illness can also precipitate porphyria, so the association with propofol may have been incidental.

Protease inhibitors

See also individual agents
Two case reports have suggested that when a protease inhibitor is used with a glucocorticoid the tendency to adverse corticosteroid effects is potentiated (969,970). Two HIV-positive patients developed severely disfiguring skin striae within 3 months of starting indinavir therapy (971).

Metabolic changes that protease inhibitors can cause after prolonged therapy include raised serum lactate, hypogonadism, hypertension and accelerated cardiovascular disease, reduced bone density, and avascular necrosis of the hip. Two large prospective studies in 1207 patients (972) and 3191 patients (973) have clarified the spectrum and incidence of metabolic changes in HAART and have explored the relative importance of protease inhibitors. In addition, data on fat redistribution from a postmarketing review of HIV-infected individuals taking indinavir have been published (974).

Blood glucose concentration

Protease inhibitors can cause a rise in blood glucose concentration, although only a few cases have been reported. Patients with a family history of diabetes mellitus may be at a greater risk, and they demand especially close monitoring, for example with both baseline and quarterly glucose determinations, at least during the first 6–12 months of treatment (975,976).

An insulin-modified frequent sampling intravenous glucose tolerance test was performed in HIV-infected children, of whom 33 were taking a protease inhibitor and 15 were not (977). The former were also taking ritonavir ($n = 10$), nelfinavir ($n = 14$), indinavir ($n = 2$), lopinavir + ritonavir ($n = 5$), ritonavir + nelfinavir ($n = 1$), and nelfinavir + saquinavir ($n = 1$). There were no differences between the two groups with respect to fasting serum insulin or C-peptide, homeostatic model assessment of insulin resistance, or a quantitative insulin sensitivity check index. In a multiple regression analysis, the insulin sensitivity index and disposition index of children taking a protease inhibitor were significantly lower than in children who were not. In those taking a protease inhibitor, insulin sensitivity correlated inversely with visceral adipose tissue area and visceral to subcutaneous adipose tissue ratio. There was mildly impaired glucose tolerance in four of 21 subjects taking a protease inhibitor. These results suggest that protease inhibitor therapy reduces insulin sensitivity in HIV-infected children but also that it impairs the beta-cell response to this reduction in insulin sensitivity and, in a subset of children, leads to the development of impaired glucose tolerance.

Dyslipidemias

While abnormal concentrations of circulating lipids are common in patients with HIV infection (usually hypercholesterolemia and moderate hypertriglyceridemia), there is no doubt that some members of this group of drugs can cause much more marked changes. The possible differences between the effects of various protease inhibitors on the lipid spectrum have been characterized in 93 HIV-infected adults taking ritonavir, indinavir, or nelfinavir, alone or in combination with saquinavir (978). There was a rise in plasma cholesterol concentration in all those who took a protease inhibitor, but it was more pronounced with ritonavir than with indinavir or nelfinavir. Plasma HDL cholesterol was unchanged. Ritonavir, but not indinavir or nelfinavir, was associated with a marked rise in plasma triglyceride concentrations. The combination of ritonavir or nelfinavir with saquinavir did not further alter plasma lipid concentrations. There was a 48% increase in plasma concentrations of lipoprotein(a) in those taking a protease inhibitor, with pretreatment values exceeding 200 µg/ml. There were similar changes in plasma lipid concentrations in six children taking ritonavir. The risk of pancreatitis and premature atherosclerosis as a consequence of such dyslipidemia remains to be established.

- A 35-year-old HIV-positive man developed a serum cholesterol concentration of 38 mmol/l and a fasting serum triglyceride concentration of 98 mmol/l after he started to take ritonavir, saquinavir, nevirapine, and didanosine (979). All other medications had been stable during this time; the condition resolved with antiretroviral drug withdrawal and lipid-lowering therapy. It was striking that the raised cholesterol and triglyceride concentrations did not recur when therapy was restarted in modified form with nelfinavir, saquinavir, nevirapine, and didanosine; the hyperlipidemia was therefore attributed to ritonavir.

In 19 consecutive HIV-positive men examined before and during treatment with a protease inhibitor (nelfinavir, ritonavir, or indinavir) and two nucleoside analogue reverse transcriptase inhibitors (NRTI), median treatment duration 22 (range 7–40) weeks, the predominant feature of dyslipidemia was an increase in triglyceride-containing lipoproteins (980). This observation is in accordance with the hypothesis of increased apoptosis of peripheral adipocytes, release of free fatty acids, and subsequent increased synthesis of VLDL cholesterol. The lipid profile, based on the ratio of total cholesterol to HDL cholesterol and the ratio HDL2 to HDL3, is significantly more atherogenic than normal.

In a cross-sectional analysis of existing databases, 17 children with HIV infection were identified as having taken protease inhibitors, either ritonavir 20–30 mg/kg/day (n = 9) or nelfinavir 60–90 mg/kg/day (n = 8) for an average of 711 days (981). They were matched with 112 apparently healthy children admitted for minor surgical procedures. Plasma concentrations of cholesterol, triglycerides, and insulin-like growth factor 1 (IGF-1) tended to be high in those who had taken a protease inhibitor. The plasma concentrations of omega-6 long-chain polyunsaturated fatty acids and in particular of the highly unsaturated 22:4 omega-6 and 22:5 omega-6, were significantly increased. Infected children also had increased delta-6 and delta-4 desaturase activities and decreased delta-5 desaturase activity. The authors concluded that these children have a metabolic syndrome associated with significant changes in plasma fatty acid composition, similar to that observed in insulin resistance.

Lipodystrophy

Soon after the introduction of highly active antiretroviral combination treatments (HAART), lipodystrophy was associated with the use of protease inhibitors, and several reports have confirmed that a syndrome of peripheral lipodystrophy, central adiposity, breast hypertrophy in women, hyperlipidemia, and insulin resistance with hyperglycemia is an adverse event associated with the use of potent combination antiretroviral therapy, particularly including HIV-1 protease inhibitors (982–987).

Peripheral lipodystrophy in patients is characterized by fat wasting of the face, limbs, buttocks, and upper trunk, while central adiposity can cause an increase in belly size ("Crix-belly" or "protease pouch") and an increase in the dorsocervical fat pad, creating the appearance of a "buffalo hump" (988–990). These effects may be related to a glucocorticoid-like action. The increase in belly size is often associated with symptoms of abdominal fullness, distension, and bloating. This is probably due to a change in body fat distribution, with selective accumulation of fat intra-abdominally (991).

Lipodystrophy is not limited to patients taking protease inhibitors (992,993). Nevertheless, protease inhibitors are strongly associated with metabolic alterations and with lipodystrophy, while NRTIs are associated with low-grade lactic acidosis and less markedly with lipodystrophy. Some reports have speculated a link between mitochondrial dysfunction and lipodystrophy. It is clear, however, that the syndrome is related to total duration of antiviral therapy and inversely related to viral load.

In a longitudinal study from an Aquitaine cohort of more than 1400 subjects, hypertriglyceridemia was significantly associated with age, low viral load, and protease inhibitors, but not NRTIs or NNRTIs. However, lipodystrophy also occurred in patients naive to protease inhibitors (994).

- "Buffalo neck" was described in a middle-aged man taking indinavir who developed a lipomatous formation in the retrocervical area; abdominal fat also increased in volume, while the subcutaneous fat on the lower limbs decreased (995).

Of 494 patients during median follow-up of 18 months, 17% developed lipodystrophy (996). Study limitations included the short time of follow-up and the lack of a standardized and accepted definition of lipodystrophy.

Pyrazinamide

Pyrazinamide interferes with the renal excretion of urate, resulting in hyperuricemia. Acute episodes of gout or arthralgia have occurred. Arthralgia responds better to NSAIDs than to uricosuric drugs (997).

Pyrazinamide can aggravate porphyria (998).

Pyritinol

Autoimmune hypoglycemia with detectable anti-insulin antibodies, probably caused by pyritinol, has been described in one patient (999). This syndrome has previously been reported in connection with other thiol compounds, (penicillamine, methimazole, and tiopronin).

Quetiapine

The effects of haloperidol and quetiapine on serum prolactin concentrations have been compared in 35 patients with schizophrenia during a drug-free period of at least 2 weeks in a randomized study (1000). There was no significant difference in prolactin concentration between the groups at the start of the study, and control prolactin concentrations were significantly lower with quetiapine than haloperidol. No patients taking quetiapine had galactorrhea.

Dose-dependent decreases in total T3 and T4 and free T4, without an increase in TSH, have been reported

(1001,1002). Such changes have not been observed with other neuroleptic drugs.

Quinine

Clinical signs and symptoms of hypoglycemia are reported occasionally; most cases are subclinical, but severe cases have been described (SEDA-13, 815). A study of the effect of quinidine on glucose homeostasis in Thai patients with malaria showed a near doubling of plasma insulin concentrations and a corresponding fall in serum glucose concentrations. An additional factor may have been impaired nutritional status and the effects of parenteral quinine in severely ill patients not taking food (SEDA-13, 815; SEDA-14, 240; SEDA-18, 288).

According to a randomized, open comparison in 113 adults with severe falciparum malaria in Thailand, hypoglycemia seems to occur less often in patients with malaria treated with artesunate (2.4 mg/kg intravenously followed by 1.2 mg/kg 12 hours later and then by 1.2 mg/kg/day intravenously or 12 mg/kg orally for 7 days) compared with those treated with quinine (20 mg/kg intravenously over 4 hours followed by 10 mg intravenously over 2 hours or orally tds for 7 days) (1003). Artesunate and quinine had comparable efficacy, but hypoglycemia was only observed in 10% of the patients treated with artesunate whereas it occurred in 28% of those treated with quinine.

Ramipril

Hypoglycemia has been attributed to several drugs in a complicated sequence of effects (1004).

- A 64-year-old man with type II diabetes, hypertension, and bilateral renal artery stenosis presented with confusion and dysarthria related to profound hypoglycemia (2.2 mmol/l). He was taking naproxen 500 mg bd, ramipril 2.5 mg/day, glibenclamide 2.5 mg bd, metformin 850 mg bd, a thiazide diuretic, terazosin, ranitidine, paracetamol, and codeine. His plasma creatinine concentration, previously 185 μmol/l, was 362 μmol/l and it fell to 210 μmol/l after the withdrawal of ramipril and naproxen.

The authors discussed the possible role of renal insufficiency, resulting from co-prescription of naproxen and ramipril in the presence of volume depletion, which may have increased the risk of hypoglycemia related to glibenclamide plus metformin.

Reboxetine

The noradrenaline re-uptake inhibitor, reboxetine, does not cause weight gain during routine clinical use and indeed has been advocated as an adjunctive treatment in the management of olanzapine-induced weight gain.

- A 44-year-old woman with bipolar disorder took lamotrigine 100 mg/day and reboxetine 12 mg/day (1005). She noted a loss of appetite but continued to eat three meals a day. However, over the next year her weight fell from 55 kg to 43 kg. There seemed to be no psychiatric explanation for the weight loss and no medical cause could be discovered. The reboxetine and lamotrigine were withdrawn and her weight returned to baseline over the next 3 months. Around that time she again took reboxetine, this time as a sole agent, and once again her weight started to fall.

The loss of weight in this patient did not seem to be due her to psychiatric condition. The authors speculated that reboxetine might have some serotonergic activity, which could have accounted for a reduction in appetite and concomitant weight loss. However, drugs that potentiate noradrenaline activity can also reduce hunger, so this adverse effect could be due to the well characterized noradrenergic effects of reboxetine.

Reserpine

In women reserpine causes a small increase in circulating concentrations of prolactin (1006), which could be related to the small increase in the risk of breast cancer. In 27 hypertensive men reserpine 0.25 mg/day for 3 months had no effect on testosterone, dihydrotestosterone, estradiol, luteinizing hormone, or prolactin (1007).

Rifamycins

In patients taking glucocorticoids for Addison's disease, rifampicin may necessitate an increase in glucocorticoid dosage. Thus, incipient adrenal insufficiency can be unmasked by rifampicin (SEDA-13, 261). The phenomenon is due to liver enzyme induction (1008).

A significantly raised concentration of TSH during therapy with rifampicin has been reported in a man taking levothyroxine; TSH concentrations returned to baseline 9 days after withdrawal of rifampicin (1009).

Rifampicin-induced hypothyroidism has been reported in three euthyroid patients (1010).

- A 62-year-old man with recurrent non-Hodgkin's lymphoma developed pulmonary tuberculosis, for which he received rifampicin. Within 2 weeks, his thyrotropin (TSH) concentration increased to 170 mU/l and the serum concentrations of thyroxine (T_4) and triiodothyronine (T_3) fell to 24 μg/l and 180 ng/l respectively. He was given thyroxine. After the course of rifampicin therapy had been completed, thyroxine was withdrawn and he remained euthyroid for 4 years.
- A 66-year-old woman with tuberculous peritonitis was given rifampicin and developed hypothyroidism (thyrotropin concentration 12.5 mU/l, T_4 48 μg/l, T_3 8.7 ng/l). She was given thyroxine for 3 months. Hypothyroidism developed again, and thyroxine was resumed for the duration of the course of rifampicin therapy and then withdrawn, after which she remained euthyroid for 42 months.
- A 56-year-old woman with liver abscesses and tuberculous lymphadenitis was given rifampicin and 2 weeks later developed a raised thyrotropin concentration of 21

mU/ml, for which she was given thyroxine. The hypothyroidism resolved on withdrawal of rifampicin. However on re-starting rifampicin she developed hypothyroidism within 4 weeks. She was again given thyroxine, which was withdrawn on completion of the course of rifampicin. She remained euthyroid for 12 months.

Hypothyroidism developed within 2 weeks of rifampicin therapy in these patients and resolved when it was withdrawn. Rifampicin increases thyroxine clearance, possibly by enhancing hepatic thyroxine metabolism and the biliary excretion of iodothyronine conjugates. In healthy volunteers rifampicin reduces circulating thyroid hormone concentrations without affecting thyrotropin, suggesting that rifampicin directly reduces thyroid hormone concentrations.

The combination of rifampicin and isoniazid reduces serum concentrations of 25-hydroxycholecalciferol. Rifampicin acts by induction of an enzyme that promotes conversion of 25-hydroxycholecalciferol to an inactive metabolite, and isoniazid acts by inhibiting 25-hydroxylation and 1-hydroxylation (SEDA-14, 258). Children or pregnant women with tuberculosis have increased calcium requirements independent of rifampicin administration (1011). In 132 children of Afro-Asian origin there was a significant increase in serum alkaline phosphatase activity. This was more pronounced in patients taking both isoniazid and rifampicin than with isoniazid alone (1012). The rise in alkaline phosphatase could reflect an effect on either liver or bone. The possibility of a link between this effect and osteomalacia is unclear.

Rifampicin-induced porphyria cutanea tarda has been described in one case, combined with altered liver function (1013).

Risperidone

Prolactin

There was a significant rise in baseline serum prolactin concentration in 10 patients after they had taken risperidone for a mean of 12 weeks compared with 10 patients who were tested after a neuroleptic drug-free wash-out period of at least 2 weeks (1014). A non-significant increase in serum prolactin has also been observed in an open comparison of risperidone with other neuroleptic drugs in 28 patients (1015). However, in a meta-analysis of two independent studies ($n = 404$), prolactin was greatly increased by risperidone (mean change 45–80 ng/ml), a larger effect than with olanzapine and haloperidol (1016).

Five patients (four women and one man, aged 30–45 years), who were evaluated for risperidone-induced hyperprolactinemia, had significant hyperprolactinemia, with prolactin concentrations of 66–209 µg/l (1017). All but one had manifestations of hypogonadism, and in these four patients, risperidone was continued and a dopamine receptor agonist (bromocriptine or cabergoline) was added; in three patients this reduced the prolactin concentration and alleviated the hypogonadism.

The relation of prolactin concentrations and certain adverse events has been explored by using data from two large randomized, double-blind studies ($n = 2725$; 813 women, 1912 men) (1018). Both risperidone and haloperidol produced dose-related increases in plasma prolactin concentrations in men and women, but they were not correlated with adverse events such as amenorrhea, galactorrhea, or reduced libido in women or with erectile dysfunction, ejaculatory dysfunction, gynecomastia, or reduced libido in men. Nevertheless, in five patients risperidone (1–8 mg/day) caused amenorrhea in association with raised serum prolactin concentrations (mean 122 ng/ml, range 61–230 ng/ml; reference range 2.7–20 ng/ml) (1019).

Furthermore, risperidone-induced galactorrhea associated with a raised prolactin has been reported (1020,1021), as have amenorrhea and sexual dysfunction (1022).

- Galactorrhea associated with a rise in prolactin occurred after a few weeks of treatment with risperidone in two women aged 24 and 39 (1021). One of them was switched to thioridazine, with an improvement in the galactorrhea, and the other continued to take risperidone owing to a robust response; her galactorrhea was partially treated with bromocriptine.
- A 34-year-old woman, who developed amenorrhea while taking risperidone, regained her normal menstrual pattern along with a marked fall in serum prolactin concentration 8 weeks after being switched to olanzapine, whereas amantadine had failed to normalize the menses and had apparently reactivated the psychotic symptoms (1023).

The authors suggested that olanzapine may offer advantages for selected patients in whom hyperprolactinemia occurs during treatment with other antipsychotic drugs.

- Galactorrhea and gynecomastia occurred in a 38-year-old hypothyroid man who took risperidone for 14 days (1024).

The authors suggested that men with primary hypothyroidism may be particularly sensitive to neuroleptic drug-induced increases in prolactin concentrations.

- A 17-year-old man developed galactorrhea and breast tenderness within weeks of starting to take risperidone.

The authors suggested that patients who have galactorrhea, amenorrhea, or both while taking risperidone should be gradually switched to olanzapine, quetiapine, or clozapine (1025). Indeed, when 20 women with schizophrenia who were taking risperidone and had menstrual disturbances, galactorrhea, and sexual dysfunction (SEDA-24, 72; SEDA-26, 65) were switched from risperidone to olanzapine over 2 weeks and then took olanzapine 5–20 mg/day for 8 further weeks, serum prolactin concentrations fell significantly (1026). Scores on the Positive and Negative Syndrome Scale, Abnormal Involuntary Movement Scale, and Simpson–Angus Scale for extrapyramidal symptoms at the end-point were also significantly reduced. There were improvements in menstrual functioning and patients' perceptions of sexual adverse effects.

The prevalence of hyperprolactinemia among women taking risperidone was 88% ($n = 42$) versus 48% ($n = 105$) in those taking conventional antipsychotic drugs; 48% of these women of reproductive age taking risperidone had abnormal menstrual cycles (1027). In the whole sample (147 women and 255 men) there were trends towards low concentrations of reproductive hormones associated with rises in prolactin; patients taking concomitant medications known to increase prolactin had been excluded. Raised prolactin concentrations were also observed in 13 (9 women and 4 men) of 20 patients (13 women and 7 men; mean age 36 years) (1028). In pre-menopausal women there was a good correlation between prolactin concentrations and age, but there was no clear correlation between duration of treatment, dose, prolactin concentration, and prolactin-related adverse effects.

In 41 schizophrenia patients who took either risperidone (11 men, 9 women; mean dose 4 mg/day) or perospirone (10 men, 11 women; mean dose 24 mg/day) for at least 4 weeks, prolactin concentrations increased only in those taking risperidone (5.3-fold in women and 4.2-fold in men) (1029).

Hyperprolactinemia was found after about 30 months in 12 premenopausal women with schizophrenia or schizoaffective disorder (aged 15–55 years) taking risperidone but not in those taking olanzapine ($n = 14$) (1030). Prolactin concentrations were significantly higher in the first group than in the second (123 ng/ml versus 26 ng/ml).

There was a high correlation between prolactin concentrations and risperidone in 14 men (mean age 53 years) (1031). In 47 men (mean age 23 years) receiving acute treatment with several neuroleptic drugs, including risperidone (mean dose 3.6, range 1–6, mg; mean duration 45 days; risperidone monotherapy in 35 subjects), there was hyperprolactinemia, defined as a prolactin concentration greater than 636 mU/l (male reference range 45–375 mIU/l), in 27 of the 37 patients who could be assessed (1032). There was neither gynecomastia nor galactorrhea. One year later, 38 of the 47 patients were reassessed (mean dose 2.3, range 1–6, mg); prolactin concentrations could be determined in 20 of these patients, and there was hyperprolactinemia in six of them. In the 35 patients taking risperidone monotherapy, two had high prolactin concentrations at baseline, but this rose to 21 of 29 patients at the end of the acute phase and fell to four of 16 after 1 year. According to the authors, the lower concentrations at 1 year might have been due to the development of tolerance to prolactin.

In a randomized, double-blind, 12-week study in 78 inpatients with schizophrenia assigned to either risperidone 6 mg/day (73% men; $n = 41$) or haloperidol 20 mg/day (81% men; $n = 37$), prolactin concentrations increased significantly in men in both groups (1033). Adjusted for haloperidol dose equivalents (risperidone 6 mg/day equivalent to haloperidol 12 mg/day), risperidone caused a significantly larger rise in prolactin than haloperidol. The study was limited by the small number of women in the sample, which allowed the comparison of prolactin concentrations by sex but without consideration of treatment; the women had a significantly larger rise in prolactin than the men.

The risk of prolactinoma in patients taking risperidone and other neuroleptic drugs, accompanied by hyperprolactinemia, amenorrhea, and galactorrhea has been discussed in the light of a case of hyperprolactinemia (1034).

- A 35-year-old woman who had taken lithium carbonate 800 mg/day for 2 years was also given risperidone 6 mg/day for a manic relapse. She missed two menstrual periods and had galactorrhea. A head CT scan showed a pituitary microadenoma and the prolactin concentration was 125 µg/l (reference range up to 20 µg/l). Risperidone withdrawal resulted in disappearance of the prolactinoma. Her other symptoms persisted and did not change with olanzapine 2.5 mg/day; however, bromocriptine 12.5 mg/day for 2 weeks relieved her symptoms and the prolactin concentration normalized.

There were no significant adverse effects on growth or sexual maturation in a retrospective study based on a sample of 700 children aged 5–15 years who had been taking risperidone (0.02–0.06 mg/kg/day) for 11 or 12 months because of disruptive behavior disorders (1035).

Galactorrhea has been reported in relation to risperidone (SEDA-25, 69; SEDA-26, 65; SEDA-27, 63), and four new cases have been published (1036). It is suggested that this condition can occur after many weeks of risperidone treatment, with small dosages (2–4 mg/day), and at times even after drug withdrawal.

Risperidone-induced hyperprolactinemia has been reported to resolve with quetiapine, a low-potency dopamine D_2 receptor antagonist (1037).

Amenorrhea presumed to have been induced by risperidone has been successfully treated with Shakuyaku-kanzo-to, a Japanese herbal medicine that contains *Peoniae radix* and *Glycyrrhizae radix* (1038).

Diabetes mellitus

There has been a report of diabetic ketoacidosis in a 42-year-old man, without a prior history of diabetes mellitus, who took risperidone (2 mg bd) (1039). The authors pointed out that in premarketing studies of risperidone, diabetes mellitus occurred in 0.01–1% of patients.

Weight gain

Pathological weight gain has been increasingly identified as a problem when atypical neuroleptic drugs are given to children (SEDA-21, 57; SEDA-22, 69). In one case, unremitting weight gain, triggered by risperidone, was eventually curbed through the use of a diet containing slowly absorbed carbohydrates and a careful balance of carbohydrates, proteins, and fats (1040).

- A 9-year-old boy with autism and overactivity was unresponsive to several drugs. Risperidone 0.5 mg bd was effective, reducing his Aberrant Behavior Checklist score from 103 to 57 by the end of the first week. Four weeks later his weight had risen from 34.6 to 37 kg. This rate of weight gain (0.6 kg/week) continued over the next 12 weeks. His weight was then contained by the use of the "Zone" diet, with an emphasis on slowly absorbed carbohydrates (examples include apples, oatmeal, kidney beans, whole-grain pasta, and sweet potatoes) in a calorie-reduced diet containing 30% proteins and 30% fats.

In 37 children and adolescent inpatients treated with risperidone for 6 months, compared with 33 psychiatric inpatients who had not taken atypical neuroleptic drugs, risperidone was associated with significant weight gain in 78% of the treated children and adolescents compared with 24% of those in the comparison group (1041). Risperidone dosage, concomitant medicaments, and other demographic characteristics (such as age, sex, pubertal status, and baseline weight and body mass index) were not associated with an increased risk of morbid weight gain.

In contrast, in a multicenter, open study in 127 elderly psychotic patients (median age 72, range 54–89 years) taking risperidone (mean dose 3.7 mg/day) there was no significant weight gain after 12 months (1042).

Risperidone-induced obesity can cause sleep apnea (1043).

- A 50-year-old man with schizophrenia gained 29 kg over 31 months and developed diabetes while taking risperidone 6 mg/day. He reported difficulty in sleeping and frequent daytime napping that left him unsatisfied, and his wife reported prominent snoring and apnea at night.

Nasal continuous positive airway pressure produced improvement.

Weight gain has been studied in 146 Chinese patients with schizophrenia (85 men and 61 women; mean age 33 years) who took risperidone in a maximum dose of 6 mg/day (1044). Mean body weight rose gradually from 61 kg at baseline to 62 kg on day 14, 63 kg on day 28, and 64 kg on day 42; the mean dose at 6 weeks was 4.3 mg/day. Weight gain was associated with a lower baseline body weight, younger age, undifferentiated subtype, a higher dosage of risperidone, and treatment response (for positive, negative, and cognitive symptoms and social functioning). However, a possible ethnic difference might contribute to the marked weight increase found in these Chinese patients, since non-white patients reported more weight gain than white patients.

Risperidone-induced weight gain varies throughout the age span, young people being the most sensitive; although preadolescents and adolescents take substantially lower daily doses and lower mg/kg doses than adults, they gain as much or more weight (corrected for age-expected growth) (1045). This effect is hardly, or not at all, experienced by those aged over 65. Furthermore, young people also had a greater percentage of drug-induced weight gain relative to baseline body weight, and the percentage increases in body mass index during risperidone treatment were consistently greater in the young.

There was weight gain of 17% (mean 5.6 kg) after risperidone treatment for 6 months in 63 autistic children and adolescents (mean age 8.6 years), taken from an initial sample of 101 outpatients; this gain exceeded the developmentally expected norms and decelerated over time (1046). Body mass index increased by 10.6% (mean

2.0 kg/m^2). Changes in serum leptin did not reliably predict risperidone-associated weight gain.

- Long-term weight gain has been described in a 35-year-old man with schizophrenia taking risperidone 4 mg/day; weight changed from 94 to 121 kg and there was also "carbohydrate craving" and persistent hunger (1047).

The underlying mechanism may involve the adipose tissue hormone leptin or immune modulators such as tumor necrosis factor alfa.

Ritodrine

Brief infusions of ritodrine (0.15 mg/minute for 4 hours) rapidly increased plasma melatonin concentrations in healthy women (1048).

There are two well-documented independent reports of severe ketoacidosis in non-diabetic pregnant subjects; both the beta-agonist therapy and inadequate dietary intake could have played a role (1049).

Roxithromycin

Roxithromycin may have anti-androgenic effects. In an in vitro model roxithromycin 5 μg/ml suppressed androgen receptor transcriptional activity by 21% (1050).

Salbutamol

Blood glucose

With inhaled salbutamol there is as a rule no significant effect on carbohydrate metabolism, but there were significant rises in blood glucose and insulin when intravenous salbutamol infusions were given to healthy pregnant women at term. The rise in blood glucose was significantly greater in pregnant women who were diabetic (SED-13, 363). Oral salbutamol 8 mg bd given for 14 days had no effect on glucose tolerance, but total cholesterol fell significantly by 9%; low-density lipoprotein cholesterol fell by 15%, and HDL increased by 10% (SEDA-21, 182).

Hypoglycemia is an adverse effect of salbutamol in newborns of mothers who have received long-term sympathomimetics as tocolytic therapy. However, hypoglycemia has also been described in children after the ingestion of high doses of salbutamol (1051).

- A three year-old boy developed initial hyperglycemia of 10.4 mmol/l (187 mg/dl) followed by hypoglycemia of 2.5 mmol/l (45 mg/dl) after the oral ingestion of 57 ml of Ventolin syrup, corresponding to 22.8 mg (1.9 mg/kg) of salbutamol (1052). He was given activated charcoal and intravenous glucose and recovered uneventfully.

The effect of nebulized salbutamol 2.5 mg on blood glucose concentration has been assessed in a double-blind, placebo-controlled study in 19 patients with insulin-dependent diabetes (9 of whom had cystic fibrosis-related diabetes) (1053). There were no significant

Lactic acidosis

Lactic acidosis can occur in adults with acute severe asthma, but there is some controversy about its significance. In a prospective study, lactic acidosis was assessed in 18 adults who presented to an emergency department with acute severe asthma and were treated with high doses of salbutamol 400 micrograms at 10-minute intervals over 2 hours (1054). At the end of treatment, mean plasma lactate concentrations were significantly higher than at baseline. Higher plasma lactate concentrations after salbutamol treatment correlated with a shorter duration of asthma attack before presentation, higher pre-treatment heart rate, lower pre-treatment SpO_2, higher pre-treatment PCO_2, and lower pre-treatment serum potassium concentration. Therefore, the hyperadrenergic state before salbutamol treatment predisposes patients to lactic acidosis. Lactic acidosis probably results from combined endogenous adrenergic stimulation and the use of beta$_2$-adrenoceptor agonists, resulting in increased conversion of pyruvate to lactate.

Transient lactic acidosis/lactatemia has been reported as an adverse effect of inhaled salbutamol. In five patients who received 5 mg salbutamol by inhalation serum lactate concentrations were 3.2–8.0 mmol/l and arterial blood pH values 7.34–7.43; after 24 hours serum lactate concentrations returned to normal without specific treatment (1055). In two other cases, high-dose salbutamol caused lactic acidosis, contributing to respiratory failure in one patient and complicating the assessment and management of acute severe asthma in the other (1056). Respiratory compensation for this primary metabolic acidosis, characterized by increased respiratory rate and effort, may be mistaken for increased respiratory distress due to asthma. Lactic acidosis in acute asthma can therefore lead to problems in asthma management, including unwarranted intensification of beta$_2$-adrenoceptor agonist therapy and the initiation of premature or unnecessary mechanical ventilation.

The pathophysiology of salbutamol-associated lactic acidosis is poorly understood and has partly been attributed to the production of lactate by overworked respiratory muscles.

- A 39-year-old woman developed salbutamol-associated lactic acidosis (peak 7.8 mmol/l) during general anesthesia for planned thoracoscopic sympathectomy (1057).

This suggests that the above mentioned mechanism is unlikely to have caused lactic acidosis in this patient. Rather, it may have resulted from beta$_2$-adrenoceptor activation, with subsequent excess glycogenolysis and lipolysis, production of pyruvate, and final conversion to lactate.

Saquinavir

Gynecomastia has been reported in a series of men taking saquinavir (1058). In these cases the association was clear (particularly since there was positive dechallenge), but this is a rare effect and has not previously been reported with either this or other protease inhibitors, although it has been associated with the nucleoside analogue reverse transcriptase inhibitor stavudine.

Triglycerides rose by 3.45 mmol/l (314 mg/dl) and total cholesterol by 1.1 mmol/l (43 mg/dl) in 11 patients taking amprenavir, saquinavir, and ritonavir (1059).

Selective serotonin re-uptake inhibitors (SSRIs)

Serotonin pathways are involved in the regulation of prolactin secretion. Amenorrhea, galactorrhea, and hyperprolactinemia have been reported in patients taking SSRIs. A similar effect would be expected with venlafaxine.

- A 38 year old woman developed galactorrhea on two separate occasions while taking venlafaxine 225 mg/day and 75 mg/day (1060). On the first occasion prolactin concentrations were modestly raised but on the second they were not.

This report confirms that, like SSRIs, venlafaxine can cause galactorrhea and also suggests, as has been observed with other drugs, that the symptom of lactation is not necessarily closely linked to plasma prolactin concentrations. This suggests that other mechanisms could be involved in the production of drug-induced galactorrhea.

Selenium

One report suggests that therapeutic use of selenium in the form of selenite could precipitate hypothyroidism, but the circumstances were complex and iodine deficiency seems to have played a major role (1061).

Sertindole

Four patients developed tardive dyskinesia while taking conventional antipsychotic drugs and were switched to sertindole; one gained 8 kg in weight (1062).

Sertraline

Serotonin pathways are involved in the regulation of prolactin secretion. Galactorrhea has also been reported in a patient taking sertraline, in whom lactation ceased after withdrawal (SEDA-18, 20) and in another case (1063).

Sirolimus

Hypothalamus–pituitary–gonad axis

The impact of sirolimus on hormone concentrations involved in the hypothalamus–pituitary–gonad axis has been investigated in 132 male heart transplant recipients (1064). There was a significant reduction in testosterone and significantly increased follicle stimulating hormone

(FSH) and increased luteinizing hormone (LH) in the sirolimus group. The duration of sirolimus treatment correlated positively with concentrations of sex hormone-binding globulin, LH, and FSH, and negatively with the unbound androgen index. Sirolimus trough concentrations correlated with LH and FSH concentrations.

Hyperlipidemia

The most striking consequence of treatment with sirolimus is dose-dependent hyperlipidemia with significant increases in both cholesterol and triglyceride serum concentrations, which resolve after dosage reduction or sirolimus withdrawal (1065).

In a 1-year follow-up of 40 renal transplant patients treated with various dosages of sirolimus ($0.5–7$ mg/m^2/day) in addition to a ciclosporin-based regimen, there were significant increases in serum cholesterol and triglycerides, and significant falls in white blood cell and platelet counts, compared with historical controls (1066). These effects correlated with sirolimus trough concentrations but not dosages. One patient had to discontinue sirolimus because of hyperlipidemia refractory to treatment.

In six patients with renal transplants treated with sirolimus, mean total plasma cholesterol, triglyceride, and apolipoprotein concentrations increased (1067). The authors suggested that sirolimus increases lipase activity in adipose tissue and reduces lipoprotein lipase activity, resulting in increased hepatic synthesis of triglycerides, increased secretion of VLDL, and increased hypertriglyceridemia.

The incidence, severity, and predisposing factors for dyslipidemia among renal transplant patients on ciclosporin with sirolimus ($n = 280$) or without sirolimus ($n = 118$) has been investigated in a retrospective study (1068). During the first 6 months after kidney transplantation there was hypercholesterolemia in 80% versus 46% and hypertriglyceridemia in 78% versus 43%. However, there was no significant difference in the incidence of cardiovascular events within 4 years after transplantation in the two groups. Thus, sirolimus-associated dyslipidemia does not seem to represent a major risk factor for the early emergence of cardiovascular complications.

In a pilot study after coronary angioplasty in 22 patients, sirolimus was given orally in a loading dose of 6 mg followed by 2 mg/day over 4 weeks. Sirolimus was withdrawn after an average of 15 days in 11 patients because of adverse effects, including hypertriglyceridemia ($n = 3$), leukopenia ($n = 3$), raised liver function tests, stomatitis, acne, flu-like symptoms, and physician preference ($n = 1$ each). The rate of coronary restenosis was 87%. Sirolimus did not benefit patients with recalcitrant stenosis and adverse effects were frequent (1069).

Hypertriglyceridemia due to sirolimus often does not respond to dosage reduction or hypolipidemic drugs. After liver transplantation ($n = 6$), significant hyperlipidemia improved after withdrawal of sirolimus (1070). The incidence of sirolimus-associated hyperlipidemia is up to 44%. After liver transplantation, there was hypercholesterolemia in 15% and hypertriglyceridemia in 10% of recipients. Sirolimus in combination with tacrolimus

and/or mycophenolate mofetil caused no higher incidence of hyperlipidemia than calcineurin inhibitors and mycophenolate mofetil (1071). After kidney transplantation, at least 60% of adult recipients develop dyslipidemia within 1 month of the start of immunosuppressive therapy; ciclosporin, sirolimus, and prednisone are mainly implicated, and the lipid profile differs between individual agents (1072).

Smallpox vaccine

Diabetes mellitus occurred in a 1-year-old child about 4 weeks after smallpox vaccination (1073).

Sorafenib

Patients with metastatic renal cell carcinoma commonly develop mild biochemical thyroid function test abnormalities while taking sorafenib. However, compared with sunitinib, which is associated with a high incidence of thyroid dysfunction, making routine monitoring necessary, patients taking sorafenib need thyroid function monitoring only if clinically indicated (1074).

Spironolactone

In an open study in 35 women with acne, mean age 21 years, spironolactone 100 mg/day on 16 days each month for 3 months had no effect on serum total testosterone concentrations but reduced serum dehydroepiandrosterone sulfate concentrations (1075).

Stavudine

Lipodystrophy, a syndrome characterized by fat redistribution, hyperglycemia/insulin resistance, and dyslipidemia, can be associated with long-term HIV infection or with highly active antiretroviral therapy (HAART). In 1035 patients, those who took stavudine were 1.35 times more likely to report lipodystrophy (1076). However, the study was retrospective, and other factors unrelated to specific drug therapy may have had a greater effect on the adjusted odds ratio.

Sulfonamides

Several sulfonamides, including co-trimoxazole in high doses, can produce hyperchloremic metabolic acidosis. This has even been seen in patients with extensive burns receiving topical mafenide (1077). Mafenide (Sulfamylon) and its metabolite *para*-sulfamoylbenzoic acid inhibit carbonic acid anhydrase, resulting in reduced reabsorption of bicarbonate and thus bicarbonate wasting.

Sunitinib

Sunitinib has been related to an increasing frequency of hypothyroidism. Screening for signs of hypothyroidism is recommended, with frequent measurements of TSH concentrations every 2–3 months in order to start levothyroxine in time.

In a prospective, observational cohort study in a tertiary-care hospital, there were abnormal serum TSH concentrations in 26 of 42 patients) who took sunitinib for renal cell carcinoma or GIST. Persistent primary hypothyroidism, isolated TSH suppression, and transient mild rises in TSH were found in 36%, 10%, and 17% of patients respectively. There appears to be a correlation between the duration of use of sunitinib and suppressed TSH concentrations as well as a risk of hypothyroidism. Whether sunitinib induces destructive thyroiditis through follicular cell apoptosis has not been fully elucidated (1078,1079,1080).

Suramin

The adrenal glands are sensitive to the toxic effects of suramin; both glucocorticoid and mineralocorticoid functions can be impaired at doses normally used, necessitating replacement therapy (1081).

Tacrolimus

Diabetes mellitus

Altered glucose metabolism and subsequent hyperglycemia or even insulin-dependent diabetes mellitus is an important issue in transplant patients, particularly in adults or patients taking high doses. In animals, high-dose tacrolimus causes glucose intolerance and reduced insulin release (1082). This resolves after withdrawal. Diabetes mellitus after transplantation is a relatively common complication in pediatric thoracic organ recipients taking tacrolimus (1083). Specific risk factors have not been identified. A switch from tacrolimus to ciclosporin for other reasons in two patients did not resolve the problem.

The risk of post-transplant diabetes mellitus is greater with tacrolimus than with ciclosporin, but this was mostly true in black patients and during the initial months after transplantation (1084). In one study, insulin sensitivity, alpha and beta cell function, and beta cell reserve were studied in 14 hepatitis C-positive patients with liver transplants, who took tacrolimus or ciclosporin maintenance for 1 year (1085). The patients were matched for low prednisolone dosage (1.1 mg/day versus 1.3 mg/day), body mass index, lean body mass, and sex, and compared with eight controls. Insulin sensitivity and insulin secretory reserve were significantly different from controls, but there was no significant difference between ciclosporin and tacrolimus.

The incidence, mechanism, and risk factors of tacrolimus-associated diabetes mellitus are still debated. In 58 patients investigated 1–3 years after liver transplantation there was a significantly higher incidence of diabetes mellitus with tacrolimus ($n = 32$) compared with ciclosporin ($n = 26$) (1086). Newly-diagnosed diabetes occurred in nine of 28 tacrolimus-treated patients, of whom six required insulin, and in none of 25 ciclosporin-treated patients. Five patients taking tacrolimus also had

islet cell-specific autoantibodies that correlated significantly with HLA risk haplotypes.

- A 32-year-old woman with previous autoimmune disorders and a susceptible HLA haplotype developed diabetes with newly positive glutamic acid decarboxylase antibody after taking tacrolimus for 5 months (1087).

Together, these reports suggest that tacrolimus does not suppress the production of autoantibodies in patients genetically prone to develop autoimmune diabetes, with induction of an autoimmune phenomenon. This also suggests that tacrolimus treatment should be undertaken cautiously in predisposed patients.

Of 834 primary adult liver transplant recipients, of whom 499 were alive and taking tacrolimus, 70% were glucocorticoid-free after 1 year; this did not change over the next 5 years (1088). However, glucocorticoid-associated adverse effects, such as hypertension, diabetes, and hyperlipidemia, were not statistically significantly less common in patients not taking glucocorticoids. This may have been because of the diabetogenic effect of tacrolimus.

The incidence of hyperglycemia or diabetes mellitus requiring insulin at some point during treatment was 10–20% in adults (2% in children), an incidence about 2–3 times higher than with ciclosporin (SEDA-20, 347). However, more recent studies and case reports have shown that children could be also very sensitive to the diabetogenic effects of tacrolimus, with an incidence possibly higher than previously thought (1089,1090). While the diabetes mellitus tends to improve or abate after the dose of tacrolimus or glucocorticoid has been reduced, glucose intolerance was more frequent in the tacrolimus group after a median of 23 months (1091). However, post-transplant diabetes mellitus requiring permanent insulin treatment was as frequent in patients with liver grafts taking ciclosporin or tacrolimus after 1 year (1092). Finally, there was a possible correlation between impaired glucose tolerance or a diabetic pattern detected by a pretransplant 75 g oral glucose tolerance test and the later development of post-transplant diabetes mellitus (1093).

In a pooled analysis of four randomized trials of tacrolimus versus ciclosporin after renal transplantation, the prevalence of post-transplant diabetes mellitus at 1 year (two studies, 532 patients) was five times higher with tacrolimus than with ciclosporin (OR = 5.0; 95% CI = 2.0, 12.4) (1094). In the opinion of the US FDA, diabetes mellitus after transplantation was a significant hazard in tacrolimus-treated patients, even though about half of the patients were no longer taking insulin at 2 years after transplantation (1095).

The exact mechanisms of tacrolimus-induced diabetes are unknown. In one renal transplant patient with genetic susceptibility, tacrolimus was associated with insulin-dependent diabetes mellitus and the simultaneous occurrence of anti-glutamic acid decarboxylase antibody (1096). Within 2 months after conversion from tacrolimus to ciclosporin, the antibody was no longer detected and the patient's insulin requirements fell dramatically. Tacrolimus-induced direct beta cell toxicity, with subsequent development of beta cell autoimmunity, was therefore suggested as a possible mechanism in patients with genetic susceptibility for type I diabetes.

Hepatitis C virus infection has been associated with diabetes and is a significant risk in patients with renal transplants. In 427 patients with renal transplants and no previous diabetes mellitus, diabetes after transplantation occurred more often in hepatitis C virus-positive than hepatitis C virus-negative patients (39 versus 9.8%) (1097). Diabetes mellitus after transplantation occurred more often in hepatitis C virus-positive patients taking tacrolimus than in those taking ciclosporin (58 versus 7.7%). In hepatitis C virus-negative patients, the rates of diabetes mellitus were similar. The authors concluded that hepatitis C is strongly associated with diabetes mellitus after renal transplantation because of the greater diabetogenicity of tacrolimus.

In 17 patients, in whom fasting blood samples were taken immediately before transplantation and at 1 and 3 months after transplantation for measurement of HbA, insulin, C-peptide, free fatty aids, lipids, urea, and creatinine, the incidence of diabetes mellitus was high (47%) (1098). Diabetes was more common in black patients, but owing to the small number of patients the difference was not statistically significant. Insulin resistance seems to be the main pathogenic mechanism involved.

In a meta-analysis of 16 studies of patients who were taking tacrolimus ($n = 1636$) or ciclosporin ($n = 1407$) the incidence of type 1 diabetes mellitus was significantly higher among those taking tacrolimus (10% versus 4.5%) (1099). The effect was observed in those with renal transplants (9.8% versus 2.7%) and those with other organ transplants (11.1% versus 6.2%), and among patients who were taking equal doses of concomitant medications in both treatment arms (12% versus 3%). Further factors associated with diabetes mellitus after kidney transplantation were older recipient age, a cadaveric organ, hepatitis C antibody status, an episode of rejection, and the use of tacrolimus (versus ciclosporin); cumulative glucocorticoid dose and calcineurin inhibitor trough concentration were not associated factors (1100).

Lipid metabolism

In contrast to its effects on glucose metabolism, tacrolimus offers potential advantages over ciclosporin for lipid disorders (1101). Compared with ciclosporin-based immunosuppressive regimens, total cholesterol and LDL cholesterol serum concentrations were lower in patients taking tacrolimus for 1 year (1102). Both findings were considered to result from a significant glucocorticoid-sparing effect of tacrolimus.

Uric acid

Hyperuricemia has been reported in association with ciclosporin and tacrolimus. In two cases there was a direct association between tacrolimus and gout after liver transplantation (1103).

- A 31-year-old male liver transplant recipient was given tacrolimus 6 mg/day and prednisolone. After 8 months,

he developed acute arthritis of the right wrist and both elbows. The serum uric concentration was 421 µmol/l and creatinine 105 µmol/l. After 16 months a mass was excised from the right forearm; histology was typical for gout.
- A 25-year-old liver transplant recipient taking tacrolimus 4 mg/day developed podagra and arthritis of the left wrist. The serum uric acid was 452 µmol/l and creatinine 190 µmol/l. The attacks of gout resolved with allopurinol.

Tenofovir

In a multicenter, double-blind, randomized study tenofovir was compared with stavudine over 3 years, both being given in combination with lamivudine and efavirenz in 602 antiviral drug-naive patients (1104). There were significantly more favorable lipid profiles with tenofovir and more patients required the addition of lipid-lowering agents with stavudine. The overall incidence of mitochondrial toxicity was significantly less among patients who took tenofovir and a higher incidence of lipodystrophy in those who took stavudine. Patients who took tenofovir had gained weight by 144 weeks, in contrast to the patients who took stavudine, who lost weight from weeks 24 to 144.

Terbutaline

The effect of terbutaline on glucose metabolism has been studied in six healthy, pregnant women, with normal glucose tolerance, between the 30th and 34th weeks of pregnancy (1105). The women took either oral terbutaline 5 mg every 6 hours for 24 hours or no medication. The study was repeated after 1 week and each subject acted as her own control. With terbutaline fasting blood glucose increased in each subject, the mean rising from 4.6 to 5.2 mmol/l (82 to 94 mg/dl). Basal serum insulin increased significantly, from 18 to 27 µU/ml. Glucagon fell from a mean of 166 to 144 pg/ml. There was a 12% rise in basal hepatic glucose production. The glucose infusion rate to maintain euglycemia fell by 33% while subjects were taking oral terbutaline. Indirect calorimetry showed that terbutaline caused a significant increase in energy expenditure. Oxygen consumption increased by 9% (270 to 294 ml/minute) and basal caloric expenditure increased by 14% (from 1.32 to 1.5 kcal/minute). Thus, oral terbutaline given for 24 hours is associated with a significant reduction in peripheral insulin sensitivity and an increase in energy expenditure. Increases in basal hepatic glucose metabolism and a reduced ability of insulin to suppress hepatic glucose output are consistent with an effect of terbutaline on maternal hepatic glucose metabolism.

Tetracyclines

See also individual agents
Hormone production in patients with "black thyroid," who had taken a tetracycline for prolonged periods, was normal (1106,1107).

Tetracyclines can increase blood urea nitrogen or serum urea concentrations without a corresponding increase in serum creatinine (that is without accompanying renal damage). The mechanism is an excess nitrogen load of metabolic origin accompanied by negative nitrogen balance. This effect is termed "anti-anabolic" (1108,1109), but is in fact the result of inhibition of protein synthesis, which affects not only microorganisms but to some degree mammalian cells also. Sodium and water depletion, due to the diuretic effect of some tetracyclines, can further enhance uremia (1109).

Tetracyclines have been associated with hypoglycemia (1110). Insulin doses may have to be reduced (1111).

Thalidomide

Hypothyroidism has occasionally been reported in patients taking thalidomide (1112,1113).

- A 44-year-old man with an initial TSH concentration within the reference range took thalidomide 400 mg/day for multiple myeloma and within 4 weeks developed cold intolerance, fatigue, depression, dizziness, and bradycardia, and had a markedly raised TSH (1114). He was given levothyroxine and the dose of thalidomide was reduced to 200 mg/day, after which he became euthyroid.

This case prompted further investigation of thyroid function in patients with multiple myeloma. TSH concentrations were measured in 174 patients who had been randomly assigned to chemotherapy plus thalidomide 400 mg/day ($n = 92$) or chemotherapy alone ($n = 82$). After 3–4 months 18 of the patients taking thalidomide had a serum TSH concentration over 5 IU/ml, including six with a concentration over 10 IU/ml (range 12–114 IU/ml), while seven receiving chemotherapy alone had a serum TSH concentration over 5 IU/ml and none had a concentration over 10 IU/ml. In 169 patients with relapsing multiple myeloma who took thalidomide 200–800 mg/day, of those with a serum TSH concentration in the reference range to begin with, 61 had increases after 2–6 months.

In a placebo-controlled study in six patients with type 2 diabetes mellitus thalidomide 150 mg/day for 3 weeks reduced insulin-stimulated glucose uptake by 31% and glycogen synthesis by 48% (1115). However, it had no effect on rates of glycolysis, carbohydrate oxidation, non-oxidative glycolysis, lipolysis, free fatty acid oxidation, or re-esterification. The authors concluded that thalidomide increases insulin resistance in obese patients with type 2 diabetes.

This effect can have clinical consequences. For example, in patients with prostate cancer, reducing the dose of thalidomide improved hyperglycemia, suggesting that thalidomide may have exacerbated it in the first place (1116).

- A 70-year-old man with no family history of diabetes or known diabetes took thalidomide 400 mg/day for refractory multiple myeloma. He developed hyperglycemia, which had to be treated with insulin and later with glipizide GITS 5 mg/day and which responded despite continuation of thalidomide (1117).

Weight gain and edema have been reported in patients taking thalidomide (1118). In 13 patients with minimally symptomatic HIV disease thalidomide for 14 days caused an increase in weight of 3.6% (1119).

Theophylline

The dangers of theophylline toxicity in hypothyroidism have been described (1120).

The metabolic effects of intravenous infusions of aminophylline have been studied in a series of healthy young subjects with regard to serum glucose, insulin, glucagon, cortisol, and free fatty acid concentrations. Infusion of aminophylline, which produced theophylline concentrations in the usual target range (10–20 µg/ml) caused only small increases in plasma glucose concentrations but rapid, pronounced, and prolonged rises in free fatty acids. Increases in free fatty acid concentrations paralleled the rise in theophylline concentrations (SEDA-6, 6).

Thiazide diuretics

Thiazide diuretics have been associated with dyslipidemia, hyperglycemia, and an increased risk of type 2 diabetes. In a community-based sample of 585 adults with essential hypertension who took monotherapy with hydrochlorothiazide 25 mg/day for 4 weeks the mean changes in response to hydrochlorothiazide were 0.16 mmol/l (6.13 mg/dl) for total cholesterol, 0.19 mmol/l (17.2 mg/dl) for triglycerides, and 0.19 mmol/l (3.5 mg/dl) for plasma glucose (1121). A range of demographic, environmental, and genetic variables taken together only accounted for 13%, 17%, and 11% of the variations in total cholesterol, triglyceride, and glucose, and less than half of this predicted variation in response was explained by measured genotypes. These studies suggest that there are no predictors of the adverse metabolic effects of thiazide-type diuretics.

Thiopental sodium

Thiopental given for cerebral protection after cardiac arrest to patients in intensive care caused altered thyroid function (1122). Five patients received 5 mg/kg as a bolus followed by 3 mg/kg/hour for 48–72 hours. Free T3 concentrations fell dramatically in three of them and remained near normal in the other two. In those in whom T3 concentrations fell they returned to near normal on withdrawal of thiopental. Reverse T3 concentrations increased in these patients. Although the study was not controlled, the authors speculated that thiopental causes conversion of T3 to reverse T3, and that this can intensify the sick euthyroid syndrome that can occur after cardiac arrest.

Tiabendazole

Instances of both hypoglycemia and hyperglycemia have been recorded in patients taking tiabendazole.

Tiagabine

Changes in body weight have been evaluated in 349 patients taking carbamazepine, phenytoin, or tiagabine. Carbamazepine add-on therapy caused a significant mean weight gain of 1.5% (1123). However, tiagabine add-on therapy to either phenytoin or carbamazepine caused no significant weight change.

Tiopronin

Autoimmune hypoglycemia with anti-insulin antibodies, a complication of penicillamine and pyritinol, has also been reported with tiopronin (1124).

- Autoimmune hypoglycemia occurred in a 49-year-old woman with regular menstrual periods accompanied by marked enlargement of the breasts, and was probably induced by tiopronin (1125). Her breasts were red and painful; histological examination showed extensive lymphocytic inflammation and edema in the connective tissue. She recovered after stopping tiopronin and taking danazol.

Topiramate

Topiramate causes a fall in body weight, ranging from a mean of 1.1 kg at 200 mg/day to 5.9 kg at 800–1000 mg/day (1126). Loss of weight may be linked to anorexia. Women tend to lose more weight than men, and weight loss is greatest in patients with the highest weight at baseline.

Weight loss with topiramate can occasionally be extensive (1127).

- A 37-year-old obese white woman with affective instability and obesity taking topiramate (up to 275 mg/day) lost 10 kg over 10 weeks, although she remained obese (BMI 52 kg/m^2). She also improved mentally.

In this case the weight loss was a beneficial collateral effect of topiramate.

In a retrospective chart review, weight loss was assessed in 214 patients with psychiatric disorders taking topiramate (1128). Patients taking either lithium or valproate gained a mean (SD) of 6.3 (9.0) kg and 6.4 (9.0) kg respectively, whereas patients taking topiramate lost 1.2 (6.3) kg. Similar statistically significant results were found in the bone mass index.

In an 8-week, double-blind, placebo-controlled study of topiramate 250 mg/day in the treatment of aggression in 42 men with borderline personality disorder there was significant weight loss of 5.0 kg (95% CI = 3.4, 6.5) (1129). There were no psychotic symptoms or other serious adverse events. Some patients complained of fatigue, dizziness, headache, or paresthesia.

In a 10-week randomized, double-blind, study in 64 women with recurrent major depressive disorder, the dosage of topiramate was titrated up to 200 mg/day (1130). There were no serious adverse effects, including psychotic symptoms and suicidal acts. Adverse effects such as headache, fatigue, dizziness, and paresthesia were rated as mild. After 10 weeks there was weight loss, which was usually regarded as beneficial.

Since topiramate can be associated with metabolic acidosis in both children and adults the incidence and magnitude of the effect of topiramate on serum bicarbonate concentrations in an adult population have been evaluated in a retrospective cohort study in 54 patients (40 women), of whom 26 had low serum bicarbonate concentrations while taking topiramate (mean concentration 18.8 mmol/l, range 13–21) (1131). However, this was not associated with any clinically significant problems.

Tricyclic antidepressants

Weight gain has long been recognized as a concomitant of antidepressant and antipsychotic drug therapy. This may in part reflect improvement in mental state, but there also appears to be a physiological component, with an increased craving for sweets (1132). No abnormalities have been found in fasting glucose and insulin concentrations or in intravenous insulin tolerance tests (1132,1133). Another possible suggestion for weight gain is that taste perception in depression improves after therapy with tricyclic antidepressants (1134). A study of 50 depressed patients attempted to address some of these issues (1135). Increased energy efficiency during antidepressant treatment has also been suggested as a reason for weight gain (SEDA-17, 8). A warning to patients with diabetes that hypoglycemia can be masked seems appropriate (1136).

The "Division of Drug Experience" of the US Department of Health and Welfare issued a note on five cases of the syndrome of inappropriate antidiuretic hormone secretion and drugs to which it has been attributed (1137). All involved drugs with a tricyclic structure; one patient was taking imipramine, three carbamazepine, and the others the closely related muscle relaxant cyclobenzaprine. The dosage of imipramine was 50 mg/day for 3 weeks and the patient was a 72-year-old woman. Other cases have been reported, involving amitriptyline (1137), imipramine, and protriptyline (SEDA-17, 17).

Tricyclic antidepressants, presumably through blocking the re-uptake of noradrenaline, can cause a crisis in a patient with a pheochromocytoma (SEDA-21, 11) (1138).

Prolactin concentrations are very rarely altered during treatment with tricyclic antidepressants, but this is more likely to occur and to produce galactorrhea or amenorrhea with clomipramine and amoxapine and when there are other contributory factors that may stimulate prolactin secretion, such as stress or electroconvulsive therapy (1139).

A striking increase in serum cholesterol was reported in 32-year-old woman during treatment with doxepin (1140).

When reboxetine was substituted for doxepin the cholesterol concentration returned to normal. Doxepin has particularly potent H_1 receptor antagonist properties, which suggests that blockade of H_1 receptors may play a role in the cholesterol raising properties of some psychotropic drugs.

Trimethoprim and co-trimoxazole

In a child, co-trimoxazole was the probable cause of growth failure (1141).

Co-trimoxazole has been suggested to have some antithyroid activity. However, whether this effect is due to trimethoprim alone is still unclear (1142,1143). Co-trimoxazole 27–31 mg/kg bd orally substantially altered serum total T4 and TSH concentrations and neutrophil counts in dogs within as short a time as a few weeks (1144), and 14–16 mg/kg orally every 12 hours for 3 weeks reduced total and free T4 concentrations and increased the TSH concentration, conditions that would be compatible with hypothyroidism (1145).

Co-trimoxazole can cause reversible hypoglycemia, which may be prolonged, particularly in patients with risk factors for hypoglycemia. Common risk factors include compromised renal function, prolonged fasting, malnutrition, and the use of excessive doses. It has been postulated that the sulfonamide mimics the action of sulfonylureas, stimulating pancreatic islet cells to secrete insulin. In elderly people, co-trimoxazole-induced hypoglycemia can cause altered mental state (1146,1147).

Metabolic acidosis has been observed in patients with AIDS after intravenous co-trimoxazole (1148). The acidosis developed 3–5 days after the start of treatment and had a favorable course. It is likely that the sulfonamide was responsible, because of renal loss of bicarbonate.

Trimethoprim 15 mg/kg/day increased urinary uric acid excretion and reduced the plasma uric acid concentration in five healthy volunteers from 333 µmol/l (5.6 mg/dl) to 226 µmol/l (3.8 mg/dl) (1149). In 90 in-patients with hypouricemia co-trimoxazole was identified as the likely cause in four patients (1150). However, since the study was limited to patients with hypouricemia and since exposure rates for co-trimoxazole were not reported for hypouricemic or non-hypouricemic patients, no conclusions about the incidence and the relevance of trimethoprim-associated hypouricemia can be made.

Tripterygium wilfordii (Celastraceae)

Tripterygium wilfordii (thundergod vine) is often used in traditional Chinese medicine, for instance to treat arthritis.

- A 36-year-old woman developed vaginal dryness, reduced libido, and hot flushes after taking *Tripterygium* for 3 months to treat psoriasis (1151). Her follicle stimulating hormone and luteinizing hormone concentrations were abnormally high, while her 17-beta-estriadol concentration was abnormally low. Her signs and symptoms normalized after the herbal remedy was withdrawn.

The authors suggested that thundergod vine has suppressive effects on both male and female gonads.

Troleandomycin

Serum TSH concentrations are moderately but significantly reduced by troleandomycin compared with josamycin or placebo given over 10 days. At the same time serum estradiol concentration was significantly increased (1152).

Tumor necrosis factor alfa

Exacerbation of hypothyroidism was noted in one patient with chronic thyroiditis who received tumor necrosis factor alfa (1153).

Metabolic effects of tumor necrosis factor alfa include a reduction in cholesterol and high-density lipoproteins, increases in triglycerides and very low-density lipoproteins, and hyperglycemia.

Valproic acid

The use of valproate in young women has been associated with an increased incidence of menstrual abnormalities (1154), polycystic ovaries, and hyperandrogenism (SEDA-18, 69; SEDA-20, 68). Of 22 valproate-treated women who underwent endocrine evaluation, 13 were obese and 11 had marked weight gain (mean 21 kg) after starting valproate (1155). There were polycystic ovaries, hyperandrogenism, or both in 64%, but the clinical relevance of these findings remains uncertain.

The syndrome of polycystic ovaries and hyperandrogenism associated with weight gain and hyperinsulinemia was reversible in 16 women with valproate-related polycystic ovaries and/or hyperandrogenism who were switched to lamotrigine (1156). While taking valproate, they had centripetal obesity with associated hyperinsulinism and unfavorable serum lipid profiles. After switching to lamotrigine, in the 12 patients available for follow-up at 1 year, body-mass index and fasting serum insulin and testosterone concentrations fell, whereas HDL cholesterol/total cholesterol ratios increased from 0.17 to 0.26. The total number of polycystic ovaries fell from 20 to 11 after 1 year of lamotrigine.

Pubertal growth arrest has been described in a 12-year-old girl who had taken valproate for 18 months (SED-13, 152) (1157).

Among 45 valproate-treated girls aged 8–18 years, hyperandrogenism (serum testosterone concentrations more than two standard deviations above the mean for healthy controls) was seen in 38% of prepubertal girls, 36% of pubertal girls, and 57% of postpubertal girls (1158). Obesity was more common in postpubertal valproate-treated girls than in controls. The authors concluded that valproate may cause hyperandrogenism in girls with epilepsy during the sensitive period of pubertal maturation.

There were increased serum androgen concentrations in 60% of those who took valproate (1155).

The endocrine consequences of valproate or carbamazepine monotherapy have been evaluated in a cross-sectional study in two groups of women with epilepsy, who were treated for at least 2 years with valproate ($n = 52$) or carbamazepine monotherapy ($n = 53$) (1159). Menstrual disturbances were reported by 29 of the women, 12 of those taking valproate and 17 of those taking carbamazepine. Polycystic ovaries were found in 28 patients, of whom 13 were taking valproate and 15 carbamazepine. Postprandial concentrations of insulin, C-peptide, and proinsulin were significantly higher with valproate than carbamazepine, but there were no differences in the fasting state. In conclusion, this study did not show an increase in the frequency of polycystic ovaries in valproate-treated women, although valproate does appear to increase glucose-stimulated pancreatic insulin secretion.

Valproate can cause hyperglycinemia and hyperglycinuria, sometimes with raised spinal fluid glycine concentrations (SED-12, 133). These changes are usually asymptomatic.

Chronic valproate treatment did not change serum concentrations of lipids, vitamin B12, or folic acid in 26 children with epilepsy (1160).

Weight gain

Weight increase, sometimes associated with increased appetite, occurs in 8–60% of patients taking valproate (1161) and may be unrelated to dose.

A randomized, double-blind study was conducted for 32 weeks to analyse weight change in patients taking lamotrigine ($n = 65$; mean age 35 years; target dosage 200 mg/day) and valproate ($n = 68$; mean age 30 years; target dosage 20 mg/kg/day) (1162). Weight remained stable in the patients taking lamotrigine. However, there was significant weight gain in the patients taking valproate by the 10th week of treatment, and weight continued to increase throughout the study. After 32 weeks, mean weight gain was significantly higher in those taking valproate (5.8 kg) compared with lamotrigine (0.6 kg). Similar proportions of patients taking lamotrigine (29%) or valproate (26%) were seizure-free. The frequencies of adverse events were similar in the two groups.

The incidence of weight gain in young patients taking valproic acid has been investigated in a series of reports. In a review of 43 patients aged 10–17 years there was a mild to moderate increase in body mass index in 25 and a fall in 16; however, the weight loss tended to be modest (1163). Six patients moved up to a potentially overweight or overweight category. Two factors tended to predict an increase in body mass index: normal cognitive status and primary generalized epilepsy.

In an open study of the effects of lamotrigine and valproic acid monotherapy on weight in 38 adolescents (18 taking lamotrigine, 20 taking valproic acid) with epilepsy treated over 8 months, weight gain and increased body mass index were greater in patients who took valproic acid than in those who took lamotrigine (1164). In contrast, in a retrospective analysis of 58 children there was no weight gain (1165).

The mechanisms involved have been assessed in 40 women with epilepsy evaluated before and after 1 year of therapy (1166). At the end of follow-up, 15 patients were obese and had higher serum leptin and insulin concentrations than patients who did not gain weight. The rise in serum leptin is consistent with that observed in other types of obesity.

In a prospective cohort study of the role of insulin and leptin (a signal factor that regulates body weight and energy expenditure) in valproate-related obesity, 81 patients with epilepsy taking valproate and 51 healthy controls were analysed (1167). Mean serum insulin concentrations were significantly higher in the valproate-treated patients than in the controls, despite similar body mass indexes. Furthermore, serum insulin concentrations were significantly higher both in lean men and lean women compared with lean controls of same sex and similar body mass indexes. This implies that the hyperinsulinemia seen in obese people taking valproate is not merely a consequence of insulin resistance induced by weight gain. Serum leptin concentrations did not differ between the valproate-treated patients and the controls. Thus, both obese and lean patients taking valproate have hyperinsulinemia, suggesting insulin resistance. This may be one of the factors that leads to weight gain during valproate treatment. Similar findings, that is increased insulin concentrations without changes in leptin concentrations, have also been published in three other reports from one center (1159,1168,1169).

Metabolic acidosis

Fanconi syndrome (metabolic acidosis secondary to malfunction of proximal renal tubules, resulting in urinary excretion of amino acids, glucose, phosphate, bicarbonate, uric acid, and other substances) secondary to long-term valproic acid has been described in an 8-year-old boy with severe developmental disability (1170). In a review of 10 previous reports of Fanconi syndrome secondary to long-term valproic acid therapy the authors found that all occurred at 4–14 years, all had taken valproic acid for 10 months to 10 years, and symptoms were fully reversible within 2–14 months after withdrawal of valproic acid. Most of the patients (9 of 11) were severely disabled, bedridden, or wheelchair-bound.

Hyperammonemia

Hyperammonemic encephalopathy has been attributed to valproate (1171).

- A 61-year-old man with epilepsy had altered consciousness after his dose of valproate was increased because of poor seizure control. Electroencephalography showed triphasic waves and high-amplitude delta-wave activity with frontal predominance. Although serum aspartate transaminase and alanine transaminase were normal, the serum ammonium concentration was high at 960 ng/ml (reference range 30–470). Serum amino acid analysis showed multiple minor abnormalities. Valproate was withdrawn. He improved within 4 days and the electroencephalogram, serum ammonium concentration, and amino acid profile were normal by day 8.

In two other cases the addition of topiramate was thought to have precipitated valproate-induced hyperammonemic encephalopathy (1172). Recovery occurred after withdrawal of valproate or topiramate. The authors suggested that topiramate may have contributed to the hyperammonemia by inhibiting carbonic anhydrase and cerebral glutamine synthetase.

Asymptomatic hyperammonemia, with ammonia concentrations as high as 140 mmol/l, has been found in up to over 50% of patients (1173) and may be due to increased renal production or inhibition of nitrogen elimination, although carnitine deficiency, nutritional influences, metabolic abnormalities secondary to increased glycine or propionic acid concentrations, and multiple drug therapy may play a role (SED-13, 149; 994). In individual patients, the condition can be associated with severe symptoms (SEDA-20, 69). Deaths have occurred after the use of valproate in patients with ornithine transcarbamylase deficiency (SED-12, 133; SED-13, 149) (1174,1175). Additional evidence points to a need for caution in patients with any enzyme disorder: an 18-year-old woman with progressive dementia and spastic paraparesis became comatose with hyperammonemia when taking valproate; moderate hyperammonemia persisted for months after drug withdrawal, coma recurred without exposure to valproate, and congenital argininemia was diagnosed (1176). Carnitine supplementation has been proposed in symptomatic hyperammonemia caused by valproate (see below).

Valproate-induced hyperammonemic encephalopathy has been reviewed (1177). Proton magnetic resonance spectroscopy was performed in a patient with valproate-induced hyperammonemic encephalopathy; there was a significant fall in the choline and myoinositol resonances and an increase in glutamine in the hyperintense basal ganglia lesions (1178). A similar pattern has been observed in other hyperammonemic encephalopathies, such as hepatic encephalopathy. In another study in seven patients with valproate-related hyperammonemia serum or cerebrospinal fluid glutamine concentrations were initially raised in most patients, sometimes in the absence of hyperammonemia (1179).

The relationship of hyperammonemia to valproic acid-associated encephalopathies has been questioned after a study of ammonia concentrations in 55 asymptomatic patients taking valproic acid showed that 29 had ammonia concentrations above the reference range, the highest being 140 µmol/l (1180).

It is difficult to establish a relation between valproate encephalopathy and increased serum ammonium concentrations. Valproate-induced hyperammonemic encephalopathy has been reported in several single case reports, but still it is difficult to ascertain whether hyperammonemia or valproic acid is the cause of the encephalopathy. In one case valproate was used in combination with lithium, which in itself could have caused encephalopathy by displacement of protein binding or other mechanisms, regardless of hyperammonemia (1181). In a second case it was also impossible to evaluate the effect of hyperammonemia on the level of consciousness, since it involved a woman who took valproic acid (30 g) in addition to

gabapentin (9 g), clonazepam (90 mg), and risperidone (120 mg) (1182). In a third case, a 62-year-old woman became encephalopathic while taking valproate (1183). Her serum ammonia concentration was three times the upper limit of the reference range, despite only mildly raised aspartate aminotransferase activity and a normal bilirubin, with a serum valproic acid concentration within the target range. Her treatment also included estradiol 1 mg/day, levothyroxine 25 micrograms/day, diazepam 20 mg/day, cyclobenzaprine 30 mg/day, paracetamol 600 mg/day, codeine 60 mg/day, and sulindac 400 mg/day. Again, other potential pharmacodynamic and pharmacokinetic interactions could have caused the reduced level of consciousness in this patient. A fourth case involved a 76-year-old woman taking sodium divalproex 2250 mg/day, who had valproic acid concentrations up to 144 µg/ml and ammonia concentrations up to 2110 µg/l (1184). Her associated medications included aspirin 325 mg/day, amlodipine 5 mg/day, atenolol 50 mg/day, losartan 50 mg/day, and pantoprazole 40 mg/day. Considering that beta-blockers can compete with valproic acid for protein binding, an increase in free valproic acid concentrations could have been another factor involved in this patient's symptoms of drug toxicity.

Carnitine deficiency

Valproate is often associated with low carnitine concentrations and occasionally with true carnitine deficiency, especially in young children with neurological disabilities taking several anticonvulsants. The condition is usually asymptomatic, but it can occasionally cause significant toxicity (1185).

- Life-threatening cardiac dysfunction in a 7-year-old boy required urgent carnitine supplementation (SEDA-17, 74).
- In one patient with acute valproate-associated encephalopathy associated with biochemical evidence of severe carnitine deficiency and a defect in valproate metabolism, L-carnitine substitution corrected the biochemical abnormalities, but the patient died (SED-13, 150) (1186).
- In another case, there was late-onset lipid storage myopathy, with secondary carnitine deficiency (SED-13, 150) (1187).

While measurement of carnitine concentrations is advisable in patients with symptoms and signs suggestive of carnitine deficiency (SED-12, 133) (1188), indiscriminate carnitine supplementation is unwarranted. A panel of pediatric neurologists recently recommended intravenous carnitine for valproate hepatotoxicity and for valproate overdose (SEDA-20, 69), whereas oral supplementation was suggested for patients with symptomatic valproate-associated hyperammonemia, multiple risk factors for valproate hepatotoxicity, and infants and young children receiving valproate (1189). It was mentioned that carnitine might be deleterious in some disorders of long-chain fatty acid oxidation. Others have considered carnitine to be valuable in valproate-induced hyperammonemia, but have suggested reserving it for patients with subnormal blood carnitine concentrations or known risk factors for carnitine deficiency (1190). In a double-blind trial in 47 children taking carbamazepine or valproate, carnitine (100 mg/kg/day for 4 weeks) was not more effective than placebo in improving subjective well-being (SEDA-19, 74).

Homocysteine

The effects of valproate 2070 mg/day and lamotrigine 250 mg/day on total plasma homocysteine, plasma and erythrocyte folate, and plasma vitamin B_{12} concentrations have been studied in 20 patients with epilepsy before and after a 32-week period of monotherapy (1191). Lamotrigine had no effect, but valproate caused a 57% increase in plasma vitamin B_{12} concentrations over baseline and a 27% fall in plasma homocysteine concentrations. The mechanisms of these changes are unknown. The data suggest that hyperhomocysteinemia may not be a serious clinical problem among patients with epilepsy taking lamotrigine or valproate.

Vancomycin

Lactic acidosis occurred in a 56-year-old woman who was given intravenous vancomycin 1 g bd for 10 days (1192).

Verapamil

There was a significant rise in serum alkaline phosphatase of skeletal origin in a group of patients taking verapamil for hypertension. It was associated with a slight increase in parathyroid hormone, indicating involvement of bone metabolism, although there was no change in the urinary excretion of calcium, phosphate, or potassium. It has yet to be shown whether verapamil causes osteopenia in man, as it does in animals (SEDA-16, 197).

Verapamil-induced hyperprolactinemia has been reported in a 74-year-old man, who presented with impotence and who was subsequently found to have a benign 6 mm pituitary microadenoma (1193). The withdrawal of verapamil was associated with the normalization of serum prolactin concentrations. Marked hyperprolactinemia has been attributed to verapamil in a 42-year-old woman who may have been hyper-susceptible to this action of verapamil (1194).

The mechanism for this adverse effect is unclear and has not been reported with other calcium channel blockers.

Vigabatrin

Weight gain occurs in as many as 40% of patients during the first 6 months of therapy.

Vinca alkaloids

A rare but well-known adverse effect of vinca alkaloids, including vinorelbine, is the syndrome of inappropriate secretion of antidiuretic hormone (SIADH) (1195–1197). The diagnosis is usually based on clinical and laboratory findings. There are falls in plasma sodium (below 120 mmol/l), chloride (below 90 mmol/l), and osmolality (below 230 mosm/kg). Further features include lethargy, anorexia, nausea, listlessness, and rarely coma, particularly when serum sodium falls below 110 mmol/l. Treatment is based on withdrawal of the causative agent and the administration of 0.9% saline and potassium (for example 40 mmol/l) at an infusion rate of 200 ml/hour. Further treatment strategies include demeclocycline (for example 300 mg bd), which can be continued for the duration of further vinca alkaloid-containing cycles. In one case demeclocycline prevented SIADH during further courses of vinorelbine (1197).

Asian patients have been proposed to be at higher risk of SIADH during treatment with vincristine. Between 1983 and 1999, 76 cases of hyponatremia and/or SIADH related to the use of vincristine were reported to the global adverse event database of Eli Lilly and Company. The average age of the patients was 36 years (range 2 weeks to 86 years) and 62% were male. Most of the patients had received vincristine for leukemia or lymphomas. Of the 76 reports, 39 included background information on race: 35 patients were Asian, three were Caucasian, and one was black. The authors concluded that there may be a correlation between race and vinca alkaloid-associated SIADH/hyponatremia; however, the reasons are still unclear (1198).

Vitamin A: Carotenoids

People with severe hypertriglyceridemia associated with Type V hyperlipoproteinemia may be at increased risk of hypervitaminosis A, even with moderate degrees of vitamin A supplementation (1199). Long-term vitamin A administration is associated with an increase in serum cholesterol and serum triglyceride concentrations (1200) and consequently might be linked with atherosclerosis (SEDA-8, 345) (1201,1202).

Vitamin A: Retinoids

Small reductions in indices of thyroid function have been observed in patients taking etretinate (1203). Thyrotoxicosis may have been triggered by isotretinoin in one patient (SEDA-12, 136).

Alterations in lipid metabolism are common and include increases in serum triglyceride and cholesterol concentrations, sometimes persisting after withdrawal of the therapy, and reductions in high-density lipoprotein cholesterol. The incidence of raised serum lipids during therapy with oral isotretinoin 1 mg/kg/day for acne has been reviewed retrospectively in 876 patients, of whom 54 had raised serum cholesterol concentrations (over 5.2 mmol/l) and 45 had triglyceride concentrations above 2.26 mmol/l (1204). In contrast, in 30 patients who had received three or more courses of isotretinoin there were no significant changes in cholesterol or triglyceride concentrations (1205).

Symptoms of hyperlipidemia and the metabolic syndrome have been investigated in a cross-sectional study in young adults who had used isotretinoin for acne for at least 4 weeks (mean dosage 0.56 mg/kg). Those in whom triglyceride concentrations increased by at least 1.0 mmol/l during therapy were termed hyper-responders (*n* = 102), and those in whom triglyceride concentrations changed by 0.1 mmol/l or less were termed non-responders (*n* = 100) (1206). Despite similar pretreatment body weights and plasma lipid concentrations, 4 years after completion of isotretinoin therapy the hyper-responders were more likely to have hypertriglyceridemia (OR = 4.8; 95% CI = 1.6, 14), hypercholesterolemia (OR = 9.1; CI = 1.9, 43), truncal obesity (OR = 11.0; CI = 2.0, 59), and hyperinsulinemia (OR = 3.0, CI = 1.6, 5.7) than non-responders. In addition, more hyper-responders had at least one parent with hypertriglyceridemia. Genotypes containing apoE ε2 and apoE ε4 alleles were over-represented among hyper-responders. Although a comparison of hyper-responders with non-responders may lead to overestimation of the risk, these data suggest that those who develop hyperlipidemia while taking isotretinoin are those who are already at risk of hyperlipidemia and the metabolic syndrome.

The consequences of hypertriglyceridemia are not well understood, but there may be an increased risk of cardiovascular disease and pancreatitis (SEDA-13, 123). Patients with an increased tendency to develop hypertriglyceridemia include those with diabetes mellitus, obesity, increased alcohol intake, and a positive family history. With a short course (16 weeks) of isotretinoin it is sufficient to ensure there is no hyperlipidemia before the start of therapy, and to determine the triglyceride response to therapy on one occasion after 4 weeks (1207).

Vitamin D analogues

A patient with psoriasis developed hypercalcemia and hypercalciuria after 28 days of treatment with tacalcitol (1208). He had been taking long-term thiazide therapy for his hypertension. When he used topical tacalcitol ointment his serum calcium concentration and urinary calcium excretion gradually increased to 3.55 mmol/l and 0.475 g/day respectively. Within 7 days of withdrawal of tacalcitol, the serum calcium concentration had normalized.

Xipamide

At equivalent therapeutic doses, the metabolic effects of xipamide are greater than those of the thiazides or furosemide (SED-11, 200).

Zidovudine

Lipodystrophy is a common adverse effect of antiretroviral drugs, particularly the NRTIs and has been reported with zidovudine (1209).

- A 42-year-old woman developed abdominal and dorsocervical fat enlargement after having taken zidovudine

for over 10 years. Zidovudine was withdrawn and the lesions improved considerably over the next 26 months.

Ziprasidone

Ziprasidone is said to be associated with less weight gain than the other atypical neuroleptic drugs and than most typical ones (1210,1211). However, weight gain can occur.

- A 12-year-old boy had significant weight gain within 3 months of starting to take ziprasidone, from 63 kg (BMI = 26.5) before treatment to 69 kg (BMI = 28.2) after treatment (1212).

Zopiclone

The syndrome of inappropriate secretion of antidiuretic hormone has been attributed to zopiclone (1213).

- A woman with a 2-week history of insomnia took zopiclone 7.5 mg nightly and over the next 9 days became confused, lethargic, and depressed, culminating in an overdose of six zopiclone tablets. Her previous medical history included hypertension and two episodes of diuretic-induced SIADH. Her serum sodium was 129 mmol/l and 4 days later fell to 113 mmol/l. Her serum osmolality was low (240 mmol/kg) and her urine sodium was 20 mmol/l. The serum sodium returned to normal 12 days after withdrawal of zopiclone.

The rapid resolution of symptoms and correction of the hyponatremia after withdrawal was consistent with an effect of zopiclone.

References

1. Modest GA, Fuller J, Hetherington SV, Lenhard JM, Powell GS. Abacavir and diabetes. N Engl J Med 2001;344(2):142–4.
2. Prince RL, Larkins RG, Alford FP. The effect of acetylsalicylic acid on plasma glucose and the response of glucose regulatory hormones to intravenous glucose and arginine in insulin treated diabetics and normal subjects. Metabolism 1981;30(3):293–8.
3. Rehm M, Orth V, Scheingraber S, Kreimeier U, Brechtelsbauer H, Finsterer U. Acid-base changes caused by 5% albumin versus 6% hydroxyethyl starch solution in patients undergoing acute normovolemic hemodilution: a randomized prospective study. Anesthesiology 2000;93(5):1174–83.
4. Vial T, Descotes J. Clinical toxicity of interleukin-2. Drug Saf 1992;7(6):417–33.
5. VanderMolen LA, Smith JW 2nd, Longo DL, Steis RG, Kremers P, Sznol M. Adrenal insufficiency and interleukin-2 therapy. Ann Intern Med 1989;111(2):185.
6. Vial T, Descotes J. Immune-mediated side-effects of cytokines in humans. Toxicology 1995;105(1):31–57.
7. Kruit WH, Bolhuis RL, Goey SH, Jansen RL, Eggermont AM, Batchelor D, Schmitz PI, Stoter G. Interleukin-2-induced thyroid dysfunction is correlated with treatment duration but not with tumor response. J Clin Oncol 1993;11(5):921–4.

8. Preziati D, La Rosa L, Covini G, Marcelli R, Rescalli S, Persani L, Del Ninno E, Meroni PL, Colombo M, Beck-Peccoz P. Autoimmunity and thyroid function in patients with chronic active hepatitis treated with recombinant interferon alpha-2a. Eur J Endocrinol 1995;132(5):587–93.

9. Vialettes B, Guillerand MA, Viens P, Stoppa AM, Baume D, Sauvan R, Pasquier J, San Marco M, Olive D, Maraninchi D. Incidence rate and risk factors for thyroid dysfunction during recombinant interleukin-2 therapy in advanced malignancies. Acta Endocrinol (Copenh) 1993;129(1):31–8.

10. Schwartzentruber DJ, White DE, Zweig MH, Weintraub BD, Rosenberg SA. Thyroid dysfunction associated with immunotherapy for patients with cancer. Cancer 1991;68(11):2384–90.

11. Jacobs EL, Clare-Salzler MJ, Chopra IJ, Figlin RA. Thyroid function abnormalities associated with the chronic outpatient administration of recombinant interleukin-2 and recombinant interferon-alpha. J Immunother 1991;10(6):448–55.

12. Pichert G, Jost LM, Zobeli L, Odermatt B, Pedia G, Stahel RA. Thyroiditis after treatment with interleukin-2 and interferon alpha-2a. Br J Cancer 1990;62(1):100–4.

13. Reid I, Sharpe I, McDevitt J, Maxwell W, Emmons R, Tanner WA, Monson JR. Thyroid dysfunction can predict response to immunotherapy with interleukin-2 and interferon-2 alpha. Br J Cancer 1991;64(5):915–8.

14. Weijl NI, Van der Harst D, Brand A, Kooy Y, Van Luxemburg S, Schroder J, Lentjes E, Van Rood JJ, Cleton FJ, Osanto S. Hypothyroidism during immunotherapy with interleukin-2 is associated with antithyroid antibodies and response to treatment. J Clin Oncol 1993;11(7):1376–83.

15. Krouse RS, Royal RE, Heywood G, Weintraub BD, White DE, Steinberg SM, Rosenberg SA, Schwartzentruber DJ. Thyroid dysfunction in 281 patients with metastatic melanoma or renal carcinoma treated with interleukin-2 alone. J Immunother Emphasis Tumor Immunol 1995;18(4):272–8.

16. Kung AW, Lai CL, Wong KL, Tam CF. Thyroid functions in patients treated with interleukin-2 and lymphokine-activated killer cells. Q J Med 1992;82(297):33–42.

17. Monig H, Hauschild A, Lange S, Folsch UR. Suppressed thyroid-stimulating hormone secretion in patients treated with interleukin-2 and interferon-alpha 2b for metastatic melanoma. Clin Investig 1994;72(12):975–8.

18. Coles AJ, Wing M, Smith S, Coraddu F, Greer S, Taylor C, Weetman A, Hale G, Chatterjee VK, Waldmann H, Compston A. Pulsed monoclonal antibody treatment and autoimmune thyroid disease in multiple sclerosis. Lancet 1999;354(9191):1691–5.

19. Kroboth PD, Salek FS, Stone RA, Bertz RJ, Kroboth FJ 3rd. Alprazolam increases dehydroepiandrosterone concentrations. J Clin Psychopharmacol 1999;19(2):114–24.

20. Deuster PA, Faraday MM, Chrousos GP, Poth MA. Effects of dehydroepiandrosterone and alprazolam on hypothalamic–pituitary responses to exercise. J Clin Endocrinol Metab 2005;90(8):4777–83.

21. Pomara N, Willoughby LM, Ritchie LC, Sidtis JJ, Greenblatt DJ, Nemeroff CB. Sex-related elevation in cortisol during chronic treatment with alprazolam associated with enhanced cognitive performance. Psychopharmacology 2005;182(3):414–9.

22. Lopez-Gonzalez MA, Delgado F, Lucas M. Aminoglycosides activate oxygen metabolites production in the cochlea of mature and developing rats. Hear Res 1999;136(1–2):165–8.

23. Sha SH, Schacht J. Stimulation of free radical formation by aminoglycoside antibiotics. Hear Res 1999;128(1–2):112–8.

24. Dobs AS, Sarma PS, Guarnieri T, Griffith L. Testicular dysfunction with amiodarone use. J Am Coll Cardiol 1991;18(5):1328–32.

25. Odeh M, Schiff E, Oliven A. Hyponatremia during therapy with amiodarone. Arch Intern Med 1999;159(21):2599–600.

26. Ikegami H, Shiga T, Tsushima T, Nirei T, Kasanuki H. Syndrome of inappropriate antidiuretic hormone secretion (SIADH) induced by amiodarone: a report on two cases. J Cardiovasc Pharmacol Ther 2002;7(1):25–8.

27. Patel GP, Kasiar JB. Syndrome of inappropriate antidiuretic hormone-induced hyponatremia associated with amiodarone. Pharmacotherapy 2002;22(5):649–51.

28. Aslam MK, Gnaim C, Kutnick J, Kowal RC, McGuire DK. Syndrome of inappropriate antidiuretic hormone secretion induced by amiodarone therapy. Pacing Clin Electrophysiol 2004;27(6 Pt 1):831–2.

29. Wolff J. Perchlorate and the thyroid gland. Pharmacol Rev 1998;50(1):89–105.

30. Wiersinga WM, Trip MD. Amiodarone and thyroid hormone metabolism. Postgrad Med J 1986;62(732):909–14.

31. Mason JW. Amiodarone. N Engl J Med 1987;316(8):455–66.

32. Kawahara C, Okada Y, Tanikawa T, Fukusima A, H, Tanaka Y. Severe hypercalcemia and hypernatremia associated with calcipotriol for treatment of psoriasis. J Bone Miner Metab 2004;22:159–62.

33. Filippi L, Bagnoli F, Margollicci M, Zammarchi E, Tronchin M, Rubaltelli FF. Pathogenic mechanism, prophylaxis, and therapy of symptomatic acid induced by acetazolamide. J Investig Med 2002;50(2):125–32.

34. Venkatesha SL, Umamaheswara Rao GS. Metabolic acidosis and hyperventilation induced by acetazolamide in patients with central nervous system pathology. Anesthesiology 2000;93(6):1546–8.

35. Morris S, Geh V, Nischal KK, Sahi S, Ahmed MA. Topical dorzolamide and metabolic acidosis in a neonate. Br J Ophthalmol 2003;87(8):1052–3.

36. Moffett BS, Moffett TI, Dickerson HA. Acetazolamide therapy for hypochloremic metabolic alkalosis in pediatric patients with heart disease. Am J Ther 2007;14:331–5.

37. Wong R, Cheung W, Stockigt JR, Topliss DJ. Heterogeneity of amiodarone-induced thyrotoxicosis: evaluation of colour-flow Doppler sonography in predicting therapeutic response. Intern Med J 2003;33:420–6.

38. Walshe CM, Cooper JD, Kossmann T, Hayes I, Iles L. Cerebral fat embolism syndrome causing brain death after long-bone fractures and acetazolamdie therapy. Crit Care Resusc 2007;9:184–6.

39. Menon GJ, Vernon SA. Topical brinzolamide and metabolic acidosis. Br J Ophthalmol 2006;90:247–8.

40. Mackie GC, Shulkin BL. Amiodarone-induced hyperthyroidism in a patient with functioning papillary carcinoma of the thyroid and extensive hepatic metastases. Thyroid 2005;15(12):1337–40.

41. Kobayacawa N, Sawaki D, Otani Y, Sekita G, Fukushima K, Takeuchi H, Aoyagi T. A case of severe diabetes mellitus occurred during management of heart failure with carvedilol and furosemide. Cardiovasc Drugs Ther 2003;17:295.

42. Brass EP, Mayer MD, Mulford DJ, Stickler TK, Hoppel CHL. Impact on carnitine homeostasis of short-term treatment with the pivalate prodrug cefditoren pivoxil. Clin Pharmacol Ther 2003;73:338–47.

43. Abrahamsson K, Melander M, Eriksson BO, Holme E, Jodal U, Jonasson A. Transient reduction of human left ventricular mass in carnitine depletion induced by antibiotics containing pivalic acid. Br Heart J 1995;74:656–9.

44. Melegh B, Kerner J, Jaszai V, Bieber L. Differential excretion of xenobiotic acylesters of carnitine due to administration of pivampicillin and valproate. Biochem Med Metabol Biol 1990;43:30–8.

45. Lokrantz CM. Eriksson B, Rosen I, Asztely F. Hyperammonemic encephalopathy induced by a combination of valproate and pivmecillinam Acta Neurol Scand 2004;109:297–301.

46. Ganapapathy ME, Huang W, Rajan DP, Carter AL, Sugawara M, Isek K, Leiback FH, Ganapathy V. Beta-lactam antibiotics as substrates for OCTN2, an organic cation/carnitine transporter. J Biol Chem 2000;275:1699–707.

47. Nezu J, Tamai I, Oku A, Ohashi R, Yabuuchi H, Hashimoto N, Nikaido H, Say Y, Koizumi A, Shoji Y, Takada G, Matsuishi T, Yoshino M, Kato A, Ohura T, Tsujimoto G, Hayakawa J, Shimane M, Tsuji A. Primary systemic carnitine deficiency is caused by mutations in a gene encoding sodium ion-dependent carnitine transporter, Nature Genet 1999;21:91–4.

48. Burwinkel B, Kreuder J, Schweitzer S, Vorgerd M, Gempel K, Gerbitz KD, Kilimann MW. Carnitine transporter OCTN2 mutations in systemic primary carnitine deficiency: a novel Arg169Gln mutation and a recurrent Arg282ter mutation associated with an unconventional splicing abnormality. Biochem Biophys Res Commun 1999;261:484–7.

49. Sharma N, Varma S. Unusual life-threatening adverse drug effects with chloroquine in a young girl. J Postgrad Med 2003;49:187.

50. Imataki O, Kim SW, Kojima R, Hori A, Hamaki T, Sakiyama M, Murashige N, Satoh M, Kami M, Makimoto A, Takaue Y. Life-threatening hypothyroidism associated with administration of cyclosporine in a patient treated with reduced-intensity hematopoietic stem-cell transplantation for metastatic renal-cell carcinoma. Transplantation 2003;75:898–907.

51. Zielinska T, Zakliczynski M, Szewczyk M, Zielinska-Kukla A, Foremny J, Kalarus Z, Religia Z, Zembala M. Influence of long term cyclosporine therapy on insulin and its precursors secretion in patients after heart transplantation. Ann Transplant 2003;8:10–12.

52. Ciancio G, Burke GW, Gaynor JJ, Mattiazzi A, Roth D, Kupin W, Nicolas M, Ruiz P, Rosen A, Miller J. A randomized long-term trial of tacrolimus/sirolimus versus tacrolimus/mycophenolate mofetil versus cyclosporine (NEORAL)/sirolimus in renal transplantation. II. Survival, function, and protocol compliance at 1 year. Transplantation 2004;77(2):252–8.

53. Chevassus H, Mourand I, Molinier N, Lacarelle B, Brun JF, Petit P. Assessment of single-dose benzodiazepines on insulin secretion, insulin sensitivity and glucose effectiveness in healthy volunteers: a double-blind, placebo-controlled, randomised, cross-over trial. BMC Clin Pharmacol 2004;4(3):1–10.

54. Howes OD, Bhatnagar A, Gaughran FP, Amiel SA, Murray RM, Pilowsky LS. A prospective study of impairment in glucose control caused by clozapine without changes in insulin resistance. Am J Psychiatry 2004;161:361–3.

55. Ball MP, Hooper ET, Skipwith DF, Cates ME. Clozapine-induced hyperlipidemia resolved after switch to aripiprazole therapy. Ann Pharmacother 2005;39:1570–2.

56. Haasen C, Lambert M, Yagdiran O, Karow A, Krausz M, Naber D. Comorbidity of schizophrenia and galactosemia: effective clozapine treatment with weight gain. Int Clin Psychopharmacol 2003;18:113–5.

57. Covell NH, Weissman EM, Essock SM. Weight gain with clozapine compared to first generation antipsychotic medications. Schizophr Bull 2004;30:229–40.

58. Tsai SJ, Yu YW, Lin CH, Wang YC, Chen JY, Hong CJ. Association study of adrenergic β3 receptor (Trp64Arg) and G-Protein β3 subunit gene (C825T) polymorphisms and weight change during clozapine treatment. Neuropsychobiology 2004;50:37–40.

59. Wang YC, Bai YM, Chen JY, Lin CC, Lai IC, Liou YJ. Polymorphism of the adrenergic receptor alpha 2a - 1291C>G genetic variation and clozapine-induced weight gain. J Neural Transm 2005;112:1463–8.

60. Bartalena L, Wiersinga WM, Tanda ML, Bogazzi F, Piantanida E, Lai A, Martino E. Diagnosis and management of amiodarone-induced thyrotoxicosis in Europe: results of an international survey among members of the European Thyroid Association. Clin Endocrinol (Oxf) 2004;61(4):494–502.

61. Dietlein M, Schicha H. Amiodarone-induced thyrotoxicosis due to destructive thyroiditis: therapeutic recommendations. Exp Clin Endocrinol Diabetes 2005;113(3):145–51.

62. Boeving A, Cubas ER, Santos CM, Carvalho GA, Graf H. [Use of lithium carbonate for the treatment of amiodarone-induced thyrotoxicosis.] Arq Bras Endocrinol Metabol 2005;49(6):991–5.

63. Diamond TH, Rajagopal R, Ganda K, Manoharan A, Luk A. Plasmapheresis as a potential treatment option for amiodarone-induced thyrotoxicosis. Intern Med J 2004;34(6):369–70.

64. Topliss DJ, Wong R, Stockigt JR A. Plasmapheresis as a potential treatment option for amiodarone-induced thyrotoxicosis. Reply. Intern Med J 2004;34(6):370–71.

65. Hermida JS, Jarry G, Tcheng E, Moullart V, Arlot S, Rey JL, Schvartz C. Prévention des récidives d'hyperthyroïdie a l'amiodarone par l'iode131. [Prevention of recurrent amiodarone-induced hyperthyroidism by iodine-131.] Arch Mal Coeur Vaiss 2004;97(3):207–13.

66. Hermida JS, Tcheng E, Jarry G, Moullart V, Arlot S, Rey JL, Delonca J, Schvartz C. Radioiodine ablation of the thyroid to prevent recurrence of amiodarone-induced thyrotoxicosis in patients with resistant tachyarrhythmias. Europace 2004;6(2):169–74.

67. Hermida JS, Jarry G, Tcheng E, Moullart V, Arlot S, Rey JL, Delonca J, Schvartz C. Radioiodine ablation of the thyroid to allow the reintroduction of amiodarone treatment in patients with a prior history of amiodarone-induced thyrotoxicosis. Am J Med 2004;116(5):345–8.

68. Ryan LE, Braverman LE, Cooper DS, Ladenson PW, Kloos RT. Can amiodarone be restarted after amiodarone-induced thyrotoxicosis? Thyroid 2004;14(2):149–53.

69. Theisen FM, Gebhardt S, Bromel T, Otto B, Heldwein W, Heinzel-Gutenbrunner M, Krieg JC, Remschmidt H, Tschop M, Hebebrand J. A prospective study of serum ghrelin levels in patients treated with clozapine. J Neural Transm 2005;112:1411–6.

70. Roy A, Bissette G, Williams R, Berman J, Gonzalez B. CSF CRH in abstinent cocaine-dependent patients. Psychiatry Res 2003;117:277–80.

71. Franzese CB, Fan CY, Stack BC. Surgical management of amiodarone-induced thyrotoxicosis. Otolaryngol Head Neck Surg 2003;129:565–70.

72. Mendelson JH, Sholar MB, Mutschler NH, Jaszyna-Gasior M, Goletiani NV, Siegel AJ, Mello NK. Effects of intravenous cocaine and cigarette smoking on luteinizing hormone, testosterone, and prolactin in men. J Pharmacol Exp Ther 2003;307:339–48.

73. Szapary PO, Wolfe ML, Bloedon LT, Cucchiara AJ, DerMarderosian AH, Cirigliano MD, Rader DJ. Guggulipid for the treatment of hypercholesterolemia: a randomised controlled trial. J Am Med Assoc 2003;290:765–72.

74. Williams M, Lo Gerfo P. Thyroidectomy using local anesthesia in critically ill patients with amiodarone-induced thyrotoxicosis: a review and description of the technique. Thyroid 2002;12(6):523–5.

75. Gheri RG, Pucci P, Falsetti C, Luisi ML, Cerisano GP, Gheri CF, Petruzzi I, Pinzani P, Salvadori B, Petruzzi E. Clinical, biochemical and therapeutical aspects of amiodarone-induced hypothyroidism (AIH) in geriatric patients with cardiac arrhythmias. Arch Gerontol Geriatr 2004;38(1):27–36.

76. Martino E, Aghini-Lombardi F, Bartalena L, Grasso L, Loviselli A, Velluzzi F, Pinchera A, Braverman LE. Enhanced susceptibility to amiodarone-induced hypothyroidism in patients with thyroid autoimmune disease. Arch Intern Med 1994;154(23):2722–6.

77. Hyatt RH, Sinha B, Vallon A, Bailey RJ, Martin A. Noncardiac side-effects of long-term oral amiodarone in the elderly. Age Ageing 1988;17(2):116–22.

78. Pollak PT, Sharma AD, Carruthers SG. Elevation of serum total cholesterol and triglyceride levels during amiodarone therapy. Am J Cardiol 1988;62(9):562–5.

79. Tubman R, Jenkins J, Lim J. Neonatal hyperthyroxinaemia associated with maternal amiodarone therapy: case report. Ir J Med Sci 1988;157(7):243.

80. De Wolf D, De Schepper J, Verhaaren H, Deneyer M, Smitz J, Sacre-Smits L. Congenital hypothyroid goiter and amiodarone. Acta Paediatr Scand 1988;77(4):616–8.

81. De Catte L, De Wolf D, Smitz J, Bougatef A, De Schepper J, Foulon W. Fetal hypothyroidism as a complication of amiodarone treatment for persistent fetal supraventricular tachycardia. Prenat Diagn 1994;14(8):762–5.

82. Jouannic J-M, Delahaye S, Fermont L, Le Bidois J, Villain E, Dumez Y, Dommergues M. Fetal supraventricular tachycardia: a role for amiodarone as second-line therapy? Prenatal Diagn 2003;23:152–6.

83. Vanbesien J, Casteels A, Bougatef A, De Catte L, Foulon W, De Bock S, Smitz J, De Schepper J. Transient fetal hypothyroidism due to direct fetal administration of amiodarone for drug resistant fetal tachycardia. Am J Perinatol 2001;18(2):113–6.

84. Bliesener N, Yokusoglu H, Quednow B, Klingmüller D, Kühn K. Usefulness of bromocriptine in the treatment of amisulpride-induced hyperprolactinemia. Pharmacopsychiatry 2004;37:189–91.

85. Fountoulakis KN, Iacovides A, Kaprinis GS. Successful treatment of Tourette's disorder with amisulpride. Ann Pharmacother 2004;38:901.

86. Perroud N, Huguelet P. A possible effect of amisulpride on a prolactinoma growth in a woman with borderline personality disorder. Pharmacol Res 2004;50:377–9.

87. Tollefson G, Lesar T. Nonketotic hyperglycemia associated with loxapine and amoxapine: case report. J Clin Psychiatry 1983;44(9):347–8.

88. Nakamura Y, Yoshimoto K, Saima S. Gynaecomastia induced by angiotensin converting enzyme inhibitor. BMJ 1990;300(6723):541.

89. Herings RM, de Boer A, Stricker BH, Leufkens HG, Porsius A. Hypoglycaemia associated with use of inhibitors of angiotensin converting enzyme. Lancet 1995;345(8959):1195–8.

90. Moore N, Kreft-Jais C, Haramburu F, Noblet C, Andrejak M, Ollagnier M, Begaud B. Reports of hypoglycaemia associated with the use of ACE inhibitors and other drugs: a case/non-case study in the French pharmacovigilance system database. Br J Clin Pharmacol 1997;44(5):513–8.

91. Thamer M, Ray NF, Taylor T. Association between antihypertensive drug use and hypoglycemia: a case-control study of diabetic users of insulin or sulfonylureas. Clin Ther 1999;21(8):1387–400.

92. Pedersen-Bjergaard U, Agerholm-Larsen B, Pramming S, Hougaard P, Thorsteinsson B. Activity of angiotensin-converting enzyme and risk of severe hypoglycaemia in type 1 diabetes mellitus. Lancet 2001;357(9264):1248–53.

93. Stolinsky DC. Sugar and saccharin content of antacids. N Engl J Med 1981;305(3):166–7.

94. Stoffel-Wagner B, Bauer J, Flugel D, Brennemann W, Klingmuller D, Elger CE. Serum sex hormones are altered in patients with chronic temporal lobe epilepsy receiving anticonvulsant medication. Epilepsia 1998;39(11):1164–73.

95. Franceschi M, Perego L, Cavagnini F, Cattaneo AG, Invitti C, Caviezel F, Strambi LF, Smirne S. Effects of long-term antiepileptic therapy on the hypothalamic–pituitary axis in man. Epilepsia 1984;25(1):46–52.

96. Luhdorf K. Endocrine function and antiepileptic treatment. Acta Neurol Scand Suppl 1983;94:15–9.

97. Elias AN, Gwinup G. Sodium valproate and Nelson's syndrome. Lancet 1981;2(8240):252–3.

98. Ostrowska Z, Buntner B, Rosciszewska D, Guz I. Adrenal cortex hormones in male epileptic patients before and during a 2-year phenytoin treatment. J Neurol Neurosurg Psychiatry 1988;51(3):374–8.

99. Masala A, Meloni T, Alagna S, Rovasio PP, Mele G, Franca V. Pituitary responsiveness to gonadotrophin-releasing and thyrotrophin-releasing hormones in children receiving phenobarbitone. BMJ 1980;281(6249):1175–7.

100. Victor A, Lundberg PO, Johansson ED. Induction of sex hormone binding globulin by phenytoin. BMJ 1977;2(6092):934–5.

101. Dana-Haeri J, Oxley J, Richens A. Reduction of free testosterone by antiepileptic drugs. BMJ (Clin Res Ed) 1982;284(6309):85–6.

102. Isojarvi JI, Repo M, Pakarinen AJ, Lukkarinen O, Myllyla VV. Carbamazepine, phenytoin, sex hormones, and sexual function in men with epilepsy. Epilepsia 1995;36(4):366–70.

103. Toone BK, Wheeler M, Fenwick PB. Sex hormone changes in male epileptics. Clin Endocrinol (Oxf) 1980;12(4):391–5.

104. Macphee GJ, Larkin JG, Butler E, Beastall GH, Brodie MJ. Circulating hormones and pituitary responsiveness in young epileptic men receiving long-term antiepileptic medication. Epilepsia 1988;29(4):468–75.

105. Duncan S, Blacklaw J, Beastall GH, Brodie MJ. Antiepileptic drug therapy and sexual function in men with epilepsy. Epilepsia 1999;40(2):197–204.

106. Rattya J, Turkka J, Pakarinen AJ, Knip M, Kotila MA, Lukkarinen O, Myllyla VV, Isojarvi JI. Reproductive effects of valproate, carbamazepine, and oxcarbazepine in men with epilepsy. Neurology 2001;56(1):31–6.

107. Rattya J, Pakarinen AJ, Knip M, Repo-Outakoski M, Myllyla VV, Isojarvi JI. Early hormonal changes during valproate or carbamazepine treatment: a 3-month study. Neurology 2001;57(3):440–4.

108. Tiihonen M, Liewendahl K, Waltimo O, Ojala M, Valimaki M. Thyroid status of patients receiving long-term anticonvulsant therapy assessed by peripheral parameters: a placebo-controlled thyroxine therapy trial. Epilepsia 1995;36(11):1118–25.

109. Isojarvi JI, Airaksinen KE, Mustonen JN, Pakarinen AJ, Rautio A, Pelkonen O, Myllyla VV. Thyroid and myocardial function after replacement of carbamazepine by oxcarbazepine. Epilepsia 1995;36(8):810–6.

110. Aanderud S, Strandjord RE. Hypothyroidism induced by anti-epileptic therapy. Acta Neurol Scand 1980;61(5):330–2.

111. Isojarvi JI, Pakarinen AJ, Ylipalosaari PJ, Myllyla VV. Serum hormones in male epileptic patients receiving anticonvulsant medication. Arch Neurol 1990;47(6):670–6.

112. Eiris-Punal J, Del Rio-Garma M, Del Rio-Garma MC, Lojo-Rocamonde S, Novo-Rodriguez I, Castro-Gago M. Long-term treatment of children with epilepsy with valproate or carbamazepine may cause subclinical hypothyroidism. Epilepsia 1999;40(12):1761–6.

113. Isojarvi JI, Turkka J, Pakarinen AJ, Kotila M, Rattya J, Myllyla VV. Thyroid function in men taking carbamazepine, oxcarbazepine, or valproate for epilepsy. Epilepsia 2001;42(7):930–4.

114. Verrotti A, Basciani F, Morresi S, Morgese G, Chiarelli F. Thyroid hormones in epileptic children receiving carbamazepine and valproic acid. Pediatr Neurol 2001;25(1):43–6.

115. Carter BL, Small RE, Mandel MD, Starkman MT. Phenytoin-induced hyperglycemia. Am J Hosp Pharm 1981;38(10):1508–12.

116. Dean JC, Penry JK. Weight gain patterns in patients with epilepsy: comparison of antiepileptic drugs. Epilepsia 1995;36:72.

117. Jallon P, Picard F. Bodyweight gain and anticonvulsants: a comparative review. Drug Saf 2001;24(13):969–78.

118. Nikkila EA, Kaste M, Ehnholm C, Viikari J. Elevation of high-density lipoprotein in epileptic patients treated with phenytoin. Acta Med Scand 1978;204(6):517–20.

119. al-Rubeaan K, Ryan EA. Phenytoin-induced insulin insensitivity. Diabet Med 1991;8(10):968–70.

120. Isojarvi JI, Pakarinen AJ, Myllyla VV. Serum lipid levels during carbamazepine medication. A prospective study. Arch Neurol 1993;50(6):590–3.

121. Isojarvi JI, Pakarinen AJ, Rautio A, Pelkonen O, Myllyla VV. Liver enzyme induction and serum lipid levels after replacement of carbamazepine with oxcarbazepine. Epilepsia 1994;35(6):1217–20.

122. Calandre EP, Rodriquez-Lopez C, Blazquez A, Cano D. Serum lipids, lipoproteins and apolipoproteins A and B in epileptic patients treated with valproic acid, carbamazepine or phenobarbital. Acta Neurol Scand 1991;83(4):250–3.

123. Larson AW, Wasserstrom WR, Felsher BF, Chih JC. Posttraumatic epilepsy and acute intermittent porphyria: effects of phenytoin, carbamazepine, and clonazepam. Neurology 1978;28(8):824–8.

124. Isobe T, Horimatsu T, Fujita T, Miyazaki K, Sugiyama T. Adult T cell lymphoma following diphenylhydantoin therapy. Nippon Ketsueki Gakkai Zasshi 1980;43(4):711–4.

125. Norohna MJ, Bevan PLT. A literature review on unwanted effects during treatment with Epilim. In: Legg NJ, editor. Clinical and Pharmacological Aspects of Sodium Valproate (Epilim) in the Treatment of Epilepsy. Tunbridge Wells, UK: MCS, 1976:61.

126. Reynolds NC Jr, Miska RM. Safety of anticonvulsants in hepatic porphyrias. Neurology 1981;31(4):480–4.

127. Rassiat E, Ragonnet D, Barriere E, Soupison A, Bernard P. Porphyrie aiguë intermittente revelée par une réaction paradoxale a une benzodiazepine. [Acute intermittent porphyria revealed by a paradoxical reaction to a benzodiazepine.] Gastroenterol Clin Biol 2001;25(8–9):832.

128. D'Alessandro R, Rocchi E, Cristina E, Cassanelli M, Benassi G, Pizzino D, Baldrati A, Baruzzi A. Safety of valproate in porphyria cutanea tarda. Epilepsia 1988;29(2):159–62.

129. Krauss GL, Hahn M, Gildemeister OS, Lambrecht RW, Pepe JA, Donohue SE, Bonkowsky HL. Porphyrinogenicity of new anticonvulsants in a liver cell culture model. Epilepsia 1996;37(Suppl 5):204.

130. Schwaninger M, Ringleb P, Winter R, Kohl B, Fiehn W, Rieser PA, Walter-Sack I. Elevated plasma concentrations of homocysteine antiepileptic drug treatment. Epilepsia 1999;40(3):345–50.

131. Botez MI, Joyal C, Maag U, Bachevalier J. Cerebrospinal fluid and blood thiamine concentrations in phenytoin-treated epileptics. Can J Neurol Sci 1982;9(1):37–9.

132. De Vivo DC, Bohan TP, Coulter DL, Dreifuss FE, Greenwood RS, Nordli DR Jr, Shields WD, Stafstrom CE, Tein I. L-carnitine supplementation in childhood epilepsy: current perspectives. Epilepsia 1998;39(11):1216–25.

133. Schwaninger M, Ringleb P, Annecke A, Winter R, Kohl B, Werle E, Fiehn W, Rieser PA, Walter-Sack I. Elevated plasma concentrations of lipoprotein(a) in medicated epileptic patients. J Neurol 2000;247(9):687–90.

134. Biton V. Effect of antiepileptic drugs on bodyweight: overview and clinical implications for the treatment of epilepsy. CNS Drugs 2003;17:781–91.

135. Kunkel G. Antihistamines reassessed. Clin Exp Allergy 1990;20:1.

136. Richards DM, Brogden RN, Heel RC, Speight TM, Avery GS. Astemizole. A review of its pharmacodynamic properties and therapeutic efficacy. Drugs 1984;28(1):38–61.

137. Lal A. Effect of a few histamine1-antagonists on blood glucose in patients of allergic rhinitis. Indian J Otolaryngol Head Neck Surg 2000;52:193–5.

138. Massip P, Marchou B, Bonnet E, Cuzin L, Montastruc JL. Lipodystrophia with protease inhibitors in HIV patients. Therapie 1997;52:615.

139. Viraben R, Aquilina C. Indinavir-associated lipodystrophy. AIDS 1998;12:F37–9.

140. Carr A, Samaras K, Chisholm DJ, Cooper DA. Pathogenesis of HIV-1-protease inhibitor-associated

peripheral lipodystrophy, hyperlipidaemia, and insulin resistance. Lancet 1998;351:1881–3.

141. Third Report of the Expert Panel on Detection, Evaluation, and Treatment of High Blood Cholesterol in Adults (Adult Treatment Panel III) http://www.nhlbi.nih.gov/guidelines/cholesterol/(accessed 20 March 2005).

142. Nolan D. Metabolic complications associated with HIV protease inhibitor therapy. Drugs 2003;63:2555–74.

143. Carr A, Samaras K, Burton S, Law M, Freund J, Chisholm DJ, Cooper DA. A syndrome of peripheral lipodystrophy, hyperlipidaemia and insulin resistance in patients receiving HIV protease inhibitors. AIDS 1998;12:F51–8.

144. Brinkman K, Smeitink JA, Romijn JA, Reiss P. Mitochondrial toxicity induced by nucleoside-analogue reverse-transcriptase inhibitors is a key factor in the pathogenesis of antiretroviral-therapy-related lipodystrophy. Lancet 1999;354:1112–5.

145. Miserez AR, Muller PY, Barella L, Schwietert M, Erb P, Vernazza PL, Battegay M; Swiss HIV Cohort Study. A single-nucleotide polymorphism in the sterol-regulatory element-binding protein 1c gene is predictive of HIV-related hyperlipoproteinaemia. AIDS 2001;15:2045–9.

146. Moyle G. Mitochondrial toxicity hypothesis for lipoatrophy: a refutation. AIDS 2001;15:413–5.

147. Murata H, Hruz PW, Mueckler M. The mechanism of insulin resistance caused by HIV protease inhibitor therapy. J Biol Chem 2000;275:20251–4.

148. Liang JS, Distler O, Cooper DA, Jamil H, Deckelbaum RJ, Ginsberg HN, Sturley SL. HIV protease inhibitors protect apolipoprotein B from degradation by the proteasome: a potential mechanism for protease inhibitor-induced hyperlipidemia. Nature Med 2001;7:1327–31.

149. Miller RF, Shahmonesh M, Hanna MG, Unwin RJ, Schapira AH, Weller IV. Polyphenotypic expression of mitochondrial toxicity caused by nucleoside reverse transcriptase inhibitors. Antivir Ther 2003;8:253–7.

150. Nolan D, Hammond E, Martin A, Taylor L, Herrmann S, McKinnon E, Metcalf C, Latham B, Mallal S. Mitochondrial DNA depletion and morphologic changes in adipocytes associated with nucleoside reverse transcriptase inhibitor therapy. AIDS 2003;17:1329–38.

151. Birkus G, Hitchcock MJ, Cihlar T. Assessment of mitochondrial toxicity in human cells treated with tenofovir: comparison with other nucleoside reverse transcriptase inhibitors. Antimicrob Agents Chemother 2002;46:716–23.

152. Garcia-Benayas T, Blanco F, de la Cruz JJ, Soriano V, Gonzalez-Lahoz J. Replacing stavudine by abacavir reduces lactate levels and may improve lipoatrophy. AIDS 2003;17:921–4.

153. Arenas-Pinto A, Grant AD, Edwards S, Weller IV. Lactic acidosis in HIV infected patients: a systematic review of published cases. Sex Transm Infect 2003;79:340–3.

154. Tashima KT. Lipid changes in patients initiating efavirenz- and indinavir-based antiretroviral regimens. 2003;4:29–36.

155. Calza L, Manfredi R, Farneti B, Chiodo F. Incidence of hyperlipidaemia in a cohort of 212 HIV-infected patients receiving a protease inhibitor-based antiretroviral therapy. Int J Antimicrob Agents 2003;22:54–9.

156. Moyle GJ, Baldwin C, Langroudi B, Mandalia S, Gazzard BG. A 48-week, randomized, open-label comparison of three abacavir-based substitution approaches in the management of dyslipidemia and peripheral lipoatrophy. J Acquir Immune Defic Syndr 2003;33:22–8.

157. John M, McKinnon EJ, James IR, Nolan DA, Herrmann SE, Moore CB, White AJ, Mallal SA. Randomized, controlled, 48-week study of switching stavudine and/or

158. Lafeuillade A, Jolly P, Chadapaud S, Hittinger G, Lambry V, Philip G. Evolution of lipid abnormalities in patients switched from stavudine- to tenofovir-containing regimens. J Acquir Immune Defic Syndr 2003;33:544–6.

159. Domingo P, Sambeat MA, Perez A, Ordonez J, Rodriguez J, Vazquez G. Fat distribution and metabolic abnormalities in HIV-infected patients on first combination antiretroviral therapy including stavudine or zidovudine: role of physical activity as a protective factor. Antivir Ther 2003;8:223–31.

160. Carr A, Samaras K, Chisholm DJ, Cooper DA. Pathogenesis of HIV-1-protease inhibitor-associated peripheral lipodystrophy, hyperlipidaemia, and insulin resistance. Lancet 1998;351:1881–3.

161. Badiou S, De Boever CM, Dupuy AM, Baillat V, Cristol JP, Reynes J. Small dense LDL and atherogenic lipid profile in HIV-positive adults: influence of lopinavir/ritonavir-containing regimen. AIDS 2003;17:772–4.

162. Noor MA, Lo JC, Mulligan K, Schwarz JM, Halvorsen RA, Schambelan M, Grunfeld C. Metabolic effects of indinavir in healthy HIV-seronegative men. AIDS 2001;15:F11–18.

163. Brambilla AM, Novati R, Calori G, Meneghini E, Vacchini D, Luzi L, Castagna A, Lazzarin A. Stavudine or indinavir-containing regimens are associated with an increased risk of diabetes mellitus in HIV-infected individuals. AIDS 2003;17:1993–5.

164. Justman JE, Benning L, Danoff A, Minkoff H, Levine A, Greenblatt RM, Weber K, Piessens E, Robison E, Anastos K. Protease inhibitor use and the incidence of diabetes mellitus in a large cohort of HIV-infected women. J Acquir Immune Defic Syndr 2003;32:298–302.

165. Zabihi E, Abdollahi M. Endocrinotoxicity induced by Coriandrum sativa: a case report. WHO Drug Inf 2002;16:15.

166. Ruffatti A, Minervini L, Romano M, Sonino N. Galactorrhea with aripiprazole. Psychother Psychosom 2005;74:391–2.

167. Newton PN, Angus BJ, Chierakul W, Dondorp A, Ruangveerayuth R, Silamut K, Teerapong P, Suputtamongkol Y, Looareesuwan S, White NJ. Randomized comparison of artesunate and quinine in the treatment of severe falciparum malaria. Clin Infect Dis 2003;37:7–16.

168. Finsterer J, Haberler C, Schmiedel J. Deterioration of Kearns–Sayre syndrome following articaine administration for local anesthesia. Clin Neuropharmacol 2005;28(3):148–9.

169. Stehr SN, Oertel R, Schindler C, Hubler M. Re: deterioration of Kearns–Sayre syndrome following articaine administration for local anesthesia. Clin Neuropharmacol 2005;28(5):253.

170. Johnston CS, Yen MF. Megadose of vitamin C delays insulin response to a glucose challenge in normoglycemic adults. Am J Clin Nutr 1994;60(5):735–8.

171. Barness LA. Safety considerations with high ascorbic acid dosage. Ann NY Acad Sci 1975;258:523–8.

172. Meschi F, di Natale B, Rondanini GF, Uderzo C, Jankovic M, Masera G, Chiumello G. Pancreatic endocrine function in leukemic children treated with L-asparaginase. Horm Res 1981;15(4):237–41.

173. Rovira A, Cordido F, Vecilla C, Bernacer M, Valverde I, Herrera Pombo JL. Study of beta-cell function and

erythrocyte insulin receptors in a patient with diabetic ketoacidosis associated with L-asparaginase therapy. Acta Paediatr Scand 1986;75(4):670–1.

174. Hsu YJ, Chen YC, Ho CL, Kao WY, Chao TY. Diabetic ketoacidosis and persistent hyperglycemia as long-term complications of L-asparaginase-induced pancreatitis. Zhonghua Yi Xue Za Zhi (Taipei) 2002;65(9):441–5.

175. Uygur-Bayramicli O, Aydin D, Ak O, Karadayi N. Hyperprolactinemia caused by azathioprine. J Clin Gastroenterol 2003;36:79–80.

176. Bruno I, Pennesi M, Marchetti F. ACE-inhibitors-induced metabolic acidosis in a child with nephrotic syndrome. Pediatr Nephrol 2003;18:1293–4.

177. Pomara N, Willoughby LM, Ritchie JC, Sidtis JJ, Greenblatt DJ, Nemeroff CB. Interdose elevation in plasma cortisol during chronic treatment with alprazolam but not lorazepam in the elderly. Neuropsychopharmacology 2004;29: 605–11.

178. Thomas DJ, Gill B, Brown P, Stubbs WA. Salbutamol-induced diabetic ketoacidosis. BMJ 1977;2(6084):438.

179. Lee ST. Hyperprolactinemia, galactorrhea, and atenolol. Ann Intern Med 1992;116(6):522.

180. Harrower AD, Fyffe JA, Horn DB, Strong JA. Thyroxine and triiodothyronine levels in hyperthyroid patients during treatment with propranolol. Clin Endocrinol (Oxf) 1977;7(1):41–4.

181. Cooper DS, Daniels GH, Ladenson PW, Ridgway EC. Hyperthyroxinemia in patients treated with high-dose propranolol. Am J Med 1982;73(6):867–71.

182. Mooradian A, Morley JE, Simon G, Shafer RB. Propranolol-induced hyperthyroxinemia. Arch Intern Med 1983;143(11):2193–5.

183. Heyma P, Larkins RG, Higginbotham L, Ng KW. D-propranolol and DL-propranolol both decrease conversion of L-thyroxine to L-triiodothyronine. BMJ 1980;281(6232): 24–5.

184. Jones DK, Solomon S. Thyrotoxic crisis masked by treatment with beta-blockers. BMJ (Clin Res Ed) 1981;283(6292):659.

185. Bakris GL, Fonseca V, Katholi RE, McGill JB, Messerli FH, Phillips RA, Raskin P, Wright JT, Oakes R, Lukas MA, Anderson KM, Bell DSH, for the GEMINI Investigators. Metabolic effects of carvedilol vs metoprolol in patients with type 2 diabetes mellitus and hypertension. A randomized controlled trial. JAMA 2004;292:2227–36.

186. Gold LA, Merimee TJ, Misbin RI. Propranolol and hypoglycemia: the effects of beta-adrenergic blockade on glucose and alanine levels during fasting. J Clin Pharmacol 1980;20(1):50–8.

187. Uusitupa M, Aro A, Pietikainen M. Severe hypoglycaemia caused by physical strain and pindolol therapy. A case report. Ann Clin Res 1980;12(1):25–7.

188. Holm G, Herlitz J, Smith U. Severe hypoglycaemia during physical exercise and treatment with beta-blockers. BMJ (Clin Res Ed) 1981;282(6273):1360.

189. Zarate A, Gelfand M, Novello A, Knepshield J, Preuss HG. Propranolol-associated hypoglycemia in patients on maintenance hemodialysis. Int J Artif Organs 1981;4(3):130–4.

190. Belton P, O'Dwyer WF, Carmody M, Donohoe J. Propranolol associated hypoglycaemia in non-diabetics. Ir Med J 1980;73(4):173.

191. Chavez H, Ozolins D, Losek JD. Hypoglycemia and propranolol in pediatric behavioral disorders. Pediatrics 1999;103(6 Pt 1):1290–2.

192. Barnett AH, Leslie D, Watkins PJ. Can insulin-treated diabetics be given beta-adrenergic blocking drugs? BMJ 1980;280(6219):976–8.

193. Wright AD, Barber SG, Kendall MJ, Poole PH. Beta-adrenoceptor-blocking drugs and blood sugar control in diabetes mellitus. BMJ 1979;1(6157):159–61.

194. Davidson NM, Corrall RJ, Shaw TR, French EB. Observations in man of hypoglycaemia during selective and non-selective beta-blockade. Scott Med J 1977;22(1):69–72.

195. Deacon SP, Barnett D. Comparison of atenolol and propranolol during insulin-induced hypoglycaemia. BMJ 1976;2(6030):272–3.

196. Blohme G, Lager I, Lonnroth P, Smith U. Hypoglycemic symptoms in insulin-dependent diabetics. A prospective study of the influence of beta-blockade. Diabete Metab 1981;7(4):235–8.

197. Shepherd AM, Lin MS, Keeton TK. Hypoglycemia-induced hypertension in a diabetic patient on metoprolol. Ann Intern Med 1981;94(3):357–8.

198. Malmberg K, Ryden L, Hamsten A, Herlitz J, Waldenstrom A, Wedel H. Mortality prediction in diabetic patients with myocardial infarction: experiences from the DIGAMI study. Cardiovasc Res 1997;34(1):248–53.

199. MacDonald TM, Butler R, Newton RW, Morris AD. Which drugs benefit diabetic patients for secondary prevention of myocardial infarction? DARTS/MEMO Collaboration. Diabet Med 1998;15(4):282–9.

200. Samuelsson O, Hedner T, Berglund G, Persson B, Andersson OK, Wilhelmsen L. Diabetes mellitus in treated hypertension: incidence, predictive factors and the impact of non-selective beta-blockers and thiazide diuretics during 15 years treatment of middle-aged hypertensive men in the Primary Prevention Trial Goteborg, Sweden. J Hum Hypertens 1994;8(4):257–63.

201. Van Brammelen P. Lipid changes induced by beta-blockers. Curr Opin Cardiol 1988;3:513.

202. Bielmann P, Leduc G, Jequier JC, et al. Changes in the lipoprotein composition after chronic administration of metoprolol and propranolol in hypertriglyceridemic-hypertensive subjects. Curr Ther Res 1981;30:956.

203. Frishman WH, Kowalski M, Nagnur S, Warshafsky S, Sica D. Cardiovascular considerations in using topical, oral, and intravenous drugs for the treatment of glaucoma and ocular hypertension: focus on beta-adrenergic blockade. Heart Dis 2001;3(6):386–97.

204. Gavalas C, Costantino O, Zuppardi E, Scaramucci S, Doronzo E, Aharrh-Gnama A, Nubile M, Di Nuzzo S, De Nicola GC. Variazioni della colesterolemia in pazienti sottoposti a terapia topica con il timololo. Ann Ottalmol Clin Ocul 2001;127:9–14.

205. Northcote RJ. Beta blockers, lipids, and coronary atherosclerosis: fact or fiction? BMJ (Clin Res Ed) 1988;296(6624):731–2.

206. Neaton JD, Grimm RH Jr, Prineas RJ, Stamler J, Grandits GA, Elmer PJ, Cutler JA, Flack JM, Schoenberger JA, McDonald R, et al. Treatment of Mild Hypertension Study. Final results. Treatment of Mild Hypertension Study Research Group. JAMA 1993;270(6):713–24.

207. Astrup AV. Fedme og diabetes som bivirkninger til beta-blokkere. [Obesity and diabetes as side-effects of beta-blockers.] Ugeskr Laeger 1990;152(40):2905–8.

208. Connacher AA, Jung RT, Mitchell PE. Weight loss in obese subjects on a restricted diet given BRL 26830A, a

new atypical beta adrenoceptor agonist. BMJ (Clin Res Ed) 1988;296(6631):1217–20.

209. Wheeldon NM, McDevitt DG, McFarlane LC, Lipworth BJ. Do beta 3-adrenoceptors mediate metabolic responses to isoprenaline. Q J Med 1993;86(9):595–600.

210. Emorine LJ, Marullo S, Briend-Sutren MM, Patey G, Tate K, Delavier-Klutchko C, Strosberg AD. Molecular characterization of the human beta 3-adrenergic receptor. Science 1989;245(4922):1118–21.

211. Sharma AM, Pischon T, Hardt S, Kunz I, Luft FC. Hypothesis: Beta-adrenergic receptor blockers and weight gain: a systematic analysis. Hypertension 2001;37(2):250–4.

212. Silverstone BZ, Marcus T. [Hypoglycemia due to ophthalmic timolol in a diabetic.]Harefuah 1990;118(12):693–4.

213. Holme E, Greter J, Jacobson CE, Lindstedt S, Nordin I, Kristiansson B, Jodal U. Carnitine deficiency induced by pivampicillin and pivmecillinam therapy. Lancet 1989;2(8661):469–73.

214. Melegh B, Kerner J, Bieber LL. Pivampicillin-promoted excretion of pivaloylcarnitine in humans. Biochem Pharmacol 1987;36(20):3405–9.

215. Abrahamsson K, Eriksson BO, Holme E, Jodal U, Jonsson A, Lindstedt S. Pivalic acid-induced carnitine deficiency and physical exercise in humans. Metabolism 1996;45(12):1501–7.

216. Holme E, Jodal U, Linstedt S, Nordin I. Effects of pivalic acid-containing prodrugs on carnitine homeostasis and on response to fasting in children. Scand J Clin Lab Invest 1992;52(5):361–72.

217. Nakashima M, Kosuge K, Ishii I, Ohtsubo M. [Influence of multiple-dose administration of cefetamet pivoxil on blood and urinary concentrations of carnitine and effects of simultaneous administration of carnitine with cefetamet pivoxil.]Jpn J Antibiot 1996;49(10):966–79.

218. Melegh B, Pap M, Molnar D, Masszi G, Kopcsanyi G. Carnitine administration ameliorates the changes in energy metabolism caused by short-term pivampicillin medication. Eur J Pediatr 1997;156(10):795–9.

219. Siegal J, Jorgensen R, Angulo P, Lindor K. Treatment with ursodeoxycholic acid is associated with weight gain in patients with primary biliary cirrhosis. J Clinical Gastroenterol 2003;37:183–5.

220. Lancaster SG, Sorkin EM. Bisoprolol. A preliminary review of its pharmacodynamic and pharmacokinetic properties, and therapeutic efficacy in hypertension and angina pectoris. Drugs 1988;36(3):256–85.

221. Russell L. Disodium pamidronate. Aust Prescr 1999;22:30.

222. Damase-Michel C, Sarrail E, Laens J, et al. Hyponatraemia in a patient treated with bromocriptine. Drug Invest 1993;5:285–7.

223. Bellet S. Caffeine and serum cholesterol. JAMA 1966;196:229.

224. Jankelson OM, Beaser SB, Howard FM, Mayer J. Effect of coffee on glucose tolerance and circulating insulin in men with maturity-onset diabetes. Lancet 1967;1(7489):527–9.

225. Rocco S, Mantero F, Boscaro M. Effects of a calcium antagonist on the pituitary–adrenal axis. Horm Metab Res 1993;25(2):114–6.

226. Malaisse WJ, Sener A. Calcium-antagonists and islet function-XII. Comparison between nifedipine and chemically related drugs. Biochem Pharmacol 1981;30(10):1039–41.

227. Giugliano D, Gentile S, Verza M, Passariello N, Giannetti G, Varricchio M. Modulation by verapamil of insulin and glucagon secretion in man. Acta Diabetol Lat 1981;18(2):163–71.

228. Donnelly T, Harrower AD. Effect of nifedipine on glucose tolerance and insulin secretion in diabetic and non-diabetic patients. Curr Med Res Opin 1980;6(10):690–3.

229. Abadie E, Passa PH. Diabetogenic effect of nifedipine. BMJ (Clin Res Ed) 1984;289(6442):438.

230. Collings WCJ, Cullen MJ, Feely J. The effect of therapy with dihydropyridine calcium channel blockers on glucose tolerance in non-insulin dependent diabetes. Br J Clin Pharmacol 1986;21:568.

231. Zezulka AV, Gill JS, Beevers DG. Diabetogenic effects of nifedipine. BMJ (Clin Res Ed) 1984;289(6442):437–8.

232. Neaton JD, Grimm RH Jr, Prineas RJ, Stamler J, Grandits GA, Elmer PJ, Cutler JA, Flack JM, Schoenberger JA, McDonald R, et al. Treatment of Mild Hypertension Study. Final results. Treatment of Mild Hypertension Study Research Group. JAMA 1993;270(6):713–24.

233. Trost BN. Glucose metabolism and calcium antagonists. Horm Metab Res Suppl 1990;22:48–56.

234. Bhatnagar SK, Amin MMA, Al-Yusuf AR. Diabetogenic effects of nifedipine. BMJ (Clin Res Ed) 1984;289:19.

235. Kolodny RC, Masters WH, Kolodner RM, Toro G. Depression of plasma testosterone levels after chronic intensive marihuana use. N Engl J Med 1974;290(16):872–4.

236. Fried PA, Watkinson B, Willan A. Marijuana use during pregnancy and decreased length of gestation. Am J Obstet Gynecol 1984;150(1):23–7.

237. Isojarvi JI, Laatikainen TJ, Pakarinen AJ, Juntunen KT, Myllyla VV. Menstrual disorders in women with epilepsy receiving carbamazepine. Epilepsia 1995;36(7):676–81.

238. Stoffel-Wagner B, Bauer J, Flugel D, Brennemann W, Klingmuller D, Elger CE. Serum sex hormones are altered in patients with chronic temporal lobe epilepsy receiving anticonvulsant medication. Epilepsia 1998;39(11):1164–73.

239. Smith DB, Mattson RH, Cramer JA, Collins JF, Novelly RA, Craft B. Results of a nationwide Veterans Administration Cooperative Study comparing the efficacy and toxicity of carbamazepine, phenobarbital, phenytoin, and primidone. Epilepsia 1987;28(Suppl 3):S50–8.

240. Hogan RE, Bertrand ME, Deaton RL, Sommerville KW. Total percentage body weight changes during add-on therapy with tiagabine, carbamazepine and phenytoin. Epilepsy Res 2000;41(1):23–8.

241. Apeland T, Mansoor MA, Strandjord RE, Vefring H, Kristensen O. Folate, homocysteine and methionine loading in patients on carbamazepine. Acta Neurol Scand 2001;103(5):294–9.

242. Werner S, Brismar K, Olsson S. Hyperprolactinaemia and liquorice. Lancet 1979;1(8111):319.

243. Donat J, Jirkalova V, Havel V, Mikulecka D. Kotazce estrogenniho ucinku digitalisu u zen po menopauze. [On the question of the estrogenic effect of digitalis in women after menopause.] Cesk Gynekol 1980;45(1):19–23.

244. Burckhardt D, Vera CA, LaDue JS. Effect of digitalis on urinary pituitary gonadotrophine excretion. A study in postmenopausal women. Ann Intern Med 1968;68(5):1069–71.

245. Stoffer SS, Hynes KM, Jiang NS, Ryan RJ. Digoxin and abnormal serum hormone levels. JAMA 1973;225(13):1643–4.

246. Neri A, Aygen M, Zukerman Z, Bahary C. Subjective assessment of sexual dysfunction of patients on long-term administration of digoxin. Arch Sex Behav 1980;9(4):343–347.

247. LeWinn EB. Gynecomastia during digitalis therapy; report of eight additional cases with liver-function studies. N Engl J Med 1953;248(8):316–20.

248. Calov WL, Whyte MH. Oedema and mammary hypertrophy: a toxic effect of digitalis leaf. Med J Aust 1954;41(1:15):556–7.

249. Navab A, Koss LG, LaDue JS. Estrogen-like activity of digitalis: its effect on the squamous epithelium of the female genital tract. JAMA 1965;194(1):30–2.

250. Stenkvist B, Bengtsson E, Eklund G, Eriksson O, Holmquist J, Nordin B, Westman-Naeser S. Evidence of a modifying influence of heart glucosides on the development of breast cancer. Anal Quant Cytol 1980;2(1):49–54.

251. Stenkvist B, Pengtsson E, Dahlqvist B, Eriksson O, Jarkrans T, Nordin B. Cardiac glycosides and breast cancer, revisited. N Engl J Med 1982;306(8):484.

252. Haux J, Lam M, Marthinsen ABL, Strickert T, Lundgren S. Digitoxin, in non toxic concentrations, induces apoptotic cell death in Jurkat cells in vitro. Z Onkol 1999;31:14–20.

253. Haux J. Digitoxin is a potential anticancer agent for several types of cancer. Med Hypotheses 1999;53(6):543–8.

254. Haux J, Solheim O, Isaksen T, Anglesen A. Digitoxin, in non toxic concentrations, inhibits proliferation and induces cell death in prostate cancer cell line. Z Onkol 2000;32:11–6.

255. Nobel CS, Aronson JK, van den Dobbelsteen DJ, Slater AF. Inhibition of Na+/K(+)-ATPase may be one mechanism contributing to potassium efflux and cell shrinkage in CD95-induced apoptosis. Apoptosis 2000;5(2):153–63.

256. Johansson S, Lindholm P, Gullbo J, Larsson R, Bohlin L, Claeson P. Cytotoxicity of digitoxin and related cardiac glycosides in human tumor cells. Anticancer Drugs 2001;12(5):475–83.

257. Spigset O, Mjorndal T. Increased glucose intolerance related to digoxin treatment in patients with type 2 diabetes mellitus. J Intern Med 1999;246(4):419–22.

258. Hannerz J. Decrease of intracranial pressure and weight with digoxin in obesity. J Clin Pharmacol 2001;41(4):465–8.

259. Saif-Ali R, Al-Qirbi A, Al-Geiry A, AL-Habori M. Effect of *Catha edulis* on plasma glucose and C-peptide in both type 2 diabetics and non-diabetics. J Ethnopharmacol 2003;86(1):45–9.

260. Anonymous. Herbal medicine. Warning: found to contain chlordiazepoxide. WHO Pharm Newslett 2001;1:2–3.

261. Petersen CS, Thomsen K. High-dose hydroxychloroquine treatment of porphyria cutanea tarda. J Am Acad Dermatol 1992;26(4):614–9.

262. Kutz DC, Bridges AJ. Bullous rash and brown urine in a systemic lupus erythematosus patient treated with hydroxychloroquine. Arthritis Rheum 1995;38(3):440–3.

263. Baler GR. Porphyria precipitated by hydroxychloroquine treatment of systemic lupus erythematosus. Cutis 1976;17(1):96–8.

264. Lefort G, Haissaguerre M, Floro J, Beauffigeau P, Warin JF, Latapie JL. Hypoglycémies au cours de surdosages par un nouvel anti-arythmique: la cibenzoline; trois observations. [Hypoglycemia caused by overdose of a new anti-arrhythmia agent: cibenzoline. 3 cases.] Presse Méd 1988;17(14):687–91.

265. Jeandel C, Preiss MA, Pierson H, Penin F, Cuny G, Bannwarth B, Netter P. Hypoglycaemia induced by cibenzoline. Lancet 1988;1(8596):1232–3.

266. Gachot BA, Bezier M, Cherrier JF, Daubeze J. Cibenzoline and hypoglycaemia. Lancet 1988;2(8605):280.

267. Takada M, Fujita S, Katayama Y, Harano Y, Shibakawa M. The relationship between risk of hypoglycemia and use of cibenzoline and disopyramide. Eur J Clin Pharmacol 2000;56(4):335–42.

268. Ogimoto A, Hamada M, Saeki H, Hiasa G, Ohtsuka T, Hashida H, Hara Y, Okura T, Shigematsu Y, Hiwada K. Hypoglycemic syncope induced by a combination of cibenzoline and angiotensin converting enzyme inhibitor. Jpn Heart J 2001;42(2):255–9.

269. Jindal RM, Sidner RA, Milgrom ML. Post-transplant diabetes mellitus. The role of immunosuppression. Drug Saf 1997;16(4):242–57.

270. Copstein LA, Zelmanovitz T, Goncalves LF, Manfro RC. Posttransplant patients: diabetes mellitus in cyclosporine-treated renal allograft a case-control study. Transplant Proc 2004;36(4):882–3.

271. Raine AE, Carter R, Mann JI, Morris PJ. Adverse effect of cyclosporin on plasma cholesterol in renal transplant recipients. Nephrol Dial Transplant 1988;3(4):458–63.

272. Ballantyne CM, Podet EJ, Patsch WP, Harati Y, Appel V, Gotto AM Jr, Young JB. Effects of cyclosporine therapy on plasma lipoprotein levels. JAMA 1989;262(1):53–6.

273. Stiller MJ, Pak GH, Kenny C, Jondreau L, Davis I, Wachsman S, Shupack JL. Elevation of fasting serum lipids in patients treated with low-dose cyclosporine for severe plaque-type psoriasis. An assessment of clinical significance when viewed as a risk factor for cardiovascular disease. J Am Acad Dermatol 1992;27(3):434–8.

274. Grossman RM, Delaney RJ, Brinton EA, Carter DM, Gottlieb AB. Hypertriglyceridemia in patients with psoriasis treated with cyclosporine. J Am Acad Dermatol 1991;25(4):648–51.

275. Hricik DE. Posttransplant hyperlipidemia: the treatment dilemma. Am J Kidney Dis 1994;23(5):766–71.

276. Massy ZA. Hyperlipidemia and cardiovascular disease after organ transplantation. Transplantation 2001;72(Suppl 6):S13–5.

277. Webb AT, Reaveley DA, O'Donnell M, O'Connor B, Seed M, Brown EA. Does cyclosporin increase lipoprotein(a) concentrations in renal transplant recipients? Lancet 1993;341(8840):268–70 Hunt BJ, Parratt R, Rose M, Yacoub M. Does cyclosporin affect lipoprotein(a) concentrations? Lancet 1994;343(8889):119–20(see also).

278. Kuster GM, Drexel H, Bleisch JA, Rentsch K, Pei P, Binswanger U, Amann FW. Relation of cyclosporine blood levels to adverse effects on lipoproteins. Transplantation 1994;57(10):1479–83.

279. Claesson K, Mayer AD, Squifflet JP, Grabensee B, Eigler FW, Behrend M, Vanrenterghem Y, van Hooff J, Morales JM, Johnson RW, Buchholz B, Land W, Forsythe JL, Neumayer HH, Ericzon BG, Muhlbacher F. Lipoprotein patterns in renal transplant patients: a comparison between FK 506 and cyclosporine A patients. Transplant Proc 1998;30(4):1292–4.

280. McCune TR, Thacker LR II, Peters TG, Mulloy L, Rohr MS, Adams PA, Yium J, Light JA, Pruett T, Gaber AO, Selman SH, Jonsson J, Hayes JM, Wright FH Jr, Armata T, Blanton J, Burdick JF. Effects of tacrolimus on hyperlipidemia after successful renal transplantation: a Southeastern Organ Procurement Foundation multicenter clinical study. Transplantation 1998;65(1):87–92.

281. Lin HY, Rocher LL, McQuillan MA, Schmaltz S, Palella TD, Fox IH. Cyclosporine-induced hyperuricemia and gout. N Engl J Med 1989;321(5):287–92.

282. Burack DA, Griffith BP, Thompson ME, Kahl LE. Hyperuricemia and gout among heart transplant recipients receiving cyclosporine. Am J Med 1992;92(2):141–6.

283. Ben Hmida M, Hachicha J, Bahloul Z, Kaddour N, Kharrat M, Jarraya F, Jarraya A. Cyclosporine-induced hyperuricemia and gout in renal transplants. Transplant Proc 1995;27(5):2722–4.

284. Pomare EW. Hyperosmolar non-ketotic diabetes and cimetidine. Lancet 1978;1(8075):1202.

285. Miller NE, Lewis B. Cimetidine and HDL cholesterol. Lancet 1983;1(8323):529–30.

286. Emmett M, Narins RG. Clinical use of the anion gap. Medicine (Baltimore) 1977;56(1):38–54.

287. Oh MS, Carroll HJ. The anion gap. N Engl J Med 1977;297(15):814–7.

288. DeMars CS, Hollister K, Tomassoni A, Himmelfarb J, Halperin ML. Citric acid ingestion: a life-threatening cause of metabolic acidosis. Ann Emerg Med 2001;38(5):588–91.

289. Jones RB, Luscombe DK, Groom GV. Plasma prolactin concentrations in normal subjects and depressive patients following oral clomipramine. Postgrad Med J 1977;53(Suppl. 4):166–71.

290. Morris AH, Harrington MH, Churchill DL, Olshan JS. Growth hormone stimulation testing with oral clonidine: 90 minutes is the preferred duration for the assessment of growth hormone reserve. J Pediatr Endocrinol Metab 2001;14(9):1657–60.

291. Houston MC. Clonidine hydrochloride. South Med J 1982;75(6):713–9.

292. Popli AP, Konicki PE, Jurjus GJ, Fuller MA, Jaskiw GE. Clozapine and associated diabetes mellitus. J Clin Psychiatry 1997;58(3):108–11.

293. Wirshing DA, Spellberg BJ, Erhart SM, Marder SR, Wirshing WC. Novel antipsychotics and new onset diabetes. Biol Psychiatry 1998;44(8):778–83.

294. Rigalleau V, Gatta B, Bonnaud S, Masson M, Bourgeois ML, Vergnot V, Gin H. Diabetes as a result of atypical anti-psychotic drugs—a report of three cases. Diabet Med 2000;17(6):484–6.

295. Wehring H, Alexander B, Perry PJ. Diabetes mellitus associated with clozapine therapy. Pharmacotherapy 2000;20(7):844–7.

296. Melkersson K, Hulting AL. Recovery from new-onset diabetes in a schizophrenic man after withdrawal of olanzapine. Psychosomatics 2002;43(1):67–70.

297. Colli A, Cocciolo M, Francobandiera F, Rogantin F, Cattalini N. Diabetic ketoacidosis associated with clozapine treatment. Diabetes Care 1999;22(1):176–7.

298. Chae BJ, Kang BJ. The effect of clozapine on blood glucose metabolism. Hum Psychopharmacol 2001;16(3):265–71.

299. Hagg S, Joelsson L, Mjorndal T, Spigset O, Oja G, Dahlqvist R. Prevalence of diabetes and impaired glucose tolerance in patients treated with clozapine compared with patients treated with conventional depot neuroleptic medications. J Clin Psychiatry 1998;59(6):294–9.

300. Yazici KM, Erbas T, Yazici AH. The effect of clozapine on glucose metabolism. Exp Clin Endocrinol Diabetes 1998;106(6):475–7.

301. Wang PS, Glynn RJ, Ganz DA, Schneeweiss S, Levin R, Avorn J. Clozapine use and risk of diabetes mellitus. J Clin Psychopharmacol 2002;22(3):236–43.

302. Frankenburg FR, Zanarini MC, Kando J, Centorrino F. Clozapine and body mass change. Biol Psychiatry 1998;43(7):520–4.

303. Bromel T, Blum WF, Ziegler A, Schulz E, Bender M, Fleischhaker C, Remschmidt H, Krieg JC, Hebebrand J. Serum leptin levels increase rapidly after initiation of clozapine therapy. Mol Psychiatry 1998;3(1):76–80.

304. Baymiller SP, Ball P, McMahon RP, Buchanan RW. Weight and blood pressure change during clozapine treatment. Clin Neuropharmacol 2002;25(4):202–6.

305. Feldman D, Goldberg JF. A preliminary study of the relationship between clozapine-induced weight gain and menstrual irregularities in schizophrenic, schizoaffective, and bipolar women. Ann Clin Psychiatry 2002;14(1):17–21.

306. Wirshing DA, Pierre JM, Wirshing WC. Sleep apnea associated with antipsychotic-induced obesity. J Clin Psychiatry 2002;63(4):369–70.

307. Borovicka MC, Fuller MA, Konicki PE, White JC, Steele VM, Jaskiw GE. Phenylpropanolamine appears not to promote weight loss in patients with schizophrenia who have gained weight during clozapine treatment. J Clin Psychiatry 2002;63(4):345–8.

308. Dursun SM, Devarajan S. Clozapine weight gain, plus topiramate weight loss. Can J Psychiatry 2000;45(2):198.

309. Ferko N, Levine MA. Evaluation of the association between St. John's wort and elevated thyroid-stimulating hormone. Pharmacotherapy 2001;21(12):1574–8.

310. Vescovi PP. Cardiovascular and hormonal responses to hyperthermic stress in cocaine addicts after a long period of abstinence. Addict Biol 2000;5:91–5.

311. Cohen S. Reinforcement and rapid delivery systems: understanding adverse consequences of cocaine. NIDA Res Monogr 1985;61:151–7.

312. Peters RS, Lehman TJ, Schwabe AD. Colchicine use for familial Mediterranean fever. Observations associated with long-term treatment. West J Med 1983;138(1):43–6.

313. Jenner C, Filshie J. Galactorrhoea following acupuncture. Acupunct Med 2002;20(2–3):107–8.

314. Walters MB. The relationship between thyroid function and anticoagulant thrapy. Am J Cardiol 1963;11:112–4.

315. Christensen F. Uricosuric effect of dicoumarol. Acta Med Scand 1964;175:461–8.

316. Basch E, Gabardi S, Ulbricht C. Bitter melon (*Momordica charantia*): a review of efficacy and safety. Am J Health Syst Pharm 2003;60(4):356–9.

317. Nord C, Fossa SD, Egeland T. Excessive annual BMI increase after chemotherapy among young survivors of testicular cancer. Br J Cancer 2003;88:36–41.

318. Perrone L, Sinisi AA, Tullio M, et al. Endocrine function in subjects treated for childhood Hodgkin's disease. J Pediatr Endocrinol 1989;3:175.

319. Kelly WK, Curley T, Slovin S, Heller G, McCaffrey J, Bajorin D, Ciolino A, Regan K, Schwartz M, Kantoff P, George D, Oh W, Smith M, Kaufman D, Small EJ, Schwartz L, Larson S, Tong W, Scher H. Paclitaxel, estramustine phosphate, and carboplatin in patients with advanced prostate cancer. J Clin Oncol 2001;19(1):44–53.

320. Halonen P, Salo MK, Makipernaa A. Fasting hypoglycemia is common during maintenance therapy for childhood acute lymphoblastic leukemia. J Pediatr 2001;138(3):428–31.

321. Kantarjian HM, Gandhi V, Kozuch P, Faderl S, Giles F, Cortes J, O' Brien S, Ibrahim N, Khuri F, Du M, Rios MB, Jeha S, McLaughlin P, Plunkett W, Keating M. Phase I clinical and pharmacology study of clofarabine in patients

with solid and hematologic cancers. J Clin Oncol 2003;6:1167–73.

322. Castro MP, VanAuken J, Spencer-Cisek P, Legha S, Sponzo RW. Acute tumor lysis syndrome associated with concurrent biochemotherapy of metastatic melanoma: a case report and review of the literature. Cancer 1999;85(5):1055–9.

323. Akasheh MS, Chang CP, Vesole DH. Acute tumour lysis syndrome: a case in AL amyloidosis. Br J Haematol 1999;107(2):387.

324. Konrad D, Sobetzko D, Schmitt B, Schoenle EJ. Insulin-dependent diabetes mellitus induced by the antitussive agent dextromethorphan. Diabetologia 2000;43(2):261–2.

325. Molnar E, Varadi A, McIlhinney RA, Ashcroft SJ. Identification of functional ionotropic glutamate receptor proteins in pancreatic beta-cells and in islets of Langerhans. FEBS Lett 1995;371(3):253–7.

326. Cooley S, Lalchandani S, Keane D. Heroin overdose in pregnancy: an unusual case report. J Obstet Gynaecol 2002;22(2):219–20.

327. Pomara N, Willoughby LM, Sidtis J, Cooper TB, Greenblatt DJ. Cortisol response to diazepam: its relationship to age, dose, duration of treatment and presence of generalised anxiety disorder. Psychopharmacology 2005;178:1–8.

328. Bergman D, Futterweit W, Segal R, Sirota D. Increased oestradiol in diazepam-related gynaecomastia. Lancet 1981;2(8257):1225–6.

329. Low LC, Yu EC, Chow OK, Yeung CY, Young RT. Hyperinsulinism in infancy. Aust Paediatr J 1989;25(3):174–7.

330. Abu-Osba YK, Manasra KB, Mathew PM. Complications of diazoxide treatment in persistent neonatal hyperinsulinism. Arch Dis Child 1989;64(10):1496–500.

331. Otsu T, Ito T, Inagaki Y, Amano I, Masamoto S, Niwa M. [Accumulation of a disopyramide metabolite in renal failure.]Nippon Jinzo Gakkai Shi 1993;35(9):1065–71Asaio J 1993;39:M609–13.

332. Series C. Hypoglycémie induite ou favorisée par le disopyramide. [Hypoglycemia induced or facilitated by disopyramide.] Rev Med Interne 1988;9(5):528–9.

333. Hasegawa J, Mori A, Yamamoto R, Kinugawa T, Morisawa T, Kishimoto Y. Disopyramide decreases the fasting serum glucose level in man. Cardiovasc Drugs Ther 1999;13(4):325–7.

334. Reynolds RM, Walker JD. Hypoglycaemia induced by disopyramide in a patient with Type 2 diabetes mellitus. Diabet Med 2001;18(12):1009–10.

335. Hoes AW, Grobbee DE, Lubsen J, Man in't Veld AJ, van der Does E, Hofman A. Diuretics, beta-blockers, and the risk for sudden cardiac death in hypertensive patients. Ann Intern Med 1995;123(7):481–7.

336. Siscovick DS, Raghunathan TE, Psaty BM, Koepsell TD, Wicklund KG, Lin X, Cobb L, Rautaharju PM, Copass MK, Wagner EH. Diuretic therapy for hypertension and the risk of primary cardiac arrest. N Engl J Med 1994;330(26):1852–7.

337. Samuelsson O, Pennert K, Andersson O, Berglund G, Hedner T, Persson B, Wedel H, Wilhelmsen L. Diabetes mellitus and raised serum triglyceride concentration in treated hypertension—are they of prognostic importance? Observational study. BMJ 1996;313(7058):660–3.

338. Kramer BK, Schweda F, Riegger GA. Diuretic treatment and diuretic resistance in heart failure. Am J Med 1999;106(1):90–6.

339. Kaplan NM. How bad are diuretic-induced hypokalemia and hypercholesterolemia? Arch Intern Med 1989;149(12):2649.

340. Weinberger MH. Selection of drugs for initial treatment of hypertension. Pract Cardiol 1989;15:81.

341. McInnes GT, Yeo WW, Ramsay LE, Moser M. Cardiotoxicity and diuretics: much speculation—little substance. J Hypertens 1992;10(4):317–35.

342. Moser M. In defense of traditional antihypertensive therapy. Hypertension 1988;12(3):324–6.

343. Thompson WG. An assault on old friends: thiazide diuretics under siege. Am J Med Sci 1990;300(3):152–8.

344. Anonymous. Potassium-sparing diuretics—when are they really needed. Drug Ther Bull 1985;23(5):17–20.

345. Ramsay LE, Yeo WW, Jackson PR. Diabetes, impaired glucose tolerance and insulin resistance with diuretics. Eur Heart J 1992;13(Suppl G):68–71.

346. Saunders A, Wilson SM. Do diuretics differ in degree of hypokalaemia, and does it matter? Aust J Hosp Pharm 1991;21:120–1.

347. Carlsen JE, Kober L, Torp-Pedersen C, Johansen P. Relation between dose of bendrofluazide, antihypertensive effect, and adverse biochemical effects. BMJ 1990;300(6730):975–8.

348. McVeigh GE, Dulie EB, Ravenscroft A, Galloway DB, Johnston GD. Low and conventional dose cyclopenthiazide on glucose and lipid metabolism in mild hypertension. Br J Clin Pharmacol 1989;27(4):523–6.

349. Ramsay LE, Yeo WW, Jackson PR. Influence of diuretics, calcium antagonists, and alpha-blockers on insulin sensitivity and glucose tolerance in hypertensive patients. J Cardiovasc Pharmacol 1992;20(Suppl 11):S49–54.

350. Weinberger MH. Mechanisms of diuretic effects on carbohydrate tolerance, insulin sensitivity and lipid levels. Eur Heart J 1992;13(Suppl G):5–9.

351. Savage PJ, Pressel SL, Curb JD, Schron EB, Applegate WB, Black HR, Cohen J, Davis BR, Frost P, Smith W, Gonzalez N, Guthrie GP, Oberman A, Rutan G, Probstfield JL, Stamler J. Influence of long-term, low-dose, diuretic-based, antihypertensive therapy on glucose, lipid, uric acid, and potassium levels in older men and women with isolated systolic hypertension: The Systolic Hypertension in the Elderly Program. SHEP Cooperative Research Group. Arch Intern Med 1998;158(7):741–51.

352. Green TP, Johnson DE, Bass JL, Landrum BG, Ferrara TB, Thompson TR. Prophylactic furosemide in severe respiratory distress syndrome: blinded prospective study. J Pediatr 1988;112(4):605–12.

353. Johnston GD. Treatment of hypertension in older adults. BMJ 1992;304:639.

354. Moser M. Diuretics and cardiovascular risk factors. Eur Heart J 1992;13(Suppl G):72–80.

355. Verdecchia P, Reboldi G, Angeli F, Borgioni C, Gattobigio R, Filippucci L, Norgiolini S, Bracco C, Porcellati C. Adverse prognostic significance of new diabetes in treated hypertensive subjects. Hypertension 2004;43(5):963–9.

356. Moser M. Diuretics should continue to be recommended as initial therapy in the treatment of hypertension. In: Puschett JB, Greenberg A, editors. Diuretics IV: Chemistry, Pharmacology and Clinical Applications. Amsterdam: Elsevier, 1993:465–76.

357. Moser M. Do different hemodynamic effects of antihypertensive drugs translate into different safety profiles? Eur J Clin Pharmacol 1990;38(Suppl 2):S134–8.

358. Waller PC, Ramsay LE. Predicting acute gout in diuretic-treated hypertensive patients. J Hum Hypertens 1989;3(6):457–61.

359. McVeigh G, Galloway D, Johnston D. The case for low dose diuretics in hypertension: comparison of low and conventional doses of cyclopenthiazide. BMJ 1988;297(6641):95–8.

360. Franse LV, Pahor M, Di Bari M, Shorr RI, Wan JY, Somes GW, Applegate WB. Serum uric acid, diuretic treatment and risk of cardiovascular events in the Systolic Hypertension in the Elderly Program (SHEP). J Hypertens 2000;18(8):1149–54.

361. Alderman MH, Cohen H, Madhavan S, Kivlighn S. Serum uric acid and cardiovascular events in successfully treated hypertensive patients. Hypertension 1999;34(1):144–50.

362. Freis ED, Papademetriou V. How dangerous are diuretics? Drugs 1985;30(6):469–74.

363. Spence JD. Effects of antihypertensive drugs on atherogenic factors: possible importance of drug selection in prevention of atherosclerosis. J Cardiovasc Pharmacol 1985;7(Suppl 2):S121–5.

364. Medical Research Council Working Party. MRC trial of treatment of mild hypertension: principal results. BMJ (Clin Res Ed) 1985;291(6488):97–104.

365. Wilhelmsen L, Berglund G, Elmfeldt D, Fitzsimons T, Holzgreve H, Hosie J, Hornkvist PE, Pennert K, Tuomilehto J, Wedel H. Beta-blockers versus diuretics in hypertensive men: main results from the HAPPHY trial. J Hypertens 1987;5(5):561–72.

366. Weinberger MH. Antihypertensive therapy and lipids. Evidence, mechanisms, and implications. Arch Intern Med 1985;145(6):1102–5.

367. Weidmann P, Ferrier C, Saxenhofer H, Uehlinger DE, Trost BN. Serum lipoproteins during treatment with antihypertensive drugs. Drugs 1988;35(Suppl 6):118–34.

368. Falch DK, Schreiner A. The effect of spironolactone on lipid, glucose and uric acid levels in blood during long-term administration to hypertensives. Acta Med Scand 1983;213(1):27–30.

369. Grimm RH Jr, Grandits GA, Prineas RJ, McDonald RH, Lewis CE, Flack JM, Yunis C, Svendsen K, Liebson PR, Elmer PJ, Stamler J. Long-term effects on sexual function of five antihypertensive drugs and nutritional hygienic treatment in hypertensive men and women. Treatment of Mild Hypertension Study (TOMHS). Hypertension 1997;29(1 Pt 1):8–14.

370. MacMahon SW, Macdonald GJ, Blacket RB. Plasma lipoprotein levels in treated and untreated hypertensive men and women. The National Heart Foundation of Australia Risk Factor Prevalence Study. Arteriosclerosis 1985;5(4):391–6.

371. Wallace RB, Hunninghake DB, Chambless LE, Heiss G, Wahl P, Barrett-Connor E. A screening survey of dyslipoproteinemias associated with prescription drug use. The Lipid Research Clinics Program Prevalence Study. Circulation 1986;73(1 Pt 2):I70–9.

372. Obermayr RP, Mayerhofer L, Knechtelsorfer M, Mersich N, Huber ER, Geyer G, Trgl K-H. The age-related downregulation of the growth hormone/insulin-like growth factor-1 axis in the elderly male is reversed considerably by donepezil, a drug for Alzheimer's disease. Exp Gerontol 2005;40:157–63.

373. Odeh M, Oliven A. Doxycycline-induced hypoglycemia. J Clin Pharmacol 2000;40(10):1173–4.

374. Basaria S, Braga M, Moore WT. Doxycycline-induced hypoglycemia in a nondiabetic young man. South Med J 2002;95(11):1353–4.

375. Haas DW, Fessel WJ, Delapenha RA, Kessler H, Seekins D, Kaplan M, Ruiz NM, Ploughman LM, Labriola DF, Manion DJ. Therapy with efavirenz plus indinavir in patients with extensive prior nucleoside reverse-transcriptase inhibitor experience: a randomized, double-blind, placebo-controlled trial. J Infect Dis 2001;183(3):392–400.

376. Manfredi R, Calza L, Chiodo F. An extremely different dysmetabolic profile between the two available nonnucleoside reverse transcriptase inhibitors: efavirenz and nevirapine. J Acquir Immune Defic Syndr 2005;38(2):236–8.

377. Castrillon JL, Mediavilla A, Mendez MA, Cavada E, Carrascosa M, Valle R. Syndrome of inappropriate antidiuretic hormone secretion (SIADH) and enalapril. J Intern Med 1993;233(1):89–91.

378. Fernandez Fernandez FJ, De la Fuente AJ, Vazquez TL, Perez FS. Síndrome de secreción inadecuada de hormona antidiurética causado por enalapril. Med Clin (Barc) 2004;123(4):159.

379. Winter WE, Funahashi M, Koons J. Encainide-induced diabetes: analysis of islet cell function. Res Commun Chem Pathol Pharmacol 1992;76(3):259–68.

380. Oyama T, Taniguchi K, Ishihara H, Matsuki A, Maeda A, Murakawa T, Kudo T. Effects of enflurane anaesthesia and surgery on endocrine function in man. Br J Anaesth 1979;51(2):141–8.

381. Buzaleh AM, Enriquez de Salamanca R, Batlle AM. Porphyrinogenic properties of the anesthetic enflurane. Gen Pharmacol 1992;23(4):665–9.

382. Wilson BE, Hobbs WN. Case report: pseudoephedrine-associated thyroid storm: thyroid hormone—catecholamine interactions. Am J Med Sci 1993;306(5):317–9.

383. Rigalleau V, Blanchetier V, Aparicio M, Baillet L, Sneed J, Dabadie H, Gin H. Erythropoietin can deteriorate glucose control in uraemic non-insulin-dependent diabetic patients. Diabetes Metab 1998;24(1):62–5.

384. Russell RP, Lindeman RD, Prescott LF. Metabolic and hypotensive effects of ethacrynic acid. Comparative study with hydrochlorothiazide. JAMA 1968;205(1):81–5.

385. Cowley AJ, Elkeles RS. Diabetes and therapy with potent diuretics. Lancet 1978;1(8056):154.

386. Maher JF, Schreiner GE. Studies on ethacrynic acid in patients with refractory edema. Ann Intern Med 1965;62:15–29.

387. Melvin KE, Farrelly RO, North JD. Ethacrynic acid: a new oral diuretic. BMJ 1963;5344:1521–4.

388. Allanore Y, Bremont C, Kahan A, Menkes CJ. Transient hyperthyroidism in a patient with rheumatoid arthritis treated by etanercept. Clin Exp Rheumatol 2001;19(3):356–7.

389. Bloom BJ. Development of diabetes mellitus during etanercept therapy in a child with systemic-onset juvenile rheumatoid arthritis. Arthritis Rheum 2000;43(11):2606–8.

390. Khanna BK, Gupta VP, Singh MP. Ethambutol-induced hyperuricaemia. Tubercle 1984;65(3):195–9.

391. Mandell GL, Sande MA. Antimicrobial agents: drugs used in the chemotherapy of tuberculosis and leprosy. In: Goodman Gilman A, Rall TW, Nies AS, Taylor P, editors.

Goodman and Gilman's The Pharmacological Basis of Therapeutics. 8th ed.. New York: Pergamon Press, 1990:1146 Chapter 49.

392. Khanna BK. Acute gouty arthritis following ethambutol therapy. Br J Dis Chest 1980;74(4):409–10.

393. Moulding T, Fraser R. Hypothyroidism related to ethionamide. Am Rev Respir Dis 1970;101(1):90–4.

394. Drucker D, Eggo MC, Salit IE, Burrow GN. Ethionamide-induced goitrous hypothyroidism. Ann Intern Med 1984;100(6):837–9.

395. Danan G, Pessayre D, Larrey D, Benhamou JP. Pyrazinamide fulminant hepatitis: an old hepatotoxin strikes again. Lancet 1981;2(8254):1056–7.

396. Filla E, Comenale D. La terapia con PAS, rifamicina ed etionamide per via endovenosa e sue ripercussioni sul ricambio glucidico in diabetici affetti da tubercolosi polmonare. [Therapy with PAS, rifamycin and ethionamide administered intravenously and its effects on glucide metabolism in diabetics affected by pulmonary tuberculosis.] Minerva Med 1965;56(103):4570–3.

397. Wagner RL, White PF, Kan PB, Rosenthal MH, Feldman D. Inhibition of adrenal steroidogenesis by the anesthetic etomidate. N Engl J Med 1984;310:1415–21.

398. Malerba G, Romano-Girard F, Cravoisy A, Dousset B, Nace L, Lévy B, Bollaert PE. Risk factors of relative adrenocortical deficiency in intensive care patients needing mechanical ventilation. Intensive Care Med 2005;31:388–92.

399. Jackson WL Jr. Should we use etomidate as an induction agent for endotracheal intubation in patients with septic shock? A critical appraisal. Chest 2005;127:1031–8.

400. Annane D. ICU physicians should abandon the use of etomidate! Intensive Care Med 2005;31:325–6.

401. Morris C, McAllister C. Etomidate for emergency anaesthesia: mad, bad and dangerous to know? Anaesthesia 2005;60(8):737–40.

402. Schenarts CL, Burton JH, Riker RR. Adrenocortical dysfunction following etomidate induction in emergency department patients. Acad Emerg Med 2001;8(1):1–7.

403. Weber MM, Lang J, Abedinpour F, Zeilberger K, Adelmann B, Engelhardt D. Different inhibitory effect of etomidate and ketoconazole on the human adrenal steroid biosynthesis. Clin Investig 1993;71(11):933–8.

404. Varga I, Racz K, Kiss R, Futo L, Toth M, Sergev O, Glaz E. Direct inhibitory effect of etomidate on corticosteroid secretion in human pathologic adrenocortical cells. Steroids 1993;58(2):64–8.

405. Vanacker B, Wiebalck A, Van Aken H, Sermeus L, Bouillon R, Amery A. Induktionsqualität und Nebennierenrindenfunktion. Ein klinischer Vergleich von Etomidat-Lipuro und Hypnomidate. [Quality of induction and adrenocortical function. A clinical comparison of Etomidate-Lipuro and Hypnomidate.] Anaesthesist 1993;42(2):81–9.

406. Crozier TA, Flamm C, Speer CP, Rath W, Wuttke W, Kuhn W, Kettler D. Effects of etomidate on the adrenocortical and metabolic adaptation of the neonate. Br J Anaesth 1993;70(1):47–53.

407. Deters M, Kirchner G, Koal T, Resch K, Kaever V. Everolimus/cyclosporine interactions on bile flow and biliary excretion of bile salts and cholesterol in rats. Dig Dis Sci 2004;49(1):30–7.

408. Oltmanns KM, Fehm HL, Peters A. Chronic fentanyl application induces adrenocortical insufficiency. J Intern Med 2005;257(5):478–80.

409. Albert SG, DeLeon MJ, Silverberg AB. Possible association between high-dose fluconazole and adrenal insufficiency in critically ill patients. Crit Care Med 2001;29(3):668–70.

410. Shibata S, Kami M, Kanda Y, Machida U, Iwata H, Kishi Y, Takeshita A, Miyakoshi S, Ueyama J, Morinaga S, Mutou Y. Acute adrenal failure associated with fluconazole after administration of high-dose cyclophosphamide. Am J Hematol 2001;66(4):303–5.

411. Magill SS, Puthanakit T, Swoboda SM, Carson KA, Salvatori R, Lipsett PA, Hendrix CW. Impact of fluconazole prophylaxis on cortisol levels in critically ill surgical Patients. Antimicrob Agents Chemother 2004;48:2471–6.

412. Strohle A, Wiedemann K. Flumazenil attenuates the pituitary response to CRH in healthy males. Eur Neuropsychopharmacol 1996;6(4):323–5.

413. Mohr JF, McKinnon PS, Peymann PJ, Kenton I, Septimus E, Okhuysen PC. A retrospective, comparative evaluation of dysglycemias in hospitalized patients receiving gatifloxacin, levofloxacin, ciprofloxacin, or ceftriaxone. Pharmacotherapy 2005;25(10):1303–9.

414. Sadoff L. Overwhelming 5-fluorouracil toxicity in patients whose diabetes is poorly controlled. Am J Clin Oncol 1998;21(6):605–7.

415. Yeh KH, Cheng AL. High-dose 5-fluorouracil infusional therapy is associated with hyperammonaemia, lactic acidosis and encephalopathy. Br J Cancer 1997;75(3):464–5.

416. Valik D, Yeh KH, Cheng AL. Encephalopathy, lactic acidosis, hyperammonaemia and 5-fluorouracil toxicity. Br J Cancer 1998;77(10):1710–2.

417. Jalil P. Toxic reaction following the combined administration of fluoxetine and phenytoin: two case reports. J Neurol Neurosurg Psychiatry 1992;55(5):412–3.

418. Fawcett J, Zajecka JM, Kravitz HM, et al. Fluoxetine versus amitriptyline in adult outpatients with major depression. Psychiatry Res 1989;45:821.

419. Peterson MC. Reversible galactorrhea and prolactin elevation related to fluoxetine use. Mayo Clin Proc 2001;76(2):215–6.

420. Schmutz JL, Barbaud A, Trechot P. Flutamide et pseudoporphyrie. [Flutamide and pseudoporphyria.] Ann Dermatol Venereol 1999;126(4):374.

421. Borroni G, Brazzelli V, Baldini F, Borghini F, Gaviglio MR, Beltrami B, Nolli G. Flutamide-induced pseudoporphyria. Br J Dermatol 1998;138(4):711–2.

422. Mantoux F, Bahadoran P, Perrin C, Bermon C, Lacour JP, Ortonne JP. Pseudo-porphyrie cutanée tardive induite par le flutamide. [Flutamide-induced late cutaneous pseudoporphyria.] Ann Dermatol Venereol 1999;126(2):150–2.

423. Peterson MC. Reversible galactorrhea and prolactin elevation related to fluoxetine use. Mayo Clin Proc 2001;76(2):215–6.

424. Morrison J, Remick RA, Leung M, Wrixon KJ, Bebb RA. Galactorrhea induced by paroxetine. Can J Psychiatry 2001;46(1):88–9.

425. Batstone GF, Alberti KG, Dewar AK. Reversible lactic acidosis associated with repeated intravenous infusions of sorbitol and ethanol. Postgrad Med J 1977;53(623):567–9.

426. Coarse JF, Cardoni AA. Use of fructose in the treatment of acute alcoholic intoxication. Am J Hosp Pharm 1975;32(5):518–9.

427. Palyza V, Bockova M. Poruchy metabolismu fruktozy a infuze. [Fructose metabolism disorders and infusions.] Vnitr Lek 1992;38(8):814–21.

428. Decaux G, Waterlot Y, Genette F, Hallemans R, Demanet JC. Inappropriate secretion of antidiuretic hormone treated with frusemide. BMJ (Clin Res Ed) 1982;285(6335):89–90.

429. Frye MA, Luckenbaugh D, Kimbrell TA, Constantino C, Grothe D, Cora-Locatelli G, Ketter TA. Possible gabapentin-induced thyroiditis. J Clin Psychopharmacol 1999;19(1):94–5.

430. DeToledo JC, Toledo C, DeCerce J, Ramsay RE. Changes in body weight with chronic, high-dose gabapentin therapy. Ther Drug Monit 1997;19(4):394–6.

431. Fischler B, Casswall TH, Malmborg P, Nemeth A. Ganciclovir treatment in infants with cytomegalovirus infection and cholestasis. J Pediatr Gastroenterol Nutr 2002;34(2):154–7.

432. Gajjar DA, LaCreta FP, Kollia GD, Stolz RR, Berger S, Smith WB, Swingle M, Grasela DM. Effect of multiple-dose gatifloxacin or ciprofloxacin on glucose homeostasis and insulin production in patients with noninsulin-dependent diabetes mellitus maintained with diet and exercise. Pharmacotherapy 2000;20(6 Pt 2):S76–86.

433. Happe MR, Mulhall BP, Maydonovitch CL, Holtzmuller KC. Gatifloxacin-induced hyperglycemia. Ann Intern Med 2004;141(12):968–9.

434. Khovidhunkit W, Sunthornyothin S. Hypoglycemia, hyperglycemia, and gatifloxacin. Ann Intern Med 2004;141(12):969.

435. Arce FC, Bhasin RS, Pasmantier R. Severe hyperglycemia during gatifloxacin therapy in patients without diabetes. Endocr Pract 2004;10(1):40–4.

436. Saraya A, Yokokura M, Gonoi T, Seino S. Effects of fluoroquinolones on insulin secretion and beta-cell ATP-sensitive K+ channels. Eur J Pharmacol 2004;497(1):111–7.

437. Frothingham R. Glucose homeostasis abnormalities associated with use of gatifloxacin. Clin Infect Dis 2005;41(9):1269–76.

438. Pichichero ME, Arguedas A, Dagan R, Sher L, Saez-Llorens X, Hamed K, Echols R. Safety and efficacy of gatifloxacin therapy for children with recurrent acute otitis media (AOM) and/or AOM treatment failure. Clin Infect Dis 2005;41(4):470–8.

439. Brogan SE, Cahalan MK. Gatifloxacin as a possible cause of serious postoperative hypoglycemia. Anesth Analg 2005;101(3):635–6.

440. Blommel AL, Lutes RA. Severe hyperglycemia during renally adjusted gatifloxacin therapy. Ann Pharmacother 2005;39(7-8):1349–52.

441. Nishiyama T, Yamashita K, Yokoyama T. Stress hormone changes in general anesthesia of long duration: isoflurane–nitrous oxide vs sevoflurane–nitrous oxide anesthesia. J Clin Anesth 2005;17(8):586–91.

442. Tanaka T, Nabatame H, Tanifuji Y. Insulin secretion and glucose utilization are impaired under general anesthesia with sevoflurane as well as isoflurane in a concentration-independent manner. J Anesth 2005;19(4):277–81.

443. Drinka PJ, Nolten WE. Effects of iodinated glycerol on thyroid function studies in elderly nursing home residents. J Am Geriatr Soc 1988;36(10):911–3.

444. Mather JL, Baycliff CD, Paterson NAM. Hypothyroidism secondary to iodinated glycerol. Can J Hosp Pharm 1993;46:177–8.

445. Oakley DE, Ellis PP. Glycerol and hyperosmolar nonketotic coma. Am J Ophthalmol 1976;81(4):469–72.

446. Sears ES. Nonketotic hyperosmolar hyperglycemia during glycerol therapy for cerebral edema. Neurology 1976;26(1):89–94.

447. Fukui M, Kitagawa Y, Nakamura N, Yoshikawa T. Glycyrrhizin and serum testosterone concentrations in male patients with type 2 diabetes. Diabetes Care 2003;26:2962.

448. Mosaddegh M, Naghibi F, Abbasi PR, Esmaeili S. The effect of liquorice extract on serum testosterone level in healthy male volunteers. J Pharm Pharmacol 2003;55 Suppl:S87–8.

449. Cawley MJ. Short-term lorazepam infusion and concern for propylene glycol toxicity: case report and review. Pharmacotherapy 2001;21(9):1140–4.

450. Anonymous. Auranofin–Diabetes situation impaired/hypoglycemia. Bull SADRAC, June/October (English version), 3.

451. Van Hoef ME, Howell A. Risk of thyroid dysfunction during treatment with G-CSF. Lancet 1992;340(8828):1169–70.

452. Duarte R, De Luis DA, Lopez-Jimenez J, Roy G, Garcia A. Thyroid function and autoimmunity during treatment with G-CSF. Clin Endocrinol (Oxf) 1999;51(1):133–4.

453. Vial T, Descotes J. Clinical toxicity of cytokines used as haemopoietic growth factors. Drug Saf 1995;13(6):371–406.

454. Hoekman K, von Blomberg-van der Flier BM, Wagstaff J, Drexhage HA, Pinedo HM. Reversible thyroid dysfunction during treatment with GM-CSF. Lancet 1991;338(8766):541–2.

455. Hansen PB, Johnsen HE, Hippe E. Autoimmune hypothyroidism and granulocyte–macrophage colony-stimulating factor. Eur J Haematol 1993;50(3):183–4.

456. Schriber JR, Negrin RS. Use and toxicity of the colony-stimulating factors. Drug Saf 1993;8(6):457–68.

457. Walter AM, Heilmeyer L. Antibiotika Fibel. In: Otten H, Siegenthaler W, editors. Antimykotica. Stuttgart: Georg Thieme Verlag, 1975:676.

458. Ziprkowski L, Szeinberg A, Crispin M, Krakowski A, Zaidman J. The effect of griseofulvin in hereditary porphyria cutanea tarda. Investigation of porphyrins and blood lipids. Arch Dermatol 1966;93(1):21–7.

459. Bickers DR. Environmental and drug factors in hepatic porphyria. Acta Dermatol Venereol Suppl (Stockh) 1982;100:29–41.

460. Shimoyama T, Nonaka S. Biochemical studies on griseofulvin-induced protoporphyria. Ann NY Acad Sci 1987;514:160–9.

461. Knasmuller S, Parzefall W, Helma C, Kassie F, Ecker S, Schulte-Hermann R. Toxic effects of griseofulvin: disease models, mechanisms, and risk assessment. Crit Rev Toxicol 1997;27(5):495–537Erratum in: Crit Rev Toxicol. 1998;28(1):102.

462. Felsher BF, Redeker AG. Acute intermittent porphyria: effect of diet and griseofulvin. Medicine (Baltimore) 1967;46(2):217–23.

463. Smith AG, De Matteis F. Drugs and the hepatic porphyrias. Clin Haematol 1980;9(2):399–425.

464. Karvonen M, Cepaitis Z, Tuomilehto J. Association between type 1 diabetes and Haemophilus influenzae type b vaccination: birth cohort study. BMJ 1999;318(7192):1169–72.

465. Classen JB, Classen DC. Association between type 1 diabetes and Hib vaccine. Causal relation is likely. BMJ 1999;319(7217):1133.

466. Classen JB, Classen DC. Clustering of cases of insulin dependent diabetes (IDDM) occurring three years after *Hemophilus influenza* B (HiB) immunization support causal relationship between immunization and IDDM. Autoimmunity 2002;35(4):247–53.

467. Peltola H, Aavitsland P, Hansen KG, Jonsdottir KE, Nokleby H, Romanus V. Perspective: a five-country analysis of the impact of four different *Haemophilus influenzae* type b conjugates and vaccination strategies in Scandinavia. J Infect Dis 1999;179(1):223–9.

468. Jefferson T. Vaccination and its adverse effects: real or perceived. Society should think about means of linking exposure to potential long term effect. BMJ 1998;317(7152):159–60.

469. Castenfors H, Allgoth AM. The effect of iodochlorohydroxyquinoline, diiodohydroxyquinoline and dichlorohydroxyquinaldine on the thyroid uptake of radio-iodine. Scand J Clin Lab Invest 1957;9(3):270–2.

470. Kleinberg DL, Davis JM, de Coster R, Van Baelen B, Brecher M. Prolactin levels and adverse events in patients treated with risperidone. J Clin Psychopharmacol 1999;19(1):57–61.

471. Zarifian E, Scatton B, Bianchetti G, Cuche H, Loo H, Morselli PL. High doses of haloperidol in schizophrenia. A clinical, biochemical, and pharmacokinetic study. Arch Gen Psychiatry 1982;39(2):212–5.

472. Jung DU, Seo YS, Park JH, Jeong CY, Conley RR, Kelly DL, Shim JC. The prevalence of hyperprolactinemia after long-term haloperidol use in patients with chronic schizophrenia. J Clin Psychopharmacol 2005;25:613–5.

473. Spitzer M, Sajjad R, Benjamin F. Pattern of development of hyperprolactinemia after initiation of haloperidol therapy. Obstet Gynecol 1998;91(5 Pt 1):693–5.

474. Feek CM, Sawers JS, Brown NS, Seth J, Irvine WJ, Toft AD. Influence of thyroid status on dopaminergic inhibition of thyrotropin and prolactin secretion: evidence for an additional feedback mechanism in the control of thyroid hormone secretion. J Clin Endocrinol Metab 1980;51(3):585–9.

475. Atmaca M, Kuloglu M, Tezcan E, Canatan H, Gecici O. Quetiapine is not associated with increase in prolactin secretion in contrast to haloperidol. Arch Med Res 2002;33(6):562–5.

476. Chae BJ, Kang BJ. The effect of clozapine on blood glucose metabolism. Hum Psychopharmacol 2001;16(3):265–71.

477. Oster JR, Singer I, Fishman LM. Heparin-induced aldosterone suppression and hyperkalemia. Am J Med 1995;98(6):575–86.

478. Levesque H, Cailleux N, Noblet C, Gancel A, Moore N, Courtois H. Hypoaldosteronisme induit par les héparines de bas poids moléculaire. [Hypoaldosteronism induced by low molecular weight heparins.] Presse Méd 1991;20(1):35.

479. Hottelart C, Achard JM, Moriniere P, Zoghbi F, Dieval J, Fournier A. Heparin-induced hyperkalemia in chronic hemodialysis patients: comparison of low molecular weight and unfractionated heparin. Artif Organs 1998;22(7):614–7.

480. Watts GF, Cameron J, Henderson A, Richmond W. Lipoprotein lipase deficiency due to long-term heparinization presenting as severe hypertriglyceridaemia in pregnancy. Postgrad Med J 1991;67(794):1062–4.

481. Wolf R, Beck OA, Hochrein H. Der Einfluss von Heparin auf die Haufigkeit von Rhythmusstorungen beim akuten Myokardinfarkt. [The effect of heparin on the incidence of arrhythmias after acute myocardial infarction.] Dtsch Med Wochenschr 1974;99(30):1549–53.

482. Chalmers TM. Clinical experience with ibuprofen in rheumatoid arthritis. Schweiz Med Wochenschr 1971;101(8):280–2.

483. Badiou S, Bellet H, Lehmann S, Cristol JP, Jaber S. Elevated plasma cysteinylglycine levels caused by cilastatin-associated antibiotic treatment. Clin Chem Lab Med 2005;43(3):332–4.

484. Stangel M, Hartung HP, Marx P, Gold R. Intravenous immunoglobulin treatment of neurological autoimmune diseases. J Neurol Sci 1998;153(2):203–14.

485. Spence JD, Huff M, Barnett PA. Effects of indapamide versus hydrochlorothiazide on plasma lipids and lipoproteins in hypertensive patients: a direct comparison. Can J Clin Pharmacol 2000;7(1):32–7.

486. Dube MP, Edmondson-Melancon H, Qian D, Aqeel R, Johnson D, Buchanan TA. Prospective evaluation of the effect of initiating indinavir-based therapy on insulin sensitivity and B cell function in HIV-infected patients. J Acquir Immune Defic Syndr 2001;27(2):130–4.

487. Young EM, Considine RV, Sattler FR, Deeg MA, Buchanan TA, Degawa-Yamauchi M, Shankar S, Edmondson-Melancon H, Hernandez J, Dube MP. Changes in thrombolytic and inflammatory markers after initiation of indinavir- or amprenavir-based antiretroviral therapy. Cardiovasc Toxicol 2004;4(2):179–86.

488. Beirne J, Jubiz W. Effect of indomethacin on the hypothalamic–pituitary–adrenal axis in man. J Clin Endocrinol Metab 1978;47(4):713–6.

489. Thack JR, Bozeman MT. Indometacin induced hyperglycemia. J Am Acad Dermatol 1982;7:502.

490. Franchimont D, Roland S, Gustot T, Quertinmont E, Toubouti Y, Gervy MC, Deviere J, Van Gossum A. Impact of infliximab on serum leptin levels in patients with Crohn's disease. J Clin Endocrinol Metab 2005;90(6):3510–6.

491. Del Monte P, Bernasconi D, De Conca V, Randazzo M, Meozzi M, Badaracco B, Mesiti S, Marugo M. Endocrine evaluation in patients treated with interferon-alpha for chronic hepatitis C. Horm Res 1995;44(3):105–9.

492. Muller H, Hiemke C, Hammes E, Hess G. Sub-acute effects of interferon-alpha 2 on adrenocorticotrophic hormone, cortisol, growth hormone and prolactin in humans. Psychoneuroendocrinology 1992;17(5):459–65.

493. Crockett DM, McCabe BF, Lusk RP, Mixon JH. Side effects and toxicity of interferon in the treatment of recurrent respiratory papillomatosis. Ann Otol Rhinol Laryngol 1987;96(5):601–7.

494. Gottrand F, Michaud L, Guimber D, Ategbo S, Dubar G, Turck D, Farriaux JP. Influence of recombinant interferon alpha on nutritional status and growth pattern in children with chronic viral hepatitis. Eur J Pediatr 1996;155(12):1031–4.

495. Levy S, Abdelli N, Diebold MD, Gross A, Thiefin G. Insuffisance surrénale réversible au cours d'un traitement par interféron alfa d'une hépatite chronique C. Gastroentérol Clin Biol 2003;27:563–4.

496. Concha LB, Carlson HE, Heimann A, Lake-Bakaar GV, Paal AF. Interferon-induced hypopituitarism. Am J Med 2003;114:161–3.

497. Farkkila AM, Iivanainen MV, Farkkila MA. Disturbance of the water and electrolyte balance during high-dose interferon treatment. J Interferon Res 1990;10(2):221–7.

498. Fentiman IS, Balkwill FR, Thomas BS, Russell MJ, Todd I, Bottazzo GF. An autoimmune aetiology for hypothyroidism following interferon therapy for breast cancer. Eur J Cancer Clin Oncol 1988;24(8):1299–303.

499. Vial T, Bailly F, Descotes J, Trepo C. Effets secondaires de l'interféron alpha. [Side effects of interferon-alpha.] Gastroenterol Clin Biol 1996;20(5):462–89.

500. Vial T, Descotes J. Immune-mediated side-effects of cytokines in humans. Toxicology 1995;105(1):31–57.

501. Fortis A, Christopoulos C, Chrysadakou E, Anevlavis E. De Quervain's thyroiditis associated with interferon-alpha-2b therapy for non-Hodgkin's lymphoma. Clin Drug Invest 1998;16:473–5.

502. Ghilardi G, Gonvers JJ, So A. Hypothyroid myopathy as a complication of interferon alpha therapy for chronic hepatitis C virus infection. Br J Rheumatol 1998;37(12):1349–51.

503. Schmitt K, Hompesch BC, Oeland K, von Staehr WG, Thurmann PA. Autoimmune thyroiditis and myelosuppression following treatment with interferon-alpha for hepatitis C. Int J Clin Pharmacol Ther 1999;37(4):165–7.

504. Papo T, Oksenhendler E, Izembart M, Leger A, Clauvel JP. Antithyroid hormone antibodies induced by interferon-alpha. J Clin Endocrinol Metab 1992;75(6):1484–6.

505. Wong V, Fu AX, George J, Cheung NW. Thyrotoxicosis induced by alpha-interferon therapy in chronic viral hepatitis. Clin Endocrinol (Oxf) 2002;56(6):793–8.

506. Carella C, Mazziotti G, Morisco F, Manganella G, Rotondi M, Tuccillo C, Sorvillo F, Caporaso N, Amato G. Long-term outcome of interferon-alpha-induced thyroid autoimmunity and prognostic influence of thyroid autoantibody pattern at the end of treatment. J Clin Endocrinol Metab 2001;86(5):1925–9.

507. Binaghi M, Levy C, Douvin C, Guittard M, Soubrane G, Coscas G. Ophtalmopathie de Basedow sévère liée a l'interféron alpha. [Severe thyroid ophthalmopathy related to interferon alpha therapy.] J Fr Ophtalmol 2002;25(4):412–5.

508. Sunbul M, Kahraman H, Eroglu C, Leblebicioglu H, Cinar T. Subacute thyroiditis in a patient with chronic hepatitis C during interferon treatment: a case report. Ondokuz Mayis Univ Tip Derg 1999;16:62–6.

509. Dalgard O, Bjoro K, Hellum K, Myrvang B, Bjoro T, Haug E, Bell H. Thyroid dysfunction during treatment of chronic hepatitis C with interferon alpha: no association with either interferon dosage or efficacy of therapy. J Intern Med 2002;251(5):400–6.

510. Preziati D, La Rosa L, Covini G, Marcelli R, Rescalli S, Persani L, Del Ninno E, Meroni PL, Colombo M, Beck-Peccoz P. Autoimmunity and thyroid function in patients with chronic active hepatitis treated with recombinant interferon alpha-2a. Eur J Endocrinol 1995;132(5):587–93.

511. Vallisa D, Cavanna L, Berte R, Merli F, Ghisoni F, Buscarini L. Autoimmune thyroid dysfunctions in hematologic malignancies treated with alpha-interferon. Acta Haematol 1995;93(1):31–5.

512. Monzani F, Caraccio N, Dardano A, Ferrannini E. Thyroid autoimmunity and dysfunction associated with type I interferon therapy. Clin Exp Med 2004;3:199–210.

513. Prummel MF, Laurberg P. Interferon-alfa and autoimmune thyroid disease. Thyroid 2003;13:547–51.

514. Marazuela M, Garcia-Buey L, Gonzalez-Fernandez B, Garcia-Monzon C, Arranz A, Borque MJ, Moreno-Otero R. Thyroid autoimmune disorders in patients with chronic hepatitis C before and during interferon-alpha therapy. Clin Endocrinol (Oxf) 1996;44(6):635–42.

515. Roti E, Minelli R, Giuberti T, Marchelli S, Schianchi C, Gardini E, Salvi M, Fiaccadori F, Ugolotti G, Neri TM, Braverman LE. Multiple changes in thyroid function in patients with chronic active HCV hepatitis treated with recombinant interferon-alpha. Am J Med 1996;101(5):482–7.

516. Barreca T, Picciotto A, Franceschini R, et al. Effects of acute administration of recombinant interferon alpha 2b on pituitary hormone secretion in patients with chronic active hepatitis. Curr Ther Res 1992;52:695–701.

517. Yamazaki K, Kanaji Y, Shizume K, Yamakawa Y, Demura H, Kanaji Y, Obara T, Sato K. Reversible inhibition by interferons alpha and beta of ^{125}I incorporation and thyroid hormone release by human thyroid follicles in vitro. J Clin Endocrinol Metab 1993;77(5):1439–41.

518. Schuppert F, Rambusch E, Kirchner H, Atzpodien J, Kohn LD, von zur Muhlen A. Patients treated with interferon-alpha, interferon-beta, and interleukin-2 have a different thyroid autoantibody pattern than patients suffering from endogenous autoimmune thyroid disease. Thyroid 1997;7(6):837–42.

519. Watanabe U, Hashimoto E, Hisamitsu T, Obata H, Hayashi N. The risk factor for development of thyroid disease during interferon-alpha therapy for chronic hepatitis C. Am J Gastroenterol 1994;89(3):399–403.

520. Fernandez-Soto L, Gonzalez A, Escobar-Jimenez F, Vazquez R, Ocete E, Olea N, Salmeron J. Increased risk of autoimmune thyroid disease in hepatitis C vs hepatitis B before, during, and after discontinuing interferon therapy. Arch Intern Med 1998;158(13):1445–8.

521. Kakizaki S, Takagi H, Murakami M, Takayama H, Mori M. HLA antigens in patients with interferon-alpha-induced autoimmune thyroid disorders in chronic hepatitis C. J Hepatol 1999;30(5):794–800.

522. Minelli R, Braverman LE, Valli MA, Schianchi C, Pedrazzoni M, Fiaccadori F, Salvi M, Magotti MG, Roti E. Recombinant interferon alpha (rIFN-alpha) does not potentiate the effect of iodine excess on the development of thyroid abnormalities in patients with HCV chronic active hepatitis. Clin Endocrinol (Oxf) 1999;50(1):95–100.

523. Carella C, Mazziotti G, Morisco F, Rotondi M, Cioffi M, Tuccillo C, Sorvillo F, Caporaso N, Amato G. The addition of ribavirin to interferon-alpha therapy in patients with hepatitis C virus-related chronic hepatitis does not modify the thyroid autoantibody pattern but increases the risk of developing hypothyroidism. Eur J Endocrinol 2002;146(6):743–9.

524. Marcellin P, Pouteau M, Renard P, Grynblat JM, Colas Linhart N, Bardet P, Bok B, Benhamou JP. Sustained hypothyroidism induced by recombinant alpha interferon in patients with chronic hepatitis C. Gut 1992;33(6):855–6.

525. Mekkakia-Benhabib C, Marcellin P, Colas-Linhart N, Castel-Nau C, Buyck D, Erlinger S, Bok B. Histoire naturelle des dysthyroïdies survenant sous interféron dans le traitement des hépatites chroniques C. [Natural history of dysthyroidism during interferon treatment of chronic hepatitis C.] Ann Endocrinol (Paris) 1996;57(5):419–27.

526. Minelli R, Braverman LE, Giuberti T, Schianchi C, Gardini E, Salvi M, Fiaccadori F, Ugolotti G, Roti E. Effects of excess iodine administration on thyroid function in euthyroid patients with a previous episode of thyroid dysfunction induced by interferon-alpha treatment. Clin Endocrinol (Oxf) 1997;47(3):357–61.

527. Calvino J, Romero R, Suarez-Penaranda JM, Arcocha V, Lens XM, Mardaras J, Novoa D, Sanchez-Guisande D.

Secondary hyperparathyroidism exacerbation: a rare side-effect of interferon-alpha? Clin Nephrol 1999;51(4):248–51.

528. Wesche B, Jaeckel E, Trautwein C, Wedemeyer H, Falorni A, Frank H, von zur Muhlen A, Manns MP, Brabant G. Induction of autoantibodies to the adrenal cortex and pancreatic islet cells by interferon alpha therapy for chronic hepatitis C. Gut 2001;48(3):378–83.

529. Fattovich G, Giustina G, Favarato S, Ruol A. A survey of adverse events in 11,241 patients with chronic viral hepatitis treated with alfa interferon. J Hepatol 1996;24(1):38–47.

530. Fraser GM, Harman I, Meller N, Niv Y, Porath A. Diabetes mellitus is associated with chronic hepatitis C but not chronic hepatitis B infection. Isr J Med Sci 1996;32(7):526–30.

531. Gori A, Caredda F, Franzetti F, Ridolfo A, Rusconi S, Moroni M. Reversible diabetes in patient with AIDS-related Kaposi's sarcoma treated with interferon alpha-2a. Lancet 1995;345(8962):1438–9.

532. Guerci AP, Guerci B, Levy-Marchal C, Ongagna J, Ziegler O, Candiloros H, Guerci O, Drouin P. Onset of insulin-dependent diabetes mellitus after interferon-alfa therapy for hairy cell leukaemia. Lancet 1994;343(8906):1167–8.

533. Mathieu E, Fain O, Sitbon M, Thomas M. Diabète autoimmun après traitement par interféron alpha. [Autoimmune diabetes after treatment with interferon-alpha.] Presse Méd 1995;24(4):238.

534. Eibl N, Gschwantler M, Ferenci P, Eibl MM, Weiss W, Schernthaner G. Development of insulin-dependent diabetes mellitus in a patient with chronic hepatitis C during therapy with interferon-alpha. Eur J Gastroenterol Hepatol 2001;13(3):295–8.

535. Recasens M, Aguilera E, Ampurdanes S, Sanchez Tapias JM, Simo O, Casamitjana R, Conget I. Abrupt onset of diabetes during interferon-alpha therapy in patients with chronic hepatitis C. Diabet Med 2001;18(9):764–7.

536. Mofredj A, Howaizi M, Grasset D, Licht H, Loison S, Devergie B, Demontis R, Cadranel JF. Diabetes mellitus during interferon therapy for chronic viral hepatitis. Dig Dis Sci 2002;47(7):1649–54.

537. Ito Y, Takeda N, Ishimori M, Akai A, Miura K, Yasuda K. Effects of long-term interferon-alpha treatment on glucose tolerance in patients with chronic hepatitis C. J Hepatol 1999;31(2):215–20.

538. Hayakawa M, Gando S, Morimoto Y, Kemmotsu O. Development of severe diabetic keto-acidosis with shock after changing interferon-beta into interferon-alpha for chronic hepatitis C. Intensive Care Med 2000;26(7):1008.

539. Fabris P, Betterle C, Greggio NA, Zanchetta R, Bosi E, Biasin MR, de Lalla F. Insulin-dependent diabetes mellitus during alpha-interferon therapy for chronic viral hepatitis. J Hepatol 1998;28(3):514–7.

540. Koivisto VA, Pelkonen R, Cantell K. Effect of interferon on glucose tolerance and insulin sensitivity. Diabetes 1989;38(5):641–7.

541. Imano E, Kanda T, Ishigami Y, Kubota M, Ikeda M, Matsuhisa M, Kawamori R, Yamasaki Y. Interferon induces insulin resistance in patients with chronic active hepatitis C. J Hepatol 1998;28(2):189–93.

542. di Cesare E, Previti M, Russo F, Brancatelli S, Ingemi MC, Scoglio R, Mazzu N, Cucinotta D, Raimondo G. Interferon-alpha therapy may induce insulin autoantibody development in patients with chronic viral hepatitis. Dig Dis Sci 1996;41(8):1672–7.

543. Schories M, Peters T, Rasenack J, Reincke M. Autoantikörper gegen Inselzellantigene und Diabetes mellitus Typ 1 unter Interferon alpha-Kombinationtherapie. Dtsch Med Wochenschr 2004;129:1120–4.

544. Fabris P, Floreani A, Tositti G, Vergani D, De Lalla F, Betterle C. Type 1 diabetes mellitus in patients with chronic hepatitis C before and after interferon therapy. Aliment Pharmacol Ther 2003;18:549–58.

545. Sasso FC, Carbonara O, Di Micco P, Coppola L, Torella R, Niglio A. A case of autoimmune polyglandular syndrome developed after interferon-alfa therapy. Br J Clin Pharmacol 2003;56:238–9.

546. Tasi TN, Hsieh CH. Development of reversible diabetes mellitus after cessation of interferon-alpha therapy for chronic hepatitis C infection. NZ Med J 2004;117:U1230.

547. Elisaf M, Tsianos EV. Severe hypertriglyceridaemia in a non-diabetic patient after alpha-interferon. Eur J Gastroenterol Hepatol 1999;11(4):463.

548. Junghans V, Runger TM. Hypertriglyceridaemia following adjuvant interferon-alpha treatment in two patients with malignant melanoma. Br J Dermatol 1999;140(1):183–4.

549. Shinohara E, Yamashita S, Kihara S, Hirano K, Ishigami M, Arai T, Nozaki S, Kameda-Takemura K, Kawata S, Matsuzawa Y. Interferon alpha induces disorder of lipid metabolism by lowering postheparin lipases and cholesteryl ester transfer protein activities in patients with chronic hepatitis C. Hepatology 1997;25(6):1502–6.

550. Yamagishi S, Abe T, Sawada T. Human recombinant interferon alpha-2a (r IFN alpha-2a) therapy suppresses hepatic triglyceride lipase, leading to severe hypertriglyceridemia in a diabetic patient. Am J Gastroenterol 1994;89(12):2280.

551. Fernandez-Miranda C, Castellano G, Guijarro C, Fernandez I, Schoebel N, Larumbe S, Gomez-Izquierdo T, del Palacio A. Lipoprotein changes in patients with chronic hepatitis C treated with interferon-alpha. Am J Gastroenterol 1998;93(10):1901–4.

552. Wong SF, Jakowatz JG, Taheri R. Management of hypertriglyceridemia in patients receiving interferon for malignant melanoma. Ann Pharmacother 2004;38:1655–9.

553. Jessner W, Der-Petrossian M, Christiansen L, Maier H, Steindl-Munda P, Gangl A, Ferenci P. Porphyria cutanea tarda during interferon/ribavirin therapy for chronic hepatitis C. Hepatology 2002;36(5):1301–2.

554. Pagliacci MC, Pelicci G, Schippa M, Liberati AM, Nicoletti I. Does interferon-beta therapy induce thyroid autoimmune phenomena? Horm Metab Res 1991;23(4):196–7.

555. Martinelli V, Gironi M, Rodegher M, Martino G, Comi G. Occurrence of thyroid autoimmunity in relapsing remitting multiple sclerosis patients undergoing interferon-beta treatment. Ital J Neurol Sci 1998;19(2):65–7.

556. Schwid SR, Goodman AD, Mattson DH. Autoimmune hyperthyroidism in patients with multiple sclerosis treated with interferon beta-1b. Arch Neurol 1997;54(9):1169–90.

557. Rotondi M, Oliviero A, Profice P, Mone CM, Biondi B, Del Buono A, Mazziotti G, Sinisi AM, Bellastella A, Carella C. Occurrence of thyroid autoimmunity and dysfunction throughout a nine-month follow-up in patients undergoing interferon-beta therapy for multiple sclerosis. J Endocrinol Invest 1998;21(11):748–52.

558. Monzani F, Caraccio N, Casolaro A, Lombardo F, Moscato G, Murri L, Ferrannini E, Meucci G. Long-term

interferon beta-1b therapy for MS: is routine thyroid assessment always useful? Neurology 2000;55(4):549–52.

559. McDonald ND, Pender MP. Autoimmune hypothyroidism associated with interferon beta-1b treatment in two patients with multiple sclerosis. Aust NZ J Med 2000;30(2):278–9.

560. Kreisler A, de Seze J, Stojkovic T, Delisse B, Combelles M, Verier A, Hautecoeur P, Vermersch P. Multiple sclerosis, interferon beta and clinical thyroid dysfunction. Acta Neurol Scand 2003;107:154–7.

561. Polman CH, Jansen PH, Jansen C, Uitdehaag BM. A rare, treatable cause of relapsing encephalopathy in an MS patient on interferon beta therapy. Neurology 2003;61:719.

562. Caraccio N, Dardano A, Manfredonia F, Manca L, Pasquali L, Iudice A, Murri L, Ferrannini E, Monzani F. Long-term follow-up of 106 multiple sclerosis patients undergoing interferon-beta 1a or 1b therapy: predictive factors of thyroid disease development and duration. J Clin Endocrinol Metab 2005;90(7):4133–7.

563. Homma Y, Kawazoe K, Ito T, Ide H, Takahashi H, Ueno F, Matsuzaki S. Chronic hepatitis C beta-interferon-induced severe hypertriglyceridaemia with apolipoprotein E phenotype E3/2. Int J Clin Pract 2000;54(4):212–6.

564. Krishnan R, Ellinwood EH Jr, Laszlo J, Hood L, Ritchie J. Effect of gamma interferon on the hypothalamic–pituitary–adrenal system. Biol Psychiatry 1987;22(9):1163–6.

565. Kurzrock R, Rohde MF, Quesada JR, Gianturco SH, Bradley WA, Sherwin SA, Gutterman JU. Recombinant gamma interferon induces hypertriglyceridemia and inhibits post-heparin lipase activity in cancer patients. J Exp Med 1986;164(4):1093–101.

566. Crown J, Jakubowski A, Kemeny N, Gordon M, Gasparetto C, Wong G, Sheridan C, Toner G, Meisenberg B, Botet J, et al. A phase I trial of recombinant human interleukin-1 beta alone and in combination with myelosuppressive doses of 5-fluorouracil in patients with gastrointestinal cancer. Blood 1991;78(6):1420–7.

567. Astwood EB. Occurrence in the sera of certain patients of large amounts of a newly isolated iodine compound. Trans Assoc Am Physicians 1957;70:183–91.

568. Fairhurst BJ, Naqvi N. Hyperthyroidism after cholecystography. BMJ 1975;3(5984):630.

569. Giroux JD, Sizun J, Rubio S, Metz C, Montaud N, Guillois B, Alix D. Hypothyroïdie transitoire après opacification iodées des cathéters epicutanéocaves au réanimation néonatale. [Transient hypothyroidism after iodine opacification of epicutaneo-caval catheters in neonatal intensive care.] Arch Fr Pediatr 1993;50 (3):273.

570. Fassbender WJ, Schluter S, Stracke H, Bretzel RG, Waas W, Tillmanns H. Schilddrusenfunktion nach gabe jodhaltigen Röntgenkontrastmittels bei Koronarangiographie—eine prospektive Untersuchung euthyreoten Patienten. [Thyroid function after iodine-containing contrast agent administration in coronary angiography: a prospective study of euthyroid patients.] Z Kardiol 2001;90(10):751–9.

571. Dembinski J, Arpe V, Kroll M, Hieronimi G, Bartmann P. Thyroid function in very low birthweight infants after intravenous administration of the iodinated contrast medium iopromide. Arch Dis Child Fetal Neonatal Ed 2000;82(3):F215–7.

572. Beckers EA, Strack van Schijndel RJ, Weijmer MC. A contrast crisis. Lancet 2000;356(9233):908.

573. van Guldener C, Blom DM, Lips P, Strack van Schijndel RJ. Hyperthyreoidie door jodiumhoudende rontgencontrastmiddelen. [Hyperthyroidism induced by iodinated roentgen contrast media.] Ned Tijdschr Geneeskd 1998;142(29):1641–4.

574. Owen PJ, Lazarus JH, Morse RE. Unusual complications of thyroid carcinoma. Postgrad Med J 2003;79:55–6.

575. Kulstad CE, Carlson A. Contrast-induced thyrotoxicosis. Ann Emerg Med 2004;44:281–2.

576. van der Molen AJ, Thomsen HS, Morcos SK, Contrast Media Safety Committee, European Society of Urogenital Radiology (ESUR). Effect of iodinated contrast media on thyroid function in adults. Eur Radiol 2004;14:902–7.

577. l'Allemand D, Gruters A, Beyer P, Weber B. Iodine in contrast agents and skin disinfectants is the major cause for hypothyroidism in premature infants during intensive care. Horm Res 1987;28(1):42–9.

578. Kelley WN. Uricosuria and X-ray contrast agents. N Engl J Med 1971;284(17):975–6.

579. Milligan A, Graham-Brown RA, Sarkany I, Baker H. Erythropoietic protoporphyria exacerbated by oral iron therapy. Br J Dermatol 1988;119(1):63–6.

580. Ivanov E, Adjarov D, Kerimova M, Naidenova E. Rare cases of porphyria cutanea tarda associated with additional iron overload. Dermatologica 1982;164(2):127–32.

581. Ferner RE. Drug-induced diabetes. Baillière's Clin Endocrinol Metab 1992;6(4):849–66.

582. Hergovich N, Singer E, Agneter E, Eichler HG, Graselli U, Simhandl C, Jilma B. Comparison of the effects of ketamine and memantine on prolactin and cortisol release in men. a randomized, double-blind, placebo-controlled trial. Neuropsychopharmacology 2001;24(5):590–3.

583. Krause W, Effendy I. Wie wirkt Ketoconazol auf den Testosteron-Stoffwechsel?. [How does ketoconazole affect testosterone metabolism?.] Z Hautkr 1985;60(14):1147–55.

584. Drouhet E, Dupont B. Evolution of antifungal agents: past, present, and future. Rev Infect Dis 1987;9(Suppl 1):S4–S14.

585. Loli P, Berselli ME, Tagliaferri M. Use of ketoconazole in the treatment of Cushing's syndrome. J Clin Endocrinol Metab 1986;63(6):1365–71.

586. Khosla S, Wolfson JS, Demerjian Z, Godine JE. Adrenal crisis in the setting of high-dose ketoconazole therapy. Arch Intern Med 1989;149(4):802–4.

587. Venturoli S, Fabbri R, Dal Prato L, Mantovani B, Capelli M, Magrini O, Flamigni C. Ketoconazole therapy for women with acne and/or hirsutism. J Clin Endocrinol Metab 1990;71(2):335–9.

588. De Pedrini P, Tommaselli A, Spano G, Montemurro G. Clinical and hormonal effects of ketoconazole on hirsutism in women. Int J Tissue React 1988;10(3):193–8.

589. Akalin S. Effects of ketoconazole in hirsute women. Acta Endocrinol (Copenh) 1991;124(1):19–22.

590. Mewasingh L, Aylett S, Kirkham F, Stanhope R. Hyponatraemia associated with lamotrigine in cranial diabetes insipidus. Lancet 2000;356(9230):656.

591. Ueberall MA. Normal growth during lamotrigine monotherapy in pediatric epilepsy patients—a prospective evaluation of 103 children and adolescents. Epilepsy Res 2001;46(1):63–7.

592. Laborde F, Loeuille D, Chary-Valckenaere I. Life-threatening hypertriglyceridemia during leflunomide therapy in

a patient with rheumatoid arthritis. Arthritis Rheum 2004;50(10):3398.

593. Anonymous. Levodopa (Larodopa). For the relief of symptoms associated with Parkinson's disease and syndrome. Clin Pharmacol Ther 1970;11(6):921–4.

594. Galea-Debono A, Jenner P, Marsden CD, Parkes JD, Tarsy D, Walters J. Plasma DOPA levels and growth hormone response to levodopa in parkinsomism. J Neurol Neurosurg Psychiatry 1977;40(2):162–7.

595. Rayfield EJ, George DT, Eichner HL, Hsu TH. L-dopa stimulation of glucagon secretion in man. N Engl J Med 1975;293(12):589–91.

596. Lamberti P, Zoccolella S, Iliceto G, Armenise E, Fraddosio A, de Mari M, Livrea P. Effects of levodopa and COMT inhibitors on plasma homocysteine in Parkinson's disease patients. Mov Disord 2005;20:69–72.

597. Friedrich LV, Dougherty R. Fatal hypoglycemia associated with levofloxacin. Pharmacotherapy 2004;24(12):1807–12.

598. Janda A, Salem C. Hypoglykämie durch Lidocain-Überdosierung. [Hypoglycemia caused by lidocaine overdosage.] Reg Anaesth 1986;9(3):88–90.

599. Kopterides P, Papadomichelakis E, Armaganidis A. Linezolid use associated with lactic acidosis. Scand J Infect Dis 2005;37(2):153–4.

600. Soriano A, Miro O, Mensa J. Mitochondrial toxicity associated with linezolid. N Engl J Med 2005;353(21):2305–6.

601. Shaikh ZH, Taylor HC, Maroo PV, Llerena LA. Syndrome of inappropriate antidiuretic hormone secretion associated with lisinopril. Ann Pharmacother 2000;34(2):176–9.

602. Bogazzi F, Bartalena L, Campomori A, Brogioni S, Traino C, De Martino F, Rossi G, Lippi F, Pinchera A, Martino E. Treatment with lithium prevents serum thyroid hormone increase after thionamide withdrawal and radioiodine therapy in patients with Graves' disease. J Clin Endocrinol Metab 2002;87(10):4490–5.

603. Bogazzi F, Bartalena L, Brogioni S, Scarcello G, Burelli A, Campomori A, Manetti L, Rossi G, Pinchera A, Martino E. Comparison of radioiodine with radioiodine plus lithium in the treatment of Graves' hyperthyroidism. J Clin Endocrinol Metab 1999;84(2):499–503.

604. Benbassat CA, Molitch ME. The use of lithium in the treatment of hyperthyroidism. Endocrinologist 1998;8:383–7.

605. Hoogenberg K, Beentjes JA, Piers DA. Lithium as an adjunct to radioactive iodine in treatment-resistant Graves' thyrotoxicosis. Ann Intern Med 1998;129(8):670.

606. Koong SS, Reynolds JC, Movius EG, Keenan AM, Ain KB, Lakshmanan MC, Robbins J. Lithium as a potential adjuvant to 131I therapy of metastatic, well differentiated thyroid carcinoma. J Clin Endocrinol Metab 1999;84(3):912–6.

607. Murphy E, Bassett JD, Meeran K, Frank JW. The efficacy of radioiodine in thyrotoxicosis is enhanced by lithium carbonate. J Nucl Med 2002;43:1280.

608. Bal CS, Kumar A, Pandey RM. A randomized controlled trial to evaluate the adjuvant effect of lithium on radioiodine treatment of hyperthyroidism. Thyroid 2002;12(5):399–405.

609. Bogazzi F, Bartalena L, Pinchera A, Martino E. Adjuvant effect of lithium on radioiodine treatment of hyperthyroidism. Thyroid 2002;12(12):1153–4.

610. Claxton S, Sinha SN, Donovan S, Greenaway TM, Hoffman L, Loughhead M, Burgess JR. Refractory amiodarone-associated thyrotoxicosis: an indication for thyroidectomy. Aust NZ J Surg 2000;70(3):174–8.

611. Muratori F, Bertini N, Masi G. Efficacy of lithium treatment in Kleine–Levin syndrome. Eur Psychiatry 2002;17(4):232–3.

612. Haden ST, Brown EM, Stoll AL, Scott J, Fuleihan GE. The effect of lithium on calcium-induced changes in adrenocorticotrophin levels. J Clin Endocrinol Metab 1999;84(1):198–200.

613. Sofuoglu S, Karaaslan F, Tutus A, Basturk M, Yabanoglu I, Esel E. Effects of short and long-term lithium treatment on serum prolactin levels in patients with bipolar affective disorder. Int J Neuropsychopharmacol 1999;2:S56.

614. Basturk M, Karaaslan F, Esel E, Sofuoglu S, Tutus A, Yabanoglu I. Effects of short and long-term lithium treatment on serum prolactin levels in patients with bipolar affective disorder. Prog Neuropsychopharmacol Biol Psychiatry 2001;25(2):315–22.

615. Turan T, Esel E, Tokgoz B, Aslan S, Sofuoglu S, Utas C, Kelestimur F. Effects of short- and long-term lithium treatment on kidney functioning in patients with bipolar mood disorder. Prog Neuropsychopharmacol Biol Psychiatry 2002;26(3):561–5.

616. Kamijo Y, Soma K, Hamanaka S, Nagai T, Kurihara K. Dural sinus thrombosis with severe hypernatremia developing in a patient on long-term lithium therapy. J Toxicol Clin Toxicol 2003;41:359–62.

617. Watson S, Young AH. Hypothalamic-pituitary-adrenal-axis function in bipolar disorder. Clin Approaches Bipolar Disorders 2002;2:57–64.

618. Bschor T, Baethge C, Adli M, Eichmann U, Ising M, Uhr M, Muller-Oerlinghausen B, Bauer M. Lithium augmentation increases post-dexamethasone cortisol in the dexamethasone suppression test in unipolar major depression. Depress Anxiety 2003;17(1):43–8.

619. Bschor T, Adli M, Baethge C, Eichmann U, Ising M, Uhr M, Modell S, Kunzel H, Muller-Oerlinghausen B, Bauer M. Lithium augmentation increases the ACTH and cortisol response in the combined DEX/CRH test in unipolar major depression. Neuropsychopharmacology 2002;27(3):470–8.

620. Lazarus JH. The effects of lithium therapy on thyroid and thyrotropin-releasing hormone. Thyroid 1998;8(10):909–13.

621. Luby ED, Singareddy RK. Long-term therapy with lithium in a private practice clinic: a naturalistic study. Bipolar Disord 2003;5(1):62–8.

622. Schiemann U, Hengst K. Thyroid echogenicity in manic-depressive patients receiving lithium therapy. J Affect Disord 2002;70(1):85–90.

623. Caykoylu A, Capoglu I, Unuvar N, Erdem F, Cetinkaya R. Thyroid abnormalities in lithium-treated patients with bipolar affective disorder. J Int Med Res 2002;30(1):80–4.

624. Deodhar SD, Singh B, Pathak CM, Sharan P, Kulhara P. Thyroid functions in lithium-treated psychiatric patients: a cross-sectional study. Biol Trace Elem Res 1999;67(2):151–63.

625. Bocchetta A, Mossa P, Velluzzi F, Mariotti S, Zompo MD, Loviselli A. Ten-year follow-up of thyroid function in lithium patients. J Clin Psychopharmacol 2001;21(6):594–8.

626. Jefferson JW. Lithium-associated clinical hypothyroidism. Int Drug Ther Newsl 2000;35:84–6.

627. Kleiner J, Altshuler L, Hendrick V, Hershman JM. Lithium-induced subclinical hypothyroidism: review of the literature and guidelines for treatment. J Clin Psychiatry 1999;60(4):249–55.

628. Kirov G. Thyroid disorders in lithium-treated patients. J Affect Disord 1998;50(1):33–40.

629. Shulman KI, Sykora K, Gill Ss, Mamdani M, Anderson G, Marras C, Wodchis WP, Lee PE, Rochon P. New thyroxine treatment in older adults beginning lithium therapy: implications for clinical practice. Am J Geriatr Psychiatry 2005;13:299–304.

630. Aliasgharpour M, Abbassi M, Shafaroodi H, Razi F. Subclinical hypothyroidism in lithium-treated psychiatric patients in Tehran, Islamic Republic of Iran. East Mediterr Health J 2005;11:329–33.

631. Baethge C, Blumentritt H, Berghöfer A, Bschor T, Gleen T, Adli M, Schlattmann P, Bauer M, Finke R. Long-term lithium treatment and thyroid antibodies: a controlled study. J Psychiatry Neurosci 2005;30:423–7.

632. Kupka RW, Nolen WA, Post RM, McElroy SL, Altshuler LL, Denicoff KD, Frye MA, Keck PE Jr, Leverich GS, Rush AJ, Suppes T, Pollio C, Drexhage HA. High rate of autoimmune thyroiditis in bipolar disorder: lack of association with lithium exposure. Biol Psychiatry 2002;51(4):305–11.

633. Kusalic M, Engelsmann F. Effect of lithium maintenance therapy on thyroid and parathyroid function. J Psychiatry Neurosci 1999;24(3):227–33.

634. Gracious BL. Elevated TSH in bipolar youth prescribed both lithium and divalproex sodium. Int Drug Ther Newsl 2001;36:94–5.

635. Gracious BL, Findling RL, McNamara NK, Youngstrom EA, Calabrese JR. Elevated TSH in bipolar youth prescribed both lithium and divalproex sodium. Bipolar Disord 2001;3(Suppl 1):38–9.

636. Kupka RW, Nolen WA, Drexhage HA, McElroy SL, Altshuler LL, Denicoff KD, Frye MA, Keck PE, Leverich GS, Rush AJ, Suppes T, Pollio C, Post RM. High rate of autoimmune thyroiditis in bipolar disorder is not associated with lithium. Bipolar Disord 2001;3(Suppl 1):44–5.

637. Henry C. Lithium side-effects and predictors of hypothyroidism in patients with bipolar disorder: sex differences. J Psychiatry Neurosci 2002;27(2):104–7.

638. Leutgeb U. Ambient iodine and lithium associated with clinical hypothyroidism. Br J Psychiatry 2000;176:495–6.

639. Bermudes RA. Psychiatric illness or thyroid disease? Don't be misled by false lab tests. Curr Psychiatry 2002;1(51–52):57–61.

640. Uchiyama Y, Nakao S, Asai T, Shingu K. [A case of atropine-resistant bradycardia in a patient on long-term lithium medication.]Masui 2001;50(11):1229–31.

641. Mira SA, Gimeno EJ, Diaz-Guerra GM, Carranza YFH. Alteraciones tiroideas y paratiroideas asociadas al tratamiento crónico con litio. A propósito de un caso. [Thyroid and parathyroid alterations associated with chronic lithium treatment. A case report.] Rev Esp Enferm Metab Oseas 2001;10:153–6.

642. Depoot I, Van Imschoot S, Lamberigts G. Lithium-geassocieerde hyperthyroïdie. [Lithium-associated hyperthyroidism.] Tijdschr Geneeskd 1998;54:413–6.

643. Calvo Romero JM, Puerto Pica JM. Crisis tirotóxica tras la retirada de tratamiento con litio. [A thyrotoxic crisis following the withdrawal of lithium treatment.] Rev Clin Esp 1998;198(11):782–3.

644. Scanelli G. Tireotossicosi da litio. Descrizione di un caso e revisione della letteratura. [Lithium thyrotoxicosis. Report of a case and review of the literature.] Recenti Prog Med 2002;93(2):100–3.

645. Ripoll Mairal M, Len Abad O, Falco Ferrer V, Fernandez de Sevilla Ribosa T. Hipertiroidismo e hypercalcemia asociados al tratamiento con litio. [Hyperthyroidism and hypercalcemia associated with lithium treatment.] Rev Clin Esp 2000;200(1):48–9.

646. Oakley PW, Dawson AH, Whyte IM. Lithium: thyroid effects and altered renal handling. J Toxicol Clin Toxicol 2000;38(3):333–7.

647. Dang AH, Hershman JM. Lithium-associated thyroiditis. Endocr Pract 2002;8(3):232–6.

648. Yamagishi S, Yokoyama-ohta M. A case of lithium-associated hyperthyroidism. Postgrad Med J 1999;75(881):188–9.

649. Miller KK, Daniels GH. Association between lithium use and thyrotoxicosis caused by silent thyroiditis. Clin Endocrinol (Oxf) 2001;55(4):501–8.

650. Obuobie K, Al-Sabah A, Lazarus JH. Subacute thyroiditis in an immunosuppressed patient. J Endocrinol Invest 2002;25(2):169–71.

651. Perrild H, Hegedus L, Baastrup PC, Kayser L, Kastberg S. Thyroid function and ultrasonically determined thyroid size in patients receiving long-term lithium treatment. Am J Psychiatry 1990;147(11):1518–21.

652. Dickstein G, Shechner C, Adawi F, Kaplan J, Baron E, Ish-Shalom S. Lithium treatment in amiodarone-induced thyrotoxicosis. Am J Med 1997;102(5):454–8.

653. Abdullah H, Bliss R, Guinea AI, Delbridge L. Pathology and outcome of surgical treatment for lithium-associated hyperparathyroidism. Br J Surg 1999;86(1):91–3.

654. Cohen O, Rais T, Lepkifker E, Vered I. Lithium carbonate therapy is not a risk factor for osteoporosis. Horm Metab Res 1998;30(9):594–7.

655. Wolf ME, Moffat M, Ranade V, Somberg JC, Lehrer E, Mosnaim AD. Lithium, hypercalcemia, and arrhythmia. J Clin Psychopharmacol 1998;18(5):420–3.

656. Sofuoglu S, Basturk M, Tutus A, Karaaslan F, Aslan SS, Gonuk AS. Lithium-induced alterations in parathormone function in patients with bipolar affective disorder. Int J Neuropsychopharmacol 1999;2:S56.

657. Turan MT, Esel E, Tutus A, Sofuoglu S, Gonuk AS. Lithium-induced alterations in parathormone function in patients with bipolar disorder. Bull Clin Psychopharmacol 2001;11:96–100.

658. Awad SS, Miskulin J, Thompson N. Parathyroid adenomas versus four-gland hyperplasia as the cause of primary hyperparathyroidism in patients with prolonged lithium therapy World J Surg 2003;27:486–8.

659. Dwight T, Kytola S, Teh BT, Theodosopoulos G, Richardson AL, Philips J, Twigg S, Delbridge L, Marsh DJ, Nelson AE, Larsson C, Robinson BG. Genetic analysis of lithium-associated parathyroid tumors. Eur J Endocrinol 2002;146(5):619–27.

660. Mak TW, Shek CC, Chow CC, Wing YK, Lee S. Effects of lithium therapy on bone mineral metabolism: a two-year prospective longitudinal study. J Clin Endocrinol Metab 1998;83(11):3857–9.

661. El Khoury A, Petterson U, Kallner G, Aberg-Wistedt A, Stain-Malmgren R. Calcium homeostasis in long-term lithium-treated women with bipolar affective disorder. Prog Neuropsychopharmacol Biol Psychiatry 2002;26(6):1063–9.

662. Morillas Arino C, Jordan Lluch M, Sola Izquierdo E, Serra Cerda M, Garzon Pastor S, Gomez Balaguer M, Hernandez Mijares YA. [Parathyroid adenoma and lithium therapy.]Endocrinol Nutr 2002;49:56–7.

663. Collumbien ECA. Een geval van therapieresistente manie. Lithium en hyperparathyreoïdie. [A case of therapy-resistant mania. Lithium and hyperparathyroidism.] Tijdschr Psychiatrie 2000;42:851–5.

664. Guirguis AF, Taylor HC. Nephrogenic diabetes insipidus persisting 57 months after cessation of lithium carbonate therapy: report of a case and review of the literature. Endocr Pract 2000;6(4):324–8.

665. Lam P, Tsai S-J, Chou Y-C. Lithium associated hyperparathyroidism with adenoma: a case report. Int Med J 2000;7:283–5.

666. Gama R, Wright J, Ferns G. An unusual case of hypercalcaemia. Postgrad Med J 1999;75(890):769–70.

667. de Celis G, Fiter M, Latorre X, Llebaria C. Oxyphilic parathyroid adenoma and lithium therapy. Lancet 1998;352(9133):1070.

668. Oakley PW, Whyte IM, Carter GL. Lithium toxicity: an iatrogenic problem in susceptible individuals. Aust NZ J Psychiatry 2001;35(6):833–40.

669. Krastins MG, Phelps KR. Nephrogenic diabetes insipidus and hyperparathyroidism in a patient receiving chronic lithium therapy. J Am Geriatr Soc 2002;50:S140.

670. Dieserud F, Brun AC, Lahne PE, Normann E. Litiumbehandling og hyperparatyreoidisme. [Lithium treatment and hyperparathyroidism.] Tidsskr Nor Laegeforen 2001;121(22):2602–3.

671. Pieri-Balandraud N, Hugueny P, Henry JF, Tournebise H, Dupont C. Hyperparathyroïdie induite par le lithium. Un nouveau cas. [Hyperparathyroidism induced by lithium. A new case.] Rev Medical Interne 2001;22(5):460–4.

672. Rifai MA, Moles JK, Harrington DP. Lithium-induced hypercalcemia and parathyroid dysfunction. Psychosomatics 2001;42(4):359–61.

673. Valeur N, Andersen RS. Lithium induceret parathyreoideahormon dysfunktion. [Lithium induced dysfunction of the parathyroid hormone.] Ugeskr Laeger 2002;164(5):639–40.

674. Catala JC, Rubio AB, Fernandez CC, Ballester YAH. Hiperparatiroidismo asociada al tratamiento con litio. Rev Esp Enferm Metab Oseas 2001;10:157–8.

675. Kanfer A, Blondiaux I. Complications rénales et métaboliques du lithium. [Renal and metabolic complications of lithium.] Nephrologie 2000;21(2):65–70.

676. Gomez Moreno R, Lobo Fresnillo T, Calvo Cebrian A, Monge Ropero N. Hiperparatiroidismo y litio. [Hyperparathyroidism and lithium.] Aten Primaria 2003;31(5):337.

677. Bilanakis N, Gibiriti M. Lithium intoxication, hypercalcemia and "accidently" induced food and water inversion: a case report. Prog Neuropsychopharmacol Biol Psychiatry 2004;28:201–3.

678. Belyavskaya NA. Lithium-induced changes in gravicurvature, statocyte ultrastructure and calcium balance of pea roots. Adv Space Res 2001;27(5):961–6.

679. Hundley JC, Woodrum DT, Saunders BD, Doherty GM, gauger PG. Revisiting lithium-associated hyperparathyroidism in the era of intraoperative parathyroid hormone monitoring. Surgery 2005;138:1027–31.

680. Cassidy F. Diabetes mellitus in manic-depressive patients. Essent Psychopharmacol 2001;4:49–57.

681. Uzu T, Ichida K, Ko M, Tsukurimichi S, Yamato M, Takahara K, Ohashi M, Yamauchi A, Nomura M. [Two cases of lithium intoxication complicated by type 2 diabetes mellitus.]J Jpn Diabetes Soc 2001;44:767–70.

682. Cyr M, Guia MA, Laizure SC. Increased lithium dose requirement in a hyperglycemic patient. Ann Pharmacother 2002;36(3):427–9.

683. Oomura S, Mukasa H, Ooji T, Mukasa H, Mukasa H, Satomura T, Tatsumoto Y. Does impaired glucose

tolerance predispose to lithium intoxication in treatment of MDI? Int J Neuropsychopharmacol 1999;2:S63.

684. Azam H, Newton RW, Morris AD, Thompson CJ. Hyperosmolar nonketotic coma precipitated by lithium-induced nephrogenic diabetes insipidus. Postgrad Med J 1998;74(867):39–41.

685. MacGregor DA, Baker AM, Appel RG, Ober KP, Zaloga GP. Hyperosmolar coma due to lithium-induced diabetes insipidus. Lancet 1995;346(8972):413–7.

686. MacGregor DA, Dolinski SY. Hyperosmolar coma. Lancet 1999;353(9159):1189.

687. Ackerman S, Nolan LJ. Bodyweight gain induced by psychotropic drugs. Incidence, mechanisms and management. CNS Drugs 1998;9:135–51.

688. Malhotra S, McElroy SL. Medical management of obesity associated with mental disorders. J Clin Psychiatry 2002;63(Suppl 4):24–32.

689. Vanina Y, Podolskaya A, Sedky K, Shahab H, Siddiqui A, Munshi F, Lippmann S. Body weight changes associated with psychopharmacology. Psychiatr Serv 2002;53(7):842–7.

690. Kelly DL, Conley RR, Love RC, Horn DS, Ushchak CM. Weight gain in adolescents treated with risperidone and conventional antipsychotics over six months. J Child Adolesc Psychopharmacol 1998;8(3):151–9.

691. Sussman N, Ginsberg D. Effects of psychotropic drugs on weight. Psychiatr Ann 1999;29:580–94.

692. Schumann C, Lenz G, Berghofer A, Muller-Oerlinghausen B. Non-adherence with long-term prophylaxis: a 6-year naturalistic follow-up study of affectively ill patients. Psychiatry Res 1999;89(3):247–57.

693. Elmslie JL, Silverstone JT, Mann JI, Williams SM, Romans SE. Prevalence of overweight and obesity in bipolar patients. J Clin Psychiatry 2000;61(3):179–84.

694. Ginsberg DL, Sussman N. Effects of mood stabilizers on weight. Primary Psychiatry 2000;7:49–58.

695. Chengappa KN, Chalasani L, Brar JS, Parepally H, Houck P, Levine J. Changes in body weight and body mass index among psychiatric patients receiving lithium, valproate, or topiramate: an open-label, nonrandomized chart review. Clin Ther 2002;24(10):1576–84.

696. Fagiolini A, Frank E, Houck PR, Mallinger AG, Swartz HA, Buysse DJ, Ombao H, Kupfer DJ. Prevalence of obesity and weight change during treatment in patients with bipolar I disorder. J Clin Psychiatry 2002;63(6):528–33.

697. Bowden CL, Calabrese JR, McElroy SL, Gyulai L, Wassef A, Petty F, Pope HG Jr, Chou JC, Keck PE Jr, Rhodes LJ, Swann AC, Hirschfeld RM, Wozniak PJDivalproex Maintenance Study Group. A randomized, placebo-controlled 12-month trial of divalproex and lithium in treatment of outpatients with bipolar I disorder. Arch Gen Psychiatry 2000;57(5):481–9.

698. Cheskin LJ, Bartlett SJ, Zayas R, Twilley CH, Allison DB, Contoreggi C. Prescription medications: a modifiable contributor to obesity. South Med J 1999;92(9):898–904.

699. Atmaca M, Kuloglu M, Tezcan E, Ustundag B. Weight gain and serum leptin levels in patients on lithium treatment. Neuropsychobiology 2002;46(2):67–9.

700. Sachs GS, Printz DJ, Kahn DA, Carpenter D, Docherty JP. The Expert Consensus Guideline Series. Medication Treatment of Bipolar Disorder 2000. Postgrad Med 2000;Special Number:1–104.

701. Kehlet H, Brandt MR, Hansen AP, Alberti KG. Effect of epidural analgesia on metabolic profiles during and after surgery. Br J Surg 1979;66(8):543–6.

702. Lund J, Stjernstrom H, Jorfeldt L, Wiklund L. Effect of extradural analgesia on glucose metabolism and gluconeogenesis. Studies in association with upper abdominal surgery. Br J Anaesth 1986;58(8):851–7.

703. Jacobs JS, Vallejo R, DeSouza GJ, TerRiet MF. Severe hypoglycemia after labor epidural analgesia. Anesth Analg 2000;90(4):892–3.

704. Gutierrez F, Padilla S, Masia M, Navarro A, Gallego J, Hernandez I, Ramos JM, Martin-Hidalgo A. Changes in body fat composition after 1 year of salvage therapy with lopinavir/ritonavir-containing regimens and its relationship with lopinavir plasma concentrations. Antivir Ther 2004;9(1):105–13.

705. Torti C, Quiros-Roldan E, Regazzi-Bonora M, De Luca A, Lo Caputo S, Di Giambenedetto S, Patroni A, Villani P, Micheli V, Carosi G; Resistance and Dosage Adapted Regimens Study Group of the MASTER Cohort. Lipid abnormalities in HIV-infected patients are not correlated with lopinavir plasma concentrations. J Acquir Immune Defic Syndr 2004;35(3):324–6.

706. Cawley MJ. Short-term lorazepam infusion and concern for propylene glycol toxicity: case report and review. Pharmacotherapy 2001;21(9):1140–4.

707. Meinertz T, Kasper W, Kersting F, Just H, Bechtold H, Jahnchen E. Lorcainide. II. Plasma concentration-effect relationship. Clin Pharmacol Ther 1979;26(2):196–204.

708. Mutti A, Bergamaschi E, Alinovi R, Lucchini R, Vettori MV, Franchini I. Serum prolactin in subjects occupationally exposed to manganese. Ann Clin Lab Sci 1996;26(1):10–7.

709. Perez OE, Henriquez N. Galactorrhea associated with maprotiline HCl. Am J Psychiatry 1983;140(5):641.

710. Nakra BR, Grossberg GT. Carbohydrate craving weight gain with maprotiline. Psychosomatics 1986;27(5):376381.

711. Fescharek R, Quast U, Maass G, Merkle W, Schwarz S. Measles–mumps vaccination in the FRG: an empirical analysis after 14 years of use. II. Tolerability and analysis of spontaneously reported side effects. Vaccine 1990;8(5):446–56.

712. Deutsche Vereinigung zur Bekampfung der Viruskrankheiten (DVV). Mumpsschutzimpfung and Diabetes mellitus (Typ I). Bundesgesundhbl 1989;237:.

713. Arze RS, Ramos JM, Rashid HU, Kerr DN. Amenorrhoea, galactorrhoea, and hyperprolactinaemia induced by methyldopa. BMJ (Clin Res Ed) 1981;283(6285):194.

714. Holtkamp K, Peters-Wallraf B, Wuller S, Pfaaffle R, Herpertz-Dahlmann B. Methylphenidate-related growth impairment. J Child Adolesc Psychopharmacol 2002;12(1):55–61.

715. Kramer JR, Loney J, Ponto LB, Roberts MA, Grossman S. Predictors of adult height and weight in boys treated with methylphenidate for childhood behavior problems. J Am Acad Child Adolesc Psychiatry 2000;39(4):517–24.

716. Madani S, Tolia V. Gynecomastia with metoclopramide use in pediatric patients. J Clin Gastroenterol 1997;24(2):79–81.

717. Shamkhani K, Azarpira M, Akbar MH. An open label crossover trial of effects of metronidazol on hyperlipidaemia. Int J Cardiol 2003;90:141–5.

718. Drouhet E, Dupont B. Evolution of antifungal agents: past, present, and future. Rev Infect Dis 1987;9(Suppl 1):S4–S14.

719. Tsokos M, Schroder S. Black thyroid. Report of an autopsy case. Int J Legal Med 2005;3:1–3.

720. Birkedal C, Tapscott WJ, Giadrosich K, Spence RK, Sperling D. Minocycline-induced black thyroid gland: medical curiosity or a marker for papillary cancer? Curr Surg 2001;58:471–1.

721. Doerge DR, Divi RL, Deck J, Taurog A. Mechanism for the anti-thyroid action of minocycline. Chem Res Toxicol 1997;10:49–58.

722. Nguyen K, Marks J. Pseudoacromegaly induced by the long-term use of minoxidil. J Am Acad Dermatol 2003;48:962–5.

723. Pardo C, Boix E, Lopez A, Pico A. Crisis addisoniana secundaria a tratamiento con mitotane. [Adrenal crisis due to mitotane therapy.] Med Clin (Barc) 2002;118(7):278.

724. Vassilopoulou-Sellin R, Samaan NA. Mitotane administration: an unusual cause of hypercholesterolemia. Horm Metab Res 1991;23(12):619–20.

725. Fujino Y, Inaba M, Imanishi Y, Nagata M, Goto H, Kumeda Y, Nakatani T, Ishimura E, Nishizawa Y. A case of SIADH induced by mizoribin administration. Nephron 2002;92(4):938–40.

726. Yoshioka K, Ohashi Y, Sakai T, Ito H, Yoshikawa N, Nakamura H, Tanizawa T, Wada H, Maki S. A multicenter trial of mizoribine compared with placebo in children with frequently relapsing nephrotic syndrome. Kidney Int 2000;58(1):317–24.

727. Dunn NR, Freemantle SN, Pearce GL, Mann RD. Galactorrhoea with moclobemide. Lancet 1998;351(9105):802.

728. Peterson JC, Pollack RW, Mahoney JJ, Fuller TJ. Inappropriate antidiuretic hormone secondary to a monoamine oxidase inhibitor. JAMA 1978;239(14):1422–3.

729. Dunleavy DL. Phenelzine and oedema. BMJ 1977;1(6072):1353.

730. Dunn NR, Freemantle SN, Pearce GL, Mann RD. Galactorrhoea with moclobemide. Lancet 1998;351(9105):802.

731. Zis AP, Haskett RF, Albala AA, Carroll BJ, Lohr NE. Prolactin response to morphine in depression. Biol Psychiatry 1985;20(3):287–92.

732. Gavin JR 3rd, Kubin R, Choudhri S, Kubitza D, Himmel H, Gross R, Meyer JM. Moxifloxacin and glucose homeostasis: a pooled-analysis of the evidence from clinical and postmarketing studies. Drug Saf 2004;27(9):671–86.

733. Islam MA, Sreedharan T. Convulsions, hyperglycemia and glycosuria from overdose of nalidixic acid. JAMA 1965;192:1100–1.

734. Leslie PJ, Cregeen RJ, Proudfoot AT. Lactic acidosis, hyperglycaemia and convulsions following nalidixic acid overdosage. Hum Toxicol 1984;3(3):239–43.

735. Suganthi AR, Ramanan AS, Pandit N, Yeshwanth M. Severe metabolic acidosis in nalidixic acid overdosage. Indian Pediatr 1993;30(8):1025–6.

736. Nogue S, Bertran A, Mas A, Nadal P, Anguita A, Milla J. Metabolic acidosis and coma due to an overdose of nalidixic acid. Intensive Care Med 1979;5(3):141–2.

737. Rubin P, Swezey S, Blaschke T. Naloxone lowers plasma-prolactin in man. Lancet 1979;1(8129):1293.

738. Antony F, Layton AM. Nabumetone-associated pseudoporphyria. Br J Dermatol 2000;142(5):1067–9.

739. Checketts SR, Morgan GJ Jr. Two cases of nabumetone induced pseudoporphyria. J Rheumatol 1999;26(12):2703–5.

740. Cron RQ, Finkel TH. Nabumetone induced pseudoporphyria in childhood. J Rheumatol 2000;27(7):1817–8.

741. Warnock JK, Biggs F. Nefazodone-induced hypoglycemia in a diabetic patient with major depression. Am J Psychiatry 1997;154(2):288–9.

742. Wood R, Phanuphak P, Cahn P, Pokrovskiy V, Rozenbaum W, Pantaleo G, Sension M, Murphy R, Mancini M, Kelleher T, Giordano M. Long-term efficacy and safety of atazanavir with stavudine and lamivudine in patients previously treated with nelfinavir or atazanavir. J Acquir Immune Defic Syndr 2004;36(2):684–92.

743. Grover SA, Coupal L, Gilmore N, Mukherjee J. Impact of dyslipidemia associated with Highly Active Antiretroviral Therapy (HAART) on cardiovascular risk and life expectancy. Am J Cardiol 2005;95(5):586–91.

744. Magharious W, Goff DC, Amico E. Relationship of gender and menstrual status to symptoms and medication side effects in patients with schizophrenia. Psychiatry Res 1998;77(3):159–66.

745. Baptista T, Kin NM, Beaulieu S. Treatment of the metabolic disturbances caused by antipsychotic drugs. Clin Pharmacokinet 2004;43:1–15.

746. Moller HJ, Kissling W, Maurach R. Beziehungen zwischen Haloperidol-Serumspiegel, Prolactin-Serumspiegel, antipsychotischen Effekt und extrapyramidalen Begleitwirkungen. [Relationship between haloperidol blood level, prolactin blood level, antipsychotic effect and extrapyramidal side effects.] Pharmacopsychiatrica 1981;14:27.

747. Zarifian E, Scatton B, Bianchetti G, Cuche H, Loo H, Morselli PL. High doses of haloperidol in schizophrenia. A clinical, biochemical, and pharmacokinetic study. Arch Gen Psychiatry 1982;39(2):212–5.

748. Meaney AM, Smith S, Howes OD, O'Brien M, Murray RM, O'Keane V. Effects of long-term prolactin-raising antipsychotic medication on bone mineral density in patients with schizophrenia. Br J Psychiatry 2004;184:503–8.

749. Brown WA, Laughren T. Low serum prolactin and early relapse following neuroleptic withdrawal. Am J Psychiatry 1981;138(2):237–9.

750. Phillips P, Shraberg D, Weitzel WD. Hirsutism associated with long-term phenothiazine neuroleptic therapy. JAMA 1979;241(9):920–1.

751. Atmaca M, Kuloglu M, Tezcan E, Canatan H, Gecici O. Quetiapine is not associated with increase in prolactin secretion in contrast to haloperidol. Arch Med Res 2002;33(6):562–5.

752. Schyve PM, Smithline F, Meltzer HY. Neuroleptic-induced prolactin level elevation and breast cancer: an emerging clinical issue. Arch Gen Psychiatry 1978;35(11):1291–301.

753. Mortensen PB. The incidence of cancer in schizophrenic patients. J Epidemiol Community Health 1989;43(1):43–7.

754. Pollock A, McLaren EH. Serum prolactin concentration in patients taking neuroleptic drugs. Clin Endocrinol (Oxf) 1998;49(4):513–6.

755. Spitzer M, Sajjad R, Benjamin F. Pattern of development of hyperprolactinemia after initiation of haloperidol therapy. Obstet Gynecol 1998;91(5 Pt 1):693–5.

756. Feek CM, Sawers JS, Brown NS, Seth J, Irvine WJ, Toft AD. Influence of thyroid status on dopaminergic inhibition of thyrotropin and prolactin secretion: evidence for an additional feedback mechanism in the control of thyroid hormone secretion. J Clin Endocrinol Metab 1980;51(3):585–9.

757. Melkersson KI, Hulting AL, Rane AJ. Dose requirement and prolactin elevation of antipsychotics in male and female patients with schizophrenia or related psychoses. Br J Clin Pharmacol 2001;51(4):317–24.

758. Kapur S, Roy P, Daskalakis J, Remington G, Zipursky R. Increased dopamine D(2) receptor occupancy and elevated prolactin level associated with addition of haloperidol to clozapine. Am J Psychiatry 2001;158(2):311–4.

759. Howes O, Smith S. Alendronic acid for antipsychotic-related osteopenia. Am J Psychiatry 2004;161:756.

760. Ali JA, Desai KD, Ali LJ. Delusions of pregnancy associated with increased prolactin concentrations produced by antipsychotic treatment. Int J Neuropsychopharmacol 2003;6:111–5.

761. O'Keane V, Meaney AM. A new risk factor for osteoporosis in young women with schizophrenia? J Clin Psychopharmacol 2005;25:26–31.

762. Bergemann N, Mundt C, Parzer P, Jannakos I Nagl I, Salbach B, Klinga K, Runnebaum B, Resch F. Plasma concentrations of estradiol in women suffering from schizophrenia treated with conventional versus atypical antipsychotics. Schizophr Res 2005;73:357–66.

763. Rao KJ, Miller M, Moses A. Water intoxication and thioridazine (Mellaril). Ann Intern Med 1975;82(1):61.

764. Meyer JM. A retrospective comparison of weight, lipid, and glucose changes between risperidone- and olanzapine-treated inpatients: metabolic outcomes after 1 year. J Clin Psychiatry 2002;63(5):425–33.

765. Bouchard RH, Demers MF, Simoneau I, Almeras N, Villeneuve J, Mottard JP, Cadrin C, Lemieux I, Despres JP. Atypical antipsychotics and cardiovascular risk in schizophrenic patients. J Clin Psychopharmacol 2001;21(1):110–1.

766. Meyer JM, Koro CE. The effects of antipsychotic therapy on serum lipids: a comprehensive review. Schizophr Res 2004;70:1–17.

767. Popli AP, Konicki PE, Jurjus GJ, Fuller MA, Jaskiw GE. Clozapine and associated diabetes mellitus. J Clin Psychiatry 1997;58(3):108–11.

768. Wirshing DA, Spellberg BJ, Erhart SM, Marder SR, Wirshing WC. Novel antipsychotics and new onset diabetes. Biol Psychiatry 1998;44(8):778–83.

769. Charatan FBE, Barlett NG. The effect of chorpromazine ("Largactil") on glucose tolerance. J Mental Sci 1955;191:351–53.

770. Hiles B. Hyperglycaemia and glycosuria following chlorpromazine therapy. J Am Med Assoc 1956;162:1651.

771. Braceland FJ, Meduna LJ, Vaichulis JA. Delayed action of insulin in schizophrenia. Am J Psychiatry 1945;102:108–10.

772. Sernyak MJ, Leslie DL, Alarcón RD, Losonczy MF, Rosenheck R. Association of diabetes mellitus with use of atypical neuroleptics in the treatment of schizophrenia. Am J Psychiatry 2002;159:561–6.

773. Buse JB, Cavazzoni P, Hornbuckle K, Hutchins D, Breier A, Jovanovic L. A retrospectivce cohort study diabetes mellitus and antipsychotic treatment in the United States. J Clin Epidemiol 2003;56:164–70.

774. Newcomer JW, Haupt DW, Fucetola R, Melson AK, Schweiger JA, Cooper BP, Selke G. Abnormalities in glucose regulation during antipsychotic treatment of schizophrenia. Arch Gen Psychiatry 2002;59(4):337–45.

775. Food and Drug Administration. www.fda.gov/medwatch/SAFETY/ 2004.

776. Gianfrancesco F, Grogg A, Mahmoud R, Wang R-H, Meletiche D. Differential effects of antipsychotic agents on the risk of development of type 2 diabetes mellitus in patients with mood disorders. Clin Ther 2003;25:1150–71.

777. García del Pozo J, Isusi L, Carvajal A, Martín I, Sáinz M, García del Pozo V, Velasco A. Evolución del consumo de fármacos antipsicóticos en Castilla y León (1990-2001). Rev Esp Salud Pública 2003;77:725–33.

778. Koro CE, Fedder DO, L'Italien GJ, Weiss SS, Magder LS, Kreyenbuhl J, Revicki DA, Buchanan RW. Assessment of independent effect of olanzapine and risperidone on risk of diabetes among patients with schizophrenia: population based nested case-control study. Br Med J 2002;325:243–7.

779. Caro JJ, Ward A, Levinton C, Robinson K. The risk of diabetes during olanzapine use compared with risperidone use: a retrospective database analysis. J Clin Psychiatry 2002;63(12):1135–9.

780. Bobes J, Rejas J, García-García M, Rico-Villademoros F, García-Portilla MP, Fernández I, Hernández G, for the EIRE Study Group. Weight gain in patients with schizophrenia treated with risperidone, olanzapine, quetiapine or haloperidol: results of the EIRE study. Schizophr Res 2003;62:77–88.

781. Sernyak MJ, Gulanski B, Leslie DL, Rosenheck R. Undiagnosed hyperglycemia in clozapine-treated patients with schizophrenia. J Clin Psychiatry 2003;64:605–8.

782. Lindenmayer J-P, Czobor P, Volavka J, Citrome L, Sheitman B, McEvoy JP, Cooper TB, Chakos M, Lieberman JA. Changes in glucose and cholesterol levels in patients with schizophrenia treated with typical or atypical antipsychotics. Am J Psychiatry 2003;160:290–6.

783. Harris MI, Flegal KM, Cowie CC, Eberhardt MS, Goldstein DE, Little RR, Wiedmeyer HM, Byrd-Holt DD. Prevalence of diabetes, impaired fasting glucose and impaired glucose tolerance in US adults. Diabetes Care 1998;21:518–24.

784. Dixon L, Weiden P, Delahanty J, Goldberg R, Postrado L, Lucksted A, Lehman A. Prevalence and correlates of diabetes in national schizophrenia samples. Schizophr Bull 2000;26:903–12.

785. Koller EA, Doraiswamy PM. Olanzapine-associated diabetes mellitus. Pharmacotherapy 2002;22:841–52.

786. Meyer JM. A retrospective comparison of weight, lipid, and glucose changes between risperidone- and olanzapine-treated inpatients metabolic outcomes after 1 year. J Clin Psychiatry 2002;63:425–33.

787. Wilson DR, D'Souza L, Sarkar N, Newton M, Hammond C. New-onset diabetes and ketoacidosis with atypical antipsychotics. Schizophr Res 2002;59:1–6.

788. Jin H, Meyer JM, Jeste DV. Phenomenology of and risk factors for new-onset diabetes mellitus and diabetes ketoacidosis associated with atypical antipsychotics: an analysis of 45 cases. Ann Clin Psychiatry 2002;14:59–64.

789. Ramankutty G. Olanzapine-induced destabilization of diabetes in the absence of weight gain. Acta Psychiatr Scand 2002;105:235–7.

790. Wirshing DA. Adverse effects of atypical antipsychotics. J Clin Psychiatry 2001;62:7–10.

791. Ebenbichler CF, Laimer M, Eder U, Mangweth B, Weiss E, Hofer A, Hummer M, Kemmler G, Lechleitner M, Patsch JR, Fleischhacker WW. Olanzapine induces insulin resistance: results from a prospective study. J Clin Psychiatry 2003;64:1436–9.

792. Henderson DC, Cagliero E, Copeland PM, Borba CP, Evins E, Hayden D, Weber MT, Anderson EJ, Allison DB, Daley TB, Schoenfeld D, Goff DC. Glucose metabolism in patients with schizophrenia treated with atypical antipsychotic agents. Arch Gen Psychiatry 2005;62:19–28.

793. Hagg S, Soderberg S, Ahren B, Olsson T, Mjornfal T. Leptin concentrations are increased in subjects treated with clozapine or conventional antipsychotics. J Clin Psychiatry 2001;62:843–8.

794. Dufresne RL. Metabolic syndrome and antipsychotic therapy: a summary of the findings. Drug Benefit Trends 2003;Suppl B:12–17.

795. Lean MEJ, Pajonk F-G. Patients on atypical antipsychotic drugs. Diabetes Care 2003;26:1597–605.

796. Liberty IF, Todder D, Umansky R, Harman-Boehm I. Atypical antipsychotics and diabetes mellitus: an association. Isr Med Assoc J 2004;6:276–9.

797. Baptista T. Body weight gain induced by antipsychotic drugs: mechanisms and management. Acta Psychiatr Scand 1999;100(1):3–16.

798. Taylor DM, McAskill R. Atypical antipsychotics and weight gain—a systematic review. Acta Psychiatr Scand 2000;101(6):416–32.

799. Gupta S, Droney T, Al-Samarrai S, Keller P, Frank B. Olanzapine-induced weight gain. Ann Clin Psychiatry 1998;10(1):39.

800. Brecher M, Geller W. Weight gain with risperidone. J Clin Psychopharmacol 1997;17(5):435–6.

801. Penn JV, Martini J, Radka D. Weight gain associated with risperidone. J Clin Psychopharmacol 1996;16(3):259–60.

802. Frankenburg FR, Zanarini MC, Kando J, Centorrino F. Clozapine and body mass change. Biol Psychiatry 1998;43(7):520–4.

803. Bustillo JR, Buchanan RW, Irish D, Breier A. Differential effect of clozapine on weight: a controlled study. Am J Psychiatry 1996;153(6):817–9.

804. Stigler KA, Potenza MN, Posey DJ, McDougle CJ. Weight gain associated with atypical antipsychotic use in children and adolescents. Pediatr Drugs 2004;6:33–44.

805. Kraepelin E. In: Dementia Praecox and Paraphrenia. Edinburgh: E & S Livingstone, 1919:87.

806. Gupta S, Droney T, Al-Samarrai S, Keller P, Frank B. Olanzapine: weight gain therapeutic efficacy. J Clin Psychopharmacol 1999;19(3):273–5.

807. Baymiller SP, Ball P, McMahon RP, Buchanan RW. Weight and blood pressure change during clozapine treatment. Clin Neuropharmacol 2002;25(4):202–6.

808. Monteleone P, Fabrazzo M, Tortorella A, La Pia S, Maj M. Pronounced early increase in circulating leptin predicts a lower weight gain during clozapine treatment. J Clin Psychopharmacol 2002;22(4):424–6.

809. Wetterling T. Bodyweight gain with atypical antipsychotics. A comparative review. Drug Saf 2001;24(1):59–73.

810. Blin O, Micallef J. Antipsychotic-associated weight gain and clinical outcome parameters. J Clin Psychiatry 2001;62(Suppl 7):11–21.

811. Allison DB, Casey DE. Antipsychotic-induced weight gain: a review of the literature. J Clin Psychiatry 2001;62(Suppl 7):22–31.

812. Kurzthaler I, Fleischhacker WW. The clinical implications of weight gain in schizophrenia. J Clin Psychiatry 2001;62(Suppl 7):32–7.

813. Casey DE, Zorn SH. The pharmacology of weight gain with antipsychotics. J Clin Psychiatry 2001;62(Suppl 7):4–10.

814. Allison DB, Mentore JL, Heo M, Chandler LP, Cappelleri JC, Infante MC, Weiden PJ. Antipsychotic-induced weight gain: a comprehensive research synthesis. Am J Psychiatry 1999;156(11):1686–96.

815. Allison DB, Mentore JL, Heo M, et al. Weight gain associated with conventional and newer antipsychotics: a meta-analysis. Boca Raton, Florida, June 10–13Presented at the New Clinical Drug Evaluation Unit 38th Annual Meeting 1998;.

816. Kelly DL, Conley RR, Lore RC, et al. Weight gain in adolescents treated with risperidone and conventional antipsychotics over six months. J Child Adolesc Psychopharmacol 1998;813:151–9.

817. Tollefson GD, Beasley CM Jr, Tran PV, Street JS, Krueger JA, Tamura RN, Graffeo KA, Thieme ME. Olanzapine versus haloperidol in the treatment of schizophrenia and schizoaffective and schizophreniform disorders: results of an international collaborative trial. Am J Psychiatry 1997;154(4):457–65.

818. Wistedt B. A depot neuroleptic withdrawal study. A controlled study of the clinical effects of the withdrawal of depot fluphenazine decanoate and depot flupenthixol decanoate in chronic schizophrenic patients. Acta Psychiatr Scand 1981;64(1):65–84.

819. Nemeroff CB. Dosing the antipsychotic medication olanzapine. J Clin Psychiatry 1997;58(Suppl 10):45–9.

820. Tran PV, Hamilton SH, Kuntz AJ, Potvin JH, Andersen SW, Beasley C Jr, Tollefson GD. Double-blind comparison of olanzapine versus risperidone in the treatment of schizophrenia and other psychotic disorders. J Clin Psychopharmacol 1997;17(5):407–18.

821. Ganguli R, Brar JS, Ayrton Z. Weight gain over 4 months in schizophrenia patients: a comparison of olanzapine and risperidone. Schizophr Res 2001;49(3):261–7.

822. Wetterling T, Mussigbrodt HE. Weight gain: side effect of atypical neuroleptics? J Clin Psychopharmacol 1999;19(4):316–21.

823. Reinstein MJ, Sirotovskaya LA, Jones LE, Mohan S, Chasanov MA. Effect of clozapine-quetiapine combination therapy on weight and glycaemic control. Clin Drug Invest 1999;18:99–104.

824. Vieweg WV, Sood AB, Pandurangi A, Silverman JJ. Newer antipsychotic drugs and obesity in children and adolescents. How should we assess drug-associated weight gain? Acta Psychiatr Scand 2005;111:177–84.

825. Owens DG. Extrapyramidal side effects and tolerability of risperidone: a review. J Clin Psychiatry 1994;55(Suppl 5):29–35.

826. Rietschel M, Naber D, Fimmers R, Moller HJ, Propping P, Nothen MM. Efficacy and side-effects of clozapine not associated with variation in the 5-HT$_{2C}$ receptor. Neuroreport 1997;8(8):1999–2003.

827. Rietschel M, Naber D, Oberlander H, Holzbach R, Fimmers R, Eggermann K, Moller HJ, Propping P, Nothen MM. Efficacy and side-effects of clozapine: testing for association with allelic variation in the dopamine D$_4$ receptor gene. Neuropsychopharmacology 1996;15(5):491–6.

828. Theisen FM, Cichon S, Linden A, Martin M, Remschmidt H, Hebebrand J. Clozapine and weight gain. Am J Psychiatry 2001;158(5):816.

829. Reynolds GP, Zhang ZJ, Zhang XB. Association of antipsychotic drug-induced weight gain with a 5-HT$_{2C}$ receptor gene polymorphism. Lancet 2002;359(9323):2086–7.

830. Allison DB, Fontaine KR, Heo M, Mentore JL, Cappelleri JC, Chandler LP, Weiden PJ, Cheskin LJ. The distribution of body mass index among individuals with and without schizophrenia. J Clin Psychiatry 1999;60(4):215–20.

831. Hummer M, Kemmler G, Kurz M, Kurzthaler I, Oberbauer H, Fleischhacker WW. Weight gain induced by clozapine. Eur Neuropsychopharmacol 1995;5(4):437–40.

832. Kohnke MD, Griese EU, Stosser D, Gaertner I, Barth G. Cytochrome P450 2D6 deficiency and its clinical relevance in a patient treated with risperidone. Pharmacopsychiatry 2002;35(3):116–8.

833. European Federation of Associations of Families of Mentally Ill People. www.eufami.org.

834. O'Keefe C, Noordsy D. Prevention and reversal of weight gain associated with antipsychotic treatment. J Clin Outcomes Manage 2002;9:575–82.

835. Rotatori AF, Fox R, Wicks A. Weight loss with psychiatric residents in a behavioral self control program. Psychol Rep 1980;46(2):483–6.

836. Floris M, Lejeune J, Deberdt W. Effect of amantadine on weight gain during olanzapine treatment. Eur Neuropsychopharmacol 2001;11(2):181–2.

837. Cohen S, Glazewski R, Khan S, Khan A. Weight gain with risperidone among patients with mental retardation: effect of calorie restriction. J Clin Psychiatry 2001;62(2):114–6.

838. Aldeen T, Wells C, Hay P, Davidson F, Lau R. Lipodystrophy associated with nevirapine-containing antiretroviral therapies. AIDS 1999;13(7):865–7.

839. Garrino MG, Plant TD, Henquin JC. Effects of putative activators of K+ channels in mouse pancreatic beta-cells. Br J Pharmacol 1989;98(3):957–65.

840. Schwartz ML. Severe reversible hyperglycemia as a consequence of niacin therapy. Arch Intern Med 1993;153(17):2050–2.

841. Capuzzi DM, Guyton JR, Morgan JM, Goldberg AC, Kreisberg RA, Brusco OA, Brody J. Efficacy and safety of an extended-release niacin (Niaspan): a long-term study. Am J Cardiol 1998;82(12A):U74–81.

842. Garg A, Grundy SM. Nicotinic acid as therapy for dyslipidemia in non-insulin-dependent diabetes mellitus. JAMA 1990;264(6):723–6.

843. Lavelle KJ, Atkinson KF, Kleit SA. Hyperlactatemia and hemolysis in G6PD deficiency after nitrofurantoin ingestion. Am J Med Sci 1976;272(2):201–4.

844. Chene G, Angelini E, Cotte L, Lang JM, Morlat P, Rancinan C, May T, Journot V, Raffi F, Jarrousse B, Grappin M, Lepeu G, Molina JM. Role of long-term nucleoside-analogue therapy in lipodystrophy and metabolic disorders in human immunodeficiency virus-infected patients. Clin Infect Dis 2002;34(5):649–57.

845. Saint-Marc T, Partisani M, Poizot-Martin I, Bruno F, Rouviere O, Lang JM, Gastaut JA, Touraine JL. A syndrome of peripheral fat wasting (lipodystrophy) in patients receiving long-term nucleoside analogue therapy. AIDS 1999;13(13):1659–67.

846. Fouty B, Frerman F, Reves R. Riboflavin to treat nucleoside analog-induced lactic acidosis. Lancet 1998;352(9124):291–2.

847. John M, Moore CB, James IR, Nolan D, Upton RP, McKinnon EJ, Mallal SA. Chronic hyperlactatemia in HIV-infected patients taking antiretroviral therapy. AIDS 2001;15(6):717–23.

848. Johri S, Alkhuja S, Siviglia G, Soni A. Steatosis–lactic acidosis syndrome associated with stavudine and lamivudine therapy. AIDS 2000;14(9):1286–7.

849. Brivet FG, Nion I, Megarbane B, Slama A, Brivet M, Rustin P, Munnich A. Fatal lactic acidosis and liver steatosis associated with didanosine and stavudine treatment: a respiratory chain dysfunction? J Hepatol 2000;32(2):364–5.

850. Mokrzycki MH, Harris C, May H, Laut J, Palmisano J. Lactic acidosis associated with stavudine administration: a report of five cases. Clin Infect Dis 2000;30(1):198–200.

851. Bharani A, Kumar H. Drug points: Diabetes inspidus induced by ofloxacin. BMJ 2001;323(7312):547.

852. Licht RW, Arngrim T, Cristensen H. Olanzapine-induced galactorrhea. Psychopharmacology (Berl) 2002;162(1):94–5.

853. Kingsbury SJ, Castelo C, Abulseoud O. Quetiapine for olanzapine-induced galactorrhea. Am J Psychiatry 2002;159(6):1061.

854. Mendhekar DN, Jiloha RC, Srivastava PK. Effect of risperidone on prolactinoma. A case report. Pharmacopsychiatry 2004;37:41–2.

855. Canuso CM, Hanau M, Jhamb KK, Green AI. Olanzapine use in women with antipsychotic-induced hyperprolactinemia. Am J Psychiatry 1998;155(10):1458.

856. Gazzola LR, Opler LA. Return of menstruation after switching from risperidone to olanzapine. J Clin Psychopharmacol 1998;18(6):486–7.

857. Potenza MN, Wasylink S, Epperson CN, McDougle CJ. Olanzapine augmentation of fluoxetine in the treatment of trichotillomania. Am J Psychiatry 1998;155(9):1299–300.

858. Popli AP, Konicki PE, Jurjus GJ, Fuller MA, Jaskiw GE. Clozapine and associated diabetes mellitus. J Clin Psychiatry 1997;58(3):108–11.

859. Wirshing DA, Spellberg BJ, Erhart SM, Marder SR, Wirshing WC. Novel antipsychotics and new onset diabetes. Biol Psychiatry 1998;44(8):778–83.

860. Ober SK, Hudak R, Rusterholtz A. Hyperglycemia and olanzapine. Am J Psychiatry 1999;156(6):970.

861. Ashim S, Warrington S, Anderson IM. Management of diabetes mellitus occurring during treatment with olanzapine: report of six cases and clinical implications. J Psychopharmacol 2004;18:128–32.

862. Folnegovic-Smalc V, Jukić V, Kozumplik O, Mimica N, Uzun S. Olanzapine use in a patient with schizophrenia and the risk of diabetes. Eur Psychiatry 2004;19:62–4.

863. Ramankutty G. Olanzapine-induced destabilization of diabetes in the absence of weight gain. Acta Psychiatr Scand 2002;105(3):235–6.

864. Fertig MK, Brooks VG, Shelton PS, English CW. Hyperglycemia associated with olanzapine. J Clin Psychiatry 1998;59(12):687–9.

865. Lindenmayer JP, Patel R. Olanzapine-induced ketoacidosis with diabetes mellitus. Am J Psychiatry 1999;156(9):1471.

866. Gatta B, Rigalleau V, Gin H. Diabetic ketoacidosis with olanzapine treatment. Diabetes Care 1999;22(6):1002–3.

867. Bettinger TL, Mendelson SC, Dorson PG, Crismon ML. Olanzapine-induced glucose dysregulation. Ann Pharmacother 2000;34(7–8):865–7.

868. Melkersson KI, Hulting AL, Brismar KE. Elevated levels of insulin, leptin, and blood lipids in olanzapine-treated patients with schizophrenia or related psychoses. J Clin Psychiatry 2000;61(10):742–9.

869. Cohn TA, Remington G, Kameh H. Hyperinsulinemia in psychiatric patients treated with olanzapine. J Clin Psychiatry 2002;63(1):75–6.

870. Bonanno DG, Davydov L, Botts SR. Olanzapine-induced diabetes mellitus. Ann Pharmacother 2001;35(5):563–5.

871. Roefaro J, Mukherjee SM. Olanzapine-induced hyperglycemic nonketotic coma. Ann Pharmacother 2001;35(3):300–2.

872. Lindenmayer JP, Smith RC, Singh A, Parker B, Chou E, Kotsaftis A. Hyperglycemia in patients with schizophrenia who are treated with olanzapine. J Clin Psychopharmacol 2001;21(3):351–3.

873. Meatherall R, Younes J. Fatality from olanzapine induced hyperglycemia. J Forensic Sci 2002;47(4):893–6.

874. Budman CL, Gayer AI. Low blood glucose and olanzapine. Am J Psychiatry 2001;158(3):500–1.

875. Bryden KE, Kopala LC. Body mass index increase of 58% associated with olanzapine. Am J Psychiatry 1999;156(11):1835–6.

876. Zullino DF, Quinche P, Hafliger T, Stigler M. Olanzapine improves social dysfunction in cluster B personality disorder. Hum Psychopharmacol 2002;17(5):247–51.

877. Gupta S, Droney T, Al-Samarrai S, Keller P, Frank B. Olanzapine-induced weight gain. Ann Clin Psychiatry 1998;10(1):39.

878. Gupta S, Droney T, Al-Samarrai S, Keller P, Frank B. Olanzapine: weight gain and therapeutic efficacy. J Clin Psychopharmacol 1999;19(3):273–5.

879. Sheitman BB, Bird PM, Binz W, Akinli L, Sanchez C. Olanzapine-induced elevation of plasma triglyceride levels. Am J Psychiatry 1999;156(9):1471–2.

880. Bronson BD, Lindenmayer JP. Adverse effects of high-dose olanzapine in treatment-refractory schizophrenia. J Clin Psychopharmacol 2000;20(3):382–4.

881. Littrell KH, Petty RG, Hilligoss NM, Peabody CD, Johnson CG. Weight loss associated with olanzapine treatment. J Clin Psychopharmacol 2002;22(4):436–7.

882. Sengupta SM, Klink R, Stip E, Baptista T, Malla A, Joober R. Weight gain and lipid metabolic abnormalities induced by olanzapine in first-episode, drug-naive patients with psychotic disorders. Schizophr Res 2005;80:131–3.

883. Haberfellner EM, Rittmannsberger H. Weight gain during long-term treatment with olanzapine: a case series. Int Clin Psychopharmacol 2004;19:251–3.

884. Vieta E, Sánchez-Moreno J, Goikolea JM, Colom F, Martínez-Arán A, Benabarre A, Corbella B, Torrent C, Comes M, Reinares M, Brugue E. Effects of weight and outcome of long-term olanzapine–topiramate combination treatment in bipolar disorder. J Clin Psychopharmacol 2004;24:374–8.

885. Gupta S, Masand PS, Virk S, Schwartz T, Hameed A, Frank BL, Lockwood K. Weight decline in patients switching from olanzapine to quetiapine. Schizophr Res 2004;70:57–62.

886. Guardia J, Segura L, Gonzalvo B, Iglesias L, Roncero C, Cardús M, Casas M. A double-blind, placebo-controlled study of olanzapine in the treatment of alcohol-dependence disorder. Alcohol Clin Exp Res 2004;28:736–45.

887. Ercan ES, Kutlu A, Varan A, Çikoğlu S, Coşkunol H, Bayraktar E. Olanzapine treatment of eight adolescent patients with psychosis. Hum Psychopharmacol Clin Exp 2004;19:53–6.

888. Barak Y, Shamir E, Mirecki I, Weizman R, Aizenberg D. Switching elderly chronic psychotic patients to olanzapine. Int J Neuropsychopharmacol 2004;7:165–9.

889. Lexchin J, Bero LA, Djulbegovic B, Clark O. Pharmaceutical industry sponsorship and research outcome and quality: systematic review. BMJ 2003;326(7400):1167–70.

890. Lasser RA, Mao L, Gharabawi G. Smokers and nonsmokers equally affected by olanzapine-induced weight gain: metabolic implications. Schizophr Res 2004;66:163–7.

891. Roerig JL, Mitchell JE, de Zwaan M, Crosby RD, Gosnell BA, Steffen KJ, Wonderlich SA. A comparison of the effects of olanzapine and risperidone versus placebo on eating behaviors. J Clin Psychopharmacol 2005;25:413–8.

892. Powers PS, Santana CA, Bannon YS. Olanzapine in the treatment of anorexia nervosa: an open label trial. Int J Eat Disord 2002;32(2):146–54.

893. Ellingrod VL, Miller D, Schultz SK, Wehring H, Arndt S. CYP2D6 polymorphisms and atypical antipsychotic weight gain. Psychiatr Genet 2002;12(1):55–8.

894. Sacchetti E, Guarneri L, Bravi D. H(2) antagonist nizatidine may control olanzapine-associated weight gain in schizophrenic patients. Biol Psychiatry 2000;48(2):167–8.

895. Cavazzoni P, Tanaka Y, Roychowdhury SM, Breier A, Allison DB. Nizatidine for prevention of weight gain olanzapine: a double-blind placebo-controlled trial. Eur Neuropsychopharmacol 2003;13:81–5.

896. Poyurovsky M, Tal V, Maayan R, Gil-Ad I, Fuchs C, Weizman A. The effect of famotidine addition on olanzapine-induced weight gain in first-episode schizophrenia patients: a double-blind placebo-controlled pilot study. Eur Neuropsychopharmacol 2004;14:332–6.

897. Littman A. Potent acid reduction and risk of enteric infection. Lancet 1990;335(8683):222.

898. Raoul JL, Bretagne JF, Ropert A, Siproudhis L, Heresbach D, Gosselin M. Zollinger–Ellison syndrome, antisecretory treatment, and body weight. Dig Dis Sci 1992;37(8):1308–9.

899. George R. Hypothalamus: anterior pituitary gland. In: Clonet DH, editor. Narcotic Drugs: Biochemical Pharmacology. New York: Plenum Press, 1971:283.

900. Raff H, Flemma RJ, Findling JW. Fast cortisol-induced inhibition of the adrenocorticotropin response to surgery in humans. J Clin Endocrinol Metab 1988;67(6):1146–8.

901. Pfeiffer A, Herz A. Endocrine actions of opioids. Horm Metab Res 1984;16(8):386–97.

902. O'Keefe SJD, Cariem AK, Levy M. The exacerbation of pancreatic endocrine dysfunction by potent pancreatic exocrine supplements in patients with chronic pancreatitis. J Clin Gastroenterol 2001;32:319–23.

903. Otsuka M, Akiba T, Okita Y, Tomita K, Yoshiyama N, Sasaoka T, Kanayama M, Marumo F. Lactic acidosis with hypoglycemia and hyperammonemia observed in two uremic patients during calcium hopantenate treatment. Jpn J Med 1990;29(3):324–8.

904. Ruvalcaba RH, Limbeck GA, Kelley VC. Acetaminophen and hypoglycemia. Am J Dis Child 1966;112(6):558–60.

905. Nakasaki H, Katayama T, Yokoyama S, Tajima T, Mitomi T, Tsuda M, Suga T, Fujii K. Complication of parenternal nutrition composed of essential amino acids and histidine in adults with renal failure. J Parenter Enteral Nutr 1993;17(1):86–90.

906. Fan BG, Salehi A, Sternby B, Axelson J, Lundquist I, Andren-Sandberg A, Ekelund M. Total parenteral nutrition influences both endocrine and exocrine function of rat pancreas. Pancreas 1997;15(2):147–53.

907. Boden G, Jadali F. Effects of lipid on basal carbohydrate metabolism in normal men. Diabetes 1991;40(6):686–92.

908. McCowen KC, Friel C, Sternberg J, Chan S, Forse RA, Burke PA, Bistrian BR. Hypocaloric total parenteral nutrition: effectiveness in prevention of hyperglycemia and infectious complications—a randomized clinical trial. Crit Care Med 2000;28(11):3606–11.

909. Lienhardt A, Rakotoambinina B, Colomb V, Souissi S, Sadoun E, Goulet O, Robert JJ, Ricour C. Insulin secretion and sensitivity in children on cyclic total parenteral nutrition. J Parenter Enteral Nutr 1998;22(6):382–6.

910. Chiolero R, Schneiter P, Cayeux C, Temler E, Jequier E, Schindler C, Tappy L. Metabolic and respiratory effects of sodium lactate during short i.v. nutrition in critically ill patients J Parenter Enteral Nutr 1996;20(4):257–63.

911. Kollef MH, McCormack MT, Caras WE, Reddy VV, Bacon D. The fat overload syndrome: successful treatment with plasma exchange. Ann Intern Med 1990;112(7):545–6.

912. Lindholm M. The ability of critically ill patients to eliminate fat emulsions. J Drug Dev 1991;4(Suppl 3):40–2.

913. Jeppesen PB, Hoy CE, Mortensen PB. Essential fatty acid deficiency in patients receiving home parenteral nutrition. Am J Clin Nutr 1998;68(1):126–33.

914. Duerksen DR, Nehra V, Palombo JD, Ahmad A, Bistrian BR. Essential fatty acid deficiencies in patients with chronic liver disease are not reversed by short-term intravenous lipid supplementation. Dig Dis Sci 1999;44(7):1342–8.

915. Hager L. Choline deficiency and TPN associated liver dysfunction: a case report. Nutrition 1998;14(1):60–2.

916. Shronts EP. Essential nature of choline with implications for total parenteral nutrition. J Am Diet Assoc 1997;97(6):639–46649.

917. Moyer RA, St John D. Acute gout precipitated by total parenteral nutrition. J Rheumatol 2003;30:849–50.

918. Bonin B, Vandel P, Sechter D, Bizouard P. Paroxetine and galactorrhea. Pharmacopsychiatry 1997;30(4):133–4.

919. Morrison J, Remick RA, Leung M, Wrixon KJ, Bebb RA. Galactorrhea induced by paroxetine. Can J Psychiatry 2001;46(1):88–9.

920. Kim EJ, Yu B-H. Increased cholesterol levels after paroxetine treatment in patients with panic disorder. J Clin Psychopharmacol 2005;25:597–9.

921. Delrieu F, Menkes CJ, Sainte-Croix A, Babinet P, Chesneau AM, Delbarre F. Myasthénie et thyroidite auto-immune au course du traitements de la polyarthrite rhumatoïde par la D-pénicillamine. Etude anatomo-clinique d'un cas. [Myasthenia gravis and autoimmune thyroiditis during the treatment of rheumatoid polyarthritis with D-penicillamine. Anatomoclinical study of 1 case.] Ann Med Interne (Paris) 1976;127(10):739–43.

922. Bertrand JL, Rousset H, Queneau P, Ollagnier M. Thyroïdite auto-immune, une complication rare du traitement à la D-pénicillamine. [Autoimmune thyroiditis. A rare complication of treatment with D-penicillamine.] Therapie 1981;36(3):333–6.

923. Addyman R, Beyeler C, Astbury C, Bird HA. Urinary glucaric acid excretion in rheumatoid arthritis: influence of disease activity and disease modifying drugs. Ann Rheum Dis 1996;55(7):478–81.

924. Benson EA, Healey LA, Barron EJ. Insulin antibodies in patients receiving penicillamine. Am J Med 1985;78(5):857–60.

925. Herranz L, Rovira A, Grande C, Suarez A, Martinez-Ara J, Pallardo LF, Gomez-Pan A. Autoimmune insulin syndrome in a patient with progressive systemic sclerosis receiving penicillamine. Horm Res 1992;37(1–2):78–80.

926. Becker RC, Martin RG. Penicillamine-induced insulin antibodies. Ann Intern Med 1986;104(1):127–8.

927. Elling P, Elling H. Penicillamine, captopril, and hypoglycemia. Ann Intern Med 1985;103(4):644–5.

928. Vardi P, Brik R, Barzilai D, Lorber M, Scharf Y. Frequent induction of insulin autoantibodies by D-penicillamine in patients with rheumatoid arthritis. J Rheumatol 1992;19(10):1527–30.

929. Faguer de Moustier B, Burgard M, Boitard C, Desplanque N, Fanjoux J, Tchobroutsky G. Syndrome hypoglycémique auto-immun induit par le pyritinol. [Auto-immune hypoglycemic syndrome induced by pyritinol.] Diabete Metab 1988;14(4):423–9.

930. Sheikh IA, Kaplan AP. Assessment of kininases in rheumatic diseases and the effect of therapeutic agents. Arthritis Rheum 1987;30(2):138–45.

931. Joyce DA. D-penicillamine pharmacokinetics and pharmacodynamics in man. Pharmacol Ther 1989;42(3):405–27.

932. Schulze E, Herrmann K, Haustein UF, Krusche U, Rothenburger I. Einfluss von Penicillin und D-Penicillamin auf die Betagalactosidaseaktivität bei Patienten met progressiver Sklerodermie. [Effect of penicillin and D-penicillamine on beta-galactosidase activity in patients with progressive scleroderma.] Dermatol Monatsschr 1988;174(11):661–6.

933. Kuperman-Beade M, Laude TA. Partial lipoatrophy in a child. Pediatr Dermatol 2000;17(4):302–3.

934. Masur H. Prevention and treatment of *Pneumocystis* pneumonia. N Engl J Med 1992;327(26):1853–60.

935. Schwarzmann E, Quast M. Kasuistische Betrachtungen zur Phenylbutazon-Struma. Dtsch Gesundheitsw 1973;28:1417.

936. Franceschi M, Perego L, Cavagnini F, Cattaneo AG, Invitti C, Caviezel F, Strambi LF, Smirne S. Effects of long–term antiepileptic therapy on the hypothalamic–pituitary axis in man. Epilepsia 1984;25(1):46–52.

937. Huang QL, Feig DS, Blackstein ME. Development of tertiary hyperparathyroidism after phosphate supplementation in oncogenic osteomalacia. J Endocrinol Invest 2000;23(4):263–7.

938. Albright F, Butler AM, Bloom E. Rickets resistant to vitamin D therapy. Am J Dis Child 1937;54:529–44.

939. Makitie O, Kooh SW, Sochett E. Prolonged high-dose phosphate treatment: a risk factor for tertiary hyperparathyroidism in X-linked hypophosphatemic rickets. Clin Endocrinol 2003;58:163–8.

940. Peet KM. Use of pizotifen in severe migraine: a long-term study. Curr Med Res Opin 1977;5(2):192–9.

941. Crowder D, Maclay WP. Pizotifen once daily in the prophylaxis of migraine: results of a multi-centre general practice study. Curr Med Res Opin 1984;9(4):280–5.

942. Bosl GJ, Bajorunas D. Pituitary and testicular hormonal function after treatment for germ cell tumours. Int J Androl 1987;10(1):381–4.

943. Gerl A, Muhlbayer D, Hansmann G, Mraz W, Hiddemann W. The impact of chemotherapy on Leydig cell function in long term survivors of germ cell tumors. Cancer 2001;91(7):1297–303.

944. Sakakura C, Hagiwara A, Kin S, Yamamoto K, Okamoto K, Yamaguchi T, Sawai K, Yamagishi H. A case of hyperosmolar nonketotic coma occurring during chemotherapy using cisplatin for gallbladder cancer. Hepatogastroenterology 1999;46(29):2801–3.

945. Hammill SC, Sorenson PB, Wood DL, Sugrue DD, Osborn MJ, Gersh BJ, Holmes DR Jr. Propafenone for the treatment of refractory complex ventricular ectopic activity. Mayo Clin Proc 1986;61(2):98–103.

946. Mateu J, Barrachina F. Hypertriglyceridaemia associated with propofol sedation in critically ill patients. Intensive Care Med 1996;22(8):834–5.

947. Sandiumenge Camps A, Sanchez-Izquierdo Riera JA, Toral Vazquez D, Sa Borges M, Peinado Rodriguez J, Alted Lopez E. Midazolam and 2% propofol in long-term sedation of traumatized critically ill patients: efficacy and safety comparison. Crit Care Med 2000;28(11):3612–9.

948. Devlin JW, Lau AK, Tanios MA. Propofol-associated hypertriglyceridemia and pancreatitis in the intensive care unit: an analysis of frequency and risk factors. Pharmacotherapy 2005;25(10):1348–52.

949. Kill C, Leonhardt A, Wulf H. Lactic acidosis after short-term infusion of propofol for anaesthesia in a child with osteogenesis imperfecta. Paediatr Anaesth 2003;13:823–6.

950. Martin PH, Murthy BV, Petros AJ. Metabolic, biochemical and haemodynamic effects of infusion of propofol for long-term sedation of children undergoing intensive care. Br J Anaesth 1997;79:276–9.

951. Hansen TG. [Propofol infusion syndrome in children.] Ugeskr Laeger 2005;167(39):3672–5.

952. Liolios A, Guerit JM, Scholtes JL, Raftopoulos C, Hantson P. Propofol infusion syndrome associated with short-term large-dose infusion during surgical anesthesia in an adult. Anesth Analg 2005;100:1804–6.

953. Kumar MA, Urrutia VC, Thomas CE, Abou-Khaled KJ, Schwartzman RJ. The syndrome of irreversible acidosis after prolonged propofol infusion. Neurocrit Care 2005;3(3):257–9.

954. Liolios A, Guerit JM, Scholtes JL, Raftopoulos C, Hantson P. Propofol infusion syndrome associated with short-term large-dose infusion during surgical anesthesia in an adult. Anesth Analg 2005;100:1804–6.

955. Betrosian AP, Papanikoleou M, Frantzeskaki F, Diakalis C, Georgiadis G. Myoglobinemia and propofol infusion. Acta Anaesthesiol Scand 2005;49:720.

956. Farag E, Deboer G, Cohen BH, Niezgoda J. Metabolic acidosis due to propofol infusion. Anesthesiology 2005;102:697–8.

957. Haase R, Sauer H, Eichler G. Lactic acidosis following short-term propofol infusion may be an early warning of propofol infusion syndrome. J Neurosurg Anesthesiol 2005;17:122–3.

958. Burow BK, Johnson ME, Packer DL. Metabolic acidosis associated with propofol in the absence of other causative factors. Anesthesiology 2004;101:239–41.

959. Salengros J-C, Velghe-Lenelle C-E, Bollens R, Engelman E, Barvais L. Lactic acidosis during propofol–remifentanil anesthesia in an adult. Anesthesiology 2004;101:243–5.

960. Funston JS, Prough DS. Two reports of propofol anesthesia associated with metabolic acidosis in adults. Anesthesiology 2004;101:6–8.

961. Withington DE, Decell MK, Al Ayed T. A case of propofol toxicity: further evidence for a causal mechanism. Pediatr Anesth 2004;14:505–8.

962. Baumeister FAM, Oberhoffer R, Liebhaber GM, Kunkel J, Eberhardt J, Holthausen H, Peters J. Fatal propofol infusion syndrome in association with ketogenic diet. Neuropediatrics 2004;35:250–2.

963. Culp KE, Augoustides JG, Ochroch AE, Milas BL. Clinical management of cardiogenic shock associated with prolonged propofol infusion. Anesth Analg 2004;99:221–6.

964. Hanna JP, Ramundo ML. Rhabdomyolysis and hypoxia associated with prolonged propofol infusion in children. Neurology 1998;50(1):301–3.

965. Cray SH, Robinson BH, Cox PN. Lactic acidemia and bradyarrhythmia in a child sedated with propofol. Crit Care Med 1998;26(12):2087–92.

966. Watanabe Y. Lactic acidosis associated with propofol in an adult patient after cardiovascular surgery. J Cardiothorac Vasc Anesth 1998;12:611–2.

967. Susla GM. Propofol toxicity in critically ill pediatric patients: show us the proof. Crit Care Med 1998;26(12):1959–60.

968. Asirvatham SJ, Johnson TW, Oberoi MP, Jackman WM. Prolonged loss of consciousness and elevated porphyrins following propofol administrations. Anesthesiology 1998;89(4):1029–31.

969. Chen F, Kearney T, Robinson S, Daley-Yates PT, Waldron S, Churchill DR. Cushing's syndrome and severe adrenal suppression in patients treated with ritonavir and inhaled nasal fluticasone. Sex Transm Infect 1999;75(4):274.

970. Hillebrand-Haverkort ME, Prummel MF, ten Veen JH. Ritonavir-induced Cushing's syndrome in a patient treated with nasal fluticasone. AIDS 1999;13(13):1803.

971. Darvay A, Acland K, Lynn W, Russell-Jones R. Striae formation in two HIV-positive persons receiving protease inhibitors. J Am Acad Dermatol 1999;41(3 Pt 1):467–9.

972. Bonfanti P, Valsecchi L, Parazzini F, Carradori S, Pusterla L, Fortuna P, Timillero L, Alessi F, Ghiselli G, Gabbuti A, Di Cintio E, Martinelli C, Faggion I, Landonio S, Quirino T. Incidence of adverse reactions in HIV patients treated with protease inhibitors: a cohort study. Coordinamento Italiano Studio Allergia e Infezione da HIV (CISAI) Group. J Acquir Immune Defic Syndr 2000;23(3):236–45.

973. Thiebaut R, Dabis F, Malvy D, Jacqmin-Gadda H, Mercie P, Valentin VD. Serum triglycerides, HIV infection, and highly active antiretroviral therapy, Aquitaine Cohort, France, 1996 to 1998. Groupe d'Epidemiologie Clinique du Sida en Aquitaine (GECSA). J Acquir Immune Defic Syndr 2000;23(3):261–5.

974. Benson JO, McGhee K, Coplan P, Grunfeld C, Robertson M, Brodovicz KG, Slater E. Fat redistribution in indinavir-treated patients with HIV infection: a review of postmarketing cases. J Acquir Immune Defic Syndr 2000;25(2):130–9.

975. Kaufman MB, Simionatto C. A review of protease inhibitor-induced hyperglycemia. Pharmacotherapy 1999;19(1):114–7.

976. Rodriguez-Rosado R, Soriano V, Blanco F, Dona C, Gonzalez-Lahoz J. Diabetes mellitus associated with protease inhibitor use. Eur J Clin Microbiol Infect Dis 1999;18(9):675–7.

977. Bitnun A, Sochett E, Dick PT, To T, Jefferies C, Babyn P, Forbes J, Read S, King SM. Insulin sensitivity and beta-cell function in protease inhibitor-treated and -naive human immunodeficiency virus-infected children. J Clin Endocrinol Metab 2005;90(1):168–74.

978. Periard D, Telenti A, Sudre P, Cheseaux JJ, Halfon P, Reymond MJ, Marcovina SM, Glauser MP, Nicod P, Darioli R, Mooser V. Atherogenic dyslipidemia in HIV-infected individuals treated with protease inhibitors. The Swiss HIV Cohort Study. Circulation 1999;100(7):700–5.

979. Echevarria KL, Hardin TC, Smith JA. Hyperlipidemia associated with protease inhibitor therapy. Ann Pharmacother 1999;33(7–8):859–63.

980. Berthold HK, Parhofer KG, Ritter MM, Addo M, Wasmuth JC, Schliefer K, Spengler U, Rockstroh JK. Influence of protease inhibitor therapy on lipoprotein metabolism. J Intern Med 1999;246(6):567–75.

981. Aldamiz-Echevarria L, Pocheville I, Sanjurjo P, Elorz J, Prieto JA, Rodriguez-Soriano J. Abnormalities in plasma fatty acid composition in human immunodeficiency virus-infected children treated with protease inhibitors. Acta Paediatr 2005;94(6):672–7.

982. Roth VR, Kravcik S, Angel JB. Development of cervical fat pads following therapy with human immunodeficiency virus type 1 protease inhibitors. Clin Infect Dis 1998;27(1):65–7.

983. Striker R, Conlin D, Marx M, Wiviott L. Localized adipose tissue hypertrophy in patients receiving human immunodeficiency virus protease inhibitors. Clin Infect Dis 1998;27(1):218–20.

984. Viraben R, Aquilina C. Indinavir-associated lipodystrophy. AIDS 1998;12(6):F37–9.

985. Toma E, Therrien R. Gynecomastia during indinavir antiretroviral therapy in HIV infection. AIDS 1998;12(6):681–2.

986. Lui A, Karter D, Turett G. Another case of breast hypertrophy in a patient treated with indinavir. Clin Infect Dis 1998;26(6):1482.

987. Walli R, Herfort O, Michl GM, Demant T, Jager H, Dieterle C, Bogner JR, Landgraf R, Goebel FD. Treatment with protease inhibitors associated with peripheral insulin resistance and impaired oral glucose tolerance in HIV-1-infected patients. AIDS 1998;12(15):F167–73.

988. Carr A, Cooper DA. Images in clinical medicine. Lipodystrophy associated with an HIV-protease inhibitor. N Engl J Med 1998;339(18):1296.

989. Carr A, Samaras K, Burton S, Law M, Freund J, Chisholm DJ, Cooper DA. A syndrome of peripheral lipodystrophy, hyperlipidaemia and insulin resistance in patients receiving HIV protease inhibitors. AIDS 1998;12(7):F51–8.

990. Lo JC, Mulligan K, Tai VW, Algren H, Schambelan M. "Buffalo hump" in men with HIV-1 infection. Lancet 1998;351(9106):867–70.

991. Miller KD, Jones E, Yanovski JA, Shankar R, Feuerstein I, Falloon J. Visceral abdominal-fat accumulation associated with use of indinavir. Lancet 1998;351(9106):871–5.

992. Carr A, Samaras K, Thorisdottir A, Kaufmann GR, Chisholm DJ, Cooper DA. Diagnosis, prediction, and natural course of HIV-1 protease-inhibitor-associated lipodystrophy, hyperlipidaemia, and diabetes mellitus: a cohort study. Lancet 1999;353(9170):2093–9.

993. Saint-Marc T, Touraine JL. Effects of metformin on insulin resistance and central adiposity in patients receiving effective protease inhibitor therapy. AIDS 1999;13(8):1000–2.

994. Thiebaut R, Daucourt V, Malvy D. Lipodystrophy, glucose and lipid metabolism dysfunctions. Aquitaine Cohort. First International Workshop on Adverse Drug Reactions and Lipodystrophy in HIV, San Diego, 1999: Abstract 17.

995. Milpied-Homsi B, Krempf M, Gueglio B, Raffi F, Stalder JF. "Bosse de bison": un effet secondaire inattendu des traitements parinhibiteurs de protéases anti-VIH. ["Buffalo neck": an unintended secondary effect of treatment with anti-HIV protease inhibitors.] Ann Dermatol Venereol 1999;126(3):254–6.

996. Martinez E, Mocroft A, Garcia-Viejo MA, Perez-Cuevas JB, Blanco JL, Mallolas J, Bianchi L, Conget I, Blanch J, Phillips A, Gatell JM. Risk of lipodystrophy in HIV-1-infected patients treated with protease inhibitors: a prospective cohort study. Lancet 2001;357(9256):592–8.

997. Patel AM, McKeon J. Avoidance and management of adverse reactions to antituberculosis drugs. Drug Saf 1995;12(1):1–25.

998. Mandell GL, Sande MA. Antimicrobial agents: drugs used in the chemotherapy of tuberculosis and leprosy. In: Goodman Gilman A, Rall TW, Nies AS, Taylor P, editors. Goodman and Gilman's The Pharmacological Basis of Therapeutics. 8th ed.. New York: Pergamon Press, 1990:1146 Chapter 49.

999. Faguer de Moustier B, Burgard M, Boitard C, Desplanque N, Fanjoux J, Tchobroutsky G. Syndrome hypoglycémique auto-immune induit par le pyritinol. [Auto-immune hypoglycemic syndrome induced by pyritinol.] Diabete Metab 1988;14(4):423–9.

1000. Atmaca M, Kuloglu M, Tezcan E, Canatan H, Gecici O. Quetiapine is not associated with increase in prolactin secretion in contrast to haloperidol. Arch Med Res 2002;33(6):562–5.

1001. Henderson DC, Nasrallah RA, Goff DC. Switching from clozapine to olanzapine in treatment-refractory schizophrenia: safety, clinical efficacy, and predictors of response. J Clin Psychiatry 1998;59(11):585–8.

1002. Sacristan JA, Gomez JC, Martin J, Garcia-Bernardo E, Peralta V, Alvarez E, Gurpegui M, Mateo I, Morinigo A, Noval D, Soler R, Palomo T, Cuesta M, Perez-Blanco F, Massip C. Pharmacoeconomic assessment of olanzapine in the treatment of refractory schizophrenia based on a pilot clinical study. Clin Drug Invest 1998;15:29–35.

1003. Newton PN, Angus BJ, Chierakul W, Dondorp A, Ruangveerayuth R, Silamut K, Teerapong P, Supputtamongkol Y, Looareesuwan S, White NJ. Randomized comparison of artesunate and quinine in the treatment of severe falciparum malaria. Clin Infect Dis 2003;37:7–16.

1004. Collin M, Mucklow JC. Drug interactions, renal impairment and hypoglycaemia in a patient with Type II diabetes. Br J Clin Pharmacol 1999;48(2):134–7.

1005. Lu T Y-T, Kupa A, Easterbrook G, Mangoni AA. Profound weight loss associated with reboxetine use in a 44 year old woman. Br J Clin Pharmacol 2005;60:218–20.

1006. Ross RK, Paganini-Hill A, Krailo MD, Gerkins VR, Henderson BE, Pike MC. Effects of reserpine on prolactin levels and incidence of breast cancer in postmenopausal women. Cancer Res 1984;44(7):3106–8.

1007. Boyden TW, Nugent CA, Ogihara T, Maeda T. Reserpine, hydrochlorothiazide and pituitary–gonadal hormones in hypertensive patients. Eur J Clin Pharmacol 1980;17(5):329–32.

1008. Kyriazopoulou V, Parparousi O, Vagenakis AG. Rifampicin-induced adrenal crisis in Addisonian patients receiving corticosteroid replacement therapy. J Clin Endocrinol Metab 1984;59(6):1204–6.

1009. Nolan SR, Self TH, Norwood JM. Interaction between rifampin and levothyroxine. South Med J 1999;92(5):529–31.

1010. Nobuyuki Takasu, Masaki Takara, Ichiro Komiya. Rifampicin induced hypothyroidism in patients with Hashimoto's thyroiditis. N Engl J Med 2005;352(5):518–9.

1011. Williams SE, Wardman AG, Taylor GA, Peacock M, Cooke NJ. Long term study of the effect of rifampicin and isoniazid on vitamin D metabolism. Tubercle 1985;66(1):49–54.

1012. Toppet M, Vainsel M, Cantraine F, Franckson M. Evolution de la phosphatase alcaline sérique sous traitement d'isoniazide et de rifampicine. [Course of serum alkaline phosphatase during treatment with isoniazid and rifampicin.] Arch Fr Pediatr 1985;42(2):79–80.

1013. Millar JW. Rifampicin-induced porphyria cutanea tarda. Br J Dis Chest 1980;74(4):405–8.

1014. Jones H, Curtis VA, Wright PA, Lucey JV. Risperidone is associated with blunting of D-fenfluramine evoked serotonergic responses in schizophrenia. Int Clin Psychopharmacol 1998;13(5):199–203.

1015. Shiwach RS, Carmody TJ. Prolactogenic effects of risperidone in male patients—a preliminary study. Acta Psychiatr Scand 1998;98(1):81–3.

1016. David SR, Taylor CC, Kinon BJ, Breier A. The effects of olanzapine, risperidone, and haloperidol on plasma prolactin levels in patients with schizophrenia. Clin Ther 2000;22(9):1085–96.

1017. Tollin SR. Use of the dopamine agonists bromocriptine and cabergoline in the management of risperidone-induced hyperprolactinemia in patients with psychotic disorders. J Endocrinol Invest 2000;23(11):765–70.

1018. Kleinberg DL, Davis JM, de Coster R, Van Baelen B, Brecher M. Prolactin levels and adverse events in patients treated with risperidone. J Clin Psychopharmacol 1999;19(1):57–61.

1019. Kim YK, Kim L, Lee MS. Risperidone and associated amenorrhea: a report of 5 cases. J Clin Psychiatry 1999;60(5):315–7.

1020. Popli A, Gupta S, Rangwani SR. Risperidone-induced galactorrhea associated with a prolactin elevation. Ann Clin Psychiatry 1998;10(1):31–3.

1021. Schreiber S, Segman RH. Risperidone-induced galactorrhea. Psychopharmacology (Berl) 1997;130(3):300–1.

1022. Keks NA, Culhane C. Risperidone (Risperdal): clinical experience with a new antipsychosis drug. Expert Opin Investig Drugs 1999;8(4):443–52.

1023. Gazzola LR, Opler LA. Return of menstruation after switching from risperidone to olanzapine. J Clin Psychopharmacol 1998;18(6):486–7.

1024. Mabini R, Wergowske G, Baker FM. Galactorrhea and gynecomastia in a hypothyroid male being treated with risperidone. Psychiatr Serv 2000;51(8):983–5.

1025. Gupta S, Frank B, Madhusoodanan S. Risperidone-associated galactorrhea in a male teenager. J Am Acad Child Adolesc Psychiatry 2001;40(5):504–5.

1026. Kim KS, Pae CU, Chae JH, Bahk WM, Jun TY, Kim DJ, Dickson RA. Effects of olanzapine on prolactin levels of female patients with schizophrenia treated with risperidone. J Clin Psychiatry 2002;63(5):408–13.

1027. Kinon BJ, Gilmore JA, Liu H, Halbreich UM. Prevalence of hyperprolactinemia in schizophrenic patients treated with conventional antipsychotic medications or risperidone. Psychoneuroendocrinology 2003;28:55–68.

1028. Brunelleschi S, Zeppegno P, Risso F, Cattaneo CI, Torre E. Risperidone-associated hyperprolactinemia: evaluation in twenty psychiatric outpatients. Pharmacol Res 2003;48:405–9.

1029. Togo T, Iseki E, Shoji M, Oyama I, Kase A, Uchikado H, Katsuse O, Kosaka K. Prolactin levels in schizophrenic patients receiving perospirone in comparison to risperidone. J Pharmacol Sci 2003;91:259–62.

1030. Becker D, Liver O, Mester R, Rapoport M, Weizman A, Weiss M. Risperidone, but not olanzapine, decreases bone mineral density in female premenopausal schizophrenia patients. J Clin Psychiatry 2003;64:761–6.

1031. Spollen JJ, Wooten RG, Cargile C, Bartztokis G. Prolactin levels and erectile function in patients treated with risperidone. J Clin Psychopharmacol 2004;24:161–6.

1032. Češková E, Přikryl R, Kašpárek T, Ondrušová M. Prolactin levels in risperidone treatment of first-episode schizophrenia. Int J Psych Clin Pract 2004;8:31–6.

1033. Zhang XY, Zhou DF, Cao LY, Zhang PY, Wu GY, Shen YC. Prolactin levels in male schizophrenic patients treated with risperidone and haloperidol: a double-blind and randomized study. Psychopharmacology 2005;178:35–40.

1034. Mendhekar DN, Jiloha RC, Srivastava PK. Effect of risperidone on prolactinoma. A case report. Pharmacopsychiatry 2004;37:41–2.

1035. Dunbar F, Kusumakar V, Daneman D, Schulz M. Growth and sexual maturation during long-term treatment with risperidone. Am J Psychiatry 2004;161:918–20.

1036. Gupta SC, Jagadheesan K, Basu S, Paul SE. Risperidone-induced galactorrhoea: a case series. Can J Psychiatry 2003;48(2):130–1.

1037. Kunwar AR, Megna JL. Resolution of risperidone-induced hyperprolactinemia with substitution of quetiapine. Ann Pharmacother 2003;37:206–8.

1038. Yamada K, Kanba S, Yagi G, Asai M. Herbal medicine (Shakuyaku-kanzo-to) in the treatment of risperidone-induced amenorrhea. J Clin Psychopharmacol 1999;19(4):380–1.

1039. Croarkin PE, Jacobs KM, Bain BK. Diabetic ketoacidosis associated with risperidone treatment? Psychosomatics 2000;41(4):369–70.

1040. Horrigan JP, Sikich L. Diet and the atypical neuroleptics. J Am Acad Child Adolesc Psychiatry 1998;37(11):1126–1127.

1041. Martin A, Landau J, Leebens P, Ulizio K, Cicchetti D, Scahill L, Leckman JF. Risperidone-associated weight gain in children and adolescents: a retrospective chart review. J Child Adolesc Psychopharmacol 2000;10(4):259–68.

1042. Barak Y. No weight gain among elderly schizophrenia patients after 1 year of risperidone treatment. J Clin Psychiatry 2002;63(2):117–9.

1043. Wirshing DA, Pierre JM, Wirshing WC. Sleep apnea associated with antipsychotic-induced obesity. J Clin Psychiatry 2002;63(4):369–70.

1044. Lane H-Y, Chang Y-C, Cheng Y-C, Liu G-C, Lin X-R, Chang W-H. Effects of patient demographics, risperidone dosage, and clinical outcome on body weight in acutely exacerbated schizophrenia. J Clin Psychiatry 2003;64:316–20.

1045. Safer DJ. A comparison of risperidone-induced weight gain across the age span. J Clin Psychopharmacol 2004;24:429–36.

1046. Martin A, Scahill L, Anderson GM, Aman M, Arnold LE, McCracken J, McDougle CJ, Tierney E, Chuang S, Vitiello B (The Research Units on Pediatric Psychopharmacology Autism Network). Weight and leptin changes among risperidone-treated youths with autism: 6-month prospective data. Am J Psychiatry 2004;161:1125–7.

1047. Ziegenbein M, Kropp S. Risperidone-induced long-term weight gain in a patient with schizophrenia. Aust NZ J Psychiatry 2004;38:175–6.

1048. Desir D, Kirkpatrick C, Fevre-Montange M, Tourniaire J. Ritodrine increases plasma melatonin in woman. Lancet 1983;1(8317):184–5.

1049. Land JM, A'Court CH, Gillmer MD, Ledingham JG. Severe non-diabetic keto-acidosis causing intrauterine death. Br J Obstet Gynaecol 1992;99(1):77–9.

1050. Inui S, Nakao T, Itami S. Modulation of androgen receptor transcriptional activity by anti-acne reagents. J Dermatol Sci 2004;36(2):97–101.

1051. Wasserman D, Amitai Y. Hypoglycemia following albuterol overdose in a child. Am J Emerg Med 1992;10:556–7.

1052. Ozdemir D, Yilmaz E, Duman M, Unal N, Tuncok Y. Hypoglycemia after albuterol overdose in a pediatric patient. Pediatr Emerg Care 2004;20:464–5.

1053. Konig P, Goldstein D, Poehlmann M, Rife D, Ge B, Hewett J. Effect of nebulized albuterol on blood glucose in patients with diabetes mellitus with and without cystic fibrosis. Pediatr Pulmonol 2005;40:105–8.

1054. Rodrigo GJ, Rodrigo C. Elevated plasma lactate level associated with high dose inhaled albuterol therapy in acute severe asthma. Emerg Med J 2005;22:404–8.

1055. Stratakos G, Kalomenidis J, Routsi C, Papiris S, Roussos C. Transient lactic acidosis as a side effect of inhaled salbutamol. Chest 2002;122(1):385–6.

1056. Prakash S, Mehta S. Lactic acidosis in asthma: report of two cases and review of the literature. Can Respir J 2002;9(3):203–8.

1057. Liem EB, Mnookin SC, Mahla ME. Albuterol-induced lactic acidosis. Anesthesiology 2003;99:505–6.

1058. Donovan B, Bodsworth NJ, Mulhall BP, Allen D. Gynaecomastia associated with saquinavir therapy. Int J STD AIDS 1999;10(1):49–50.

1059. Corbett AH, Eron JJ, Fiscus SA, Rezk NL, Kashuba AD. The pharmacokinetics, safety, and initial virologic response of a triple-protease inhibitor salvage regimen containing amprenavir, saquinavir, and ritonavir. J Acquir Immune Defic Syndr 2004;36(4):921–8.

1060. Sternbach H. Venlafaxine-induced galactorrhea. J Clin Psychopharmacol 2003;23:109.

1061. Hofbauer LC, Spitzweg C, Magerstadt RA, Heufelder AE. Selenium-induced thyroid dysfunction. Postgrad Med J 1997;73(856):103–4.

1062. Perquin LN. Treatment with the new antipsychotic sertindole for late-occurring undesirable movement effects. Int Clin Psychopharmacol 2005;20:335–8.

1063. Lesaca TG. Sertraline and galactorrhea. J Clin Psychopharmacol 1996;16(4):333–4.

1064. Kaczmarek I, Groetzner J, Adamidis I, Landwehr P, Mueller M, Vogeser M, Gerstorfer M, Uberfuhr P, Meiser B, Reichart B. Sirolimus impairs gonadal function in heart transplant recipients. Am J Transplant 2004;4(7):1084–8.

1065. Brattstrom C, Wilczek H, Tyden G, Bottiger Y, Sawe J, Groth CG. Hyperlipidemia in renal transplant recipients treated with sirolimus (rapamycin). Transplantation 1998;65(9):1272–4.

1066. Kahan BD, Podbielski J, Napoli KL, Katz SM, Meier-Kriesche HU, Van Buren CT. Immunosuppressive effects and safety of a sirolimus/cyclosporine combination regimen for renal transplantation. Transplantation 1998;66(8):1040–6.

1067. Morrisett JD, Abdel-Fattah G, Hoogeveen R, Mitchell E, Ballantyne CM, Pownall HJ, Opekun AR, Jaffe JS, Oppermann S, Kahan BD. Effects of sirolimus on plasma lipids, lipoprotein levels, and fatty acid metabolism in renal transplant patients. J Lipid Res 2002;43(8):1170–80.

1068. Chueh SC, Kahan BD. Dyslipidemia in renal transplant recipients treated with a sirolimus and cyclosporine-based immunosuppressive regimen: incidence, risk factors, progression, and prognosis. Transplantation 2003;76:375–82.

1069. Brara PS, Moussavian M, Grise MA, Reilly JP, Fernandez M, Schatz RA, Teirstein PS. Pilot trial of oral rapamycin for recalcitrant restenosis. Circulation 2003;107:1722–4.

1070. Firpi RJ, Tran TT, Flores P, Nissen N, Colquhoun S, Shackleton C, Martin P, Vierling JM, Poordad FF. Sirolimus-induced hyperlipidaemia in liver transplant recipients is not dose-dependent. Aliment Pharmacol Ther 2004;19(9):1033–9.

1071. Kniepeiss D, Iberer F, Schaffellner S, Jakoby E, Duller D, Tscheliessnigg K. Dyslipidemia during sirolimus therapy in patients after liver transplantation. Clin Transplant 2004;18(6):642–6.

1072. Mathis AS, Dave N, Knipp GT, Friedman GS. Drug-related dyslipidemia after renal transplantation. Am J Health Syst Pharm 2004;61(6):565–85.

1073. Schneider H. Diabetesmanifestation nach Pockenimpfung. [Manifestation of diabetes after smallpox vaccination.] Kinderarztl Prax 1975;43(3):101–7.

1074. Tamaskar IR, Unnithan J, Garcia JA, Dreicer R, Wood L, Iochimescu A, Bukowski R, Rini B. Thyroid function test (TFT) abnormalities in patients (pts) with metastatic renal cell carcinoma (RCC) treated with sorafenib. ASCO Annual Meeting Proceedings. J Clin Oncol 2007;25 (June 20 Suppl):5048.

1075. Yemisci A, Gorgulu A, Piskin S. Effects and side-effects of spironolactone therapy in women with acne. J Eur Acad Dermatol Venereol 2005;19(2):163–6.

1076. Heath KV, Hogg RS, Chan KJ, Harris M, Montessori V, O'Shaughnessy MV, Montanera JS. Lipodystrophy-associated morphological, cholesterol and triglyceride abnormalities in a population-based HIV/AIDS treatment database. AIDS 2001;15(2):231–9.

1077. White MG, Asch MJ. Acid-base effects of topical mafenide acetate in the burned patient. N Engl J Med 1971;284(23):1281–6.

1078. Desai J, Yassa L, Marqusee E, George S, Frates MC, Chen MH, Morgan JA, Dychter SS, Larsen PR, Demetri GD, Alexander EK. Hypothyroidism after sunitinib treatment for patients with gastrointestinal stromal tumors. Ann Intern Med 2006;145:660–4.

1079. de Groot JW, Links TP, van der Graaf WT. Tyrosine kinase inhibitors causing hypothyroidism in a patient on levothyroxine. Ann Oncol 2006;17:1719–20.

1080. Rini BI, Tamaskar I, Shaheen P, Salas R, Garcia J, Wood L, Reddy S, Dreicer R, Bukowski RM. Hypothyroidism in patients with metastatic renal cell carcinoma treated with sunitinib. J Natl Cancer Inst 2007;99:81–3.

1081. Kobayashi K, Weiss RE, Vogelzang NJ, Vokes EE, Janisch L, Ratain MJ. Mineralocorticoid insufficiency due to suramin therapy. Cancer 1996;78(11):2411–20.

1082. Tze WJ, Tai J, Murase N, Tzakis A, Starzl TE. Effect of FK 506 on glucose metabolism and insulin secretion in normal rats. Transplant Proc 1991;23(6):3158–60.

1083. Paolillo JA, Boyle GJ, Law YM, Miller SA, Lawrence K, Wagner K, Pigula FA, Griffith BP, Webber SA. Posttransplant diabetes mellitus in pediatric thoracic organ recipients receiving tacrolimus-based immunosuppression. Transplantation 2001;71(2):252–6.

1084. Weir MR, Fink JC. Risk for posttransplant diabetes mellitus with current immunosuppressive medications. Am J Kidney Dis 1999;34(1):1–13.

1085. Fernandez LA, Lehmann R, Luzi L, Battezzati A, Angelico MC, Ricordi C, Tzakis A, Alejandro R. The effects of maintenance doses of FK506 versus cyclosporin A on glucose and lipid metabolism after orthotopic liver transplantation. Transplantation 1999;68(10):1532–41.

1086. Lohmann T, List C, Lamesch P, Kohlhaw K, Wenzke M, Schwarz C, Richter O, Hauss J, Seissler J. Diabetes mellitus and islet cell specific autoimmunity as adverse effects of immunsuppressive therapy by FK506/tacrolimus. Exp Clin Endocrinol Diabetes 2000;108(5):347–52.

1087. Kawai T, Shimada A, Kasuga A. FK506-induced autoimmune diabetes. Ann Intern Med 2000;132(6):511.

1088. Jain A, Kashyap R, Marsh W, Rohal S, Khanna A, Fung JJ. Reasons for long-term use of steroid in primary adult liver transplantation under tacrolimus. Transplantation 2001;71(8):1102–6.

1089. Furth S, Neu A, Colombani P, Plotnick L, Turner ME, Fivush B. Diabetes as a complication of tacrolimus (FK506) in pediatric renal transplant patients. Pediatr Nephrol 1996;10(1):64–6.

1090. Moxey-Mims MM, Kay C, Light JA, Kher KK. Increased incidence of insulin-dependent diabetes mellitus in pediatric renal transplant patients receiving tacrolimus (FK506). Transplantation 1998;65(5):617–9.

1091. Krentz AJ, Dmitrewski J, Mayer D, McMaster P, Buckels J, Dousset B, Cramb R, Smith JM, Nattrass M. Postoperative glucose metabolism in liver transplant recipients. A two-year prospective randomized study of cyclosporine versus FK506. Transplantation 1994;57(11):1666–9.

1092. Jindal RM, Popescu I, Schwartz ME, Emre S, Boccagni P, Miller CM. Diabetogenicity of FK506 versus cyclosporine in liver transplant recipients. Transplantation 1994;58(3):370–2.

1093. Tanabe K, Koga S, Takahashi K, Sonda K, Tokumoto T, Babazono T, Yagisawa T, Toma H, Kawai T, Fuchinoue S, Teraoka S, Ota K. Diabetes mellitus after renal transplantation under FK 506 (tacrolimus) as primary immunosuppression. Transplant Proc 1996;28(3):1304–5.

1094. Knoll GA, Bell RC. Tacrolimus versus cyclosporin for immunosuppression in renal transplantation: meta-analysis of randomised trials. BMJ 1999;318(7191):1104–7.

1095. Cavaille-Coll MW, Elashoff MR. Commentary on a comparison of tacrolimus and cyclosporine for immunosuppression after cadaveric renal transplantation. Transplantation 1998;65(1):142–5.

1096. Yoshioka K, Sato T, Okada N, Ishii T, Imanishi M, Tanaka S, Kim T, Sugimoto T, Fujii S. Post-transplant diabetes with anti-glutamic acid decarboxylase antibody during tacrolimus therapy. Diabetes Res Clin Pract 1998;42(2):85–9.

1097. Bloom RD, Rao V, Weng F, Grossman RA, Cohen D, Mange KC. Association of hepatitis C with posttransplant diabetes in renal transplant patients on tacrolimus. J Am Soc Nephrol 2002;13(5):1374–80.

1098. Panz VR, Bonegio R, Raal FJ, Maher H, Hsu HC, Joffe BI. Diabetogenic effect of tacrolimus in South African patients undergoing kidney transplantation. Transplantation 2002;73(4):587–90.

1099. Heisel O, Heisel R, Balshaw R, Keown P. New onset diabetes mellitus in patients receiving calcineurin inhibitors: a systematic review and meta-analysis. Am J Transplant 2004;4(4):583–95.

1100. Gourishankar S, Jhangri GS, Tonelli M, Wales LH, Cockfield SM. Development of diabetes mellitus following kidney transplantation: a Canadian experience. Am J Transplant 2004;4(11):1876–82.

1101. Gomez E, Aguado S, Rodriguez M, Alvarez-Grande J. Kaposi's sarcoma after renal transplantation—disappearance after reduction of immunosuppression and reappearance 7 years later after start of mycophenolate mofetil treatment. Nephrol Dial Transplant 1998;13(12):3279–80.

1102. Abouljoud MS, Levy MF, Klintmalm GBUS Multicenter Study Group. Hyperlipidemia after liver transplantation:

long-term results of the FK506/cyclosporine a US Multicenter trial. Transplant Proc 1995;27(1):1121–3.

1103. Gerster JC, Dudler M, Halkic N, Gillet M. Gout in liver transplant patients receiving tacrolimus. Ann Rheum Dis 2004;63(7):894–5.

1104. Gallant JE, Staszewski S, Pozniak AL, DeJesus E, Suleiman JM, Miller MD, Coakley DF, Lu B, Toole JJ, Cheng AK; 903 Study Group. Efficacy and safety of tenofovir DF vs stavudine in combination therapy in anti-retroviral-naive patients: a 3-year randomized trial. JAMA 2004;292(2):191–201.

1105. Smigaj D, Roman-Drago NM, Amini SB, Caritis SN, Kalhan SC, Catalano PM. The effect of oral terbutaline on maternal glucose metabolism and energy expenditure in pregnancy. Am J Obstet Gynecol 1998;178(5):1041–7.

1106. Billano RA, Ward WQ, Little WP. Minocycline and black thyroid. JAMA 1983;249(14):1887.

1107. Reid JD. The black thyroid associated with minocycline therapy. A local manifestation of a drug-induced lyso-some/substrate disorder. Am J Clin Pathol 1983;79(6):738–46.

1108. Korkelia J. Antianabolic effect of tetracyclines. Lancet 1971;1(7706):974–5.

1109. Morgan T, Ribush N. The effect of oxytetracycline and doxycycline on protein metabolism. Med J Aust 1972;1(2):55–8.

1110. Seltzer HS. Drug-induced hypoglycemia. A review based on 473 cases. Diabetes 1972;21(9):955–66.

1111. Garbitelli VP. Tetracycline reduces the need for insulin. NY State J Med 1987;87(10):576.

1112. Simpson JA. Myxoedema after thalidomide. BMJ 1962;1:55.

1113. Lillicrap DA. Myxoedema after thalidomide (Distaval). BMJ 1962;1:477.

1114. Badros AZ, Siegel E, Bodenner D, Zangari M, Zeldis J, Barlogie B, Tricot G. Hypothyroidism in patients with multiple myeloma following treatment with thalidomide. Am J Med 2002;112(5):412–3.

1115. Iqbal N, Zayed M, Boden G. Thalidomide impairs insulin action on glucose uptake and glycogen synthesis in patients with type 2 diabetes. Diabetes Care 2000;23(8):1172–6.

1116. Figg WD, Arlen P, Gulley J, Fernandez P, Noone M, Fedenko K, Hamilton M, Parker C, Kruger EA, Pluda J, Dahut WL. A randomized phase II trial of doc-etaxel (Taxotere) plus thalidomide in androgen-independent prostate cancer. Semin Oncol 2001;28(4 Suppl 15):62–6.

1117. Pathak RD, Jayaraj K, Blonde L. Thalidomide-associated hyperglycemia and diabetes: case report and review of literature. Diabetes Care 2003;26(4):1322–3.

1118. Tseng S, Pak G, Washenik K, Pomeranz MK, Shupack JL. Rediscovering thalidomide: a review of its mechanism of action, side effects, and potential uses. J Am Acad Dermatol 1996;35(6):969–79.

1119. Haslett P, Hempstead M, Seidman C, Diakun J, Vasquez D, Freedman VH, Kaplan G. The metabolic and immunologic effects of short-term thalidomide treat-ment of patients infected with the human immunodefi-ciency virus. AIDS Res Hum Retroviruses 1997;13(12):1047–54.

1120. Aderka D, Shavit G, Garfinkel D, Santo M, Gitter S, Pinkhas J. Life-threatening theophylline intoxication in a hypothyroid patient. Respiration 1983;44(1):77–80.

1121. Maitland-van der Zee AH, Turner ST, Schwartz GL, Chapman AB, Klungel OH, Boerwinkle E.

1122. Demographic, environmental, and genetic predictors of metabolic side effects of hydrochlorothiazide treatment in hypertensive subjects. Am J Hypertens 2005;18:1077–83.

1122. Kotake Y, Matsumoto M, Takeda J. Thiopental intensi-fies the euthyroid sick syndrome after cardiopulmonary resuscitation. J Anesth 2000;14(1):38–41.

1123. Hogan RE, Bertrand ME, Deaton RL, Sommerville KW. Total percentage body weight changes during add-on therapy with tiagabine, carbamazepine and phenytoin. Epilepsy Res 2000;41(1):23–8.

1124. Faguer de Moustier B, Burgard M, Boitard C, Desplanque N, Fanjoux J, Tchobroutsky G. Syndrome hypoglycémique auto-immune induit par le pyritinol. [Auto-immune hypoglycemic syndrome induced by pyr-itinol.] Diabete Metab 1988;14(4):423–9.

1125. Gregoir C, Hilliquin P, Acar F, Lessana-Leibowitch M, Renoux M, Menkes CJ. Mastite aiguë au cours d'une polyarthrite rhumatoïde avec syndrome de Gougerot–Sjögren traitée par tiopronine (acadione). [Acute mastitis in rheumatoid polyarthritis with Gougerot–Sjögren syn-drome treated with tiopronin (Acadione).] Rev Rhum Mal Osteoartic 1991;58(3):203–6.

1126. Shorvon SD. Safety of topiramate: adverse events and relationships to dosing. Epilepsia 1996;37(Suppl 2):S18–22.

1127. Teter CJ, Early JJ, Gibbs CM. Treatment of affective disorder and obesity with topiramate. Ann Pharmacother 2000;34(11):1262–5.

1128. Chengappa KN, Chalasani L, Brar JS, Parepally H, Houck P, Levine J. Changes in body weight and body mass index among psychiatric patients receiving lithium, valproate, or topiramate: an open-label, nonrandomized chart review. Clin Ther 2002;24(10):1576–84.

1129. Nickel MK, Nickel C, Kaplan P, Lahmann C, Muhlbacher M, Tritt K, Krawczyk J, Leiberich PK, Rother WK, Loew TH. Treatment of aggression with topiramate in male borderline patients: a double-blind, placebo-controlled study. Biol Psychiatry 2005;57:495–89.

1130. Nickel C, Lahmann C, Tritt K, Muehlbacher M, Kaplan P, Kettler C, Krawczyk J, Loew TH, Rother WK, Nickel MK. Topiramate in treatment of depressive and anger symptoms in female depressive patients: a randomized, double-blind, placebo-controlled study. J Affect Disord 2005;87:243–52.

1131. Garris SS, Oles KS. Impact of topiramate on serum bicar-bonate concentration in adults. Ann Pharmacother 2005;39:424–6.

1132. Paykel ES, Mueller PS, De la Vergne PM. Amitriptyline, weight gain and carbohydrate craving: a side effect. Br J Psychiatry 1973;123(576):501–7.

1133. Nakra BR, Rutland P, Verma S, Gaind R. Amitriptyline and weight gain: a biochemical and endocrinological study. Curr Med Res Opin 1977;4(8):602–6.

1134. Steiner JE, Rosenthal-Zifroni A, Edelstein EL. Taste perception in depressive illness. Isr Ann Psychiatr Relat Discip 1969;7(2):223–32.

1135. Fernstrom MH, Krowinski RL, Kupfer DJ. Appetite and food preference in depression: effects of imipramine treatment. Biol Psychiatry 1987;22(5):529–39.

1136. Sherman KE, Bornemann M. Amitriptyline and asympto-matic hypoglycemia. Ann Intern Med 1988;109(8):683–4.

1137. Luzecky MH, Burman KD, Schultz ER. The syndrome of inappropriate secretion of antidiuretic hormone asso-ciated with amitriptyline administration. South Med J 1974;67(4):495–7.

1138. Kuhs H. Demaskierung eines Phäochromozytoms durch Amitriptylin. [Unmasking pheochromocytoma by amitriptyline.] Nervenarzt 1998;69(1):76–7.

1139. Anand VS. Clomipramine-induced galactorrhoea and amenorrhoea. Br J Psychiatry 1985;147:87–8.

1140. Roessner MD, Demling J, Bleich S. Doxepin increases serum cholesterol levels. Can J Psychiatry 2004;49:74–5.

1141. Murphy JL, Griswold WR, Reznik VM, Mendoza SA. Trimethoprim/sulfamethoxazole-induced renal tubular acidosis. Child Nephrol Urol 1990;10(1):49–50.

1142. Cohen HN, Pearson DW, Thomson JA, Ratcliffe WA, Beastall GH. Trimethoprim and thyroid function. Lancet 1981;1(8221):676–7.

1143. Smellie JM, Bantock HM, Thompson BD. Co-trimoxazole and the thyroid. Lancet 1982;2(8289):96.

1144. Williamson NL, Frank LA, Hnilica KA. Effects of short-term trimethoprim–sulfamethoxazole administration on thyroid function in dogs. J Am Vet Med Assoc 2002;221(6):802–6.

1145. Frank LA, Hnilica KA, May ER, Sargent SJ, Davis JA. Effects of sulfamethoxazole–trimethoprim on thyroid function in dogs. Am J Vet Res 2005;66(2):256–9.

1146. Fox GN. Trimethoprim–sulfamethoxazole-induced hypoglycemia. J Am Board Fam Pract 2000;13(5):386.

1147. Mathews WA, Manint JE, Kleiss J. Trimethoprim–sulfamethoxazole-induced hypoglycemia as a cause of altered mental status in an elderly patient. J Am Board Fam Pract 2000;13(3):211–2.

1148. Porras MC, Lecumberri JN, Castrillon JL. Trimethoprim–sulfamethoxazole and metabolic acidosis in HIV-infected patients. Ann Pharmacother 1998;32(2):185–9.

1149. Don BR. The effect of trimethoprim on potassium and uric acid metabolism in normal human subjects. Clin Nephrol 2001;55:45–52.

1150. Bairaktari ET, Kakafika AI, Pritsivelis N, Hatzidimou KG, Tsianos EV, Seferiadis KI, Elisaf MS. Hypouricemia in individuals admitted to an inpatient hospital-based facility. Am J Kidney Dis 2003;41:1225–32.

1151. Edmonds SE, Montgomery JC. Reversible ovarian failure induced by a Chinese herbal medicine: lei gong teng. Br J Obstet Gynaecol 2003;110:77–8.

1152. Uzzan B, Nicolas P, Perret G, Vassy R, Tod M, Petitjean O. Effects of troleandomycin and josamycin on thyroid hormone and steroid serum levels, liver function tests and microsomal monooxygenases in healthy volunteers: a double blind placebo-controlled study. Fundam Clin Pharmacol 1991;5(6):513–26.

1153. Miyakoshi H, Ohsawa K, Yokoyama H, Nagai Y, Ieki Y, Bando YI, Kobayashi K. Exacerbation of hypothyroidism following tumor necrosis factor-alpha infusion. Intern Med 1992;31(2):200–3.

1154. Margraf JW, Dreifuss FE. Amenorrhea following initiation of therapy with valproic acid. Neurology 1981;31:159.

1155. Isojarvi JI, Laatikainen TJ, Knip M, Pakarinen AJ, Juntunen KT, Myllyla VV. Obesity and endocrine disorders in women taking valproate for epilepsy. Ann Neurol 1996;39(5):579–84.

1156. Isojarvi JI, Rattya J, Myllyla VV, Knip M, Koivunen R, Pakarinen AJ, Tekay A, Tapanainen JS. Valproate, lamotrigine, and insulin-mediated risks in women with epilepsy. Ann Neurol 1998;43(4):446–51.

1157. Cook JS, Bale JF Jr, Hoffman RP. Pubertal arrest associated with valproic acid therapy. Pediatr Neurol 1992;8(3):229–31.

1158. Vainionpaa LK, Rattya J, Knip M, Tapanainen JS, Pakarinen AJ, Lanning P, Tekay A, Myllyla VV, Isojarvi JI. Valproate-induced hyperandrogenism during pubertal maturation in girls with epilepsy. Ann Neurol 1999;45(4):444–50.

1159. Luef G, Abraham I, Haslinger M, Trinka E, Seppi K, Unterberger I, Alge A, Windisch J, Lechleitner M, Bauer G. Polycystic ovaries, obesity and insulin resistance in women with epilepsy. A comparative study of carbamazepine and valproic acid in 105 women. J Neurol 2002;249(7):835–41.

1160. Geda G, Caksen H, Icagasioglu D. Serum lipids, vitamin B12 and folic acid levels in children receiving long-term valproate therapy. Acta Neurol Belg 2002;102(3):122–6.

1161. Davis R, Peters DH, McTavish D. Valproic acid. A reappraisal of its pharmacological properties and clinical efficacy in epilepsy. Drugs 1994;47(2):332–72.

1162. Biton V, Mirza W, Montouris G, Vuong A, Hammer AE, Barrett PS. Weight change associated with valproate and lamotrigine monotherapy in patients with epilepsy. Neurology 2001;56(2):172–7.

1163. Wirrell EC. Valproic acid-associated weight gain in older children and teens with epilepsy. Pediatr Neurol 2003;28:126–9.

1164. Biton V, Levisohn P, Hoyler S, Vuong A, Hammer AE. Lamotrigine versus valproate monotherapy-associated weight change in adolescents with epilepsy: results from a post hoc analysis of a randomized, double-blind clinical trial. J Child Neurol 2003;18:133–9.

1165. Bosnak M, Dikici B, Haspolat K, Dagli A, Dikici S. Do epileptic children treated with valproate have a risk of excessive weight gain? J Child Neurol 2003;18:306.

1166. Verrotti A, Basciani F, Morresi S, de Martino M, Morgese G, Chiarelli F. Serum leptin changes in epileptic patients who gain weight after therapy with valproic acid. Neurology 1999;53(1):230–2.

1167. Pylvanen V, Knip M, Pakarinen A, Kotila M, Turkka J, Isojarvi JI. Serum insulin and leptin levels in valproate-associated obesity. Epilepsia 2002;43(5):514–7.

1168. Luef G, Abraham I, Hoppichler F, Trinka E, Unterberger I, Bauer G, Lechleitner M. Increase in postprandial serum insulin levels in epileptic patients with valproic acid therapy. Metabolism 2002;51(10):1274–8.

1169. Luef G, Abraham I, Trinka E, Alge A, Windisch J, Daxenbichler G, Unterberger I, Seppi K, Lechleitner M, Kramer G, Bauer G. Hyperandrogenism, postprandial hyperinsulinism and the risk of PCOS in a cross sectional study of women with epilepsy treated with valproate. Epilepsy Res 2002;48(1–2):91–102.

1170. Knorr M, Schaper J, Harjes M, Mayatepek E, Rosenbaum T. Fanconi syndrome caused by antiepileptic therapy with valproic acid. Epilepsia 2004;45(7):868–71.

1171. Kifune A, Kubota F, Shibata N, Akata T, Kikuchi S. Valproic acid-induced hyperammonemic encephalopathy with triphasic waves. Epilepsia 2000;41(7):909–12.

1172. Hamer HM, Knake S, Schomburg U, Rosenow F. Valproate-induced hyperammonemic encephalopathy in the presence of topiramate. Neurology 2000;54(1):230–2.

1173. Murphy JV, Marquardt K. Asymptomatic hyperammonemia in patients receiving valproic acid. Arch Neurol 1982;39(9):591–2.

1174. Kay JD, Hilton-Jones D, Hyman N. Valproate toxicity and ornithine carbamoyltransferase deficiency. Lancet 1986;2(8518):1283–4.

1175. Hjelm M, de Silva LV, Seakins JW, Oberholzer VG, Rolles CJ. Evidence of inherited urea cycle defect in a case of fatal valproate toxicity. BMJ (Clin Res Ed) 1986;292(6512):23–4.

1176. Christmann R. Valproate-induced coma in a patient with urea cycle enzyme deficiency. Epilepsia 1990;31:228.

1177. Verrotti A, Trotta D, Morgese G, Chiarelli F. Valproate-induced hyperammonemic encephalopathy. Metab Brain Dis 2002;17(4):367–73.

1178. Ziyeh S, Thiel T, Spreer J, Klisch J, Schumacher M. Valproate-induced encephalopathy: assessment with MR imaging and ^{1}H MR spectroscopy. Epilepsia 2002;43(9):1101–5.

1179. Vossler DG, Wilensky AJ, Cawthon DF, Kraemer DL, Ojemann LM, Caylor LM, Morgan JD. Serum and CSF glutamine levels in valproate-related hyperammonemic encephalopathy. Epilepsia 2002;43(2):154–9.

1180. Murphy JV. Valproate-induced hyperammonemic encephalopathy. Epilepsia 2003;44:268.

1181. Yehya N, Saldarini CT, Koski ME, Davanzo P. Valproate-induced hyperammonemic encephalopathy. J Am Acad Child Adolesc Psychiatry 2004;43(8):926–7.

1182. García D, Nogué S, Sanjurjo E, Espígol G. Hiperamonemia aguda secundaria a intoxicación aguda por ácido valproico. Rev Toxicol 2003;20:43–5.

1183. McCall M, Bourgeois JA. Valproic acid-induced hyperammonemia: a case report. J Clin Psychopharmacol 2004;24(5):521–6.

1184. Mallet L, Babin S, Morais JA. Valproic acid-induced hyperammonemia and thrombocytopenia in an elderly woman. Ann Pharmacother 2004;38(10):1643–7.

1185. Coulter DL. Carnitine, valproate, and toxicity. J Child Neurol 1991;6(1):7–14.

1186. Murakami K, Sugimoto T, Nishida N, Kobayashi Y, Kuhara T, Matsumoto I. Abnormal metabolism of carnitine and valproate in a case of acute encephalopathy during chronic valproate therapy. Brain Dev 1992;14(3):178–81.

1187. Papadimitriou A, Servidei S. Late onset lipid storage myopathy due to multiple acyl CoA dehydrogenase deficiency triggered by valproate. Neuromuscul Disord 1991;1(4):247–52.

1188. Gram L. Valproate. In: Dam M, Gram L, editors. Comprehensive Epileptology. New York: Raven Press, 1990:537.

1189. De Vivo DC, Bohan TP, Coulter DL, Dreifuss FE, Greenwood RS, Nordli DR Jr, Shields WD, Stafstrom CE, Tein I. L-carnitine supplementation in childhood epilepsy: current perspectives. Epilepsia 1998;39(11):1216–25.

1190. Coulter DL. Carnitine deficiency in epilepsy: Risk factors and treatment. J Child Neurol 1995;10(Suppl. 2):S32–9.

1191. Gidal BE, Tamura T, Hammer A, Vuong A. Blood homocysteine, folate and vitamin B12 concentrations in patients with epilepsy receiving lamotrigine or sodium valproate for initial monotherapy. Epilepsy Res 2005;64:161–6.

1192. Gavazzi C, Stacchiotti S, Cavalletti R, Lodi R. Confusion after antibiotics. Lancet 2001;357(9266):1410.

1193. Dombrowski RC, Romeo JH, Aron DC. Verapamil-induced hyperprolactinemia complicated by a pituitary incidentaloma. Ann Pharmacother 1995;29(10):999–1001.

1194. Krysiak R, Okopien B, Herman ZS. Hiperprolaktynemia spowodowana przez werapamil. Opis przypadku. Arch Med Wewn 2005;113(2):155–8.

1195. Cutting HO. Inappropriate secretion of antidiuretic hormone secondary to vincristine therapy. Am J Med 1971;51(2):269–71.

1196. Stahel RA, Oelz O. Syndrome of inappropriate ADH secretion secondary to vinblastine. Cancer Chemother Pharmacol 1982;8(2):253–4.

1197. Garrett CA, Simpson TA Jr. Syndrome of inappropriate antidiuretic hormone associated with vinorelbine therapy. Ann Pharmacother 1998;32(12):1306–9.

1198. Hammond IW, Ferguson JA, Kwong K, Muniz E, Delisle F. Hyponatremia and syndrome of inappropriate anti-diuretic hormone reported with the use of vincristine: an over-representation of Asians? Pharmacoepidemiol Drug Saf 2002;11(3):229–34.

1199. Ellis JK, Russell RM, Makrauer FL, Schaefer EJ. Increased risk for vitamin A toxicity in severe hypertriglyceridemia. Ann Intern Med 1986;105(6):877–9.

1200. Pastorino U, Chiesa G, Infante M, Soresi E, Clerici M, Valente M, Belloni PA, Ravasi G. Safety of high-dose vitamin A. Randomized trial on lung cancer chemoprevention. Oncology 1991;48(2):131–7.

1201. Gerber LE, Erdman JW Jr. Changes in lipid metabolism during retinoid administration. J Am Acad Dermatol 1982;6(4 Pt 2 Suppl):664–74.

1202. Warrell RP Jr, de The H, Wang ZY, Degos L. Acute promyelocytic leukemia. N Engl J Med 1993;329(3): 177–89.

1203. Fontan B, Bonafe JL, Moatti JP. Toxic effects of the aromatic retinoid etretinate. Arch Dermatol 1983;119(3):187–8.

1204. Alcalay J, Landau M, Zucker A. Analysis of laboratory data in acne patients treated with isotretinoin: is there really a need to perform routine laboratory tests? J Dermatol Treat 2001;12(1):9–12.

1205. Baxter K, Ling T, Barth J, Cunliffe W. Retrospective survey of serum lipids in patients receiving more than three courses of isotretinoin. J Dermatol Treat 2003;14:216–8.

1206. Rodondi N, Darioli R, Ramelet AA, Hohl D, Lenain V, Perdrix J, Wietlisbach V, Riesen WF, Walther T, Medinger L, Nicod P, Desvergne B, Mooser V. High risk for hyperlipidemia and the metabolic syndrome after an episode of hypertriglyceridemia during 13-cis retinoic acid therapy for acne: a pharmacogenetic study. Ann Intern Med 2002;136(8):582–9.

1207. Barth JH, Macdonald-Hull SP, Mark J, Jones RG, Cunliffe WJ. Isotretinoin therapy for acne vulgaris: a re-evaluation of the need for measurements of plasma lipids and liver function tests. Br J Dermatol 1993;129(6):704–7.

1208. Kawaguchi M, Mitsuhashi Y, Kondo S. Iatrogenic hypercalcemia due to vitamin D3 ointment (1,24 OH2D3) combined with thiazide diuretics in a case of psoriasis. J Dermatol 2003;30:801–4.

1209. Garcia-Benayas T, Blanco F, Gomez-Viera JM, Barrios A, Soriano V, Gonzalez-Lahoz J. Lipodystrophy body-shape changes in a patient undergoing zidovudine monotherapy. AIDS 2002;16(7):1087–9.

1210. Buckley PF. Ziprasidone: pharmacology, clinical progress and therapeutic promise. Drugs Today 2000;36:583–9.

1211. Daniel DG, Copeland LF. Ziprasidone: comprehensive overview and clinical use of a novel antipsychotic. Expert Opin Investig Drugs 2000;9(4):819–28.

1212. Jaworowski S, Hauser S, Mergui J, Hirsch H. Ziprasidone and weight gain. Clin Neuropharmacol 2004;27:99–100.

1213. Cubbin SA, Ali IM. Inappropriate antidiuretic hormone secretion associated with zopiclone. Psychiatr Bull 1999;23:306–7.

Index of drug names

Note: The letter '*t*' with the locater refers to tables.

Printed in the United States
By Bookmasters